THE WA...
OF MEDICAL THERAPEUTICS

37th Edition

THE WASHINGTON MANUAL®
OF MEDICAL THERAPEUTICS

37th Edition

Editors

Siri Ancha, MD

Christine Auberle, MD

Devin Cash, MD, PhD

Mohit Harsh, MD

John Hickman, MD

Carole Kounga, MD, PharmD

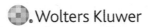

Philadelphia · Baltimore · New York · London
Buenos Aires · Hong Kong · Sydney · Tokyo

Acquisitions Editor: Joe Cho
Development Editor: Thomas Celona/Ariel S. Winter
Editorial Coordinator: Anthony Gonzales
Production Project Manager: Kirstin Johnson
Marketing Manager: Kirsten Watrud
Manager, Graphic Arts & Design: Stephen Druding
Manufacturing Coordinator: Beth Welsh
Prepress Vendor: TNQ Technologies

9 8 7 6 5 4 3 2 1

Printed in Mexico.

Library of Congress Cataloging-in- Publication Data

ISBN-13: 978-1-975190-62-0

Cataloging in Publication data available on request from publisher.

shop.lww.com

We thank our families for their love and support and our mentors for their guidance and dedication.

Siri: To my family Dr. Sudhakar Ancha, Rani, Suma, and Jack; to my mentors Dr. Osama Altayar and Dr. Jeff Crippin.

Christine: To my family Dr. Jacob Beck, Melissa and Jake Studer, Maryanne Tsivitse, and Dr. Jim Auberle; to my mentor Dr. Amanda Cashen.

Devin: To my family Sherrie, Tim, Derek, Therese, Josephine, and Daphne Cash; to my mentors Dr. Cynthia Cornelissen, Dr. Stephanie Call, Dr. Patrick Aguilar, and Dr. Nickole Forget.

Mohit: To my parents and brother. To all of my mentors: Dr. Gerome Escota, Dr. Reza Manesh, Dr. Bob Centor, and Dr. James Jensen. To my academic partners Dr. Lucas Bracero, Dr. Keegan Mullins, and Dr. Eamonn Maher. To my MUSOM family and my college squad. To all of my patients who teach and humble me.

John: To Alex, Joanna, and Elliot; Zachariah and Frank; Dr. Janet and Dr. Robert Hickman; Allison; Dr. Steve Bus; and Dr. Peggie Findlay.

Carole: To the Tabouta family, Dr. Kounga, Drs. Djoko, Papa Maurice, Maman Rebecca, Anne, Melaine, Maggie, Laure, Valery, and my teammate Armand. To my friends, especially Dr. Briana McLaughlin. To my mentors Dr. Battle, Dr. Maynard, Dr. D. Brown, Dr. A. Brown, Dr. Bauch, Dr. Faddis, and Dr. Lenihan.

To the Department of General Medicine Staff: Dr. Ann Ahrens, Jen Bogovich, Julie Byington, Jenae Davis, Megan Dietrich, Amy Foyil, Kirsten Jones, Bethany Millar, Rachel Noon, and Katie Sidler.

Preface

We have the privilege and honor to introduce the 37th edition of *The Washington Manual® of Medical Therapeutics*. *The Manual* began as a simple assortment of "Therapeutic Notes" collected by a senior resident, Wayland MacFarlane, in 1943 at the Washington University School of Medicine in St. Louis. That collection of notes has become one of the most successful medical reference manuals in the history of medicine. During the mid-1960s, *The Manual* grew in popularity with the publishing of 4000 copies of the 16th edition by Robert Packman, MD, making it available to numerous medical schools across the United States for the first time. The subsequent edition grew to 25,000 copies sold. *The Manual* has since expanded to incorporate the broad depth of medical knowledge in its increasing complexity. *The Manual* has sold more than 1 million electronic and print copies worldwide and has been translated into more than 20 languages. Despite the growth of *The Manual*, the initial mission remains steadfast: to provide relevant, evidence-based clinical support to physicians at the bedside and to positively impact patient care.

With the advent of the COVID-19 pandemic, the editors appreciate the speed at which medical knowledge can advance through interprofessional and global collaboration. This edition of *The Manual* was compiled through the efforts of generations of physicians and learners who sought to contribute to that growing knowledge.

This edition is foremost a tribute to the Washington University in St. Louis Internal Medicine housestaff, fellows, medical students, and attendings with whom we work daily. Their role modeling, mentoring, compassion, teaching, brilliance, and hard work are an unlimited source of enthusiasm, inspiration, and dedication. We consider ourselves very lucky and grateful to have trained alongside them, in service to our patients.

We have great appreciation for the substantial support and direction that Dr. Thomas Ciesielski, the executive editor, provided in the creation of this edition. We also sincerely thank Katie Sharp and the editorial staff at Wolters Kluwer for their assistance and guidance in this effort.

We have had the distinction of serving as chief residents in the Department of Medicine at the Washington University School of Medicine in St. Louis, and our accomplishments would not have been possible without our larger departmental team. We would like to acknowledge the support and collaboration we have experienced from our Associate Program Directors, Drs. Thomas Ciesielski, Geoffrey Cislo, Anthony Dao, Amber Deptola, Michael DeVita, Patricia Kao, Mary Clare McGregor, Jennifer Schmidt, and Megan Wren. Our Program Director, Dr. Dominique Cosco, has provided us with guidance and immense support during the course of this year. The Chair of the Department of Medicine, Dr. Victoria Fraser, has served as an excellent role model and mentor and holds our sincere admiration.

Department Chair's Note

Medicine and health care delivery continue to evolve based on the significant advances in biomedical science, improvements in patient safety and quality, and diversity of health care settings. It has become more important than ever for physicians to have rapid access to new evidence to guide clinical practice. Tremendous advances in science have led to new molecular diagnostics, more sensitive biomarkers, and novel therapies that improve patient outcomes. *The Washington Manual® of Medical Therapeutics* provides an excellent source of information focused on practical clinical approaches to the diagnosis, investigation, and treatment of common medical conditions regularly encountered by internists. The online and in-print versions of *The Washington Manual®* ensure that it will continue to be of enormous assistance to interns, residents, medical students, and other practitioners. *The Washington Manual®* provides an important resource of medical information and efficient approaches to transfer new knowledge into evidenced-based patient care.

I am very grateful to the authors, who include outstanding house officers, fellows, and attendings at Washington University/Barnes-Jewish Hospital. Their efforts and exceptional skills are evident in the quality of the final product. In particular, I am proud of our editors: Drs. Siri Ancha, Christine Auberle, Devin Cash, Mohit Harsh, John Hickman, and Carole Kounga, and Executive Editor Thomas M. Ciesielski, who have produced another outstanding edition of *The Washington Manual® of Medical Therapeutics*. I also thank Dr. Dominique Cosco for her leadership of our residency training program. I am confident that this edition will meet its desired goal of providing practical knowledge that will be directly applied to improving patient care.

Victoria J. Fraser, MD
Adolphus Busch Professor of Medicine
Chair, Department of Medicine
Washington University School of Medicine
St. Louis, Missouri

Contents

Contributors

Samantha E. Adamson, MD, PhD
Fellow
Division of Endocrinology

Siri Ancha, MD
Instructor in Medicine
Division of General Medicine

Lolwa Al-Obaid, MD
Fellow
Division of Gastroenterology

Crystal Atwood, MD
Assistant Professor of Medicine
Division of Hospital Medicine

Kevin Baumgartner, MD
Assistant Professor of Medicine
Department of Emergency Medicine

Amanda Cashen, MD
Professor of Medicine
Divisions of Hematology and Oncology

Murali Chakinala, MD
Professor of Medicine
Division of Pulmonary and Critical
  Care Medicine

Miguel A. Chavez, MD, MSc
Instructor in Medicine
Division of Hospital Medicine

Alexander Chen, MD
Associate Professor of Medicine and
  Surgery
Division of Pulmonary and Critical
  Care Medicine

Steven Cheng, MD
Professor of Medicine
Division of Nephrology

Praveen Chenna, MD
Associate Professor
Division of Pulmonary and Critical
  Care Medicine

Joseph N. Cherabie, MD, MSc
Instructor in Medicine
Division of Infectious Diseases

William E. Clutter, MD
Associate Professor of Medicine
Division of Endocrinology, Metabolism,
  and Lipid Research

Daniel H. Cooper, MD
Associate Professor
Cardiovascular Division

Zachary D. Crees, MD
Fellow
Divisions of Hematology and Oncology

Jeffrey Crippen, MD
Professor of Medicine
Division of Gastroenterology

Siddhartha Devarakonda, MD
Assistant Professor of Medicine
Division of Medical Oncology

Jason Devgun, MD
Assistant Professor of Emergency
  Medicine
Department of Emergency Medicine

Katherine Dittman, DO
Fellow
Division of Pulmonary and Critical
  Care Medicine

Lauren East, MD
Resident
Department of Internal Medicine

Mitchell N. Faddis, MD, PhD
Professor of Medicine
Cardiovascular Division

Brian F. Gage, MD
Professor of Medicine
Division of General Medical Sciences

James A. Giles, MD
Fellow
Division of Neurology

Anne C. Goldberg, MD
Professor of Medicine
Division of Endocrinology, Metabolism,
and Lipid Research

Seth Goldberg, MD
Associate Professor of Medicine
Division of Nephrology

Ramaswamy Govindan, MD
Professor of Medicine
Division of Medical Oncology

Martin H. Gregory, MD
Fellow
Division of Gastroenterology

Rodrigo Vazquez Guillamet, MD
Associate Professor of Medicine
Division of Pulmonary and Critical
Care Medicine

C. Prakash Gyawali, MD
Professor of Medicine
Division of Gastroenterology

Laura Halverson, MD
Assistant Professor of Medicine
Division of Pulmonary and Critical
Care Medicine

Katrina Han, MD
Fellow
Division of Endocrinology, Metabolism,
and Lipid Research

Justin C. Hartupee, MD
Assistant Professor of Medicine
Cardiovascular Division

Cynthia J. Herrick, MD, MPHS
Associate Professor of Medicine
Division of Endocrinology, Metabolism,
and Lipid Research

SueLin Hilbert, MD, MPH
Associate Professor of Emergency
Medicine
Department of Emergency Medicine

Wut Yi Hninn, MD, MBBS
Fellow
Transplant Nephrology

Daniel T. Ilges, PharmD, BCIDP
Pharmacy Resident
Division of Infectious Diseases

Eric Johnson, MD
Assistant Professor of Medicine
Division of Hospital Medicine

Kai Jones, MD
Resident
Department of Internal Medicine

Paul Kannarkat, MD
Instructor in Medicine
Division of Pulmonary and Critical
Care Medicine

Phillip M. King, MD
Fellow
Cardiovascular Division

Nigar Kirmani, MD
Professor of Medicine
Division of Infectious Diseases

Marin H. Kollef, MD
Professor of Medicine
Division of Pulmonary and Critical
Care Medicine

James G. Krings, MD, MSCI
Assistant Professor
Division of Pulmonary and Critical
Care Medicine

Mark D. Levine, MD
Associate Professor of Emergency
Medicine
Department of Emergency Medicine

Stephen Y. Liang, MD, MPHS
Associate Professor of Medicine
Division of Infectious Diseases

Michael Lin, MD
Associate Professor
Division of Hospital Medicine

Caline Mattar, MD
Assistant Professor of Medicine
Division of Infectious Diseases

Janet B. McGill, MD
Professor of Medicine
Division of Endocrinology, Metabolism,
and Lipid Research

Carlos Mejia-Chew, MD
Assistant Professor of Medicine
Division of Infectious Diseases

Jennifer M. Monroy, MD
Associate Professor of Medicine
Division of Allergy and Immunology

Daniel Morgensztern, MD
Professor of Medicine
Division of Medical Oncology

Nathaniel Moulton, MD
Fellow
Division of Pulmonary and Critical
Care Medicine

Michael E. Mullins, MD
Associate Professor of Emergency
Medicine
Department of Emergency Medicine

Blessing Osondu, MD
Fellow
Division of Pulmonary and Critical
Care Medicine

Bindiya G. Patel, MD
Fellow
Division of Medical Oncology

Mary E. Petrulis, MD
Clinical Fellow
Division of Neurology

Rachel M. Presti, MD, PhD
Associate Professor of Medicine
Division of Infectious Diseases

Nishath Quader, MD
Associate Professor of Medicine
Cardiovascular Division

Andrea Ramirez Gomez, MD
Fellow
Division of Rheumatology

Dominic Reeds, MD
Professor of Medicine
Division of Geriatrics and Nutritional
Science

Sana Saif Ur Rehman, MD
Assistant Professor
Division of Hematology

Hilary E. L. Reno, MD, PhD
Associate Professor of Medicine
Division of Infectious Diseases

Amy E. Riek, MD
Assistant Professor of Medicine
Division of Endocrinology, Metabolism,
and Lipid Research

David J. Ritchie, PharmD
Clinical Pharmacist Specialist
Infectious Diseases
Barnes-Jewish Hospital

Rebecca Roediger, MD
Fellow
Division of Gastroenterology

David B. Rose, MD
Fellow
Division of Pulmonary and Critical
Care Medicine

Tonya D. Russell, MD
Professor of Medicine
Division of Pulmonary and Critical
Care Medicine

Maryam Saleem, MD
Fellow
Division of Nephrology

Kristen M. Sanfilippo, MD
Assistant Professor of Medicine
Division of Hematology

Rowena Delos Santos, MD
Associate Professor of Medicine
Division of Nephrology

Evan S. Schwarz, MD
Associate Professor of Medicine
Department of Emergency Medicine

Gabriel Schroeder, MD
Fellow
Division of Pulmonary and Critical
Care Medicine

Deepali Sen, MD
Associate Professor of Medicine
Division of Rheumatology

Parth Shah, MD
Fellow
Division of Gastroenterology

Adrian Shifren, MD
Assistant Professor of Medicine
Division of Pulmonary and Critical
Care Medicine

Marc A. Sintek, MD
Assistant Professor of Medicine
Cardiovascular Division

Sandeep S. Sodhi, MD, MBA
Assistant Professor of Medicine
Cardiovascular Division

Kaharu Sumino, MD
Associate Professor of Medicine
Division of Pulmonary and Critical
Care Medicine

Justin M. Vader, MD
Associate Professor of Medicine
Cardiovascular Division

Dayne Voelker, MD
Fellow
Division of Allergy and Immunology

Tzu-Fei Wang, MD
Assistant Professor of Internal Medicine
Division of Hematology
The Ohio State University

Dominique S. Williams, MD
Assistant Professor of Medicine
Cardiovascular Division

Noah N. Williford, MD
Fellow
Cardiovascular Division

Bin Q. Yang, MD
Fellow
Cardiovascular Division

Roger D. Yusen, MD, MPH
Associate Professor of Medicine
Division of Pulmonary and Critical
Care Medicine

Ray Zhang, MD, PhD
Assistant Professor of Medicine
Department of Pathology &
Immunology
Division of Laboratory & Genomic
Medicine

Amy Zhou, MD
Assistant Professor of Medicine
Division of Medical Oncology

1 Inpatient Care in Internal Medicine

Michael Lin, Eric Johnson, and Crystal Atwood

General Care of the Hospitalized Patient

GENERAL PRINCIPLES

- Although a general approach to common problems can be outlined, **therapy must be individualized.** All diagnostic and therapeutic procedures should be explained carefully to the patient, including the potential risks, benefits, and alternatives.
- The period of hospitalization represents a complex interplay of multiple caregivers that subjects the patient to potential harm by **medical errors and iatrogenic complications.** Every effort must be made to minimize these risks. Basic measures include the following:
  - Use of standardized abbreviations and dose designations
  - Excellent communication between physicians and other caregivers
  - Institution of appropriate prophylactic precautions
  - Prevention of nosocomial infections, including attention to hygiene and discontinuation of unnecessary catheters
  - Medicine reconciliation at all transfers of care
- **Hospital orders**
  - Admission orders should be entered promptly after evaluation of a patient.
  - Daily rounds should include assessment for ongoing need of IV fluids, telemetry, catheters, and supplemental oxygen, all of which can limit mobility.
  - The need for daily labs should be reassessed each day while patients are admitted in the hospital.
- **Discharge**
  - **Discharge planning** begins at the time of admission. Assessment of the patient's social situation and potential discharge needs should be planned.
  - **Early coordination** with nursing, social work, and case coordinators facilitates efficient discharge and a complete postdischarge plan.
  - **Patient education** should occur regarding changes in medications and other new therapies. Adherence is influenced by the patient's understanding of the treatment plan.
  - **Prescriptions** should be written for all new medication, and the patient should be provided with a complete medication list including instructions and indications.
  - **Communication** with physicians who will be resuming care of the patient is important for optimal follow-up care and should be a component of the discharge process.

PROPHYLACTIC MEASURES

Venous Thromboembolism Prophylaxis

GENERAL PRINCIPLES

Epidemiology

Venous thromboembolism (VTE) is a preventable cause of death in hospitalized patients. In the largest observational study to date attempting to risk-stratify medical patients, 1.2% of medical patients developed VTE within 90 days of admission. A total of 10%–31% of patients were deemed to be at high risk for VTE, defined as having **two or more points** by weighted risk factors listed below[1]:
* Three points: previous VTE, thrombophilia
* One point: cancer, age >60 years

Prevention

* **Ambulation** several times a day should be encouraged.
* **Pharmacologic prophylaxis** results in a 50% decrease in VTE risk. No overall mortality benefit from prophylaxis has been demonstrated.
* Acutely ill patients at high risk of VTE, without bleeding or high risk of bleeding, can be treated with low-dose unfractionated heparin (UFH) or low-molecular-weight heparin (LMWH) such as enoxaparin, dalteparin, or fondaparinux.[1]
* Betrixaban and rivaroxaban are the only direct oral anticoagulant approved for deep venous thrombosis DVT prophylaxis in nonsurgical hospitalized patients.[2]
* Aspirin alone is not sufficient for prophylaxis in hospitalized patients.[3]
* At-risk patients with contraindications to anticoagulation prophylaxis may receive mechanical prophylaxis with intermittent pneumatic compression or graded compression stockings, although evidence of benefit is lacking.[4]

Decubitus Ulcers

GENERAL PRINCIPLES

Epidemiology

Decubitus ulcers typically occur within the first 2 weeks of hospitalization and can develop within 2–6 hours. Once they develop, decubitus ulcers are difficult to heal and have been associated with increased mortality.[5] The most important risk factors for the development of decubitus ulcers are immobility, malnutrition, reduced skin perfusion, and sensory loss.

Prevention

Prevention is key to management of decubitus ulcers. It is recognized that not all decubitus ulcers are avoidable. Preventative measures include the following:
* **Advanced static mattresses** or overlays should be used in at-risk patients.[6]
* **Skin care** includes daily inspection with particular attention to bony prominences including heels, minimizing exposure to moisture, and applying moisturizers to dry sacral skin.
* **Nutritional supplements** may be provided to patients at risk.
* **Frequent repositioning** (minimum of every 2 hours) is suggested.
* **Multilayer foam dressings** have been shown to reduce the rates of pressure injuries.[7]

DIAGNOSIS

National Pressure Ulcer Advisory Panel Staging:
- **Suspected deep tissue injury:** Localized area of purple or maroon intact skin or blood-filled blister because of damage of underlying soft tissue from pressure and/ or shear.
- **Stage I:** Intact skin with nonblanching redness of a localized area usually over a bony prominence. Darkly pigmented skin may obscure findings.
- **Stage II:** Partial thickness loss of dermis presenting as a shallow open ulcer with a red pink wound bed without slough. May also present as a blister.
- **Stage III:** Full-thickness tissue loss. Subcutaneous fat may be visible, but the bone, tendon, or muscle is not exposed. Slough may be present but does not obscure the depth of tissue loss. May include undermining and tunneling.
- **Stage IV:** Full-thickness tissue loss with exposed bone, tendon, or muscle. Slough or eschar may be present on some parts of the wound bed. Often includes undermining and tunneling.
- **Unstageable:** Full-thickness tissue loss in which the base of the ulcer is covered by slough (yellow, tan, gray, green, or brown) and/or eschar (tan, brown, or black) in the wound bed.

TREATMENT

Optimal treatment of pressure ulcers remains poorly defined. There is evidence to support the following:[8]
- **Hydrocolloid or foam** dressings may reduce wound size.
- **Electrical stimulation** may accelerate healing.
- **Other adjunctive therapies** with less supporting evidence include radiant heat, negative pressure, and platelet-derived growth factor. Topical agents (Santyl, Xenaderm) may optimize healing or lead to minor slough débridement.

OTHER PRECAUTIONS

- **Fall precautions** should be written for patients who are at high risk of a fall (e.g., dementia, weakness, orthostasis). Falls are the most common accident in hospitalized patients, frequently leading to injury. **Fall risk should not be equated with bed rest,** which may lead to debilitation and higher risk of future falls.
- **Seizure precautions,** which include padded bed rails and an oral airway at the bedside, should be considered for patients with a history of seizures or those at risk of seizing.
- **Restraint orders** are written for patients who are at risk of injuring themselves or interfering with their treatment because of disruptive or dangerous behaviors. Physical restraints may exacerbate agitation. Bed alarms, sitters, and sedatives are alternatives in appropriate settings.

ACUTE INPATIENT CARE

An approach to selected common complaints is presented in this section. An evaluation should generally include a directed history and physical examination, review of the medical problem list, review of medications with attention to recent medication changes, and consideration of recent procedures.

Chest Pain

GENERAL PRINCIPLES

Common causes of chest pain range from life-threatening causes such as myocardial infarction (MI) and pulmonary embolism (PE) to other causes including esophageal reflux, peptic ulcer disease, pneumonia, costochondritis, shingles, trauma, and anxiety.

DIAGNOSIS

History and Physical Examination

- History should include previous cardiac or vascular disease history, cardiac risk factors, and risk factors for VTE.
- Physical examination is ideally conducted during an episode of pain and includes vital signs (bilateral blood pressure [BP] measurements if considering aortic dissection), cardiopulmonary and abdominal examination, and inspection and palpation of the chest.

Diagnostic Testing

Assessment of oxygenation status, CXR, and ECG is appropriate in most patients. Serial cardiac biomarkers should be obtained if there is suspicion of ischemia. Spiral CT and ventilation/perfusion scans can be used to diagnose PE.

TREATMENT

- If cardiac ischemia is a concern, see Chapter 4, Ischemic Heart Disease, for details.
- Musculoskeletal pain typically responds to acetaminophen or NSAID therapy.
- Prompt treatment is necessary if there is high suspicion for MI or PE.

Dyspnea

GENERAL PRINCIPLES

Dyspnea is most commonly caused by a cardiopulmonary abnormality, such as congestive heart failure (CHF), cardiac ischemia, bronchospasm, PE, infection, mucus plugging, and aspiration. Dyspnea must be promptly and carefully evaluated.

DIAGNOSIS

History and Physical Examination

- Initial evaluation should include a review of the medical history for underlying pulmonary or cardiovascular disease and a detailed history of present illness.
- A detailed cardiopulmonary examination should take place.

Diagnostic Testing

- Oxygen assessment by pulse oximetry and CXR are useful in most patients.
- Other diagnostic measures should be directed by the findings in the initial evaluation.

TREATMENT

Oxygen should be administered promptly if needed. Other therapeutic measures should be directed by the findings in the initial evaluation.

Acute Hypertensive Episodes

GENERAL PRINCIPLES

- Acute hypertensive episodes in the hospital are most often caused by inadequately treated essential hypertension. If there is evidence of end organ damage, IV medications are indicated. Oral agents are more appropriate for hypertensive urgency without end organ damage.
- Hypertension associated with withdrawal syndromes (e.g., alcohol, cocaine) and rebound hypertension associated with sudden withdrawal of antihypertensive medications (e.g., clonidine, α-adrenergic antagonists) should be considered.
- Volume overload and pain may exacerbate hypertension and should be recognized appropriately and treated.

Fever

GENERAL PRINCIPLES

Fever accompanies many illnesses and is a valuable marker of disease activity. Infection is a primary concern. Drug reaction, malignancy, VTE, vasculitis, central fever, and tissue infarction are other possibilities but are diagnoses of exclusion.

DIAGNOSIS

History and Physical Examination

- History should include chronology of the fever and associated symptoms, medications, potential exposures, and a complete social and travel history.
- In the hospitalized patient, special attention should be paid to any IV lines, asymmetric edema, a thorough skin examination, and indwelling devices such as urinary catheters.

Diagnostic Testing

- Testing includes blood and urine cultures, complete blood count (CBC) with differential, and serum chemistries with liver function tests.
- Diagnostic evaluation generally includes CXR.
- Cultures of abnormal fluid collections, sputum, cerebrospinal fluid, urine, and stool should be sent if clinically indicated. Cultures are ideally obtained prior to initiation of antibiotics; however, antibiotics should not be delayed if serious infection is suspected.

TREATMENT

- Antipyretic drugs may be given to decrease associated discomfort.
- Empiric antibiotics should be considered in hemodynamically unstable patients in whom infection is a primary concern, as well as in neutropenic and asplenic patients.
- Heat stroke and malignant hyperthermia are medical emergencies that require prompt recognition and treatment (see Chapter 26, Medical Emergencies).

Pain

GENERAL PRINCIPLES

Pain is subjective and therapy must be individualized. Chronic pain may not be associated with any objective physical findings. Pain scales can be employed for quantitation.

TREATMENT

- Acute pain usually requires short-term therapy and often improves with acetaminophen- or NSAID-based regimens.
- **Chronic pain requires multimodality management to keep opioid use to a minimum to prevent risk of dependence and subsequent escalation of opioid doses.** Higher doses of opioids have been shown to increase the risk of overdose without providing increased pain relief.[9]
- If pain is refractory to medical therapy, then nonpharmacologic modalities, such as nerve blocks, sympathectomy, and cognitive behavioral therapy, may be appropriate.

Opioid Analgesics

- Effects: Opioid analgesics are pharmacologically similar to opium or morphine and are indicated for moderate to severe pain.
- Dosage: Table 1-1 lists equianalgesic dosages.
- For acute pain management, the **lowest effective dose of immediate-release opioids** should be given. Patients with demonstrated tolerance often require higher doses.
- Use of nonopioid pain medications and nonpharmacological pain management strategies to minimize opioid needs is encouraged.
- Both parenteral and transdermal administration are useful in the setting of dysphagia, emesis, or decreased gastrointestinal (GI) absorption.
- Patient-controlled analgesia often is used to control pain in a postoperative or terminally ill patient. Opioid-naïve patients should not have basal rates prescribed due to risk of overdose.

TABLE 1-1	Equipotent Doses of Opioid Analgesics			
Drug	Onset (min)	Duration (h)	IM/IV/SC (mg)	PO (mg)
Fentanyl	7–8	1–2	0.1	NA
Levorphanol	30–90	4–6	2	4
Hydromorphone	15–30	2–4	1.5–2.0	7.5
Methadone	30–60	4–12	10	20
Morphine	15–30	2–4	10	30[a]
Oxycodone	15–30	3–4	NA	20
Codeine	15–30	4–6	120	200

[a]An IM:PO ratio of 1:2–1:3 used for repetitive dosing.
Note: Equivalences are based on single-dose studies.
NA, not applicable.

- If a patient requires continuous (basal) analgesia, supplementary PRN doses for breakthrough pain of roughly 5%–15% of the daily basal dose can be provided. If frequent PRN doses are required, the maintenance dose should be increased, or the dosing interval should be decreased.
- Severe pain uncontrolled with large doses of opiates, particularly while using patient-controlled analgesia with basal rates, may warrant consultation with a pain specialist.
  - Opioids are relatively contraindicated in acute disease states in which the pattern and degree of pain are important diagnostic signs (e.g., head injuries). They also may increase intracranial pressure.
  - Opioid dosage should be adjusted for patients with impaired hepatic or renal function.
  - Drugs that potentiate the adverse effects of opioids include phenothiazines, antidepressants, benzodiazepines, and alcohol.
  - Tolerance develops with chronic use and coincides with the development of physical dependence, which is characterized by a withdrawal syndrome when the drug is stopped abruptly. It may occur after only 2 weeks of therapy.
  - Administration of an opioid antagonist may precipitate withdrawal after only 3 days of therapy.
  - The quantity of opioid tablets prescribed at discharge should not exceed the expected duration of pain. A quantity to cover 3 days or less should be sufficient. **Prescribing a quantity at discharge to cover more than 7 days duration of pain should not be necessary and is discouraged.**[9]
- Adverse and toxic effects
  - Central nervous system effects include sedation, euphoria, and pupillary constriction.
  - **Respiratory depression** is dose related and pronounced after IV administration.
  - Cardiovascular effects include **peripheral vasodilation** and hypotension.
  - GI effects include **constipation, nausea,** and **vomiting.** Stool softeners and laxatives should be prescribed to prevent constipation. Opioids may precipitate toxic megacolon in patients with inflammatory bowel disease.
  - Genitourinary effects include **urinary retention.**
  - **Pruritus** occurs most commonly with spinal administration.
  - **Opioid overdose**
    - Naloxone, an opioid antagonist, should be readily available for administration in the case of accidental or intentional overdose.
    - Naloxone home rescue kits have been shown to reduce opioid overdose mortality.[10] **Patients being discharged home on more than 50 morphine milligram equivalents per day have a higher risk of overdose** and may benefit from a prescription for intranasal naloxone at discharge.

Altered Mental Status

GENERAL PRINCIPLES

Mental status changes have a broad differential diagnosis that includes neurologic (e.g., stroke, seizure, delirium), metabolic (e.g., hypoxemia, hypoglycemia), toxic (e.g., drug effects, alcohol withdrawal), and other etiologies. Infection is a common cause of mental status changes in the elderly and in patients with underlying neurologic disease. Sundown syndrome refers to the appearance of worsening confusion in the evening and is associated with dementia, delirium, and unfamiliar environments.

DIAGNOSIS

History and Physical Examination

• Focus particularly on medications, underlying dementia, cognitive impairment, neurologic or psychiatric disorders, and a history of alcohol and/or drug use.
• Physical examination generally includes vital signs, a search for sites of infection, a complete cardiopulmonary examination, and a detailed neurologic examination including mental status evaluation.

Diagnostic Testing

• Testing includes blood glucose, serum electrolytes, creatinine, CBC, urinalysis, and oxygen assessment.
• Other evaluation, including lumbar puncture, toxicology screen, cultures, thyroid function tests, noncontrast head CT, electroencephalogram, CXR, or ECG, should be directed by initial findings.

TREATMENT

Management of specific disorders is discussed in Chapter 27, Neurologic Disorders.

Medications

Agitation and psychosis may be features of a change in mental status. The antipsychotic haloperidol and the benzodiazepine lorazepam are commonly used in the acute management of these symptoms. Second-generation antipsychotics (risperidone, olanzapine, quetiapine, clozapine, ziprasidone, aripiprazole, paliperidone) are alternative agents that may lead to decreased incidence of extrapyramidal symptoms. All of these agents pose risks to elderly patients and those with dementia if given long term.

• Haloperidol is the initial drug of choice for acute management of agitation and psychosis. It has fewer active metabolites and fewer anticholinergic, sedative, and hypotensive effects than other antipsychotics but may have more extrapyramidal side effects.
• In low dosages, haloperidol rarely causes hypotension, cardiovascular compromise, or excessive sedation.
• Postural hypotension may occasionally be acute and severe after administration. IV fluids should be given initially for treatment.
• Use should be discontinued with prolongation of QTc >450 ms or 25% above baseline.
• Neuroleptic malignant syndrome (see Chapter 27, Neurologic Disorders).
• Lorazepam can also be used for agitation. Lorazepam has a short duration of action and few active metabolites. Excessive sedation and respiratory depression can occur.

Nonpharmacologic Therapies

Patients with delirium of any etiology often respond to frequent reorientation, observance of the day–night light cycle, and maintenance of a familiar environment. **These methods should be trialed before the use of the above medications if the patient is not a threat to themselves or care teams.**

PERIOPERATIVE MEDICINE

The role of the medical consultant is to estimate the level of risk associated with a given procedure, determine the need for further evaluation based on this risk estimate, and prescribe interventions to mitigate risk.

Preoperative Cardiac Evaluation

GENERAL PRINCIPLES

Perioperative cardiac complications are generally defined as cardiac death, MIs (both ST and non-ST elevation), CHF, and clinically significant rhythm disturbances.

DIAGNOSIS

Clinical Presentation

History

Patient factors and comorbid conditions that affect perioperative cardiac risk include the following:
- Clinical risk factors for coronary artery disease (CAD)
- Preexisting, stable CAD
- Unstable coronary syndromes
- Recent MI (defined as >7 but <30 days)
- Decompensated CHF (New York Heart Association class IV, worsening or new-onset heart failure [HF])
- Arrhythmias
- Severe valvular disease
- Compensated or prior CHF
- Diabetes mellitus
- Prior cerebrovascular accident (CVA) or transient ischemic attack (TIA)
- Chronic kidney disease
- Poorly controlled hypertension
- Abnormal ECG (e.g., left ventricular hypertrophy, left bundle branch block, ST–T wave abnormalities)
- Age >70 years identified in several studies as a significant risk factor but not uniformly accepted as independent.[11,12]

Physical Examination

Specific attention should be paid to the following:
- Vital signs, in particular elevated BP. Systolic blood pressure (SBP) <180 mm Hg and diastolic blood pressure (DBP) <110 mm Hg are generally considered permissible. The management of stage III hypertension (SBP >180 mm Hg or DBP >110 mm Hg) is controversial. Though postposing elective surgery to allow adequate BP control in this setting seems reasonable, how long to wait after treatment implementation to proceed remains unclear. Evidence of **decompensated CHF** (elevated jugular venous pressure, rales, S_3, edema).
- **Murmurs suggestive of significant valvular lesions.** According to the 2014 American Heart Association (AHA)/American College of Cardiology (ACC) Guideline for the Management of Patients with Valvular Heart Disease, the risk of noncardiac surgery is increased in all patients with significant valvular heart disease, although symptomatic aortic stenosis (AS) is thought to carry the greatest risk. The estimated rate of cardiac complications in patients with undiagnosed severe AS undergoing noncardiac surgery is 10%–30%. However, aortic valve replacement is also associated with considerable risk. Risk–benefit analysis appears to favor proceeding to intermediate-risk elective noncardiac surgery (see below) with appropriate intra- and postoperative hemodynamic monitoring (including intraoperative

right heart catheter or transesophageal echocardiogram) as opposed to prophylactic aortic valve replacement in the context of asymptomatic severe disease. The same recommendations (albeit with less supporting evidence) apply to asymptomatic severe mitral regurgitation, asymptomatic severe aortic regurgitation with normal ejection fraction, and asymptomatic severe mitral stenosis (assuming valve morphology is not amenable to percutaneous balloon mitral commissurotomy, which should otherwise be considered to optimize cardiac status prior to proceeding to surgery). Symptomatic severe valvular disease of any type should prompt preoperative cardiology consultation.

Diagnostic Criteria

The 2014 ACC/AHA Guideline on Perioperative Cardiovascular Evaluation and Management of Patients Undergoing Noncardiac Surgery offers a stepwise approach to preoperative evaluation and risk stratification (Figure 1-1).

* Step 1: Establish the urgency of surgery. Many surgeries are unlikely to allow for a time-consuming evaluation.
* Step 2: Assess for active cardiac conditions (see "History," above).
* Step 3: Determine the surgery-specific risk as follows:
  ○ Low-risk surgeries (<1% expected risk of adverse cardiac events) include superficial procedures, cataract/breast surgery, endoscopic procedures, and most procedures that can be performed in an ambulatory setting.
  ○ Intermediate-risk surgeries (1%–5% risk of adverse cardiac events) include carotid endarterectomy, intraperitoneal/intrathoracic surgery, orthopedic surgery, head and neck surgery, and prostate surgery.
  ○ Vascular surgery involving extremity revascularization or aortic repair generally carries the highest risk (>5% risk of adverse cardiac events).
* Step 4: Assess the patient's functional capacity.

  Poor functional capacity (<4 metabolic equivalents [METs]) is associated with an increased risk of perioperative cardiac events.[13,14] Although exercise testing is the gold standard, functional capacity can be reliably estimated by patient self-report.[15] Examples of activities that suggest at least moderate functional capacity (>4 METs) include climbing one to two flights of stairs or walking a block at a brisk pace. Patients with a functional capacity of >4 METs without symptoms can proceed to surgery with relatively low risk.
* Step 5: Assess the patient's clinical risk factors.
  ○ The number of risk factors combined with the surgery-specific risk (intermediate vs. vascular) determines further management. The following risk factors are adapted from the Revised Cardiac Risk Index (RCRI):[16]
    ■ Ischemic heart disease
    ■ History of TIA or CVA
    ■ History of CHF
    ■ Preoperative serum creatinine ≥2 mg/dL
    ■ Diabetes mellitus requiring insulin
  ○ Patients with no clinical risk factors are at inherently low risk (<1% risk of cardiac events) and may proceed to surgery without further testing. Patients with one or two clinical risk factors are generally at intermediate risk and may proceed to surgery, although stress testing might help refine risk assessment in selected cases. Patients with three or more clinical risk factors are at high risk of adverse cardiac events, particularly when undergoing vascular surgery. In this population especially, stress testing may provide a better estimate of cardiovascular risk and may be considered if knowledge of this increased risk would change management.[17]

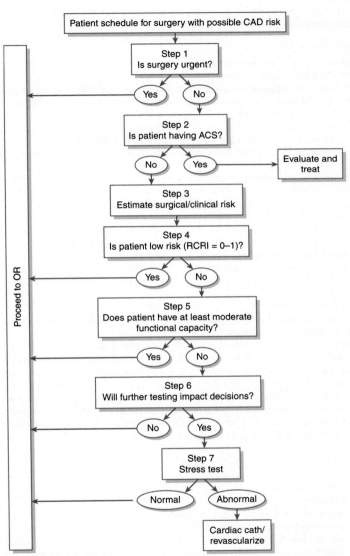

Figure 1-1. Cardiac evaluation algorithm for noncardiac surgery. ACS, acute coronary syndrome; CAD, coronary artery disease; OR, operating room; RCRI, Revised Cardiac Risk Index. (Modified from Fleisher LA, Fleischmann KE, Auerbach AD, et al. 2014 ACC/AHA guideline on perioperative cardiovascular evaluation and management of patients undergoing noncardiac surgery: a report of the American College of Cardiology/American Heart Association Task Force on Practice Guidelines. *Circulation.* 2014;130(24):e278-e333.)

A positive stress test in a high-risk patient portends a substantially increased risk of a perioperative cardiac event, whereas a negative study suggests a lower risk than that predicted by clinical factors alone.[11]

Diagnostic Testing

- **12-Lead ECG.** The value of a routine ECG is controversial. Per the 2014 ACC/AHA guidelines (level of evidence: B):
  - ECG is "reasonable" in patients with known CAD, significant arrhythmia, peripheral arterial disease, cerebrovascular disease, or other significant structural heart disease prior to intermediate-risk surgery and above (class IIa);
  - "May be considered" for asymptomatic patients without known coronary heart disease prior to intermediate- and high-risk surgery (class IIb);
  - Is "not useful" for asymptomatic patients undergoing low-risk surgical procedures (class III).
- **Resting echocardiogram.** In general, the indications for preoperative echocardiographic evaluation are no different from those in the nonoperative setting. Murmurs found on physical examination suggestive of significant underlying valvular disease (see above) should be evaluated by echocardiogram. Assessment of left ventricular function should be considered when there is clinical concern for underlying undiagnosed CHF or if there is concern for deterioration since the last examination.
- **Noninvasive stress testing.** The decision to pursue a stress evaluation should be guided by an assessment of preoperative risk as detailed above. For further details on stress testing, see Chapter 4, Ischemic Heart Disease.

Special Considerations

- Patients with drug-eluting coronary stents: See "Perioperative Anticoagulation and Antithrombotic Management."
- Multiple studies have reported a correlation between delayed repair of hip fracture and increased morbidity and mortality.[18,19] For urgent surgical procedures (i.e., those that should be done within 48 hours of diagnosis), the value of additional testing is typically outweighed by the risk of worsened short- and long-term outcomes incurred with surgical delay. Unnecessary preoperative cardiac testing may be an independent risk factor for postoperative complications in hip fracture patients.[20] In such cases, it is advisable to optimize the patient's medical status and modifiable risk factors and then proceed to the operating room.

TREATMENT

Medications

- **β-Blockers**
  - Multiple studies have provided support for perioperative β-blockade in patients with or at risk for CAD undergoing noncardiac surgeries. The most pronounced benefit has been observed in high-risk patients undergoing vascular surgery where β-blocker dose was titrated to heart rate control.[17,21] However, a subsequent analysis has called into question the role of dose titration.[22] Although reduction in perioperative cardiac events has been observed consistently, it warrants mentioning that few data support the effectiveness of perioperative β-blockade in reducing mortality.
  - According to the 2014 ACC/AHA guidelines:
    - In patients with three or more RCRI risk factors (see above) or evidence of myocardial ischemia on preoperative stress testing, starting preoperative β-blockade is reasonable (level of evidence: B).

- β-Blockade should not be started on the day of surgery, as it is at minimum ineffective level and may actually be harmful (level of evidence: B).
  - Patients already taking β-blockers should be continued on their medication (level of evidence: B).
- **Statins**
  - Multiple trials have shown a decrease in perioperative cardiac events and/or mortality with statin use in patients undergoing vascular surgery. Moreover, a recent cohort study of statin therapy in patients undergoing intermediate-risk noncardiac, nonvascular surgery revealed a fivefold reduced risk of 30-day all-cause mortality along with a statistically significant reduction in the composite end point of 30-day all-cause mortality, atrial fibrillation (AF), and nonfatal MI.[23]
  - Per the 2014 ACC/AHA guidelines:
    - Patients currently taking statins should be maintained on therapy (level of evidence: B).
    - Patients undergoing vascular surgery, and those with risk factors undergoing intermediate-risk surgery, may benefit from initiation of statin therapy perioperatively (level of evidence: B and C, respectively). Optimal dose, duration of therapy, and target low-density lipoprotein levels for perioperative risk reduction are unclear.
- **Aspirin**
  For discussion, see "Perioperative Anticoagulation and Antithrombotic Management."

Revascularization

- The best available data on preoperative revascularization come from the Coronary Artery Revascularization Prophylaxis (CARP) trial, a prospective study of patients scheduled to undergo vascular surgery.[24] Patients with proven significant CAD were randomized to revascularization versus no revascularization. There was no difference between the groups in the occurrence of MI or death at 30 days or in mortality with long-term follow-up. Patients with three or more clinical risk factors and extensive ischemia on stress testing were evaluated in a separate small study.[25] High event rates were seen in both study arms, and no benefit was seen with revascularization. Taken together, these studies suggest that the risk of adverse cardiac events is not altered by attempts at preoperative revascularization, even in high-risk populations. Patients with left main disease, who appeared to have benefited from preoperative revascularization in a subset analysis of the CARP trial data, are a notable possible expectation.[26]
- Based on these cumulative results, a strategy of routinely pursuing coronary revascularization as a method of decreasing perioperative cardiac risk cannot be recommended. However, careful screening of patients is still essential to identify those high-risk subsets who may obtain a survival benefit from revascularization independent of their need for noncardiac surgery.

MONITORING/FOLLOW-UP

Postoperative Infarction and Surveillance

- Most events will occur within 48–72 hours of surgery, with the majority in the first 24 hours.[27] Most are also **clinically silent**.[28] Although overall 30-day mortality has been linked to postoperative troponin elevation, the cause of death is not predictable, and no specific course of therapy may be offered.[29]

- The 2014 ACC/AHA guidelines offer the following[30]:
  - Routine postoperative ECGs and troponins are not recommended.
  - The benefit of troponin measurements and ECGs in high cardiac risk patients is uncertain.
  - Symptomatic infarctions should be addressed according to standard therapy of acute coronary syndromes (see Chapter 4, Ischemic Heart Disease). The major caveat is that bleeding risk with anticoagulants must be carefully considered.

Perioperative Anticoagulation and Antithrombotic Management

GENERAL PRINCIPLES

- Patients on chronic anticoagulation for AF, VTE, or mechanical heart valves often need to undergo procedures that pose risk of bleeding.
- The indication for anticoagulation and risk of interruption must be weighed against the risk of bleeding of the procedure (including possible neuraxial anesthesia).

TREATMENT

- Recommended management varies according to the indication for anticoagulation, medication used, and surgical bleeding risk.
- For patients being treated with vitamin K antagonists (VKA) such as warfarin:
  - **Low bleeding risk** procedures permit continuation of **oral anticoagulation** through the perioperative period (e.g., minor dental and dermatologic procedures, cataract extraction, endoscopy without biopsy, arthrocentesis). Pacemaker and implantable cardioverter defibrillator (ICD) placement lead to less hematoma if anticoagulation is not interrupted.[31]
  - **Significant bleeding risk procedures** require the anticoagulation to be discontinued.
    - Although the international normalized ratio (INR) at which surgery can be safely performed is subjective, an INR of <1.5 is typically a reasonable goal.
    - The VKA will typically need to be stopped 5 days preoperatively.
    - The INR should be checked the day before surgery. If a level <1.5 is not obtained, 1–2.5 mg oral vitamin K effectively achieves an INR <1.5 on the day of surgery.
    - The VKA can generally be resumed 12–24 hours postoperatively if postoperative bleeding has been controlled.[32]
- **High bleeding risk procedures** (e.g., intracranial or spinal) with potential catastrophic outcomes because of bleeding will preclude any anticoagulation in the perioperative period. Resumption of anticoagulation should be delayed at least 48 hours for other procedures with high bleeding risk (e.g., sessile polypectomy, bowel resection; kidney, liver, or spleen biopsy; extensive orthopedic or plastic surgery).
- **Bridging therapy** refers to the administration of an alternative anticoagulation during the time the INR is anticipated to be below the therapeutic range. The potential decrease in thrombosis must be weighed against the increased risk of bleeding.[33]
- **High thrombotic risk patients** with the following conditions should typically be treated with bridging therapy:
  - Mechanical mitral valve
  - Older-generation mechanical valve (e.g., Starr-Edwards ball-in-cage valve)

- Any mechanical valve with a history of cardioembolism within the preceding 6 months
- Nonvalvular AF with either a history of embolism in the last 3 months or $CHADS_2$ score ≥5
- Valvular AF
- Recent VTE (<3 months)
- Known thrombophilic state (e.g., protein C deficiency)
- For **moderate thrombotic risk patients** as below, bridging may be considered in patients with low bleeding risk. DVT prophylaxis dosing is acceptable.
  - Mechanical aortic valve (bileaflet) with one or more associated risk factors: AF, CHF, hypertension, age ≥75 years, diabetes mellitus, and prior CVA or TIA
  - History of VTE within preceding 3–12 months
  - Non–high-risk thrombophilia (e.g., heterozygous factor V Leiden mutation)
  - History of recurrent VTE
  - Active malignancy
- **Low thrombotic risk** patients are **not** believed to require bridging therapy. Treatment with DVT prophylaxis doses of LMWH or UFH is an alternative. This group includes patients with:
  - Mechanical aortic valve (bileaflet) without associated risk factors, as above
  - AF with a $CHADS_2$ score <4, or history of prior embolism[34]
  - Prior VTE >12 months prior (without history of recurrent VTE or known hypercoagulable state)
- **Choices for bridging therapy** are generally the LMWHs and UFH, including patients with mechanical heart valves.[31] There is less experience in this setting with other agents (e.g., fondaparinux), and their use cannot be considered routine.
  - **LMWHs** have the advantages of relatively predictable pharmacokinetics and ability to be administered SC. Monitoring of anticoagulant effect is typically not required. Renal dosing is available for patients not on dialysis. Subcutaneous administration allows for outpatient therapy in appropriate patients. This decreases the length and cost of hospitalization. The last dose should be given 24 hours prior to surgery.
  - **UFH** is the agent of choice for patients with end-stage renal disease (ESRD). It is typically administered IV and requires frequent monitoring of the activated partial thromboplastin time. UFH should be stopped at least 4 hours prior to the planned surgical procedure to allow the anticoagulant effect to wane. Fixed-dose subcutaneous UFH has been proven efficacious for treatment of VTE and may be considered as an option.[35]
  - **Direct oral anticoagulants** have relatively short half-lives (dabigatran = 14 hours, rivaroxaban = 9 hours, apixaban = 12 hours), obviating the need for bridging anticoagulation. Agents should be held for two or three half-lives for low bleed risk procedures and three or four half-lives for high bleed risk procedures, keeping in mind the effects of renal function on clearance.
  - **Reversal agents** may be used if urgent surgery is required before this washout period.
    - **Idarucizumab** reverses dabigatran, and **andexanet alfa** reverses all Xa inhibitors.
- **Patients being treated with antiplatelet agents**
  - Continuing antiplatelet therapy perioperatively carries a risk of bleeding, whereas discontinuation may increase cardiovascular events. Irreversible agents must be withheld for 5–7 days before effects fully abate. Clinicians are again left with little evidence and sometimes conflicting guidelines.

- **Low bleeding risk procedures** (e.g., minor dermatologic or dental procedures) allow continuation of aspirin (acetylsalicylic acid [ASA]) being given for secondary prevention of cardiovascular disease.
- **Noncardiac surgery patients** should generally have clopidogrel (or other thienopyridines) held 5 days preoperatively. Prompt reinitiation with a loading dose of 300 mg should take place postoperatively. Further stratification drives decisions regarding ASA:
    - **Moderate to high cardiac risk,** in which case ASA should be continued perioperatively
    - **Low cardiac risk,** in which case ASA should be held 7 days preoperatively
- **Coronary artery bypass graft** candidates should generally continue ASA perioperatively and have clopidogrel held 5 days preoperatively.
- **Coronary stents** pose a particular risk of in-stent thrombosis and infarction if dual antiplatelet therapy is prematurely withheld. Whenever possible, surgery should be deferred until the minimum period of dual antiplatelet therapy is completed (balloon angioplasty without stent, 14 days; drug-eluting stents, 6 months; bare metal stents, 30 days).
- **Urgent surgeries** within the previous time frames should proceed with continued dual antiplatelet treatment, if possible. If the bleeding risk is felt to be high, ASA alone should be continued. Heparin bridging has not been shown to be of benefit. Bridging with IV glycoprotein IIb/IIIa antagonists or reversible oral agents (e.g., ticagrelor) is not routinely recommended.[36]

PERIOPERATIVE MANAGEMENT OF SPECIFIC CONDITIONS

Hypertension

GENERAL PRINCIPLES

- Antihypertensive agents that the patient has taken prior to admission for surgery may have an impact on the perioperative period.
    - When the patient is receiving β-blockers or clonidine chronically, withdrawal of these medications may result in tachycardia and rebound hypertension, respectively.
    - Evidence suggests that holding angiotensin-converting enzyme inhibitors and angiotensin II receptor blockers on the day of surgery may reduce perioperative hypotension.[37] These agents should not be held if given for HFrEF.

TREATMENT

- Hypertension in the postoperative period is a common problem with multiple possible causes.
    - All **reversible causes of hypertension**, such as pain, agitation, hypercarbia, hypoxia, hypervolemia, and bladder distention, should be excluded or treated.
    - Poor control of hypertension secondary to discontinuing medications the patient was previously taking in the immediate postoperative period is not uncommon; thus, reviewing the patient's home medication list is recommended.
- Many parenteral antihypertensive medications are available for patients who are unable to take medications orally. Transdermal clonidine also is an option, but the onset of action is delayed.

Pacemakers and ICDs

GENERAL PRINCIPLES

- The use of electrocautery intraoperatively can have adverse effects on the function of implanted cardiac devices.
- A variety of errors can occur, from resetting the device to inadvertent discharge of an ICD.
- Complications are rare but are more likely with abdominal and thoracic surgeries.
- The type of device (i.e., pacemaker or ICD) and manufacturer should be determined along with initial indication for placement and the patient's underlying rhythm. History and ECG review should suffice.
- The device should be interrogated within 3–6 months of a significant surgical procedure.

TREATMENT

- **If the patient is pacemaker dependent, the device should be reprogrammed to an asynchronous mode (e.g., VOO, DOO) for the surgery.**
- The application of a magnet will cause most pacemakers to revert to an asynchronous pacing mode; however, if this is the planned management, it should be tested preoperatively, especially in the pacemaker-dependent patient.
- It should be noted that the effect of a magnet on ICDs is typically different from the effect on pacemakers in that it affects the antitachycardia function but does not alter the pacing function of most models. If the pacing function of an ICD needs to be altered perioperatively, the device will need to be reprogrammed.
- The antitachycardia function of an ICD will typically need to be programmed off for surgical procedures in which electrocautery may cause interference with device function, leading to the potential for unintentional discharge. The effect of a magnet on this function is variable, so programming is the preferred management. Continuous monitoring for arrhythmia is essential during the period when this function is suspended.
- Postoperative interrogation may be necessary, particularly if the device settings were changed perioperatively or if the patient is pacemaker dependent.
- **Consultation with an electrophysiologist** is strongly recommended if there is any uncertainty regarding the perioperative management of a device.

Pulmonary Disease and Preoperative Pulmonary Evaluation

GENERAL PRINCIPLES

Clinically significant pulmonary complications include atelectasis, pneumonia, bronchospasm, exacerbation of preexisting chronic lung disease, and respiratory failure.[38] Postoperative respiratory failure, defined as ventilator dependency for more than 48 hours or unplanned reintubation, carries a 30-day mortality rate as high as 26.5%.[39]

Risk Factors

- **Surgical site** is generally considered the greatest determinant of risk of pulmonary complications, with proximity to the diaphragm correlating with increasing risk.[40] Neurosurgery and surgeries involving the mouth and palate also impart increased risk.[39,41]
- **Duration of surgery** also correlates strongly with risk.[42-44]
- Regional anesthesia may reduce risk of pneumonia and respiratory failure as compared with **general anesthesia**.[45-47] Prolonged **neuromuscular blockade** is also strongly associated with postoperative pulmonary complications.[48]
- **COPD** is a well-known risk factor, with disease severity associated with risk of serious complications.[49]
- **Interstitial lung disease** places patients at elevated risk for surgical lung biopsy and resection of malignancy but is not as well studied in patients undergoing general surgery.[50-52]
- **Pulmonary hypertension** is associated with significant morbidity in patients undergoing surgery.[53,54]
- Conversely, treated asthma and restrictive physiology associated with obesity do not appear to be significant risk factors.[55,56]
- **CHF** may increase the risk of pulmonary complications to an even greater degree than that seen with COPD.[57]
- Multiple indices of general health status including **degree of functional dependence** and **American Society of Anesthesiologists (ASA) class** have been linked to poor pulmonary outcomes.[56,57] Odds ratios for postoperative respiratory failure of 2.53 and 2.29 were observed for **hypoalbuminemia** (<3 g/dL) and **azotemia** (BUN > 30 mg/dL), respectively, in a large cohort.[41]
- **Age >50 years** has been identified as an independent predictor of postoperative pulmonary complications. Risk increases linearly with age.
- **Smoking** is a well-established risk factor for both postoperative pulmonary and nonpulmonary complications. As with malignancy, risk appears to be dose-dependent and associated with active use.[44,58,59]
- **Obstructive sleep apnea** (OSA) increases the odds of postoperative complications two- to fourfold.[60] Unrecognized OSA may pose an even greater risk; it is estimated that over 50% of patients with OSA presenting for surgery are undiagnosed.[61-63]

Risk Stratification

- Several validated risk indices have been developed for quantitating risk of postoperative pulmonary complications. Of these, the Arozullah respiratory failure index offers both practicality and ease of use. It consists of six factors for which point scores are assigned based on multivariate analysis to stratify patients into five classes of postoperative respiratory failure risk (ranging from 0.5% to 26.6%).[41]

DIAGNOSIS

Clinical Presentation

History

Preoperative pulmonary evaluation should focus on the abovementioned patient-dependent risk factors.

- Is there a history of lung disease? If so, what is the patient's baseline (e.g., level of exertional tolerance, degree of hypoxemia)? Is there evidence of recent deterioration (e.g., increased cough, sputum production)? Though not an absolute

contraindication to surgery, it may be prudent to postpone an elective procedure until an exacerbation is treated or a superimposed upper respiratory tract infection has resolved.
- A full smoking history should be obtained.
- Screening for OSA should be undertaken. The STOP-Bang questionnaire (see Chapter 10, Obstructive Sleep Apnea) can be implemented to determine risk of OSA.
- As nonpulmonary comorbidities impact the likelihood of pulmonary complications, a review of other organ systems is mandatory.

Physical Examination
- Vital signs can be helpful in determining pulmonary risk. Both **body mass index (BMI)** and **BP** are components of the STOP-Bang questionnaire. **Oxygen saturation by pulse oximetry** may assist in risk stratification.[64]
- High **Mallampati score** may corroborate clinical suspicion for OSA. A study of 137 adults being evaluated for OSA found that every 1-point increase in Mallampati score increased the odds of OSA by 2.5.[65]
- **Stigmata of chronic lung disease** (e.g., increased anteroposterior dimension of the thorax, digital clubbing, adventitious lung sounds) should be actively sought along with **signs of decompensated HF** (jugular venous distention, rales, pretibial edema).

Diagnostic Testing
- Routine laboratory testing
  As mentioned earlier, underlying chronic kidney disease and hypoalbuminemia portend increased risk of postoperative pulmonary complications. The addition of **serum bicarbonate 28 mmol/L or above** to a STOP-Bang score of three or above increases the specificity for detecting moderate to severe OSA from 30% to 82%, though sensitivity is accordingly reduced.[66]
- CXR
  As many findings deemed abnormal on routine CXR are chronic and do not alter management, imaging is recommended only if signs or symptoms (e.g., unexplained dyspnea) warrant investigation.[67,68]
- Arterial blood gas (ABG) analysis
  No data exist that suggest that ABG results contribute to risk estimation beyond the variables delineated earlier.
- Pulmonary function testing (PFTs)
  The value of preoperative PFTs is at best debatable outside of lung resection surgery, where its role is relatively well defined. However, they may be considered in further evaluation of selected patients with unexplained dyspnea or exertional impairment or for those with known lung disease with unclear baseline.

TREATMENT
- Preoperative treatment should focus on modifiable risk factors.
- The effect of preoperative smoking cessation on pulmonary complications has been largely described in cardiothoracic surgeries, where a **benefit to quitting smoking at least 2 months prior to surgery** has been shown.[69] Though the effect on a general surgical population is less clear, pooled data show a significant reduction in pulmonary complications.[70] Maximizing the preoperative smoking cessation period appears to minimize complications. Though it is unknown whether smoking cessation is beneficial within 2 weeks of surgery, previous concerns about a paradoxical increase in complications appear unfounded.[71]

- COPD and asthma therapy should be optimized (see Chapter 9, Obstructive Lung Disease), and respiratory tract infections should be treated. Indeed, risk of postoperative pulmonary complications is increased in the month following a respiratory tract infection.[72] Nonemergent surgery may need postponement to allow recovery of pulmonary function to baseline.
- OSA should be treated prior to elective high-risk surgery when feasible. A cohort study revealed a significant reduction in cardiovascular complications (primarily cardiac arrest and shock) between undiagnosed and diagnosed OSA after prescription of continuous positive airway pressure (CPAP).[73] However, a subsequent meta-analysis of 904 patients failed to show a significant difference in postoperative adverse events despite statistically significant reduction in apnea–hypopnea index with postoperative use of CPAP, a finding attributed to overall poor adherence.[74] Patients with known OSA should be continued on CPAP perioperatively.[75]
- Alternative procedures with reduced pulmonary risk should be considered for high-risk patients. Laparoscopic procedures may yield fewer pulmonary complications; regional nerve block appears to be associated with decreased risk as well.[76,77] If general anesthesia (particularly with neuromuscular blockade) is absolutely necessary, duration should be minimized to the degree possible.

Anemia and Transfusion Issues in Surgery

GENERAL PRINCIPLES

There is no standardized preoperative evaluation for anemia.
- For low-risk procedures, there is no evidence that routine testing of asymptomatic individuals before low-risk procedures increases safety.[78]
- For higher risk procedures, particularly those with higher bleeding risk, a baseline CBC and coagulation profile are typically obtained. Further testing should be performed as indicated.

DIAGNOSIS

- A history of anemia, hematologic disease, or bleeding diathesis should be noted on history or review of medical records.
- Any clinical signs of anemia (e.g., pallor) or coagulopathy (e.g., petechiae) should prompt further evaluation.

TREATMENT

Volume resuscitation and control of active bleeding are the initial therapy of anemia, particularly in the perioperative period when acute blood loss is a common occurrence.

A restrictive red blood cell (RBC) transfusion threshold of **8 g/dL** is recommended for patients undergoing orthopedic surgery and cardiac surgery and those with pre-existing cardiovascular disease.[79] In most other circumstances, a transfusion threshold of **7 g/dL** suffices.

SPECIAL CONSIDERATIONS

Patients with sickle cell anemia should generally be transfused to a hemoglobin level of **10 g/dL** preoperatively to decrease the incidence of complications.[80]

Liver Disease

GENERAL PRINCIPLES

Patients with liver disease face increased operative morbidity and mortality in comparison to those with normal hepatic function. Not only does the stress of surgery place them at risk for acute hepatic decompensation, the myriad systemic effects of liver disease result in an increased frequency of complications to multiple other organs as well.

Classification

- Both the older Child–Turcotte–Pugh (CTP) and more recent Model for End-stage Liver Disease (MELD) classification schemes (see Chapter 19, Liver Diseases) are well-validated statistical models for predicting surgical risk in patients with cirrhosis.
  - Two different studies separated by 13 years revealed strikingly similar results: a mortality rate of 10% for patients with CTP class A, 30% for class B, and 76%–82% for class C cirrhosis.[81,82] Accordingly, it has been suggested that patients with CTP class A cirrhosis can safely undergo elective surgery in general, and those with class C cirrhosis should not under any circumstances.[83] However, the distinction is less clear for class B cirrhosis, and the inherent subjectivity of the CTP system limits its discriminatory ability.[84]
  - MELD offers several advantages for calculation of 30-day mortality:
    - Variables are both objective and weighted.
    - It includes serum creatinine, which has been shown to correlate with postoperative mortality.[85]
    - Predictive performance is equal to if not better than that of CTP.[86-88]
  - Because CTP includes ascites, which is also correlated with poor prognosis in general surgical patients, the two scoring systems could be considered complementary rather than mutually exclusive.[89,90]
- American Society of Anesthesiologists (ASA) class appears to be the strongest predictor of 7-day mortality in cirrhotic patients undergoing surgery.[91] All 10 patients with ASA class V disease died, indicating that ASA class V should be a contraindication to surgery other than liver transplantation.[92]

DIAGNOSIS

Clinical Presentation

Significant hepatic disease that greatly impacts surgical risk (e.g., acute liver failure, advanced cirrhosis) is usually clinically obvious (scleral icterus, abdominal distention from ascites, florid encephalopathy). For milder disease, however, more subtle findings such as spider angiomas, palmar erythema, and testicular atrophy may be the only clues. Historical details such as family history of hepatic disease, current or prior alcohol and/or IV drug abuse, and transfusion history may increase clinical suspicion. See Chapter 19, Liver Diseases, for further details.

Diagnostic Testing

- Because of the exceedingly low yield of laboratory testing (0.14% in one prospective study enrolling 7620 patients), routine preoperative assessment of hepatic function is not recommended unless clinical findings dictate.[83,93]
- Those with suspected or known hepatic disease should undergo thorough laboratory evaluation including hepatic enzyme levels, albumin and bilirubin

measurement, and coagulation studies along with renal function and electrolytes. If significant laboratory abnormalities (e.g., unexplained transaminase elevation > three times upper limit of normal) are found in patients without known liver disease, surgical intervention may need to be postponed to allow further workup, as the incidence of undiagnosed cirrhosis in this population may be 6% or even higher.[83,94]

TREATMENT

- Historically, patients with acute viral or alcoholic hepatitis have been observed to tolerate surgery poorly and delaying surgery until clinical and biochemical recovery is recommended.[83,95,96]
- Patients with mild chronic hepatitis without associated cirrhosis generally tolerate surgery well.[97]
- For patients with cirrhosis, several steps should be taken to optimize preoperative status:
  - ○ Coagulopathy should be treated to minimize risk of hemorrhage. Vitamin K supplementation may be helpful if the INR is elevated. However, in the context of marked hepatic synthetic dysfunction, administration of fresh frozen plasma and/or cryoprecipitate may be necessary. Severe thrombocytopenia should be corrected via transfusion. (See Chapter 20, Disorders of Hemostasis and Thrombosis, under Liver Disease.)
  - ○ As cirrhosis is associated with renal dysfunction, intravascular hypovolemia, and extravascular fluid retention, careful attention to volume status is crucial. Nephrotoxic agents should be used with extreme caution if at all, and free water restriction may be required in patients with serum sodium below 130 mEq/L. However, judicious use of diuretics and/or timely paracentesis may be required to control ascites, particularly if abdominal surgery is being considered.[98] Administration of large amounts of crystalloid should be avoided. Despite theoretical benefits, strong evidence for preoperative transjugular intrahepatic portosystemic shunt to reduce portal hypertension prior to major abdominal surgery remains lacking but may be considered in select circumstances.[90]
  - ○ Close attention to nutritional status is warranted in light of the very high incidence of malnutrition in this population.[99]
  - ○ Lastly, encephalopathy frequently complicates surgical intervention.[100] Lactulose should be titrated to three to four bowel movements per day, and concurrent rifaximin therapy should be strongly considered.[101] Opioid use should be minimized to avoid constipation and ileus, and dose reduction should be considered in light of expected reduced hepatic clearance.

Diabetes Mellitus

GENERAL PRINCIPLES

- Medical and surgical patients with hyperglycemia are at increased risk for poor outcomes.[102]
- The fact that hyperglycemia is a marker for poor outcomes appears to be relatively clear. However, whether aggressive management truly improves outcomes is uncertain. Trial results have been mixed.

TREATMENT

- Elective surgery in patients with uncontrolled diabetes mellitus should preferably be scheduled after acceptable glycemic control has been achieved. If possible, the operation should be scheduled for early morning to minimize prolonged fasting. Frequent monitoring of blood glucose levels is required in all situations.
- **Type 1 diabetes**
  - **Some form of basal insulin is required to prevent ketosis.**
  - On the evening prior to surgery, the regularly scheduled basal insulin should be continued. If taken in the morning, it is still recommended to give the regularly scheduled basal insulin without dose adjustment.[103] However, patients who are tightly controlled may be at increased risk for hypoglycemia and will need to be monitored closely. A decrease in the last preoperative basal insulin dose may be considered in this circumstance.
  - Glucose infusions (e.g., D5-containing fluids) can be administered to avoid hypoglycemia while the patient is NPO and until tolerance of oral intake postoperatively is established.
  - For complex procedures and procedures requiring a prolonged NPO status, a continuous insulin infusion will likely be necessary.
  - **Caution should be exercised with the use of subcutaneous insulin** in the intraoperative and critical care settings, as alterations in tissue perfusion may result in variable absorption.
- **Type 2 diabetes**
  - Treatment of type 2 diabetics varies according to their preoperative requirements and the complexity of the planned procedure.[104]
  - **Diet-controlled type 2 diabetes** can generally be managed without insulin therapy. Glucose values should be checked regularly (four times daily at minimum). Elevated levels (>180 mg/dL) can be treated with intermittent doses of short-acting insulin.
  - **Type 2 diabetes managed with oral therapy**
    - **Short-acting sulfonylureas and other oral agents** should be withheld on the operative day.
    - **Metformin** should be withheld 1 day before planned surgical procedures. Metformin is generally held for 48 hours postoperatively provided there is no acute renal injury. Other oral agents can be resumed when patients are tolerating their preprocedure diet.
    - Glucose values should be checked regularly and elevated levels (>180 mg/dL) can be treated with intermittent doses of short-acting insulin.
  - **Type 2 diabetes managed with insulin**
    - Long-acting insulin (e.g., glargine insulin) can be given at 50% of the usual dose the day of surgery.
    - Intermediate-acting insulin (e.g., Neutral Protamine Hagedorn) can be given at one-half to two-thirds of the usual morning dose.
    - Dextrose-containing IV fluids may be required to avoid hypoglycemia.
    - The usual insulin treatment can be reintroduced once oral intake is established postoperatively.
- **Target glucose levels**
  - There are no generally agreed-upon target glucose levels applicable to the entire postsurgical population. Pending further research, a goal of maintaining glucose levels <180 mg/dL in the postoperative setting seems reasonable. It should be noted that this may still require intensive treatments such as insulin infusion.

- In patients treated with sliding scale insulin, it is essential to monitor the response to therapy. Patients who are hyperglycemic consistently are unlikely to have adequate glucose control with intermittent treatment alone, and a basal/bolus regimen should be introduced if hyperglycemia is persistent.[105]

Adrenal Insufficiency and Corticosteroid Management

GENERAL PRINCIPLES

- Surgery is a potent activator of the hypothalamic–pituitary axis, and patients with adrenal insufficiency may lack the ability to respond appropriately to surgical stress.
- Patients receiving corticosteroids as anti-inflammatory therapy may rarely develop postoperative adrenal insufficiency.
- The dose and duration of exogenous corticosteroids required to produce clinically significant tertiary adrenal insufficiency is highly variable, but general principles can be outlined.[104]
  - Daily therapy with 5 mg or less of prednisone (or its equivalent), alternate-day corticosteroid therapy, and any dose given for <3 weeks should not result in clinically significant adrenal suppression.
  - Patients receiving >20 mg/d prednisone (or equivalent) for >3 weeks and patients who are clinically "cushingoid" in appearance can be expected to have significant suppression of adrenal responsiveness.
  - The function of the hypothalamic–pituitary axis cannot be readily predicted in patients receiving doses of prednisone 5–20 mg for >3 weeks.

DIAGNOSIS

Cosyntropin stimulation test may also be performed to determine adrenal responsiveness, measuring a single cortisol level at 60 minutes after 250 µg of cosyntropin. This can be done any time of day and baseline cortisol is not needed. Levels >18 µg/dL at 60 minutes generally suggest an intact hypothalamic–pituitary axis.

TREATMENT

- If there is concern for secondary adrenal insufficiency, it is reasonable **to simply continue prior steroid dosing** perioperatively.[106] It may be prudent to switch to an IV formulation to ensure it is not withheld while the patient is NPO.
- For patients with primary adrenal insufficiency, a stress stratification scheme has been developed, based on expert opinion.

Chronic Renal Insufficiency and ESRD

GENERAL PRINCIPLES

- **Chronic renal insufficiency (CRI)** is an independent risk factor for **perioperative cardiac complications**, so all patients with renal disease need appropriate cardiac risk stratification.[11]
- **Patients with ESRD** have a substantial mortality risk when undergoing surgery.[107]
- Most general anesthetic agents have no appreciable nephrotoxicity or effect on renal function other than that mediated through hemodynamic changes.[108]

TREATMENT

- **Volume status**
  - Every effort should be made to **achieve euvolemia** preoperatively to reduce the incidence of volume-related complications intraoperatively and postoperatively.[109]
  - Patients with CRI not receiving hemodialysis may require treatment with loop diuretics.
  - Patients being treated with **hemodialysis** should undergo dialysis preoperatively, which is commonly performed on the day prior to surgery. Hemodialysis can be performed on the day of surgery as well, but the possibility should be considered that transient electrolyte abnormalities and hemodynamic changes post dialysis can occur.
- **Electrolyte abnormalities**
  - **Hyperkalemia** in the preoperative setting should be treated, particularly because tissue breakdown associated with surgery may elevate the potassium level further postoperatively.
    - For patients on dialysis, preoperative dialysis should be undertaken.
    - For patients with CRI not undergoing dialysis, alternative methods of potassium excretion will be necessary.
      - □ **Loop diuretics** can be used, particularly if the patient is also hypervolemic.
      - □ **Sodium zirconium cyclosilicate** is an option if volume status is not an issue.
  - Although chronic **metabolic acidosis** has not been associated with elevated perioperative risk, some local anesthetics have reduced efficacy in acidotic patients. Preoperative metabolic acidosis should be corrected with sodium bicarbonate infusions or dialysis.
- **Bleeding diathesis**
  - **Platelet dysfunction** has long been associated with uremia.
    - The value of a preoperative bleeding time in predicting postoperative bleeding has been questioned.[110] A preoperative bleeding time is, therefore, not recommended.
    - Patients with evidence of perioperative bleeding should, however, be treated.
      - □ **Dialysis** for patients with ESRD will improve platelet function.
      - □ **Desmopressin** (0.3 µg/kg IV or intranasally) can be utilized.
      - □ **Cryoprecipitate,** 10 units over 30 minutes IV, is an additional option.
      - □ In patients with coexisting anemia, **RBC transfusions** can improve uremic bleeding.
      - □ For patients **with a history of prior uremic bleeding**, preoperative desmopressin or **conjugated estrogens** (0.5 mg/kg/d IV for 5 days) should be considered.
  - **Heparin** given with dialysis can increase bleeding risk. Heparin-free dialysis should be discussed with the patient's nephrologist when surgery is planned.

Acute Renal Failure

GENERAL PRINCIPLES

Surgery has been associated with an increased risk of **acute renal failure (ARF).**[109]
- Patients with **CRI** are at increased risk of ARF.
- ARF among patients with normal preoperative renal function is a relatively rare event but is associated with increased mortality when it occurs.[111]

DIAGNOSIS

- The approach to ARF in the perioperative setting is not substantially different from that in the nonoperative setting (see Chapter 13, Renal Diseases).
- However, certain additional factors have to be considered when evaluating the cause in the perioperative setting:
  - **Intraoperative hemodynamic changes,** particularly hypotension, should be investigated. Intraoperative vasopressor and diuretic administration have been associated with postoperative ARF.

TREATMENT

For a detailed discussion regarding the management of ARF, please refer to Chapter 13, Renal Diseases.

REFERENCES

1. Spyropoulos AC, Anderson FA, FitzGerald G, et al. Predictive and associative models to identify hospitalized medical patients at risk for VTE. *Chest.* 2011;140(3):706-714. doi:10.1378/chest.10-1944
2. Gibson CM, Halaby R, Korjian S, et al. The safety and efficacy of full- versus reduced-dose betrixaban in the Acute Medically Ill VTE (Venous Thromboembolism) Prevention With Extended-Duration Betrixaban (APEX) trial. *Am Heart J.* 2017;185:93-100. doi:10.1016/j.ahj.2016.12.004
3. Kahn SR, Lim W, Dunn AS, et al. Prevention of VTE in nonsurgical patients: antithrombotic therapy and prevention of thrombosis, 9th ed. American College of Chest Physicians evidence-based clinical practice guidelines. *Chest.* 2012;141(2 suppl):e195S-e226S. doi:10.1378/chest.11-2296
4. Qaseem A, Chou R, Humphrey LL, Starkey M, Shekelle P; Clinical Guidelines Committee of the American College of Physicians. Venous thromboembolism prophylaxis in hospitalized patients: a clinical practice guideline from the American College of Physicians. *Ann Intern Med.* 2011;155(9):625-632. doi:10.7326/0003-4819-155-9-201111010-00011
5. Berlowitz DR, Brandeis GH, Anderson J, Du W, Brand H. Effect of pressure ulcers on the survival of long-term care residents. *J Gerontol A Biol Sci Med Sci.* 1997;52(2):M106-M110.
6. Qaseem A, Mir TP, Starkey M, Denberg TD; Clinical Guidelines Committee of the American College of Physicians. Risk assessment and prevention of pressure ulcers: a clinical practice guideline from the American College of Physicians. *Ann Intern Med.* 2015;162(5):359-369. doi:10.7326/M14-1567.
7. Padula WV. Effectiveness and value of prophylactic 5-layer foam sacral dressings to prevent hospital-acquired pressure injuries in acute care hospitals: an observational cohort study. *J Wound Ostomy Continence Nurs.* 2017;44(5):413-419. doi:10.1097/WON.0000000000000358
8. Qaseem A, Humphrey LL, Forciea MA, Starkey M, Denberg TD; Clinical Guidelines Committee of the American College of Physicians. Treatment of pressure ulcers: a clinical practice guideline from the American College of Physicians. *Ann Intern Med.* 2015;162(5):370-379. doi:10.7326/M14-1568
9. Dowell D, Haegerich TM, Chou R. CDC guideline for prescribing opioids for chronic pain – United States, 2016. *MMWR Recomm Rep.* 2016;65(1):1-49. doi:10.15585/mmwr.rr6501e1
10. Wheeler E, Jones TS, Gilbert MK, Davidson PJ; Centers for Disease Control and Prevention (CDC). Opioid overdose prevention programs providing naloxone to laypersons – United States, 2014. *MMWR Morb Mortal Wkly Rep.* 2015;64(23):631-635.
11. Boersma E, Poldermans D, Bax JJ, et al. Predictors of cardiac events after major vascular surgery: role of clinical characteristics, dobutamine echocardiography, and beta-blocker therapy. *J Am Med Assoc.* 2001;285(14):1865-1873.
12. McFalls EO, Ward HB, Moritz TE, et al. Predictors and outcomes of a perioperative myocardial infarction following elective major vascular surgery in patients with documented coronary artery disease: results of the CARP trial. *Eur Heart J.* 2008;29(3):394-401. doi:10.1093/eurheartj/ehm620
13. Reilly DF, McNeely MJ, Doerner D, et al. Self-reported exercise tolerance and the risk of serious perioperative complications. *Arch Intern Med.* 1999;159(18):2185-2192.
14. Older P, Hall A, Hader R. Cardiopulmonary exercise testing as a screening test for perioperative management of major surgery in the elderly. *Chest.* 1999;116(2):355-362.
15. Hlatky MA, Boineau RE, Higginbotham MB, et al. A brief self-administered questionnaire to determine functional capacity (the Duke Activity Status Index). *Am J Cardiol.* 1989;64(10):651-654.

16. Lee TH, Marcantonio ER, Mangione CM, et al. Derivation and prospective validation of a simple index for prediction of cardiac risk of major noncardiac surgery. *Circulation.* 1999;100(10):1043-1049.

17. Poldermans D, Bax JJ, Schouten O, et al. Should major vascular surgery be delayed because of preoperative cardiac testing in intermediate-risk patients receiving beta-blocker therapy with tight heart rate control? *J Am Coll Cardiol.* 2006;48(5):964-969. doi:10.1016/j.jacc.2006.03.059

18. Villar RN, Allen SM, Barnes SJ. Hip fractures in healthy patients: operative delay versus prognosis. *Br Med J.* 1986;293(6556):1203-1204.

19. Kenzora JE, McCarthy RE, Lowell JD, Sledge CB. Hip fracture mortality. Relation to age, treatment, preoperative illness, time of surgery, and complications. *Clin Orthop Relat Res.* 1984;(186):45-56.

20. Cluett J, Caplan J, Yu W. Preoperative cardiac evaluation of patients with acute hip fracture. *Am J Orthop.* 2008;37(1):32-36.

21. Feringa HHH, Bax JJ, Boersma E, et al. High-dose beta-blockers and tight heart rate control reduce myocardial ischemia and troponin T release in vascular surgery patients. *Circulation.* 2006;114(1 suppl):I344-I349. doi:10.1161/CIRCULATIONAHA.105.000463

22. Wijeysundera DN, Duncan D, Nkonde-Price C, et al. Perioperative beta blockade in noncardiac surgery: a systematic review for the 2014 ACC/AHA guideline on perioperative cardiovascular evaluation and management of patients undergoing noncardiac surgery. A report of the American College of Cardiology/American Heart Association Task Force on practice guidelines. *J Am Coll Cardiol.* 2014;64(22):2406-2425. doi:10.1016/j.jacc.2014.07.939.

23. Raju MG, Pachika A, Punnam SR, et al. Statin therapy in the reduction of cardiovascular events in patients undergoing intermediate-risk noncardiac, nonvascular surgery. *Clin Cardiol.* 2013;36(8):456-461. doi:10.1002/clc.22135

24. McFalls EO, Ward HB, Moritz TE, et al. Coronary-artery revascularization before elective major vascular surgery. *N Engl J Med.* 2004;351(27):2795-2804. doi:10.1056/NEJMoa041905.

25. Poldermans D, Schouten O, Vidakovic R, et al. A clinical randomized trial to evaluate the safety of a noninvasive approach in high-risk patients undergoing major vascular surgery: the DECREASE-V Pilot Study. *J Am Coll Cardiol.* 2007;49(17):1763-1769. doi:10.1016/j.jacc.2006.11.052

26. Garcia S, Moritz TE, Ward HB, et al. Usefulness of revascularization of patients with multivessel coronary artery disease before elective vascular surgery for abdominal aortic and peripheral occlusive disease. *Am J Cardiol.* 2008;102(7):809-813. doi:10.1016/j.amjcard.2008.05.022

27. Devereaux PJ, Goldman L, Yusuf S, Gilbert K, Leslie K, Guyatt GH. Surveillance and prevention of major perioperative ischemic cardiac events in patients undergoing noncardiac surgery: a review. *Can Med Assoc J.* 2005;173(7):779-788. doi:10.1503/cmaj.050316.

28. Mangano DT. Perioperative cardiac morbidity. *Anesthesiology.* 1990;72(1):153-184.

29. Vascular Events In Noncardiac Surgery Patients Cohort Evaluation (VISION) Study Investigators, Devereaux PJ, Chan MTV, et al. Association between postoperative troponin levels and 30-day mortality among patients undergoing noncardiac surgery. *J Am Med Assoc.* 2012;307(21):2295-2304. doi:10.1001/jama.2012.5502

30. Fleisher LA, Fleischmann KE, Auerbach AD, et al. 2014 ACC/AHA guideline on perioperative cardiovascular evaluation and management of patients undergoing noncardiac surgery: executive summary. A report of the American College of Cardiology/American Heart Association Task Force on Practice Guidelines. *Circulation.* 2014;130(24):2215-2245. doi:10.1161/CIR.0000000000000105

31. Birnie DH, Healey JS, Wells GA, et al. Pacemaker or defibrillator surgery without interruption of anticoagulation. *N Engl J Med.* 2013;368(22):2084-2093. doi:10.1056/NEJMoa1302946.

32. Douketis JD, Spyropoulos AC, Spencer FA, et al. Perioperative management of antithrombotic therapy: antithrombotic therapy and prevention of thrombosis, 9th ed. American College of Chest Physicians evidence-based clinical practice guidelines. *Chest.* 2012;141(2 suppl):e326S-e350S. doi:10.1378/chest.11-2298

33. Siegal D, Yudin J, Kaatz S, Douketis JD, Lim W, Spyropoulos AC. Periprocedural heparin bridging in patients receiving vitamin K antagonists: systematic review and meta-analysis of bleeding and thromboembolic rates. *Circulation.* 2012;126(13):1630-1639. doi:10.1161/CIRCULATIONAHA.112.105221

34. Douketis JD, Spyropoulos AC, Kaatz S, et al. Perioperative bridging anticoagulation in patients with atrial fibrillation. *N Engl J Med.* 2015;373(9):823-833. doi:10.1056/NEJMoa1501035

35. Metzger NL, Chesson MM. Subcutaneous unfractionated heparin for treatment of venous thromboembolism in end-stage renal disease. *Ann Pharmacother.* 2010;44(12):2023-2027. doi:10.1345/aph.1P403

36. Levine GN, Bates ER, Bittl JA, et al. 2016 ACC/AHA guideline focused update on duration of dual antiplatelet therapy in patients with coronary artery disease: a report of the American College of Cardiology/American Heart Association Task Force on clinical practice guidelines. *J Am Coll Cardiol.* 2016;68(10):1082-1115. doi:10.1016/j.jacc.2016.03.513

37. Jammer I, Wickboldt N, Sander M, et al. Standards for definitions and use of outcome measures for clinical effectiveness research in perioperative medicine. European Perioperative Clinical Outcome (EPCO) definitions: a statement from the ESA-ESICM joint taskforce on perioperative outcome measures. *Eur J Anaesthesiol.* 2015;32(2):88-105. doi:10.1097/EJA.0000000000000118

38. Johnson RG, Arozullah AM, Neumayer L, Henderson WG, Hosokawa P, Khuri SF. Multivariable predictors of postoperative respiratory failure after general and vascular surgery: results from the patient safety in surgery study. *J Am Coll Surg.* 2007;204(6):1188-1198. doi:10.1016/j.jamcollsurg.2007.02.070

39. Hollmann C, Fernandes NL, Biccard BM. A systematic review of outcomes associated with withholding or continuing angiotensin-converting enzyme inhibitors and angiotensin receptor blockers before noncardiac surgery. *Anesth Analg.* 2018;127(3):678-687. doi:10.1213/ANE.0000000000002837.

40. Smetana GW. Preoperative pulmonary evaluation. *N Engl J Med.* 1999;340(12):937-944. doi:10.1056/NEJM199903253401207

41. Arozullah AM, Daley J, Henderson WG, Khuri SF. Multifactorial risk index for predicting postoperative respiratory failure in men after major noncardiac surgery. The National Veterans Administration Surgical Quality Improvement Program. *Ann Surg.* 2000;232(2):242-253.

42. Brooks-Brunn JA. Predictors of postoperative pulmonary complications following abdominal surgery. *Chest.* 1997;111(3):564-571.

43. Møller AM, Maaløe R, Pedersen T. Postoperative intensive care admittance: the role of tobacco smoking. *Acta Anaesthesiol Scand.* 2001;45(3):345-348.

44. McAlister FA, Khan NA, Straus SE, et al. Accuracy of the preoperative assessment in predicting pulmonary risk after nonthoracic surgery. *Am J Respir Crit Care Med.* 2003;167(5):741-744. doi:10.1164/rccm.200209-985BC

45. Wijeysundera DN, Beattie WS, Austin PC, Hux JE, Laupacis A. Epidural anaesthesia and survival after intermediate-to-high risk non-cardiac surgery: a population-based cohort study. *Lancet.* 2008;372(9638):562-569. doi:10.1016/S0140-6736(08)61121-6

46. Hausman MS, Jewell ES, Engoren M. Regional versus general anesthesia in surgical patients with chronic obstructive pulmonary disease: does avoiding general anesthesia reduce the risk of postoperative complications? *Anesth Analg.* 2015;120(6):1405-1412. doi:10.1213/ANE.0000000000000574

47. Smith LM, Cozowicz C, Uda Y, Memtsoudis SG, Barrington MJ. Neuraxial and combined neuraxial/general anesthesia compared to general anesthesia for major truncal and lower limb surgery: a systematic review and meta-analysis. *Anesth Analg.* 2017;125(6):1931-1945. doi:10.1213/ANE.0000000000002069

48. Berg H, Roed J, Viby-Mogensen J, et al. Residual neuromuscular block is a risk factor for postoperative pulmonary complications. A prospective, randomised, and blinded study of postoperative pulmonary complications after atracurium, vecuronium and pancuronium. *Acta Anaesthesiol Scand.* 1997;41(9):1095-1103.

49. Kroenke K, Lawrence VA, Theroux JF, Tuley MR, Hilsenbeck S. Postoperative complications after thoracic and major abdominal surgery in patients with and without obstructive lung disease. *Chest.* 1993;104(5):1445-1451.

50. Han Q, Luo Q, Xie JX, et al. Diagnostic yield and postoperative mortality associated with surgical lung biopsy for evaluation of interstitial lung diseases: a systematic review and meta-analysis. *J Thorac Cardiovasc Surg.* 2015;149(5):1394.e1-1401.e1. doi:10.1016/j.jtcvs.2014.12.057

51. Watanabe A, Miyajima M, Mishina T, et al. Surgical treatment for primary lung cancer combined with idiopathic pulmonary fibrosis. *Gen Thorac Cardiovasc Surg.* 2013;61(5):254-261. doi:10.1007/s11748-012-0180-6

52. Choi SM, Lee J, Park YS, et al. Postoperative pulmonary complications after surgery in patients with interstitial lung disease. *Respiration.* 2014;87(4):287-293. doi:10.1159/000357046

53. Ramakrishna G, Sprung J, Ravi BS, Chandrasekaran K, McGoon MD. Impact of pulmonary hypertension on the outcomes of noncardiac surgery: predictors of perioperative morbidity and mortality. *J Am Coll Cardiol.* 2005;45(10):1691-1699. doi:10.1016/j.jacc.2005.02.055

54. Lai HC, Lai HC, Wang KY, Lee WL, Ting CT, Liu TJ. Severe pulmonary hypertension complicates postoperative outcome of non-cardiac surgery. *Br J Anaesth.* 2007;99(2):184-190. doi:10.1093/bja/aem126

55. Woods BD, Sladen RN. Perioperative considerations for the patient with asthma and bronchospasm. *Br J Anaesth.* 2009;103(suppl 1):i57-i65. doi:10.1093/bja/aep271

56. Smetana GW, Lawrence VA, Cornell JE; American College of Physicians. Preoperative pulmonary risk stratification for noncardiothoracic surgery: systematic review for the American College of Physicians. *Ann Intern Med.* 2006;144(8):581-595.

57. Fernandez-Bustamante A, Frendl G, Sprung J, et al. Postoperative pulmonary complications, early mortality, and hospital stay following noncardiothoracic surgery: a multicenter study by the Perioperative Research Network Investigators. *JAMA Surg.* 2017;152(2):157-166. doi:10.1001/jamasurg.2016.4065

58. Grønkjær M, Eliasen M, Skov-Ettrup LS, et al. Preoperative smoking status and postoperative complications: a systematic review and meta-analysis. *Ann Surg.* 2014;259(1):52-71. doi:10.1097/SLA.0b013e3182911913

59. Bluman LG, Mosca L, Newman N, Simon DG. Preoperative smoking habits and postoperative pulmonary complications. *Chest.* 1998;113(4):883-889.

60. Kaw R, Chung F, Pasupuleti V, Mehta J, Gay PC, Hernandez AV. Meta-analysis of the association between obstructive sleep apnoea and postoperative outcome. *Br J Anaesth.* 2012;109(6):897-906. doi:10.1093/bja/aes308

61. Gupta RM, Parvizi J, Hanssen AD, Gay PC. Postoperative complications in patients with obstructive sleep apnea syndrome undergoing hip or knee replacement: a case-control study. *Mayo Clin Proc.* 2001;76(9):897-905. doi:10.4065/76.9.897

62. Singh M, Liao P, Kobah S, Wijeysundera DN, Shapiro C, Chung F. Proportion of surgical patients with undiagnosed obstructive sleep apnoea. *Br J Anaesth.* 2013;110(4):629-636. doi:10.1093/bja/aes465

63. Lockhart EM, Willingham MD, Abdallah AB, et al. Obstructive sleep apnea screening and postoperative mortality in a large surgical cohort. *Sleep Med.* 2013;14(5):407-415. doi:10.1016/j.sleep.2012.10.018

64. Canet J, Gallart L, Gomar C, et al. Prediction of postoperative pulmonary complications in a population-based surgical cohort. *Anesthesiology.* 2010;113(6):1338-1350. doi:10.1097/ALN.0b013e3181fc6e0a

65. Nuckton TJ, Glidden DV, Browner WS, Claman DM. Physical examination: Mallampati score as an independent predictor of obstructive sleep apnea. *Sleep.* 2006;29(7):903-908.

66. Chung F, Chau E, Yang Y, Liao P, Hall R, Mokhlesi B. Serum bicarbonate level improves specificity of STOP-Bang screening for obstructive sleep apnea. *Chest.* 2013;143(5):1284-1293. doi:10.1378/chest.12-1132

67. Joo HS, Wong J, Naik VN, Savoldelli GL. The value of screening preoperative chest x-rays: a systematic review. *Can J Anaesth.* 2005;52(6):568-574. doi:10.1007/BF03015764

68. den Harder AM, de Heer LM, de Jong PA, Suyker WJ, Leiner T, Budde RPJ. Frequency of abnormal findings on routine chest radiography before cardiac surgery. *J Thorac Cardiovasc Surg.* 2018;155(5):2035-2040. doi:10.1016/j.jtcvs.2017.12.124

69. Warner MA, Offord KP, Warner ME, Lennon RL, Conover MA, Jansson-Schumacher U. Role of preoperative cessation of smoking and other factors in postoperative pulmonary complications: a blinded prospective study of coronary artery bypass patients. *Mayo Clin Proc.* 1989;64(6):609-616.

70. Mills E, Eyawo O, Lockhart I, Kelly S, Wu P, Ebbert JO. Smoking cessation reduces postoperative complications: a systematic review and meta-analysis. *Am J Med.* 2011;124(2):144.e8-154.e8. doi:10.1016/j.amjmed.2010.09.013

71. Myers K, Hajek P, Hinds C, McRobbie H. Stopping smoking shortly before surgery and postoperative complications: a systematic review and meta-analysis. *Arch Intern Med.* 2011;171(11):983-989. doi:10.1001/archinternmed.2011.97

72. Mazo V, Sabaté S, Canet J, et al. Prospective external validation of a predictive score for postoperative pulmonary complications. *Anesthesiology.* 2014;121(2):219-231. doi:10.1097/ALN.0000000000000334

73. Mutter TC, Chateau D, Moffatt M, Ramsey C, Roos LL, Kryger M. A matched cohort study of postoperative outcomes in obstructive sleep apnea: could preoperative diagnosis and treatment prevent complications? *Anesthesiology.* 2014;121(4):707-718. doi:10.1097/ALN.0000000000000407

74. Nagappa M, Mokhlesi B, Wong J, Wong DT, Kaw R, Chung F. The effects of continuous positive airway pressure on postoperative outcomes in obstructive sleep apnea patients undergoing surgery: a systematic review and meta-analysis. *Anesth Analg.* 2015;120(5):1013-1023. doi:10.1213/ANE.0000000000000634

75. Chung F, Nagappa M, Singh M, Mokhlesi B. CPAP in the perioperative setting: evidence of support. *Chest.* 2016;149(2):586-597. doi:10.1378/chest.15-1777

76. Owen RM, Perez SD, Lytle N, et al. Impact of operative duration on postoperative pulmonary complications in laparoscopic versus open colectomy. *Surg Endosc.* 2013;27(10):3555-3563. doi:10.1007/s00464-013-2949-9

77. Oshikiri T, Yasuda T, Kawasaki K, et al. Hand-assisted laparoscopic surgery (HALS) is associated with less-restrictive ventilatory impairment and less risk for pulmonary complication than open laparotomy in thoracoscopic esophagectomy. *Surgery.* 2016;159(2):459-466. doi:10.1016/j.surg.2015.07.026

78. Benarroch-Gampel J, Sheffield KM, Duncan CB, et al. Preoperative laboratory testing in patients undergoing elective, low-risk ambulatory surgery. *Ann Surg.* 2012;256(3):518-528. doi:10.1097/SLA.0b013e318265bcdb

79. Carson JL, Guyatt G, Heddle NM, et al. Clinical practice guidelines from the AABB: red blood cell transfusion thresholds and storage. *J Am Med Assoc.* 2016;316(19):2025-2035. doi:10.1001/jama.2016.9185

CHAPTER 1

80. Howard J, Malfroy M, Llewelyn C, et al. The Transfusion Alternatives Preoperatively in Sickle Cell Disease (TAPS) study: a randomised, controlled, multicentre clinical trial. *Lancet.* 2013;381(9870):930-938. doi:10.1016/S0140-6736(12)61726-7

81. Garrison RN, Cryer HM, Howard DA, Polk HC. Clarification of risk factors for abdominal operations in patients with hepatic cirrhosis. *Ann Surg.* 1984;199(6):648-655.

82. Mansour A, Watson W, Shayani V, Pickleman J. Abdominal operations in patients with cirrhosis: still a major surgical challenge. *Surgery.* 1997;122(4):730-735; discussion 735-736.

83. Hanje AJ, Patel T. Preoperative evaluation of patients with liver disease. *Nat Clin Pract Gastroenterol Hepatol.* 2007;4(5):266-276. doi:10.1038/ncpgasthep0794

84. Friedman LS. The risk of surgery in patients with liver disease. *Hepatology.* 1999;29(6):1617-1623. doi:10.1002/hep.510290639

85. Wait RB, Kahng KU. Renal failure complicating obstructive jaundice. *Am J Surg.* 1989;157(2):256-263.

86. Farnsworth N, Fagan SP, Berger DH, Awad SS. Child-Turcotte-Pugh versus MELD score as a predictor of outcome after elective and emergent surgery in cirrhotic patients. *Am J Surg.* 2004;188(5):580-583. doi:10.1016/j.amjsurg.2004.07.034

87. Befeler AS, Palmer DE, Hoffman M, Longo W, Solomon H, Di Bisceglie AM. The safety of intra-abdominal surgery in patients with cirrhosis: model for end-stage liver disease score is superior to Child-Turcotte-Pugh classification in predicting outcome. *Arch Surg.* 2005;140(7):650-654; discussion 655. doi:10.1001/archsurg.140.7.650

88. Neeff H, Mariaskin D, Spangenberg HC, Hopt UT, Makowiec F. Perioperative mortality after non-hepatic general surgery in patients with liver cirrhosis: an analysis of 138 operations in the 2000s using Child and MELD scores. *J Gastrointest Surg.* 2011;15(1):1-11. doi:10.1007/s11605-010-1366-9

89. Ziser A, Plevak DJ, Wiesner RH, Rakela J, Offord KP, Brown DL. Morbidity and mortality in cirrhotic patients undergoing anesthesia and surgery. *Anesthesiology.* 1999;90(1):42-53.

90. Bhangui P, Laurent A, Amathieu R, Azoulay D. Assessment of risk for non-hepatic surgery in cirrhotic patients. *J Hepatol.* 2012;57(4):874-884. doi:10.1016/j.jhep.2012.03.037

91. Teh SH, Nagorney DM, Stevens SR, et al. Risk factors for mortality after surgery in patients with cirrhosis. *Gastroenterology.* 2007;132(4):1261-1269. doi:10.1053/j.gastro.2007.01.040

92. O'Leary JG, Friedman LS. Predicting surgical risk in patients with cirrhosis: from art to science. *Gastroenterology.* 2007;132(4):1609-1611. doi:10.1053/j.gastro.2007.03.016

93. Schemel WH. Unexpected hepatic dysfunction found by multiple laboratory screening. *Anesth Analg.* 1976;55(6):810-812.

94. Hultcrantz R, Glaumann H, Lindberg G, Nilsson LH. Liver investigation in 149 asymptomatic patients with moderately elevated activities of serum aminotransferases. *Scand J Gastroenterol.* 1986;21(1):109-113.

95. Harville DD, Summerskill WH. Surgery in acute hepatitis. Causes and effects. *J Am Med Assoc.* 1963;184:257-261.

96. Greenwood SM, Leffler CT, Minkowitz S. The increased mortality rate of open liver biopsy in alcoholic hepatitis. *Surg Gynecol Obstet.* 1972;134(4):600-604.

97. Runyon BA. Surgical procedures are well tolerated by patients with asymptomatic chronic hepatitis. *J Clin Gastroenterol.* 1986;8(5):542-544.

98. Im GY, Lubezky N, Facciuto ME, Schiano TD. Surgery in patients with portal hypertension: a preoperative checklist and strategies for attenuating risk. *Clin Liver Dis.* 2014;18(2):477-505. doi:10.1016/j.cld.2014.01.006

99. Maharshi S, Sharma BC, Srivastava S. Malnutrition in cirrhosis increases morbidity and mortality. *J Gastroenterol Hepatol.* 2015;30(10):1507-1513. doi:10.1111/jgh.12999

100. Yoshimura Y, Kubo S, Shirata K, et al. Risk factors for postoperative delirium after liver resection for hepatocellular carcinoma. *World J Surg.* 2004;28(10):982-986. doi:10.1007/s00268-004-7344-1

101. Neff GW, Jones M, Broda T, et al. Durability of rifaximin response in hepatic encephalopathy. *J Clin Gastroenterol.* 2012;46(2):168-171. doi:10.1097/MCG.0b013e318231faae

102. Umpierrez GE, Isaacs SD, Bazargan N, You X, Thaler LM, Kitabchi AE. Hyperglycemia: an independent marker of in-hospital mortality in patients with undiagnosed diabetes. *J Clin Endocrinol Metab.* 2002;87(3):978-982. doi:10.1210/jcem.87.3.8341

103. Clement S, Braithwaite SS, Magee MF, et al. Management of diabetes and hyperglycemia in hospitals. *Diabetes Care.* 2004;27(2):553-591.

104. Schiff RL, Welsh GA. Perioperative evaluation and management of the patient with endocrine dysfunction. *Med Clin North Am.* 2003;87(1):175-192.

105. Umpierrez GE, Smiley D, Zisman A, et al. Randomized study of basal-bolus insulin therapy in the inpatient management of patients with type 2 diabetes (RABBIT 2 trial). *Diabetes Care.* 2007;30(9):2181-2186. doi:10.2337/dc07-0295

106. Marik PE, Varon J. Requirement of perioperative stress doses of corticosteroids: a systematic review of the literature. *Arch Surg.* 2008;143(12):1222-1226. doi:10.1001/archsurg.143.12.1222

107. Kellerman PS. Perioperative care of the renal patient. *Arch Intern Med.* 1994;154(15):1674-1688.
108. Wagener G, Brentjens TE. Renal disease: the anesthesiologist's perspective. *Anesthesiol Clin.* 2006;24(3):523-547.
109. Joseph AJ, Cohn SL. Perioperative care of the patient with renal failure. *Med Clin North Am.* 2003;87(1):193-210.
110. Lind SE. The bleeding time does not predict surgical bleeding. *Blood.* 1991;77(12):2547-2552.
111. Kheterpal S, Tremper KK, Englesbe MJ, et al. Predictors of postoperative acute renal failure after non-cardiac surgery in patients with previously normal renal function. *Anesthesiology.* 2007;107(6):892-902. doi:10.1097/01.anes.0000290588.29668.38

Nutrition Support

Kai Jones, Dominic Reeds, and Katrina Han

NUTRIENT REQUIREMENTS

General Principles

ENERGY

- **Total daily energy expenditure (TEE)** is composed of resting energy expenditure (normally ~70% of TEE), the thermic effect of food (normally ~10% of TEE), and energy expenditure of physical activity (normally ~20% of TEE).
- Use of predictive equations can provide a reasonable estimate of **daily energy requirements** that should be modified based on the factors that affect the patient's metabolic rate.
- **Malnutrition and hypocaloric feeding** may decrease resting energy expenditure to 15%–20% below expected for actual body size, whereas metabolic stressors, such as inflammatory diseases or trauma, often increase energy requirements by ~30%–50%.
- The **Harris–Benedict equation** provides a reasonable estimate of resting energy expenditure (in kilocalories [kcal] per day) in healthy adults. It takes into account the effects of body size and lean tissue mass (which are influenced by gender and age) on energy requirements and can be used to estimate total daily energy needs in hospitalized patients (where W is the weight in kilograms, H the height in centimeters, and A is the age in years).[1]
  - Men = $66 + (13.7 \times W) + (5 \times H) - (6.8 \times A)$
  - Women = $665 + (9.6 \times W) + (1.8 \times H) - (4.7 \times A)$
- Energy requirements per kilogram of body weight are inversely related to body mass index (BMI) (Table 2-1). The lower range within each category should be considered in insulin-resistant, critically ill patients unless they are depleted in body fat.
- **Ideal body weight** can be estimated based on height
  - For men: 106 + 6 lb for each inch over 5 ft
  - For women, 100 + 5 lb for each inch over 5 ft

PROTEIN

- Protein intake of 0.8 g/kg/d meets the requirements of 97% of the adult population.
- Protein requirements are affected by several factors, including the amount of nonprotein calories provided, overall energy requirements, protein quality, baseline nutritional status, and the presence of inflammation and metabolic stressors (Table 2-2).
- Inadequate amounts of any essential amino acid results in inefficient utilization.

TABLE 2-1	Estimated Energy Requirements for Hospitalized Patients Based on Body Mass Index
Body Mass Index (kg/m²)	Energy Requirements (kcal/kg/d)
15	35–40
15–19	30–35
20–24	20–25
25–29	15–20
≥30	<15

Note: These values are recommended for critically ill patients and all obese patients; add 20% of total calories in estimating energy requirements in non–critically ill patients.

TABLE 2-2	Recommended Daily Protein Intake
Clinical Condition	Protein Requirements (g/kg IBW/d)[a]
Normal	0.8
Metabolic stress (illness/injury)	1.0–1.5
Acute renal failure (undialyzed)	0.8–1.0
Hemodialysis	1.2–1.4
Peritoneal dialysis	1.3–1.5

IBW, ideal body weight.
[a]Additional protein intake may be needed to compensate for excess protein loss in specific patient populations such as those with burn injury, open wounds, and protein-losing enteropathy or nephropathy. Lower protein intake may be necessary in patients with chronic renal insufficiency who are not treated by dialysis and certain patients with hepatic encephalopathy.

- Illness increases the efflux of amino acids from skeletal muscle; however, increasing protein intake to >1.2 g/kg/d of prehospitalization body weight in critically ill patients may not reduce the loss of lean body mass.[2]

ESSENTIAL FATTY ACIDS

- Humans lack the desaturase enzyme needed to produce the ω-3 and ω-6 fatty acids. Therefore, linoleic acid should constitute at least 2% and linolenic acid at least 0.5% of the daily caloric intake to prevent deficiency.
- The plasma pattern of increased triene-to-tetraene ratio (>0.4) can be used to detect essential fatty acid deficiency.

CARBOHYDRATE

Certain tissues, such as bone marrow, erythrocytes, leukocytes, renal medulla, eye tissues, and peripheral nerves, cannot metabolize fatty acids and require glucose (~40 g/d) as a fuel. Endogenous protein and glycerol from lipid stores can undergo gluconeogenesis to supply glucose-requiring organs.

MAJOR MINERALS

Major minerals such as sodium, potassium, and chloride are important for ionic equilibrium, water balance, and normal cell function.

MICRONUTRIENTS (TRACE ELEMENTS AND VITAMINS)

Trace elements and vitamins are essential constituents of enzyme complexes. The recommended dietary intake for trace elements, fat-soluble vitamins, and water-soluble vitamins is set at two standard deviations above the estimated mean as to meet the needs of 97% of the healthy population.

See Table 2-3 for specifics regarding the assessment of micronutrient nutritional states as well as signs and symptoms of micronutrient deficiency and toxicity.

SPECIAL CONSIDERATIONS

- Both the amount and location of prior gut resection influence nutrient needs. Patients with a reduced length of functional small bowel may require additional vitamins and minerals if they are not receiving parenteral nutrition. Table 2-4 provides guidelines for supplementation in these patients.
- Ileal inflammation, resection, inflammatory bowel disease (IBD), and bypass (ileojejunal bypass) can cause B_{12} deficiency and bile salt loss. Diarrhea in this setting may be improved with oral cholestyramine.
- Proximal gut resection (stomach or duodenum) via partial gastrectomy, Billroth I and II, duodenal switch/biliopancreatic diversion, Roux-en-Y gastric bypass, pancreaticoduodenectomy (Whipple), and sleeve gastrectomy may impair absorption of divalent cations such as iron, calcium, and copper. Copper deficiency is extremely common in post–gastric bypass patients who do not receive routine supplementation.[3]
- Patients with excessive gastrointestinal (GI) tract losses require additional fluids and electrolytes. An assessment of fluid losses due to diarrhea, ostomy output, and fistula volume should be made to help determine fluid requirements. Intestinal mineral losses may be calculated by multiplying the volume of fluid loss by the fluid electrolyte concentration (Table 2-5).
- Hyperammonemic encephalopathy is an uncommon but serious complication of Roux-en-Y gastric bypass with an estimated mortality rate of 50%.[4] Laboratory hallmarks include elevated ammonia, elevated plasma glutamate, hypoalbuminemia, nutritional and essential amino acid deficiencies, and low zinc.[5] It does not appear to resolve with replacement of trace elements. Some reports suggest improvement with total parental nutrition after several months; however, data remain limited.[6]

ASSESSMENT OF NUTRITIONAL STATUS

General Principles

- Patients should be assessed for protein–energy malnutrition as well as specific nutrient deficiencies.
- A thorough history and physical examination combined with appropriate laboratory studies is the best approach to evaluate nutritional status.

TABLE 2-3	Trace Minerals, Fat-Soluble Vitamins, and Water-Soluble Vitamins: Recommended Daily Intake, Deficiency, At-Risk Populations, Toxicity, and Status Evaluation				
Nutrient	Recommended Daily Enteral Intake[32]/ *Parenteral Intake*[33]	Signs and Symptoms of Deficiency[34-45]	Populations at Risk for Deficiency	Signs and Symptoms of Toxicity	Status Evaluation[32]
Chromium (Cr^{3+})	30–35 µg/***10–15 µg***	Glucose intolerance, peripheral neuropathy[a]	None[a,34]	PO: gastritis IV: skin irritation Cr^{6+}: (steel, welding) lung carcinogen if inhaled	Chromium$_s$
Copper (Cu^{2+})	900 µg/***300–500 µg***	Hypochromic normocytic or macrocytic anemia (rarely microcytic), neutropenia, thrombocytopenia, diarrhea, osteoporosis/pathologic fractures[a] Intrinsic: Menkes disease[46]	Chronic diarrhea, high-zinc/low-protein diets[47,48]	PO: gastritis, nausea, vomiting, coma, movement/neurologic abnormalities, hepatic necrosis Intrinsic: Wilson disease	Copper$_{s,u}$ Ceruloplasmin$_p$
Iodine (I^-)	150 µg/***70–140 µg (not routinely added)***	Thyroid hyperplasia (goiter) + functional hypothyroidism Intrinsic in utero: cretinism, poor CNS development, hypothyroidism	Those without access to fortified salt, grain, milk, or cooking oil[49]	Deficiency: causes hypothyroidism Excess: acutely causes hypothyroidism; chronic excess: hyperthyroidism	TSH$_s$, iodine$_u$ (24-h iodine and iodine: Cr ratio are more representative than a single sample) Thyroglobulin$_s$[35,49]

(continued)

TABLE 2-3	Trace Minerals, Fat-Soluble Vitamins, and Water-Soluble Vitamins: Recommended Daily Intake, Deficiency, At-Risk Populations, Toxicity, and Status Evaluation *(continued)*				
Nutrient	Recommended Daily Enteral Intake[33] / Parenteral Intake[34]	Signs and Symptoms of Deficiency[35-46]	Populations at Risk for Deficiency	Signs and Symptoms of Toxicity	Status Evaluation[33]
Iron ($Fe^{2+,3+}$)	8 mg/**1.0–1.5 µg (not routinely added)**	Fatigue, hypochromic microcytic anemia, glossitis, koilonychia	Reproductive-age females, pregnant females, chronic anemias, hemoglobinopathies, post-gastric bypass/duodenectomy, alcoholics	PO or IV: hemosiderosis, followed by deposition in liver, pancreas, heart, and glands Intrinsic: hereditary hemochromatosis	$Ferritin_s$, $TIBC_s$, % transferrin saturation[c], $iron_s$
Manganese (Mn^{2+})	2.3 mg/**60–100 µg**	Hypercholesterolemia, dermatitis, dementia, weight loss[b]	Chronic liver disease, iron-deficient populations	PO: none[b] Inhalation: hallucination, Parkinsonian-type symptoms[50]	No reliable markers Manganese[s] does not reflect bodily stores, especially in the CNS
Selenium (SeO_4^{2-})	55 µg/**20–60 µg**	Myalgias, cardiomyopathy[a] Intrinsic: Keshan disease (Chinese children), Kashin–Beck disease, myxedematous endemic cretinism[51]	Endemic areas of low soil content include certain parts of China and New Zealand[39]	PO: nausea, diarrhea, AMS, irritability, fatigue, peripheral neuropathy, hair loss, white splotchy nails, halitosis (garlic-like odor)	$Selenium_s$, glutathione peroxidase activity[b]

Zinc (Zn^{2+})	11 mg/*2.5–5.0 mg*	Poor wound healing, diarrhea (high fistula risk), dysgeusia, teratogenicity, hypogonadism, infertility, acrofacial and oral skin lesions (glossitis, alopecia), behavioral changes Intrinsic: acrodermatitis enteropathica	Chronic diarrhea, cereal-based diets, alcoholics, chronic liver disease, sickle cell, HIV, pancreatic insufficiency/any intestinal malabsorptive states, fistulas/ostomies, nephrotic syndrome, diabetes, post-gastric bypass/duodenectomy, anorexia, pregnancy[48] Intrinsic: acrodermatitis enteropathica	PO: nausea, vomiting, gastritis, diarrhea, low HDL, gastric erosions Competition with GI absorption can precipitate Cu^{2+} *deficiency* Inhaled: hyperpnea, weakness, diaphoresis	$Zinc_{s,p}$, alkaline phosphatase$_s$ (good for those on TPN, but in general $Zinc_{s,p}$ hair, RBC, WBC levels can be misleading) Zinc radioisotope studies (most accurate tests at present; limited by cost and availability)[36]
Vitamin A *Retinol*	900 µg/*3300 IU*	Conjunctival xerosis, keratomalacia, follicular hyperkeratosis, night blindness, *Bitot spots*, corneal + retinal dysfunction	Any malabsorptive state involving proximal small bowel, vegetarians, chronic liver disease	Acute: teratogenic, skin exfoliation, intracranial hypertension, hepatocellular necrosis Chronic: alopecia, ataxia, cheilitis, dermatitis, conjunctivitis, pseudotumor cerebri, hyperlipidemia, hyperostosis	$Retinol_s$, retinol esters$_p$, electroretinogram, liver biopsy (diagnostic for toxicity), retinol binding protein (useful in ESRD; accurately assesses blood levels)[52]

(continued)

CHAPTER 2

TABLE 2-3 Trace Minerals, Fat-Soluble Vitamins, and Water-Soluble Vitamins: Recommended Daily Intake, Deficiency, At-Risk Populations, Toxicity, and Status Evaluation *(continued)*

Nutrient	Recommended Daily Enteral Intake[33] / *Parenteral Intake*[34]	Signs and Symptoms of Deficiency[35-46]	Populations at Risk for Deficiency	Signs and Symptoms of Toxicity	Status Evaluation[33]
Vitamin D *Ergocalciferol*	5–15 µg/*200 IU*	Rickets/osteomalacia	Any malabsorptive state involving proximal small bowel, chronic liver disease Of note: those with higher skin melanin content (i.e., darker skin) have low baseline 25-OH vitamin D levels; it is unclear whether this merits their inclusion as an "at-risk" population[52]	Hypercalcemia, hyperphosphatemia, which can lead to $CaPO_4$ precipitation, systemic calcification +/− AMS +/− AKI	25-OH vitamin D_s Of note: lively debate between IOM and Endocrine Society regarding definitions of deficiency, goal serum 25-OH levels, and at-risk populations[53,54]
Vitamin E (α, γ)- *Tocopherol*	15 mg/*10 IU*	Hemolytic anemia, posterior column degeneration, ophthalmoplegia, peripheral neuropathy Seen in severe malabsorption, abetalipoproteinemia	Any malabsorptive state involving proximal small bowel, chronic liver disease	Possible increased risk in hemorrhagic CVA, functional inhibition of vitamin K–mediated procoagulants	Tocopherol Must account for cholesterol/triglyceride ratio: otherwise, higher cholesterol/triglyceride ratio overestimates vitamin E, lower cholesterol/triglyceride ratio underestimates vitamin E[45,c]

Vitamin	Dose	Deficiency	At-risk populations	Toxicity	Laboratory test
Vitamin K *Phylloquinone*	120 µg/**150 IU**	Hemorrhagic disease of newborn, coagulopathy	Any malabsorptive state involving proximal small bowel, chronic liver disease	In utero: hemolytic anemia, hyperbilirubinemia, kernicterus; IV: flushing, dyspnea, hypotension (possibly related to dispersal agent)	Prothrombin time$_p$
Vitamin B$_1$ *Thiamine*	1.2 mg/**6 mg**	Irritability, fatigue, headache; *Wernicke encephalopathy, Korsakoff psychosis, "wet" beriberi, "dry" beriberi*	Alcoholics, severely malnourished	IV: lethargy and ataxia	RBC transketolase activity$_b$, thiamine$_{b,u}$
Vitamin B$_2$ *Riboflavin*	1.3 mg/**3.6 mg**	Cheilosis, angular stomatitis, glossitis, seborrheic dermatitis, normocytic normochromic anemia	Alcoholics, severely malnourished	None[b]	RBC glutathione reductase activity$_p$
Vitamin B$_3$ *Niacin*	16 mg/**40 mg**	*Pellagra dysesthesias,* glossitis, stomatitis, vaginitis, vertigo; Intrinsic: Hartnup disease	Alcoholics, malignant carcinoid syndrome, severely malnourished	Flushing, hyperglycemia, hyperuricemia, hepatocellular injury[b]	N-methyl-nicotinamide$_u$
Vitamin B$_5$ *Pantothenic acid*	5 mg/**15 mg**	Fatigue, abdominal pain, vomiting, insomnia, paresthesias[b]	Alcoholics[32]	PO: diarrhea	Pantothenic acid$_u$

(continued)

CHAPTER 2

TABLE 2-3 Trace Minerals, Fat-Soluble Vitamins, and Water-Soluble Vitamins: Recommended Daily Intake, Deficiency, At-Risk Populations, Toxicity, and Status Evaluation *(continued)*

Nutrient	Recommended Daily Enteral Intake[33]/ *Parenteral Intake[34]*	Signs and Symptoms of Deficiency[35-46]	Populations at Risk for Deficiency	Signs and Symptoms of Toxicity	Status Evaluation[33]
Vitamin B_6 *Pyridoxine*	1.3–1.7 mg/*6 mg*	Cheilosis, stomatitis, glossitis, irritability, depression, confusion, normochromic normocytic anemia	Alcoholics, diabetics, celiac sprue, chronic isoniazid or penicillamine use[44]	Peripheral neuropathy, photosensitivity	Pyridoxal phosphate$_p$
Vitamin B_7 *Biotin*	30 μg/*60 μg*	Mental status changes, myalgias, hyperesthesias, anorexia[c,55] (excessive egg white consumption results in avidin-mediated biotin inactivation)	Alcoholics	None[b,55]	Biotin$_p$, methylcitrate$_u$, 3-methylcrotonylglycine$_u$, 3-hydroxyisovalerate$_u$
Vitamin B_9 *Folic acid*	400 μg/*600 μg*	Bone marrow suppression, macrocytic megaloblastic anemia, glossitis, diarrhea. Can be precipitated by sulfasalazine + phenytoin	Alcoholics, celiac or tropical sprue, chronic sulfasalazine use	PO: may lower seizure threshold in those taking anticonvulsants	Folic acid$_s$, RBC folic acid$_p$

Vitamin B₁₂ Cobalamin	2.4 µg/**5 µg**	Bone marrow suppression, macrocytic megaloblastic anemia, glossitis, diarrhea, posterolateral column demyelination, AMS, depression, psychosis	Vegetarians, atrophic gastritis, pernicious anemia, celiac sprue, Crohn disease, patients postgastrectomy or ileal resection	None[b]	Cobalamin (B₁₂)s, methylmalonic acids,p
Vitamin C Ascorbic acid	90 mg/**200 mg**	*Scurvy*, ossification abnormalities / Tobacco lowers plasma and WBC vitamin C[42] / Sudden cessation of high-dose vitamin C can precipitate scurvy	Fruit-deficient diet, smokers,[42] ESRD[56]	Nausea, diarrhea, increased oxalate synthesis (theoretical nephrolithiasis risk)	Ascorbic acidp, leukocyte ascorbic acid

AKI, acute kidney injury; AMS, altered mental status; CNS, central nervous system; CVA, cerebrovascular accident; ESRD, end-stage renal disease; IOM, Institute of Medicine; GI, gastrointestinal; HDL, high-density lipoprotein (cholesterol); RBC, red blood cell; TIBC, total iron bonding capacity; TPN, total parenteral nutrition; TSH, thyroid-stimulating hormone; WBC, white blood cell.

Subscript: b, blood; c, calculated; p, plasma; s, serum; u, urine.

[a]Only reported in patients on long-term TPN.

[b]Never demonstrated in humans.

[c]Only able to induce under experimental conditions and/or only been able to induce in animals.

TABLE 2-4	Guidelines for Vitamin and Mineral Supplementation in Patients with Severe Malabsorption	
Supplement	Dose	Route
Prenatal multivitamin with minerals[a]	1 tablet daily	PO
Vitamin D[a]	50,000 units 2–3 times per week	PO
Calcium[a]	500 mg elemental calcium tid–qid	PO
Vitamin B_{12}[b]	1 mg daily	PO
–	100–500 µg q1–2 mo	SC
Vitamin A[b]	10,000–50,000 units daily	PO
Vitamin K[b]	5 mg/d	PO
–	5–10 mg/wk	SC
Vitamin E[b]	30 units/d	PO
Magnesium gluconate[b]	108–169 mg elemental magnesium qid	PO
Magnesium sulfate[b]	290 mg elemental magnesium 1–3 times per week	IM/IV
Zinc gluconate or zinc sulfate[b]	25 mg elemental zinc daily plus 100 mg elemental zinc per liter intestinal output	PO
Ferrous sulfate[b]	60 mg elemental iron tid	PO
Iron dextran[b]	Daily dose based on formula or table	IV

[a]Recommended routinely for all patients.
[b]Recommended for patients with documented nutrient deficiency or malabsorption.

TABLE 2-5	Electrolyte Concentrations in Gastrointestinal Fluids			
Location	Na (mEq/L)	K (mEq/L)	Cl (mEq/L)	HCO_3 (mEq/L)
Stomach	65	10	100	–
Bile	150	4	100	35
Pancreas	150	7	80	75
Duodenum	90	15	90	15
Mid–small bowel	140	6	100	20
Terminal ileum	140	8	60	70
Rectum	40	90	15	30

Diagnosis

HISTORY

• Assess for changes in diet pattern (size, number, and content of meals) and if present, the reason(s) for altered food intake.
• Unintentional weight loss of >10% body weight in the prior 6 months is associated with a poor clinical outcome. This may not be due directly to malnutrition but rather to the underlying illness.[7,8]
• Look for evidence of **malabsorption** (diarrhea, weight loss).

- For symptoms of specific **nutrient deficiencies**, see Table 2-3.
- Consider factors that may increase metabolic stress (e.g., infection, inflammatory disease, malignancy).
- Assess the patient's functional status (e.g., bedridden, suboptimally active).

PHYSICAL EXAMINATION

- By World Health Organization (WHO) criteria, patients can be classified by BMI as underweight (<18.5 kg/m^2), normal weight (18.5–24.9 kg/m^2), overweight (25.0–29.9 kg/m^2), class I obesity (30.0–34.9 kg/m^2), class II obesity (35.0–39.9 kg/m^2), or class III obesity (≥40.0 kg/m^2).[9]
- Patients who are **extremely underweight** (BMI <15 kg/m^2) or those **with rapid, severe weight loss** (even with supranormal BMI) have a high risk of death and should be considered for admission to the hospital for nutritional support.
- Look for **tissue depletion** (loss of body fat and skeletal muscle atrophy).
- Assess **muscle function** (strength testing of individual muscle groups).
- **Fluid status:** Evaluate patients for dehydration (e.g., hypotension, tachycardia, mucosal xerosis) or excess body fluid (edema or ascites).
- Evaluate patients for sources of protein or nutrient losses: large wounds, burns, nephrotic syndrome, surgical drains, etc. Quantify the volume of drainage and the concentration of fat and protein content in the fluid losses.

DIAGNOSTIC TESTING

- Perform laboratory studies to determine specific nutrient deficiencies only when clinically indicated because the plasma concentration of many nutrients may not accurately reflect body stores (Table 2-3).
- Plasma albumin and prealbumin concentrations should **not** be used to assess patients for malnutrition or to monitor the adequacy of nutrition support. Although levels of these plasma proteins correlate with clinical outcome, inflammation and injury can alter their synthesis and degradation, limiting their usefulness for nutritional assessment.[9-12]

ENTERAL NUTRITION

General Principles

Whenever possible, **oral/enteral** feeding is preferred to **parenteral** feeding because it limits mucosal atrophy, maintains IgA secretion, and prevents cholelithiasis. Additionally, oral/enteral feeds are less expensive than parenteral nutrition and have a lower likelihood of infectious complications.

TYPES OF FEEDINGS

Hospital diets include a regular diet and those modified in either nutrient content (amount of fiber, fat, protein, or sodium) or consistency (liquid, puréed, soft). There are ways that food intake can often be increased:
- Aid at mealtime.
- Allow relatives and friends to supply food.

CHAPTER 2

- Limit missed meals for medical tests and procedures.
- Avoid unpalatable diets. Milk-based formulas (e.g., Carnation Instant Breakfast™) contain milk as a source of protein and fat and are more palatable than many other formula diets.
- Use of calorically dense supplements (e.g., Ensure™, Boost™).

Defined Liquid Formulas (Table 2-6)

- **Polymeric formulas** (e.g., Osmolite™, Jevity™) are appropriate for most patients. They contain nitrogen in the form of whole proteins and include blenderized food, milk-based, and lactose-free formulas. Other formulas are available with modified content including high-nitrogen, high-calorie, fiber-enriched, and low-potassium/phosphorus/magnesium.
- **Semielemental *oligomeric* formulas** (e.g., Peptamen™) contain hydrolyzed protein in the form of small peptides and free amino acids. Although these formulas may have benefit in those with exocrine pancreatic insufficiency or short gut, pancreatic enzyme replacement is a less expensive and an equally effective intervention in most patients.
- **Elemental monomeric formulas** (e.g., Vivonex™, Glutasorb™) contain nitrogen in the form of free amino acids and small amounts of fat (<5% of total calories) and are hyperosmolar (550–650 mOsm/kg). These formulas are not palatable and therefore require either tube feeding or mixing with other foods or flavorings for oral ingestion. Furthermore, these formulas have not been shown to be clinically superior to oligomeric or polymeric formulas in patients with adequate pancreatic digestive function and are much more expensive than polymeric formulas.
- **Oral rehydration solutions** stimulate sodium and water absorption via the sodium–glucose cotransporter present in the brush border of intestinal epithelium. Oral rehydration therapy (using 90–120 mEq/L solutions to avoid intestinal sodium secretion and negative sodium and water balance) can be especially useful in patients with short bowel syndrome.[13] The characteristics of several oral rehydration solutions are listed in Table 2-6.

Tube Feeding

- Tube feeding is useful in patients who have a **functional GI tract** but cannot ingest adequate nutrients.
- The type of feeding tube selected (nasogastric, nasoduodenal, nasojejunal, gastrostomy, jejunostomy, pharyngostomy, and esophagostomy tubes) depends on physician experience, clinical prognosis, gut patency and motility, risk of aspirating gastric contents, patient preference, and anticipated duration of feeding.
- Short-term (<6 weeks) tube feeding can be achieved using a soft, small-bore nasogastric or nasoenteric feeding tube. Although nasogastric feeding is usually the most appropriate route, orogastric feeding may be needed in those who are intubated or those with nasal injury or deformity. Nasoduodenal and nasojejunal feeding tubes can be placed at the bedside; however, ~2% of tubes can be misplaced and the use of electromagnetic, carbon dioxide sensing (capnography), or direct camera visualization devices is recommended. Confirmation of placement, usually by using radiography, is mandatory prior to use. Auscultation should **not** be used to confirm placement.
- Long-term (>6 weeks) tube feeding usually requires a gastrostomy or jejunostomy tube that can be placed percutaneously by endoscopic or radiographic assistance. Alternatively, they can be placed surgically, depending on the clinical situation and local expertise.

TABLE 2-6	Enteral Feeding Formulas: Comparing Composition							
Formula	kcal/mL	% Protein	% Lipid	% Carbohydrate	K⁺ (mEq/L)	PO_4^{3-} (mg/L)	Purpose/Niche
Osmolite	1.0	16.7	29	54.3	40.2	760	Standard polymeric
Jevity	1.5	17	29	53.6	40.2	1200	Standard polymeric
TwoCal HN	2	16.7	40.1	43.2	62.6	1050	Volume restricted
Nepro with Carb Steady	1.8	18	48	34	27.2	700	ESRD
Glucerna	1.5	22	45	33	64.6	1000	Glucose intolerance/ diabetes
Promote	1.0	25	23	52	50.8	1200	High protein
Vital AF	1.2	25	39	36	43.2	844	Short gut, exocrine pancreatic insufficiency
Vivonex RTF	1.0	20	10	70	31	668	Fat malabsorption
Pivot 1.5	1.5	25	30	45	51.3	1000	SIRS, ARDS, sepsis

ARDS, acute respiratory distress syndrome; ESRD, end-stage renal disease; SIRS, systemic inflammatory response syndrome.
Adapted from Barnes-Jewish Hospital Enteral Nutrition Formulary (2019).

CHAPTER 2

Feeding Schedules

Patients who have feeding tubes in the stomach can often tolerate intermittent bolus or gravity feedings, in which the total amount of daily formula is divided into four to six equal portions.

- **Bolus feedings** are given by syringe as rapidly as tolerated.
- **Gravity feedings** are infused over 30–60 minutes.
- The patient's upper body should be elevated by 30–45 degrees during feeding and for at least 2 hours afterward. Tubes should be flushed with water after each feeding. Intermittent feedings are useful for patients who cannot be positioned with continuous head-of-the-bed elevation or who require greater freedom from feeding. Patients who experience nausea and early satiety with bolus gravity feedings may require continuous infusion at a slower rate.
- **Continuous feeding** can often be started at 20–30 mL/h and advanced by 10 mL/h every 6 hours until the feeding goal is reached. Patients who have gastroparesis often tolerate gastric tube feedings when they are started at a slow rate (e.g., 10 mL/h) and advanced by small increments (e.g., 10 mL/h every 8–12 hours). Patients with severe gastroparesis may require passage of the feeding tube tip past the ligament of Treitz. Continuous feeding should always be used when feeding directly into the duodenum or jejunum to avoid distention, abdominal pain, and dumping syndrome.
- Jejunal feeding may be possible in closely monitored patients with mild to moderate acute pancreatitis.[14] RCTs comparing jejunal and gastric feeding in severe acute pancreatitis showed no differences in tolerance, complication rates, and mortality rates. Early initiation of enteral nutrition within 24–72 hours of admission is associated with decreased mortality, organ failure, and infectious complications compared with delayed enteral nutrition.[15]

CONTRAINDICATIONS TO ENTERAL FEEDING

The intestinal tract cannot be used effectively in some patients because of the following:
- Persistent nausea or vomiting
- Postprandial abdominal pain or diarrhea
- Mechanical obstruction or severe hypomotility
- Malabsorption
- Presence of high-output fistula

COMPLICATIONS

- Mechanical complications
  - Nasogastric feeding tube misplacement, including intubation of the tracheobronchial tree, occurs more often in unconscious patients. Intracranial placement can occur in patients with skull fractures.
  - Erosive tissue damage can lead to nasopharyngeal erosions, pharyngitis, sinusitis, otitis media, pneumothorax, and GI tract perforation.
  - Tube occlusion is often caused by inspissated feedings or pulverized medications given through small-diameter (<#10 French) tubes. Frequent flushing of the tube with 30–60 mL of water and avoiding administration of pill fragments or viscous medications help to prevent occlusion. The techniques used

to unclog tubes include the use of a small-volume syringe (10 mL) to flush warm water or pancreatic enzymes (Viokase™ dissolved in water) through the tube.

- Hyperglycemia
  - ADA/AACE guidelines recommend a blood glucose target between 140 and 180 mg/dL for most hospitalized patients. In patients with severe comorbidities and terminal illness, less stringent targets are appropriate.[16,17]
  - The majority of non–critically ill inpatients will require basal insulin while receiving enteral nutrition to achieve and maintain reasonable glucose control.[18]
  - Long-duration insulin (e.g., detemir, glargine) can be used for basal coverage, while short-acting (e.g., lispro™) can be used to cover prandial and correctional needs.
  - Patients receiving bolus feeds should be given short-acting insulin at the time of each feed with an approximate dose of 1 unit of short-acting insulin per 10–15 g carbohydrate, plus a correctional dose if needed.
  - Patients receiving continuous (24 hours per day) feeding should receive basal and bolus insulin when clinically stable.
  - For patients receiving nocturnal tube feeding, intermediate-duration insulin (e.g., NPH) administered with initiation of feeding is a reasonable approach; however, care should be taken to avoid nocturnal hypoglycemia.
  - If tube feeds are interrupted and insulin has been given, an infusion of dextrose-containing fluid should be started at a rate to match the infusion rate of the scheduled tube feeds until the insulin has worn off.
- Pulmonary complications
  - The etiology of **pulmonary aspiration** is often difficult to discern in tube-fed patients as it can occur both from refluxed tube feedings or oropharyngeal secretions unrelated to feedings. Recent evidence suggests that oral secretions play a far greater role in the development of ventilator-associated pneumonia than aspiration of tube feedings.[19]
  - Gastric residuals are poorly predictive of aspiration risk.[20]
  - Prevention of reflux: Decrease gastric acid secretion with H2 blockers or proton pump inhibitors, elevate head of bed during feeds, and avoid gastric feeding in high-risk patients (e.g., those with gastroparesis, frequent vomiting, gastric outlet obstruction).
- GI complications
  - Nausea, vomiting, and abdominal pain are common.
  - Diarrhea is often associated with antibiotic therapy and the use of liquid medications that contain nonabsorbable carbohydrates, such as sorbitol. If diarrhea from tube feeding persists after proper evaluation of possible causes, a trial of antidiarrheal agents or fiber is warranted. Diarrhea is common in patients who receive tube feeding and occurs in up to 50% of critically ill patients. Supplementation with fiber or switching to a fiber-enriched feed has not yielded consistent results. A change to an elemental feeding formula is rarely needed and likely will not resolve the issue unless significant impairment in absorption is well-documented.[21]
  - Diarrhea in patients with short gut, who do not have other causes such as *Clostridioides difficile* infection, may be minimized using small, frequent meals that do not contain concentrated sweets (e.g., soda). Intestinal transit time should be maximized to optimize nutrient absorption using a tincture of opium, loperamide, or diphenoxylate. Low-dose clonidine (0.025–0.05 mg orally bid) may be

used to reduce diarrhea in hemodynamically stable patients with short bowel syndrome.[22] Intestinal ischemia/necrosis has been reported in patients receiving tube feeds. These cases have occurred predominantly in critically ill patients receiving vasopressors for blood pressure support in conjunction with enteral feeding. There are no reliable clinical signs for diagnosis, and the mortality rate is high. **Caution should be used when enterally feeding critically ill patients requiring vasopressors.**

PARENTERAL NUTRITION

General Principles

Parenteral nutrition should be considered if energy intake cannot, or it is anticipated that it cannot, be met by enteral nutrition (<50% of daily requirements) for more than 7–10 days. This guideline originates from two intensive care unit (ICU)-focused meta-analyses citing increased complications and increased overall mortality in ICU patients receiving early parenteral nutrition (i.e., within 7 days of admission), compared with those receiving no nutrition support.[23,24] Recent studies have found that critically ill patients who are unable to meet caloric goals by enteral nutrition alone for the first 8 days of hospitalization have longer durations of stay and greater mortality rates than those in whom total parenteral nutrition (TPN) is withheld for the first 8 days after admission.[24]

CENTRAL PARENTERAL NUTRITION

- The infusion of hyperosmolar (usually >1500 mOsm/L) nutrient solutions requires a large-bore, high-flow vessel to minimize vessel irritation and damage.
- Percutaneous subclavian vein catheterization and peripherally inserted central venous catheterization (PICC) are the most common techniques for central parenteral nutrition (CPN) access. The internal jugular, saphenous, and femoral veins are also used, although they are less desirable due to patient discomfort and difficulty in maintaining sterility. Tunneled catheters are preferred in patients likely to receive >8 weeks of TPN in order to decrease the risk of mechanical failure.
- PICCs are increasingly used to provide CPN in patients with adequate antecubital vein access. They should not be used in patients requiring CPN for an extended time (>6 months).

CPN MACRONUTRIENT SOLUTIONS

- Crystalline **amino acid solutions** consisting of 40%–50% essential and 50%–60% nonessential amino acids (usually with little or no glutamine, glutamate, aspartate, asparagine, tyrosine, and cysteine) are used to provide protein needs (Table 2-2). Infused amino acids are oxidized and should be included in the estimate of energy provided as part of the parenteral formulation.
- Some amino acid solutions have been modified for specific disease states such as those enriched in branched-chain amino acids for use in patients with hepatic

encephalopathy and those that contain mostly essential amino acids for use in patients with renal insufficiency.

- **Glucose** (dextrose) in IV solutions is hydrated; each gram of dextrose monohydrate provides 3.4 kcal. Although there is no absolute requirement for glucose in most patients, providing >150 g of glucose per day maximizes protein balance.
- **Lipid emulsions** are available as a 10% (1.1 kcal/mL) or 20% (2.0 kcal/mL) solution and provide energy as well as serve as a source of essential fatty acids. Lipid emulsions are as effective as glucose in conserving body nitrogen economy once absolute tissue requirements for glucose are met. The optimal percentage of calories that should be infused as fat is not known, but 20%–30% of total calories are reasonable for most patients. The infusion rate should not exceed 1.0 kcal/kg/h (0.11 g/kg/h) as most complications reported have occurred when providing more than this amount.[25] A rate of 0.03–0.05 g/kg/h is adequate for most patients receiving continuous CPN. Lipid emulsions should not be used in patients with triglyceride concentrations >400 mg/dL. Moreover, patients at risk for hypertriglyceridemia should have serum triglyceride concentrations checked at least once during lipid emulsion infusion to ensure adequate clearance. Underfeeding obese patients by the amount of lipid calories that would normally be given (e.g., 20%–30% of calories) facilitates mobilization of endogenous fat stores for fuel and may improve insulin sensitivity. IV lipids should still be administered twice weekly to these patients to provide essential fatty acids. A recent meta-analysis of 49 RCTs demonstrated that use of ω-3 fatty-acid-enriched parenteral nutrition compared to standard parenteral nutrition leads to reduction in infection, sepsis, and ICU and hospital stay length.[26]

PERIPHERAL PARENTERAL NUTRITION

- Peripheral parenteral nutrition is of limited utility due to high risk of thrombophlebitis.
- Appropriate management of peripheral parenteral nutrition can increase the life of a single infusion site to >10 days. The following guidelines are recommended:
  - Provide at least 50% of total energy as a lipid emulsion piggybacked with the dextrose–amino acid solution.
  - Add 500–1000 units of heparin and 5 mg of hydrocortisone per liter (to decrease phlebitis).
  - Place a fine-bore 22- or 23-gauge polyvinylpyrrolidone-coated polyurethane catheter in as large a vein as possible in the proximal forearm using sterile technique.
  - Place a 5-mg glycerol trinitrate ointment patch (or 0.25 in of 2% nitroglycerin ointment) over the infusion site.
  - Infuse the solution with a volumetric pump.
  - Keep the total infused volume <3500 mL/d.
  - Filter the solution with an inline 1.2-m filter.

LONG-TERM HOME PARENTERAL NUTRITION

- Long-term home parenteral nutrition is usually given through a tunneled catheter or an implantable subcutaneous port inserted in the subclavian vein.

- Nutrient formulations can be infused overnight to permit daytime activities in patients who are able to tolerate the fluid load. IV lipids may not be necessary in patients who are able to ingest and absorb adequate amounts of fat.
- Appropriate patient selection for home TPN is crucial due to high complication rates (~50% at 6 months). Risk factors for complications include the use of a non-tunneled or multilumen catheter, use of the catheter for blood draws, infusion of nonparenteral medications, use of lipid infusions, anticoagulation, older age, and open wounds.[27]

COMPLICATIONS

Mechanical Complications

- Complications at time of line placement include pneumothorax, air embolism, arterial puncture, hemothorax, and brachial plexus injury.
- Thrombosis and pulmonary embolism: Radiologically evident subclavian vein thrombosis occurs commonly; however, clinical manifestations (upper extremity edema, superior vena cava syndrome) are rare. Fatal microvascular pulmonary emboli can be caused by nonvisible precipitate in parenteral nutrition solutions. Inline filters should be used with all solutions to minimize the risk of emboli.

Metabolic Complications

- Fluid overload.
- Hypertriglyceridemia.
- Hypercalcemia.
- Specific nutrient deficiencies. Consider providing supplemental **thiamine** (100 mg for 3–5 days) during initiation of CPN in patients at risk of thiamine deficiency (e.g., alcoholism).
- Hypoglycemia.
- Hyperglycemia. In most patients, a blood glucose concentration of 140–180 mg/dL should be targeted during TPN infusion. Management of patients with hyperglycemia or type 2 diabetes can be performed in several ways:
  ○ If blood glucose is >200 mg/dL, consider improving blood glucose control before starting CPN.
  ○ If CPN is started, (1) limit dextrose to <200 g/d, (2) add 0.1 unit of regular insulin for each gram of dextrose in CPN solution (e.g., 15 units for 150 g), (3) discontinue other sources of IV dextrose, and (4) order routine, regular insulin with blood glucose monitoring by finger stick every 4–6 hours or IV regular insulin infusion with blood glucose monitoring by finger stick every 1–2 hours.
  ○ In outpatients who use insulin, an estimate of the reduction in blood sugar that will be caused by the administration of 1 unit of insulin may be calculated by dividing 1500 by the total daily insulin dose (e.g., for a patient receiving 50 units of insulin as an outpatient, 1 unit of insulin may be predicted to reduce plasma glucose concentration by 1500/50 = 30 mg/dL).
  ○ If blood glucose remains >200 mg/dL and the patient has been requiring SC insulin, add 50% of the supplemental short-acting insulin given in the last 24 hours to the next day's CPN solution and double the amount of SC insulin sliding-scale dose for blood glucose values >200 mg/dL.
  ○ The insulin-to-dextrose ratio in the CPN formulation should be maintained while the CPN dextrose content is changed.

Infectious Complications

- Catheter-related sepsis is the most common life-threatening complication in patients receiving CPN. The responsible microorganisms are most often skin flora: *Staphylococcus epidermidis* and *Staphylococcus aureus.*
- In **immunocompromised patients** and those receiving CPN for >2 weeks, *Enterococcus, Candida* species, *Escherichia coli, Pseudomonas, Klebsiella, Enterobacter, Acinetobacter, Proteus,* and *Xanthomonas* should be considered.
- The principles of **evaluation and management** of suspected catheter-related infection are outlined in Chapter 14, Treatment of Infectious Diseases.
- Use of sterile technique during connection of TPN, avoiding access of the TPN lumen of the central catheter for other purposes, and ensuring that TPN is never disconnected and restarted can reduce the risk of infection. Microorganisms can form biofilms on the intraluminal surface of the catheter and once attached they are difficult to eliminate. In patients on home TPN, ethanol lock therapy has been shown to be effective in reducing the rate of catheter-related infection.[28]

Hepatobiliary Complications

Although these abnormalities are usually benign and transient, more serious and progressive disease may develop in a subset of patients, usually after 16 weeks of CPN therapy or in those with short bowel syndrome.

- Biochemical: Elevated aminotransferases and alkaline phosphatase are commonly seen.
- Histologic alterations: Steatosis, steatohepatitis, lipidosis, phospholipidosis, cholestasis, fibrosis, and cirrhosis have all been seen.
- Biliary complications as listed below usually occur in patients who receive CPN for >3 weeks:
  ○ Acalculous cholecystitis
  ○ Gallbladder sludge
  ○ Cholelithiasis
- Strategies to prevent hepatobiliary complications in patients receiving long-term CPN include providing a portion (20%–40%) of calories as fat, cycling CPN so that the glucose infusion is stopped for at least 8–10 hours per day, encouraging enteral intake to stimulate gallbladder contraction and maintain mucosal integrity, and avoiding excess calories and hyperglycemia.
- If biochemical or other evidence of liver damage occurs, evaluation for other causes of liver disease should ensue.
- If mild hepatobiliary complications develop, parenteral nutrition should not necessarily be discontinued. Rather, the same principles used in preventing hepatic complications can be applied therapeutically.
- When cholestasis is present, copper and manganese should be removed from the CPN formula to prevent accumulation in the liver and basal ganglia. A 4-week trial of metronidazole or ursodeoxycholic acid can be helpful in some patients.

Metabolic Bone Disease

- Metabolic bone disease has been observed in patients receiving CPN for >3 months
- Patients may be asymptomatic. Clinical manifestations include bone fractures and pain. Demineralization may be seen on radiologic studies. Osteopenia, osteomalacia, or both may be present.
- The precise causes of metabolic bone disease are not known, but several mechanisms have been proposed, including aluminum toxicity, vitamin D toxicity, and negative calcium balance.

CHAPTER 2

- Several therapeutic options should be considered in patients who have evidence of bone abnormalities.
- Remove vitamin D from the CPN formulation if parathyroid hormone and 1,25-hydroxy vitamin D levels are low.
- Reduce protein to <1.5 g/kg/d as amino acids can cause hypercalciuria.
- Maintain normal magnesium status because magnesium is necessary for normal parathormone action and renal conservation of calcium.
- Provide oral calcium supplements of 1–2 g/d.
- Consider bisphosphonate therapy to decrease bone resorption.

SPECIAL CONSIDERATIONS

- Monitoring nutrition support
  - Adjustment of the nutrient formulation is often needed as medical therapy or clinical status changes.
  - When nutrition support is initiated, other sources of **glucose** (e.g., peripheral IV dextrose infusions) should be stopped and the volume of other IV fluids adjusted to account for CPN.
  - Vital signs should be checked every 8 hours.
  - In certain patients, body weight, fluid intake, and fluid output should be followed daily.
  - Serum electrolytes (including phosphorus) should be measured every 1–2 days after CPN is started until the values are stable and then rechecked weekly.
  - Serum glucose should be checked up to every 4–6 hours by finger stick until blood glucose concentrations are stable and then rechecked weekly.
  - If lipid emulsions are being given, **serum triglycerides** should be measured during lipid infusion in patients at risk for hypertriglyceridemia to demonstrate adequate clearance (triglyceride concentrations should be <400 mg/dL).
- Careful attention to the catheter and catheter site can help to prevent **catheter-related infections.**
  - Gauze dressings should be changed every 48–72 hours or when contaminated or wet. Transparent dressings can be changed weekly.
  - Tubing that connects the parenteral solutions with the catheter should be changed every 24 hours.
  - A 0.22-μm filter should be inserted between the IV tubing and the catheter when **lipid-free CPN** is infused and should be changed with the tubing.
  - A 1.2-μm filter should be used when a total nutrient admixture containing a **lipid emulsion** is infused.
  - When a **single-lumen** catheter is used to deliver CPN, the catheter should not be used to infuse other solutions/medications (apart from compatible antibiotics) or to monitor central venous pressure.
  - When a **triple-lumen** catheter is used, the distal port should be reserved solely for the administration of CPN.

REFEEDING THE SEVERELY MALNOURISHED PATIENT

Refeeding syndrome may occur after initiating nutritional therapy in patients who are severely malnourished and have had minimal nutrient intake.
- **Hypophosphatemia, hypokalemia, and hypomagnesemia:** Rapid and marked decreases in these electrolytes occur during initial refeeding because

of insulin-stimulated increases in cellular mineral uptake from extracellular fluid. For example, plasma phosphorus concentration can fall below 1 mg/dL and cause death within hours of initiating nutritional therapy if not adequately replaced. Suggested replacement guidelines are reviewed in several sources.[29-31]

- **Fluid overload and congestive heart failure** are associated with decreased cardiac function and insulin-induced increases in sodium and water reabsorption in conjunction with nutritional therapy containing water, glucose, and sodium. Renal mass may be reduced, limiting the ability to excrete salt or water loads.
- **Cardiac arrhythmias:** Patients who are severely malnourished often have bradycardia. Sudden death from ventricular tachyarrhythmias can occur during the first week of refeeding in severely malnourished patients and may be associated with a prolonged QT interval and electrolyte abnormalities. Patients with ECG changes should be monitored on telemetry, possibly in an ICU.
- **Glucose intolerance:** Starvation causes insulin resistance such that refeeding with high-carbohydrate meals or large amounts of parenteral glucose can cause marked elevations in blood glucose concentration, glycosuria, dehydration, and hyperosmolar coma. In addition, carbohydrate refeeding in patients who are depleted in thiamine can precipitate Wernicke encephalopathy.

MANAGEMENT OF SEVERE MALNUTRITION

- Careful **evaluation** of cardiovascular function and plasma electrolytes (history, physical examination, ECG, and blood tests) and correction of abnormal plasma electrolytes are **important before initiation of feeding**.
- Refeeding by the oral or enteral route involves frequent or continuous administration of small amounts of food or an isotonic liquid formula.
- Parenteral supplementation or complete parenteral nutrition may be necessary if the intestine cannot tolerate feeding.
- During initial refeeding, fluid intake should be limited to approximately 800 mL/d plus insensible losses. Adjustments in fluid and sodium intake are needed in patients who have evidence of fluid overload or dehydration.
- Changes in body weight provide a useful guide for evaluating the efficacy of fluid administration. Weight gain >0.25 kg/d or 1.5 kg/wk probably represents fluid accumulation in excess of tissue repletion. Initially, approximately 15 kcal/kg (containing approximately 100 g carbohydrate and 1.5 g protein per kilogram of actual body weight) should be given daily.
- The rate at which caloric intake can be increased depends on the severity of malnutrition and tolerance to feeding. In general, increasing by 2–4 kcal/kg every 24–48 hours is appropriate.
- Sodium should be restricted to approximately 50 mEq/m^2 body surface area/day, but liberal amounts of phosphorus, potassium, and magnesium should be given to patients with normal renal function.
- All other nutrients should be given in amounts needed to meet the recommended dietary intake (Table 2-7).
- Body weight, fluid intake, urine output, plasma glucose, and electrolyte values should be **monitored daily** during early refeeding (first 3–7 days) so that nutritional therapy can be appropriately modified when necessary.

TABLE 2-7   Major Mineral Daily Requirements, Deficiency, Toxicity, and Diagnostic Evaluation

Mineral	Recommended Daily Enteral Intake/Parenteral Intake[33]	Signs and Symptoms of Deficiency	Signs and Symptoms of Toxicity	Diagnostic Evaluation
Sodium	1.2–1.5 g[a]/**1–2 mEq/kg**	Encephalopathy, seizure, weakness, dehydration, cerebral edema[31]	Encephalopathy, seizure	$Sodium_p$ (correct for hyperglycemia) $Sodium_u$ (will often only provide a rough estimate [i.e., too low, too high])
Potassium	4700 mg[(47)][a]/**1–2 mEq/kg**	Abdominal cramping, diarrhea, paresthesias, QT prolongation, weakness	QRS widening, QT shortening (sine wave morphology in extreme cases), peaked T waves	$Potassium_{w,b}$
Calcium	1000–1200 mg/**10–15 mEq**	QRS widening, paresthesias (Trousseau sign), tetany (Chvostek sign), osteomalacia	Encephalopathy, headache, abdominal pain, nephrolithiasis, metastatic calcification	$Calcium_{w,b}$, 24-h $calcium_u$ (correct for $albumin_s$)
Magnesium	420 mg/**8–20 mEq**	Tachyarrhythmia, weakness, muscle cramping, peripheral and central nervous system overstimulation (seizure, tetany)	Hyporeflexia, nausea, vomiting, weakness, encephalopathy, decreased respiratory drive, hypocalcemia, hyperkalemia, heart block	$Magnesium_s$, $magnesium_u$
Phosphorus	700 mg/**20–40 mmol**	Weakness, fatigue, increased cell membrane fragility (hemolytic anemias, leukocyte + platelet dysfunction), encephalopathy	Metastatic calcification, theoretic higher risk of nephrolithiasis, secondary hyperparathyroidism	$Phosphorus_p$

Subscript: b, blood; p, plasma; s, serum; u, urine; w, whole blood.
[a]*Note*: Adequate daily intake.

REFERENCES

1. Harris JA, Benedict FG. A biometric study of human basal metabolism. *Proc Natl Acad Sci.* 1918;4(12):370-373. doi:10.1073/pnas.4.12.370
2. Ishibashi N, Plank LD, Sando K, Hill GL. Optimal protein requirements during the first 2 weeks after the onset of critical illness. *Crit Care Med.* 1998;26(9):1529-1535. doi:10.1097/00003246-199809000-00020
3. Gletsu-Miller N, Broderius M, Frediani JK, et al. Incidence and prevalence of copper deficiency following roux-en-y gastric bypass surgery. *Int J Obes (Lond).* 2012;36(3):328-335. doi:10.1038/ijo.2011.159
4. Fenves AZ, Shchelochkov OA, Mehta A. Hyperammonemic syndrome after Roux-en-Y gastric bypass. *Obesity.* 2015;23(4):746-749. doi:10.1002/oby.21037
5. Nagarur A, Fenves AZ. Late presentation of fatal hyperammonemic encephalopathy after roux-en-Y gastric bypass. *Proc (Bayl Univ Med Cent).* 2017;30(1):41-43. doi:10.1080/08998280.2017.11929521
6. Hu WT, Kantarci OH, Merritt JL, et al. Ornithine transcarbamylase deficiency presenting as encephalopathy during adulthood following bariatric surgery. *Arch Neurol.* 2007;64(1):126-128. doi:10.1001/archneur.64.1.126
7. Clinical guidelines on the identification, evaluation, and treatment of overweight and obesity in adults - the evidence report. *Obes Res.* 1998;6(suppl 2):51S-2019S.
8. Dewys WD, Begg C, Lavin PT, et al. Prognostic effect of weight loss prior tochemotherapy in cancer patients. *Am J Med.* 1980;69(4):491-497. doi:10.1016/S0149-2918(05)80001-3
9. Apelgren KN, Rombeau JL, Twomey PL, Miller RA. Comparison of nutritional indices and outcome in critically ill patients. *Crit Care Med.* 1982;10(5):305-307. doi:10.1097/00003246-198205000-00003
10. Klein S. The myth of serum albumin as a measure of nutritional status. *Gastroenterology.* 1990;99(6):1845-1846. doi:10.1016/0016-5085(90)90500-Z
11. McClave SA, Taylor BE, Martindale RG, et al. Guidelines for the provision and assessment of nutrition support therapy in the adult critically ill patient. *J Parenter Enter Nutr.* 2016;40(2):159-221. doi:10.1177/0148607115621863
12. Evans DC, Corkins MR, Malone A, et al. The use of visceral proteins as nutrition markers: an ASPEN position paper. *Nutr Clin Pract.* 2021;36(1):22-28. doi:10.1002/ncp.10588
13. Lennard-Jones JE. Oral rehydration solutions in short bowel syndrome. *Clin Ther.* 1990;12(suppl A):129-137.
14. Simpson WG, Marsano L, Gates L. Enteral nutritional support in acute alcoholic pancreatitis. *J Am Coll Nutr.* 1995;14(6):662-665. doi:10.1080/07315724.1995.10718557
15. McClave SA, Taylor BE, Martindale RG. ESPEN guidelines on nutritional support for polymorbid internal medicine patients. *Clin Nutr.* 2018;37(1):336-353.
16. American Diabetes Association. Diabetes care in the hospital: standards of medical care in diabetes-2021. *Diabetes Care.* 2021;44(suppl 1):S211-S220. doi:10.2337/dc21-s015
17. Moghissi ES, Korytkowski MT, DiNardo M, et al. American association of clinical endocrinologists and american diabetes association consensus statement on inpatient glycemic control. *Endocr Pract.* 2009;15(4):353-369. doi:10.4158/EP09102.RA
18. Korytkowski MT, Salata RJ, Koerbel GL, et al. Insulin therapy and glycemic control in hospitalized patients with diabetes during enteral nutrition therapy. *Diabetes Care.* 2009;32(4):594-596. doi:10.2337/dc08-1436
19. Reignier J, Mercier E, Le Gouge A, et al. Effect of not monitoring residual gastric volume on risk of ventilator-associated pneumonia in adults receiving mechanical ventilation and early enteral feeding: a randomized controlled trial. *J Am Med Assoc.* 2013;309(3):249-256. doi:10.1001/jama.2012.196377
20. Metheny NA, Schallom L, Oliver DA, Clouse RE. Gastric residual volume and aspiration in critically ill patients receiving gastric feedings. *Am J Crit Care.* 2008;17(6):512-520. doi:10.4037/ajcc2008.17.6.512
21. Gavi S, Hensley J, Cervo F, Nicastri Z, Fields S. Management of feeding tube complications in the long-term care resident. *Ann Long Term Care.* 2008;16:28-32.
22. McDoniel K, Taylor B, Huey W, et al. Use of clonidine to decrease intestinal fluid losses in patients with high-output short-bowel syndrome. *J Parenter Enter Nutr.* 2004;28(4):265-268. doi:10.1177/0148607104028004265
23. Braunschweig CL, Levy P, Sheean PM, Wang X. Enteral compared with parenteral nutrition: a meta-analysis. *Am J Clin Nutr.* 2001;74(4):534-542. doi:10.1093/ajcn/74.4.534
24. Casaer MP, Mesotten D, Hermans G, et al. Early versus late parenteral nutrition in critically ill adults. *N Engl J Med.* 2011;365(6):506-517. doi:10.1056/nejmoa1102662
25. Miles JM. Intravenous fat emulsions in nutritional support. *Curr Opin Gastroenterol.* 1991;7(2):306-311. doi:10.1097/00001574-199104000-00018
26. Pradelli L, Mayer K, Klek S, et al. ω-3 fatty-acid enriched parenteral nutrition in hospitalized patients: systematic review with meta-analysis and trial sequential analysis. *JPEN J Parenter Enteral Nutr.* 2020;44(1):44-57. doi:10.1002/jpen.1672
27. Durkin MJ, Dukes JL, Reeds DN, Mazuski JE, Camins BC. A descriptive study of the risk factors associated with catheter-related bloodstream infections in the home parenteral nutrition population. *JPEN J Parenter Enter Nutr.* 2016;40(7):1006-1013. doi:10.1177/0148607114567899

CHAPTER 2

28. Gundogan K, Dave NJ, Griffith DP, et al. Ethanol lock therapy markedly reduces catheter-related blood stream infections in adults requiring home parenteral nutrition: a retrospective study from a tertiary medical center. *JPEN J Parenter Enter Nutr.* 2020;44(4):661-667. doi:10.1002/jpen.1698

29. Boateng AA, Sriram K, Meguid MM, Crook M. Refeeding syndrome: treatment considerations based on collective analysis of literature case reports. *Nutrition.* 2010;26(2):156-167. doi:10.1016/j.nut.2009.11.017

30. Higdon J, Drake V, Pao-Hwa L. *Micronutrient Information Center: Potassium.* Linus Pauling Institute: Micronutrient Research for Optimum Health. Accessed September 20, 2021. http://lpi.oregonstate.edu/infocenter/minerals/potassium/

31. Higdon J, Drake V, Obarzanek E. *Micronutrient Information Center: Sodium (Chloride).* Linus Pauling Institute: Micronutrient Research for Optimum Health. Accessed September 20, 2021. http://lpi.oregonstate.edu/infocenter/minerals/potassium/

32. Trumbo P, Yates AA, Schlicker S, Poos M. Dietary reference intakes: vitamin A, vitamin K, arsenic, boron, chromium, copper, iodine, iron, manganese, molybdenum, nickel, silicon, vanadium, and zinc. *J Am Diet Assoc.* 2001;101(3):294-301. doi:10.1016/S0002-8223(01)00078-5

33. Mirtallo J, Canada T, Johnson D, et al. Safe practices for parenteral nutrition. *JPEN J Parenter Enter Nutr.* 2004;28(6):S39-S70. doi:10.1177/0148607104028006s39

34. NIH Office of Dietary Supplements. *Chromium - Fact Sheet for Health Professionals.* Published 2020. https://ods.od.nih.gov/factsheets/chromium-HealthProfessional/

35. NIH Office of Dietary Supplements. *Iodine – Fact Sheet for Health Professionals.* Published 2020. https://ods.od.nih.gov/factsheets/iodine-HealthProfessional/

36. NIH Office of Dietary Supplements. *Zinc – Fact Sheet for Health Professionals.* Published 2021. https://ods.od.nih.gov/factsheets/zinc-HealthProfessional/

37. Uauy R, Olivares M, Gonzalez M. Essentiality of copper in humans. *Am J Clin Nutr.* 1998;67(5 suppl):952S-959S. doi:10.1093/ajcn/67.5.952S

38. NIH Office of Dietary Supplements. *Iron – Fact Sheet for Health Professionals.* Published 2020. https://ods.od.nih.gov/factsheets/iron-HealthProfessional/

39. NIH Office of Dietary Supplements. *Selenium – Fact Sheet for Health Professionals.* Published 2021. https://ods.od.nih.gov/factsheets/selenium-HealthProfessional/

40. NIH Office of Dietary Supplements. *Vitamin A – Fact Sheet for Health Professionals.* Published 2021. https://ods.od.nih.gov/factsheets/vitamina-HealthProfessional/

41. NIH Office of Dietary Supplements. *Vitamin B12 – Fact Sheet for Health Professionals.* Published 2020. https://ods.od.nih.gov/factsheets/vitaminb12-HealthProfessional/

42. NIH Office of Dietary Supplements. *Vitamin C – Fact Sheet for Health Professionals.* Published 2021. https://ods.od.nih.gov/factsheets/vitaminC-HealthProfessional/

43. NIH Office of Dietary Supplements. *Vitamin D – Fact Sheet for Health Professionals.* Published 2021. https://ods.od.nih.gov/factsheets/vitamind-HealthProfessional/

44. NIH Office of Dietary Supplements. *Vitamin B6 – Fact Sheet for Health Professionals.* Published 2021. https://ods.od.nih.gov/factsheets/VitaminB6-HealthProfessional/

45. NIH Office of Dietary Supplements. *Vitamin E – Fact Sheet for Health Professionals.* Published 2021. https://ods.od.nih.gov/factsheets/vitamine-HealthProfessional/

46. Stern BR. Essentiality and toxicity in copper health risk assessment: overview, update and regulatory considerations. *J Toxicol Environ Health A.* 2010;73(2):114-127. doi:10.1080/15287390903337100

47. Abumrad NN, Schneider AJ, Steel D, Rogers LS. Amino acid intolerance during prolonged total parenteral nutrition reversed by molybdate therapy. *Am J Clin Nutr.* 1981;34(11):2551-2559. doi:10.1093/ajcn/34.11.2551

48. Semrad CE. Zinc and intestinal function. *Curr Gastroenterol Rep.* 1999;1(5):398-403. doi:10.1007/s11894-999-0021-7

49. Zimmermann MB. Iodine deficiency. *Endocr Rev.* 2009;30(4):376-408. doi:10.1210/er.2009-0011

50. Santamaria AB, Sulsky SI. Risk assessment of an essential element: Manganese. *J Toxicol Environ Health A.* 2010;73(2):128-155. doi:10.1080/15287390903337118

51. Fairweather-Tait SJ, Collings R, Hurst R. Selenium bioavailability: current knowledge and future research requirements. *Am J Clin Nutr.* 2010;91(5):1484S-1491S. doi:10.3945/ajcn.2010.28674J

52. Mahmood K, Samo AH, Jairamani KL, Ali G, Talib A, Qazmi W. Serum retinol binding protein as an indicator of vitamin A status in cirrhotic patients with night blindness. *Saudi J Gastroenterol.* 2008;14(1):7-11. doi:10.4103/1319-3767.37794

53. Rosen J, Spatz ES, Gaaserud AMJ, et al. A new approach to developing cross-cultural communication skills. *Med Teach.* 2004;26(2):126-132. doi:10.1080/01421590310001653946

54. Holick MF, Binkley NC, Bischoff-Ferrari HA, et al. Evaluation, treatment, and prevention of vitamin D deficiency: an endocrine society clinical practice guideline. *J Clin Endocrinol Metab.* 2011;96(7):1911-1930. doi:10.1210/jc.2011-0385

55. Said HM. Intestinal absorption of water-soluble vitamins in health and disease. *Biochem J.* 2011;437(3):357-372. doi:10.1042/BJ20110326

56. Deicher R, Hörl WH. Vitamin C in chronic kidney disease and hemodialysis patients. *Kidney Blood Press Res.* 2003;26(2):100-106. doi:10.1159/000070991

Preventive Cardiology

Lauren East, Dominique S. Williams, and
Anne C. Goldberg

Hypertension

GENERAL PRINCIPLES

Hypertension is defined as the presence of blood pressure (BP) elevation to a level that places patients at increased risk for target organ damage in several vascular beds including the retina, brain, heart, kidneys, and large conduit arteries (Table 3-1 and Table 3-2).

Classification

- The following definitions and recommendations are based on the 2017 American College of Cardiology (ACC)/American Heart Association (AHA) guidelines. The 2018 European Society of Cardiology and European Society of Hypertension (ESC/ESH) guidelines and 2019 National Institute for Health and Care Excellence (NICE) guidelines do differ, particularly in terms of treatment thresholds.[1,3]
- **Normal BP** is defined as systolic blood pressure (SBP) <120 mm Hg and diastolic blood pressure (DBP) <80 mm Hg; pharmacologic intervention is not indicated.
- **Elevated blood pressure** is defined as SBP of 120–129 mm Hg and DBP of >80 mm Hg. These patients should engage in comprehensive lifestyle modifications to delay progression or prevent the development of hypertension. Blood pressure should be reassessed in 3–6 months.

TABLE 3-1	Manifestations of Target Organ Disease
Organ System	**Manifestation**
Large vessel	Aneurysmal dilation
	Accelerated atherosclerosis
	Aortic dissection
Cardiac	*Acute:* Pulmonary edema, myocardial infarction
	Chronic: Clinical or ECG evidence of CAD; LVH by ECG or echocardiogram
Cerebrovascular	*Acute:* Intracerebral bleeding, coma, seizures, mental status changes, TIA, stroke
	Chronic: TIA, stroke
Renal	*Acute:* Hematuria, azotemia
	Chronic: Serum creatinine >1.5 mg/dL, proteinuria >1+ on dipstick
Retinopathy	*Acute:* Papilledema, hemorrhages
	Chronic: Hemorrhages, exudates, arterial nicking

CAD, coronary artery disease; LVH, left ventricular hypertrophy; TIA, transient ischemic attack.

TABLE 3-2	Classification of Blood Pressure for Adults Age 18 Years and Older[a]	
Category	Systolic Pressure (mm Hg)	Diastolic Pressure (mm Hg)
Normal	<120	<80
Elevated blood pressure	120–129	<80
Hypertension, stage 1	130–139	80–89
Hypertension, stage 2	≥140	≥90

[a]Not taking antihypertensive drugs and not acutely ill. When systolic and diastolic pressures fall into different categories, the higher category should be selected to classify the individual's blood pressure status.
Data from Whelton PK, Carey RM, Aronow WS, et al. 2017 ACC/AHA/AAPA/ABC/ACPM/AGS/APhA/ASH/ASPC/NMA/PCNA guideline for the prevention, detection, evaluation, and management of high blood pressure in adults: a report of the American College of Cardiology/American Heart Association task force on clinical practice guidelines. *J Am Coll Cardiol.* 2018;71:e127-e248.

- **In stage 1 hypertension** (SBP 130–139 mm Hg or DBP 80–89 mm Hg), low-risk adults (no atherosclerotic cardiovascular disease [ASCVD] and 10-year cardiovascular disease [CVD] risk of <10%) should start with nonpharmacologic therapy and comprehensive lifestyle modifications. Blood pressure should be reassessed in 3–6 months. If not at goal, pharmacological therapy should be considered. In those with ASCVD or a 10-year CVD risk of ≥10%, pharmacologic therapy should be initiated in addition to lifestyle modification. Blood pressure should be reassessed in 1 month with a target of <130/80 mm Hg. If at goal, reassess every 3–6 months. If not at goal, assess for adherence and consider intensification of therapy.[1,4]
- **In stage 2 hypertension** (SBP ≥140 mm Hg or DBP ≥90 mm Hg), pharmacologic therapy should be initiated in addition to lifestyle modification to lower BP to <130/80 mm Hg. Patients with BP levels >20/10 mm Hg above their treatment target will often require more than one medication to achieve adequate control, and a two-drug regimen may be initiated as initial therapy. Blood pressure should be reassessed in 1 month. If at goal, reassess every 3–6 months. If not at goal, assess for adherence and consider intensification of therapy.
- If there is a disparity in category between systolic and diastolic blood pressures, individuals should be designated to the higher BP category.[1,5]
- **Hypertensive emergency** is the association of substantially elevated blood pressure with evidence of acute end-organ damage (retina, brain, heart, large arteries, kidneys). It usually develops in patients with a previous history of elevated BP but may arise in those who were previously normotensive. Appropriate treatment of hypertensive emergency lowers blood pressure to prevent continued end-organ damage but does so slowly and gradually to prevent ischemic damage. Mean arterial pressure should be reduced by 10%–20% in the first hour and a further 5%–15% over the next 23 hours. Exceptions to gradual blood pressure lowering include acute ischemic stroke, acute aortic dissection, and intracerebral hemorrhage.[6-8]
  - **Malignant hypertension** is severe blood pressure elevation (largely BP >200/120) with associated advanced bilateral retinopathy.
  - **Hypertensive encephalopathy** is severe blood pressure elevation associated with lethargy, seizures, cortical blindness, and coma in the absence of other possible etiologies.

- ○ Other examples of clinical presentations of hypertensive emergencies include hypertensive thrombotic microangiopathy, acute coronary syndrome, acute stroke, cerebral hemorrhage, flash pulmonary edema, and aortic aneurysm/dissection.
- Patients with severe asymptomatic hypertension who lack acute hypertension-mediated organ damage are not considered to have hypertensive emergency. Treatment with oral antihypertensive therapy in these patients is often appropriate as there is no proven benefit from rapid reduction of blood pressure in patients with severe asymptomatic hypertension.[6,9,11]
- **Isolated systolic hypertension,** defined as an SBP ≥140 mm Hg and DBP <90, occurs frequently in the elderly (beginning after the fifth decade and increasing with age). Nonpharmacologic therapy should be initiated with medications added as needed and tolerated to lower SBP.
- **Resistant hypertension** is defined as BP ≥130/80 in hypertensive patients on ≥3 antihypertensive agents, one of which is a diuretic, or controlled BP on ≥4 antihypertensive agents. All agents should be prescribed at maximally recommended (or maximally tolerated) doses. Causes of pseudoresistance should be ruled out prior to diagnosis with resistant hypertension (inaccuracy in BP measurement, white coat hypertension, poor adherence, or poor regimen).[12,13] Potential causes of resistant hypertension include ingestion of exogenous substances (e.g., decongestants, oral contraceptives, appetite suppressants, sympathomimetics, venlafaxine, tricyclic antidepressants, monoamine oxidase inhibitors [MAOIs], chlorpromazine, some herbal supplements [e.g.: ma huang], steroids, NSAIDs, cyclosporine, caffeine, thyroid hormones, cocaine, alcohol use, erythropoietin) and secondary causes of hypertension.[1]
- **White coat hypertension** is defined as blood pressure that is consistently elevated by office readings but does not meet diagnostic criteria for hypertension based on out-of-office readings.
- **Masked hypertension** is defined as blood pressure that is consistently elevated by out-of-office measurements but does not meet the criteria for hypertension based on office readings.

Epidemiology

- The **public health burden** of hypertension is enormous. According to recent estimates from the National Health and Nutrition Examination Survey (NHANES) through the Centers for Disease Control and Prevention (CDC), hypertension affects an estimated 116 million American adults, up from 103 million per ACC/AHA guidelines in 2017.[14,15] Of the population with hypertension, 73.9% of people with hypertension in the United States have uncontrolled hypertension. For nonhypertensive individuals aged 55–65 years, the lifetime risk of developing hypertension is 90%.[16]
- Data derived from the Framingham Study have shown that hypertensive patients have a *fourfold* increase in cerebrovascular accidents and a *sixfold* increase in congestive heart failure (CHF) when compared with normotensive control subjects.[16]
- Disease-associated morbidity and mortality, including ASCVD, stroke, heart failure (HF), and renal insufficiency, increase with higher levels of SBP and DBP. Elevated blood pressure is the strongest modifiable risk factor for CVD worldwide.[17]
- Over the last 3 decades, aggressive treatment of hypertension has resulted in a substantial decrease in death rates from stroke and coronary heart disease (CHD). Although the incidence of end-stage renal disease (ESRD) has stabilized and hospitalizations for CHF have overall decreased,[18] BP control rates remain poor, with 53% of treated hypertensive patients having BP above target goal.[15]

CHAPTER 3

Etiology

- BP rises with age. Other contributing factors include obesity, decreased physical activity, increased dietary sodium intake, increased alcohol consumption, and lower dietary intake of fruits, vegetables, and potassium.
- Of all hypertensive patients, more than 90% have primary or essential hypertension. The remainder have secondary hypertension due to renal parenchymal disease, renovascular disease, pheochromocytoma, Cushing syndrome, primary hyperaldosteronism, coarctation of the aorta, obstructive sleep apnea, and uncommon autosomal dominant or autosomal recessive diseases of the adrenal–renal axis, which result in salt retention.

DIAGNOSIS

Clinical Presentation

- BP elevation is usually discovered in asymptomatic individuals during routine health visits. However, appropriately measured out-of-office BP measurements should be used in complement with office readings for purposes of confirming the diagnosis of hypertension, titatring BP-lowering medication, and excluding white coat and masked hypertension.[1,2,19]
- Optimal detection and evaluation of hypertension require accurate noninvasive BP measurement, which should be obtained in a seated patient with the arm resting at heart level. The patient should be relaxed and sitting in the chair with their feet on the floor and back supported for more than 5 minutes prior to obtaining the blood pressure reading. They should avoid caffeine, exercise, and smoking for at least 30 minutes before measurement and should have an empty bladder. A calibrated, appropriately fitting BP cuff (inflatable bladder encircling at least 80% of the arm) should be used because falsely high readings can be obtained if the cuff is too small. Neither the patient nor the observer should talk during measurement.
- Two readings should be taken, separated by 2 minutes on two separate occasions. SBP should be noted with the appearance of Korotkoff sounds (phase I) and DBP with the disappearance of sounds (phase V).
- In certain patients, the Korotkoff sounds do not disappear but are present at 0 mm Hg. In this case, the initial muffling of Korotkoff sounds (phase IV) should be taken as the DBP. One should be careful to avoid reporting spuriously low BP readings because of an auscultatory gap, which is caused by the disappearance and reappearance of Korotkoff sounds in hypertensive patients and may account for up to a 25-mm Hg gap between true and measured SBP.
- Hypertension should be confirmed in both arms, and the higher reading should be used.

History

- History should seek to discover secondary causes of hypertension and note the presence of medications and supplements that can affect BP (see examples of substances above under "Resistant hypertension" definition).
- A diagnosis of secondary hypertension should be considered in the following situations:
  - Age at onset younger than 30 years
  - Onset of diastolic hypertension in persons older than 65 years
  - Hypertension that is difficult to control after therapy has been initiated
  - Stable hypertension that becomes difficult to control
  - Resistant hypertension
  - Clinical occurrence of a hypertensive emergency

- ○ The presence of signs or symptoms of a secondary cause such as hypokalemia or metabolic alkalosis that is not explained by diuretic therapy
- In patients who present with significant hypertension at a young age, a careful family history may give clues to forms of hypertension that follow simple Mendelian inheritance.
- The 2011 ACC/AHA and 2017 ACC/AHA guidelines for peripheral vascular disease recommend diagnostic testing for renal artery stenosis in individuals with onset of hypertension at <30 years of age, or new-onset diastolic hypertension after the age of 55, unexplained deterioration of kidney function during antihypertensive therapy, severe hypertension in patients with diffuse atherosclerosis, and/or systolic-diastolic bruit that lateralizes to one side (low sensitivity, high specificity).[1,20]
- A newer body of evidence suggests that primary aldosteronism is part of a spectrum of aldosterone excess states and found that aldosterone excess is much more common even in primary hypertension than previously thought (plasma aldosterone/renin ratios had poor sensitivity and negative predictive value), suggesting that further investigation of aldosterone excess in those with uncontrolled or resistant hypertension may be warranted.[21,22]

Physical Examination
Physical examination should include measurement of blood pressure in both extremities, and investigation for target organ damage or a secondary cause of hypertension by noting the presence of carotid bruits, an S_3 or S_4, cardiac murmurs, neurologic deficits, elevated jugular venous pressure, rales, retinopathy, unequal pulses, enlarged or small kidneys, cushingoid features, and abdominal bruits.

Differential Diagnosis

- Hypertension may be partly due to withdrawal from drugs, including alcohol, cocaine, and opioid analgesics. Rebound increases in BP may be seen in patients who abruptly discontinue antihypertensive therapy, particularly β-adrenergic antagonists and central α_2-agonists (see "Complications").
- Cocaine and other sympathomimetic drugs (e.g., amphetamines, phencyclidine hydrochloride) can produce hypertension in the setting of acute intoxication and when the agents are discontinued abruptly after chronic use. Hypertension in these cases is often complicated by other end-organ insults, such as ischemic heart disease, stroke, and seizures. Phentolamine (a nonselective α-adrenergic antagonist) is effective in acute management, and sodium nitroprusside or nitroglycerin can be used as an alternative. β-Adrenergic antagonists should be avoided because of the risk of unopposed α-adrenergic activity, which can exacerbate hypertension.

Diagnostic Testing

- Tests are needed to help identify patients with possible target organ damage, to assess cardiovascular risk, and to provide a baseline for monitoring the adverse effects of therapy.
- Basic laboratory data should include urinalysis, hematocrit, plasma glucose, serum potassium, serum creatinine, calcium, uric acid, hemoglobin A1c, and fasting lipid levels.
- Other testing includes ECG and chest radiography. Echocardiography may be of value for certain patients to assess cardiac function or detection of left ventricular hypertrophy (LVH) or other structural abnormalities such as valvular diseases.
- Ambulatory blood pressure monitoring can also be particularly useful in evaluating those with suspected white coat hypertension or possible drug resistance after initiation of pharmacologic therapy.[1]

CHAPTER 3

TREATMENT

- The goal of treatment is to prevent long-term sequelae (i.e., target organ damage) while controlling other modifiable cardiovascular risk factors. BP should be reduced to a goal of <130/80 mm Hg for most patients. Discretion is warranted in prescribing medication to lower BP that may affect cardiovascular risk adversely in other ways (e.g., glucose control, lipid metabolism, uric acid levels).
- Lifestyle modifications should be encouraged in all hypertensive patients regardless of whether they require medication (Table 3-3). These changes may have beneficial effects on other cardiovascular risk factors.
- Barring an overt need for immediate pharmacologic therapy, or diagnosis of stage 2 hypertension, most patients should be given the opportunity to achieve a reduction in BP over an interval of a month by applying nonpharmacologic modifications prior to initiation of pharmacologic therapies.

MONITORING/FOLLOW-UP

- BP measurements should be performed on multiple occasions under nonstressful circumstances (e.g., rest, sitting with legs uncrossed, empty bladder, comfortable temperature) to obtain an accurate assessment of BP in a given patient.
- Hypertension should not be diagnosed based on one measurement alone, unless it is >180/120 mm Hg or accompanied by target organ damage (i.e., hypertension urgency or emergency). Two or more abnormal readings should be obtained, preferably over a period of several weeks, before therapy is considered.
- Care should also be used to exclude pseudohypertension, which usually occurs in elderly individuals with stiff, noncompressible vessels. A palpable artery that persists after cuff inflation (Osler sign) should alert the physician to this possibility.
- Home and ambulatory BP monitoring can be used to assess a patient's true average BP, which correlates better with target organ damage.[23-25]

Medications

- Initial drug therapy.
- Drug interactions, cost, and coexistent factors such as age, race, angina, HF, renal insufficiency, LVH, obesity, hyperlipidemia, gout, and bronchospasm should be considered in initial drug choice. The amount of blood pressure reduction is the major determinant of reduction in cardiovascular risk, not the choice of antihypertensive

TABLE 3-3	Lifestyle Modifications and Effects
Modification	Approximate SBP Reduction (mm Hg)
Weight reduction (for every 10-kg weight loss)	5–20
Adoption of DASH eating plan	8–14
Dietary sodium reduction (intake <2 g/d)	2–8
Physical activity (150 min/wk)	4–9
Moderation of alcohol consumption (intake <2 drinks/d)	2–4

DASH, Dietary Approaches to Stop Hypertension; SBP, systolic blood pressure.

drug. The BP response is usually consistent within a given class of agents; therefore, if a drug fails to control BP, another agent from the same class is unlikely to be effective. At times, however, a change within drug class may be useful in reducing adverse effects. The lowest possible effective dosage should be used to control BP, adjusted every 1–2 months as needed (Table 3-4).

TABLE 3-4	Commonly Used Antihypertensive Agents by Functional Class		
Drugs by Class	Properties	Initial Dose	Dosage Range (mg)
β-Adrenergic Antagonists			
Atenolol[a]	Selective	50 mg PO daily	25–100
Betaxolol[a]	Selective	10 mg PO daily	5–40
Bisoprolol[a]	Selective	5 mg PO daily	2.5–20
Metoprolol	Selective	50 mg PO bid	50–450
Metoprolol XL	Selective	50–100 mg PO daily	50–400
Nebivolol[a]	Selective with vasodilatory properties	5 mg PO daily	5–40
Nadolol[a]	Nonselective	40 mg PO daily	20–240
Propranolol	Nonselective	40 mg PO bid	40–240
Propranolol LA	Nonselective	80 mg PO daily	60–240
Timolol	Nonselective	10 mg PO bid	20–40
Pindolol	ISA	5 mg PO daily	10–60
Labetalol	α- and β-antagonist properties	100 mg PO bid	200–1200
Carvedilol	α- and β-antagonist properties	6.25 mg PO bid	12.5–50
Carvedilol CR	α- and β-antagonist properties	10 mg PO daily	10–80
Acebutolol[a]	ISA, selective	200 mg PO bid, 400 mg PO daily	200–1200
Calcium Channel Antagonists			
Amlodipine	DHP	5 mg PO daily	2.5–10
Diltiazem		30 mg PO qid	90–360
Diltiazem LA		180 mg PO daily	120–540
Diltiazem CD		180 mg PO daily	120–480
Diltiazem XR		180 mg PO daily	120–540
Diltiazem XT		180 mg PO daily	120–480
Isradipine	DHP	2.5 mg PO bid	2.5–10

CHAPTER 3

(continued)

TABLE 3-4	Commonly Used Antihypertensive Agents by Functional Class *(continued)*		
Drugs by Class	**Properties**	**Initial Dose**	**Dosage Range (mg)**
Nicardipine	DHP	20 mg PO tid	60–120
Nifedipine	DHP	10 mg PO tid	30–120
Nifedipine XL (or CC)	DHP	30 mg PO daily	30–90
Nisoldipine	DHP	20 mg PO daily	20–40
Verapamil		80 mg PO tid	80–480
Verapamil SR		120 mg PO daily	120–480
Angiotensin-Converting Enzyme Inhibitors[c]			
Benazepril		10 mg PO bid	10–40
Captopril		25 mg PO bid–tid	12.5–450
Enalapril		5 mg PO daily	2.5–40
Fosinopril		10 mg PO daily	10–40
Lisinopril		10 mg PO daily	5–40
Moexipril		7.5 mg PO daily	7.5–30
Quinapril		10 mg PO daily	5–80
Ramipril		2.5 mg PO daily	1.25–20
Trandolapril		1–2 mg PO daily	1–4
Perindopril		4 mg PO daily	2–16
Angiotensin II Receptor Blockers[c]			
Azilsartan[b]		40 mg daily	40–80
Candesartan		8 mg PO daily	8–32
Eprosartan		600 mg PO daily	600–800
Irbesartan		150 mg PO daily	150–300
Olmesartan		20 mg PO daily	20–40
Losartan		50 mg PO daily	25–100
Telmisartan		40 mg PO daily	20–80
Valsartan		80 mg PO daily	80–320
Direct Renin Inhibitor[c]			
Aliskiren		150 mg PO daily	150–300
Angiotensin Receptor–Neprilysin Inhibitor[c]			
Sacubitril/valsartan[b]		24/26 mg PO BID	24/26–97/103
Diuretics[c]			
Chlorthalidone	Thiazide diuretic	25 mg PO daily	12.5–50
Hydrochlorothiazide	Thiazide diuretic	12.5 mg PO daily	12.5–50
Hydroflumethiazide[b]	Thiazide diuretic	50 mg PO daily	50–100

TABLE 3-4	Commonly Used Antihypertensive Agents by Functional Class (continued)		
Drugs by Class	**Properties**	**Initial Dose**	**Dosage Range (mg)**
Indapamide	Thiazide diuretic	1.25 mg PO daily	2.5–5
Methyclothiazide	Thiazide diuretic	2.5 mg PO daily	2.5–5
Metolazone	Thiazide diuretic	2.5 mg PO daily	1.25–5
Bumetanide	Loop diuretic	0.5 mg PO daily (or IV)	0.5–5
Ethacrynic acid	Loop diuretic	50 mg PO daily (or IV)	25–100
Furosemide	Loop diuretic	20 mg PO daily (or IV)	20–320
Torsemide	Loop diuretic	5 mg PO daily (or IV)	5–10
Amiloride	Potassium-sparing diuretic	5 mg PO daily	5–10
Triamterene	Potassium-sparing diuretic	50 mg PO bid	50–200
Eplerenone	Aldosterone antagonist	25 mg PO daily	25–100
Spironolactone	Aldosterone antagonist	25 mg PO daily	25–100
α-Adrenergic Antagonists			
Doxazosin		1 mg PO daily	1–16
Prazosin		1 mg PO bid–tid	1–20
Terazosin		1 mg PO at bedtime	1–20
Centrally Acting Adrenergic Agents			
Clonidine		0.1 mg PO bid	0.1–1.2
Clonidine patch		TTS 1/wk (equivalent to 0.1 mg/d release)	0.1–0.3
Guanfacine		1 mg PO daily	1–3
Guanabenz		4 mg PO bid	4–64
Methyldopa[a]		250 mg PO bid–tid	250–2000
Direct-Acting Vasodilators			
Hydralazine[a]		10 mg PO qid	50–300
Minoxidil		5 mg PO daily	2.5–100
Miscellaneous			
Reserpine		0.5 mg PO daily	0.1–0.25

DHP, dihydropyridine; ISA, intrinsic sympathomimetic activity; TTS, transdermal therapeutic system.
[a]Adjusted in renal failure.
[b]Available only in brand name. Assume all drugs are available in generic form unless otherwise denoted by superscript "b."
[c]Renal function should be considered before initiation.

- Thiazide or thiazide-like diuretics, calcium channel blockers (CCBs), angiotensin-converting enzyme (ACE) inhibitors, and angiotensin receptor blockers (ARBs) should be considered as first-line therapy for the general population (except for those from African descent), including those with diabetes. Multiple large randomized controlled trials have shown comparable effects on decreasing overall cardiovascular and cerebrovascular mortality for all four drug classes.[5]
- In patients from African descent, including those with diabetes, a thiazide or thiazide-like diuretic or CCB can be considered for first-line therapy. Data from the ALLHAT trial have shown decreased cardiovascular and cerebrovascular morbidity and mortality with the use of thiazide diuretics or CCB over an ACE inhibitor.[26]
- In patients with chronic kidney disease (CKD) stage 3 or higher, or CKD with albuminuria (>300 mg/d), initial or combination therapy with an ACE inhibitor or ARB is recommended.[1]
- **Additional therapy:** When a second drug is needed, it should generally be chosen from among the other first-line agents.
- **Adjustments of a therapeutic regimen:** Before considering a modification of therapy because of inadequate response to the current regimen, other possible contributing factors should be investigated. Poor patient compliance, use of antagonistic drugs (examples provided above), inappropriately high sodium intake, or increased alcohol consumption may be the cause of inadequate BP response. Secondary causes of hypertension should be considered when a previously effective regimen becomes inadequate and other confounding factors are absent.
- **Diuretics** (see Table 3-4) are effective agents in the therapy of hypertension and have been shown to reduce the incidence of stroke and cardiovascular events. Several classes of diuretics are available, generally categorized by their site of action in the kidney.
  - **Thiazides** and thiazide-like diuretics (e.g., hydrochlorothiazide, chlorthalidone) block sodium reabsorption predominantly in the distal convoluted tubule by inhibition of the thiazide-sensitive sodium/chloride (Na/Cl) cotransporter. Thiazide diuretics can cause weakness, muscle cramps, and impotence. Metabolic side effects include hypokalemia, hypomagnesemia, hyperlipidemia (increased in low-density lipoproteins [LDLs] and triglyceride levels), hypercalcemia, hyperglycemia, hyperuricemia, hyponatremia, and rarely azotemia. Thiazide-induced pancreatitis has also been reported. Metabolic side effects may be limited when thiazides are used in low doses (e.g., hydrochlorothiazide, 12.5–25 mg/d). Chlorthalidone and indapamide, thiazide-like diuretics, are often the preferred diuretics for management of hypertension due to their longer duration of action. Thiazide-like diuretics are particularly useful in patients with osteoporosis, edema, and calcium nephrolithiasis with hypercalcemia. It should be noted that chlorthalidone is associated with greater risks of hypokalemia, glucose intolerance, and new-onset diabetes than hydrochlorothiazide.[27]
  - **Loop diuretics** (e.g., furosemide, bumetanide, ethacrynic acid, torsemide) block sodium reabsorption in the thick ascending limb of the loop of Henle through inhibition of the Na/K/2Cl cotransporter and are the most effective agents in patients with renal insufficiency (estimated glomerular filtration rate [GFR] <35 mL/min/1.73 m^2). Loop diuretics can cause electrolyte abnormalities such as hypomagnesemia, hypocalcemia, and hypokalemia and can also produce irreversible ototoxicity (usually dose related and more common with parenteral use).
  - **Spironolactone and eplerenone, potassium-sparing agents,** act by competitively inhibiting the actions of aldosterone on the kidney. Triamterene and amiloride are

potassium-sparing drugs that inhibit the epithelial Na^+ channel in the distal nephron to inhibit reabsorption of Na^+ and secretion of potassium ions. Potassium-sparing diuretics are weak agents when used alone; thus, they are often combined with a thiazide for added potency. Aldosterone antagonists reduce morbidity and mortality in HF with reduced ejection fraction and may have an additional benefit in improving myocardial function; this effect may be independent of its effect on renal transport mechanisms. Spironolactone or eplerenone are recommended for BP control in patients with resistant hypertension.[1,13] Spironolactone and eplerenone can produce hyperkalemia. The gynecomastia that may occur in men and breast tenderness in women are not seen with eplerenone. Triamterene (usually in combination with hydrochlorothiazide) can cause renal tubular damage and renal calculi. Unlike thiazides, potassium-sparing and loop diuretics do not cause adverse lipid effects. Of note finerenone is a nonsteroidal mineralocorticoid receptor antagonist recently approved for HF management but not indicated for hypertension.

- **Calcium channel antagonists** (see Table 3-4) generally have no significant central nervous system (CNS) side effects and can be used to treat coexisting diseases, such as angina pectoris. **Short-acting dihydropyridine calcium channel antagonists may increase the number of ischemic cardiac events, and therefore are not indicated for hypertension management**[28]; long-acting agents are considered safe in the management of hypertension.[29,30]

  ○ **Classes of calcium channel antagonists** include diphenylalkylamines (e.g., verapamil), benzothiazepines (e.g., diltiazem), and dihydropyridines (e.g., nifedipine). The dihydropyridines include many newer second-generation drugs (e.g., amlodipine, felodipine, isradipine, and nicardipine), which are more vasoselective and have longer plasma half-lives than nifedipine. Verapamil and diltiazem have negative cardiac inotropic and chronotropic effects. Nifedipine also has a negative inotropic effect, but in clinical use, this effect is much less pronounced than that of verapamil or diltiazem because of peripheral vasodilation and reflex tachycardia. The second-generation dihydropyridines have observed less negative inotropic effects. All calcium channel antagonists are metabolized in the liver; thus, in patients with cirrhosis, the dosing interval should be adjusted accordingly. Some of these drugs also inhibit the metabolism of other hepatically cleared medications (e.g., cyclosporine). Verapamil and diltiazem should be used with caution in patients with cardiac conduction abnormalities, and they can worsen HF in patients with decreased left ventricular function.

  ○ **Side effects** of verapamil include constipation, nausea, headache, and orthostatic hypotension. Diltiazem can cause nausea, headache, and rash. Dihydropyridines can cause lower extremity edema, flushing, headache, and rash. Calcium channel antagonists can also cause gingival hyperplasia. They have no significant effects on glucose tolerance, electrolytes, or lipid profiles.

- **Inhibitors of the renin–angiotensin system** (see Table 3-4) include ACE inhibitors, ARBs, a direct renin inhibitor, and an angiotensin receptor-neprilysin inhibitor (ARNI).

  ○ **ACE inhibitors** have beneficial effects in patients with concomitant HF or kidney disease. One study has also suggested that ACE inhibitors (ramipril) may significantly reduce the rate of death, MI, and stroke in patients without HF or low ejection fraction.[31] Additionally, they can reduce hypokalemia, hypercholesterolemia, hyperglycemia, and hyperuricemia caused by diuretic therapy and are particularly effective in states of hypertension associated with a high renin state (e.g., scleroderma renal crisis). **Side effects** associated with the use of ACE inhibitors are infrequent.

They can cause a dry cough (up to 20% of patients), angioneurotic edema, and hypotension, but they do not affect levels of lipids, glucose, or uric acid. ACE inhibitors that contain a sulfhydryl group (e.g., captopril) may cause taste disturbance, leukopenia, and a glomerulopathy with proteinuria. Patients who have decreased renal perfusion or preexisting severe renal insufficiency may end up with worsening renal function because ACE inhibitors cause preferential vasodilation of the efferent arteriole in the kidney. ACE inhibitors can cause hyperkalemia and should be used with caution in patients with a decreased GFR who are taking potassium supplements or who are receiving potassium-sparing diuretics.

- **ARBs** are a class of antihypertensive drugs that are effective in diverse patient populations.[32] ARBs are useful alternatives in patients with HF who are unable to tolerate ACE inhibitors.[33] **Side effects** of ARBs occur rarely but include angioedema, allergic reaction, and rash. Patients should not be prescribed both an ACE inhibitor and an ARB as this puts patients at high risk of vascular events or renal dysfunction.
- The **direct renin inhibitor** class consists of a single agent, aliskiren, which is indicated solely for the treatment of hypertension (see Table 3-4). It may be used in combination with other antihypertensive agents; however, combined use with ACE inhibitors or ARBs is contraindicated in patients with diabetes and increases the risk of hyperkalemia[34,35] (Food and Drug Administration [FDA] Drug Safety Communication, April 2012).
- ARNI (sacubitril–valsartan) is a drug combination of a neprilysin inhibitor plus an ARB. ARNI act by both blocking effects of the renin–angiotensin–aldosterone system and raising levels of potentially beneficial endogenous vasoactive peptides. ARNI is particularly useful in patients with HF, as sacubitril–valsartan reduces all-cause mortality as well as cardiovascular mortality and hospitalization rate for HF compared with enalapril (ACE inhibitor).[36] ARNI therapy also likely has beneficial effects on renal function and glucose control, based on recent emerging data.[37-39] Patients are often transitioned from an ACE inhibitor or ARB to an ARNI. ARNIs should not be administered within 36 hours of switching to or from an ACE inhibitor. ARNIs also should not be used with aliskiren in patients with diabetes or reduced renal function (eGFR <60 mL/min/1.73 m^2).

- **β-Adrenergic antagonists** (see Table 3-4) are part of medical regimens that have been proven to decrease the incidence of stroke, MI, and HF. β-Adrenergic antagonists work via competitive inhibition of the effects of catecholamines at β-adrenergic receptors, which decreases heart rate and cardiac output. These agents also decrease plasma renin and cause a resetting of baroreceptors to accept a lower level of BP. β-Adrenergic antagonists cause release of vasodilatory prostaglandins, decrease plasma volume, and may also have a CNS-mediated antihypertensive effect.
  - **Classes of β-adrenergic antagonists** can be subdivided into those that are cardioselective, with primarily β_1-blocking effects, and those that are nonselective, with β_1- and β_2-blocking effects. At low doses, the cardioselective agents can be given with caution to patients with mild chronic obstructive pulmonary disease, diabetes, or peripheral vascular disease. At higher doses, these agents lose their β_1 selectivity and may cause unwanted effects in these patients. β-Adrenergic antagonists can also be categorized according to the presence or absence of partial agonist or intrinsic sympathomimetic activity (ISA). β-Adrenergic antagonists with ISA cause less bradycardia than do those without it. In addition, there are agents with mixed properties having both α- and β-adrenergic antagonist actions (labetalol and carvedilol). Nebivolol is a highly selective β-adrenergic antagonist that has vasodilatory properties through an unclear mechanism.

- ○ **Side effects** include high-degree atrioventricular block, HF, Raynaud phenomenon, and impotence. Lipophilic β-adrenergic antagonists, such as propranolol, have a higher incidence of CNS side effects including insomnia and depression. Propranolol can also cause nasal congestion. β-Adrenergic antagonists can cause adverse effects on the lipid profile; increased triglyceride and decreased high-density lipoprotein (HDL) levels occur mainly with nonselective β-adrenergic antagonists but generally do not occur when β-adrenergic antagonists with ISA are used. Pindolol, a selective β-adrenergic antagonist with ISA, may increase HDL and nominally increase triglycerides. Side effects of labetalol include hepatocellular damage, postural hypotension, a positive antinuclear antibody (ANA) test, a lupus-like syndrome, tremors, and potential hypotension in the setting of halothane anesthesia. Carvedilol appears to have a similar side effect profile to other β-adrenergic antagonists. Both labetalol and carvedilol have negligible effects on lipids. Rarely, reflex tachycardia may occur due to the initial vasodilatory effect of labetalol and carvedilol. Since β-receptor density is increased with chronic antagonism, abrupt withdrawal of these agents can precipitate angina pectoris, increases in BP, and other effects attributable to an increase in adrenergic tone.
- **Selective α-adrenergic antagonists** such as prazosin, terazosin, and doxazosin have replaced nonselective α-adrenergic antagonists such as phenoxybenzamine (see Table 3-4) in the treatment of essential hypertension. Based on the ALLHAT trial, these drugs appear to be less efficacious than diuretics, CCBs, and ACE inhibitors in reducing primary end points of CVD when used as monotherapy.[26] **Side effects** of these agents include a "first-dose effect," which results from a greater decrease in BP with the first dose than with subsequent doses. Selective α_1-adrenergic antagonists can cause syncope, orthostatic hypotension, dizziness, headache, and drowsiness. In most cases, side effects are self-limited and do not recur with continued therapy. Selective α_1-adrenergic antagonists may improve lipid profiles by decreasing total cholesterol and triglyceride levels and increasing HDL levels. Additionally, these agents can improve the negative effects on lipids induced by thiazide diuretics and β-adrenergic antagonists. Doxazosin specifically may be less effective at lowering SBP than thiazide diuretics and may be associated with a higher risk of HF and stroke in patients with hypertension and at least one additional risk factor for coronary artery disease (CAD).[26]
- **Centrally acting adrenergic agents** (see Table 3-4) are potent antihypertensive agents. In addition to its oral dosage forms, clonidine is available as a transdermal patch that is applied weekly. **Side effects** may include bradycardia, drowsiness, dry mouth, orthostatic hypotension, galactorrhea, and sexual dysfunction. Transdermal clonidine causes a rash in up to 20% of patients. These agents can precipitate HF in patients with decreased left ventricular function, and abrupt cessation can precipitate an acute withdrawal syndrome (AWS) of elevated BP, tachycardia, and diaphoresis. Methyldopa produces a positive direct antibody (Coombs) test in up to 25% of patients, but significant hemolytic anemia is much less common. If hemolytic anemia develops secondary to methyldopa, the drug should be withdrawn. Severe cases of hemolytic anemia may require treatment with glucocorticoids. Methyldopa also causes positive ANA test results in approximately 10% of patients and can cause an inflammatory reaction in the liver that is indistinguishable from viral hepatitis; fatal hepatitis has been reported. Guanabenz and guanfacine decrease total cholesterol levels, and guanfacine can also decrease serum triglyceride levels.
- **Direct-acting vasodilators** are potent antihypertensive agents (see Table 3-4) now reserved for refractory hypertension or specific circumstances such as the use of hydralazine in pregnancy.

- ○ Hydralazine in combination with nitrates is useful in treating patients with hypertension and specific subsets of patients with HF with reduced ejection fraction (see Chapter 5, Heart Failure and Cardiomyopathy). **Side effects** of hydralazine therapy may include headache, nausea, emesis, tachycardia, and postural hypotension. Asymptomatic patients may have a positive ANA test result, and a hydralazine-induced systemic lupus-like syndrome may develop in approximately 10% of patients. Patients at greater risk for the latter complication include those treated with excessive doses (e.g., >400 mg/d), those with impaired renal or cardiac function, and those with the slow acetylation phenotype. Hydralazine should be discontinued if clinical evidence of a lupus-like syndrome develops and a positive ANA test result is present. The syndrome usually resolves with discontinuation of the drug, leaving no adverse long-term effects.
  - ○ **Side effects** of minoxidil include weight gain, hypertrichosis, hirsutism, ECG abnormalities, and pericardial effusions.
- • **Reserpine, guanethidine, and guanadrel** (see Table 3-4) were among the first effective antihypertensive agents available. Currently, these drugs are not regarded as first- or second-line therapy because of their significant side effects. **Side effects** of reserpine include severe depression in approximately 2% of patients. Sedation and nasal stuffiness also are potential side effects. Guanethidine can cause severe postural hypotension through a decrease in cardiac output, a decrease in peripheral resistance, and venous pooling in the extremities. Patients who are receiving guanethidine with orthostatic hypotension should be cautioned to arise slowly and to wear support hose. Guanethidine can also cause ejaculatory failure and diarrhea.
- • **Parenteral antihypertensive agents** are indicated for the immediate reduction of BP in patients with hypertensive emergencies. Judicious administration of these agents (Table 3-5) may also be appropriate in patients with hypertension complicated by HF or MI. These drugs are also indicated for individuals who have perioperative severe hypertension or need an emergency surgery. If possible, an accurate baseline BP should be determined before the initiation of therapy. In the setting of hypertensive emergency, the patient should be admitted to an intensive care unit for close monitoring, and an intra-arterial monitor should be used when available. Although parenteral agents are indicated as a first-line treatment in hypertensive emergencies, oral agents may also be effective in this group; the choice of drug and route of administration must be individualized. If parenteral agents are used initially, oral medications should be administered shortly thereafter to facilitate rapid weaning from parenteral therapy.
  - ○ **Sodium nitroprusside,** a direct-acting arterial and venous vasodilator, is the drug of choice for most hypertensive emergencies (see Table 3-5). It reduces BP rapidly and is easily titratable, and its action is short lived when discontinued. Patients should be monitored very closely to avoid an exaggerated hypotensive response. Therapy for more than 48–72 hours with a high cumulative dose or renal insufficiency may cause accumulation of thiocyanate, a toxic metabolite. Thiocyanate toxicity may cause paresthesias, tinnitus, blurred vision, delirium, or seizures. Serum thiocyanate levels should be kept at <10 mg/dL. Patients on high doses (>2–3 µg/kg/min) or those with renal dysfunction should have serum levels of thiocyanate drawn after 48–72 hours of therapy. In patients with normal renal function or those receiving lower doses, levels can be drawn after 5–7 days. Hepatic dysfunction may result in accumulation of cyanide, which can cause lactic acidosis, dyspnea, vomiting, dizziness, ataxia, and syncope. Hemodialysis should be considered for thiocyanate poisoning. Nitrites and thiosulfate can be administered intravenously for cyanide poisoning.

TABLE 3-5	Parenteral Antihypertensive Drug Preparations				
Drug	Administration	Onset	Duration of Action	Dosage	Adverse Effects and Comments
Fenoldopam	IV infusion	<5 min	30 min	0.1–0.3 µg/kg/min	Tachycardia, nausea, vomiting
Sodium nitroprusside	IV infusion	Immediate	2–3 min	0.5–10 µg/kg/min (initial dose, 0.25 µg/kg/min for eclampsia and renal insufficiency)	Hypotension, nausea, vomiting, apprehension; risk of thiocyanate and cyanide toxicity is increased in renal and hepatic insufficiency, respectively; levels should be monitored; must shield from light
Diazoxide	IV bolus	15 min	6–12 h	50–100 mg q5–10 min, up to 600 mg	Hypotension, tachycardia, nausea, vomiting, fluid retention, hyperglycemia; may exacerbate myocardial ischemia, heart failure, or aortic dissection
Labetalol	IV bolus	5–10 min	3–6 h	20–80 mg q5–10min, up to 300 mg	Hypotension, heart block, heart failure, bronchospasm, nausea, vomiting, scalp tingling, paradoxical pressor response; may not be effective in patients receiving α- or β-antagonists
	IV infusion			0.5–2 mg/min	
Nitroglycerin	IV infusion	1–2 min	3–5 min	5–250 µg/min	Headache, nausea, vomiting. Tolerance may develop with prolonged use
Esmolol	IV bolus	1–5 min	10 min	500 µg/kg/min for first 1 min	Hypotension, heart block, heart failure, bronchospasm
	IV infusion			50–300 µg/kg/min	

(continued)

CHAPTER 3

TABLE 3-5	Parenteral Antihypertensive Drug Preparations	(continued)			
Drug	Administration	Onset	Duration of Action	Dosage	Adverse Effects and Comments
Phentolamine	IV bolus	1–2 min	3–10 min	5–10 mg q5–15 min	Hypotension, tachycardia, headache, angina, paradoxical pressor response
Hydralazine (for treatment of eclampsia)	IV bolus	10–20 min	3–6 h	10–20 mg q20min (if no effect after 20 mg, try another agent)	Hypotension, fetal distress, tachycardia, headache, nausea, vomiting, local thrombophlebitis. Infusion site should be changed after 12 h
Methyldopate (for treatment of eclampsia)	IV bolus	30–60 min	10–16 h	250–500 mg	Hypotension
Nicardipine	IV infusion	1–5 min	3–6 h	5 mg/h, increased by 1–2.5 mg/h q15min, up to 15 mg/h	Hypotension, headache, tachycardia, nausea, vomiting
Clevidipine	IV infusion	2–4 min	5–15 min	1–2 mg/h, double dose every 90 s up to 16 mg/h	Hypotension, reflex tachycardia
Enalaprilat	IV bolus	5–15 min	1–6 h	0.6255 mg q6h	Hypotension

○ **Nitroglycerin** given as a continuous IV infusion (see Table 3-5) may be appropriate in situations in which sodium nitroprusside is relatively contraindicated, such as in patients with severe coronary insufficiency or advanced renal or hepatic disease. It is the preferred agent for patients with moderate hypertension in the setting of acute coronary ischemia or after coronary artery bypass surgery because of its more favorable effects on pulmonary gas exchange and collateral coronary blood flow. In patients with severely elevated BP, sodium nitroprusside remains the agent of choice. Nitroglycerin reduces preload more than afterload and should be used with caution or avoided in patients who have inferior MI with right ventricular infarction and are often dependent on preload to maintain cardiac output.

○ **Labetalol** can be administered parenterally (see Table 3-5) in hypertensive crisis, even in patients in the early phase of an acute MI, and is the drug of choice in hypertensive emergencies that occur during pregnancy. When given intravenously, the β-adrenergic antagonist effect is greater than the α-adrenergic antagonist effect. Nevertheless, symptomatic postural hypotension may occur with IV use; thus, patients should be treated in a supine position. Labetalol may be particularly beneficial during adrenergic excess (e.g., clonidine withdrawal, pheochromocytoma, post–coronary bypass grafting). Because the half-life of labetalol is 5–8 hours, intermittent IV bolus dosing may be preferable to IV infusion. IV infusion can be discontinued before oral labetalol is begun. When the supine DBP begins to rise, oral dosing can be initiated at 200 mg PO, followed in 6–12 hours by 200–400 mg PO, depending on the BP response.

○ **Esmolol** is a parenteral, short-acting, cardioselective β-adrenergic antagonist (see Table 3-5) that can be used in the treatment of hypertensive emergencies in patients in whom β-blocker intolerance is a concern. Esmolol is also useful for the treatment of aortic dissection. β-Adrenergic antagonists may be ineffective when used as monotherapy in the treatment of severe hypertension and are frequently combined with other agents (e.g., with sodium nitroprusside in the treatment of aortic dissection).

○ **Nicardipine** is an effective IV calcium channel antagonist preparation (see Table 3-5). Side effects include headache, flushing, reflex tachycardia, and venous irritation. Nicardipine should be administered via a central venous line. If it is given peripherally, the IV site should be changed q12h. Fifty percent of the peak effect is seen within the first 30 minutes, but the full peak effect is not achieved until after 48 hours of administration. **Clevidipine**, an IV calcium channel antagonist, has a quicker onset of action and shorter half-life than nicardipine.

○ **Enalaprilat** is the active de-esterified form of enalapril (see Table 3-5) that results from hepatic conversion after an oral dose. Enalaprilat (as well as other ACE inhibitors) has been used effectively in cases of severe and malignant hypertension. However, variable and unpredictable results have also been reported. ACE inhibition can cause rapid BP reduction in hypertensive patients with high renin states such as renovascular hypertension, concomitant use of vasodilators, and scleroderma renal crisis; thus, enalaprilat should be used cautiously to avoid precipitating hypotension. Therapy can be changed to an oral preparation when IV therapy is no longer necessary.

○ **Diazoxide and hydralazine** are only rarely used in hypertensive crises and offer little or no advantage to the agents discussed previously. It should be noted, however, that hydralazine is a useful agent in pregnancy-related hypertensive emergencies because of its established safety profile.

○ **Fenoldopam** is a selective agonist to peripheral dopamine-1 receptors, and it produces vasodilation, increases renal perfusion, and enhances natriuresis.

CHAPTER 3

Fenoldopam has a short duration of action; the elimination half-life is <10 minutes. The drug has important application as parenteral therapy for high-risk hypertensive surgical patients and the perioperative management of patients undergoing organ transplantation.

SPECIAL CONSIDERATIONS

- **Hypertensive emergency and severe asymptomatic hypertension:** In hypertensive emergency, control of acute or ongoing end-organ damage is more important than the absolute level of BP. Appropriate treatment of hypertensive emergency lowers blood pressure to prevent continued end-organ damage but does so slowly and gradually to prevent ischemic damage. Mean arterial pressure should be reduced by 10%–20% in the first hour and a further 5%–15% over the next 23 hours. Exceptions to gradual blood pressure lowering include acute ischemic stroke, acute aortic dissection, and intracerebral hemorrhage.[6-8] A precipitous fall in BP may occur in patients who are elderly, volume depleted, or receiving other antihypertensive agents. BP control in severe asymptomatic hypertension without evidence of end-organ damage can be accomplished more slowly and with use of oral antihypertensives. Excessive or rapid decreases in BP should be avoided to minimize the risk of cerebral hypoperfusion or coronary insufficiency. Normal BP can be attained gradually over several days as tolerated by the individual patient as there is no proven benefit from rapid reduction of blood pressure in patients with severe asymptomatic hypertension.[6,9-11]
- **Aortic dissection**
  - All patients with aortic dissection, including those treated surgically, require acute and chronic antihypertensive therapy to provide initial stabilization and to prevent complications (e.g., aortic rupture, continued dissection). Medical therapy of chronic stable aortic dissection should seek to maintain SBP ≤120 mm Hg and heart rate <60 bpm if tolerated.[40] Antihypertensive agents with negative inotropic properties, including calcium channel antagonists, β-adrenergic antagonists, methyldopa, clonidine, and reserpine, are preferred for management in the post–acute phase.
  - **β-Blockers** are considered the initial drug of choice and should precede vasodilator therapy. β-Blockers are effective in lowering the heart rate and counteracting the reflex tachycardia and increased inotropy seen with vasodilator therapy. **IV labetalol** has been used successfully as a single agent in the treatment of acute aortic dissection. Labetalol produces a dose-related decrease in BP and lowers contractility. It has the advantage of allowing for oral administration after the successful acute stage of dissection management. **Esmolol**, a cardioselective class intravenous β-adrenergic antagonist with a very short duration of action, may be preferable, especially in patients with relative contraindications to β-antagonists. If esmolol is tolerated, a longer-acting β-adrenergic antagonist should be used. In patients who are β-blockade-intolerant, CCBs such as diltiazem and verapamil may be used.
  - **Vasodilator therapy** in combination with β-blockade allows for more effective and rapid reduction in BP. **Sodium nitroprusside** is considered the initial vasodilator drug of choice because of the predictability of response and absence of tachyphylaxis. Nitroprusside alone causes an increase in left ventricular contractility and subsequent arterial shearing forces, which contribute to ongoing intimal dissection. Thus, when using sodium nitroprusside, adequate simultaneous **β-adrenergic antagonist therapy** is essential. Nicardipine, clevidipine, nitroglycerin, enalaprilat, and fenoldopam may also be used.

- **The elderly hypertensive patient** (age >65 years) is generally characterized by increased vascular resistance, decreased plasma renin activity, and greater LVH than in younger patients. Often, elderly hypertensive patients have coexisting medical problems that must be considered when initiating antihypertensive therapy. SBP <140 mm Hg has been associated with decreased major adverse cardiovascular events.[41,42] Drug doses should be increased slowly to avoid adverse effects and hypotension. Diuretics as initial therapy have been shown to decrease the incidence of stroke, fatal MI, and overall mortality in this age group.[43] Calcium channel antagonists decrease vascular resistance, have no adverse effects on lipid levels, and are also good choices for elderly patients. ACE inhibitors and ARBs may be effective agents in this population.
- **Hypertensive patients of African descent** generally have a lower plasma renin level, higher plasma volume, and higher vascular resistance than do Caucasian patients. Thus, patients of African descent respond well to diuretics, particularly thiazides or thiazide-like diuretics, alone or in combination with calcium channel antagonists. ACE inhibitors, ARBs, and β-adrenergic antagonists are also effective agents in this population, particularly when combined with a diuretic.
- **The hypertensive patient with obesity** is characterized by more modest elevations in vascular resistance, higher cardiac output, expanded intravascular volume, and lower plasma renin activity at any given level of arterial pressure. Weight reduction is the primary goal of therapy and is effective in reducing BP and causing regression of LVH.
- **The diabetic patient** with nephropathy may have significant proteinuria and renal insufficiency, which can complicate management (see Chapter 13, Renal Diseases). Control of BP is the most important intervention shown to slow down additional loss of renal function. In the setting of proteinuria, ACE inhibitors should be used as first-line therapy because they have been shown to decrease proteinuria and to slow down progressive loss of renal function independent of their antihypertensive effects. Hyperkalemia is a common side effect in diabetic patients treated with ACE inhibitors, especially in those with moderate to severe renal impairment. ARBs are also effective antihypertensive agents and have been shown to slow down the rate of progression to ESRD, thus supporting a renal protective effect.[44]
- **The patient with chronic renal insufficiency** has hypertension that is usually partially volume dependent. Retention of sodium and water exacerbates the existing hypertensive state, and diuretics are important in the management of this problem. When estimated GFR is <30–35 mL/min/1.73 m^2, loop diuretics are the most effective class. In the presence of proteinuria, ACE inhibitors/ARBs should be considered because higher urinary excretion of protein is associated with a more rapid decline in GFR, regardless of the cause of renal insufficiency. More recently, an updated Kidney Disease Improving Global Outcomes BP guideline recommended more intensive BP control with a systolic target of <120 mm Hg for all patients with CKD not on dialysis.[45] Data from the SPRINT trial seemed to indicate higher rates of acute kidney injury with intensive treatment for patients with stage 3 or 4 CKD.[46] However, subsequent analyses of SPRINT and findings from a substudy have shown that these changes were likely benign and hemodynamic rather than causing permanent injury.[47-49] Longer-term data are needed for clarification and confirmation of these findings.
- **The hypertensive patient with LVH** is at increased risk for sudden death, MI, and all-cause mortality. Although there is no direct evidence, regression of LVH could be expected to reduce the risk for subsequent complications. Aggressive BP control and renin–angiotensin system blockade with ACE inhibitors/ARBs appear to have the greatest effect on the regression.[50-52]

CHAPTER 3

- **The hypertensive patient with CAD** is at increased risk for unstable angina (UA) and MI. β-Adrenergic antagonists can be used as first-line agents in these patients because they can decrease cardiac mortality and subsequent reinfarction in the setting of acute MI and can decrease progression to MI in those who present with UA. β-Adrenergic antagonists also have a role in secondary prevention of cardiac events and increasing long-term survival after an MI. Care should be exercised in those with cardiac conduction system disease. ACE inhibitors are beneficial in patients with CAD and decrease mortality in individuals who present with acute MI, especially those with left ventricular dysfunction.[53-56]

- **The hypertensive patient with heart failure with reduced ejection fraction (HFrEF)** is at risk for progressive left ventricular dilatation and sudden death. Patients should be prescribed guideline-directed medical therapy to attain a BP <130/80 mm Hg (see Chapter 5, Heart Failure and Cardiomyopathy). In this population, ACE inhibitors decrease mortality,[54] and in the setting of acute MI, they decrease the risk of recurrent MI, hospitalization for HF, and mortality.[57] ARBs have similar beneficial effects, and they appear to be an effective alternative in patients who do not tolerate an ACE inhibitor.[33] Several recent studies have supported the use of ARNI over ACE inhibitors or ARBs in HFrEF patients as sacubitril–valsartan (ARNI) was shown to reduce all-cause and cardiovascular mortality and HF hospitalization rate when compared head-to-head to enalapril (ACE inhibitor).[36] ARNI therapy also likely has beneficial effects on renal function and glucose control, based on recent emerging data.[37-39] β-Adrenergic antagonist therapy has also been shown to decrease morbidity and mortality. Agents shown to have proven benefit include metoprolol succinate, carvedilol, and bisoprolol.[29,58,59] Nitrates and hydralazine also decrease mortality in specific subsets of patients with HF irrespective of hypertension, but hydralazine can cause reflex tachycardia and worsening ischemia in patients with unstable coronary syndromes and should be used with caution. Mineralocorticoid receptor antagonists have been shown to decrease mortality in patients with HFrEF. Nondihydropyridine calcium channel antagonists should generally be avoided.

- **The hypertensive patient with heart failure with preserved ejection fraction (HFpEF)** may present with signs of volume overload and thus diuretics may be used as initial therapy. The optimal treatment regimen for hypertension in patients with HFpEF is unclear. ACE inhibitors/ARBs have the greatest effect on regression of LVH and thus may improve diastolic function.[60]

- **In the pregnant patient with hypertension,** there is concern for potential maternal and fetal morbidity and mortality associated with elevated BP and the clinical syndromes of preeclampsia and eclampsia. The possibility of teratogenic or other adverse effects of antihypertensive medications on fetal development should also be considered.

  ○ **Classification of hypertension** during pregnancy has been proposed by the American College of Obstetrics and Gynecology.[61]

    ■ **Preeclampsia–eclampsia:** Diagnosis is established if there is **new-onset** hypertension after 20 weeks of gestation and the presence of proteinuria. Elevated SBP ≥ 140 mm Hg or DBP ≥90 mm Hg on two occasions at least 4 hours apart or a one-time measurement of SBP ≥160 mm Hg or DBP ≥110 mm Hg qualifies as hypertension. If no proteinuria is present, then hypertension along with one of the following qualifies: platelets <100,000/μL, creatinine >1.1 mg/dL (or doubling from baseline), liver transaminases greater than twice the normal, pulmonary edema, or cerebral/visual symptoms. Eclampsia encompasses these parameters in addition to generalized seizures.

- **Chronic (preexisting) hypertension:** This disorder is defined as hypertension diagnosed or present before pregnancy or 20 weeks of gestation (traditionally, a BP ≥140/90 mm Hg with at least two determinations at least 4 hours apart is used).
- **Chronic hypertension with superimposed preeclampsia:** This classification is used when a woman with chronic hypertension develops worsening hypertension and new proteinuria and/or other features of preeclampsia as outlined previously.
- **Gestational hypertension:** This disorder is defined by a BP ≥140/90 mm Hg after the 20th week of pregnancy without proteinuria or other features of preeclampsia.
  - **Therapy:** Treatment of hypertension in pregnancy is recommended when SBP is ≥160 mm Hg or DBP is ≥100 mm Hg; however, clinical judgment should be used in determining treatment in pregnant women with comorbid conditions such as CVD or CKD.
    - Nonpharmacologic therapy, such as weight reduction and vigorous exercise, is not recommended during pregnancy.
    - Alcohol and tobacco use should be strongly discouraged.
    - Pharmacologic intervention with labetalol, nifedipine, or methyldopa is recommended as first-line therapy because of their proven safety.
    - ACE inhibitors and ARB have been proven to be teratogenic and increase fetal morbidity or mortality.
    - β-Blockers may be used in pregnancy; however, atenolol should not be used due to increased risk of fetal growth restriction.
    - If a patient is suspected of having preeclampsia or eclampsia, urgent evaluation is recommended.
- **MAOIs:** MAOIs used in association with certain drugs or foods can produce a catecholamine excess state and accelerated hypertension. Interactions are common with tricyclic antidepressants, meperidine, methyldopa, levodopa, sympathomimetic agents, and antihistamines. Tyramine-containing foods that can lead to this syndrome include certain cheeses, red wine, beer, chocolate, chicken liver, processed meat, herring, broad beans, canned figs, and yeast. Nitroprusside, labetalol, and phentolamine have been used effectively in the treatment of accelerated hypertension associated with MAOI use (see Table 3-5).

COMPLICATIONS

Withdrawal syndrome associated with discontinuation of antihypertensive therapy: When substituting therapy in patients with moderate to severe hypertension, it is reasonable to increase doses of the new medication in small increments while tapering the previous medication to avoid excessive BP fluctuations. On occasion, an antihypertensive withdrawal syndrome (AWS) develops, usually within the first 24–72 hours, when BP rises to levels that are much higher than those of baseline values. The most severe complications of AWS include encephalopathy, stroke, MI, and sudden death. AWS is most commonly associated with centrally acting adrenergic agents (particularly clonidine) and β-adrenergic antagonists but has been reported with other agents as well, including diuretics. Discontinuation of antihypertensive medications should be done with caution in patients with preexisting cerebrovascular or cardiac disease. Management of AWS by reinstitution of the previously administered drug is generally effective.

Dyslipidemia

GENERAL PRINCIPLES

- Lipids are sparingly soluble macromolecules that include cholesterol, fatty acids, and their derivatives.
- Plasma lipids are transported by lipoprotein particles composed of **apolipoproteins, phospholipids, free cholesterol, cholesterol esters,** and **triglycerides.**
- Human plasma lipoproteins are separated into **five major classes** based on density:
  - Chylomicrons (least dense)
  - Very-low-density lipoproteins (VLDLs)
  - Intermediate-density lipoproteins (IDLs)
  - Low-density lipoproteins (LDLs)
  - High-density lipoproteins (HDLs)
- A sixth class, lipoprotein(a) [Lp(a)], resembles LDL in lipid composition and has a density that overlaps LDL and HDL.
- Physical properties of plasma lipoproteins are summarized in Table 3-6.
- Nearly 90% of patients with congestive heart disease (CHD) have some form of dyslipidemia. Increased levels of LDL cholesterol (LDL-C), remnant lipoproteins, Lp(a), and decreased levels of HDL cholesterol have all been associated with an increased risk of premature vascular disease.[62,63] In addition, dyslipidemia is highly prevalent in children with nonalcoholic fatty liver disease and may play a role in its pathophysiology.[64]
- **Clinical dyslipoproteinemias**
  - Most dyslipidemias are multifactorial in etiology and reflect the effects of genetic influences coupled with diet, inactivity, smoking, alcohol use, and comorbid conditions such as obesity and diabetes (DM).
  - Differential diagnosis of the major lipid abnormalities is summarized in Table 3-7.

TABLE 3-6	Physical Properties of Plasma Lipoproteins[a]		
Lipoprotein	Lipid Composition	Origin	Apolipoproteins
Chylomicrons	TG, 85%; chol, 3%	Intestine	A-I, A-IV; B-48; C-I, C-II, C-III; E
VLDL	TG, 55%; chol, 20%	Liver	B-100; C-I, C-II, C-III; E
IDL	TG, 25%; chol, 35%	Metabolic product of VLDL	B-100; C-I, C-II, C-III; E
LDL	TG, 5%; chol, 60%	Metabolic product of IDL	B-100
HDL	TG, 5%; chol, 20%	Liver, intestine	A-I, A-II; C-I, C-II, C-III; E
Lp(a)	TG, 5%; chol, 60%	Liver	B-100; Apo(a)

Chol, cholesterol; HDL, high-density lipoprotein; IDL, intermediate-density lipoprotein; LDL, low-density lipoprotein; Lp(a), lipoprotein(a); TG, triglyceride; VLDL, very-low-density lipoprotein.
[a]Remainder of particle is composed of phospholipid and protein.

- ○ The major genetic dyslipoproteinemias are reviewed in Table 3-8.[65,66]
  - Familial hypercholesterolemia (FH) and familial combined hyperlipidemia are disorders that contribute significantly to premature CVD.
  - FH is an underdiagnosed, autosomal co-dominant condition with a prevalence of approximately 1 in 200 people that causes elevated LDL-C levels from birth.[67,68] It is associated with significantly increased risk of early CVD.[69]
  - Familial combined hyperlipidemia has a prevalence of 1%–2% and typically presents in adulthood, although obesity and high dietary fat and sugar intake have led to increased presentation in childhood and adolescence.[69]
- **Standards of care for hyperlipidemia**
  - ○ LDL-C–lowering therapy, particularly with hydroxymethylglutaryl-coenzyme A (HMG-CoA) reductase inhibitors (commonly referred to as statins), lowers the risk of CHD-related death, morbidity, and revascularization procedures in patients *with* (secondary prevention) *or without* (primary prevention) known CHD.[70-77] LDL-lowering therapy has proven beneficial even in patients at low risk for vascular disease.[78]
  - ○ Prevention of ASCVD is the primary goal of the 2018 ACC/AHA guidelines. These guidelines address risk assessment, lifestyle modifications, evaluation and treatment of obesity, and evaluation and management of blood cholesterol and aim for a more personalized and shared decision-making approach to risk management.[79]

TABLE 3-7	Differential Diagnosis of Major Lipid Abnormalities	
Lipid Abnormality	**Primary Disorders**	**Secondary Disorders**
Hypercholesterolemia	Polygenic, familial hypercholesterolemia, familial defective apo B-100; PCSK9 gain-of-function mutation	Hypothyroidism, nephrotic syndrome, anorexia nervosa
Hypertriglyceridemia	Lipoprotein lipase deficiency, apo C-II deficiency, apo A-V deficiency, familial hypertriglyceridemia, dysbetalipoproteinemia	Diabetes mellitus, obesity, metabolic syndrome, alcohol use, oral estrogen, renal failure, hypothyroidism, retinoic acid, lipodystrophies
Combined hyperlipidemia	Familial combined hyperlipidemia, dysbetalipoproteinemia	Diabetes mellitus, obesity, metabolic syndrome, nephrotic syndrome, hypothyroidism, lipodystrophies
Low HDL	Familial hypoalphalipoproteinemia, Tangier disease (ABCA1 deficiency), apoA1 mutations, lecithin–cholesterol acyltransferase deficiency	Diabetes mellitus, obesity, metabolic syndrome, hypertriglyceridemia, smoking, anabolic steroids

apo, apolipoprotein; HDL, high-density lipoprotein.

CHAPTER 3

TABLE 3-8	Review of Major Genetic Dyslipoproteinemias			
Type of Genetic Dyslipidemia	Typical Lipid Profile	Type of Inheritance Pattern	Phenotypic Features	Other Information
Familial hypercholesterolemia	• Increased LDL cholesterol (>190 mg/dL) • Homozygous form or compound heterozygous form (rare) can have LDL cholesterol >500 mg/dL	Autosomal dominant (prevalence of 1 in 200–250 for heterozygote form and 1 in 250,000 for homozygous form)	• Premature CAD • Tendon xanthomas • Premature arcus corneae (full arc before age 40) • Homozygous form: planar and tendon xanthomas and CAD in childhood and adolescence	Mutations of the LDL receptor, apolipoprotein B-100, and gain-of-function mutations of proprotein convertase/kexin subtype 9 (PCSK9) lead to impaired uptake and degradation of LDL
Familial combined hyperlipidemia	• High levels of VLDL, LDL, or both • LDL apo B-100 level >130 mg/dL	Autosomal dominant (prevalence of 1%–2%)	• Premature CAD • Patients do *not* develop tendon xanthomas	Genetic and metabolic defects are not established
Familial dysbetalipoproteinemia	• Symmetric elevations of cholesterol and triglycerides (300–500 mg/dL) • Elevated VLDL-to-triglyceride ratio (>0.3)	Autosomal recessive	• Premature CAD • Tuberous or tuberoeruptive xanthomas • Planar xanthomas of the palmar creases are essentially pathognomonic	Mutation of ApoE gene Many homozygotes are normolipidemic, and emergence of hyperlipidemia often requires a secondary metabolic factor such as diabetes mellitus, hypothyroidism, or obesity

TABLE 3-8	Review of Major Genetic Dyslipoproteinemias (continued)			
Type of Genetic Dyslipidemia	Typical Lipid Profile	Type of Inheritance Pattern	Phenotypic Features	Other Information
Familial hypertriglyceridemia (can result in chylomicronemia syndrome)	• Most patients have triglyceride levels in the range of 150–500 mg/dL • Clinical manifestations may occur when triglyceride levels exceed 1500 mg/dL	• Familial hypertriglyceridemia is an autosomal dominant disorder caused by overproduction of VLDL triglycerides and manifests in adults	• Eruptive xanthomas • Lipemia retinalis • Pancreatitis • Hepatosplenomegaly	Patients may develop the chylomicronemia syndrome in the presence of secondary factors such as obesity, alcohol use, or diabetes
Familial hyperchylomicronemia	• Similar to familial hypertriglyceridemia	• Onset before puberty indicates deficiency of lipoprotein lipase or apo C-II, both autosomal recessive	• Similar to familial hypertriglyceridemia	Homozygosity for mutations in apoAV, LMF, and GHIHBP1 also found (rare)

CAD, coronary artery disease; GHIHBP1, glycosylphosphatidylinositol-anchored high-density lipoprotein–binding protein 1; LDL, low-density lipoprotein; VLDL, very-low-density lipoprotein.

Screening

- Screening for hypercholesterolemia should be done **in all adults age 20 years or older**.[79]
- Screening is best performed with a lipid profile (total cholesterol, LDL-C, HDL cholesterol, and triglycerides) obtained after a 12-hour fast.
- If a fasting lipid panel cannot be obtained, total and HDL cholesterol should be measured. Non-HDL cholesterol ≥220 mg/dL may indicate a genetic or secondary cause. A fasting lipid panel is required if non-HDL cholesterol is ≥220 mg/dL or triglycerides are ≥500 mg/dL.
- If the patient does not have an indication for LDL-lowering therapy, screening can be performed every 4–6 years between ages 40 and 75.[79]
- Patients hospitalized for an acute coronary syndrome or coronary revascularization should have a lipid panel obtained within 24 hours of admission if lipid levels are unknown.
- Individuals with hyperlipidemia should be evaluated for potential **secondary causes**, including hypothyroidism, DM, obstructive liver disease, chronic renal disease such as nephrotic syndrome, and medications such as estrogens, progestins, anabolic steroids/androgens, corticosteroids, cyclosporine, retinoids, atypical antipsychotics, and antiretrovirals (particularly protease inhibitors).

Risk Assessment

- The 2018 guidelines emphasize risk stratification based on predicted future risk, with further stratification using risk-enhancing factors to identify groups in whom the benefits of LDL-C–lowering therapy with HMG-CoA reductase inhibitors (statins) clearly outweigh the risks and to aim for certain goals in the reduction of LDL-C. The more LDL-C is reduced, the greater the subsequent risk reduction.[79] In all individuals, a heart healthy lifestyle should be encouraged as it reduces ASCVD risk at all ages.
- Areas in which treatment with statin therapy is recommended include the following:
  ○ Patients with clinical ASCVD
  ○ Patients with LDL-C ≥190 mg/dL
  ○ Patients with DM age 40–75
  ○ Patients age 40–75 with a calculated ASCVD risk ≥7.5% if a discussion of treatment options favors statin therapy
- For patients **without** clinical ASCVD or an LDL-C ≥190 mg/dL, the guidelines advise having a clinician–patient risk discussion before starting statin therapy. This includes calculating a patient's risk for ASCVD based on age, sex, ethnicity, total and HDL cholesterol, SBP (treated or untreated), presence of DM, and current smoking status in addition to the presence of risk-enhancing factors.[79]
- The ACC/AHA risk calculator is available at tools.acc.org/ASCVD-Risk-Estimator-Plus/.
  ○ For patients of ethnicities other than African American or non-Hispanic white, risk cannot be well assessed with the risk calculator. Use of the non-Hispanic white risk calculation is suggested, with the understanding that risk may be lower than calculated in East Asian Americans and Hispanic Americans and higher in American Indians and South Asians.
  ○ Ten-year risk should be calculated beginning at age 40 in patients without ASCVD or LDL-C ≥190 mg/dL.
  ○ Lifetime risk may be calculated in patients age 20–39 and patients age 40–59 with a 10-year risk <7.5% to inform decisions regarding lifestyle modification.

TREATMENT

- The 2018 guidelines recognize lifestyle factors, including diet and weight management as an important component of risk reduction for all patients.[79]
- Patients should be advised to adopt a diet that is high in fruits and vegetables, whole grains, fish, lean meat, low-fat dairy, legumes, and nuts, with lower intake of red meat, saturated and trans fats, sweets, and sugary beverages (Table 3-9). Saturated fat should comprise no more than 5%–6% of total calories.[80]
- Efforts should be made to replace dietary saturated fat with polyunsaturated and monounsaturated fats, as this has been shown to lower LDL-C and triglycerides. Polyunsaturated fat intake has been shown to promote atherosclerosis regression.[81]
- Physical activity, including aerobic and resistance exercise, is recommended in all patients.[70]
- The 2019 ACC/AHA guidelines recommend that adults engage in at least 150 minutes per week of moderate-intensity or 75 minutes per week of vigorous-intensity physical exercise.[82]
- For all obese patients (body mass index ≥30) and for overweight patients (body mass index ≥25) who have additional risk factors, sustained weight loss of 5%–10% of initial weight, achieved through lifestyle changes, has been shown to improve the lipid profile, lower BP, delay the onset of type 2 diabetes (T2DM), and improve glycemic control in those with T2DM.[82]
- Consultation with a registered dietitian nutritionist may be helpful to plan, start, and maintain a saturated fat–restricted and weight loss–promoting diet.
- Prior to the start of treatment, there should be a risk discussion between the patient and the clinician. Topics for discussion include the following:
  ○ Potential for ASCVD risk reduction benefits
  ○ Potential for adverse effects and drug–drug interactions

CHAPTER 3

TABLE 3-9	Nutrient Composition of the Therapeutic Lifestyle Change Diet[54]
Nutrient	**Recommended Intake**
Saturated fat[a]	<5%–6% of total calories
Polyunsaturated fat	Up to 10% of total calories
Monounsaturated fat	Up to 20% of total calories
Total fat	25%–35% of total calories
Carbohydrate[b]	50%–60% of total calories
Fiber	20–30 g/d
Protein	Approximately 15% of total calories
Cholesterol	<200 mg/d
Total calories (energy)[c]	Balance energy intake and expenditure to maintain desirable body weight/prevent weight gain

[a]Trans fatty acids are another low-density lipoprotein–raising fat that should be kept at a low intake.
[b]Carbohydrates should be derived predominantly from foods rich in complex carbohydrates, including grains (especially whole grains), fruits, and vegetables.
[c]Daily energy expenditure should include at least moderate physical activity (contributing approximately 200 kcal/d).

- ○ Heart healthy lifestyle and management of other risk factors
- ○ Patient preferences
- Aspirin should be used infrequently in the *primary* prevention of ASCVD because of lack of net benefit.[82]
- All adults should be assessed for tobacco use. Those who smoke should be strongly advised to quit and provided assistance in this pursuit.[82]
- **Clinical ASCVD**
  - ○ Clinical ASCVD includes acute coronary syndromes, history of MI, stable angina, arterial revascularization (coronary or otherwise), stroke, transient ischemic attack, or atherosclerotic peripheral arterial disease.
  - ○ Secondary prevention is an indication for high-intensity statin therapy, which has been shown to reduce events more than moderate-intensity statin therapy. Statin regimens are listed in Table 3-10. Goal is reduction of LDL-C by >50%.
  - ○ If high-dose statin therapy is contraindicated, poorly tolerated, or there are significant risks to high-intensity therapy (including age >75 years), the maximally tolerated statin therapy is an option.
  - ○ In patients with very-high-risk ASCVD, use an LDL-C threshold of 70 mg/dL (1.8 mmol/L) to consider addition of nonstatins to statin therapy. If proprotein convertase subtilisin/kexin type 9 (PCSK9) inhibitor is considered, add ezetimibe to maximal statin before adding PCSK9 inhibitor. Very-high-risk ASCVD includes a history of multiple major ASCVD events or one major ASCVD event and multiple high-risk conditions (major ASCVD events are recent acute coronary syndrome [past 12 months], history of MI, history of ischemic stroke, symptomatic peripheral arterial disease).
  - ○ High-risk conditions include age >65 years, heterozygous FH, history of prior coronary bypass surgery or percutaneous intervention outside the major ASCVD event, DM, hypertension, CKD (eGFR 15–59 mL/min/1.73 m^2), current smoking, persistently elevated LDL-C (>100 mg/dL) despite maximally tolerated statin therapy and ezetimibe, history of CHF.
  - ○ In patients with T2DM and known ASCVD, consider starting an SGLT2 inhibitor or GLP-1 RA for cardiovascular and renal benefits.[82-84]
- **LDL-C ≥190 mg/dL**
  - ○ These individuals have elevated lifetime risk because of long-term exposure to very high LDL-C levels, and the risk calculator does not account for this.

TABLE 3-10	Statin Therapy Regimens by Intensity[53]	
High Intensity (↓ LDL ≥50%)	**Medium Intensity** (↓ LDL 30%–49%)	**Low Intensity** (↓ LDL <30%)
Atorvastatin 40–80 mg	Atorvastatin 10–20 mg	Fluvastatin 20–40 mg
Rosuvastatin 20–40 mg	Fluvastatin 40 mg bid, 80 mg XL	Lovastatin 20 mg
	Lovastatin 40 mg	Pravastatin 10–20 mg
	Pitavastatin 1–4 mg	Simvastatin 10 mg
	Pravastatin 40–80 mg	
	Rosuvastatin 5–10 mg	
	Simvastatin 20–40 mg	

LDL, low-density lipoprotein; ↓, decreased.

○ LDL-C should be reduced with high-intensity statin therapy. If high-intensity therapy is not tolerated, maximum tolerated intensity should be used.

○ If LDL-C on statin therapy remains >100 mg/dL (>2.6 mmol/L), adding ezetimibe is reasonable.

○ If the LDL-C level on statin plus ezetimibe remains >100 mg/dL (>2.6 mmol/L) and the patient has multiple factors that increase subsequent risk of ASCVD event, a PCSK9 inhibitor may be considered, although the long-term safety (>3 years) is uncertain.

○ LDL apheresis is an optional therapy in patients with homozygous FH and those with severe heterozygous FH with insufficient response to medication. Lomitapide, a microsomal triglyceride transfer protein inhibitor, and mipomersen, an apolipoprotein B antisense oligonucleotide, are medications indicated for the treatment of patients with homozygous FH.[66]

○ Because hyperlipidemia of this degree is often genetically determined, discuss screening of other family members (including children) to identify candidates for treatment. In addition, screen for and treat secondary causes of hyperlipidemia.[67]

• **Patients with diabetes, aged 40–75, LDL-C >70 mg/dL**

○ Moderate-intensity statin therapy is indicated regardless of estimated 10-year ASCVD risk.

○ In patients with DM at higher risk, especially those with multiple risk factors or those aged 50–75, it is reasonable to use a high-intensity statin to reduce the LDL-C by >50%.

○ Diabetes-specific risk enhancers: long duration (>10 years for T2DM or >20 years for T1DM), albuminuria (>30 μg of albumin/mg creatinine), eGFR <60 mL/min/1.73 m^2, retinopathy, neuropathy, ankle-brachial index (ABI) <0.9.

○ In adults with DM and 10-year ASCVD risk of 20% or higher, it may be reasonable to add ezetimibe to maximally tolerated statin therapy to reduce LDL-C by 50% or more.

○ The JACC 2020 Expert Consensus Decision Pathway on Novel Therapies for Cardiovascular Risk Reduction in patients with T2DM recommends considering the use of an sodium–glucose transport protein 2 (SGLT2) inhibitor or glucagon-like peptide-1 receptor agonists (GLP-1 RA) for patients with T2DM who are at high risk for clinical ASCVD for cardiovascular and renal benefits. The 2019 AHA/ACC preventative cardiology guidelines recommend metformin first-line and then consideration of an SGLT2 inhibitor or GLP-1 RA as well.[82-84]

• **Patients without diabetes, aged 40–75, LDL-C between 70 and 189 mg/dL**

○ Using the AHA/ACC risk calculator, calculate 10-year risk of an ASCVD event in these patients (categories: >20%, ≥7.5% to <20%, 5.0%–7.5%, and <5.0%).

○ "Borderline risk": A 10-year risk between 5.0% and 7.5% and risk-enhancing factors are indications for moderate-intensity statin therapy if a discussion of options favors statin therapy.

○ "Intermediate risk": A 10-year risk ≥7.5% to <20% is an indication for moderate-intensity statin to reduce LDL-C by 30%–49%.

○ "High risk": A 10-year risk of >20% favors initiating statin therapy to reduce LDL-C by at least 50%.[82]

○ Risk-enhancing factors include family history of premature ASCVD, persistently elevated LDL-C levels (>160 mg/dL), metabolic syndrome, CKD, history of pre-eclampsia or premature menopause (<40 years), chronic inflammatory disorders (e.g., rheumatoid arthritis, psoriasis, or chronic HIV), high-risk ethnic groups (e.g., South Asian), persistent elevations of triglycerides >175 mg/dL, and, if measured in selected individuals, apolipoprotein B >130 mg/dL, high-sensitivity C-reactive protein >2.0 mg/L, ABI <0.9, and Lp(a) >50 mg/dL or 125 nmol/L.

CHAPTER 3

- In intermediate-risk adults in whom high-intensity statins are advisable to reach goal reduction, but not acceptable or tolerated, it is reasonable to add a nonstatin drug (ezetimibe or bile acid sequestrant) to moderate-intensity statin.
- **Other patient populations**
  - If a 10-year ASCVD risk is >7.5%–19.9% and decision about statin therapy is uncertain, consider measuring coronary artery calcium (CAC) to help identify risk. If the CAC is zero, it is reasonable to withhold statin therapy and reassess in 5–10 years, as long as higher risk conditions are absent. If CAC score is 1–99, it is reasonable to initiate statin therapy for patients >55 years. If CAC score is >100 and/or greater than 75th percentile, it is reasonable to initiate statin therapy.
  - Patients with stage 3–5 CKD are high risk for ASCVD[85] and the use of LDL-lowering therapy is indicated in patients with nondialysis-dependent CKD.[86]
  - Use of statin therapy should be individualized for patients older than 75. In randomized controlled trials, patients older than 75 continued to have benefit from statin therapy, particularly for secondary prevention.[73,87] In addition, many ASCVD events occur in this age group, and patients without other comorbidities may benefit substantially from cardiovascular risk reduction.
  - In adults >75 years it may be reasonable to stop statin therapy when functional decline (physical or cognitive), multimorbidity, frailty, or reduced life expectancy limits the potential benefits of statin therapy.
  - In adults with advanced kidney disease that requires dialysis treatment who are currently on LDL-lowering therapy with a statin, it may be reasonable to continue the statin.
  - In adults with advanced kidney disease who require dialysis treatment, initiation of a statin is not recommended.
  - In patients with HF with reduced ejection fraction attributable to ischemic heart disease who have a reasonable life expectancy (3–5 years) and are not already on a statin because of ASCVD, clinicians may consider initiation of moderate-intensity statin therapy to reduce the occurrence of ASCVD events.[66]
- **LDL-C reduction beyond statin therapy**
  - When statins are insufficient for LDL-C reduction, further therapy with non-statins may be indicated. This would generally include ezetimibe, bile acid sequestrants, and PCSK9 monoclonal antibodies.[88]
- **Hypertriglyceridemia**
  - Hypertriglyceridemia may be an independent cardiovascular risk factor.[65,89-91]
  - Hypertriglyceridemia is often observed in the metabolic syndrome,[91] and there are many potential etiologies for hypertriglyceridemia, including obesity, DM, renal insufficiency, genetic dyslipidemias, and therapy with oral estrogen, glucocorticoids, β-blockers, tamoxifen, cyclosporine, antiretrovirals, and retinoids.
  - The classification of serum triglyceride levels is as follows: normal: <150 mg/dL; borderline high: 150–199 mg/dL; high: 200–499 mg/dL; very high: ≥500 mg/dL; severe: 1000–1999 mg/dL (greatly increases the risk of pancreatitis); and very severe: ≥2000 mg/dL.[69,91]
  - Treatment of hypertriglyceridemia depends on the degree of severity.
    - For patients with very high triglyceride levels, triglyceride reduction through a very-low-fat diet (≤15% of calories), exercise, weight loss, and drugs (fibrates, ω-3 fatty acids) is the primary goal of therapy to prevent acute pancreatitis.
    - When patients have a lesser degree of hypertriglyceridemia, controlling the LDL-C level is the primary aim of initial therapy. Lifestyle changes are indicated to lower triglyceride levels.[69]

- **Low HDL cholesterol**
  - Low HDL cholesterol is an **independent ASCVD risk factor** that is identified as a non–LDL-C risk and is included as a component of the ACC/AHA ASCVD risk scoring algorithm.[92]
  - Etiologies of low HDL cholesterol include genetic conditions, physical inactivity, obesity, insulin resistance, DM, hypertriglyceridemia, cigarette smoking, high-carbohydrate (>60% of calories) diets, and certain medications (β-blockers, anabolic steroids/androgens, progestins). Acquired low HDL can also occur with plasma cell dyscrasias due to interference of paraproteins with the assay.[93]
  - Because therapeutic interventions for low HDL cholesterol are of limited efficacy, the guidelines recommend considering low HDL cholesterol as a component of overall risk, rather than a specific therapeutic target.
  - There are no clinical trial data showing a benefit of pharmacologic methods of elevating HDL cholesterol.
- **Starting and monitoring therapy**
  - Before starting therapy, guidelines recommend checking alanine aminotransferase (ALT), hemoglobin A1C (if diabetes status is unknown), labs for secondary causes (if indicated), and creatine kinase (if indicated).
  - Evaluate for patient characteristics that increase the risk of adverse events from statins, including impaired hepatic and renal function, history of statin intolerance, history of muscle disorders, unexplained elevations of ALT >3× the upper limit of normal, drugs affecting statin metabolism, Asian ethnicity, and age >75 years.[79]
  - **A repeat fasting lipid panel** is indicated 4–12 weeks after starting therapy to assess adherence, with reassessment every 3–12 months as indicated.
  - In patients without the anticipated level of LDL-C reduction based on intensity of statin therapy (≥50% for high intensity, 30%–50% for moderate intensity), assess adherence to therapy and lifestyle modifications, evaluate for intolerance, and consider secondary causes. After evaluation, if the therapeutic response is still insufficient on maximally tolerated statin therapy, it is reasonable to consider adding a nonstatin agent.[88]
  - Creatine kinase should not be routinely checked in patients on statin therapy but is reasonable to measure in patients with muscle symptoms.
  - In 2012, the FDA stated that liver enzyme tests should be performed before starting statin therapy and only as clinically indicated thereafter. The FDA concluded that serious liver injury with statins is rare and unpredictable and that routine monitoring of liver enzymes does not appear to be effective in detecting or preventing serious liver injury. Elevations of liver transaminases 2–3× the upper limit of normal are dose-dependent, may decrease on repeat testing even with continuation of statin therapy, and are reversible with discontinuation of the drug.

Treatment of Elevated LDL Cholesterol

- **HMG-CoA reductase inhibitors (statins)**
  - Statins (see Table 3-10) are the treatment of choice for elevated LDL-C and usually lower levels by 30%–50% with moderate-intensity and ≥50% with high-intensity statin therapy.[79,94,95]
  - The lipid-lowering effect of statins appears within the first week of use and becomes stable after approximately 4 weeks of use.
  - Statin therapy is effective in both men and women.[96]
  - Common side effects (5%–10% of patients) include gastrointestinal upset (e.g., abdominal pain, diarrhea, bloating, constipation) and muscle pain or weakness,

which can occur without creatine kinase elevations. Other potential side effects include malaise, fatigue, headache, and rash.[95,97-99]

- ○ Myalgias are the most common cause of statin discontinuation and are often dose-dependent. They occur more often with increasing age and number of medications and decreasing renal function and body size.[98-100]
  - ■ Discontinue statins in patients who develop muscle symptoms until they can be evaluated. For severe symptoms, a creatine kinase level can be measured.[79]
  - ■ For mild to moderate symptoms, evaluate for conditions increasing the risk of muscle symptoms, including renal or hepatic impairment, hypothyroidism, vitamin D deficiency, rheumatologic disorders, and primary muscle disorders. Statin-induced myalgias are likely to resolve within 2 months of discontinuing the drug.
  - ■ If symptoms resolve, the same or lower dose of the statin can be reintroduced.
  - ■ If symptoms recur, use a low dose of a different statin and increase as tolerated.
  - ■ If the cause of symptoms is determined to be unrelated, restart the original statin.
- ○ Statins have been associated with an increased incidence of DM. However, the total benefit of statin use usually outweighs the potential adverse effects from an increase in blood sugar.[101]
- ○ There is no aggregated evidence that statins have any negative impact on cognitive function.[102]
- ○ Because a number of drug interactions are possible depending on the statin and other medications being used, drug interaction programs and package inserts should be consulted.[103]
- ○ Because some statins undergo metabolism by the cytochrome P450 enzyme system, taking these statins in combination with other drugs metabolized by this enzyme system increases the risk of **rhabdomyolysis**.[95,97,98] Among these drugs are fibrates (greater risk with gemfibrozil), itraconazole, ketoconazole, erythromycin, clarithromycin, cyclosporine, nefazodone, and protease inhibitors.[98]
- ○ Statins may also interact with large quantities of grapefruit juice to increase the risk of myopathy.
- ○ Simvastatin can increase the levels of warfarin and digoxin and has significant dose-limiting interactions with amlodipine, amiodarone, dronedarone, verapamil, diltiazem, and ranolazine. Rosuvastatin may also increase warfarin levels.
- ○ The use of statins is contraindicated during pregnancy and lactation.
- • **Bile acid sequestrant resins**
  - ○ Currently available bile acid sequestrant resins include the following:
    - ■ **Cholestyramine:** 4–24 g/d PO in divided doses before meals.
    - ■ **Colestipol:** tablets, 2–16 g/d PO; granules, 5–30 g/d PO in divided doses before meals.
    - ■ **Colesevelam:** 625 mg tablets, three tablets PO bid or six tablets PO daily (maximum of seven tablets daily) with food, or one packet of oral suspension daily.
  - ○ Bile acid sequestrants typically lower LDL-C levels by 15%–30% and thereby lower the incidence of CHD.[95,104]
  - ○ These agents should not be used as monotherapy in patients with triglyceride levels >250 mg/dL because they can raise triglyceride levels. They may be combined with statins or nicotinic acid.
  - ○ Common side effects of resins include constipation, abdominal pain, bloating, nausea, and flatulence.
  - ○ Bile acid sequestrants may decrease oral absorption of many other drugs, including warfarin, digoxin, thyroid hormone, thiazide diuretics, amiodarone, glipizide, and statins.

- Colesevelam interacts with fewer drugs than do the older resins but can affect the absorption of thyroxine.
- Other medications should be given at least 1 hour before or 4 hours after resins.
- **Nicotinic acid (niacin)**
  - Niacin can lower LDL-C levels by ≥15%, lower triglyceride levels by 20%–50%, and raise HDL cholesterol levels by up to 35%.[89,105] The use of niacin is limited by its side effect profile.
  - Crystalline niacin is given 1–3 g/d PO in two to three divided doses with meals. Extended-release niacin is dosed at night, with a starting dose of 500 mg PO, and the dose may be titrated monthly in 500 mg increments to a maximum of 2000 mg PO (administer dose with milk, applesauce, or crackers).
  - Common side effects of niacin include flushing, pruritus, headache, nausea, and bloating. Other potential side effects include elevation of liver transaminases, hyperuricemia, and hyperglycemia.
    - Flushing may be decreased with the use of aspirin 325 mg 30 minutes before the first few doses.
    - Hepatotoxicity associated with niacin is partially dose-dependent and appears to be more prevalent with some over-the-counter time-release preparations.
  - Avoid use of niacin in patients with gout, liver disease, active peptic ulcer disease, and uncontrolled DM.
    - Niacin can be used with care in patients with well-controlled DM (hemoglobin A1C level ≤7%).
    - Serum transaminases, glucose, and uric acid levels should be monitored every 6–8 weeks during dose titration and then every 4 months
  - The use of niacin in patients with well-controlled LDL-C levels (with statins) has not been shown to be of benefit in clinical trials.[106,107] Niacin can be useful as an additional agent in patients with severely elevated LDL-C levels.
- **Ezetimibe**
  - Ezetimibe is currently the only available cholesterol-absorption inhibitor. It appears to act at the brush border of the small intestine and inhibits cholesterol absorption.
  - Ezetimibe may provide an additional 25% mean reduction in LDL-C when combined with a statin and provides an approximately 18% decrease in LDL-C when used as monotherapy.[107-111]
  - The recommended dosing is 10 mg PO once daily. No dosage adjustment is required for renal insufficiency and mild hepatic impairment or in elderly patients. It is not recommended for use in patients with moderate to severe hepatic impairment.
  - Side effects are infrequent and include gastrointestinal symptoms (e.g., diarrhea, abdominal pain) and myalgias.
  - In clinical trials, there was no excess of rhabdomyolysis or myopathy when compared with statin or placebo alone.
  - Liver enzymes should be monitored when used in conjunction with fenofibrate but are not required in monotherapy or with a statin.
  - A clinical outcome trial showed decreased reduction of cardiovascular events with the combination of simvastatin and ezetimibe compared with placebo in patients with chronic renal failure.[112] The IMPROVE-IT trial showed a reduction in cardiovascular end points when ezetimibe was added to simvastatin in high-risk patients with already low LDL levels.[113]
  - Ezetimibe is useful in patients with FH who do not achieve adequate LDL-C reductions with statin therapy alone.[114]

CHAPTER 3

- **Bempedoic acid**
  - Bempedoic acid is an inhibitor of adenosine triphosphate citrate lyase, an enzyme upstream of the target of statins (3-hydroxy-3-methylglutaryl-CoA reductase) in the cholesterol biosynthesis pathway.
  - Bempedoic acid alone or in combination with a statin or ezetimibe (combination bempedoic acid-ezetimibe tablet with FDA approval is available) safely lowers LDL-C as shown in the CLEAR Harmony and CLEAR Wisdom randomized controlled trials in 2019.[115,116]
  - In patients with gout, serum uric acid levels should be measured and stabilized prior to initiation.
- **PCSK9 inhibitors**
  - Monoclonal antibodies have been developed that lower LDL-C. They work by inhibiting the PCSK9 enzyme, which is involved in breaking down the LDL-C receptor. Their use increases the number of available cell surface LDL receptors and subsequently remove more LDL from circulation. Major studies have shown significant reduction in LDL-C when PCSK9 inhibitors were added to statin therapy.[117]
  - These agents have shown great ability in further reducing LDL-C in high-risk patients and are approved for use as adjuncts in patients with clinical ASCVD and heterozygous FH and as monotherapy for homozygous FH.
  - Two PCSK9 inhibitors are approved for clinical use, evolocumab and alirocumab. Evolocumab is dosed at 140 mg subcutaneously every 2 weeks or 420 mg every 4 weeks. Alirocumab is dosed at 75 or 150 mg every 2 weeks or 300 mg every 4 weeks.
  - Evolocumab has been shown to decrease major cardiovascular events.[117] The more recent ODYSSEY OUTCOMES trial showed alirocumab significantly reduces ischemic events, all-cause mortality, and MI among patients with an acute coronary syndrome event within the preceding 1–12 months.[118]
- Evinacumab
  - Evinacumab is a human monoclonal antibody against ANGPTL3, a angiopoietin-like protein (ANGPTLs) that regulates lipoprotein metabolism.
  - A recent phase 2 trial in 2020 showed reduction in hepatic VLDL-C production and secretion and consequently lowered LDL-C when safely used in combination with a PCSK9 inhibitor and statin, with or without ezetimibe.[119]

Treatment of Hypertriglyceridemia

- **Nonpharmacologic treatment**
- Nonpharmacologic treatments are important in the therapy of hypertriglyceridemia. Approaches include the following:
  - Changing oral estrogen replacement to transdermal estrogen
  - Decreasing alcohol intake
  - Encouraging weight loss and exercise
  - Controlling hyperglycemia in patients with DM
  - Avoiding simple sugars and very-high-carbohydrate diets[69,91]
- **Pharmacologic treatment**
  - Pharmacologic treatment of severe hypertriglyceridemia consists of fibric acid derivative (fibrates), niacin, or ω-3 fatty acids.
  - Patients with severe hypertriglyceridemia (>1000 mg/dL) should be treated with pharmacotherapy in addition to reduction of dietary fat, alcohol, and simple carbohydrates to decrease the risk of pancreatitis.
  - Statins may be effective for patients with mild to moderate hypertriglyceridemia and concomitant LDL-C elevation.[69,91,120]

- Fibric acid derivatives
  - Currently available fibric acid derivatives include the following (bezafibrate is not available in the United States):
    - **Gemfibrozil:** 600 mg PO bid before meals
    - **Fenofibrate:** available in several forms, dosage typically 48–145 mg/d PO
  - Fibrates generally lower triglyceride levels by 30%–50% and increase HDL cholesterol levels by 10%–35%. They can lower LDL-C levels by 5%–25% in patients with normal triglyceride levels but may actually increase LDL-C levels in patients with elevated triglyceride levels.[120,121]
  - Common side effects include dyspepsia, abdominal pain, cholelithiasis, rash, and pruritus.
  - Fibrates may potentiate the effects of warfarin.[95] Gemfibrozil given in conjunction with statins may increase the risk of rhabdomyolysis.[99,122-124]
- ω-3 fatty acids
  - High doses of ω-3 fatty acids from fish oil can lower triglyceride levels.[125,126]
  - The active ingredients are eicosapentaenoic acid (EPA) and docosahexaenoic acid (DHA).
  - To lower triglyceride levels, 1–6 g of ω-3 fatty acids, either EPA alone or with DHA, is needed daily.
  - Main side effects are burping, bloating, and diarrhea.
  - Prescription forms of ω-3 fatty acids are available and are indicated for triglyceride levels >500 mg/dL. One preparation contains EPA and DHA; four tablets contain about 3.6 g of ω-3 acid ethyl esters and can lower triglyceride levels by 30%–40%. Other preparations contain only EPA or contain unesterified EPA and DHA.
  - Three recent large cardiovascular outcomes trials (ASCEND, VITAL, REDUCE-IT) showed clear benefits for ω-3 fatty acid intake for CVD, including risk reduction for heart attack, other major cardiovascular events, and death from CVD.[127-130]
  - Applying the results of these trials to clinical practice, the addition of 4 g/d of EPA should be considered for statin-treated patients who have CVD or diabetes plus elevated triglycerides. All adults should consume at least one to two servings of fish/seafood per week, with additional primary prevention benefits conferred by consuming 1 g/d of EPA and DHA.
  - In addition, EPA and DHA may help preserve physical function in CAD patients.[131]
  - The combination of ω-3 fatty acids plus a statin has the advantage of avoiding the risk of myopathy seen with statin–fibrate combinations.[132,133]

Treatment of Low HDL Cholesterol

- Low HDL cholesterol often occurs in the setting of hypertriglyceridemia and metabolic syndrome. Management of accompanying high LDL-C, hypertriglyceridemia, and the metabolic syndrome may result in improvement of HDL cholesterol.[134]
- Nonpharmacologic therapies are the mainstay of treatment, including the following:
  - Smoking cessation
  - Exercise
  - Weight loss
- In addition, medications known to lower HDL levels, such as β-blockers (except carvedilol), progestins, and androgenic compounds, should be avoided if possible.
- No clinical outcomes trials have shown a clear benefit to pharmacologic treatment for raising HDL cholesterol.

CHAPTER 3

REFERENCES

1. Whelton PK, Carey RM, Aronow WS, et al. 2017 ACC/AHA/AAPA/ABC/ACPM/AGS/APhA/ASH/ASPC/NMA/PCNA guideline for the prevention, detection, evaluation, and management of high blood pressure in adults: a report of the American College of Cardiology/American Heart Association task force on clinical practice guidelines. *J Am Coll Cardiol.* 2018;71:e127-e248.

2. Williams B, Mancia G, Spiering W, et al. 2018 ESC/ESH guidelines for the management of arterial hypertension. *Eur Heart J.* 2018;39:3021-3104.

3. National Institute for Health and Care Excellence. *Hypertension in Adults: Diagnosis and Management.* NICE Guideline 136. August, 2019. https://www.nice.org.uk/guidance/ng136

4. Jones DW, Whelton PK, Allen N, et al. Management of stage 1 hypertension in adults with a low 10-year risk for cardiovascular disease: filling a guidance gap—a scientific statement from the American Heart Association. *Hypertension.* 2021;77:e58-e67.

5. James PA, Oparil S, Carter BL, et al. 2014 Evidence-based guideline for the management of high blood pressure in adults: report from the panel members appointed to the Eighth Joint National Committee (JNC 8). *JAMA.* 2014;311:507-520.

6. Unger T, Borghi C, Charchar F, et al. 2020 International society of hypertension global hypertension practice guidelines. *Hypertension.* 2020;75:1334-1357.

7. Elliott WJ. Clinical features in the management of selected hypertensive emergencies. *Prog Cardiovasc Dis.* 2006;48:316-325.

8. Alshami A, Romero C, Avila A, Varon J. Management of hypertensive crises in the elderly. *J Geriatr Cardiol.* 2018;15:504-512.

9. Amraoui F, Van Der Hoeven NV, Van Valkengoed IG, et al. Mortality and cardiovascular risk in patients with a history of malignant hypertension: a case-control study. *J Clin Hypertens (Greenwich).* 2014;16:122-126.

10. Patel KK, Young L, Howell EH, et al. Characteristics and outcomes of patients presenting with hypertensive urgency in the office setting. *JAMA Intern Med.* 2016;176:981-988.

11. Levy PD, Mahn JJ, Miller J, et al. Blood pressure treatment and outcomes in hypertensive patients without acute target organ damage: a retrospective cohort. *Am J Emerg Med.* 2015;33:1219-1224.

12. Siddiqui M, Judd EK, Dudenbostel T, et al. Antihypertensive medication adherence and confirmation of true refractory hypertension. *Hypertension.* 2020;75:510-515.

13. Carey RM, Calhoun DA, Bakris GL, et al; AHA Professional/Public Education and Publications Committee of the Council on Hypertension; Council on Cardiovascular and Stroke Nursing; Council on Clinical Cardiology; Council on Genomic and Precision Medicine; Council on Peripheral Vascular Disease; Council on Quality of Care and Outcomes Research; and Stroke Council. Resistant hypertension: detection, evaluation, and management – a scientific statement from the American Heart Association. *Hypertension.* 2018;72:e53-e90.

14. Centers for Disease Control and Prevention. *Hypertension cascade: Hypertension Prevalence, Treatment and Control Estimates Among US Adults Aged 18 Years and Older Applying the Criteria from the ACC/AHA's 2017 Hypertension Guideline—NHANES 2015-2018.* US Department of Health and Human Services. 2021.

15. Muntner P, Carey RM, Gidding S, et al. Potential U.S. population impact of the 2017 ACC/AHA high blood pressure guideline. *J Am Coll Cardiol.* 2018;71:109-118.

16. Vasan RS, Beiser A, Seshadri S, et al. Residual lifetime risk for developing hypertension in middle-aged women and men: the Framingham Heart Study. *JAMA.* 2002;287:1003-1010.

17. Olsen MH, Angell SY, Asma S, et al. A call to action and a lifecourse strategy to address the global burden of raised blood pressure on current and future generations: the Lancet Commission on hypertension. *Lancet.* 2016;388:2665-2712.

18. Akintoye E, Briasoulis A, Egbe A, et al. National trends in admission and in-hospital mortality of patients with heart failure in the United States (2001-2014). *J Am Heart Assoc.* 2017;6:e006955.

19. Nerenberg KA, Zarnke KB, Leung AA, et al. Hypertension Canada's 2018 guidelines for diagnosis, risk assessment, prevention, and treatment of hypertension in adults and children. *Can J Cardiol.* 2018;34:506-525.

20. Rooke TW, Hirsch AT, Misra S, et al. 2011 ACCF/AHA Focused update of the guideline for the management of patients with peripheral artery disease (updating the 2005 guideline): a report of the American College of Cardiology Foundation/American Heart Association Task Force on Practice Guidelines. *J Am Coll Cardiol.* 2011;58:2020-2045.

21. Brown JM, Siddiqui M, Calhoun DA, et al. The unrecognized prevalence of primary aldosteronism: a cross-sectional study. *Ann Intern Med.* 2020;173:10-20.

22. Cohen JB, Cohen DL, Herman DS, et al. Testing for primary aldosteronism and mineralocorticoid receptor antagonist use among U.S. veterans: a retrospective cohort study. *Ann Intern Med.* 2021;174:289-297.

23. Stergiou GS, Bliziotis IA. Home blood pressure monitoring in the diagnosis and treatment of hypertension: a systematic review. *Am J Hypertens.* 2011;24:123-134.

24. Ohkubo T, Imai Y, Tsuji I, et al. Home blood pressure measurement has a stronger predictive power for mortality than does screening blood pressure measurement: a population-based observation in Ohasama, Japan. *J Hypertens*. 1998;16:971-975.
25. Niiranen TJ, Hanninen MR, Johansson J, et al. Home-measured blood pressure is a stronger predictor of cardiovascular risk than office blood pressure: the Finn-Home study. *Hypertension*. 2010;55:1346-1351.
26. ALLHAT Collaborative Research Group. Major outcomes in high-risk hypertensive patients randomized to angiotensin-converting enzyme inhibitor or calcium channel blocker vs diuretic: the Antihypertensive and Lipid-Lowering Treatment to Prevent Heart Attack Trial (ALLHAT). *JAMA*. 2002;288:2981-2997.
27. Messerli FH, Bangalore S, Julius S. Risk/benefit assessment of beta-blockers and diuretics precludes their use for first-line therapy in hypertension. *Circulation*. 2008;117:2706-2715.
28. Psaty BM, Heckbert SR, Koepsell TD, et al. The risk of myocardial infarction associated with antihypertensive drug therapies. *JAMA*. 1995;274:620-625.
29. Packer M, Bristow MR, Cohn JN, et al. The effect of carvedilol on morbidity and mortality in patients with chronic heart failure. U.S. Carvedilol Heart Failure Study Group. *N Engl J Med*. 1996;334:1349-1355.
30. The Danish Study Group on Verapamil in Myocardial Infarction. Effect of verapamil on mortality and major events after acute myocardial infarction (the Danish Verapamil Infarction Trial II–DAVIT II). *Am J Cardiol*. 1990;66:779-785.
31. Yusuf S, Sleight P, Pogue J, et al. Effects of an angiotensin-converting-enzyme inhibitor, ramipril, on cardiovascular events in high-risk patients. *N Engl J Med*. 2000;342:145-153.
32. Goodfriend TL, Elliott ME, Catt KJ. Angiotensin receptors and their antagonists. *N Engl J Med*. 1996;334:1649-1654.
33. Cohn JN, Tognoni G. A randomized trial of the angiotensin-receptor blocker valsartan in chronic heart failure. *N Engl J Med*. 2001;345:1667-1675.
34. Harel Z, Gilbert C, Wald R, et al. The effect of combination treatment with aliskiren and blockers of the renin-angiotensin system on hyperkalaemia and acute kidney injury: systematic review and meta-analysis. *BMJ*. 2012;344:e42.
35. Parving HH, Brenner BM, McMurray JJ, et al. Cardiorenal end points in a trial of aliskiren for type 2 diabetes. *N Engl J Med*. 2012;367:2204-2213.
36. McMurray JJ, Packer M, Desai AS, et al. Angiotensin-neprilysin inhibition versus enalapril in heart failure. *N Engl J Med*. 2014;371:993-1004.
37. Habibi J, Aroor AR, Das NA, et al. The combination of a neprilysin inhibitor (sacubitril) and angiotensin-II receptor blocker (valsartan) attenuates glomerular and tubular injury in the Zucker Obese rat. *Cardiovasc Diabetol*. 2019;18:40.
38. Packer M, Claggett B, Lefkowitz MP, et al. Effect of neprilysin inhibition on renal function in patients with type 2 diabetes and chronic heart failure who are receiving target doses of inhibitors of the renin-angiotensin system: a secondary analysis of the PARADIGM-HF trial. *Lancet Diabetes Endocrinol*. 2018;6:547-554.
39. Seferovic JP, Claggett B, Seidelmann SB, et al. Effect of sacubitril/valsartan versus enalapril on glycaemic control in patients with heart failure and diabetes: a post-hoc analysis from the PARADIGM-HF trial. *Lancet Diabetes Endocrinol*. 2017;5:333-340.
40. Erbel R, Aboyans V, Boileau C, et al. 2014 ESC guidelines on the diagnosis and treatment of aortic diseases: document covering acute and chronic aortic diseases of the thoracic and abdominal aorta of the adult. The task force for the diagnosis and treatment of aortic diseases of the European Society of Cardiology. *Eur Heart J*. 2014;35:2873-2926.
41. Williamson JD, Supiano MA, Applegate WB, et al. Intensive vs standard blood pressure control and cardiovascular disease outcomes in adults aged ≥75 years: a randomized clinical trial. *JAMA*. 2016;315:2673-2682.
42. Bavishi C, Bangalore S, Messerli FH. Outcomes of intensive blood pressure lowering in older hypertensive patients. *J Am Coll Cardiol*. 2017;69:486-493.
43. SHEP Cooperative Research Group. Prevention of stroke by antihypertensive drug treatment in older persons with isolated systolic hypertension. Final results of the Systolic Hypertension in the Elderly Program (SHEP). *JAMA*. 1991;265:3255-3264.
44. Brenner BM, Cooper ME, de Zeeuw D, et al. Effects of losartan on renal and cardiovascular outcomes in patients with type 2 diabetes and nephropathy. *N Engl J Med*. 2001;345:861-869.
45. Kidney Disease: Improving Global Outcomes (KDIGO) Work Group. KDIGO 2021 clinical practice guideline for the management of blood pressure in chronic kidney disease. *Kidney Int*. 2021;99:S1-S87.
46. Cheung AK, Rahman M, Reboussin DM, et al; SPRINT Research Group. Effects of intensive BP control in CKD. *J Am Soc Nephrol*. 2017;28:2812-2823.
47. Beddhu S, Rocco MV, Toto R, et al; SPRINT Research Group. Effects of intensive systolic blood pressure control on kidney and cardiovascular outcomes in persons without kidney disease: a secondary analysis of a randomized trial. *Ann Intern Med*. 2017;167:375-383.
48. Malhotra R, Katz R, Jotwani V, et al. Urine markers of kidney tubule cell injury and kidney function decline in SPRINT Trial Participants with CKD. *Clin J Am Soc Nephrol*. 2020;15:349-358.

CHAPTER 3

49. Nadkarni GN, Chauhan K, Rao V, et al. Effect of intensive blood pressure lowering on kidney tubule injury: findings from the ACCORD Trial Study Participants. *Am J Kidney Dis.* 2019;73:31-38.

50. Schlaich MP, Schmieder RE. Left ventricular hypertrophy and its regression: pathophysiology and therapeutic approach—focus on treatment by antihypertensive agents. *Am J Hypertens.* 1998;11:1394-1404.

51. Klingbeil AU, Schneider M, Martus P, et al. A meta-analysis of the effects of treatment on left ventricular mass in essential hypertension. *Am J Med.* 2003;115:41-46.

52. Soliman EZ, Byington RP, Bigger JT, et al. Effect of intensive blood pressure lowering on left ventricular hypertrophy in patients with diabetes mellitus: action to control cardiovascular risk in diabetes blood pressure trial. *Hypertension.* 2015;66:1123-1129.

53. Swedberg K, Kjekshus J, Snapinn S. Long-term survival in severe heart failure in patients treated with enalapril. Ten year follow-up of CONSENSUS I. *Eur Heart J.* 1999;20:136-139.

54. Yusuf S, Pitt B, Davis CE, et al. Effect of enalapril on survival in patients with reduced left ventricular ejection fractions and congestive heart failure. *N Engl J Med.* 1991;325:293-302.

55. ISIS-4 (Fourth International Study of Infarct Survival) Collaborative Group. ISIS-4: a randomised factorial trial assessing early oral captopril, oral mononitrate, and intravenous magnesium sulphate in 58,050 patients with suspected acute myocardial infarction. *Lancet.* 1995;345:669-685.

56. Gruppo Italiano per lo Studio della Sopravvivenza nell'infarto Miocardico. GISSI-3: effects of lisinopril and transdermal glyceryl trinitrate singly and together on 6-week mortality and ventricular function after acute myocardial infarction. *Lancet.* 1994;343:1115-1122.

57. Pfeffer MA, Braunwald E, Moye LA, et al. Effect of captopril on mortality and morbidity in patients with left ventricular dysfunction after myocardial infarction. Results of the survival and ventricular enlargement trial. The SAVE investigators. *N Engl J Med.* 1992;327:669-677.

58. Hjalmarson A, Goldstein S, Fagerberg B, et al. Effects of controlled-release metoprolol on total mortality, hospitalizations, and well-being in patients with heart failure: the Metoprolol CR/XL Randomized Intervention Trial in congestive heart failure (MERIT-HF). MERIT-HF study group. *JAMA.* 2000;283:1295-1302.

59. Leizorovicz A, Lechat P, Cucherat M, et al. Bisoprolol for the treatment of chronic heart failure: a meta-analysis on individual data of two placebo-controlled studies–CIBIS and CIBIS II. Cardiac insufficiency bisoprolol study. *Am Heart J.* 2002;143:301-307.

60. Wachtell K, Bella JN, Rokkedal J, et al. Change in diastolic left ventricular filling after one year of antihypertensive treatment: the Losartan Intervention for Endpoint reduction in hypertension (LIFE) study. *Circulation.* 2002;105:1071-1076.

61. Hypertension in pregnancy. Report of the American College of obstetricians and Gynecologists' task force on hypertension in pregnancy. *Obstet Gynecol.* 2013;122:1122-1131.

62. Genest JJ Jr, Martin-Munley SS, McNamara JR, et al. Familial lipoprotein disorders in patients with premature coronary artery disease. *Circulation.* 1992;85:2025-2033.

63. Kugiyama K, Doi H, Motoyama T, et al. Association of remnant lipoprotein levels with impairment of endothelium-dependent vasomotor function in human coronary arteries. *Circulation.* 1998;97:2519-2526.

64. Dowla S, Aslibekyan S, Goss A, et al. Dyslipidemia is associated with pediatric nonalcoholic fatty liver disease. *J Clin Lipidol.* 2018;12:981-987.

65. Hegele RA, Ginsberg HN, Chapman MJ, et al. The polygenic nature of hypertriglyceridaemia: implications for definition, diagnosis, and management. *Lancet Diabetes Endocrinol.* 2014;2:655-666.

66. Nordestgaard BG, Chapman MJ, Humphries SE, et al. Familial hypercholesterolaemia is underdiagnosed and undertreated in the general population—guidance for clinicians to prevent coronary heart disease:consensus statement of the European Atherosclerosis Society. *Eur Heart J.* 2013;34:3478-3490a.

67. Haase A, Goldberg AC. Identification of people with heterozygous familial hypercholesterolemia. *Curr Opin Lipidol.* 2012;23:282-289.

68. Goldberg AC, Hopkins PN, Toth PP, et al. Familial hypercholesterolemia: screening, diagnosis and management of pediatric and adult patients – clinical guidance from the National Lipid Association Expert Panel on Familial Hypercholesterolemia. *J Clin Lipidol.* 2011;5:133-140.

69. Berglund L, Brunzell JD, Goldberg AC, et al. Evaluation and treatment of hypertriglyceridemia: an endocrine society clinical practice guideline. *J Clin Endocrinol Metab.* 2012;97:2969-2989.

70. Randomised trial of cholesterol lowering in 4444 patients with coronary heart disease: the Scandinavian Simvastatin Survival Study (4S). *Lancet.* 1994;344:1383-1389.

71. Sacks FM, Pfeffer MA, Moye LA, et al. The effect of pravastatin on coronary events after myocardial infarction in patients with average cholesterol levels. Cholesterol and recurrent events trial investigators. *N Engl J Med.* 1996;335:1001-1009.

72. The Long-Term Intervention with Pravastatin in Ischaemic Disease (LIPID) Study Group. Prevention of cardiovascular events and death with pravastatin in patients with coronary heart disease and a broad range of initial cholesterol levels. *N Engl J Med.* 1998;339:1349-1357.

73. Heart Protection Study Collaborative Group. MRC/BHF heart protection study of cholesterol lowering with simvastatin in 20,536 high-risk individuals: a randomised placebo-controlled trial. *Lancet.* 2002;360:7-22.

74. Shepherd J, Cobbe SM, Ford I, et al. Prevention of coronary heart disease with pravastatin in men with hypercholesterolemia. West of Scotland coronary prevention study group. *N Engl J Med.* 1995;333:1301-1307.

75. Downs JR, Clearfield M, Weis S, et al. Primary prevention of acute coronary events with lovastatin in men and women with average cholesterol levels: results of AFCAPS/TexCAPS. Air Force/Texas Coronary Atherosclerosis Prevention Study. *JAMA.* 1998;279:1615-1622.

76. Sever PS, Dahlof B, Poulter NR, et al. Prevention of coronary and stroke events with atorvastatin in hypertensive patients who have average or lower-than-average cholesterol concentrations, in the Anglo-Scandinavian Cardiac Outcomes Trial–Lipid Lowering Arm (ASCOT-LLA): a multicentre randomised controlled trial. *Lancet.* 2003;361:1149-1158.

77. Colhoun HM, Betteridge DJ, Durrington PN, et al. Primary prevention of cardiovascular disease with atorvastatin in type 2 diabetes in the Collaborative Atorvastatin Diabetes Study (CARDS): multicentre randomised placebo-controlled trial. *Lancet.* 2004;364:685-696.

78. Mihaylova B, Emberson J, Blackwell L, et al. The effects of lowering LDL cholesterol with statin therapy in people at low risk of vascular disease: meta-analysis of individual data from 27 randomised trials. *Lancet.* 2012;380:581-590.

79. Grundy SM, Stone NJ, Bailey AL, et al. AHA/ACC/AACVPR/AAPA/ABC/ACPM/ADA/AGS/APhA/ASPC/NLA/PCNA guideline on the management of blood cholesterol: executive summary – a report of the American College of Cardiology/American Heart Association task force on clinical practice guidelines. *J Am Coll Cardiol.* 2019;73:3168-3209.

80. Eckel RH, Jakicic JM, Ard JD, et al. 2013 AHA/ACC guideline on lifestyle management to reduce cardiovascular risk: a report of the American College of Cardiology/American Heart Association task force on practice guidelines. *Circulation.* 2014;129:S76-S99.

81. Jensen MD, Ryan DH, Apovian CM, et al. 2013 AHA/ACC/TOS guideline for the management of overweight and obesity in adults: a report of the American College of Cardiology/American Heart Association task force on practice guidelines and the obesity society. *Circulation.* 2014;129:S102-S138.

82. Arnett DK, Blumenthal RS, Albert MA, et al. 2019 ACC/AHA Guideline on the primary prevention of cardiovascular disease: a report of the American College of Cardiology/American Heart Association task force on clinical practice guidelines. *Circulation.* 2019;140:e596-e646.

83. Das SR, Everett BM, Birtcher KK, et al. 2020 Expert consensus decision pathway on novel therapies for cardiovascular risk reduction in patients with Type 2 Diabetes: a report of the American College of Cardiology solution set oversight committee. *J Am Coll Cardiol.* 2020;76:1117-1145.

84. Wiviott SD, Raz I, Bonaca MP, et al. Dapagliflozin and cardiovascular outcomes in type 2 diabetes. *N Engl J Med.* 2019;380:347-357.

85. Matsushita K, van der Velde M, Astor BC, et al. Association of estimated glomerular filtration rate and albuminuria with all-cause and cardiovascular mortality in general population cohorts: a collaborative meta-analysis. *Lancet.* 2010;375:2073-2081.

86. Palmer SC, Navaneethan SD, Craig JC, et al. HMG CoA reductase inhibitors (statins) for people with chronic kidney disease not requiring dialysis. *Cochrane Database Syst Rev.* 2014;2014:CD007784.

87. Shepherd J, Blauw GJ, Murphy MB, et al. Pravastatin in elderly individuals at risk of vascular disease (PROSPER): a randomised controlled trial. *Lancet.* 2002;360:1623-1630.

88. Lloyd-Jones DM, Morris PB, Ballantyne CM, et al. 2017 Focused update of the 2016 ACC expert consensus decision pathway on the role of non-statin therapies for LDL-cholesterol lowering in the management of atherosclerotic cardiovascular disease risk: a report of the American College of Cardiology task force on expert consensus decision pathways. *J Am Coll Cardiol.* 2017;70:1785-1822.

89. Sarwar N, Danesh J, Eiriksdottir G, et al. Triglycerides and the risk of coronary heart disease: 10,158 incident cases among 262,525 participants in 29 Western prospective studies. *Circulation.* 2007;115:450-458.

90. Tirosh A, Rudich A, Shochat T, et al. Changes in triglyceride levels and risk for coronary heart disease in young men. *Ann Intern Med.* 2007;147:377-385.

91. Miller M, Stone NJ, Ballantyne C, et al. Triglycerides and cardiovascular disease: a scientific statement from the American Heart Association. *Circulation.* 2011;123:2292-2333.

92. Goff DC Jr, Lloyd-Jones DM, Bennett G, et al. 2013 ACC/AHA guideline on the assessment of cardiovascular risk: a report of the American College of Cardiology/American Heart Association task force on practice guidelines. *Circulation.* 2014;129:S49-S73.

93. van Gorselen EO, Diekman T, Hessels J, et al. Artifactual measurement of low serum HDL-cholesterol due to paraproteinemia. *Clin Res Cardiol.* 2010;99:599-602.

94. Robinson JG, Goldberg AC. Treatment of adults with familial hypercholesterolemia and evidence for treatment: recommendations from the National Lipid association expert panel on familial hypercholesterolemia. *J Clin Lipidol.* 2011;5:S18-S29.

95. Knopp RH. Drug treatment of lipid disorders. *N Engl J Med.* 1999;341:498-511.

96. Fulcher J, O'Connell R, Voysey M, et al. Efficacy and safety of LDL-lowering therapy among men and women: meta-analysis of individual data from 174,000 participants in 27 randomised trials. *Lancet.* 2015;385:1397-1405.

CHAPTER 3

97. Chong PH. Lack of therapeutic interchangeability of HMG-CoA reductase inhibitors. *Ann Pharmacother.* 2002;36:1907-1917.
98. Pasternak RC, Smith SC Jr, Bairey-MerzCN, et al. ACC/AHA/NHLBI clinical advisory on the use and safety of statins. *Circulation.* 2002;106:1024-1028.
99. Thompson PD, Panza G, Zaleski A, et al. Statin-associated side effects. *J Am Coll Cardiol.* 2016;67:2395-2410.
100. Venero CV, Thompson PD. Managing statin myopathy. *Endocrinol Metab Clin North Am.* 2009;38:121-136.
101. Sattar N, Preiss D, Murray HM, et al. Statins and risk of incident diabetes: a collaborative meta-analysis of randomised statin trials. *Lancet.* 2010;375:735-742.
102. Collins R, Reith C, Emberson J, et al. Interpretation of the evidence for the efficacy and safety of statin therapy. *Lancet.* 2016;388:2532-2561.
103. Kellick KA, Bottorff M, Toth PP, et al. A clinician's guide to statin drug-drug interactions. *J Clin Lipidol.* 2014;8:S30-S46.
104. The lipid research clinics coronary primary prevention trial results. I. Reduction in incidence of coronary heart disease. *JAMA.* 1984;251:351-364.
105. Illingworth DR, Stein EA, Mitchel YB, et al. Comparative effects of lovastatin and niacin in primary hypercholesterolemia. A prospective trial. *Arch Intern Med.* 1994;154:1586-1595.
106. Boden WE, Probstfield JL, Anderson T, et al. Niacin in patients with low HDL cholesterol levels receiving intensive statin therapy. *N Engl J Med.* 2011;365:2255-2267.
107. HPS2-THRIVE Collaborative Group. HPS2-THRIVE randomized placebo-controlled trial in 25 673 high-risk patients of ER niacin/laropiprant: trial design, pre-specified muscle and liver outcomes, and reasons for stopping study treatment. *Eur Heart J.* 2013;34:1279-1291.
108. Dujovne CA, Ettinger MP, McNeer JF, et al. Efficacy and safety of a potent new selective cholesterol absorption inhibitor, ezetimibe, in patients with primary hypercholesterolemia. *Am J Cardiol.* 2002;90:1092-1097.
109. Knopp RH, Gitter H, Truitt T, et al. Effects of ezetimibe, a new cholesterol absorption inhibitor, on plasma lipids in patients with primary hypercholesterolemia. *Eur Heart J.* 2003;24:729-741.
110. Gagne C, Bays HE, Weiss SR, et al. Efficacy and safety of ezetimibe added to ongoing statin therapy for treatment of patients with primary hypercholesterolemia. *Am J Cardiol.* 2002;90:1084-1091.
111. Goldberg AC, Sapre A, Liu J, et al. Efficacy and safety of ezetimibe coadministered with simvastatin in patients with primary hypercholesterolemia: a randomized, double-blind, placebo-controlled trial. *Mayo Clin Proc.* 2004;79:620-629.
112. Baigent C, Landray MJ, Reith C, et al. The effects of lowering LDL cholesterol with simvastatin plus ezetimibe in patients with chronic kidney disease (Study of Heart and Renal Protection): a randomised placebo-controlled trial. *Lancet.* 2011;377:2181-2192.
113. Cannon CP, Blazing MA, Giugliano RP, et al. Ezetimibe added to statin therapy after acute coronary syndromes. *N Engl J Med.* 2015;372:2387-2397.
114. Ito MK, McGowan MP, Moriarty PM. Management of familial hypercholesterolemias in adult patients: recommendations from the National Lipid Association expert panel on familial hypercholesterolemia. *J Clin Lipidol.* 2011;5:S38-S45.
115. Ray KK, Bays HE, Catapano AL, et al. Safety and efficacy of bempedoic acid to reduce LDL cholesterol. *N Engl J Med.* 2019;380:1022-1032.
116. Goldberg AC, Leiter LA, Stroes ESG, et al. Effect of bempedoic acid vs placebo added to maximally tolerated statins on low-density lipoprotein cholesterol in patients at high risk for cardiovascular disease: the CLEAR Wisdom Randomized Clinical Trial. *JAMA.* 2019;322:1780-1788.
117. Sabatine MS, Giugliano RP, Keech AC, et al. Evolocumab and clinical outcomes in patients with cardiovascular disease. *N Engl J Med.* 2017;376:1713-1722.
118. Schwartz GG, Steg PG, Szarek M, et al. Alirocumab and cardiovascular outcomes after acute coronary syndrome. *N Engl J Med.* 2018;379:2097-2107.
119. Banerjee P, Chan KC, Tarabocchia M, et al. Functional analysis of LDLR (low-density lipoprotein receptor) variants in patient lymphocytes to assess the effect of evinacumab in homozygous familial hypercholesterolemia patients with a spectrum of LDLR activity. *Arterioscler Thromb Vasc Biol.* 2019;39:2248-2260.
120. Brunzell JD. Clinical practice. Hypertriglyceridemia. *N Engl J Med.* 2007;357:1009-1017.
121. Keech A, Simes RJ, Barter P, et al. Effects of long-term fenofibrate therapy on cardiovascular events in 9795 people with type 2 diabetes mellitus (the FIELD study): randomised controlled trial. *Lancet.* 2005;366:1849-1861.
122. Rosenson RS. Current overview of statin-induced myopathy. *Am J Med.* 2004;116:408-416.
123. Alsheikh-Ali AA, Kuvin JT, Karas RH. Risk of adverse events with fibrates. *Am J Cardiol.* 2004;94:935-938.
124. Jones PH, Davidson MH. Reporting rate of rhabdomyolysis with fenofibrate + statin versus gemfibrozil + any statin. *Am J Cardiol.* 2005;95:120-122.

125. Nestel PJ, Connor WE, Reardon MF, et al. Suppression by diets rich in fish oil of very low density lipoprotein production in man. *J Clin Invest.* 1984;74:82-89.
126. Harris WS, Connor WE, Illingworth DR, et al. Effects of fish oil on VLDL triglyceride kinetics in humans. *J Lipid Res.* 1990;31:1549-1558.
127. Kris-Etherton PM, Richter CK, Bowen KJ, et al. Recent clinical trials shed new light on the cardiovascular benefits of omega-3 fatty acids. *Methodist Debakey Cardiovasc J.* 2019;15:171-178.
128. Manson JE, Cook NR, Lee IM, et al. Marine n-3 fatty acids and prevention of cardiovascular disease and cancer. *N Engl J Med.* 2019;380:23-32.
129. Bowman L, Mafham M, Wallendszus K, et al. Effects of n-3 fatty acid supplements in Diabetes Mellitus. *N Engl J Med.* 2018;379:1540-1550.
130. Bhatt DL, Steg PG, Miller M, et al. Cardiovascular risk reduction with icosapent ethyl for hypertriglyceridemia. *N Engl J Med.* 2019;380:11-22.
131. Alfaddagh A, Elajami TK, Saleh M, et al. The effect of eicosapentaenoic and docosahexaenoic acids on physical function, exercise, and joint replacement in patients with coronary artery disease: a secondary analysis of a randomized clinical trial. *J Clin Lipidol.* 2018;12:937-947.e2.
132. Maki KC, McKenney JM, Reeves MS, et al. Effects of adding prescription omega-3 acid ethyl esters to simvastatin (20 mg/day) on lipids and lipoprotein particles in men and women with mixed dyslipidemia. *Am J Cardiol.* 2008;102:429-433.
133. Barter P, Ginsberg HN. Effectiveness of combined statin plus omega-3 fatty acid therapy for mixed dyslipidemia. *Am J Cardiol.* 2008;102:1040-1045.
134. Ballantyne CM, Olsson AG, Cook TJ, et al. Influence of low high-density lipoprotein cholesterol and elevated triglyceride on coronary heart disease events and response to simvastatin therapy in 4S. *Circulation.* 2001;104:3046-3051

4 Ischemic Heart Disease

Noah N. Williford and Marc A. Sintek

Coronary Heart Disease and Stable Angina

GENERAL PRINCIPLES

Definition

- Coronary artery disease (CAD) refers to the luminal narrowing of a coronary artery, usually due to atherosclerosis. CAD is the leading contributor to ischemic heart disease (IHD). IHD includes angina pectoris, myocardial infarction (MI), and silent myocardial ischemia.
- Cardiovascular disease (CVD) includes IHD, cardiomyopathy, heart failure (HF), arrhythmia, hypertension, cerebrovascular accident (CVA), diseases of the aorta, peripheral vascular disease (PVD), valvular heart disease, and congenital heart disease.
- Stable angina is defined as angina symptoms or angina equivalent symptoms that are reproduced by consistent levels of activity and relieved by rest.
- American Heart Association/American College of Cardiology (AHA/ACC) guidelines provide a more thorough overview of stable IHD.[1,2]

Epidemiology

- The lifetime risk of IHD at age 40 is one in two for men and one in three for women.
- There are more than 15 million Americans with IHD, 50% of whom have chronic angina.
- CVD has become an important cause of death worldwide, accounting for nearly 30% of all deaths and has become increasingly significant in developing nations.[3]

Etiology

- CAD most commonly results from luminal accumulation of atheromatous plaque.
- Other causes of obstructive CAD include congenital coronary anomalies, myocardial bridging, vasculitis, and prior radiation therapy.

Pathophysiology

- Stable angina results from progressive luminal obstruction of angiographically visible epicardial coronary arteries or, less commonly, obstruction of the microvasculature, which results in a mismatch between myocardial oxygen supply and demand.
- Atherosclerosis is an inflammatory process, initiated by lipid deposition in the arterial intima layer followed by recruitment of inflammatory cells and proliferation of arterial smooth muscle cells to form an atheroma.
  - The coronary lesions responsible for stable angina differ from the vulnerable plaques associated with acute MI. The stable angina lesion is fixed and is less prone to fissuring, hence producing symptoms that are more predictable.[4]
  - All coronary lesions are eccentric and do not uniformly alter the inner circumference of the artery.

- Epicardial coronary lesions causing less than 40% luminal narrowing generally do not significantly impair coronary flow.
- Moderate angiographic lesions (40%–70% obstruction) may interfere with flow and are routinely underestimated on coronary angiograms given the eccentricity of CAD.

Risk Factors

- Of IHD events, >90% can be attributed to elevations in at least one major risk factor.[5]
- Assessment of traditional CVD risk factors includes:
  - Age
  - Blood pressure (BP)
  - Blood glucose (Note: Diabetes is considered an IHD risk equivalent.)
  - Lipid profile (low-density lipoprotein [LDL], high-density lipoprotein [HDL], triglycerides); direct LDL for nonfasting samples or very high triglycerides
  - Tobacco use (Note: Smoking cessation restores the risk of IHD to that of a non-smoker within approximately 15 years.)[6]
  - Family history of premature CAD: Defined as first-degree male relative with IHD before age 55 years or female relative before age 65 years
  - Measures for obesity, particularly central obesity; body mass index goal is between 18.5 and 24.9 kg/m^2; waist circumference goal is <40 in for men and <35 in for women
- As of 2013, AHA/ACC guidelines recommend assessing 10-year atherosclerotic cardiovascular disease (ASCVD) risk for patients aged 40–79 years using new race and age-specific pooled cohort equations.[7]
  - The ASCVD risk calculator is available online (http://tools.cardiosource.org/ASCVD-Risk-Estimator/).
  - If there remains uncertainty about lower risk estimates, high-sensitivity C-reactive protein (≥2 mg/dL), coronary artery calcium score (≥300 Agatston units or ≥75th percentile), or ankle-brachial index (<0.9) may be obtained to revise risk estimates upward.
  - Traditional risk factors noted above should be assessed in patients younger than 40 years and every 4–6 years after 40; 10-year ASCVD risk should be calculated every 4–6 years in patients 40–79 years of age.
  - Lifetime risk can be assessed using the ASCVD risk calculator and may be helpful in the setting of counseling patients about lifestyle modifications.

Prevention

Primary prevention: See Chapter 3, Preventive Cardiology.

Clinical Presentation

History

- **Typical angina** has three features: (1) substernal chest discomfort with a characteristic quality and duration that is (2) provoked by stress or exertion and (3) relieved by rest or nitroglycerin.
  - **Atypical angina** has two of these three characteristics.
  - **Noncardiac chest pain** meets one or none of these characteristics.
- Chronic stable angina is reproducibly precipitated in a predictable manner by exertion or emotional stress and relieved within 5–10 minutes by sublingual nitroglycerin or rest.

TABLE 4-1	Canadian Cardiovascular Society (CCS) Classification System
Class	Definition
CCS 1	Angina with strenuous or prolonged activity
CCS 2	Angina with moderate activity (walking greater than two level blocks or one flight of stairs)
CCS 3	Angina with mild activity (walking less than two level blocks or one flight of stairs)
CCS 4	Angina that occurs with any activity or at rest

Anginal symptoms may include typical chest discomfort or anginal equivalents.
Data from Sangareddi V, Anand C, Gnanavelu G, et al. Canadian Cardiovascular Society classification of effort angina: an angiographic correlation. *Coron Artery Dis.* 2004;15(2):111-114.

- The severity of angina may be quantified using the Canadian Cardiovascular Society (CCS) classification system (Table 4-1).
- Associated symptoms may include dyspnea, diaphoresis, nausea, vomiting, dizziness, jaw pain, and left arm pain.
- Female patients and those with diabetes or chronic kidney disease may have minimal or atypical symptoms that serve as anginal equivalents. Such symptoms include dyspnea (most common), epigastric pain, and nausea.
- The clinician's assessment of the pretest probability of IHD is the important driver for further diagnostic testing in patients without known CAD and is largely ascertained from the clinical history (Table 4-2). Patients with a low pretest probability (<5%) of CAD are unlikely to benefit from further diagnostic testing aimed at detecting CAD.

TABLE 4-2	Pretest Probability of Coronary Artery Disease by Age, Gender, and Symptoms							
Age (y)	Asymptomatic		Nonanginal Chest Pain		Atypical/ Probable Angina Pectoris		Typical/ Definite Angina Pectoris	
Gender	Women	Men	Women	Men	Women	Men	Women	Men
30–39	<5	<5	2	4	12	34	26	76
40–49	<5	<10	3	13	22	51	55	87
50–59	<5	<10	7	20	31	65	73	93
60–69	<5	<5	14	27	51	72	86	94
	Very low < 5%		Low < 10%		Intermediate 10%–80%		High > 80%	

Data from Gibbons RJ, Balady GJ, Bricker JT, et al. (Committee Members). ACC/AHA 2002 guideline update for exercise testing – summary article: a report of the American College of Cardiology/American Heart Association Task Force on Practice Guidelines (Committee to Update the 1997 Exercise Testing Guidelines). *Circulation.* 2002;106(14):1883-1892.

TABLE 4-3	Differential Diagnosis of Chest Pain Excluding Epicardial Atherosclerosis
Diagnosis	**Comments**
Cardiovascular	
Aortic stenosis	Anginal episodes can occur with severe aortic stenosis.
HCM	Subendocardial ischemia may occur with exercise and/or exertion.
Prinzmetal angina	Coronary vasospasm that may be elicited by exertion or emotional stress.
Pericarditis	Pleuritic chest pain associated with pericardial inflammation from infectious or autoimmune disease.
Aortic dissection	May mimic anginal pain and/or involve the coronary arteries.
Cocaine use	Results in coronary vasospasm and/or thrombus formation.
Other	
Anemia	Marked anemia can result in a myocardial O_2 supply–demand mismatch.
Thyrotoxicosis	Increase in myocardial demand may result in an O_2 supply–demand mismatch.
Esophageal disease	GERD and esophageal spasm can mimic angina (responsive to NTG).
Biliary colic	Gallstones can usually be visualized on abdominal sonography.
Respiratory diseases	Pneumonia with pleuritic pain, pulmonary embolism, pulmonary hypertension.
Musculoskeletal	Costochondritis, cervical radiculopathy.

GERD, gastroesophageal reflux disease; HCM, hypertrophic cardiomyopathy; NTG, nitroglycerin.

Differential Diagnosis

- A wide range of disorders may manifest with chest discomfort and may include both cardiovascular and noncardiovascular etiologies (Table 4-3).
- A careful history focused on cardiac risk factors, physical exam, and initial laboratory evaluation usually narrows the differential diagnosis.
- In patients with established IHD, always look for exacerbating factors that contribute to ischemia.
- Any process that reduces myocardial oxygen supply or increases demand can cause or exacerbate angina (Table 4-4).

Diagnostic Testing

- **General diagnostic testing**
  - A resting ECG can be helpful in determining the presence of prior infarcts or conduction system disease and may alert the clinician to the possibility of CAD in patients with chest pain.
  - A transthoracic echocardiogram (TTE) can be useful in determining presence of left ventricular (LV) dysfunction or valvular heart disease that may affect the

CHAPTER 4

TABLE 4-4	Conditions That May Provoke or Exacerbate Ischemia/ Angina Independent of Worsening Atherosclerosis
Increased Oxygen Demand	**Decreased Oxygen Supply**
Noncardiac	
Hyperthermia	Anemia
Hyperthyroidism	Sickle cell disease
Sympathomimetic toxicity (i.e., cocaine use)	Hypoxemia
	Pneumonia
Hypertension	*Asthma exacerbation*
Anxiety	*Chronic obstructive pulmonary disease*
	Pulmonary hypertension
	Pulmonary fibrosis
	Obstructive sleep apnea
	Pulmonary embolus
	Sympathomimetic toxicity (i.e., cocaine use, pheochromocytoma)
	Hyperviscosity
	Polycythemia
	Leukemia
	Thrombocytosis
	Hypergammaglobulinemia
Cardiac	
Hypertrophic cardiomyopathy	Aortic stenosis
Aortic stenosis	Elevated left ventricular end-diastolic pressure
Dilated cardiomyopathy	Hypertrophic cardiomyopathy
Tachycardia	Microvascular disease
Ventricular	
Supraventricular	

Modified from Fihn SD, Gardin JM, Abrams J, et al. 2012 ACCF/AHA/ACP/AATS/PCNA/ SCAI/STS Guideline for the diagnosis and management of patients with stable ischemic heart disease: a report of the American College of Cardiology Foundation/American Heart Association Task Force on Practice Guidelines, and the American College of Physicians, American Association for Thoracic Surgery, Preventive Cardiovascular Nurses Association, Society for Cardiovascular Angiography and Interventions, and Society of Thoracic Surgeons. *J Am Coll Cardiol.* 2012;60(24):e44-e164. Copyright © 2012 American College of Cardiology Foundation and the American Heart Association, Inc. With permission.

management and diagnosis of IHD. TTE can also be used to assess for resting wall motion abnormalities that may be the result of prior MI.
  ○ Evidence of vascular disease or prior MI on the diagnostic testing modalities noted above should raise the pretest probability of IHD in patients presenting with chest pain.
• **Stress testing overview**
  ○ All stress testing requires (1) a cardiovascular stress and (2) a way of evaluating cardiac changes consistent with ischemia. The latter is always done with continuous ECG; however, it can be done either with or without an imaging modality.
  ○ Many stress testing modalities provide not only detection of ischemia/CAD but also prognostic information based on the burden of ischemia.
  ○ Table 4-5 provides an overview of the sensitivity and specificity for each stress and imaging modality along with advantages and disadvantages for the clinician to consider.

TABLE 4-5	Diagnostic Accuracy of Common Stress Testing Modalities in Patients Without Known Ischemic Heart Disease			
Test Type	Sensitivity	Specificity	Advantages	Disadvantages
ECG				
Exercise	61%	70%–77%	• Easy to perform • Inexpensive	• Less diagnostic accuracy, especially in women • No viability assessment
Pharmacologic	—	—		
Echocardiography				
Exercise	70%–85%	77%–89%	• Gather other important information on diastolic function, valvular disorders, and pulmonary pressures • Can assess viability with pharmacologic stress	• Limited by image quality • Diagnostic accuracy reduced with resting wall motion abnormalities
Pharmacologic (dobutamine)	85%–90%	79%–90%		
Nuclear Perfusion Imaging				
Exercise	82%–88%	70%–88%	• More sensitive for small areas of ischemia/infarct • Very accurate ejection fraction assessment • Easy to compare to prior studies	• Significant radiation • May underestimate severe balanced ischemia • No other valve or other structural information • Viability may require separate testing
Pharmacologic (adenosine, regadenoson, or dobutamine)	82%–91%	75%–90%		
Cardiac MRI				
Exercise	—	—	• Excellent assessment of viability • Anatomic detail of heart and great vessels superb	• Expensive • Requires closed MRI • Exercise option not typically available
Pharmacologic[a]	91%	81%		

All diagnostic accuracies unadjusted for referral bias.[1,2]
[a]Vasodilator stress only; dobutamine has sensitivity of 83% and specificity of 86%.

CHAPTER 4

- **Stress testing indications**
  - See the ACCF 2013 Multimodality Appropriate Use Criteria for the Detection and Risk Assessment of Stable Ischemic Heart Disease[10] for a comprehensive list of the indications for stress testing.
  - The following are some of the more common indications:
    - Patients without known CAD:
      - Patients with anginal symptoms who are intermediate risk
      - Asymptomatic intermediate-risk patients who plan on beginning a vigorous exercise program or working in a high-risk occupation (e.g., airline pilot)
      - Atypical symptoms in patients with a high risk of IHD (i.e., diabetes or vascular disease patients)
    - Patients with known CAD:
      - Post-MI risk stratification (see section on ST-segment elevation MI)
      - Preoperative risk assessment if it will change management prior to surgery
      - Recurrent anginal symptoms despite medical therapy or revascularization
- **Contraindications to stress testing**
  - Acute MI within 2 days
  - Unstable angina not previously stabilized by medical therapy
  - Cardiac arrhythmias causing symptoms or hemodynamic compromise
  - Symptomatic severe aortic stenosis
  - Symptomatic HF
  - Acute pulmonary embolus, myocarditis, pericarditis, or aortic dissection
- **Stress modalities**
  - **Exercise stress testing**
    - The stress modality of choice for evaluating most patients of intermediate risk for CAD (see Table 4-2).
    - Bruce protocol: Consists of 3-minute stages of increasing treadmill speed and incline. BP, heart rate, and ECG are monitored throughout the study and the recovery period.
    - The ECG portion of the study is considered positive if:
      - New ST-segment depressions of >1 mm in multiple contiguous leads
      - Hypotensive response to exercise
      - Sustained ventricular arrhythmias are precipitated by exercise
    - The Duke Treadmill Score provides prognostic information for patients presenting with chronic angina (Table 4-6).
    - When exercise testing is combined with imaging (e.g., echocardiography), and the test is normal at the target heart rate for age, the risk of infarction or death from CVD is <1% annually in patients with no prior history of IHD.
    - In patients who cannot exercise and require pharmacologic testing, the annual risk of infarction or death in a normal study, doubles (i.e., 2% per year). This underscores the inability to perform physical activity as a marker of increased cardiovascular risk.
  - **Pharmacologic stress testing**
    - In patients who are unable to exercise, pharmacologic stress testing may be preferable.
    - Pharmacologic stress is preferred in patients with left bundle branch block (LBBB) or a paced rhythm on ECG. This is due to the increased incidence of false-positive stress tests seen with either exercise or dobutamine infusion.
    - Dipyridamole, adenosine, and regadenoson are vasodilators commonly used in conjunction with myocardial perfusion scintigraphy. Relative ischemia across a coronary vascular bed is elucidated as healthy vessels dilate more than diseased

TABLE 4-6	Exercise Stress Testing: Duke Treadmill Score[11]	

Duke Treadmill Score (DTS) = Minutes exercised − [5 × maximum ST-segment deviation] − [4 × angina score]. Angina score: 0 = none, 1 = not test limiting, 2 = test limiting

DTS

5	Annual mortality 0.25%	Low-risk study
−10 to 4	Annual mortality 1.25%	Intermediate-risk study
<−10	Annual mortality >5%	High-risk study

In general, β-blockers, other nodal blocking agents, and nitrates should be discontinued prior to stress testing.[11]

vessels with fixed obstruction. This in turn leads to relative changes in perfusion that are reflected in the postvasodilator images.
  - Dobutamine is a positive inotrope commonly used with echocardiographic stress tests and may be augmented with atropine to achieve target heart rate for age.
- **Stress testing with imaging**
  - Recommended for patients with the following baseline ECG abnormalities:
    - Preexcitation (Wolf-Parkinson-White syndrome)
    - LVH
    - LBBB or paced rhythm
    - Intraventricular conduction delay
    - Resting ST-segment or T-wave changes
    - Patients unable to exercise or who do not have an interpretable ECG at rest or with exercise
    - May be considered in patients with high pretest probability of IHD who have not met the threshold of invasive angiography
- **Imaging modalities**
  - **Myocardial perfusion imaging (MPI):** Both PET (positron emission tomography) and SPECT (single-photon emission tomography) use tracers that emit radiation detected by a camera in conjunction with exercise or pharmacologic stress. PET has better contrast and spatial resolution than SPECT, but PET is much more expensive and less widely available. Perfusion imaging compares rest perfusion to stress perfusion images to discern areas of ischemia or infarct. It can be limited by body habitus, breast attenuation, and quality of the acquisition and processing of images. Severe CAD may cause balanced reduction in perfusion and an underestimation of ischemic burden.
  - **Echocardiographic imaging:** Exercise or dobutamine stress testing can be performed with echocardiography to aid in the diagnosis of CAD. Echocardiography adds to the sensitivity and specificity of the test by revealing areas with wall motion abnormalities. The technical quality of this study can be limited by imaging quality (i.e., obesity).
  - **Magnetic resonance perfusion imaging:** MRI sequences obtained with contrast and vasodilator stress testing (and very rarely exercise testing) provides viability assessment without additional testing, as well as evaluation for other causes of myocardial dysfunction that may mimic IHD (i.e., sarcoidosis or infiltrative cardiomyopathies). Can be performed in patients with implanted cardiac devices (i.e., defibrillators and pacemakers).

CHAPTER 4

Diagnostic Procedures
- **Coronary angiography**
  - The gold standard for evaluating epicardial coronary anatomy because it quantifies the presence and severity of atherosclerotic lesions, which has prognostic value.
  - Coronary angiography is invasive and associated with a small risk of death, MI, CVA, bleeding, arrhythmia, and vascular complications. Therefore, it is reserved for patients whose risk–benefit ratio favors an invasive approach such as:
    - ST-segment elevation MI (STEMI) patients
    - Most unstable angina (UA)/non–ST-segment elevation MI (NSTEMI) patients
    - Symptomatic patients with high-risk stress tests who are expected to benefit from revascularization
    - Class III and IV angina despite medical therapy (see Table 4-1)
    - Survivors of sudden cardiac death or those with serious ventricular arrhythmias
    - Signs or symptoms of HF or decreased LV function
    - Angina that is inadequately controlled with medical therapy for the patient's lifestyle
    - Previous coronary artery bypass grafting (CABG) or percutaneous coronary intervention (PCI)
    - Suspected or known left main (≥50% stenosis) or severe three-vessel CAD
    - To diagnose CAD in patients with angina who have not undergone stress testing due to a high pretest probability of having CAD (see Table 4-2)
  - Can be used to evaluate patients who are suspected of having a nonatherosclerotic cause of ischemia (e.g., coronary anomaly, coronary dissection, radiation vasculopathy).
  - Functional significance of intermediate stenotic lesions (50%–70% narrowing) can further be assessed by fractional flow reserve (FFR) or instantaneous wave-free ratio (iFR).
    - Both FFR and iFR are calculated by determining the ratio of pressure distal to the coronary obstruction to that of the aortic pressure (flow) using slightly different methods.
      - An FFR ≤ 0.8 or iFR ≤ 0.89 is considered flow limiting, and PCI decreases the need for urgent revascularization for UA or MI, as well as risk of recurrent MI.[12]
      - Whether PCI in stable IHD improves cardiovascular outcomes or symptoms compared to medical therapy is controversial.[13]
        - An early invasive strategy did not reduce death, death from cardiovascular causes, MI, or a composite of the three in stable IHD.[14] These patients did have decreased angina and improved quality of life.
          - Patients with recent acute coronary syndrome (ACS), severe angina, left main disease, or left ventricular ejection fraction (LVEF) < 35% were excluded.
          - Physiological studies (FFR) were performed in only 20% of cases, and use of intravascular imaging (intravascular ultrasound, optical coherence tomography) was not reported.
            - The use of physiological studies and intravascular imaging is associated with better outcomes in PCI.[15,16]
          - 21% of patients assigned to a conservative strategy eventually underwent revascularization.

▲ PCI for stable IHD did not improve survival, but was associated with decreased nonprocedural MI, unstable angina, and angina in a meta-analysis. However, there was an increased incidence of procedural MI.[17]

○ Measurement of LV filling pressures (diastolic function) and aortic and mitral valve gradients, assessment of regional wall motion and LV function, and assessment for certain aortopathies can be accomplished by placing a catheter in the LV cavity or aorta directly and making the appropriate pressure measurements and/or injection of contrast.

○ Contrast-induced nephropathy (CIN) occurs after 24–48 hours in up to 5% of patients undergoing coronary angiography. In most patients, creatinine returns to baseline within 7 days.[18] The following are considerations in the prevention of CIN:
  ▪ The volume of contrast media used should be minimized.
  ▪ All patients should receive some CIN prophylactic therapy: oral hydration, IV hydration, held IV diuretics, and statin therapy have proven benefit.
  ▪ We recommend a 3 mL/kg bolus of normal saline at least 6 hours prior to the procedure with a 1 mL/kg continuous infusion rate until procedure start.
  ▪ N-Acetyl-L-cysteine has no advantage over simple hydration for prevention of CIN.

- **Coronary CT angiography**
  ○ A noninvasive technique used to establish a diagnosis of CAD. Like cardiac angiography, it exposes the patient to both radiation and contrast material.
  ○ Uses arterial phase contrast CT images to evaluate coronary stenosis. Where available, a proprietary software package can calculate intracoronary hemodynamics akin to FFR.
  ○ CT has a high negative predictive value, so it is better suited to rule out disease for symptomatic patients with a low pretest probability for CAD, such as a patient with repeated emergency room admissions for chest pain or patients with equivocal stress test results.
    ▪ The 2021 AHA/ACC/ASE/CHEST/SAEM/SCCT/SCMR Guideline for the Evaluation and Diagnosis of Chest Pain gives CT a class I indication for use in intermediate risk patients with acute chest pain, without known CAD, to exclude obstructive CAD.[19]
  ○ May assist in identification of congenital anomalies of the coronary arteries.
  ○ Due to diminished study quality, it is not useful in patients with extensive coronary calcification (e.g., elderly, or advanced CKD), coronary stents, or small-caliber vessels.

TREATMENT

- The major goal of treatment is to reduce symptoms.
- An absolute reduction in incidence of MI or cardiac death in patients with stable IHD is accomplished mainly through medical therapy and not revascularization.
- A combination of lifestyle modification, medical therapy, and coronary revascularization can be used. A recommended strategy for the evaluation and management of the patient with stable angina can be found in Figure 4-1.
- Medical treatment is aimed at improving myocardial oxygen supply, reducing myocardial oxygen demand, controlling exacerbating factors (e.g., anemia), and limiting the development of further atherosclerotic disease.
- Medical treatment often is sufficient to control anginal symptoms in chronic stable angina.

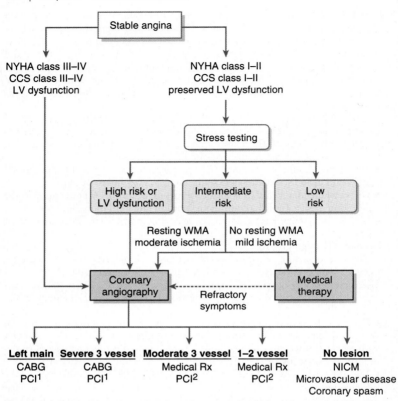

Figure 4-1. Approach to the evaluation and management of the patient with stable ischemic heart disease based on the ISCHEMIA trial. Of note, patients with severe limiting angina, clinical heart failure, or left ventricle (LV) dysfunction should proceed directly to coronary angiography to define underlying coronary artery disease. Patients without these features may first undergo medical optimization with guideline-directed medical therapies (GDMT). If the patient is satisfied with their symptoms on optimal GDMT and is tolerating treatment without significant side effects, coronary CTA should then be obtained to rule out significant left main disease. If no significant left main disease is present, the patient may continue medical therapy without further testing or intervention. If significant left main disease is present, the patient should undergo cardiac catheterization. Patients who are not satisfied with the outcome of optimal GDMT may proceed directly to cardiac catheterization. Information obtained from cardiac catheterization should then be used by a multidisciplinary team to determine whether continued medical therapy, PCI, or CABG should be pursued. [1]CABG generally preferred due to known survival advantage over medical therapy alone; however, if the coronary lesions are not complex, PCI may offer similar results to CABG but with a higher need for future revascularizations. [2]PCI should be reserved for patients who have high-grade lesions, have severe ischemia, and are refractory to medical therapy. CABG, coronary artery bypass grafting; CCS, Canadian Cardiovascular Society Classification (angina); CTA, computed tomography angiography; NICM, nonischemic cardiomyopathy; NYHA, New York Heart Association; PCI, percutaneous coronary intervention; WMA, wall motion abnormality.

Medications

- **Anti-ischemic therapy**
  - ○ **β-Adrenergic antagonists** (Table 4-7) control anginal symptoms by decreasing heart rate and myocardial work, leading to reduced myocardial oxygen demand.
    - ▪ β-Blockers with intrinsic sympathomimetic activity should be avoided.
    - ▪ Dosage can be adjusted to result in a resting heart rate of 50–60 bpm.
    - ▪ Use with caution or avoid in patients with active bronchospasm, atrioventricular (AV) block, resting bradycardia, or poorly compensated HF.
  - ○ **Calcium channel blockers** can be used either in conjunction with or in lieu of β-blockers in the presence of contraindications or adverse effects as a second-line agent (Table 4-8).
    - ▪ Calcium antagonists are often used in conjunction with β-blockers if the latter are not fully effective at relieving anginal symptoms. Both long-acting dihydropyridines and nondihydropyridine agents can be used.
    - ▪ Calcium channel blockers are effective agents for the treatment of coronary vasospasm.
    - ▪ Nondihydropyridine agents (verapamil/diltiazem) should be avoided in patients with systolic dysfunction due to their negative inotropic effects.
  - ○ **Nitrates**, either long-acting formulations for chronic use or sublingual/topical preparations for acute anginal symptoms, are more often used as adjunctive antianginal agents (Table 4-9).
    - ▪ Sublingual preparations should be used at the first indication of angina or prophylactically before engaging in activities that are known to precipitate angina. Patients should seek prompt medical attention if angina occurs at rest or fails to respond to the third sublingual dose.
    - ▪ Nitrate tolerance resulting in reduced therapeutic response may occur with all nitrate preparations. The institution of a nitrate-free period of 10–12 hours (usually at night) can enhance treatment efficacy.
    - ▪ For patients with CAD, nitrates have not shown a mortality benefit.

TABLE 4-7	β-Blockers Commonly Used for Ischemic Heart Disease	
Drug	β-Receptor Selectivity	Dose
Propranolol	β_1 and β_2	20–80 mg bid
Metoprolol	β_1	50–200 mg bid
Atenolol	β_1	50–200 mg daily
Nebivolol	β_1	5–40 mg daily
Nadolol	β_1 and β_2	40–80 mg daily
Timolol	β_1 and β_2	10–30 mg tid
Acebutolol[a]	β_1	200–600 mg bid
Bisoprolol	β_1	10–20 mg daily
Esmolol (IV)	β_1	50–300 µg/kg/min
Labetalol	Combined α, β_1, β_2	200–600 mg bid
Pindolol[a]	β_1 and β_2	2.5–7.5 mg tid
Carvedilol	Combined α, β_1, β_2	3.125–25 mg bid

[a]β-Blockers with intrinsic sympathomimetic activity.

CHAPTER 4

TABLE 4-8	Calcium Channel Blockers Commonly Used for Ischemic Heart Disease	
Drug	**Duration of Action**	**Usual Dosage**
Dihydropyridines		
Nifedipine	Long	30–180 mg daily
Amlodipine	Long	5–10 mg daily
Felodipine (SR)	Long	5–10 mg daily
Isradipine	Medium	2.5–10 mg daily
Nicardipine	Short	20–40 mg tid
Nondihydropyridines		
Diltiazem		
Immediate release	Short	30–90 mg qid
Slow release	Long	120–360 mg daily
Verapamil		
Immediate release	Short	80–160 mg tid
Slow release	Long	120–480 mg daily

- ▪ Nitrates are contraindicated (even in patients with ACS) for use in patients who are on phoshodiesterase-5 inhibitors due to risk of severe hypotension. A washout period of 24 hours for sildenafil and vardenafil and 48 hours for tadalafil is required prior to nitrate use.
  - ○ **Ranolazine** is indicated for angina refractory to standard medical therapy and has shown benefit in improving symptoms and quality of life. Ranolazine interacts with simvastatin metabolism and should not be used together.
- • **Secondary prevention medications**
  - ○ **Acetylsalicylic acid (ASA)** (75–162 mg/d) reduces cardiovascular events, including repeat revascularization, MI, and cardiac death, by approximately 33%.[20]

TABLE 4-9	Nitrate Preparations Commonly Used for Ischemic Heart Disease		
Preparation	**Dosage**	**Onset (min)**	**Duration**
Sublingual nitroglycerin	0.3–0.6 mg PRN	2–5	10–30 min
Aerosol nitroglycerin	0.4 mg PRN	2–5	10–30 min
Oral isosorbide dinitrate	5–40 mg tid	30–60	4–6 h
Oral isosorbide mononitrate	10–20 mg bid	30–60	6–8 h
Oral isosorbide mononitrate SR	30–120 mg daily	30–60	12–18 h
2% Nitroglycerin ointment	0.5–2 in tid	20–60	3–8 h
Transdermal nitroglycerin patches	5–15 mg daily	>60	12 h
Intravenous nitroglycerin	10–200 µg/min	<2	During infusion

- ASA 81 mg appears to be sufficient for most patients.
- ASA desensitization may be performed in patients with ASA allergy.
- **Clopidogrel** (75 mg/d) can be used in those allergic or intolerant of ASA.
○ **Angiotensin-converting enzyme inhibitors (ACE inhibitors) and angiotensin receptor blockers (ARBs)** have cardiovascular protective effects that reduce the recurrence of ischemic events.
  - ACE inhibitor therapy, or ARBs in those with ACE inhibitors intolerance, should be used in all patients with an LVEF <40%, hypertension, diabetes, or chronic kidney disease.
○ **Statins** have a marked effect in secondary prevention, and all patients with IHD who can tolerate therapy should be on a high-potency statin (see Chapter 3, Preventive Cardiology).
  - In secondary prevention of coronary heart disease, statins have the most evidence demonstrating a robust mortality benefit.
○ **Proprotein convertase subtilisin/kexin type 9 (PCSK9) inhibitors** confer a mortality benefit to patients with IHD whose LDL levels remain >70 mg/dL despite high-intensity statins. Currently, expense and insurance coverage limit the use of this class of medications.[21]
○ **Ezetimibe** also improves cardiovascular outcomes among patients with IHD whose LDL remains >100 mg/dL despite high-intensity statin therapy.[22]
○ **Influenza vaccination** is recommended for all patients with IHD.

Revascularization
- **Coronary revascularization**
○ In general, medical therapy with at least two classes of antianginal agents should be attempted before medical therapy is considered a failure and coronary revascularization pursued in stable angina.
○ Relief of angina symptoms is the most common objective of all revascularization procedures for stable angina.
○ The indication for all revascularization procedures should consider the acuity of presentation, the extent of ischemia, and the ability to achieve full revascularization. The selection of revascularization should be tailored to the individual patient and, in complex cases, include the use of a multidisciplinary heart team.
○ The choice between PCI and CABG surgery is dependent on the coronary anatomy, medical comorbidities, and patient preference.
  - In general, patients with complex and diffuse disease or diabetes do better with CABG, whereas PCI in select patients with the proper coronary anatomy can provide comparable results as CABG.[23]
  - The Syntax Score is a validated angiographic model that can aid the clinician in determining outcomes after PCI or CABG. In general, patients with a low or intermediate Syntax Score do as well or better with PCI compared to CABG[24] (available at http://www.syntaxscore.com/).
  - The Society of Thoracic Surgeons (STS) score can help determine the risk of mortality and morbidity associated with CABG and should be determined for all patients when considering surgical revascularization (available at http://riskcalc.sts.org/).
○ Revascularization is shown to **improve survival** in the following circumstances as compared to medical therapy:
  - CABG for >50% left main CAD that has not been grafted (unprotected). PCI is a reasonable alternative for patients with left main disease if the patient is a poor

surgical candidate (STS score > 5) and has a favorable morphology for PCI (low Syntax Score). PCI, in the right clinical context, can offer rates of MI, CVA, or death similar to CABG.[25]

- CABG for three-vessel disease or two-vessel disease that includes the proximal left anterior descending (LAD) artery.
- CABG for patients with two-vessel disease, not including the LAD artery, if there is extensive ischemia (>20% myocardium at risk) or in patients with isolated proximal LAD artery disease when an internal mammary artery revascularization is performed.
- CABG, as compared to PCI or medical therapy, in patients with multivessel disease and diabetes, if a left internal mammary artery to the LAD artery can be placed.[26] PCI *may* offer similar survival outcomes in diabetics with multivessel disease and a low Syntax Score (<22) but does have a higher need for repeat revascularization.[27]
- PCI or CABG in patients who have survived sudden cardiac death due to ischemic ventricular tachycardia (VT).

○ Due to the morbidity of a repeat CABG, PCI is often used to improve symptoms in patients with recurrent angina after CABG.

○ The use of internal mammary artery grafts is associated with 90% graft patency at 10 years, compared with 40%–50% for saphenous vein grafts. The long-term patency of a radial artery graft is 80% at 5 years. After 10 years of follow-up, 50% of patients develop recurrent angina or other adverse cardiac events related to late vein graft failure or progression of native CAD.

○ The risks of elective PCI include <1% mortality, a 2%–5% rate of nonfatal MI, and <1% need for emergent CABG for an unsuccessful procedure. Patients undergoing PCI have shorter hospitalizations but require more frequent repeat revascularization procedures compared to CABG.

○ Elderly patients represent a unique population when considering revascularization due to comorbidities, frailty, the physiology of aging as it relates to drug metabolism and cardiopulmonary function, and concern over polypharmacy. In general, this population has been underrepresented in most trials but still derives benefit from revascularization to relieve symptoms. Frailty should be heavily considered when considering a procedure or counseling about the benefits of revascularization.

○ It is reasonable to revascularize selected patients with severe LV dysfunction (EF < 35%), as evidenced by the long-term mortality benefit seen with CABG in the STICHES trial.[28]

○ Viability testing (nuclear perfusion imaging or MRI) may provide some assistance to the clinician when trying to determine the possible benefit of revascularization in patients with prior MI or severe LV dysfunction but is still largely unproven.

MONITORING/FOLLOW-UP

- Close patient follow-up is a critical component of the treatment of CAD because lifestyle modification and secondary risk factor reduction require serial reassessment and interventions.
- All patients should be aggressively treated for the traditional risk factors mentioned above.
- Relatively minor changes in anginal symptoms can be safely treated with titration and/or addition of antianginal medications.

- Significant changes in anginal complaints (frequency, severity, or time to onset with activity) should be evaluated by either stress testing (usually in conjunction with an imaging modality) or cardiac angiography as warranted.
- Cardiac rehabilitation or an exercise program should be offered or instituted.

Acute Coronary Syndromes, Unstable Angina, and Non–ST-Segment Elevation Myocardial Infarction

GENERAL PRINCIPLES

Definition

- NSTEMI and UA are closely related conditions whose pathogenesis and clinical presentations are similar but differ in severity.
- If coronary flow is not severe enough or the occlusion does not persist long enough to cause myocardial necrosis (as indicated by positive cardiac biomarkers), the syndrome is labeled UA.
- NSTEMI is defined by an elevation of cardiac biomarkers and the absence of ST-segment elevation on the ECG.
- NSTEMI, like STEMI, can lead to cardiogenic shock.
- AHA/ACC guidelines provide a more thorough overview of NSTEMI/UA.[29,30]

Epidemiology

- The annual incidence of ACS is >780,000 events, with 70% being NSTEMI/UA.
- Among patients with ACS, approximately 60% have UA and 40% have MI (one-third of MIs present with an acute STEMI).
- At 1 year, patients with UA/NSTEMI are at considerable risk for death (~6%), recurrent MI (~11%), and need for revascularization (~50%–60%). It is important to note that although the short-term mortality of STEMI is greater than that of NSTEMI, the long-term mortality is similar.[31,32]
- Patients with NSTEMI/UA tend to have more comorbidities, both cardiac and noncardiac, than STEMI patients.
- Women with NSTEMI/UA have worse short-term and long-term outcomes and more complications compared to men. Much of this has been attributed to delays in recognition of symptoms and underutilization of guideline-directed medical therapy and invasive management.

Etiology and Pathophysiology

- Myocardial ischemia results from decreased myocardial oxygen supply and/or increased demand. In the majority of cases, NSTEMI is due to a sudden decrease in blood supply via partial occlusion of the affected vessel. In some cases, markedly increased myocardial oxygen demand may lead to NSTEMI (demand ischemia), as seen in severe anemia, hypertensive crisis, acute decompensated HF, surgery, or any other significant physiologic stressor.
- Plaque rupture may be triggered by local and/or systemic inflammation as well as shear stress. Rupture allows exposure of lipid-rich subendothelial components to circulating platelets and inflammatory cells, serving as a potent substrate for thrombus formation. A thin fibrous cap (thin-cap fibroatheroma) is felt to be more vulnerable to rupture and is most frequently represented as only moderate stenosis on angiography.

CHAPTER 4

- Less common causes include dynamic obstruction of the coronary artery due to vasospasm (Prinzmetal angina, cocaine use), coronary artery dissection (more common in women), coronary vasculitis, and embolus.

Clinical Presentation

History
- The three principal presentations for UA are **rest angina** (angina occurring at rest and prolonged, usually >20 minutes), **new-onset angina**, and **progressive angina** (previously diagnosed angina that has become more frequent, lasts longer, or occurs with less exertion). New-onset and progressive angina should occur with at least mild to moderate activity, CCS class III severity.
  - Female sex, diabetes, HF, end-stage kidney disease, and older age are traits that have been associated with a greater likelihood of atypical ACS symptoms. However, the most common presentation in these populations is still typical anginal chest pain.
  - Jaw, neck, arm, back, or epigastric pain and/or dyspnea can be anginal equivalents.
  - Pleuritic pain, pain that radiates down the legs or originates in the mid/lower abdomen, pain that can be reproduced by extremity movement or palpation, and pain that lasts seconds in duration are unlikely to be related to ACS.

Physical Examination
- Physical examination should be directed at identifying hemodynamic instability, pulmonary congestion, and other causes of acute chest discomfort.
- Objective evidence of HF, including peripheral hypoperfusion, heart murmur (particularly mitral regurgitation [MR] murmur), elevated jugular venous pulsation, pulmonary edema, hypotension, and peripheral edema worsen the prognosis.
- Killip classification can be useful to risk stratify and identify patients with features of cardiogenic shock (Table 4-10).
- Examination may also give clues to other causes of ischemia such as thyrotoxicosis or aortic dissection (see Table 4-4).

Diagnostic Testing

Electrocardiography
- Prior to or immediately on arrival to the emergency department, a baseline ECG should be obtained in all patients with suspected ACS. A normal tracing does not exclude the presence of disease.
- The presence of Q waves, ST-segment changes, or T-wave inversions is suggestive of CAD.

TABLE 4-10	Killip Classification[33]	
Class	Definition	Mortality[a] (%)
I	No signs or symptoms of heart failure	6
II	Heart failure: S_3 gallop, rales, or JVD	17
III	Severe heart failure: pulmonary edema	38
IV	Cardiogenic shock: SBP < 90 mm Hg and signs of hypoperfusion and/or signs of severe heart failure	81

JVD, jugular venous distention; SBP, systolic blood pressure.
[a]In-hospital mortality of patients in 1965–1967 with no reperfusion therapy ($n = 250$).[33]

- Isolated Q waves in lead III only are a normal finding.
- Serial ECGs should be obtained to assess for dynamic ischemic changes.
- Comparison to prior ECGs is important when evaluating an ECG for dynamic changes.
- The posterior circulation (i.e., circumflex coronary artery distribution) is poorly assessed with standard ECG lead placement and should always be considered when evaluating patients with ACS. Posterior leads or urgent echocardiography may more accurately assess the presence of ischemia when the suspicion is high.
- Approximately 50% of patients with UA/NSTEMI have significant ECG abnormalities, including transient ST-segment elevations, ST depressions, and T-wave inversions.[32,34]
  - ST-segment depression in two contiguous leads is a sensitive indicator of myocardial ischemia, especially if dynamic and associated with symptoms.
    - Threshold value for abnormal J-point depression should be 0.5 mm in leads V_2 and V_3 and 1 mm in all other leads.
    - ST-segment depression in multiple leads plus ST-segment elevation in aVR and/or V_1 suggests ischemia due to multivessel or left main disease.
  - Biphasic or deeply inverted T waves (>5 mm) with QT prolongation in leads V_2 to V_4 in the setting of stuttering chest pain within the past 24 hours suggests a critical lesion in the LAD artery distribution (Wellens syndrome).[34]
  - Nonspecific ST-segment changes or T-wave inversions (those that do not meet voltage criteria) are nondiagnostic and unhelpful in management of acute ischemia but are associated with a higher risk for future cardiac events.

Laboratories
- A complete blood count, basic metabolic panel, fasting glucose, and lipid profile should be obtained in all patients with suspected CAD. Other conditions may be found to be contributing to ischemia (e.g., anemia) or mimicking ischemia (e.g., hyperkalemia-related ECG changes) or may alter management (e.g., severe thrombocytopenia).
- **Troponin** is the recommended biomarker for assessment of myocardial necrosis.
  - Troponin T and I assays are highly specific and sensitive markers of myocardial necrosis. Serum troponin levels are usually undetectable in normal individuals, and any elevation is considered abnormal.
  - In patients with troponin below the detectable limit of the assay within 6 hours of the onset of pain, a second sample should be drawn 8–12 hours after symptom onset.
  - MI size and prognosis are directly proportional to magnitude of increase in troponin.[34]
- Creatine kinase (CK)-MB is no longer a recommended marker for the initial diagnosis of NSTEMI. It lacks specificity because it is present in both skeletal and cardiac muscle cells.
  - CK-MB may be a useful assay for detecting postinfarct ischemia because a fall and subsequent rise in enzyme levels suggests reinfarction if accompanied by recurrent ischemic symptoms or ECG changes.
- Brain natriuretic peptide (BNP) can be a useful biomarker of myocardial stress in patients with ACS, and elevations are associated with worse outcomes.[35] Severe elevations of BNP in the setting of ACS in patients without known HF should raise concern for a large infarction and urgent angiography.

CHAPTER 4

TREATMENT

- Acute treatment aims to reduce the symptoms of chest pain and risk of recurrent MI or death.
- Risk stratification can be helpful in determining the appropriate testing, pharmacologic interventions, and timing or need for coronary angiography.
  - Risk of death or MI progression is elevated with the following **high-risk ACS characteristics,** which should prompt **urgent coronary angiography (<2 hours)** with intent to revascularize:
    - Recurrent/accelerating angina despite adequate medical therapy
    - Signs or symptoms of new HF, pulmonary edema, or shock (high Killip Classification)
    - New or worsening MR
    - New LBBB
    - VT
  - Several clinical tools can estimate a patient's risk of recurrent MI and cardiac mortality, such as the Thrombolysis in Myocardial Infarction (TIMI) and Global Registry of Acute Coronary Events (GRACE) risk scores. The TIMI risk score can be used to determine the risk of death or nonfatal MI up to 1 year after an ACS event (Figure 4-2).
- In the stabilized patient, two treatment strategies are available: the **ischemia-driven approach** (formerly termed *conservative*) versus the **routine invasive approach** (*early* defined as <24 hours of presentation or *delayed* >24 hours).
  - The planned approach should always be individualized to the patient (Figure 4-3). All patients should receive aggressive antithrombotic, antiplatelet, and ischemic medical therapy no matter the final revascularization strategy. Table 4-11 summarizes the selection approach.
  - In ACS, as opposed to stable IHD, a routine invasive approach with possible PCI has been shown to **reduce the incidence of recurrent MI, hospitalizations, and death.** In general, patients with ACS should undergo a routine invasive strategy unless it is clear that the risk outweighs the possible benefit in a given patient.
  - In the **ischemia-driven approach,** if the patient does not develop high-risk ACS features, has normal subsequent cardiac biomarkers, has no dynamic ECG changes, and responds to medical therapy, a noninvasive stress test should be obtained for further risk stratification.
    - Patients should be angina free for at least 12 hours prior to stress testing.
    - If a patient with positive cardiac biomarkers is selected for noninvasive testing, a submaximal or pharmacologic stress test 72 hours after the peak value may be performed.
    - Coronary angiography is reserved for patients who develop high-risk ACS features, have a high-risk stress test, develop angina at low levels of stress, or are noted to have an LVEF < 40%.
  - In the **routine invasive strategy,** the patient is planned for a coronary angiography with intent to revascularize. An early (<24 hours from presentation) invasive approach is recommended for patients with high-risk scores or other high-risk features (see Table 4-11).
    - Note: Refractory chest pain, hemodynamic instability, or serious ventricular arrhythmias are indications for an urgent/emergent invasive strategy similar to STEMI; this is not to be confused with a routine invasive strategy.

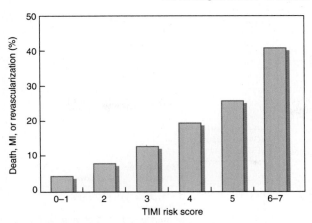

TIMI risk score (1 point for each)
1. Age > 65 y
2. Known CAD (stenosis > 50%)
3. 2+ episodes of chest pain in 24 h
4. ST-segment or T-wave changes
5. Elevated cardiac biomarkers
6. ASA in the last 7 d
7. 3+ CAD risk factors

| Ischemia driven strategy | Routine invasive strategy |

β-Blocker, nitrates, oxygen⟶
UFH, LMWH ⟶
ASA ⟶
Dual antiplatelet therapy ⟶
Triple antiplatelet therapy ⟶

TIMI risk score

Figure 4-2. Fourteen-day rates of death, MI, or urgent revascularization from the TIMI 11B and ESSENCE trials based on increasing TIMI risk score. Coronary artery disease (CAD) risk factors include family history of CAD, diabetes, hypertension, hyperlipidemia, and tobacco use. ASA, aspirin; LMWH, low–molecular-weight heparin; MI, myocardial infarction; TIMI, Thrombolysis in Myocardial Infarction; UFH, unfractionated heparin.[36]

- ○ An early invasive strategy is also warranted in low- or intermediate-risk patients with repeated ACS presentations despite appropriate therapy.
- ○ A routine invasive strategy is not recommended for the following:
  - ▪ Patients with severe comorbid illnesses such as advanced chronic kidney disease, end-stage liver or lung disease, or metastatic/uncontrolled cancer whereby the

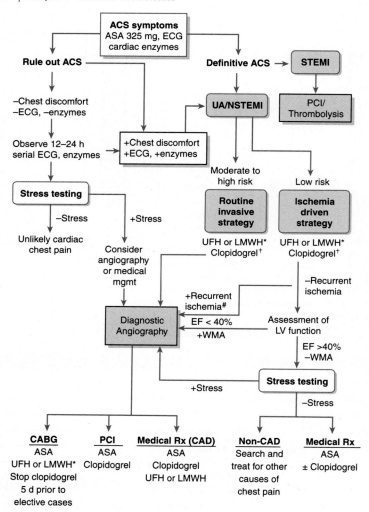

Figure 4-3. Diagnostic and therapeutic approach to patients presenting with acute coronary syndrome (ACS) focusing on antiplatelet and antithrombotic therapy. *Bivalirudin is an appropriate alternative to UFH and LMWH, or at time of PCI, patients on UFH may be switched to bivalirudin. †Choose either clopidogrel, ticagrelor, or prasugrel as the second antiplatelet agent. #Indicators of recurrent ischemia include worsening chest pain, increasing cardiac biomarkers, heart failure signs/symptoms, arrhythmia (VT/VF), and dynamic ECG changes. 1UFH for 48 hours or LMWH until discharge or up to 8 days and clopidogrel or ticagrelor for 1 year. ASA, aspirin; CABG, coronary artery bypass grafting; CAD, coronary artery disease; EF, ejection fraction; LMWH, low–molecular-weight heparin; NSTEMI, non–ST-segment elevation myocardial infarction; PCI, percutaneous coronary intervention; Rx, treatment; STEMI, ST-segment elevation myocardial infarction; UA, unstable angina; UFH, unfractionated heparin; VT/VF, ventricular tachycardia/ventricular fibrillation; WMA, wall motion abnormality.[31,37]

TABLE 4-11 Appropriate Selection of Routine Invasive Versus Ischemia-Driven Revascularization Strategy in Patients With NSTEMI/UA

Immediate/urgent invasive (within 2 h)	Refractory Angina Worsening Signs or Symptoms of heart failure or Mitral regurgitation Hemodynamic instability or Shock Sustained VT or VF
Ischemia-driven	Low-risk score (TIMI ≤ 1 or GRACE < 109) Low-risk biomarker-negative female patients Patient or clinician preference in the absence of high-risk features
Early invasive (within 24 h)	None of the above but a high-risk score (TIMI ≥ 3 or GRACE > 140) Rapid rate of rise in biomarkers New or presumably new ST depressions
Delayed invasive (24–72 h)	None of the above but presence of diabetes Renal insufficiency (GFR < 60) LV ejection fraction <40% Early postinfarction angina Prior PCI within 6 months Prior CABG TIMI score ≥2 or GRACE score 109–140 and no indication for early invasive strategy

CABG, coronary artery bypass graft; GFR, glomerular filtration rate; GRACE, Global Registry of Acute Coronary Events; LV, left ventricular; NSTEMI, non–ST-segment elevation myocardial infarction; PCI, percutaneous coronary intervention; TIMI, Thrombolysis in Myocardial Infarction; UA, unstable angina; VF, ventricular fibrillation; VT, ventricular tachycardia.

benefits of the procedure are likely outweighed by the risk from the routine invasive procedure
- Acute chest pain with a low likelihood of ACS and negative biomarkers, especially in women

Medications
- Patients presenting with UA/NSTEMI should receive medications that reduce myocardial ischemia through reduction in myocardial oxygen demand, improvement in coronary perfusion, and prevention of further thrombus formation.
- This approach should include antiplatelet, anticoagulant, and antianginal medications.
- Supplemental oxygen should be provided if the patient is hypoxemic (<SpO₂ 90%) or having difficulty breathing. Routine use of oxygen is not needed and possibly harmful.[38]
- **Antiplatelet therapy**
  ○ Table 4-12 summarizes available agents and dosing recommendations for use in ACS.
  ○ Early dual antiplatelet therapy (DAPT) with aspirin plus a P2Y₁₂ inhibitor is strongly recommended for patients with NSTEMI/UA without a contraindication

TABLE 4-12	Antiplatelet Agents in UA/NSTEMI	
Medication	**Dosage**	**Comments**
Aspirin (ASA)	162–325 mg initial, then 75–100 mg daily	In patients taking ticagrelor, the maintenance dose of ASA *should not* exceed 100 mg.
Clopidogrel	300–600 mg loading dose, 75 mg daily	In combination with ASA, clopidogrel (300–600 mg loading dose, then 75 mg/d) decreased the composite end point of cardiovascular death, MI, or stroke by 18%–30% in patients with UA/NSTEMI.[39-41]
Ticagrelor	180 mg loading dose, then 90 mg bid	Ticagrelor reduced incidence of vascular death, MI, or CVA (9.8% vs. 11.0%) but with higher major bleeding not related to CABG (4.5% vs. 3.8%) as compared to clopidogrel.[42,43]
Prasugrel	60 mg loading dose, then 10 mg daily	Prasugrel has increased antiplatelet potency compared to clopidogrel.
		Prasugrel reduced the incidence of cardiovascular death, MI, and stroke (9.9% vs. 12.1%) at the expense of increased major (2.4% vs. 1.1%) and fatal bleeding (0.4% vs. 0.1%), compared to clopidogrel.[44]
Cangrelor	30 µg/kg IV bolus, then 4 µg/kg/min	Currently FDA approved only for patients undergoing PCI. Expense and modest evidence of benefit compared to other $P2Y_{12}$ inhibitors limit use.
Eptifibatide	180 µg/kg IV bolus, then 2 µg/kg/min[a]	Eptifibatide reduces the risk of death or MI in patients with ACS undergoing either invasive or noninvasive therapy in combination with ASA and heparin.[45,46]
		Compared to abciximab and tirofiban, eptifibatide has the most consistent effects on platelet inhibition with shortest on-time and drug half-life.[47]
Tirofiban	0.4 µg/kg IV bolus, then 0.1 µg/kg/min[a]	Tirofiban reduces the risk of death or MI in patients with ACS undergoing either invasive or noninvasive therapy in combination with ASA and heparin.[48-50]
Abciximab	0.25 mg/kg IV bolus, then 10 µg/min[b]	Abciximab reduces the risk of death or MI in patients with ACS undergoing coronary intervention.[51-53] It should not be used in patients in whom percutaneous intervention is not planned.[54]
		Platelet inhibition may be reversed by platelet transfusion.

ACS, acute coronary syndrome; CABG, coronary artery bypass grafting; CVA, cerebrovascular accident; ESRD, end-stage renal disease; GFR, glomerular filtration rate; HD, hemodialysis; MI, myocardial infarction; NSTEMI, non–ST-segment elevation myocardial infarction; UA, unstable angina.
[a]Infusion doses should be decreased by 50% in patients with a GFR < 30 mL/min and avoided in patients on HD.
[b]Abciximab may be used in patients with ESRD because it is not cleared by the kidney.

(e.g., uncontrolled severe bleeding, recent neuraxial surgery or trauma, recent hemorrhagic stroke, or intra-cranial or spinal metastases).

○ DAPT should ideally be continued for 12 months from the index ACS event, regardless of whether revascularization is performed or not. See the 2016 ACC/AHA Guideline Focused Update on Duration of Dual Antiplatelet Therapy in Patients With Coronary Artery Disease for specific recommendations tailored to stent type, bleeding risk, and other considerations.

○ **Aspirin** blocks platelet aggregation within minutes.

   ■ A chewable 162- to 325-mg dose of ASA should be administered immediately at symptom onset or at first medical contact unless a contraindication exists. This should be followed by ASA 81 mg daily indefinitely.

   ■ If an ASA allergy is present, clopidogrel may be a substitution. An allergy consultation should be obtained for possible desensitization, preferably prior to the need for a coronary stent.

   ■ After PCI, ASA 81 mg is the current recommended dose in the setting of DAPT.

○ **Clopidogrel** is a prodrug whose metabolite blocks the $P2Y_{12}$ receptor and inhibits platelet activation and aggregation by blocking the adenosine diphosphate receptor site on platelets.

   ■ The addition of clopidogrel to ASA reduced cardiovascular mortality and recurrent MI both acutely and at 11 months of follow-up.[39]

   ■ A loading dose of 600 mg should always be given in naïve patients.

   ■ In patients unable to take oral medications or unable to absorb oral medications due to ileus, rectal administration is unproven but has been reported. Alternatively, parenteral agents (e.g., cangrelor or eptifibatide) may be considered.

   ■ Can be used as part of the protocol in both the ischemia-driven and routinely invasive strategies.

○ **Prasugrel** is also a prodrug that blocks the $P2Y_{12}$ adenosine receptor; its conversion to its active metabolite occurs faster and to a greater extent than clopidogrel.

   ■ Results in faster, greater, and more uniform platelet inhibition compared to clopidogrel at the expense of higher risk of bleeding.[55]

   ■ It decreases risk of CVD death, MI, CVA, and acute stent thrombosis as compared to clopidogrel in ACS patients, including STEMI patients.

   ■ It should be used with caution or avoided in patients older than 75 years and who weigh less than 60 kg. It is contraindicated in those with prior stroke or transient ischemic attack (TIA).

   ■ Used **only in the invasive approach of ACS** and only after coronary anatomy is known and PCI is planned. There is no benefit over clopidogrel when tested before initiation of PCI.

   ■ Prasugrel may be superior to ticagrelor with regards to the composite of MI, stroke, and death.[56]

○ **Ticagrelor** is not a prodrug and blocks the $P2Y_{12}$ adenosine receptor directly.

   ■ Reduces the risk of death, MI, CVA, and stent thrombosis as compared to clopidogrel in ACS patients, including STEMI patients.[42]

   ■ After the loading dose of ASA, the maintenance dose of ASA must be <100 mg.

   ■ Can be used as part of the protocol in both the ischemia-driven and early invasive strategies.

   ■ Barring any contraindication, ticagrelor is the preferred $P2Y_{12}$ inhibitor of choice due to the mortality advantage over other medications in this class.[43]

   ■ Relative contraindications include baseline bradycardia, severe reactive airways disease, and prior hemorrhagic stroke.

- **Cangrelor** is a parenteral, direct, and reversible inhibitor of the $P2Y_{12}$ adenosine receptor.
  - It has a uniquely rapid onset (<2 minutes), potency (>90% platelet inhibition), and short duration of action after cessation (normal platelet function after 1 hour).
  - Reduces the risk of death, MI, urgent revascularization, or stent thrombosis among patients undergoing PCI.[57]
  - FDA approved only for patients undergoing PCI, and currently very expensive. Thus, it is not yet recommended for routine use in either ischemia-guided or invasive strategy. Thus, we recommend consulting a cardiologist before the use of cangrelor.
  - Sometimes used as a bridging strategy in patients who have had recent PCI and require surgery where DAPT is prohibited. This approach is of unproven benefit.
- **Glycoprotein IIb/IIIa (GPIIb/IIIa) antagonists** (abciximab, eptifibatide, or tirofiban) block the interaction between platelets and fibrinogen, thus targeting the final common pathway for platelet aggregation.
  - GPIIb/IIIa inhibitors play a limited role in ACS management with the introduction of more potent oral antiplatelet agents.
  - Routine use of GPIIb/IIIa antagonists on initial presentation, before angiography, in patients undergoing the invasive approach *should be avoided* due to increased risk of major bleeding and a lack of improvement in outcomes.
  - GPIIb/IIIa agents may be considered in scenarios of worsening ischemia despite DAPT, complex PCI, or bridging strategy in patients with an indication for DAPT (e.g., recent PCI) but require surgery.
  - Thrombocytopenia, which can be severe, is an uncommon complication of these agents and should prompt discontinuation.
- **Other concerns with antiplatelet agents**
  - Timing of CABG
    - Due to increased risk of bleeding, it is currently recommended that clopidogrel be withheld for at least 5 days prior to CABG, prasugrel 7 days prior, ticagrelor 5 days prior, and cangrelor 1–6 hours prior.
    - Cangrelor or GPIIb/IIIa antagonists can be used as an alternative to clopidogrel, ticagrelor, and prasugrel in appropriate patients with UA/NSTEMI who are known to require surgical revascularization.
    - In general, DAPT should not be withheld during the initial management of ACS (i.e., prior to angiography) out of concern for the potential need for surgical revascularization. There is a larger risk of withholding beneficial therapy to patients in this setting than causing harm by delaying surgical revascularization.
  - Proton pump inhibitors (PPIs)
    - PPIs should be used in patients on DAPT with a prior history of gastrointestinal bleeding or increased risk of bleeding (e.g., elderly, known ulcers or *Helicobacter pylori* infection, or coprescribed warfarin, steroids, or NSAIDs).[58]
    - Pharmacologic studies have raised concerns about the potential of PPIs to blunt the efficacy of clopidogrel. However, in a prospective randomized trial, no apparent cardiovascular interaction was noted between PPIs and clopidogrel.[59]
  - Triple therapy
    - Many patients requiring DAPT after PCI have a preexisting indication for oral anticoagulation (OAC), such as atrial fibrillation or recent venous thromboembolism.
    - The most recent guidelines have not yet made specific recommendations, but generally support tailoring selection of triple therapy (DAPT plus OAC) or

SAPT (single antiplatelet therapy) plus OAC to the patient by comparing the risk of bleeding to the risk of ischemic events.[60-62]

  ▲ In the AUGUSTUS trial, patients with atrial fibrillation and recent ACS or PCI treated with a P2Y$_{12}$ inhibitor and apixaban, without aspirin, had fewer bleeding events and fewer hospitalizations without significantly increased ischemic events versus regimens including warfarin, aspirin, or both.[63]

  □ In patients with an average risk of bleeding and average risk of ischemic events, we recommend triple therapy (e.g., aspirin, clopidogrel, and warfarin) for 4 weeks followed by SAPT plus OAC (e.g., clopidogrel and warfarin) for at least 1 year.

  □ In patients with either high risk of bleeding or high risk of ischemic events, we recommend consultation with a cardiologist to tailor therapy.

- **Anticoagulant therapy**
  ○ See Table 4-13 for recommended use and dosing in ACS.
  ○ Anticoagulation accompanied by DAPT is required for all UA/NSTEMI patients, whether along the early invasive or conservative pathway.
  ○ **Unfractionated heparin (UFH)** works by binding antithrombin III, which catalyzes the inactivation of thrombin and other clotting factors.
    ▪ Most commonly used and easily monitored but also most inconsistent in its anticoagulation and metabolism.
    ▪ Heparin-induced thrombocytopenia (HIT) is a concern with prior use.
    ▪ Easily reversed in the event of a severe hemorrhagic complication.
    ▪ Always requires aggressive bolus dosing and anticoagulation monitoring in the setting of ACS.
    ▪ Recommended anticoagulant to be used in the setting of ACS.
  ○ **Low–molecular-weight heparin (LMWH)** inhibits mostly factor Xa but also affects thrombin activity and offers an ease of administration (weight-based, twice-daily subcutaneous dose). The risk of HIT is lower but not absent.
    ▪ As compared to UFH, LMWH has a more predictable anticoagulant effect.
    ▪ It has a similar efficacy as UFH but is associated with a higher risk of postprocedural bleeding.[68]
    ▪ LMWH must be adjusted for renal dysfunction and should be avoided in patients with severe impairments.
    ▪ Enoxaparin 0.3 mg/kg IV should be administered at the time of PCI in patients who have received less than two therapeutic doses or if the last dose was received more than 8 hours before PCI.
  ○ **Fondaparinux** is a synthetic polysaccharide that selectively inhibits factor X and can be subcutaneously administered on a daily routine.
    ▪ Associated with an increased risk of thrombosis during PCI and should not be used without additional antithrombin anticoagulation; as such, it is not recommended for the routine management of ACS.
    ▪ In patients not undergoing invasive management, fondaparinux may significantly reduce bleeding and improve outcomes compared to LMWH.[69]
  ○ **Bivalirudin** is a direct thrombin inhibitor given as a continuous IV infusion and requires partial thromboplastin time (PTT) monitoring when used for >4 hours.
    ▪ It does not cause HIT and is used in the treatment of patients who develop HIT or patients with ACS who have history of HIT.
    ▪ Bivalirudin can be given in conjunction with ASA and clopidogrel in patients presenting with UA/NSTEMI who will undergo a routine invasive strategy.
    ▪ Bivalirudin alone compared to UFH/LMWH + GPIIb/IIIa inhibitor was associated with less bleeding.[70]

CHAPTER 4

TABLE 4-13	Anticoagulant Medications	
Medication	Dosage	Comments
Heparin (UFH)	60 units/kg IV bolus (maximum dose: 4000 units), 12–14 units/kg/h	Heparin therapy, when used in conjunction with ASA, has been shown to reduce the early rate of death or MI by up to 60%.[64] The aPTT should be adjusted to maintain a value of 1.5–2.0 times control.
Enoxaparin (LMWH)	1 mg/kg Sub-Q bid[a]	LMWH is at least as efficacious as UFH and may further reduce the rate of death, MI, or recurrent angina.[65] LMWH may increase the rate of bleeding[62] and cannot be reversed in the setting of refractory bleeding. LMWH does not require monitoring for clinical effect.
Fondaparinux	2.5 mg Sub-Q daily	Fondaparinux has efficacy similar to that of LMWH with possibly reduced bleeding rates.[66]
Bivalirudin[b]	0.75 mg/kg IV bolus, 1.75 mg/kg/h	When used in conjunction with ASA and clopidogrel, bivalirudin is at least as effective as the combination of ASA, UFH, clopidogrel, and GPIIb/IIIa antagonists with decreased bleeding rates.[67] May increase risk for stent thrombosis. Monitoring is required with a goal aPTT of 1.5–2.5 times control.

aPTT, activated partial thromboplastin time; ASA, aspirin; GFR, glomerular filtration rate; GP, glycoprotein; LMWH, low–molecular-weight heparin; MI, myocardial infarction; UFH, unfractionated heparin.

[a]LMWH should be given at reduced dose (50%) in patients with a serum creatinine >2 mg/dL or GFR < 30 mL/min.

[b]Bivalirudin requires dosage adjustment in patients with a GFR less than 30 mL/min or those on hemodialysis.

- Recent evidence has shown that in ACS without significant GPIIb/IIIa inhibitor use, bivalirudin is associated with increased risk of stent thrombosis and target lesion revascularization.[71]
- Caution should be used with routine use of bivalirudin in ACS unless there is a high risk of bleeding.
- **Anti-ischemic therapy** (please also refer to Treatment section of stable angina)
  - **Nitroglycerin**
    - Treatment can be initiated at the time of presentation with sublingual nitroglycerin. **NOTE:** 40% of patients with chest pain *not* due to CAD will get relief with nitroglycerin[62] (see Table 4-9).
    - Patients with ongoing ischemic symptoms or those who require additional agents to control significant hypertension can be treated with IV nitroglycerin until pain relief, hypertension control, or both are achieved.

- Rule out right ventricular (RV) infarct prior to administration of nitrates because this can precipitate profound hypotension.
  - **β-Adrenergic blockers (BBs)** (please also refer to the Treatment section for stable angina)
    - Oral therapy should be started early in the absence of contraindications.
    - Treatment with an IV preparation should be reserved for treatment of arrhythmia, ongoing chest pain, or advanced hypertension rather than routine use.
    - Routine use of IV BBs is associated with increased risk of cardiogenic shock and should be avoided.
    - Contraindications to BB therapy include advanced AV block, active bronchospasm, decompensated HF, cardiogenic shock, hypotension, and bradycardia.
  - **Morphine** 2–4 mg IV may be used as an adjunct to BB, nitrates, and calcium channel blockers. Care must be used not to mask further clinical evaluation by heavy use of narcotic medications.
- **Adjunctive medical therapy**
  - **ACE inhibitors** (refer to Treatment section for stable angina) are effective antihypertensive agents and have been shown to reduce mortality in patients with CAD and LV systolic dysfunction. ACE inhibitors should be used in patients with LV dysfunction (EF < 40%), hypertension, or diabetes presenting with ACS. **ARBs** are appropriate in patients who cannot tolerate ACE inhibitors.
  - **Aldosterone antagonists** should be added, if there are no contraindications (potassium > 5 mEq/L or creatinine clearance [CrCl] < 30 mL/min), after initiation of ACE inhibitors to patients with diabetes or an LVEF < 40%.
  - **3-Hydroxy-3-methylglutaryl–coenzyme A (HMG-CoA) reductase inhibitors (statins)** are potent lipid-lowering agents that reduce the incidence of ischemia, MI, and death in patients with CAD. High-intensity statins should be routinely administered within 24 hours of presentation in patients presenting with ACS. A lipid profile should be obtained in all patients.
    - Aggressive statin therapy reduces the risk of recurrent ischemia, MI, and death in patients presenting with ACS.[62]
    - A reduction in adverse CVD outcomes following early initiation of a high-dose statin with achievement of an LDL < 70 mg/dL can be seen as early as 30 days following initial presentation with ACS.[72] Aggressive LDL lowering also reduces the incidence of periprocedural MI following PCI.[67,73]
  - **NSAIDs** are associated with an increased risk of death, MI, myocardial rupture, hypertension, and HF in large meta-analyses.[74] Adverse outcomes have been observed for both nonselective and selective cyclooxygenase-2 (COX-2) agents. NSAIDs should be discontinued in patients presenting with UA/NSTEMI.
  - **Blood glucose** should not be tightly controlled in diabetic patients who have suffered ACS because it may increase mortality. Goal is <180 mg/dL while avoiding hypoglycemia at all costs.

Revascularization

- **PCI**
  - Please see "Revascularization" section under Stable Angina for invasive management strategies.
- **CABG**
  - The indications for PCI versus CABG in patients with UA/NSTEMI are similar to those for individuals with chronic stable angina (please see "Revascularization" section under Stable Angina).

CHAPTER 4

○ The urgency of revascularization should weigh heavily in the decision for CABG; patients in cardiogenic shock may benefit from PCI and mechanical support compared to emergency cardiac surgery.

○ NSTEMI in the setting of critical left main CAD should prompt urgent surgical revascularization and consideration of intra-aortic balloon pump (IABP) for stabilization prior to the induction of anesthesia.

MONITORING/FOLLOW-UP

The highest rate of progression to MI or development of recurrent MI is in the first 2 months after presentation with the index episode. Beyond that time, most patients have a clinical course similar to those with chronic stable angina.

• Patients should be discharged on dual antiplatelet, BB, and statin therapy.
• Most patients should be discharged on ACE inhibitors.
• Patients should be evaluated for the need of aldosterone antagonists.
• Screen for life stressors and depression. Refer for depression treatment as needed.
• Smoking cessation and risk factor modification should be stressed.
• Referral to cardiac rehabilitation should also be pursued.

ST-Segment Elevation Myocardial Infarction

GENERAL PRINCIPLES

Definition

• STEMI is defined as a clinical syndrome of myocardial ischemia in association with persistent ECG ST elevations (see "Diagnostic Testing" section).
• STEMI is a medical emergency.
• Compared to UA/NSTEMI, STEMI is associated with a higher in-hospital and 30-day morbidity and mortality. Left untreated, the mortality rate of STEMI can exceed 30%, and the presence of mechanical complications (papillary muscle rupture, ventricular septal defect [VSD], and free wall rupture) increases the mortality rate to 90%.
• Ventricular fibrillation (VF) accounts for approximately 50% of mortality and often occurs within the first hour from symptom onset.
• Keys to treatment of STEMI include rapid recognition and diagnosis, coordinated mobilization of health care resources, and prompt reperfusion therapy.
• Mortality is directly related to total ischemia time.
• AHA/ACC guidelines provide a more thorough overview of STEMI.[75]

Epidemiology

• STEMI accounts for approximately 25%–30% of ACS cases annually, and the incidence has been declining.
• Over the last several decades, there has been a dramatic improvement in short-term mortality to the current rate of 6%–10%.
• Approximately 30% of STEMI presentations occur in women, but outcomes and complications continue to be worse compared with male counterparts.

Pathophysiology

• STEMI is caused by acute, total occlusion of an epicardial coronary artery, most often due to atherosclerotic plaque rupture/erosion and subsequent thrombus formation.
• As compared to NSTEMI/UA, thrombotic occlusion is complete such that there is total transmural ischemia/infarct in the distribution of the large, occluded artery.

DIAGNOSIS

Clinical Presentation

History

- Severe tearing chest pain or focal neurologic deficits should raise concern for aortic dissection. Aortic dissection can mimic ACS; in addition, dissections of the ascending aorta may involve the right coronary artery and cause ST elevations on the ECG.
- STEMI may have an atypical presentation particularly in female, elderly, and postoperative patients, as well as those with diabetes and chronic or end-stage kidney disease. Such patients may experience atypical or no chest pain and may instead present with confusion, dyspnea, unexplained hypotension, or HF.
- STEMI should always be considered as an etiology when any patient is hemodynamically compromised (i.e., postoperative, delirium, or shock).
- The initial history by the clinician should always include an inquiry about prior cardiac procedures or surgery. Prior PCI or CABG can have profound implications for acute revascularization management.
- The clinician should assess for absolute and relative contraindications to thrombolytic therapy (see the following text) and potential issues complicating primary PCI (IV contrast allergy, PVD/peripheral revascularization, renal dysfunction, central nervous system disease, pregnancy, bleeding diathesis, or severe comorbidity).
- Inquire about recent cocaine use. In this setting, aggressive medical therapy with nitroglycerin, coronary vasodilators, and benzodiazepines should be administered before reperfusion therapy is considered.

Physical Examination

Physical examination should be directed at identifying hemodynamic instability, pulmonary congestion, mechanical complications of MI, and other causes of acute chest discomfort.

- The identification of a new systolic murmur may suggest the presence of ischemic MR or a VSD.
- A limited neurologic exam to detect baseline cognitive and motor deficits and a vascular examination (lower extremity pulses and bruits) will aid in determining candidacy and planning for reperfusion treatment.
- Cardiogenic shock due to right ventricular MI (RVMI) may be clinically suspected by the presence of hypotension, elevated jugular venous pressure, and absence of pulmonary congestion.
- Bilateral arm BPs should be obtained to assess for the presence of aortic dissection.

Diagnostic Testing

Electrocardiography

The ECG is paramount to the diagnosis of STEMI and should be obtained within 10 minutes of presentation. If the diagnosis of STEMI is in doubt, serial ECGs may help elucidate the diagnosis. Classic findings include the following:

- Peaked upright T waves are the first ECG manifestation of myocardial injury.
- ST elevations correlate with the territory of injured myocardium (Table 4-14).
- **Diagnostic ECG criteria for STEMI**[76]
  - When ST elevations reach threshold values in two or more anatomically contiguous leads, a diagnosis of STEMI can be made.
  - In men > 40 years of age, threshold value for abnormal ST-segment elevation at the J point is ≥2 mm in leads V_2 and V_3 and >1 mm in all other leads. In men < 40 years of age, threshold value for abnormal ST-segment elevation at the J point in leads V_2 and V_3 is >2.5 mm.

CHAPTER 4

TABLE 4-14	Electrocardiogram-Based Anatomic Distribution	
ST Elevation	**Myocardial Territory**	**Coronary Artery**
V_1–V_6 or LBBB	Anterior and septal walls	Proximal LAD or left main
V_1–V_2	Septum	Proximal LAD or septal branch
V_2–V_4	Anterior wall	LAD
V_5–V_6	Lateral wall	LCX
II, III, aVF	Inferior wall	RCA or LCX
I, aVL	High lateral wall	Diagonal or proximal LCX

LAD, left anterior descending artery; LBBB, left bundle branch block; LCX, left circumflex artery; RCA, right coronary artery.

- In women, the threshold value of abnormal ST-segment elevation at the J point is >1.5 mm in leads V_2 and V_3 and >1 mm in all other leads.
- In right-sided leads (V_3R and V_4R), the threshold for abnormal ST elevation at the J point is 0.5 mm, except in males <30 years in whom it is 1 mm. Right-sided leads should be obtained in all patients with evidence of inferior wall ischemia to rule out RV ischemia. RV infarction can occur with proximal right coronary artery (RCA) lesions.
- In posterior leads (V_7, V_8, and V_9), the threshold for abnormal ST elevation at the J point is 0.5 mm.
  - All patients with ST-segment depression in leads V_1–V_3, inferior wall ST elevation, or tall R waves in V_1–V_3 should have posterior leads placed in order to diagnose a posterior wall MI. Posterior STEMIs are usually due to occlusion of the circumflex artery and are often misdiagnosed as UA/NSTEMI. R waves in V_1 or V_2 represent Q waves of the posterior territory.
  - Ischemia of the circumflex artery may also be electrocardiographically silent.
- The presence of reciprocal ST-segment depression opposite of the infarct territory increases the specificity for acute MI.
- New LBBB suggests a large anterior wall MI with a worse prognosis.
- ECG criteria for STEMI in patients with preexisting LBBB or RV pacing can be found in Table 4-15. Above criteria do not apply.
- **ECG changes that mimic MI.** ST-segment elevation and Q waves may result from numerous etiologies other than acute MI, including prior MI with aneurysm formation, aortic dissection, LV hypertrophy, pericarditis, myocarditis, pulmonary embolism, or they may be a normal finding (Table 4-16). It is critical to obtain prior ECGs to clarify the diagnosis.
- **Q waves.** Development of new pathologic Q waves is considered diagnostic for transmural MI but may occur in patients with prolonged ischemia or poor collateral supply. The presence of Q waves only is not an indication for acute reperfusion therapy; however, it is very helpful to have an old ECG to compare to in order to determine chronicity. Diagnostic criteria include the following:
  - In leads V_2 and V_3, a pathologic Q wave is ≥0.02 second or a QS complex in V_2 or V_3. An isolated Q wave in lead V_1 or lead III is normal.
  - In leads other than V_1 through V_3, presence of a Q wave ≥0.03 second and ≥0.1 mV deep or a QS complex in any two contiguous leads suggests prior MI.
  - R wave ≥0.04 second in V_1 and V_2 and R/S ratio ≥1 with a positive T wave suggest prior posterior MI (in the absence of RV hypertrophy or right bundle branch block [RBBB]).

TABLE 4-15	Criteria for ST-Segment Elevation for Prior LBBB or RV-Paced Rhythm
ECG Change	
ST-segment elevation >1 mm in the presence of a positive QRS complex (concordant with the QRS)	
ST-segment elevation >5 mm in the presence of a negative QRS complex (disconcordant with the QRS)	
ST-segment depression >1 mm in V_1–V_3	

LBBB, left bundle branch block; RV, right ventricular.
Sgarbossa's (GUSTO) criteria: *Am J Cardiol.* 1996;77:423; *N Engl J Med.* 1996;334:481; *Pacing Clin Electrophysiol.* 2001;24:1289.

Laboratories and Imaging
- STEMI diagnosis and initiation of treatment are done in a patient who reports prolonged chest discomfort or anginal equivalent with qualifying ECG findings. Attempting to wait for results of cardiac biomarkers will add unnecessary delay.
- Blood samples should be sent for cardiac biomarkers (troponin), complete blood cell count, coagulation studies (aPTT, prothrombin time [PT], international normalized ratio [INR]), creatinine, electrolytes including magnesium, and type and screen. A lipid profile should be obtained in all patients with STEMI for secondary prevention (note however, that lipid levels may be falsely lowered during the acute phase of MI).
- Initial cardiac biomarkers (including troponin assays) may be normal, depending on the time in relation to symptom onset.
- The risk of subsequent cardiac death is directly proportional to the increase in cardiac-specific troponins. Measuring biomarkers until the peak level has been attained can be used to determine infarct size.
- Routine use of cardiac noninvasive imaging is not recommended for the initial diagnosis of STEMI. When the diagnosis is in question, a TTE can be performed to document regional wall motion abnormalities. If not adequately evaluated by TTE,

TABLE 4-16	Differential Diagnosis of ST-Segment Elevation on ECG Excluding STEMI	
Cardiac Etiologies		**Other Etiologies**
Prior MI with aneurysm formation		Pulmonary embolism
Aortic dissection with coronary involvement		Hyperkalemia
Pericarditis		
Myocarditis		
LV hypertrophy or aortic stenosis (with strain)[a]		
Hypertrophic cardiomyopathy		
Coronary vasospasm (cocaine, Prinzmetal angina)		
Early repolarization (normal variant)		
Brugada syndrome		

LV, left ventricular; MI, myocardial infarction; ST-segment elevation myocardial infarction.
[a]Strain may occur in numerous settings including systemic hypertension, hypotension, tachycardia, exercise, and sepsis.

CHAPTER 4

a transesophageal echocardiogram (TEE) can be obtained to assess for acute complications of MI and presence of aortic dissection.
• A portable chest radiograph is useful to assess for pulmonary edema and evaluate for other causes of chest pain including aortic dissection. Importantly, a normal mediastinal width does not exclude aortic dissection, especially if clinically suspected.

TREATMENT

• Prompt treatment should be initiated as soon as the diagnosis is suspected, as mortality and risk of subsequent HF are directly related to ischemia time (Figure 4-4).
• All medical centers should have in place and use an AHA/ACC guideline–based STEMI protocol. Centers that are not primary PCI capable should have protocols

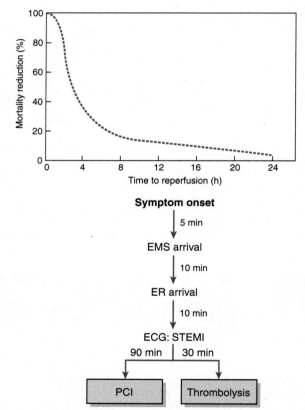

Figure 4–4. The benefit of coronary reperfusion is inversely related to ischemia time. **Top.** Graphic representation of mortality benefit of coronary reperfusion as a function of ischemia time.[77] **Bottom.** Recommended timeline of events following chest pain onset according to AHA/ACC guidelines.[78] AHA/ACC, American Heart Association/American College of Cardiology; ECG, electrocardiogram; EMS, emergency medical service; ER, emergency room; PCI, percutaneous coronary intervention; STEMI, ST-segment elevation myocardial infarction.

in place to meet accepted time-to-therapy guidelines, with either rapid transfer to a PCI-capable facility or administration of thrombolytics with subsequent transfer to a PCI center.

- **In the emergency department**, an acute MI protocol should be activated that includes a targeted clinical examination and a 12-lead ECG completed within 10 minutes of arrival.
- The goal of immediate management in patients with STEMI is to identify candidates for reperfusion therapy and to immediately initiate that process. Other priorities include relief of ischemic pain, as well as recognition and treatment of hypotension, pulmonary edema, and arrhythmia.
  - ○ Supplemental oxygen should be administered if saturations are <90%. If necessary, institution of mechanical ventilation decreases the work of breathing and reduces myocardial oxygen demand.
  - ○ Serial ECGs should be obtained for patients who do not have ST-segment elevation on the initial ECG but experience ongoing chest discomfort as they may have an evolving STEMI. Telemetry should be placed to monitor for arrhythmias.

Medications

Upstream medical therapy should include administration of ASA, a second antiplatelet agent, an anticoagulant, and agents that reduce myocardial ischemia (Table 4-17).

- **ASA** 162–325 mg should be given orally (chewed) or rectally immediately to *all* patients with suspected acute MI; 325 mg is preferred for those who are ASA naïve. After PCI, the subsequent dose of ASA is 81 mg/d indefinitely.[80]

TABLE 4-17	Upstream Medical Therapy	
Medication	Dosage	Comments
Aspirin (ASA)	162–325 mg	Non–enteric-coated formulations (chewed or crushed) given orally or rectally facilitate rapid drug absorption and platelet inhibition.
Clopidogrel	600 mg loading dose, 75–150 mg/d	600 mg loading dose followed by 150 mg maintenance dose for 7 d may reduce the incidence of stent thrombosis and MI compared to the standard 300 mg loading dose and 75 mg maintenance dose.
		Caution should be used in the elderly because clinical trials validating clopidogrel use in STEMI either did not include elderly patients or did not use a loading dose.
Prasugrel	60 mg loading dose, 10 mg/d	Compared to clopidogrel, prasugrel is a quicker acting and more potent antiplatelet agent with improved efficacy but did significantly increase CABG bleeding rates.
		Prasugrel should not be used in patients >75 y old, <60 kg, or with a history of stroke/TIA.

CHAPTER 4

TABLE 4-17	Upstream Medical Therapy *(continued)*	
Medication	**Dosage**	**Comments**
Ticagrelor	180 mg loading, then 90 mg bid	ASA dose should not exceed 100 mg. Ticagrelor has shown mortality benefit over clopidogrel at the expense of higher bleeding rates.
Cangrelor	30 µg/kg IV bolus, then 4 µg/kg/min	Currently FDA-approved only for patients undergoing PCI. Expense and modest evidence of benefit compared to other $P2Y_{12}$ inhibitors limit use.
Unfractionated heparin (UFH)	60 units/kg IV bolus, then 12 units/kg/h	UFH should be given to all patients undergoing PCI and those receiving thrombolytics with the exception of streptokinase. The maximum IV bolus is 4000 units.
Enoxaparin (LMWH)	30 mg IV bolus, then 1 mg/kg Sub-Q bid	Patients >75 y old should not be given a loading dose and receive 0.75 mg/kg SC bid.
		An additional loading dose of 0.3 mg/kg should be given if the last dose of LMWH was >8 h prior to PCI. The use of LMWH is only validated in thrombolysis and rescue PCI.
Bivalirudin	0.75 mg/kg IV bolus, then 1.75 mg/kg/h	Bivalirudin has been validated in patients undergoing PCI and has not been studied in conjunction with thrombolysis.
		Patients who received a heparin bolus prior to bivalirudin had a lower incidence of stent thrombosis than those who only received bivalirudin.
Fondaparinux	2.5 mg IV bolus, 2.5 mg Sub-Q daily	Shown to be superior to UFH when used during thrombolysis with decreased bleeding rates.
		Fondaparinux increases the risk of catheter thrombosis when used during PCI.[79]
Nitroglycerin	0.4 mg SL or aerosol infusion; 10–200 µg/min IV	Sublingual or aerosol nitroglycerin can be given every 5 min for a total of three doses in the absence of hypotension. IV nitroglycerin can be used for uncontrolled chest discomfort.
Metoprolol	25 mg PO qid, uptitrate as needed	β-Blockers should be avoided in patients with evidence of heart failure, hemodynamic instability, marked first-degree AV block, advanced heart block, and bronchospasm.

AV, atrioventricular; CABG, coronary artery bypass graft; LMWH, low–molecular-weight heparin; MI, myocardial infarction; PCI, percutaneous coronary intervention; SL, sublingual; STEMI, ST-segment elevation myocardial infarction; TIA, transient ischemic attack.

- **P2Y$_{12}$ inhibitor** loading dose should be given to all STEMI patients, as part of DAPT, as soon as possible after presentation. Cost and bleeding risk should be taken into consideration when choosing an agent. (Please also refer to the antiplatelet section on UA/NSTEMI for background information and dosing on agents listed in the following text.)
  - If the patient is going for PCI, **one** of the following should be added to ASA and anticoagulant:
    - **Ticagrelor** 180 mg loading dose, then 90 mg bid (Note: maintenance ASA must be <100 mg daily) for a minimum of 12 months. It is the preferred P2Y$_{12}$ inhibitor for ACS due to its mortality advantage over others in this class.
    - **Clopidogrel** 600 mg loading dose, then 75 mg daily for 12 months.
    - **Prasugrel** 60 mg loading dose, then 10 mg daily for minimum of 12 months (contraindicated in patients with prior CVA/TIA or active pathological bleeding and avoided in those >75 years and with weight < 60 kg). **Prasugrel should only be given after diagnostic angiography** (or within an hour of PCI) given a higher incidence of bleeding compared to clopidogrel.[81]
  - If the patient is to receive fibrinolytic therapy, along with ASA and an anticoagulant, patients should receive:
    - Clopidogrel 300 mg loading dose if given during the first 24 hours of therapy; if started 24 hours after administration of fibrinolytics, a 600-mg loading dose is preferred. Maintenance is 75 mg/d.
    - Patients older than 75 years should not be given the loading dose.
- **GPIIb/IIIa inhibitors** do not have a routine role in the initial presentation of STEMI patients or as part of adjunctive therapy with thrombolytics.
- **Anticoagulant therapy** should be initiated on presentation in all patients with STEMI regardless of the choice of PCI or thrombolytic therapy. *Please also refer to the Medications section for UA/NSTEMI for background information on agents listed in the following text.*
  - **Anticoagulant choice for patients who will receive primary PCI:**
    - **UFH** is often preferred during PCI by many operators due to the availability and real-time therapeutic monitoring with activating clotting times (ACTs) in the catheterization laboratory. Additional bolus doses of UFH are given at PCI, with the dose and ACT goal dependent on whether a GPIIb/IIIa antagonist has been given.
    - **Enoxaparin** use in STEMI patients as an anticoagulant for PCI is unclear, and we generally do not recommend it.
    - **Bivalirudin** can be given to patients already treated with ASA and clopidogrel on presentation.
      - Bivalirudin is an acceptable alternative to the use of combined heparin and GPIIb/IIIa inhibitor during PCI with lower bleeding rates but higher rate of stent thrombosis.[82,83]
      - It is the agent of choice in patients with known HIT.
      - It can be given with or without prior treatment with UFH. If patient is being treated with UFH, discontinue UFH for 30 minutes prior to starting bivalirudin.
      - Dose is 0.75 mg/kg bolus, then 1.75 mg/kg/h infusion.
  - **Patients who will receive fibrinolytic therapy should be started on either:**
    - **UFH** with monitoring to ensure the activated PTT is twice the upper limit of normal. UFH should be continued for at least 48 hours after fibrinolysis. If angiography with intent to perform PCI is anticipated to occur early after fibrinolysis, then UFH may be preferable.

- **Enoxaparin**, if the serum creatinine is <2.5 mg/dL in men or 2 mg/dL in women, an initial 30-mg IV bolus is given followed 15 minutes later with 1 mg/kg Sub-Q bid. Give for the entirety of the index hospitalization but not to exceed 8 days.
- **Bivalirudin** can be used for HIT-positive patients but has not been studied extensively in STEMI patients or patients with fibrinolysis.
- **Anti-ischemic therapy** (also refer to the Medications section for UA/NSTEMI for background information on agents listed here).
  - **Nitroglycerin** should be administered to patients with ischemic chest pain, to aid in control of hypertension, or as part of the management of HF. Nitroglycerin should either be avoided or used with caution in patients with:
    - Hypotension (systolic BP [SBP] < 90 mm Hg)
    - RV infarct
    - Heart rate > 100 bpm or <50 bpm
    - Documented use of phosphodiesterase inhibitors (e.g., sildenafil) in previous 48 hours
  - **Morphine** (2–4 mg IV) can be used for refractory chest pain that is not responsive to nitroglycerin. Adequate analgesia decreases levels of circulating catecholamines and reduces myocardial oxygen consumption.
  - **BBs** improve myocardial ischemia, limit infarct size, and reduce major adverse cardiac events including mortality, recurrent ischemia, and malignant arrhythmias.
    - Oral BBs should be started in all patients with STEMI within the first 24 hours who do not have signs of new HF, evidence of cardiogenic shock (Killip class II or greater), age older than 70 years, SBP < 120 mm Hg, pulse > 110 or <60 bpm, or advanced heart block.[84]
    - IV BBs can increase mortality in patients with STEMI and should be reserved for management of arrhythmias or acute treatment of accelerated hypertension in patients without the earlier mentioned features. Sinus tachycardia in the setting of a STEMI may be a compensatory response to maintain cardiac output and should not prompt IV BB use.

Acute Coronary Reperfusion

- The majority of patients who suffer an acute STEMI have thrombotic occlusion of a coronary artery. Early restoration of coronary perfusion limits infarct size, preserves LV function, and reduces mortality.
- All other therapies are secondary and should not delay the timely goal of achieving coronary reperfusion.
- Unless spontaneous resolution of ischemia occurs (as determined by resolution of chest discomfort and normalization of ST elevation), the choice of reperfusion strategy includes thrombolysis, primary PCI, or emergent CABG (Figure 4-5).
  - Normalization of the ECG and symptoms should not preclude the patient being referred for urgent diagnostic angiography. Morphine may mask ongoing ischemic symptoms.
  - Note: Ongoing symptoms are not required criteria for treatment of STEMI in the first 12 hours of symptom onset. Patients who arrive within 12 hours of their symptoms, despite symptom resolution, but with continued ECG changes of STEMI are still candidates for immediate reperfusion (either primary PCI or fibrinolytics). We recommend angiography with intent for PCI/CABG in such a circumstance.

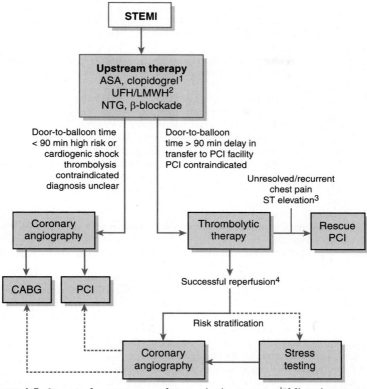

Figure 4-5. Strategies for coronary reperfusion and risk assessment. [1]If fibrinolytics are to be given, use clopidogrel only. If primary PCI is planned, give ticagrelor, prasugrel, or clopidogrel. [2]UFH may be used with either PCI or thrombolytic therapy, whereas bivalirudin has only been studied with PCI and LMWH has only been validated for fibrinolytic therapy and rescue PCI. In patients who are to receive fibrinolysis, LMWH and fondaparinux are preferred to UFH. [3]Patients who do not experience chest pain relief, have recurrent chest pain, have unstable arrhythmias, develop heart failure, or have ST-segment elevations that do not normalize 60–90 minutes following fibrinolysis should undergo rescue PCI. [4]Signs of successful reperfusion include chest pain relief, 50% reduction in ST-segment elevation, and idioventricular rhythm. $P2Y_{12}$ inhibitors include antiplatelet agents: clopidogrel, prasugrel, and ticagrelor. ASA, aspirin; CABG, coronary artery bypass graft; LMWH, low–molecular-weight heparin; NTG, nitroglycerin; PCI, percutaneous coronary intervention; STEMI, ST-segment elevation myocardial infarction; UFH, unfractionated heparin.

- The choice of reperfusion therapy should be considered of secondary importance to the overall goal of achieving reperfusion in a timely manner.
  - **Primary PCI**
    - Primary PCI is the preferred reperfusion strategy when available within 90 minutes of first medical contact. Compared to fibrinolytic therapy, PCI offers superior vessel patency and perfusion (TIMI 3 flow) with less reinfarction, less risk of intracranial hemorrhage, and improved survival regardless of lesion location

or patient age. STEMI patients with symptom onset <12 hours prior have a better prognosis and outcome after PCI. PCI should still be routinely offered to patients with STEMI who have ongoing symptoms that began 12–24 hours prior to presentation.

- PCI may also be considered, although evidence of benefit is limited, in patients who are now asymptomatic but had symptoms in the previous 12- to 24-hour period.
- Asymptomatic patients who are hemodynamically and electrically stable without evidence of ischemia and whose symptoms began more than 24 hours prior should not be offered PCI of a totally occluded infarct artery.[85]
- **PCI** is always preferred over fibrinolysis in the following situations:
  □ Patients who present with severe HF or cardiogenic shock should receive primary PCI (even if transfer to a PCI center may cause delays beyond current time goals for reperfusion). Patients with Killip class III/IV or TIMI risk score ≥5 represent high-risk groups where PCI is preferred despite a potential time delay.[86,87]
  □ Have a contraindication to fibrinolytic therapy.
  □ Have had recent PCI or prior CABG.
  □ PCI is generally preferred to fibrinolysis in patients with symptom onset >12 hours prior.[88,89]
- Coronary stenting is superior to balloon angioplasty alone and reduces the rates of target vessel revascularization.
- If the infarct-related artery is successfully treated and patients have lesions in non–infarct-related arteries that are amenable to PCI, complete revascularization results in a decrease in the composite of cardiovascular death and MI, as well as a decrease in future need for revascularization.[90] Timing, prior to discharge or return in the outpatient setting, should depend on the clinical stability of the patient and comorbid illnesses (i.e., renal function). Both are acceptable strategies for revascularization of nonculprit pathology.
- Previously, it was thought to be advantageous for patients in shock to have significant lesions in non–infarct-related arteries intervened on if feasible. However, in the CULPRIT-SHOCK trial, culprit-lesion only PCI resulted in a reduction in all-cause mortality and need for renal replacement therapy.[91]
- Transradial approach in STEMI reduces bleeding and may have a mortality benefit compared to transfemoral access.
  □ Dorsal radial artery access is another alternative.
- Facilitated PCI, a strategy of reduced dose of GPIIb/IIIa inhibitors and/or fibrinolytic agent just prior to PCI, should not be routinely used because it does not improve efficacy and significantly increases bleeding rates.

○ **Fibrinolytic therapy**
- Fibrinolytic therapy has the main advantages of widespread availability and ease of delivery. The primary disadvantages of fibrinolytic therapy are the risk of intracranial hemorrhage, uncertainty of whether normal coronary flow has been restored, and risk of re-occlusion of the infarct-related artery.
- Fibrinolysis is indicated when primary PCI is not available in a timely fashion (i.e., delay > 120 minutes or time-to-transfer > 120 minutes). Transfer to a PCI-capable facility should occur regardless of whether fibrinolytics are given or not.
- Fibrinolytic therapy is indicated for use if given within 12 hours of the symptom onset with qualifying ECG changes of ST elevation, new LBBB, or true posterior MI. When given, it should be administered within 30 minutes of initial patient contact. Fibrinolytic therapy is most successful when given in the first 3 hours of symptom onset, after which the benefit tapers.

- Patients presenting to a hospital without PCI capability should be transferred for primary PCI, rather than being given fibrinolytics, if time from first medical contact to PCI will not be >120 minutes. This seems particularly relevant to patients arriving 3–12 hours from symptom onset.
- In patients transferred for PCI, primary PCI significantly lowered the incidence of death, MI, or stroke compared to on-site thrombolysis.[91-94]
- All patients should be transferred to a PCI-capable facility after fibrinolysis (early routine angiography); this should occur urgently if patients are in shock or have failed reperfusion.
- Available thrombolytic agents include the fibrin-selective agents such as **alteplase (recombinant tissue plasminogen activator [rt-PA]), reteplase (r-PA), and tenecteplase** (TNK-tPA). **Streptokinase** is the only nonselective agent in use. Further details and dosing information can be found in Table 4-18.
  - □ TNK-tPA is the current agent of choice due to similar efficacy, lower risk of bleeding, and convenient single bolus administration as compared to rt-PA. Streptokinase is the cheapest and still widely used worldwide.
  - □ Fibrin-selective agents should be used in combination with anticoagulant therapy, ASA, and clopidogrel (see earlier). GPIIb/IIIa inhibitors should not be used in conjunction. Prasugrel and ticagrelor have not been studied for use with fibrinolytics.
- Fibrinolytic therapy is contraindicated:
  - □ In patients with ECG evidence of ST-segment depressions (unless posterior MI suspected).
  - □ In those who are asymptomatic with initial symptoms occurring >24 hours prior (*this is in contrast to patients who are asymptomatic with symptom onset <12 hours prior; see earlier*).
  - □ In patients with other contraindications to fibrinolysis (Table 4-19).
  - □ In patients with presence of five or more risk factors for intracranial hemorrhage.
- Any patient who experiences a sudden change in neurologic status should undergo urgent head CT, and all anticoagulant and thrombolytic therapies should be discontinued. Neurologic and neurosurgical consultation should be obtained immediately.
- Major bleeding complications that require blood transfusion occur in approximately 10% of patients.
- **Postfibrinolysis care**
  - □ All patients should receive appropriate DAPT and at least 48 hours of anticoagulation after fibrinolysis.
  - □ Routine coronary angiography within 24 hours of thrombolysis has reduced adverse cardiac events compared to rescue PCI.[99]
  - □ Immediate transfer for angiography (3–24 hours after fibrinolysis) at a PCI-capable facility is also proven to be beneficial.[100]
  - □ Evidence for successful fibrinolysis includes:
    - ▲ Relief of chest pain or angina symptoms
    - ▲ >50% reduction in ST-segment elevations at 90 minutes
    - ▲ Reperfusion arrhythmia (i.e., accelerated idioventricular rhythm) up to 2 hours after completion of infusion
  - ○ **Emergency CABG** is a high-risk procedure that should be considered only if the patient has severe left main disease or refractory ischemia in the setting of failed PCI or coronary anatomy that is not amenable to PCI. Emergency surgery should also be considered for patients with acute mechanical complications of MI including papillary muscle rupture, severe ischemic MR, VSD, ventricular aneurysm formation in the setting of intractable ventricular arrhythmias, or ventricular free wall rupture.

CHAPTER 4

TABLE 4-18	Fibrinolytic Agents	
Medication	**Dosage**	**Comments**
Streptokinase (SK)	1.5 million units IV over 60 min	Produces a generalized fibrinolytic state (not clot specific). SK reduces mortality following STEMI: 18% relative risk reduction and 2% absolute risk reduction.[95] Allergic reactions including skin rashes, fever, and anaphylaxis may be seen in 1%–2% of patients. Isolated hypotension occurs in 10% of patients and usually responds to volume expansion. Because of the development of antibodies, patients who were previously treated with SK should be given an alternate thrombolytic agent.
Recombinant tissue plasminogen activator (rt-PA)	15 mg IV bolus 0.75 mg/kg over 30 min (maximum 50 mg) 0.5 mg/kg over 60 min (maximum 35 mg)	Fibrin-selective agent with improved clot specificity compared to SK. Does not cause allergic reactions or hypotension. Mortality benefit compared to SK at the expense of an increased risk of intracranial hemorrhage.[96,97]
Reteplase (r-PA)	Two 10-unit IV boluses administered 30 min apart	Fibrin selective agent with a longer half-life but reduced clot specificity compared to rt-PA. Mortality benefit equivalent to that of rt-PA.[97]
Tenecteplase (TNK-tPA)	0.5 mg/kg IV bolus (total dose 30–50 mg)	Genetically engineered variant of rt-PA with slower plasma clearance, improved fibrin specificity, and higher resistance to PAI-1. Mortality benefit equivalent to that of rt-PA with reduced bleeding rates.[98] Monitoring is required with a goal aPTT of 1.5–2.5 times control.

aPTT, activated partial thromboplastin time; PAI-1, plasminogen activator inhibitor-1; STEMI, ST-segment elevation myocardial infarction.

Peri-Infarct Management

- **The coronary care unit (CCU)** was the first major advance in the modern era of treatment of acute MI. All patients with STEMI should be observed in a specialized CCU or intensive care unit setting for at least 24 hours after STEMI.
- Patients should have continuous telemetry monitoring to detect for recurrent ischemia and arrhythmias.

TABLE 4-19	Contraindications to Thrombolytic Therapy
Absolute Contraindications	**Relative Contraindications**
History of intracranial hemorrhage or hemorrhagic stroke	Prior ischemic stroke > 3 mo ago
Ischemic stroke within 3 mo	Allergy or previous use of streptokinase (>5 d ago)[a]
Known structural cerebrovascular lesion (AVMs, aneurysms, tumor)	Recent internal bleeding (2–4 wk)
Closed head injury within 3 mo	Prolonged/traumatic CPR more than 10 min
Aortic dissection	Major surgery within 3 weeks
Severe uncontrolled hypertension (SBP > 180 mm Hg, DBP > 110 mm Hg)	Active peptic ulcer disease
	Noncompressible vascular punctures
Active bleeding or bleeding diathesis	History of intraocular bleeding
Acute pericarditis	Pregnancy
	Uncontrolled hypertension
	Use of oral anticoagulants

AVM, arteriovenous malformation; CPR, cardiopulmonary resuscitation; DBP, diastolic blood pressure; SBP, systolic blood pressure.
[a]Thrombolytics other than streptokinase may be used.

- Daily evaluation should include assessment for recurrent chest discomfort, new HF symptoms, and routine ECGs. Physical exam should focus on new murmurs and any evidence of HF.
- A baseline echocardiogram should be obtained to document EF, wall motion abnormalities, valvular lesions, and presence of ventricular thrombus.
- **Cardiac pacing** may be required in the setting of an acute MI. Rhythm disturbance may be transient in nature, in which case temporary pacing is sufficient until a stable rhythm returns (see the following text). As compared to inferior wall MIs where AV block is transient and stable, AV block with anterior wall MIs can be unstable with wide QRS escape rhythms with 80% mortality and usually requires temporary and then permanent pacemakers.

Post-STEMI Medical Therapy
- See also Medications section for UA/NSTEMI.
- **ASA** should be continued indefinitely. Dose of 81 mg/d has been shown to be effective after PCI; however, the range of 75–162 mg/d has also been endorsed.
- **Clopidogrel** (75 mg/d), **prasugrel** (10 mg/d), or **ticagrelor** (90 mg bid) should be given for a minimum of 12 months regardless of whether a bare metal stent (BMS) or drug-eluting stent (DES) was used (*this is in contrast to non-ACS patients who receive a BMS and the minimum duration of therapy is 1 month*).
- **BBs** confer a mortality benefit following acute MI. Treatment should begin as soon as possible (preferably within the first 24 hours) and continued indefinitely unless contraindicated.
- **ACE inhibitors** provide a reduction in short-term mortality, incidence of HF, and recurrent MI when initiated within the first 24 hours of an acute MI.[101,102]
  - Patients with EF < 40%, large anterior MI, and prior MI derive the most benefit from ACE inhibitor therapy.
  - Contraindications include hypotension, history of angioedema with use, pregnancy, acute renal failure, and hyperkalemia.
  - ARBs can be used in patients who are intolerant of ACE inhibitors.

- **HMG-CoA reductase inhibitors** should be started in all patients in the absence of contraindications. Several trials have shown the benefit of early and aggressive use of high-dose statins following acute MI. The goal is at least 50% reduction in LDL or LDL <70 mg/dL. Patients unable to achieve LDL < 70 mg/dL despite a high intensity should be evaluated for adjunctive therapy with a PCSK9 inhibitor or ezetimibe.
- **Aldosterone receptor antagonists (spironolactone and eplerenone)** have shown benefit in post-MI patients with LVEF < 40% and in diabetics.[103,104] Caution should be used in patients with hyperkalemia and renal insufficiency.
- **Warfarin** should not be routinely prescribed to patients with apical hypokinesis in the setting of an anterior MI in the absence of LV thrombus or other indications for anticoagulation. Such therapy is associated with increased bleeding and death. The actual risk of developing LV thrombus is low because many patients will have recovery of hypokinesis.[105]

SPECIAL CONSIDERATIONS

- **Special clinical situations**
  - **RVMI** is seen in patients with an acute inferior MI secondary to complete occlusion of the proximal RCA. RV function is very preload dependent, and frequently, hypotension responds to fluid resuscitation.
    - The clinical triad of hypotension, elevated jugular venous pressure, and clear lung fields in the setting of STEMI should prompt an evaluation for RV infarct or massive pulmonary embolism.
    - One-mm ST elevations in the V_1 or V_4R leads are the most sensitive marker of RV involvement.
    - Initial therapy is IV fluids. If hypotension persists, inotropic support with dobutamine and/or IABP may be necessary. Right-sided mechanical support devices are available when pharmacologic support fails.
    - Invasive hemodynamic monitoring is critical in the persistently hypotensive patient because it guides volume status and the need for inotropic and mechanical support.
    - In patients with heart block and AV dyssynchrony, sequential AV pacing has a marked beneficial effect.
  - **Restenosis and stent thrombosis** are disease entities unique to patients who have previously undergone PCI.
    - **Restenosis** is a result of neointimal hyperplasia and occurs more frequently in patients with BMS placement, diabetics, patients with long areas of prior stenting, and patients with stenting in small arteries.
    - **Stent thrombosis** is the thrombotic occlusion of a previously placed coronary stent and presents as ACS or sudden cardiac death. Stent thrombosis is associated with a high mortality rate and poor prognosis.[106,107]
      - Acute stent thrombosis occurs within 24 hours and is due to mechanical procedural complications as well as inadequate anticoagulation and antiplatelet therapies.
      - Subacute stent thrombosis (24 hours–30 days) is a consequence of inadequate platelet inhibition and mechanical stent complications. Cessation of $P2Y_{12}$ inhibitor therapy during this time yields a 30- to 100-fold risk of stent thrombosis.
      - Late (30 days–1 year) stent thrombosis and very late stent thrombosis occurs principally with DESs.
      - Neoatherosclerosis is atherosclerotic plaque unique to prior PCI, occurs in previously placed stents, and can predispose a patient to angina or plaque rupture with subsequent ACS.

○ **Ischemic MR** is a poor prognostic indicator following MI. Papillary muscle rupture is associated with inferior and posterior infarcts. The anterior papillary muscle has a dual blood supply and is less vulnerable to rupture. The mechanism of chronic MR after STEMI includes papillary muscle dysfunction or leaflet tethering due to posterior wall akinesis.

- Acute MR from papillary muscle rupture is a severe complication of MI associated with high mortality (see below).
- Progressive MR following MI may develop as a result of LV chamber dilation, apical remodeling, or posterior wall dyskinesis. These changes lead to leaflet tethering or mitral annular dilation.
- Echocardiography is the diagnostic modality of choice.
- Initial treatment of MR involves aggressive afterload reduction and revascularization. *Stable* patients should receive a trial of medical therapy and undergo surgery only if they fail to improve.

○ **STEMI** in the setting of recent **cocaine use** presents a unique and challenging management situation.[108] ST elevation can result from myocardial ischemia due to coronary vasospasm, in situ thrombus formation, and/or increased myocardial oxygen demand. The common pathophysiology is excessive stimulation of α- and β-adrenergic receptors. Chest pain due to cocaine use usually occurs within 3 hours but may be seen several days following use.

- Oxygen, ASA, and heparin (UFH or LMWH) should be administered to all patients with cocaine-associated STEMI.
- Nitrates should be used preferentially to treat vasospasm. Additionally, benzodiazepines may confer additional relief by decreasing sympathetic tone.
- BBs are contraindicated; both selective and nonselective BBs should be avoided.
- Phentolamine (α-adrenergic antagonist) and calcium channel blockers may reverse coronary vasospasm and are recommended as second-line agents.
- The use of reperfusion therapy is controversial and should be reserved for those patients whose symptoms persist despite initial medical therapy.
  □ Primary PCI is the preferred approach for the patient with persistent symptoms and ECG changes despite aggressive medical therapy. It is important to note that coronary angiography and intervention carry a significant risk of worsening vasospasm.
  □ Fibrinolytic therapy should be reserved for patients who are clearly having a STEMI and who cannot undergo PCI.

COMPLICATIONS

Myocardial damage predisposes the patient to several potential adverse consequences and complications that should be considered if the patient experiences new clinical signs and/or symptoms. These include recurrent chest pain, cardiac arrhythmias, cardiogenic shock, and mechanical complications of MI.

- **Recurrent chest pain** may be due to ischemia in the territory of the original infarction, pericarditis, myocardial rupture, or pulmonary embolism.
  ○ Recurrent angina is experienced by 20%–30% of patients after MI who receive fibrinolytic therapy and up to 10% of patients in the early time period following percutaneous revascularization. These symptoms may represent recurrence of ischemia or infarct extension.
    - Assessment of the patient may include evaluation for new murmurs or friction rubs, ECG to assess for new ischemic changes, cardiac biomarkers (troponin and CK-MB), echocardiography, and repeat coronary angiography if indicated.

CHAPTER 4

- Patients with recurrent chest pain should continue to receive ASA, $P2Y_{12}$ inhibition, anticoagulants, nitroglycerin, and BB therapy.
- If recurrent angina is refractory to medical treatment, urgent repeat coronary angiography and intervention should be considered.

○ **Acute pericarditis** occurs 24–96 hours after MI in approximately 10%–15% of patients. The associated chest pain is often pleuritic and may be relieved in the upright position. A friction rub may be noted on clinical examination, and the ECG may show diffuse ST-segment elevation and PR-segment depression. Lead AVR may have PR elevation. Treatment is directed at pain management.

  - High-dose ASA (up to 650 mg qid maximum) is generally considered a first-line agent. NSAIDs such as ibuprofen may be used if ASA is not effective but should be avoided early after acute MI.
  - Colchicine along with ASA may also be beneficial for recurrent symptoms and may also be superior to each agent alone.
  - Glucocorticoids (prednisone 1 mg/kg daily) may be useful if symptoms are severe and refractory to initial therapy. Steroids should be used sparingly because they may lead to an increased risk of recurrence of pericarditis. Use should also be deferred until at least 4 weeks after acute MI due to their adverse impact on infarct healing and risk of ventricular aneurysm.
  - Heparin should be avoided in the setting of pericarditis with or without pericardial effusion because it may lead to pericardial hemorrhage.

○ **Dressler syndrome** is thought to be an autoimmune process characterized by malaise, fever, pericardial pain, leukocytosis, elevated erythrocyte sedimentation rate, and often a pericardial effusion. In contrast to acute pericarditis, Dressler syndrome occurs 1–8 weeks after MI. Treatment is identical to acute pericarditis.

○ **Arrhythmias.** Cardiac rhythm abnormalities are common following MI and may include conduction block, atrial arrhythmias, and ventricular arrhythmias. Arrhythmias that result in hemodynamic compromise require prompt, aggressive intervention. If the arrhythmia precipitates refractory angina or HF, urgent therapy is warranted. For all rhythm disturbances, exacerbating conditions should be addressed, including electrolyte imbalances, hypoxia, acidosis, and adverse drug effects. Refer to section on Cardiac Arrhythmia management for further details. **Atropine** should be attempted for all bradyarrhythmias in the setting of STEMI. Bradycardia is a common complication of intense vagal input to the AV node as a result of baroreceptor activation in the myocardium (also called Bezold-Jarisch reflex).

○ **Transcutaneous and transvenous pacing.** Conduction system disease that progresses to complete heart block or results in symptomatic bradycardia can be effectively treated with cardiac pacing. A transcutaneous pacing device can be used under emergent circumstances; however, a temporary transvenous system should be used for longer duration therapy.

  - Absolute indications for temporary transvenous pacing include asystole, symptomatic bradycardia, recurrent sinus pauses, complete heart block, and incessant polymorphic VT.
  - Temporary transvenous pacing may also be warranted for new trifascicular block, new Mobitz II block, and patients with LBBB who require a pulmonary artery catheter, given the risk of developing complete heart block.

○ **Implantable cardioverter-defibrillators (ICDs)** should not routinely be implanted in patients with reduced LV function following MI or those with VT/VF in the setting of ischemia or immediately following reperfusion (<48 hours).

  - Routine insertion of ICDs into patients with reduced LV function immediately following MI does not improve outcomes.[109-111]

- In patients with LVEF <35% less than 40 days post MI, consideration of a wearable cardioverter defibrillation (e.g., Zoll LifeVest) as a bridge to reevaluation for recovery of EF is reasonable.[112,113]
- ICD therapy is also indicated for patients with recurrent episodes of sustained VT or VF after >48 hours following coronary reperfusion.
- **Cardiogenic shock** is an infrequent, but serious, complication of MI and is defined as hypotension in the setting of inadequate ventricular function to meet the metabolic needs of the peripheral tissue. Risk factors include prior MI, older age, diabetes, and anterior infarction. Organ hypoperfusion may manifest as progressive renal failure, dyspnea, diaphoresis, or mental status changes. Hemodynamic monitoring reveals elevated filling pressures (wedge pressure >20 mm Hg), depressed cardiac index (<2.5 L/min/m^2), and hypotension.
  - Patients with cardiogenic shock in the setting of MI have a mortality rate in excess of 50%.
  - **Dobutamine and milrinone** are the most frequently used medications for inotropic support. They both possess vasodilatory properties (i.e., afterload reducing) and are arrhythmogenic. Milrinone should be avoided in the setting of renal insufficiency.
  - **Dopamine** can be used as both a vasopressor and inotrope but increases the risk of atrial arrhythmias in patients with shock and is not a preferred first-line agent.
  - **Norepinephrine and phenylephrine** may be required to maintain systemic BP. The use of any vasoconstrictive agents in the setting of cardiogenic shock should prompt an evaluation for mechanical circulatory support.
  - **Epinephrine** is a potent vasopressor and inotrope and is frequently used as an adjunct to other medical therapies. There may be some preferential benefit to RV function, and thus, epinephrine may be used for shock secondary to RV infarct or severe RV dysfunction.
  - **Mechanical circulatory support** includes both temporary and durable support devices. Temporary support devices include IABP, Impella catheter, or extracorporeal membrane oxygenation (ECMO). Temporary support is offered as bridge to recovery or as bridge to decision about long-term durable mechanical support such as an LV assist device (see Chapter 5, Heart Failure and Cardiomyopathy). The choice of temporary support device is not always clear and should be made by a team familiar with the management of cardiogenic shock.
  - All patients with cardiogenic shock should undergo echocardiography to evaluate for mechanical complications of MI (see the following text).
  - **LV thrombus** occurs most often in setting of anterior MI and should be treated with anticoagulation. Warfarin is the recommended long-term anticoagulation agent; direct oral anticoagulants (e.g., rivaroxaban, apixaban) have led to conflicting results regarding safety and efficacy compared to warfarin.[114,115] Patients should receive warfarin for 3–6 months unless other indications warrant its continued use. You may repeat a TTE to confirm resolution of the LV thrombus.
- **Mechanical complications**
  - **Aneurysm.** After MI, the affected area of the myocardium may undergo infarct expansion and thinning, forming an aneurysm. The wall motion may become dyskinetic, making the endocardial surface susceptible to mural thrombus formation.
    - LV aneurysm is suggested by persistent ST elevation on the ECG and may be diagnosed by imaging studies including ventriculography, echocardiography, and MRI.
    - Anticoagulation is warranted to lower the risk of embolic events, especially if a mural thrombus is present.

CHAPTER 4

- Surgical intervention may be appropriate if the aneurysm results in HF or ventricular arrhythmias that are not satisfactorily managed with medical therapy.
  - **Ventricular pseudoaneurysm.** Incomplete rupture of the myocardial free wall can result in formation of a ventricular pseudoaneurysm. In this case, blood escapes through the myocardial wall and is contained within the visceral pericardium. In the post-CABG patient, hemorrhage from frank ventricular rupture may be contained within the fibrotic pericardial space producing a pseudoaneurysm.
    - Echocardiography (TTE with contrast or TEE) is the preferred diagnostic test to assess for a pseudoaneurysm, often allowing differentiation from a true aneurysm.
    - Prompt surgical intervention for pseudoaneurysms is advised because of the high incidence of myocardial rupture.
  - **Free wall rupture** represents a rare but catastrophic complication of STEMI in the modern early-reperfusion era. Rupture typically occurs within the first week after MI and presents with sudden hemodynamic collapse. This complication can occur after anterior or inferior MI and is more commonly seen in hypertensive women with their first large transmural MI, in patients receiving late therapy with fibrinolytics, and patients given NSAIDs or glucocorticoids.
    - Echocardiography may identify patients with particularly thinned ventricular walls at risk for rupture.
    - Despite optimal intervention, mortality of free wall rupture remains >90%.
  - **Papillary muscle rupture** (*please also refer to earlier MR section*) is a rare complication after MI and is associated with abrupt clinical deterioration. The posterior medial papillary muscle is most commonly affected due to its isolated vascular supply, but anterolateral papillary muscle rupture has been reported. Of note, papillary muscle rupture may be seen in the setting of a relatively small acute MI or even NSTEMI.
    - The diagnostic test of choice is echocardiography with Doppler imaging and/or TEE because physical exam reveals a murmur in only ~50% of cases.
    - Initial medical therapy should include aggressive afterload reduction. Patients with refractory HF and those with hemodynamic instability may require inotropic support with dobutamine and/or IABP. Surgical repair is indicated in the majority of patients.
  - **Ventricular septal rupture** is most commonly associated with anterior MI occurring 3–5 days after MI. The perforation may follow a direct course between the ventricles or a serpiginous route through the septal wall.
    - Diagnosis can be made by echocardiography with Doppler imaging and often requires TEE.
    - Diagnosis should be suspected in the postinfarct patient who develops HF symptoms and a new holosystolic murmur.
    - Stabilization with afterload reduction, inotropic support, and/or IABP may be necessary for hemodynamically unstable patients until definitive therapy with surgical repair can be performed.
    - In hemodynamically stable patients, surgery is best deferred for at least a week to improve patient outcome. Left untreated, mortality approaches 90%.
    - Percutaneous device closure in the cardiac catheterization laboratory can be performed in select patients with an unacceptable surgical risk.

REFERENCES

1. Fihn SD, Gardin JM, Abrams J, et al. 2012 ACCF/AHA/ACP/AATS/PCNA/SCAI/STS guideline for the diagnosis and management of patients with stable ischemic heart disease: a report of the American College of Cardiology Foundation/American Heart Association Task Force on Practice Guidelines, and the American College of Physicians, American Association for Thoracic Surgery, Preventive Cardiovascular Nurses Association, Society for Cardiovascular Angiography and Interventions, and Society of Thoracic Surgeons. *J Am Coll Cardiol.* 2012;60(24):e44-e164.

2. Fihn SD, Blankenship JC, Alexander KP, et al. 2014 ACC/AHA/AATS/PCNA/SCAI/STS focused update of the guideline for the diagnosis and management of patients with stable ischemic heart disease: a report of the American College of Cardiology/American Heart Association Task Force on Practice Guidelines, and the American Association for Thoracic Surgery, Preventive Cardiovascular Nurses Association, Society for Cardiovascular Angiography and Interventions, and Society of Thoracic Surgeons. *J Am Coll Cardiol.* 2014;64(18):1929-1949.

3. Go AS, Mozaffarian D, Roger VL, et al. Heart disease and stroke statistics—2013 update: a report from the American Heart Association [published correction appears in *Circulation.* 2013 Jan 1;127(1):doi:10.1161/CIR.0b013e31828124ad] [published correction appears in *Circulation.* 2013 Jun 11;127(23):e841]. *Circulation.* 2013;127(1):e6-e245.

4. Arbab-Zadeh A, Nakano M, Virmani R, Fuster V. Acute coronary events. *Circulation.* 2012;125(9):1147-1156.

5. Greenland P, Knoll MD, Stamler J, et al. Major risk factors as antecedents of fatal and nonfatal coronary heart disease events. *JAMA.* 2003;290(7):891-897.

6. Kawachi I, Colditz GA, Stampfer MJ, et al. Smoking cessation and time course of decreased risks of coronary heart disease in middle-aged women. *Arch Intern Med.* 1994;154(2):169-175.

7. Goff DC Jr, Lloyd-Jones DM, Bennett G, et al. 2013 ACC/AHA guideline on the assessment of cardiovascular risk: a report of the American College of Cardiology/American Heart Association Task Force on Practice Guidelines [published correction appears in *J Am Coll Cardiol.* 2014 Jul 1;63(25 Pt B):3026]. *J Am Coll Cardiol.* 2014;63(25 pt B):2935-2959.

8. Sangareddi V, Chockalingam A, Gnanavelu G, Subramaniam T, Jagannathan V, Elangovan S. Canadian Cardiovascular Society classification of effort angina: an angiographic correlation. *Coron Artery Dis.* 2004;15(2):111-114.

9. Gibbons RJ, Balady GJ, Bricker JT, et al. ACC/AHA 2002 guideline update for exercise testing – summary article: a report of the American College of Cardiology/American Heart association task force on practice guidelines (committee to update the 1997 exercise testing guidelines). *Circulation.* 2002;106(14):1883-1892.

10. Wolk MJ, Bailey SR, Doherty JU, et al. ACCF/AHA/ASE/ASNC/HFSA/HRS/SCAI/SCCT/SCMR/STS 2013 multimodality appropriate use criteria for the detection and risk assessment of stable ischemic heart disease: a report of the American College of Cardiology Foundation Appropriate Use Criteria Task Force, American Heart Association, American Society of Echocardiography, American Society of Nuclear Cardiology, Heart Failure Society of America, Heart Rhythm Society, Society for Cardiovascular Angiography and Interventions, Society of Cardiovascular Computed Tomography, Society for Cardiovascular Magnetic Resonance, and Society of Thoracic Surgeons. *J Am Coll Cardiol.* 2014;63(4):380-406.

11. Mark DB, Shaw L, Harrell FE Jr, et al. Prognostic value of a treadmill exercise score in outpatients with suspected coronary artery disease. *N Engl J Med.* 1991;325(12):849-853.

12. Fearon WF, Nishi T, De Bruyne B, et al. Clinical outcomes and cost-effectiveness of fractional flow reserve-guided percutaneous coronary intervention in patients with stable coronary artery disease: three-year follow-up of the FAME 2 trial (fractional flow reserve versus angiography for multivessel evaluation). *Circulation.* 2018;137(5):480-487.

13. Al-Lamee R, Thompson D, Dehbi HM, et al. Percutaneous coronary intervention in stable angina (ORBITA): a double-blind, randomised controlled trial [published correction appears in *Lancet.* 2018 Jan 6;391(10115):30]. *Lancet.* 2018;391(10115):31-40.

14. Maron DJ, Hochman JS, Reynolds HR, et al. Initial invasive or conservative strategy for stable coronary disease. *N Engl J Med.* 2020;382(15):1395-1407.

15. Serruys PW, Kogame N, Katagiri Y, et al. Clinical outcomes of state-of-the-art percutaneous coronary revascularisation in patients with three-vessel disease: two-year follow-up of the SYNTAX II study. *EuroIntervention.* 2019;15(3):e244-e252. Published 2019 Jun 12.

16. Jeremias A, Davies JE, Maehara A, et al. Blinded physiological assessment of residual ischemia after successful angiographic percutaneous coronary intervention: the DEFINE PCI study. *JACC Cardiovasc Interv.* 2019;12(20):1991-2001.

17. Bangalore S, Maron DJ, Stone GW, Hochman JS. Routine revascularization versus initial medical therapy for stable ischemic heart disease: a systematic review and meta-analysis of randomized trials. *Circulation.* 2020;142(9):841-857.

CHAPTER 4

18. Tsai TT, Patel UD, Chang TI, et al. Validated contemporary risk model of acute kidney injury in patients undergoing percutaneous coronary interventions: insights from the National Cardiovascular Data Registry Cath-PCI Registry. *J Am Heart Assoc.* 2014;3(6):e001380.

19. Gulati M, Levy PD, Mukherjee D, et al. 2021 AHA/ACC/ASE/CHEST/SAEM/SCCT/SCMR guideline for the evaluation and diagnosis of chest pain: executive summary—a report of the American College of Cardiology/American heart association joint committee on clinical practice guidelines. *Circulation.* 2021;144(22):e368-e454. doi: 10.1161/CIR.0000000000001030. Epub 2021 Oct 28. PMID: 34709928.

20. Juul-Möller S, Edvardsson N, Jahnmatz B, Rosén A, Sørensen S, Omblus R. Double-blind trial of aspirin in primary prevention of myocardial infarction in patients with stable chronic angina pectoris. The Swedish Angina Pectoris Aspirin Trial (SAPAT) Group. *Lancet.* 1992;340(8833):1421-1425.

21. Sabatine MS, Giugliano RP, Keech AC, et al. Evolocumab and clinical outcomes in patients with cardiovascular disease. *N Engl J Med.* 2017;376(18):1713-1722.

22. Cannon CP, Blazing MA, Giugliano RP, et al. Ezetimibe added to statin therapy after acute coronary syndromes. *N Engl J Med.* 2015;372(25):2387-2397.

23. Head SJ, Milojevic M, Daemen J, et al. Mortality after coronary artery bypass grafting versus percutaneous coronary intervention with stenting for coronary artery disease: a pooled analysis of individual patient data [published correction appears in *Lancet.* 2018 Aug 11;392(10146):476]. *Lancet.* 2018;391(10124):939-948.

24. Kappetein AP, Feldman TE, Mack MJ, et al. Comparison of coronary bypass surgery with drug-eluting stenting for the treatment of left main and/or three-vessel disease: 3-year follow-up of the SYNTAX trial. *Eur Heart J.* 2011;32(17):2125-2134.

25. Serruys PW, Morice MC, Kappetein AP, et al. Percutaneous coronary intervention versus coronary-artery bypass grafting for severe coronary artery disease [published correction appears in *N Engl J Med.* 2013 Feb 7;368(6):584]. *N Engl J Med.* 2009;360(10):961-972.

26. Bypass Angioplasty Revascularization Investigation (BARI) Investigators. Comparison of coronary bypass surgery with angioplasty in patients with multivessel disease [published correction appears in *N Engl J Med* 1997 Jan 9;336(2):147]. *N Engl J Med.* 1996;335(4):217-225.

27. Banning AP, Westaby S, Morice MC, et al. Diabetic and nondiabetic patients with left main and/or 3-vessel coronary artery disease: comparison of outcomes with cardiac surgery and paclitaxel-eluting stents. *J Am Coll Cardiol.* 2010;55(11):1067-1075.

28. Velazquez EJ, Lee KL, Jones RH, et al. Coronary-artery bypass surgery in patients with ischemic cardiomyopathy. *N Engl J Med.* 2016;374(16):1511-1520.

29. Amsterdam EA, Wenger NK, Brindis RG, et al. 2014 AHA/ACC guideline for the management of patients with non-ST-elevation acute coronary syndromes: a report of the American College of Cardiology/American Heart Association Task Force on Practice Guidelines [published correction appears in *J Am Coll Cardiol.* 2014 Dec 23;64(24):2713-2714. Dosage error in article text]. *J Am Coll Cardiol.* 2014;64(24):e139-e228.

30. Anderson JL, Adams CD, Antman EM, et al. ACC/AHA 2007 guidelines for the management of patients with unstable angina/non-ST-Elevation myocardial infarction: a report of the American College of Cardiology/American Heart Association Task Force on Practice Guidelines (Writing Committee to Revise the 2002 Guidelines for the Management of Patients With Unstable Angina/Non-ST-Elevation Myocardial Infarction) developed in collaboration with the American College of Emergency Physicians, the Society for Cardiovascular Angiography and Interventions, and the Society of Thoracic Surgeons endorsed by the American Association of Cardiovascular and Pulmonary Rehabilitation and the Society for Academic Emergency Medicine [published correction appears in *J Am Coll Cardiol.* 2008 Mar 4;51(9):974]. *J Am Coll Cardiol.* 2007;50(7):e1-e157.

31. Stone PH, Thompson B, Anderson HV, et al. Influence of race, sex, and age on management of unstable angina and non-Q-wave myocardial infarction: the TIMI III registry. *JAMA.* 1996;275(14):1104-1112.

32. Ohman EM, Armstrong PW, Christenson RH, et al. Cardiac troponin T levels for risk stratification in acute myocardial ischemia. GUSTO IIA Investigators. *N Engl J Med.* 1996;335(18):1333-1341.

33. Killip TIIIrd, Kimball JT. Treatment of myocardial infarction in a coronary care unit. A two-year experience with 250 patients. *Am J Cardiol.* 1967;20(4):457-464.

34. Newby LK, Christenson RH, Ohman EM, et al. Value of serial troponin T measures for early and late risk stratification in patients with acute coronary syndromes. The GUSTO-IIa investigators. *Circulation.* 1998;98(18):1853-1859.

35. Sabatine MS, Morrow DA, de Lemos JA, et al. Multimarker approach to risk stratification in non-ST elevation acute coronary syndromes: simultaneous assessment of troponin I, C-reactive protein, and B-type natriuretic peptide. *Circulation.* 2002;105(15):1760-1763.

36. Antman EM, Cohen M, Bernink PJ, et al. The TIMI risk score for unstable angina/non-ST elevation MI: a method for prognostication and therapeutic decision making. *JAMA.* 2000;284(7):835-842.

37. Anderson JL, Adams CD, Antman EM, et al. ACC/AHA 2007 guidelines for the management of patients with unstable angina/non ST-elevation myocardial infarction: a report of the American College of Cardiology/American heart association Task Force on Practice guidelines (writing committee to revise

the 2002 guidelines for the management of patients with unstable Angina/non ST-elevation myocardial infarction)—developed in collaboration with the American College of emergency Physicians, the Society for cardiovascular angiography and interventions, and the Society of Thoracic Surgeons – endorsed by the American association of cardiovascular and pulmonary rehabilitation and the Society for academic emergency medicine [published correction appears in *Circulation*. 2008 Mar 4;117(9):e180]. *Circulation*. 2007;116(7):e148-e304.

38. Wijesinghe M, Perrin K, Ranchord A, Simmonds M, Weatherall M, Beasley R. Routine use of oxygen in the treatment of myocardial infarction: systematic review. *Heart*. 2009;95(3):198-202.

39. Yusuf S, Zhao F, Mehta SR, et al. Effects of clopidogrel in addition to aspirin in patients with acute coronary syndromes without ST-segment elevation [published correction appears in *N Engl J Med* 2001 Dec 6;345(23):1716] [published correction appears in *N Engl J Med* 2001 Nov 15;345(20):1506]. *N Engl J Med*. 2001;345(7):494-502.

40. Mehta SR, Yusuf S, Peters RJ, et al. Effects of pretreatment with clopidogrel and aspirin followed by long-term therapy in patients undergoing percutaneous coronary intervention: the PCI-CURE study. *Lancet*. 2001;358(9281):527-533.

41. Steinhubl SR, Berger PB, Mann JTIIIrd, et al. Early and sustained dual oral antiplatelet therapy following percutaneous coronary intervention: a randomized controlled trial [published correction appears in *JAMA*. 2003 Feb 26;289(8):987.]. *JAMA*. 2002;288(19):2411-2420.

42. Wallentin L, Becker RC, Budaj A, et al. Ticagrelor versus clopidogrel in patients with acute coronary syndromes. *N Engl J Med*. 2009;361(11):1045-1057.

43. Mahaffey KW, Wojdyla DM, Carroll K, et al. Ticagrelor compared with clopidogrel by geographic region in the Platelet Inhibition and Patient Outcomes (PLATO) trial. *Circulation*. 2011;124(5):544-554.

44. Wiviott SD, Braunwald E, McCabe CH, et al. Prasugrel versus clopidogrel in patients with acute coronary syndromes. *N Engl J Med*. 2007;357(20):2001-2015.

45. Platelet Glycoprotein IIb/IIIa in Unstable Angina: Receptor Suppression Using Integrilin Therapy (PURSUIT) Trial Investigators. Inhibition of platelet glycoprotein IIb/IIIa with eptifibatide in patients with acute coronary syndromes. *N Engl J Med*. 1998;339(7):436-443.

46. Kleiman NS, Lincoff AM, Flaker GC, et al. Early percutaneous coronary intervention, platelet inhibition with eptifibatide, and clinical outcomes in patients with acute coronary syndromes. PURSUIT investigators. *Circulation*. 2000;101(7):751-757.

47. Batchelor WB, Tolleson TR, Huang Y, et al. Randomized COMparison of platelet inhibition with abciximab, tiRofiban and eptifibatide during percutaneous coronary intervention in acute coronary syndromes: the COMPARE trial. Comparison of Measurements of Platelet aggregation with Aggrastat, Reopro, and Eptifibatide. *Circulation*. 2002;106(12):1470-1476

48. Effects of platelet glycoprotein IIb/IIIa blockade with tirofiban on adverse cardiac events in patients with unstable angina or acute myocardial infarction undergoing coronary angioplasty. The RESTORE Investigators. Randomized Efficacy Study of Tirofiban for Outcomes and REstenosis. *Circulation*. 1997;96(5):1445-1453.

49. Martinelli I, Sacchi E, Landi G, Taioli E, Duca F, Mannucci PM. High risk of cerebral-vein thrombosis in carriers of a prothrombin-gene mutation and in users of oral contraceptives. *N Engl J Med*. 1998;338(25):1793-1797.

50. Platelet Receptor Inhibition in Ischemic Syndrome Management in Patients Limited by Unstable Signs and Symptoms (PRISM-PLUS) Study Investigators. Inhibition of the platelet glycoprotein IIb/IIIa receptor with tirofiban in unstable angina and non-Q-wave myocardial infarction [published correction appears in *N Engl J Med* 1998 Aug 6;339(6):415]. *N Engl J Med*. 1998;338(21):1488-1497.

51. EPIC Investigators. Use of a monoclonal antibody directed against the platelet glycoprotein IIb/IIIa receptor in high-risk coronary angioplasty. *N Engl J Med*. 1994;330(14):956-961.

52. EPILOG Investigators. Platelet glycoprotein IIb/IIIa receptor blockade and low-dose heparin during percutaneous coronary revascularization. *N Engl J Med*. 1997;336(24):1689-1696.

53. Randomised placebo-controlled trial of abciximab before and during coronary intervention in refractory unstable angina: the CAPTURE study [published correction appears in *Lancet* 1997 Sep 6;350(9079):744]. *Lancet*. 1997;349(9063):1429-1435.

54. Simoons ML; GUSTO IV-ACS Investigators. Effect of glycoprotein IIb/IIIa receptor blocker abciximab on outcome in patients with acute coronary syndromes without early coronary revascularisation: the GUSTO IV-ACS randomised trial. *Lancet*. 2001;357(9272):1915-1924.

55. Wiviott SD, Trenk D, Frelinger AL, et al. Prasugrel compared with high loading and maintenance-dose clopidogrel in patients with planned percutaneous coronary intervention: the Prasugrel in Comparison to Clopidogrel for Inhibition of Platelet Activation and Aggregation-Thrombolysis in Myocardial Infarction 44 trial. *Circulation*. 2007;116(25):2923-2932.

56. Schüpke S, Neumann FJ, Menichelli M, et al. Ticagrelor or prasugrel in patients with acute coronary syndromes. *N Engl J Med*. 2019;381(16):1524-1534.

57. Bhatt DL, Stone GW, Mahaffey KW, et al. Effect of platelet inhibition with cangrelor during PCI on ischemic events. *N Engl J Med*. 2013;368(14):1303-1313.

CHAPTER 4

58. Abraham NS, Hlatky MA, Antman EM, et al. ACCF/ACG/AHA 2010 Expert Consensus Document on the concomitant use of proton pump inhibitors and thienopyridines—a focused update of the ACCF/ACG/AHA 2008 expert consensus document on reducing the gastrointestinal risks of antiplatelet therapy and NSAID use: a report of the American College of Cardiology Foundation Task Force on Expert Consensus Documents. *Circulation.* 2010;122(24):2619-2633.

59. Bhatt DL, Cryer BL, Contant CF, et al. Clopidogrel with or without omeprazole in coronary artery disease. *N Engl J Med.* 2010;363(20):1909-1917.

60. Sambola A, Mutuberría M, García Del Blanco B, et al. Effects of triple therapy in patients with non-valvular atrial fibrillation undergoing percutaneous coronary intervention regarding thromboembolic risk stratification. *Circ J.* 2016;80(2):354-362.

61. Levine GN, Bates ER, Bittl JA, et al. 2016 ACC/AHA guideline focused update on duration of dual antiplatelet therapy in patients with coronary artery disease: a report of the American College of Cardiology/American heart association Task Force on clinical Practice guidelines—an update of the 2011 ACCF/AHA/SCAI guideline for percutaneous coronary intervention, 2011 ACCF/AHA guideline for coronary artery bypass graft surgery, 2012 ACC/AHA/ACP/AATS/PCNA/SCAI/STS guideline for the diagnosis and management of patients with stable ischemic heart disease, 2013 ACCF/AHA guideline for the management of ST-elevation myocardial infarction, 2014 AHA/ACC guideline for the management of patients with non-ST-elevation acute coronary syndromes, and 2014 ACC/AHA guideline on Perioperative cardiovascular evaluation and management of patients undergoing noncardiac surgery [published correction appears in *Circulation.* 2016 Sep 6;134(10):e192-4]. *Circulation.* 2016;134(10):e123-e155.

62. Lopes RD, Heizer G, Aronson R, et al. Antithrombotic therapy after acute coronary syndrome or PCI in atrial fibrillation. *N Engl J Med.* 2019;380(16):1509-1524.doi: 10.1056/NEJMoa1817083. Epub 2019 Mar 17. PMID: 30883055.

63. Ferguson JJ, Califf RM, Antman EM, et al. Enoxaparin vs unfractionated heparin in high-risk patients with non-ST-segment elevation acute coronary syndromes managed with an intended early invasive strategy: primary results of the SYNERGY randomized trial. *JAMA.* 2004;292(1):45-54.

64. Oler A, Whooley MA, Oler J, Grady D. Adding heparin to aspirin reduces the incidence of myocardial infarction and death in patients with unstable angina. A meta-analysis. *JAMA.* 1996;276(10):811-815.

65. Cohen M, Demers C, Gurfinkel EP, et al. A comparison of low-molecular-weight heparin with unfractionated heparin for unstable coronary artery disease. Efficacy and Safety of Subcutaneous Enoxaparin in Non-Q-Wave Coronary Events Study Group. *N Engl J Med.* 1997;337(7):447-452.

66. Fifth Organization to Assess Strategies in Acute Ischemic Syndromes Investigators; Yusuf S, Mehta SR, et al. Comparison of fondaparinux and enoxaparin in acute coronary syndromes. *N Engl J Med.* 2006;354(14):1464-1476.

67. Cannon CP, Braunwald E, McCabe CH, et al. Intensive versus moderate lipid lowering with statins after acute coronary syndromes [published correction appears in *N Engl J Med.* 2006 Feb 16;354(7):778]. *N Engl J Med.* 2004;350(15):1495-1504.

68. Szummer K, Oldgren J, Lindhagen L, et al. Association between the use of fondaparinux vs low-molecular-weight heparin and clinical outcomes in patients with non-ST-segment elevation myocardial infarction. *JAMA.* 2015;313(7):707-716.

69. Stone GW, McLaurin BT, Cox DA, et al. Bivalirudin for patients with acute coronary syndromes. *N Engl J Med.* 2006;355(21):2203-2216.

70. Shahzad A, Kemp I, Mars C, et al. Unfractionated heparin versus bivalirudin in primary percutaneous coronary intervention (HEAT-PPCI): an open-label, single centre, randomised controlled trial [published correction appears in *Lancet.* 2014 Nov 22;384(9957):1848]. *Lancet.* 2014;384(9957):1849-1858.

71. Henrikson CA, Howell EE, Bush DE, et al. Chest pain relief by nitroglycerin does not predict active coronary artery disease. *Ann Intern Med.* 2003;139(12):979-986.

72. Schwartz GG, Olsson AG, Ezekowitz MD, et al. Effects of atorvastatin on early recurrent ischemic events in acute coronary syndromes: the MIRACL study—a randomized controlled trial. *JAMA.* 2001;285(13):1711-1718.

73. Patti G, Pasceri V, Colonna G, et al. Atorvastatin pretreatment improves outcomes in patients with acute coronary syndromes undergoing early percutaneous coronary intervention: results of the ARMYDA-ACS randomized trial. *J Am Coll Cardiol.* 2007;49(12):1272-1278.

74. Gislason GH, Jacobsen S, Rasmussen JN, et al. Risk of death or reinfarction associated with the use of selective cyclooxygenase-2 inhibitors and nonselective nonsteroidal antiinflammatory drugs after acute myocardial infarction. *Circulation.* 2006;113(25):2906-2913.

75. O'Gara PT, Kushner FG, Ascheim DD, et al. 2013 ACCF/AHA guideline for the management of ST-elevation myocardial infarction: a report of the American College of Cardiology Foundation/American Heart Association Task Force on practice guidelines. *J Am Coll Cardiol.* 2013;61(4):e78-e140.

76. Wagner GS, Macfarlane P, Wellens H, et al. AHA/ACCF/HRS recommendations for the standardization and interpretation of the electrocardiogram: part VI—acute ischemia/infarction—a scientific statement from the American heart association electrocardiography and arrhythmias committee, council on clinical Cardiology; the American College of Cardiology Foundation; and the heart rhythm

Society. Endorsed by the international Society for computerized electrocardiology. *J Am Coll Cardiol.* 2009;53(11):1003-1011.

77. Gersh BJ, Stone GW, White HD, Holmes DR Jr. Pharmacological facilitation of primary percutaneous coronary intervention for acute myocardial infarction: is the slope of the curve the shape of the future? *JAMA.* 2005;293(8):979-986.

78. Antman EM, Hand M, Armstrong PW, et al. 2007 focused update of the ACC/AHA 2004 guidelines for the management of patients with ST-elevation myocardial infarction: a report of the American College of Cardiology/American heart association Task Force on Practice guidelines—developed in collaboration with the Canadian cardiovascular Society endorsed by the American academy of family Physicians—2007 writing group to review new evidence and update the ACC/AHA 2004 guidelines for the management of patients with ST-elevation myocardial infarction, writing on behalf of the 2004 writing committee [published correction appears in *Circulation.* 2008 Feb 12;117(6):e162]. *Circulation.* 2008;117(2):296-329.

79. Yusuf S, Mehta SR, Chrolavicius S, et al. Effects of fondaparinux on mortality and reinfarction in patients with acute ST-segment elevation myocardial infarction: the OASIS-6 randomized trial. *JAMA.* 2006;295(13):1519-1530.

80. Jolly SS, Pogue J, Haladyn K, et al. Effects of aspirin dose on ischaemic events and bleeding after percutaneous coronary intervention: insights from the PCI-CURE study. *Eur Heart J.* 2009;30(8):900-907.

81. Montalescot G, Wiviott SD, Braunwald E, et al. Prasugrel compared with clopidogrel in patients undergoing percutaneous coronary intervention for ST-elevation myocardial infarction (TRITON-TIMI 38): double-blind, randomised controlled trial. *Lancet.* 2009;373(9665):723-731.

82. Stone GW, Witzenbichler B, Guagliumi G, et al. Bivalirudin during primary PCI in acute myocardial infarction. *N Engl J Med.* 2008;358(21):2218-2230.

83. Lincoff AM, Bittl JA, Harrington RA, et al. Bivalirudin and provisional glycoprotein IIb/IIIa blockade compared with heparin and planned glycoprotein IIb/IIIa blockade during percutaneous coronary intervention: REPLACE-2 randomized trial [published correction appears in *JAMA.* 2003 Apr 2;289(13):1638]. *JAMA.* 2003;289(7):853-863.

84. Chen ZM, Pan HC, Chen YP, et al. Early intravenous then oral metoprolol in 45,852 patients with acute myocardial infarction: randomised placebo-controlled trial. *Lancet.* 2005;366(9497):1622-1632.

85. Hochman JS, Reynolds HR, Dzavík V, et al. Long-term effects of percutaneous coronary intervention of the totally occluded infarct-related artery in the subacute phase after myocardial infarction. *Circulation.* 2011;124(21):2320-2328.

86. Tarantini G, Razzolini R, Napodano M, Bilato C, Ramondo A, Iliceto S. Acceptable reperfusion delay to prefer primary angioplasty over fibrin-specific thrombolytic therapy is affected (mainly) by the patient's mortality risk: 1 h does not fit all. *Eur Heart J.* 2010;31(6):676-683.

87. Thune JJ, Hoefsten DE, Lindholm MG, et al. Simple risk stratification at admission to identify patients with reduced mortality from primary angioplasty. *Circulation.* 2005;112(13):2017-2021.

88. Global Use of Strategies to Open Occluded Coronary Arteries in Acute Coronary Syndromes (GUSTO IIb) Angioplasty Substudy Investigators. A clinical trial comparing primary coronary angioplasty with tissue plasminogen activator for acute myocardial infarction [published correction appears in *N Engl J Med* 1997 Jul 24;337(4):287]. *N Engl J Med.* 1997;336(23):1621-1628.

89. Keeley EC, Boura JA, Grines CL. Primary angioplasty versus intravenous thrombolytic therapy for acute myocardial infarction: a quantitative review of 23 randomised trials. *Lancet.* 2003;361(9351):13-20.

90. Mehta SR, Wood DA, Storey RF, et al. Complete revascularization with multivessel PCI for myocardial infarction. *N Engl J Med.* 2019;381(15):1411-1421.

91. Thiele H, Akin I, Sandri M, et al. One-year outcomes after PCI strategies in cardiogenic shock. *N Engl J Med.* 2018;379(18):1699-1710.

92. Andersen HR, Nielsen TT, Rasmussen K, et al. A comparison of coronary angioplasty with fibrinolytic therapy in acute myocardial infarction. *N Engl J Med.* 2003;349(8):733-

93. Grines CL, Westerhausen DR Jr, Grines LL, et al. A randomized trial of transfer for primary angioplasty versus on-site thrombolysis in patients with high-risk myocardial infarction: the Air Primary Angioplasty in Myocardial Infarction study. *J Am Coll Cardiol.* 2002;39(11):1713-1719.

94. Widimský P, Groch L, Zelízko M, Aschermann M, Bednár F, Suryapranata H. Multicentre randomized trial comparing transport to primary angioplasty vs immediate thrombolysis vs combined strategy for patients with acute myocardial infarction presenting to a community hospital without a catheterization laboratory. The PRAGUE study. *Eur Heart J.* 2000;21(10):823-831.

95. Long-term effects of intravenous thrombolysis in acute myocardial infarction: final report of the GISSI study. Gruppo Italiano per lo Studio della Streptochi-nasi nell'Infarto Miocardico (GISSI). *Lancet.* 1987;2(8564):871-874.

96. Global Use of Strategies to Open Occluded Coronary Arteries (GUSTO III) Investigators. A comparison of reteplase with alteplase for acute myocardial infarction. *N Engl J Med.* 1997;337(16):1118-1123.

97. GUSTO investigators. An international randomized trial comparing four thrombolytic strategies for acute myocardial infarction. *N Engl J Med.* 1993;329(10):673-682.

CHAPTER 4

98. Assessment of the Safety and Efficacy of a New Thrombolytic (ASSENT-2) Investigators; Van De Werf F, Adgey J, et al. Single-bolus tenecteplase compared with front-loaded alteplase in acute myocardial infarction: the ASSENT-2 double-blind randomised trial. *Lancet*. 1999;354(9180):716-722.

99. Fernandez-Avilés F, Alonso JJ, Castro-Beiras A, et al. Routine invasive strategy within 24 hours of thrombolysis versus ischaemia-guided conservative approach for acute myocardial infarction with ST-segment elevation (GRACIA-1): a randomised controlled trial. *Lancet*. 2004;364(9439):1045-1053.

100. Di Mario C, Dudek D, Piscione F, et al. Immediate angioplasty versus standard therapy with rescue angioplasty after thrombolysis in the Combined Abciximab REteplase Stent Study in Acute Myocardial Infarction (CARESS-in-AMI): an open, prospective, randomised, multicentre trial. *Lancet*. 2008;371(9612):559-568.

101. GISSI-3: effects of lisinopril and transdermal glyceryl trinitrate singly and together on 6-week mortality and ventricular function after acute myocardial infarction. Gruppo Italiano per lo Studio della Sopravvivenza nell'infarto Miocardico. *Lancet*. 1994;343(8906):1115-1122.

102. ISIS-4: a randomised factorial trial assessing early oral captopril, oral mononitrate, and intravenous magnesium sulphate in 58,050 patients with suspected acute myocardial infarction. ISIS-4 (Fourth International Study of Infarct Survival) Collaborative Group. *Lancet*. 1995;345(8951):669-685.

103. Pitt B, Zannad F, Remme WJ, et al. The effect of spironolactone on morbidity and mortality in patients with severe heart failure. Randomized aldactone evaluation study investigators. *N Engl J Med*. 1999;341(10):709-717.

104. Pitt B, Remme W, Zannad F, et al. Eplerenone, a selective aldosterone blocker, in patients with left ventricular dysfunction after myocardial infarction [published correction appears in *N Engl J Med*. 2003 May 29;348(22):2271]. *N Engl J Med*. 2003;348(14):1309-1321.

105. Le May MR, Acharya S, Wells GA, et al. Prophylactic warfarin therapy after primary percutaneous coronary intervention for anterior ST-segment elevation myocardial infarction. *JACC Cardiovasc Interv*. 2015;8(1 pt B):155-162.

106. Iakovou I, Schmidt T, Bonizzoni E, et al. Incidence, predictors, and outcome of thrombosis after successful implantation of drug-eluting stents. *JAMA*. 2005;293(17):2126-2130.

107. van Werkum JW, Heestermans AA, Zomer AC, et al. Predictors of coronary stent thrombosis: the Dutch stent thrombosis registry. *J Am Coll Cardiol*. 2009;53(16):1399-1409.

108. McCord J, Jneid H, Hollander JE, et al. Management of cocaine-associated chest pain and myocardial infarction: a scientific statement from the American heart association acute cardiac care committee of the council on clinical cardiology. *Circulation*. 2008;117(14):1897-1907.

109. Hohnloser SH, Kuck KH, Dorian P, et al. Prophylactic use of an implantable cardioverter-defibrillator after acute myocardial infarction. *N Engl J Med*. 2004;351(24):2481-2488.

110. Bardy GH, Lee KL, Mark DB, et al. Amiodarone or an implantable cardioverter-defibrillator for congestive heart failure [published correction appears in *N Engl J Med*. 2005 May 19;352(20):2146]. *N Engl J Med*. 2005;352(3):225-237.

111. Moss AJ, Zareba W, Hall WJ, et al. Prophylactic implantation of a defibrillator in patients with myocardial infarction and reduced ejection fraction. *N Engl J Med*. 2002;346(12):877-883.

112. Olgin JE, Pletcher MJ, Vittinghoff E, et al. Wearable cardioverter-defibrillator after myocardial infarction. *N Engl J Med*. 2018;379(13):1205-1215.

113. Masri A, Altibi AM, Erqou S, et al. Wearable cardioverter-defibrillator therapy for the prevention of sudden cardiac death: a systematic review and meta-analysis. *JACC Clin Electrophysiol*. 2019;5(2):152-161.

114. Alcalai R, Butnaru A, Moravsky G, et al. Apixaban versus warfarin in patients with left ventricular thrombus, a prospective multicenter randomized clinical trial [published online ahead of print, 2021 Jul 19]. *Eur Heart J Cardiovasc Pharmacother*. 2021;pvab057. doi:10.1093/ehjcvp/pvab057.

115. Camaj A, Fuster V, Giustino G, et al. Left ventricular thrombus following acute myocardial infarction: JACC state-of-the-art review. *J Am Coll Cardiol*. 2022;79:1010-1022.

5 Heart Failure and Cardiomyopathy

Bin Q. Yang, Justin C. Hartupee, and Justin M. Vader

HEART FAILURE

General Principles

DEFINITION

Heart failure (HF) is a **clinical syndrome** in which either structural or functional abnormalities of the heart impair its ability to fill with or eject blood, resulting in dyspnea, fatigue, and fluid retention.[1,2] HF is a progressive disorder and is associated with high morbidity and mortality.

CLASSIFICATION

- HF may be due to abnormalities in myocardial contraction (systolic dysfunction), relaxation and filling (diastolic dysfunction), or both.
- Left ventricular (LV) ejection fraction (EF) is used to subdivide HF patients into groups for therapeutic and prognostic purposes.[3] These groups are:
  - EF ≤40%: HF with reduced EF (HFrEF)
  - EF 41%–49%: HF with mildly reduced EF (HFmrEF)
  - EF ≥50%: HF with preserved EF (HFpEF)
  - EF with baseline ≤40%, a ≥10-point increase from baseline EF, and a second measurement of LVEF >40%: HF with improved EF (HFimpEF).
- HF is classified in terms of natural history by American College of Cardiology/ American Heart Association (ACC/AHA) HF stage and in terms of symptom status by New York Heart Association (NYHA) Functional Class (Tables 5-1 and 5-2).

EPIDEMIOLOGY

- In the United States, over 6.5 million adults over 20 years of age are living with HF and this number is expected to exceed 8 million by 2030.[4]
- Approximately 1 million new cases of HF are diagnosed each year.
- HF accounts for approximately 1 million hospitalizations per year.
- Estimated 1- and 5-year mortality rates are 22% and 42.3%, respectively.[5]

ETIOLOGY

See Table 5-3.

TABLE 5-1	American College of Cardiology/American Heart Association Guidelines of Evaluation and Management of Chronic Heart Failure in Adults	
Stage	Description	Treatment
A	No structural heart disease and no symptoms but risk factors: CAD, HTN, DM, cardio toxins, familial cardiomyopathy	Lifestyle modification—diet, exercise, smoking cessation; treat hyperlipidemia and use ACE inhibitor for HTN
B	Abnormal LV systolic function, MI, valvular heart disease, but no HF symptoms	Lifestyle modifications, ACE inhibitor, β-adrenergic blockers
C	Structural heart disease and HF symptoms	Lifestyle modifications, ACE inhibitor, β-adrenergic blockers, diuretics, digoxin
D	Refractory HF symptoms to maximal medical management	Therapy listed under A, B, and C, and mechanical assist device, heart transplantation, continuous IV inotropic infusion, hospice care in selected patients

ACE, angiotensin-converting enzyme; CAD, coronary artery disease; DM, diabetes mellitus; HF, heart failure; HTN, hypertension; LV, left ventricular; MI, myocardial infarction.
Adapted from Yancy CW, Jessup M, Bozkurt B, et al. 2017 ACC/AHA/HFSA focused update of the 2013 ACCF/AHA guideline for the management of heart failure: a report of the American College of Cardiology/American Heart Association Task Force on Clinical Practice Guidelines and the Heart Failure Society of America. *Circulation.* 2017;136(6):e137-e161.

PATHOPHYSIOLOGY

• HF begins with an initial insult leading to myocardial injury.
• Regardless of etiology, the myocardial injury leads to a pathologic remodeling, which manifests as an increase in LV volume (dilatation) and/or mass (hypertrophy).

TABLE 5-2	New York Heart Association (NYHA) Functional Classification
NYHA Class	Symptoms
I (Mild)	No symptoms or limitation while performing ordinary physical activity (walking, climbing stairs, etc.).
II (Mild)	Mild symptoms (mild shortness of breath, palpitations, fatigue, and/or angina) and slight limitation during ordinary physical activity.
III (Moderate)	Marked limitation in activity because of symptoms, even during less than ordinary activity (walking short distances [20–100 m]). Comfortable only at rest.
IV (Severe)	Severe limitations with symptoms even while at rest. Mostly bedbound patients.

TABLE 5-3	Heart Failure Etiology
Ischemic Cardiomyopathy	**Nonischemic Cardiomyopathy**
• Severe angiographic coronary artery disease, post–myocardial infarction, or evidence of hibernating myocardium • Other risk factors include tobacco use, hypertension, diabetes, and obesity • Ischemic cardiomyopathy is the most common cause of heart failure	• Idiopathic • Familial • Myocarditis (infectious or autoimmune) • Infiltrative (amyloidosis, sarcoidosis, hemochromatosis) • Peripartum • Valvular heart disease • Toxin-induced (e.g., alcohol, amphetamine, chemotherapy) • Tachycardia-induced • High-output (peripheral shunt, chronic anemia) • Generalized myopathy (e.g., muscular dystrophy)

- Compensatory adaptations initially maintain cardiac output; specifically, there is activation of the renin–angiotensin–aldosterone system (RAAS) and vasopressin (antidiuretic hormone), which leads to increased sodium retention and peripheral vasoconstriction. The sympathetic nervous system is also activated (Figure 5-1), with increased levels of circulating catecholamines, resulting in increased myocardial contractility. Over time, these neurohormonal pathways result in direct cellular toxicity, fibrosis, arrhythmias, and pump failure.

Diagnosis

CLINICAL PRESENTATION

History
- Afflicted patients most commonly present with the following symptoms:
  - Dyspnea (on exertion and/or at rest)
  - Fatigue
  - Exercise intolerance
  - Orthopnea, paroxysmal nocturnal dyspnea
  - Bendopnea (dyspnea when leaning forward)
  - Systemic or pulmonary venous congestion (lower extremity swelling or cough/wheezing)
  - Presyncope, palpitations, and angina may also be present
- Other possible presentations include incidental detection of asymptomatic cardiomegaly or symptoms related to coexisting arrhythmia, conduction disturbance, thromboembolic complications, or sudden death.
- Clinical manifestations of HF vary depending on the severity and rapidity of cardiac decompensation, underlying etiology, age, and comorbidities of the patient.
- Extreme decompensation may present as cardiogenic shock (resulting from both low arterial and high venous pressures), characterized by hypoperfusion of vital organs, renal failure (decreased urine output), mental status changes (confusion and lethargy), or "shock liver" (elevated liver function tests).

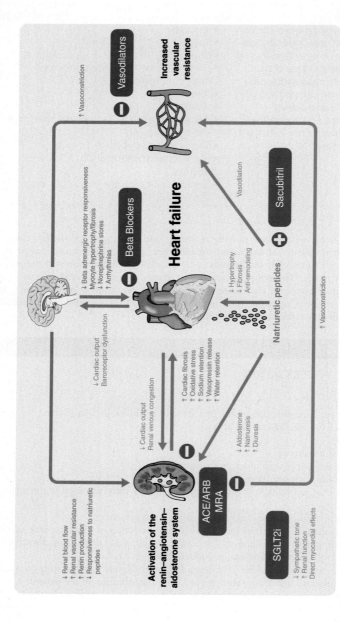

Figure 5-1. Activation of the sympathetic nervous system. ACE, angiotensin-converting enzyme; ARB, angiotensin II receptor blocker; SGLT2i; sodium–glucose cotransporter 2 inhibitor.

Physical Examination

- The goal of the physical examination in HF is to estimate intracardiac pressures, cardiac output, and end-organ perfusion.
- Elevated right-sided pressures result in lower extremity edema, jugular venous distension (JVD), abdominojugular reflux, pleural and pericardial effusions, hepatic congestion, and ascites.
- JVD is the most specific and reliable physical examination indicator of right-sided volume overload and is representative of left-sided filling pressures except in cases of disproportionate right heart dysfunction (e.g., pulmonary hypertension, severe tricuspid regurgitation, and pericardial disease).
- JVD is best visualized with oblique light and the patient at 45 degrees. Venous pulsations are differentiated from carotid pulsation by their biphasic nature, respiratory variability, and compressibility.
- Abdominojugular reflux suggests an impaired ability of the right ventricle to handle augmented preload and may be due to constriction or pulmonary hypertension in addition to myocardial disease.
- Elevated left-sided pressures may result in pulmonary rales, but rales are absent in the majority of HF patients with elevated left-sided filling pressures.
- In the setting of systolic dysfunction, a third (S_3) or fourth (S_4) heart sound as well as the holosystolic murmurs of tricuspid or mitral regurgitation (MR) may be present; carotid upstrokes may also be diminished.
- Low cardiac output is suggested by a proportional pulse pressure (pulse pressure/diastolic blood pressure) ≤25%, diminished carotid upstroke, and cool extremities.

DIAGNOSTIC TESTING

Laboratories

- Initial laboratory studies should include complete blood count, basic metabolic panel, magnesium, liver function tests, lipid profile, and thyroid function tests.
- B-type natriuretic peptide (BNP) and the biologically inactive cleavage product N-terminal prohormone BNP (NT-proBNP) are released by myocytes in response to stretch, volume overload, and increased filling pressures. Natriurietic peptides serve as a natural compensatory mechanism to enhance natriuresis.
  - Elevated BNP/NT-proBNP is present in patients with asymptomatic LV dysfunction as well as symptomatic HF.
  - BNP/NT-proBNP levels have been shown to correlate with HF severity and to predict survival.[6] A serum BNP >400 pg/mL is consistent with HF; however, specificity is reduced in patients with renal dysfunction and levels may be low in the setting of obesity. A serum BNP level <100 pg/mL has a good negative predictive value to exclude HF in patients presenting with dyspnea.[7] Age-specific cut points have also been identified; for example, NT-proBNP levels of 450, 900, and 1800 pg/mL optimally identified acute HF for patients age <50, 50–75, and >75, respectively.[8]
- Additional laboratory testing in a patient with new-onset HF without coronary artery disease (CAD) may include diagnostic tests for HIV, hepatitis, and hemochromatosis. When clinically suspected, serum tests for rheumatologic diseases (antinuclear antibody, antineutrophil cytoplasmic antibody, etc.), amyloidosis (serum protein electrophoresis, urine protein electrophoresis), or pheochromocytoma (catecholamines) should be considered.

Electrocardiography

An ECG should be performed to look for evidence of ischemia (ST-T wave abnormalities), hypertrophy (increased voltage), infiltration (reduced voltage), previous myocardial infarction (MI) (Q waves), conduction block (PR interval), interventricular conduction delays (prolonged QRS), and arrhythmias (supraventricular and ventricular).

Imaging

- Chest radiography should be performed to evaluate the presence of pulmonary edema or cardiomegaly and rule out other etiologies of dyspnea (e.g., pneumonia, pneumothorax). Although chest radiograph findings of cephalization and interstitial edema are highly specific for identifying patients presenting with acute HF (specificity of 98% and 99%, respectively), they have limited sensitivity (41% and 27%, respectively).[9]
- An echocardiogram should be performed to assess right ventricular (RV) and LV systolic and diastolic function, valvular structure and function, and chamber size and to exclude cardiac tamponade.
- LV function may also be evaluated using radionuclide ventriculography (i.e., multigated acquisition [MUGA] scan) or cardiac catheterization with ventriculography and invasive hemodynamics.
- Cardiac MRI may be useful in assessing ventricular function and evaluating the presence of intracardiac shunting, valvular heart disease, infiltrative cardiomyopathy, myocarditis, and/or previous MI.
- Cardiac positron emission tomography (PET) may be useful in the diagnosis and surveillance of cardiac sarcoidosis.
- Bone scintigraphy (99m technetium-labeled pyrophosphate scan) should be considered if there is clinical suspicion for transthyretin (TTR) amyloidosis once immunoglobulin light chain (AL) amyloidosis has been ruled out.

Diagnostic Procedures

- Coronary angiography should be performed in patients with angina or evidence of ischemia, unless the patient is not a candidate for revascularization.
- Stress nuclear imaging or echocardiography may be an acceptable alternative for assessing ischemia in patients presenting with HF who have known CAD and no angina, unless they are ineligible for revascularization.
- Right heart catheterization with placement of a pulmonary artery catheter may help guide therapy in patients with hypotension and evidence of shock.
- Cardiopulmonary exercise testing with measurement of peak oxygen consumption (VO_2) is useful in assessing functional capacity and in identifying candidates for heart transplantation.[10]
- Endomyocardial biopsy should be considered when seeking a specific diagnosis that would influence therapy, specifically in patients with rapidly progressive and unexplained cardiomyopathy; those in whom active myocarditis, especially giant cell myocarditis, is considered; and those with possible infiltrative processes such as cardiac amyloidosis and sarcoidosis.[11]

Treatment of Heart Failure

PHARMACOTHERAPY

- In general, pharmacologic therapy in chronic HF is aimed at blocking the neurohormonal pathways that contribute to cardiac remodeling and the progression of HF resulting in reduced symptoms, hospitalizations, and mortality.

- The cornerstone of medical therapy for HF includes β-adrenergic blockade, neprilysin and RAAS inhibition, and diuretic therapy to improve symptoms of volume overload.
- Pharmacotherapy is determined by the presence of a preserved or reduced LVEF. Several pharmacotherapies for HFrEF have been demonstrated to reduce death and hospitalization and improve quality of life in HF. No pharmacotherapy has been unequivocally demonstrated to improve mortality in patients with HFpEF.

Chronic Medical Therapy with Reduced Ejection Fraction (Figure 5-2)

- **First-line therapies—all patients with HFrEF should be placed on a β-blocker, angiotensin receptor–neprilysin inhibitor (ARNI) (or angiotensin-converting enzyme [ACE] inhibitor or angiotensin II receptor blocker [ARB]), mineralocorticoid receptor antagonist (MRA), and sodium-glucose cotransporter 2 (SGLT2) inhibitor.**
- **β-Adrenergic receptor antagonists (β-blockers)** (Table 5-4). β-Blockers are a critical component of HF therapy and work by blocking the effects of chronic adrenergic stimulation on the heart.
  - Large randomized trials have documented the beneficial effects of β-blockers on functional status, disease progression, and survival in patients with NYHA class II–IV symptoms.[12]
  - Typically, 2–3 months of therapy is required to observe significant effects on LV function, but reduction of cardiac arrhythmia and incidence of sudden cardiac death (SCD) may occur much earlier.[13]
  - β-Blockers should be instituted at a low dose and titrated with careful attention to blood pressure and heart rate. Some patients experience volume retention and worsening HF symptoms that typically respond to transient increases in diuretic therapy.

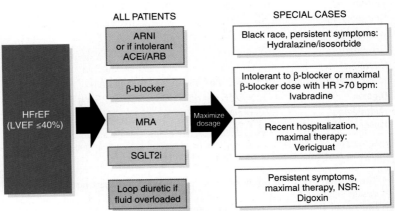

Figure 5-2. Chronic medical therapies for heart failure with reduced ejection fraction (HFrEF). ACEi, angiotensin-converting enzyme inhibitor; ARB, angiotensin II receptor blocker; ARNI, angiotensin receptor–neprilysin inhibitor; bpm, beats per minute; HR, heart rate; LVEF, left ventricular ejection fraction; NSR, normal sinus rhythm; SGLT2i, sodium–glucose cotransporter 2 inhibitor.

TABLE 5-4	Drugs Commonly Used for Treatment of Heart Failure	
Drug	Initial Dose	Target
Angiotensin-Converting Enzyme Inhibitors		
Captopril	6.25–12.5 mg tid	50 mg tid
Enalapril	2.5 mg bid	10 mg bid
Lisinopril	2.5–5.0 mg daily; can use bid	10–20 mg bid
Ramipril	1.25–2.5 mg bid	5 mg bid
Angiotensin Receptor Blockers		
Valsartan[a]	40 mg bid	160 mg bid
Losartan	25 mg daily; can use bid	25–100 mg daily
Candesartan[a]	2–16 mg daily	2–32 mg daily
Angiotensin Receptor–Neprilysin Inhibitor		
Entresto (sacubitril/valsartan)	24/26 mg bid	97/103 mg bid
IKf Channel Inhibitor		
Ivabradine	5 mg bid	7.5 mg bid
Thiazide Diuretics		
Hydrochlorothiazide	25–50 mg daily	25–50 mg daily
Metolazone	2.5–5.0 mg daily or bid	10–20 mg total daily
Loop Diuretics		
Bumetanide	0.5–1.0 mg daily or bid	10 mg total daily (maximum)
Furosemide	20–40 mg daily or bid	400 mg total daily (maximum)
Torsemide	10–20 mg daily or bid	200 mg total daily (maximum)
Aldosterone Antagonists		
Eplerenone	25 mg daily	50 mg daily
Spironolactone	12.5–25.0 mg daily	25 mg daily
β-Blockers		
Bisoprolol	1.25 mg daily	10 mg daily
Carvedilol	3.125 mg bid	25–50 mg bid
Metoprolol succinate	12.5–25.0 mg daily	200 mg daily
Digoxin	0.125–0.25 mg daily	0.125–0.25 mg daily
Hydralazine/Isosorbide Dinitrate	37.5 mg/20 mg tid	75 mg/40 mg TID

[a]Valsartan and candesartan are the only U.S. Food and Drug Administration–approved angiotensin II receptor blockers in the treatment of heart failure.

- The survival benefit of β-blockers is proportional to the heart rate reduction and dosage achieved.
- Individual β-blockers have unique properties, and the beneficial effects of β-blockers are not a class effect. Therefore, one of the three β-blockers with proven benefit on mortality in large clinical trials should be used:
  - Carvedilol[14,15]
  - Metoprolol succinate[16]
  - Bisoprolol[17]

- **Angiotensin receptor–neprilysin inhibitor. Sacubitril/valsartan** is a combination of the neprilysin inhibitor (sacubitril) and ARB (valsartan).
  - Neprilysin is a neutral endopeptidase involved in the degradation of vasoactive peptides including the natriuretic peptides, bradykinin, and adrenomedullin. Inhibition of neprilysin increases the availability of these peptides, which exert favorable effects in HF.
  - Sacubitril/valsartan was shown to be *superior* to enalapril in reducing death and rehospitalization among NYHA class II–IV patients with HFrEF who were stably tolerant of ACE inhibitor or ARB therapy.[18]
  - Sacubitril/valsartan is approved for use in patients with HFrEF and NYHA class II–IV symptoms.
  - Rates of angioedema are increased with sacubitril/valsartan compared with ACE inhibitors (0.5% vs. 0.2%) and **require a 36-hour ACE inhibitor washout** prior to initiation. Angioedema rates were comparatively higher in African-Americans (2.4% vs. 0.5%).
- **ACE inhibitors and ARBs** target the compensatory RAAS activation and attenuate vasoconstriction, vital organ hypoperfusion, hyponatremia, hypokalemia, and fluid retention. These medications should be used as second-line therapy if patients cannot tolerate or afford ARNI.
  - **ACE inhibitors**
    - Multiple large clinical trials have clearly demonstrated that ACE inhibitors improve symptoms and survival in patients with LV systolic dysfunction.[1]
    - ACE inhibitors may also prevent the development of HF in patients with asymptomatic LV dysfunction and in those at high risk of developing structural heart disease or HF symptoms (e.g., patients with CAD, diabetes mellitus, hypertension).
    - No consensus exists on optimal dosing of ACE inhibitors in HF. Higher doses have been shown to reduce morbidity without improving overall survival.[19]
    - Most ACE inhibitors are excreted by the kidneys, necessitating careful dose titration in patients with renal insufficiency. ACE inhibitors should be used cautiously in the presence of renal dysfunction and use should be avoided in patients with bilateral renal artery stenosis. Renal function and potassium levels should be monitored with dose adjustment and periodically with chronic use.
    - A rise in serum creatinine up to 30% above baseline may be seen when initiating an ACE inhibitor and should not result in reflexive discontinuation of therapy.[20]
    - Additional adverse effects may include cough, rash, angioedema, dysgeusia, hyperkalemia, and leukopenia.
    - Oral potassium supplements, potassium salt substitutes, and potassium-sparing diuretics should be used with caution during treatment with an ACE inhibitor.
    - **ACE inhibitors are contraindicated in pregnancy. Enalapril and captopril may be safely used by breastfeeding mothers.**
  - **ARBs**
    - ARBs reduce morbidity and mortality associated with HF in patients who are not receiving an ACE inhibitor[21-23] and therefore should be instituted when ACE inhibitors are not tolerated.
    - In contrast to ACE inhibitors, ARBs do not increase bradykinin levels and therefore are not associated with cough.
    - Renal precautions and monitoring for ARB use are similar to ACE inhibitor use.
    - Use of ARBs is contraindicated in patients taking both ACE inhibitors and aldosterone antagonists due to a high risk for hyperkalemia.
    - **ARBs are contraindicated in pregnancy and breastfeeding.**

- **MRAs** attenuate aldosterone-mediated sodium retention, vascular reactivity, oxidant stress, inflammation, and fibrosis.
  - MRAs are recommended for use in patients with NYHA class II–IV HF and acceptable renal function (serum creatinine is <2.5 mg/dL in men or <2.0 mg/dL in women, and potassium is <5.0 mEq/L).
  - **Spironolactone** is a nonselective aldosterone receptor antagonist that has been shown to improve survival and decrease hospitalizations in NYHA class III–IV patients with low EF.[24]
  - **Eplerenone** is a selective aldosterone receptor antagonist without the estrogenic side effects of spironolactone. It has proven beneficial in patients with HF following MI[25] and in less symptomatic HF patients (NYHA class II) with reduced EF.[26]
  - Life-threatening hyperkalemia may occur with the use of these agents. Serum potassium must be monitored closely after initiation; concomitant use of ACE inhibitors and NSAIDs and the presence of renal insufficiency increase the risk of hyperkalemia.
  - Gynecomastia may develop in 10%–20% of men treated with spironolactone; eplerenone should be used in this case.
- **SGLT2 inhibitors** promote osmotic diuresis and natriuresis and exert beneficial pleiotropic effects on the heart, vasculature, and metabolic profile.
  - **Dapagliflozin** and **empagliflozin** have been shown to decrease cardiovascular mortality and HF hospitalizations when added to standard therapy in patients with HFrEF with or without diabetes.[27,28]
  - **Canagliflozin** has been shown to decrease the composite outcome of cardiovascular mortality, nonfatal MI, or nonfatal stroke in patients with type 2 diabetes and elevated cardiovascular risk. Post-hoc analysis showed canagliflozin reduced cardiovascular mortality and HF hospitalizations across a range of subgroups.[29]
  - **Sotagliflozin** is a dual SGLT1 and SGLT2 inhibitor that has been shown to reduce cardiovascular death and HF hospitalizations or urgent visits when initiated shortly before or after inpatient discharge in patients with HF and diabetes irrespective of EF.[30]
  - Currently, the U.S. Food and Drug Administration (FDA) has approved dapagliflozin and empagliflozin for treatment of HFrEF independent of diabetes.
- **Diuretic therapy** in conjunction with restriction of dietary sodium and fluids often leads to clinical improvement in patients with symptomatic HF. Frequent assessment of the patient's weight and careful observation of fluid intake and output are essential during initiation and maintenance of therapy.
  - Complications of therapy include hypokalemia, hyponatremia, hypomagnesemia, volume contraction alkalosis, intravascular volume depletion, and hypotension. Therefore, serum electrolytes, BUN, and creatinine levels should be monitored after institution of diuretic therapy.
  - Hypokalemia may be life threatening in patients who are receiving digoxin or are predisposed to ventricular arrhythmias.
  - **Loop diuretics (furosemide, torsemide, bumetanide, ethacrynic acid)** should be used in patients who require significant diuresis and in those with markedly decreased renal function.
    - Furosemide reduces preload acutely by causing direct venodilation when administered intravenously, making it useful for managing severe HF or acute pulmonary edema.
    - Use of loop diuretics may be complicated by hyperuricemia, hypocalcemia, ototoxicity, rash, and vasculitis. Furosemide, torsemide, and bumetanide are sulfa

derivatives and may rarely cause drug reactions in sulfa-sensitive patients; ethacrynic acid can be used in such patients.

- Dose equivalence of oral loop diuretics is approximately 50 mg ethacrynic acid = 40 mg furosemide = 20 mg torsemide = 1 mg bumetanide.
- Torsemide and bumetanide have >80% oral bioavailability as compared to ~50% bioavailability of furosemide. In patients requiring increased dosage of furosemide, transition to torsemide or bumetanide should be considered.
  - ○ **Thiazide diuretics (hydrochlorothiazide, chlorthalidone)** can be used as initial agents in patients with normal renal function in whom only a mild diuresis is desired.
    - **Metolazone**, unlike other oral thiazides, exerts its action at the proximal and distal tubule and may be useful in combination with a loop diuretic in patients with a low glomerular filtration rate.
  - ○ **Potassium-sparing diuretics (amiloride, triamterene)** do not exert a potent diuretic effect when used alone.
- **Second-line therapies**—In patients who have ongoing symptoms despite maximization of the four cornerstone medications mentioned above or have intolerance/contraindications preventing use of certain agents, additional therapies may provide benefit.
  - ○ **Vasodilator therapy** alters preload and afterload to improve cardiac output.
    - **Hydralazine** acts directly on arterial smooth muscle cells to produce vasodilation and reduce afterload. Reflex tachycardia and increased myocardial oxygen consumption may occur in the setting of hydralazine use, requiring cautious use in patients with ischemic heart disease.
    - **Nitrates** are predominantly venodilators and help relieve symptoms of congestion. They also reduce myocardial ischemia by decreasing ventricular filling pressures and by directly dilating coronary arteries. Nitrate therapy may precipitate hypotension, especially in patients who have low preload or are taking phosphodiesterase inhibitors.
    - **A combination of hydralazine and isosorbide dinitrate** (starting dose: 37.5/20 mg three times daily), when added to β-blockers and ACEi/ARB, was shown to reduce mortality in African-American patients.[31]
    - In the absence of ACEi/ARBs, MRAs, and β-blockers, the combination of nitrates and hydralazine improves survival in patients with HFrEF[32] and should therefore be considered for use in HFrEF patients unable to tolerate RAAS blockade.
  - ○ **Vericiguat** is a soluble guanylate cyclase stimulator that increases cyclic guanosine monophosphate, leading to vasodilation and improved endothelial function.
    - Vericiguat was shown to reduce cardiovascular death and HF hospitalization in patients with HFrEF and worsening symptoms or recent decompensation.[33] It is indicated for use in this population as an addition to background therapy with ACE/ARB/ARNI, MRAs, and β-blockers.
  - ○ **Ivabradine** is an inhibitor of the IKf channel involved in generating "pacemaker" currents in cardiac tissue.
    - Ivabradine was shown to reduce HF hospitalization and HF death in outpatients with HFrEF and is indicated for the reduction of HF hospitalization in patients with EF <35%, stable HF symptoms, and sinus rhythm with a resting heart rate ≥70 bpm who are already taking β-blockers at the highest tolerated dose.[34]
  - ○ **Digitalis glycosides (digoxin)** increase myocardial contractility and may attenuate the neurohormonal activation associated with HF.

- Digoxin has been shown to decrease rates of HF hospitalizations without improving overall mortality.[35]
- Digoxin has a **narrow therapeutic index**, and serum levels should be followed closely, particularly in patients with unstable renal function.
- The usual daily dose is 0.125–0.25 mg and should be decreased in patients with renal insufficiency.
- Women and patients with higher serum digoxin levels (1.2–2.0 ng/mL) have an increased mortality risk.[36,37]
- Discontinuation of digoxin in patients who are stable on a regimen of digoxin, diuretics, and an ACE inhibitor may result in clinical deterioration.[38]
- Drug interactions with digoxin are common and may lead to toxicity. Agents that may increase levels include erythromycin, tetracycline, quinidine, verapamil, flecainide, and amiodarone. Electrolyte abnormalities (particularly hypokalemia), hypoxemia, hypothyroidism, renal insufficiency, and volume depletion may also exacerbate toxicity.
- Digoxin is not dialyzable, and toxicity is only treatable by the administration of digoxin immune Fab.

- **Therapies with unproven benefit**
  - **α-Adrenergic receptor antagonists** have not been shown to improve survival in HF, and hypertensive patients treated with doxazosin as first-line therapy are at increased risk of developing HF.
  - **Calcium channel blockers** have no favorable effects on mortality in HFrEF.
    - Dihydropyridine calcium channel blockers such as amlodipine may be used in hypertensive HF patients already on maximal guideline-directed medical therapy (GDMT); however, these agents do not improve mortality.[39,40]
    - Nondihydropyridine calcium channel blockers should be avoided in HFrEF because their negative inotropic effects may potentiate worsening HF.

- **Sympathomimetic agents** are reserved for the treatment of severe HF. Beneficial and adverse effects are mediated by stimulation of myocardial β-adrenergic receptors. The most important adverse effects are related to arrhythmias and exacerbation of myocardial ischemia. Patients with refractory chronic HF may benefit symptomatically from continuous ambulatory administration of parenteral inotropes as palliative therapy or as a bridge to mechanical ventricular support or cardiac transplantation. Risks include life-threatening arrhythmias or catheter-related infections.
  - **Dobutamine** (see Table 5-5) is a synthetic analog of dopamine with predominantly β_1-adrenoreceptor activity. It increases cardiac output, lowers cardiac filling pressures, and generally has a neutral effect on systemic blood pressure. Dobutamine tolerance has been described, and several studies have demonstrated increased mortality in patients treated with continuous dobutamine. Dobutamine has no significant role in the treatment of HF resulting from diastolic dysfunction or a high-output state.
  - **Phosphodiesterase inhibitors** increase myocardial contractility and produce vasodilation by increasing intracellular cyclic adenosine monophosphate. **Milrinone** is indicated for treatment of refractory HF. Hypotension may develop in patients who receive vasodilator therapy or have intravascular volume contraction, or both. Milrinone may improve hemodynamics in patients who are treated concurrently with dobutamine or dopamine. Data suggest that in-hospital short-term milrinone administration in addition to standard medical therapy does not reduce the length of hospitalization or the 60-day mortality or rehospitalization rate when compared with placebo.[41]

TABLE 5-5	Inotropic/Sympathomimetic Agents[a]		
Drug	Dose	Mechanism	Effects/Side Effects
Dopamine	1–3 µg/kg/min	Dopaminergic receptors	Splanchnic vasodilation
	2–8 µg/kg/min	β_1-Receptor agonist	+Inotropic
	7–10 µg/kg/min	α-Receptor agonist	↑ SVR
Dobutamine	2.5–15.0 µg/kg/min	β_1- > β_2- > α-receptor agonist	+Inotropic, ↓ SVR, tachycardia
Epinephrine	0.05–1 µg/kg/min; titrate to desired mean arterial pressure. May adjust dose every 10–15 min by 0.05–0.2 µg/kg/min to achieve desired blood pressure goal	$\beta_1 > \alpha_1$ Low doses = β High doses = α	+Inotropic, ↑ SVR
Milrinone[b]	50-µg/kg bolus IV over 10 min, 0.375–0.75 µg/kg/min	↑ cAMP	+Inotropic, ↓ SVR

cAMP, cyclic adenosine monophosphate; SVR, systemic vascular resistance; ↑, increased; ↓, decreased.
[a]Increased risk of atrial and ventricular tachyarrhythmias.
[b]Needs dose adjustment for creatinine clearance.

- **Oral inotropes**
  Omecamtiv mecarbil binds cardiac myosin and directly augments cardiac sarcomere function. Use of omecamtiv mecarbil in addition to guideline medical therapy in patients with NYHA II-IV HF resulted in lower rates of the composite outcome of HF events or cardiovascular death.[42] This agent is not yet FDA approved.

Chronic Medical Therapy With Preserved Ejection Fraction (Figure 5-3)

- No pharmacotherapy has been definitively shown to improve mortality in HFpEF.
  - The use of ACE inhibitors, ARBs, spironolactone, and β-blockers is reasonable and may be associated with a small reduction in HF hospitalization rates.
  - **Sacubitril/valsartan** did not reduce cardiovascular mortality or HF hospitalizations compared to valsartan in patients with HFpEF and EF >45%. However, sacubitril/valsartan did have a beneficial effect in patients who had less than normal LVEF. **Therefore, FDA has approved sacubitril/valsartan for use in all patients with HFpEF,** with benefit most likely in patients with less than normal LV systolic function.[43,44]
  - **Spironolactone** reduced HF hospitalization in patients with HFpEF in a large randomized trial, but mortality was not reduced.[45]

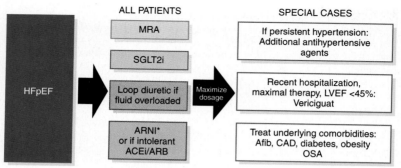

Figure 5-3. Chronic medical therapies for heart failure with preserved ejection fraction (HFpEF). ACEi, angiotensin-converting enzyme inhibitor; Afib, atrial fibrillation; ARB, angiotensin II receptor blocker; ARNI, angiotensin receptor–neprilysin inhibitor; CAD, coronary artery disease; LVEF, left ventricular ejection fraction; OSA, obstructive sleep apnea; SGLT2i, sodium–glucose cotransporter 2 inhibitor.

- ○ **SGLT2 inhibitors** have the most extensive data for improved outcomes in HFpEF. Empagliflozin reduced the composite outcome of HF hospitalizations and cardiac death in patients with HFpEF, independent of diabetes, driven by decrease in HF hospitalizations.[46] In a prespecified, pooled analysis from two placebo-controlled trials of type 2 diabetics with HF, **sotagliflozin** reduced cardiovascular death and HF hospitalizations or urgent visits, irrespective of EF.[30,47] **SGLT2 inhibitors should be considered in all patients with HFpEF.**
- Control of blood pressure, treatment of atrial fibrillation (AF), and treatment of coronary disease through pharmacotherapy and/or revascularization in accordance with practice guidelines is recommended.

Antiarrhythmic Therapy

- Suppression of asymptomatic ventricular premature beats or nonsustained ventricular tachycardia (NSVT) using antiarrhythmic drugs in patients with HF does not improve survival and may increase mortality as a result of the proarrhythmic effects of the drugs.[48]
- For patients with AF as a suspected cause of new-onset HF, a rhythm control strategy should be pursued. For patients with preexisting HF who develop AF, despite evidence suggesting improved symptom status in patients treated with rhythm control, the use of antiarrhythmic drug therapy for the maintenance of sinus rhythm has not been shown to improve mortality.[49]
- Agents recommended for the maintenance of sinus rhythm in HF with reduced LVEF include dofetilide and amiodarone. Sotalol may also be considered in patients with mildly depressed LVEF. These agents require close monitoring of the QT interval. In patients with severe LV systolic dysfunction and HF, dronedarone should not be used.[50]
- Catheter ablation for AF in patients with HF as compared with medical therapy was associated with a lower rate of mortality in one randomized trial, but guideline consensus for use has not been formalized.[51]

Anticoagulant and Antiplatelet Therapy

- Although patients with HF are at relatively greater risk for thromboembolic events, the absolute risk is modest, and routine anticoagulation is not recommended in HF patients in the absence of AF, prior thromboembolism, or a cardioembolic source.
- In patients with AF, use of the CHADS2 or CHA2DS2-VASc risk score is recommended for determining when to use anticoagulant therapies.
- The direct oral anticoagulants dabigatran, rivaroxaban, and apixaban have been shown to be effective in HF patients with nonvalvular AF.
- There are insufficient data to support the routine use of aspirin in patients with HF who do not have coronary disease or atherosclerosis.

NONPHARMACOLOGIC THERAPIES FOR HEART FAILURE

- **Coronary revascularization** reduces ischemia and may improve systolic function in patients with CAD and HF.
- Surgical or percutaneous revascularization is recommended in HF patients with angina and suitable anatomy (class I recommendation) and may be considered in patients without angina who have suitable anatomy, whether in the presence of viable myocardium (class IIa recommendation) or nonviable myocardium (class IIb recommendation).[1]
- In a large, randomized trial of HF patients with CAD and LVEF <35% comparing medical therapy to medical therapy plus coronary artery bypass graft surgery (CABG), there was no difference in the primary outcome of death from any cause at 5 years. At longer follow-up intervals of up to 10 years, the rates of death from any cause and death from cardiovascular causes were significantly lower in patients who underwent CABG in addition to medical therapy than those receiving medical therapy alone.[52,53]
- **Cardiac resynchronization therapy (CRT)** or **biventricular pacing** (see Chapter 7, Cardiac Arrhythmias) can improve quality of life and reduce the risk of death in certain patients with an EF of ≤35%, NYHA class II–IV HF, and conduction abnormalities (left bundle branch block [LBBB] and atrioventricular delay).[54,55]
- CRT can also be useful (class IIA recommendation) in the following situations:
  - LVEF ≤35%, sinus rhythm, a non-LBBB pattern with a QRS ≥150 ms, and NYHA class III/ambulatory class IV symptoms on GDMT.
  - LVEF ≤35%, sinus rhythm, LBBB with a QRS 120–149 ms, and NYHA class II, III, or ambulatory IV symptoms on GDMT.
  - AF and LVEF ≤35% on GDMT if the patient requires ventricular pacing and atrioventricular nodal ablation or rate control allows near 100% ventricular pacing with CRT.
  - Patients on GDMT who have LVEF ≤35% and are undergoing new or replacement device implantation with anticipated frequent ventricular pacing (>40% of the time).
  - Factors most strongly favoring response to CRT include female sex, QRS duration ≥150 ms, LBBB, body mass index <30 kg/m², nonischemic cardiomyopathy, and a small left atrium.[56]
- **Implantable cardioverter-defibrillator (ICD)** placement for primary prevention of SCD is recommended for selected HF patients with a persistently reduced LVEF ≤35%.
  - SCD occurs six to nine times more often in patients with HF compared with the general population and is the leading cause of death in ambulatory HF patients.

CHAPTER 5

○ Multiple large, randomized trials have demonstrated a survival benefit of 1%–1.5% per year in patients with both ischemic and nonischemic cardiomyopathy.

○ Patients should receive at least 3–6 months of optimal GDMT prior to reassessment of EF and implantation of an ICD.

○ Following an acute MI or revascularization, LVEF should be assessed after 40 days of GDMT prior to ICD implantation.

○ ICD therapy should be reserved for patients expected to otherwise live >1 year with good functional capacity. ICD therapy should not be used in end-stage HF patients who are not candidates for transplantation or durable mechanical circulatory support (MCS).

• **CardioMEMS™** is an implantable hemodynamic monitoring system delivered into the pulmonary artery that can be used to monitor a patient's ambulatory pulmonary artery pressures and allow clinicians to adjust medications accordingly. It has been shown to reduce hospitalization in patients with NYHA class III HF, irrespective of LVEF.[57]

SURGICAL MANAGEMENT

• **Surgical or nonsurgical replacement or repair** of the mitral valve in the setting of a reduced LVEF and severe MR is discussed elsewhere (see Chapter 6, Pericardial and Valvular Heart Disease).

In select patients who are on maximally tolerated medical therapy with symptomatic moderate to severe MR, Mitraclip™ resulted in lower mortality and HF hospitalizations.[58]

• **Left ventricular assist devices (LVADs)** are surgically implanted pumps that draw blood from the left ventricle, energize flow through a motor unit, and deliver the energized blood to the aorta, resulting in augmented cardiac output and lower intracardiac filling pressures. These devices may be temporary (CentriMag, percutaneous LVADs) or durable (HeartWare, HeartMate II, HeartMate III). Due to clinical inferiority, HeartWare and HeartMate II are no longer manufactured. **HeartMate 3** is the only durable LVAD commercially available in the United States.

○ Temporary MCS is indicated for patients with severe HF after cardiac surgery or individuals with intractable cardiogenic shock after acute MI.

○ Durable MCS is indicated as a "bridge to transplantation" for patients awaiting heart transplantation or as "destination" therapy for select patients ineligible for transplant with refractory end-stage HF and HF-related life expectancy with therapy of <2 years.[59]

○ Complications of durable LVADs include RV dysfunction, gastrointestinal bleeding, driveline infections, aortic insufficiency, pump thrombosis, hemolysis, and strokes. Newer magnetic levitation technology offers less risk of pump thrombosis and disabling stroke.[60,61]

○ The decision to institute MCS must be made in consultation with a HF cardiologist and a cardiac surgeon who have experience with this technology.

• **Cardiac transplantation** is an option for selected patients with severe end-stage HF refractory to aggressive medical therapy and for whom no other conventional treatment options are available.

○ Approximately 3700 transplants were performed in the United States in 2020 and the number of heart transplants has been slowly increasing.

○ Candidates considered for transplantation should generally be <65 years old (although selected older patients may also benefit), have advanced HF (NYHA class IV), have a strong psychosocial support system, have exhausted all other therapeutic options, and be free of irreversible extracardiac organ dysfunction that would limit functional recovery or predispose them to posttransplant complications.[62]

○ Survival rates after heart transplant are approximately 90%, 75%, and 50% at 1, 5, and 10 years, respectively. Annual statistics can be found on the United Network for Organ Sharing website (www.unos.org).

○ **Posttransplant complications** may include acute or chronic rejection, typical and atypical infections, and adverse effects of immunosuppressive agents. Surgical complications and acute rejection are the major causes of death in the first post-transplant year. Cardiac allograft vasculopathy and malignancy are the leading causes of death after the first posttransplant year.

LIFESTYLE/RISK MODIFICATION

• Dietary counseling for sodium and fluid restriction should be provided. Daily intake of approximately 2 g of sodium per day for most patients and fluid restriction <1.5 L/d for patients with hyponatremia (serum sodium <130 mEq/L) are reasonable.
• Smoking cessation should be strongly encouraged.
• Abstinence from alcohol is recommended in symptomatic HF patients with low EF.
• Exercise training is recommended in stable HF patients as an adjunct to pharmacologic treatment. Exercise training in patients with HF has been shown to improve exercise capacity (peak VO_2 max as well as 6-minute walk time), improve quality of life, and decrease neurohormonal activation. Treatment programs should be individualized and include a warm-up period, 20–30 minutes of exercise at the desired intensity, and a cool-down period.
• Weight loss should be recommended in obese HF patients.

Special Considerations

• **Minimization of medications** with deleterious effects in HF should be emphasized.
  ○ **Negative inotropes** (e.g., verapamil, diltiazem) should be avoided in patients with impaired ventricular contractility, as should over-the-counter β stimulants (e.g., compounds containing ephedra, pseudoephedrine hydrochloride).
  ○ **NSAIDs**, which antagonize the effect of ACE inhibitors and diuretic therapy, should be avoided if possible.
• **Administration of supplemental oxygen** may relieve dyspnea, improve oxygen delivery, reduce the work of breathing, and limit pulmonary vasoconstriction in patients with hypoxemia but is not routinely recommended in patients without measurable hypoxemia.
• **Sleep apnea** has a prevalence rate as high as 50% in the HF population. Treatment of obstructive sleep apnea with nocturnal positive airway pressure improves symptoms and EF.[63] However, treatment of *central* sleep apnea with adaptive servo-ventilation in patients with HFrEF was associated with increased mortality.[64]
• **Dialysis** or **ultrafiltration** may be beneficial in patients with severe HF and renal dysfunction who cannot respond adequately to fluid and sodium restriction and diuretics.[65] Ultrafiltration is not superior to a scaled diuretic regimen in patients with acute HF and cardiorenal syndrome and is associated with higher rate of adverse events.[66] Other mechanical methods of fluid removal such as therapeutic thoracentesis and paracentesis may provide temporary symptomatic relief of dyspnea. Care must be taken to avoid rapid fluid removal and hypotension.

CHAPTER 5

- **End-of-life considerations** should be strongly considered in patients with advanced HF who are refractory to therapy. Discussions regarding the disease course, treatment options, survival, functional status, and advance directives should be addressed early in the treatment of the patient with HF. For those with end-stage disease (stage D, NYHA class IV) with multiple hospitalizations and severe decline in their functional status and quality of life, hospice and palliative care is recommended.[67]

Acute Heart Failure and Cardiogenic Pulmonary Edema

GENERAL PRINCIPLES

Acute heart failure (AHF) results from a sudden increase in intracardiac pressure or acute myocardial dysfunction leading to decreased peripheral perfusion and cardiogenic pulmonary edema (CPE). CPE occurs when the pulmonary capillary pressure exceeds the forces that maintain fluid within the vascular space (serum oncotic pressure and interstitial hydrostatic pressure).
- Increased pulmonary capillary pressure may be caused by LV failure of any cause, obstruction to transmitral flow (e.g., mitral stenosis, atrial myxoma), or rarely, pulmonary veno-occlusive disease.
- Alveolar flooding and impairment of gas exchange follow accumulation of fluid in the pulmonary interstitium.

DIAGNOSIS

Clinical Presentation
- Clinical manifestations of AHF and CPE may occur rapidly and include dyspnea, anxiety, cough, and restlessness.
- The patient may expectorate pink frothy fluid.
- Physical signs of decreased peripheral perfusion, pulmonary congestion, hypoxemia, use of accessory respiratory muscles, and wheezing are often present.

Diagnostic Testing
- Radiographic abnormalities include cardiomegaly, interstitial and perihilar vascular engorgement, Kerley B lines, and pleural effusions.
- The radiographic abnormalities may follow the development of symptoms by several hours, and their resolution may be out of phase with clinical improvement.

TREATMENT

- Placing the patient in a sitting position improves pulmonary function.
- Bed rest, pain control, and relief of anxiety can decrease cardiac workload.
- **Noninvasive positive-pressure ventilation** is preferred and may have particularly favorable effects in the setting of pulmonary edema.[68] **Mechanical ventilation** is indicated if oxygenation is inadequate or hypercapnia occurs.
- **Precipitating factors** should be identified and corrected because resolution of pulmonary edema can often be accomplished with correction of the underlying process. The most common precipitants are:
  - Severe hypertension
  - MI or myocardial ischemia (particularly if associated with MR)

○ Acute valvular regurgitation
○ New-onset tachyarrhythmias or bradyarrhythmias
○ Volume overload in the setting of severe LV dysfunction

Medications

- **Furosemide** is a venodilator that decreases pulmonary congestion within minutes of IV administration, well before its diuretic action begins. An initial dose of 40–80 mg IV should be given over several minutes and can be increased based on response to a maximum of 200 mg in subsequent doses.
- **Nitroglycerin** is a venodilator that can potentiate the effect of furosemide. IV administration is preferable to oral and transdermal forms because it can be rapidly titrated.
- **Supplemental oxygen** should be administered initially to raise the arterial oxygen tension to >60 mm Hg.
- **Inotropic agents** may be necessary for treatment of AHF and CPE in patients with concomitant hypotension or shock.
  - **Dobutamine** and **milrinone** are positive inotropes, chronotropes, and arterial vasodilators. Major drawbacks include arrhythmias and hypotension.
  - **Norepinephrine**, rather than **dopamine** (Table 5-5), should be used for stabilization of the hypotensive HF patient. Although a large randomized trial found no mortality difference between dopamine and norepinephrine in a cohort of undifferentiated shock patients, there were more adverse events (primarily arrhythmic) in the dopamine group, and subgroup analysis of those with cardiogenic shock showed an increased rate of death at 28 days in the dopamine group.[69]
- **Parenteral vasodilators** such as **sodium nitroprusside** should be reserved for patients with severe HF not responding to oral medications. **Sodium nitroprusside** is a direct arterial vasodilator with less potent venodilatory properties. It is particularly effective in patients who have concomitant hypertension or severe aortic/mitral valve insufficiency.
  - Sodium nitroprosside should be used carefully in patients with myocardial ischemia because of potential reduction in regional myocardial blood flow (coronary steal).
  - Parenteral agents should be started at low doses, titrated to the desired hemodynamic effect, and discontinued slowly to avoid rebound vasoconstriction. Continuous hemodynamic monitoring should be utilized to help guide therapy.
  - The initial dose of **0.25 μg/kg/min** can be titrated (**maximum dose of 10 μg/kg/min**) to the desired hemodynamic effect or until hypotension develops.
  - The half-life of nitroprusside is 1–3 minutes, and its metabolism results in the release of cyanide, which is metabolized by the liver to thiocyanate and is then excreted via the kidney.
  - Toxic levels of thiocyanate (>10 mg/dL) may develop in patients with renal insufficiency. Thiocyanate toxicity may manifest as nausea, paresthesias, mental status changes, abdominal pain, and seizures.
  - **Methemoglobinemia** is a rare complication of treatment with nitroprusside.
- **Epinephrine** may be considered in patients with refractory cardiogenic shock; however, its use has been associated with increased mortality. Escalation of therapy to include epinephrine should prompt consideration of MCS.

SPECIAL CONSIDERATIONS

- **Right heart catheterization** (e.g., Swan-Ganz catheter) may be helpful in cases where a prompt response to therapy does not occur by allowing differentiation between cardiogenic and noncardiogenic causes of pulmonary edema via measurement of central hemodynamics and cardiac output. It may then be used to guide subsequent therapy. The *routine* use of right heart catheterization in acute HF patients is not beneficial.[70]
- An **intra-aortic balloon pump (IABP)** can be considered for temporary hemodynamic support in patients who have failed pharmacologic therapies and have transient myocardial dysfunction or are awaiting a definitive procedure such as an LVAD or transplantation. Severe aortoiliac atherosclerosis and moderate to severe aortic valve insufficiency are contraindications to IABP placement.
- **Percutaneous LVADs** provide short-term hemodynamic support for patients in cardiogenic shock. These devices have been shown to provide superior hemodynamic effects compared with IABP. However, use of percutaneous LVADs compared with IABP did not improve 30-day survival in critically ill patients.[71]

CARDIOMYOPATHY

Dilated Cardiomyopathy

GENERAL PRINCIPLES

Definition

Dilated cardiomyopathy (DCM) is a disease of cardiac muscle characterized by dilation of the cardiac chambers and reduction in ventricular contractile function.

Epidemiology

DCM is the most common form of nonischemic cardiomyopathy and is responsible for approximately 10,000 deaths and 46,000 hospitalizations each year. The lifetime incidence of DCM is about 30 cases per 100,000 persons.

Pathophysiology

- DCM may be secondary to progression of any process that affects the myocardium, and dilation is directly related to neurohormonal activation. Familial DCM accounts for up to 50% of cases and is likely underestimated.[4,72]
- Dilation of the cardiac chambers and varying degrees of hypertrophy are anatomic hallmarks. Tricuspid and mitral regurgitation are common because of the effect of chamber dilation on the valvular apparatus.
- **Atrial and ventricular arrhythmias** are present in as many as one-half of these patients and contribute to the high incidence of sudden death in this population.

DIAGNOSIS

Clinical Presentation

Patients most often present with typical features of heart failure.

Diagnostic Testing

Imaging
Diagnosis of DCM can be confirmed with echocardiography or cardiac MRI.

Diagnostic Procedures
Endomyocardial biopsy provides little information that affects treatment of patients with DCMs and is not routinely recommended.[11] Endomyocardial biopsy for DCM is recommended in clinical scenarios that may result in the diagnosis of a treatable form of acute myocarditis, including:
- New-onset HF of <2 weeks in duration with normal-sized or dilated left ventricle and hemodynamic compromise.
- New-onset HF of 2 weeks to 3 months in duration associated with a dilated left ventricle and new ventricular arrhythmias, high-grade atrioventricular block (type II second-degree or third-degree), and failure to respond to usual care.

TREATMENT

Medications
- The medical management of symptomatic patients is identical to that for HFrEF from other causes. This consists of controlling total body sodium and volume and pharmacotherapy including β-blockers, ARNI (or ACE inhibitors or ARBs), MRAs, and SGLT2 inhibitors.
- Immunosuppressive therapy with agents such as prednisone, azathioprine, and cyclosporine for biopsy-proven myocarditis has been advocated by some, but efficacy has not been established, with the possible exception of the very rare patient with giant cell myocarditis.[73]

Nonpharmacologic Therapies
Nonpharmacologic therapies for DCM are identical to those for HFrEF in general and, when indicated by practice guidelines, include ICD implantation, CRT, and temporary MCS.

Surgical Management
- Cardiac transplantation should be considered for selected patients with HF due to DCM that is refractory to medical therapy.
- LVAD placement may be necessary for stabilization of patients in whom cardiac transplantation is an option or in select patients who are not eligible for transplantation.

Heart Failure With Preserved Ejection Fraction

GENERAL PRINCIPLES

Definition
- HFpEF, also called diastolic HF, refers to the clinical syndrome of HF in the presence of preserved systolic function (LVEF ≥50%).
- Diastolic dysfunction refers to an abnormality in the mechanical function of the heart during the relaxation phase of the cardiac cycle, resulting in elevated filling pressures and impairment of ventricular filling.

CHAPTER 5

Epidemiology

- Almost half of patients admitted to the hospital with HF have a normal or near-normal EF.
- HFpEF is most prevalent in older women, most of whom have hypertension and/or diabetes mellitus. Many of these patients also have CAD and/or AF.

Etiology

- The vast majority of patients with HFpEF have hypertension and LV hypertrophy.
- Myocardial disorders associated with HFpEF include restrictive cardiomyopathy, obstructive and nonobstructive hypertrophic cardiomyopathy, infiltrative cardiomyopathies, and constrictive pericarditis.

Pathophysiology

- Reduced ventricular compliance and elastance play a major role in the pathophysiology of HFpEF.
- Factors contributing to the clinical HFpEF syndrome include abnormal sodium handling by the kidneys, atrial dysfunction, autonomic dysfunction, increased arterial stiffness, pulmonary hypertension, sarcopenia, obesity, deconditioning, and other comorbidities.

DIAGNOSIS

Diagnosis is based on echocardiographic criteria and Doppler findings of normal LVEF and impaired diastolic relaxation and elevated filling pressures. More sensitive echocardiographic parameters of systolic function, such as LV strain, may be abnormal in patients with HFpEF.

TREATMENT

- No pharmacologic therapy has been shown in a randomized controlled trial to reduce mortality in HFpEF patients. Treatments that reduce the combined outcome of cardiac death and HF hospitalization include ARNI, MRA, and SGLT2 inhibitors.
- Practice guidelines for HFpEF emphasize blood pressure control, heart rate control or restoration of sinus rhythm in symptomatic patients, judicious diuretic use, and treatment of ischemic heart disease.

Hypertrophic Cardiomyopathy

GENERAL PRINCIPLES

Definition

Hypertrophic cardiomyopathy (HCM) can be defined broadly as the presence of increased LV wall thickness that is not solely explained by abnormal loading conditions. More specifically, HCM is a genetically determined disease wherein sarcomere mutations lead to LV hypertrophy associated with nondilated ventricular chambers in the absence of another disease that would be capable of causing the magnitude of hypertrophy present in a given individual.[74-76]

Epidemiology

- HCM is the most commonly inherited heart defect, occurring in 1 out of 500 individuals.
- Approximately 500,000 people have HCM in the United States, although many are unaware. An estimated 36% of young athletes who die suddenly have probable or definite HCM, making it the leading cause of SCD in young people in the United States.

Pathophysiology

- HCM results from a mutation in a gene encoding one of the proteins involved in essential myocardial sarcomere functions.
- Over 50% of clinically affected patients have an identified mutation.[77]
- The most common mutations involve myosin binding protein C (*MYBPC3*) and myosin heavy chain 7 (*MYH7*).
- The histopathologic change in HCM consists of hypertrophied myocytes arranged in a disorganized manner with interstitial fibrosis.
- These changes lead grossly to myocardial hypertrophy that is typically predominant in the ventricular septum (asymmetric septal hypertrophy) but may involve any and all ventricular segments. HCM can be classified clinically according to the presence or absence of LV outflow tract (LVOT) obstruction. When present, it is termed **hypertrophic obstructive cardiomyopathy.**
- LVOT obstruction may occur at rest but is enhanced by factors that increase LV contractility (exercise), decrease ventricular volume (e.g., Valsalva maneuver, volume depletion, large meal), or decrease afterload (vasodilators).
- Delayed ventricular diastolic relaxation and decreased compliance are common and, along with MR, may lead to pulmonary congestion.
- Myocardial ischemia is common, secondary to a myocardial oxygen supply–demand mismatch.
- Systolic anterior motion of the anterior leaflet of the mitral valve is often associated with MR and likely determines the severity of LVOT obstruction.

DIAGNOSIS

HCM is usually diagnosed by maximal LV wall thickness ≥15 mm in the absence of another disease that could account for the degree of hypertrophy.

Clinical Presentation

- Presentation varies but may include exertional dyspnea, angina, fatigue, dizziness, syncope, palpitations, or sudden death.
- Sudden death is most common in children and young adults between the ages of 10 and 35 years and often occurs during or immediately after periods of strenuous exertion.

Physical Examination

- Coarse **systolic outflow murmur** localized along the left sternal border that is **accentuated by maneuvers that decrease preload** (e.g., standing, Valsalva maneuver) and may be associated with a forceful double or triple apical impulse.
- Bisferiens (double peak per cardiac cycle) carotid pulse may occur in the presence of obstruction.

CHAPTER 5

Diagnostic Testing

Electrocardiography

The ECG of HCM is usually abnormal and invariably so in symptomatic patients with LVOT obstruction. The most common abnormalities are ST-segment and T-wave abnormalities, followed by evidence of LV hypertrophy. The ECG in apical-variant HCM is characterized by large, inverted T waves across the precordial leads.

Imaging

- Two-dimensional echocardiography and Doppler flow studies can establish the presence of a significant LV outflow gradient at rest or with provocation.
- Additional risk stratification should be pursued with 24- to 48-hour Holter monitoring and exercise testing.
- Cardiac MRI is indicated in patients with suspected HCM in whom the diagnosis cannot be confirmed with echocardiography. Delayed gadolinium enhancement on MRI indicates increased risk of SCD.

Genetic Testing

Genetic testing for HCM is commercially available. Genetic testing can be used to confirm the diagnosis of HCM when the clinical presentation is unclear or to facilitate family screening to determine at-risk first-degree relatives of an index patient.[78]

TREATMENT

- Management is directed toward relief of symptoms and prevention of sudden death.
- Infective endocarditis prophylaxis remains controversial, and prophylactic antibiotics are no longer recommended by guidelines.
- Treatment in asymptomatic individuals is controversial, and no conclusive evidence has been found that medical therapy is beneficial.
- Mild- to moderate-intensity recreational exercise is beneficial.
- Participation in high-intensity recreational activities or moderate- to high-intensity competitive sports may increase the risk of sudden death. These activities should only be considered after a comprehensive evaluation and shared discussion.

Medications

- Nonvasodilating β-blockers are first-line agents to reduce symptoms of HCM by reducing myocardial contractility and heart rate.
- Nondihydropyridine calcium channel antagonists (verapamil and diltiazem) may improve the symptoms of HCM by reducing myocardial contractility and heart rate. Therapy should be initiated at low doses, with careful titration in patients with outflow obstruction. The dose should be increased gradually over several days to weeks if symptoms persist.
- Disopyramide, a negative inotropic agent that results in lowering of the LVOT gradient, may be added for HCM patients who remain symptomatic despite the use of β-blockers and calcium channel blockers (alone or in combination). Use requires monitoring of the QT interval, and concomitant use of other antiarrhythmic drugs should be avoided.
- Diuretics may improve pulmonary congestive symptoms in patients with elevated pulmonary venous pressures. These agents should be used cautiously in patients with LVOT obstruction because excessive preload reduction worsens the obstruction.
- Vasodilators should be avoided, due to the risk of increasing the LVOT gradient.

- **Atrial and ventricular arrhythmias** occur commonly in patients with HCM. Supraventricular tachyarrhythmias are tolerated poorly. Cardioversion is indicated if hemodynamic compromise develops.
- **Digoxin is relatively contraindicated** because of its positive inotropic properties and potential for exacerbating ventricular outflow obstruction.
- AF should be converted to sinus rhythm when possible, and anticoagulation is recommended if paroxysmal or chronic AF develops.
- **Diltiazem, verapamil, or β-blockers** can be used to control the ventricular response. Procainamide, disopyramide, or amiodarone (see Chapter 7, Cardiac Arrhythmias) may be effective in the chronic suppression of AF.
- ICD implantation is recommended for patients with HCM and prior cardiac arrest, ventricular fibrillation, or hemodynamically significant ventricular tachycardia.
- ICD implantation is reasonable in high-risk patients with the following:
  - Prior cardiac arrest
  - Unexplained syncope
  - LV maximal wall thickness >30 mm
  - Sudden death attributed to HCM in one or more first-degree relatives
  - LV apical aneurysm
  - LV systolic dysfunction with LVEF <50%
  - NSVT
  - Extensive delayed gadolinium enhancement on MRI

Nonpharmacologic Therapies for HCM

Dual-chamber pacing (see Chapter 7, Cardiac Arrhythmias) improves symptoms in some patients with HCM. Alteration of the ventricular activation sequence via RV pacing may minimize LVOT obstruction secondary to asymmetric septal hypertrophy. Only 10% of patients with HCM meet the criteria for pacemaker implantation, and the effect on decreasing the LVOT gradient is only 25%. A subset of patients with HCM may derive symptomatic benefit from dual-chamber pacing without an effect on survival.[78]

Surgical Management

- Septal reduction therapy (surgical myectomy or catheter-based alcohol septal ablation) is recommended for those with LVOT obstruction and severe symptoms despite medical therapy.
- Septal myectomy is the most commonly performed surgical intervention in HCM. In experienced centers, it is associated with symptom improvement in 95% of patients with <1% operative mortality.[79] Concomitant mitral valve intervention (mitral valve repair or replacement) is rarely required in experienced centers because MR generally responds well to septal reduction.
- Alcohol septal ablation, a catheter-based alternative to surgical myectomy, also provides relief of obstruction and symptomatic benefit with low procedural mortality, although it can be associated with heart block, requiring pacemaker placement in up to 20% of patients.[80]
- Cardiac transplantation should be considered for patients with refractory symptoms and end-stage HCM.

PATIENT EDUCATION

Genetic counseling and clinical screening are recommended for first-degree relatives of patients with HCM because it is transmitted as an autosomal dominant trait.

Restrictive Cardiomyopathy

GENERAL PRINCIPLES

Definition

- Restrictive cardiomyopathy (RCM) is characterized by a rigid heart with poor ventricular filling but generally a nondilated LV and normal LVEF. Right HF symptoms often predominate.
- RCM may be primary, including conditions such as idiopathic RCM, endomyocardial fibrosis, and Löeffler endocarditis, or secondary to either infiltrative conditions (amyloidosis, sarcoidosis, hypereosinophilic syndrome) or storage diseases (Fabry disease, hemochromatosis, and the glycogen storage diseases).
- Constrictive pericarditis may present similarly to RCM but is a disease wherein the pericardium limits diastolic filling. Constriction carries a different prognosis and therapy, and the distinction between constriction and RCM is essential.

Pathophysiology

- In amyloidosis, misfolded protein (amyloid) deposits in the cardiac interstitium, interrupting the normal myocardial contractile units and causing restriction. Most commonly, the misfolded protein is either AL or TTR.
- In sarcoidosis, granulomatous infiltration of the myocardium is often subclinical and more commonly presents with arrhythmias or conduction system disease; however, in up to 5% of sarcoidosis cases, restriction occurs.
- In hemochromatosis, excess iron is deposited in the cardiomyocyte sarcoplasm, ultimately overcoming antioxidant capacity and resulting in lipid peroxidation and membrane permeability. Injury occurs initially in the epicardium and then later in the myocardium and endocardium, with systolic function initially preserved.
- Fabry disease, an X-linked genetic disorder, is characterized by deficient activity of the lysosomal enzyme α-galactosidase A, resulting in lysosomal accumulation of globotriaosylceramide in tissues. More than half of patients develop cardiomyopathy, typically with LV hypertrophy and RCM.

DIAGNOSIS

Diagnostic Testing

Electrocardiography

The classic ECG finding in amyloidosis is low voltage (despite echocardiographic evidence of ventricular thickening) with poor R-wave progression. In sarcoidosis, conduction disease is often present.

Imaging

- In RCM, echocardiography with Doppler analysis often demonstrates thickened myocardium with normal or abnormal systolic function, abnormal diastolic filling patterns, and evidence of elevated intracardiac pressure. Compared with constrictive pericarditis, respiratory variation is less marked and tissue Doppler velocities are reduced.
- Cardiac MRI and PET are useful diagnostic tools for patients with cardiac sarcoidosis because granulomas, inflammation, and edema may be seen, which appear to improve with therapy.[81] Cardiac MRI is also useful in the diagnosis of amyloidosis.
- Bone-seeking radiotracers have strong avidity for TTR-variant amyloid, and bone scintigraphy with 99m technetium-labeled pyrophosphate is highly sensitive and specific for TTR-cardiac amyloidosis.

Diagnostic Procedures

- On cardiac catheterization, elevated and equalized RV and LV filling pressures are seen with a classic "dip-and-plateau" pattern in the RV and LV pressure tracing. Although pericardial constriction may produce similar findings, absence of ventricular interdependence identifies RCM as opposed to constriction.[82]
- RV endomyocardial biopsy should be considered in patients in whom a diagnosis is not established or where characterization of a protein species will alter therapy, as in cardiac amyloidosis.

TREATMENT

- Specific therapy aimed at amelioration of the underlying cause should be initiated.
- In patients with AL cardiac amyloidosis, chemotherapy to reduce AL production should be pursued in conjunction with a hematologist.
- In patients with TTR amyloidosis, tafamidis has been shown to reduce all-cause mortality and HF hospitalizations and improve functional status and quality of life.[83]
- Heart or heart-liver transplantation may be considered for treatment refractory cardiac amyloidosis.
- Cardiac hemochromatosis may respond to reduction of total body iron stores via phlebotomy or chelation therapy with deferoxamine.[84]
- Cardiac sarcoidosis may respond to glucocorticoid therapy or other immunomodulatory therapies.
- Fabry disease may be treated with recombinant α-galactosidase A enzyme replacement therapy.[85,86]
- Digoxin should be avoided in patients with AL cardiac amyloidosis because digoxin is bound extracellularly by amyloid fibrils and may cause hypersensitivity and toxicity.[87] β-Blockers should be avoided in patients with cardiac amyloidosis.

Peripartum Cardiomyopathy

GENERAL PRINCIPLES

Definition

Peripartum cardiomyopathy (PPCM) is defined as LV systolic dysfunction diagnosed in the last month of pregnancy up to 5 months postpartum, with an incidence 1 in 1000–4000 pregnancies in the United States.[88]

Etiology

The exact etiology of PPCM remains unclear. There is evidence to support viral, nutritional, and autoimmune contributors. Animal model and epidemiologic data suggest that **vascular dysfunction and toxicity** incited by the peripartum hormonal environment plays a central role in PPCM.[89-91]

Risk Factors

Risk factors that predispose a woman to PPCM include advanced maternal age, multiparity, multiple pregnancies, preeclampsia, and gestational hypertension. There is a higher risk in African-American women, but this may be confounded by the higher prevalence of hypertension in this population.

CHAPTER 5

DIAGNOSIS

Clinical Presentation

- Women with PPCM typically present with NYHA III and IV HF, although mild cases and sudden cardiac arrest also occur.
- Because dyspnea on exertion and lower extremity edema are common in late pregnancy, PPCM may be difficult to recognize. Cough, orthopnea, and paroxysmal nocturnal dyspnea are warning signs that PPCM may be present, as is the presence of a displaced apical impulse and a new MR murmur on examination.

Diagnostic Testing

Electrocardiography

On ECG, LV hypertrophy is often present, as are ST-T–wave abnormalities.

Imaging

Diagnosis requires an echocardiogram with a newly depressed EF and/or LV dilatation.

TREATMENT

Medications

- Therapy in the postpartum patient mirrors GDMT for HFrEF. Most agents are safe in lactation. Data for sacubitril/valsartan and ivabradine are lacking.
- During pregnancy, ACE/ARB/ARNI, MRA, and ivabradine should be avoided. β-Blockers, loop diuretics, hydralazine/nitrates, and digoxin are safe.
- In patients with thromboembolism, **low molecular weight heparin** is required, followed by **warfarin** after delivery.

OUTCOME/PROGNOSIS

- The prognosis in PPCM is better than that seen in other forms of nonischemic cardiomyopathy.
- The extent of ventricular recovery at 6 months after delivery can predict overall recovery, although continued improvement has been seen up to 2–3 years after diagnosis.
- Subsequent pregnancies in patients with PPCM may be associated with significant deterioration in LV function and can even result in death, particularly in women who do not recover normal LV function after the first insult. Women who do not recover LV function should be encouraged to consider foregoing future pregnancy.

REFERENCES

1. Yancy CW, Jessup M, Bozkurt B, et al. 2017 ACC/AHA/HFSA focused update of the 2013 ACCF/AHA guideline for the management of heart failure: a report of the American College of Cardiology/American Heart Association Task Force on clinical practice guidelines and the Heart Failure Society of America. *Circulation.* 2017;136(6):e137-e161.
2. Writing Committee, Maddox TM, Januzzi JL Jr, et al. 2021 update to the 2017 ACC expert consensus decision pathway for optimization of heart failure treatment. Answers to 10 pivotal issues about heart failure with reduced ejection fraction: a report of the American College of Cardiology Solution Set Oversight Committee. *J Am Coll Cardiol.* 2021;77(6):772-810.
3. Bozkurt B, Coats AJ, Tsutsui H, et al. Universal definition and classification of heart failure: a report of the Heart Failure Society of America, Heart Failure Association of the European Society of Cardiology, Japanese Heart Failure Society and Writing Committee of the Universal Definition of Heart Failure. *J Card Fail.* 2021:S1071-9164(21)00050-6.

4. Benjamin EJ, Virani SS, Callaway CW, et al. Heart disease and stroke statistics-2018 update: a report from the American Heart Association. *Circulation.* 2018;137:e67-e492.
5. Loehr LR, Rosamond WD, Chang PP, et al. Heart failure incidence and survival (from the Atherosclerosis Risk in Communities Study). *Am J Cardiol.* 2008;101:1016-1022.
6. Maisel AS, Krishnaswamy P, Nowak RM, et al. Rapid measurement of B-type natriuretic peptide in the emergency diagnosis of heart failure. *N Engl J Med.* 2002;347:161-167.
7. Januzzi JL, van Kimmenade R, Lainchbury J, et al. NT-proBNP testing for diagnosis and short-term prognosis in acute destabilized heart failure. An international pooled analysis of 1256 patients: the International Collaborative of NT-proBNP Study. *Eur Heart J.* 2006;27:330-337.
8. Roberts E, Ludman AJ, Dworzynski K, et al. The diagnostic accuracy of the natriuretic peptides in heart failure: systematic review and diagnostic meta-analysis in the acute care setting. *Br Med J.* 2015;350:h910.
9. Knudsen CW, Omland T, Clopton P, et al. Diagnostic value of B-Type natriuretic peptide and chest radiographic findings in patients with acute dyspnea. *Am J Med.* 2004;116:363-368.
10. Mancini DM, Eisen H, Kussmaul W, et al. Value of peak exercise oxygen consumption for optimal timing of cardiac transplantation in ambulatory patients with heart failure. *Circulation.* 1991;83:778-786.
11. Cooper LT, Baughman KL, Feldman AM, et al. The role of endomyocardial biopsy in the management of cardiovascular disease: a scientific statement from the American Heart Association, the American College of Cardiology, and the European Society of Cardiology. *Circulation.* 2007;116:2216-2233.
12. Cleland JGF, Bunting KV, Flather MD, et al; Beta-Blockers in Heart Failure Collaborative Group. Beta-blockers for heart failure with reduced, mid-range, and preserved ejection fraction: an individual patient-level analysis of double-blind randomized trials. *Eur Heart J.* 2018;39(1):26-35.
13. Krum H, Roecker EB, Mohacsi P, et al. Effects of initiating carvedilol in patients with severe chronic heart failure: results from the COPERNICUS study. *J Am Med Assoc.* 2003;289:712-718.
14. Packer M, Coats AJ, Fowler MB, et al. Effect of carvedilol on survival in severe chronic heart failure. *N Engl J Med.* 2001;344:1651-1658.
15. Poole-Wilson PA, Swedberg K, Cleland JG, et al. Comparison of carvedilol and metoprolol on clinical outcomes in patients with chronic heart failure in the Carvedilol Or Metoprolol European Trial (COMET): randomised controlled trial. *Lancet.* 2003;362:7-13.
16. Hjalmarson A, Goldstein S, Fagerberg B, et al. Effects of controlled-release metoprolol on total mortality, hospitalizations, and well-being in patients with heart failure: the Metoprolol CR/XL Randomized Intervention Trial in congestive heart failure (MERIT-HF). MERIT-HF Study Group. *J Am Med Assoc.* 2000;283:1295-1302.
17. CIBIS-II Investigators and Committees. The cardiac insufficiency Bisoprolol study II (CIBIS-II): a randomised trial. *Lancet.* 1999;353:9-13.
18. McMurray JJ, Packer M, Desai AS, et al. Angiotensin-neprilysin inhibition versus enalapril in heart failure. *N Engl J Med.* 2014;371:993-1004.
19. Packer M, Poole-Wilson PA, Armstrong PW, et al. Comparative effects of low and high doses of the angiotensin-converting enzyme inhibitor, lisinopril, on morbidity and mortality in chronic heart failure. ATLAS Study Group. *Circulation.* 1999;100:2312-2318.
20. Palmer BF. Renal dysfunction complicating the treatment of hypertension. *N Engl J Med.* 2002;347:1256-1261.
21. Pitt B, Poole-Wilson PA, Segal R, et al. Effect of losartan compared with captopril on mortality in patients with symptomatic heart failure: randomised trial–the Losartan Heart Failure Survival Study ELITE II. *Lancet.* 2000;355:1582-1587.
22. Cohn JN, Tognoni G. A randomized trial of the angiotensin-receptor blocker valsartan in chronic heart failure. *N Engl J Med.* 2001;345:1667-1675.
23. Yusuf S, Pfeffer MA, Swedberg K, et al. Effects of candesartan in patients with chronic heart failure and preserved left-ventricular ejection fraction: the CHARM-preserved trial. *Lancet.* 2003;362:777-781.
24. Pitt B, Zannad F, Remme WJ, et al. The effect of spironolactone on morbidity and mortality in patients with severe heart failure. Randomized Aldactone Evaluation Study Investigators. *N Engl J Med.* 1999;341:709-717.
25. Pitt B, Remme W, Zannad F, et al. Eplerenone, a selective aldosterone blocker, in patients with left ventricular dysfunction after myocardial infarction. *N Engl J Med.* 2003;348:1309-1321.
26. Zannad F, McMurray JJ, Krum H, et al. Eplerenone in patients with systolic heart failure and mild symptoms. *N Engl J Med.* 2011;364:11-21.
27. McMurray JJV, Solomon SD, Inzucchi SE, et al; DAPA-HF Trial Committees and Investigators. Dapagliflozin in patients with heart failure and reduced ejection fraction. *N Engl J Med.* 2019;381(21):1995-2008.
28. Packer M, Anker SD, Butler J, et al; EMPEROR-Reduced trial Investigators. Cardiovascular and renal outcomes with empagliflozin in heart failure. *N Engl J Med.* 2020;383(15):1413-1424.
29. Neal B, Perkovic V, Mahaffey KW, et al; CANVAS Program Collaborative Group. Canagliflozin and cardiovascular and renal events in type 2 diabetes. *N Engl J Med.* 2017;377(7):644-657.

CHAPTER 5

30. Bhatt DL, Szarek M, Steg PG, et al; SOLOIST-WHF Trial Investigators. Sotagliflozin in patients with diabetes and recent worsening heart failure. *N Engl J Med.* 2021;384(2):117-128.

31. Taylor AL, Ziesche S, Yancy C, et al. Combination of isosorbide dinitrate and hydralazine in blacks with heart failure. *N Engl J Med.* 2004;351:2049-2057.

32. Cohn JN, Archibald DG, Ziesche S, et al. Effect of vasodilator therapy on mortality in chronic congestive heart failure. Results of a Veterans Administration Cooperative Study. *N Engl J Med.* 1986;314:1547-1552.

33. Armstrong PW, Pieske B, Anstrom KJ, et al; VICTORIA Study Group. Vericiguat in patients with heart failure and reduced ejection fraction. *N Engl J Med.* 2020;382(20):1883-1893.

34. Swedberg K, Komajda M, Bohm M, et al. Ivabradine and outcomes in chronic heart failure (SHIFT): a randomised placebo-controlled study. *Lancet.* 2010;376:875-885.

35. Digitalis Investigation Group. The effect of digoxin on mortality and morbidity in patients with heart failure. *N Engl J Med.* 1997;336:525-533.

36. Rathore SS, Wang Y, Krumholz HM. Sex-based differences in the effect of digoxin for the treatment of heart failure. *N Engl J Med.* 2002;347:1403-1411.

37. Rathore SS, Curtis JP, Wang Y, et al. Association of serum digoxin concentration and outcomes in patients with heart failure. *J Am Med Assoc.* 2003;289:871-878.

38. Packer M, Gheorghiade M, Young JB, et al. Withdrawal of digoxin from patients with chronic heart failure treated with angiotensin-converting-enzyme inhibitors. RADIANCE Study. *N Engl J Med.* 1993;329:1-7.

39. Packer M, O'Connor CM, Ghali JK, et al. Effect of amlodipine on morbidity and mortality in severe chronic heart failure. Prospective Randomized Amlodipine Survival Evaluation Study Group. *N Engl J Med.* 1996;335:1107-1114.

40. Packer M, Carson P, Elkayam U, et al. Effect of amlodipine on the survival of patients with severe chronic heart failure due to a nonischemic cardiomyopathy: results of the PRAISE-2 study (prospective randomized amlodipine survival evaluation 2). *JACC Heart Fail.* 2013;1:308-314.

41. Cuffe MS, Califf RM, Adams KF Jr, et al. Short-term intravenous milrinone for acute exacerbation of chronic heart failure: a randomized controlled trial. *J Am Med Assoc.* 2002;287:1541-1547.

42. Teerlink JR, Diaz R, Felker GM, et al; GALACTIC-HF Investigators. Cardiac myosin activation with omecamtiv mecarbil in systolic heart failure. *N Engl J Med.* 2021;384(2):105-116.

43. Solomon SD, McMurray JJV, Anand IS, et al; PARAGON-HF Investigators and Committees. Angiotensin-neprilysin inhibition in heart failure with preserved ejection fraction. *N Engl J Med.* 2019;381(17):1609-1620.

44. Solomon SD, Vaduganathan M, Claggett BL, et al. Sacubitril/valsartan across the Spectrum of ejection fraction in heart failure. *Circulation.* 2020;141(5):352-361.

45. Pitt B, Pfeffer MA, Assmann SF, et al. Spironolactone for heart failure with preserved ejection fraction. *N Engl J Med.* 2014;370:1383-1392.

46. Anker SD, Butler J, Filippatos G, et al; EMPEROR-Preserved Trial Investigators. Empagliflozin in heart failure with a preserved ejection fraction. *N Engl J Med.* 2021;385(16):1451-1461. doi:10.1056/NEJMoa2107038

47. Bhatt DL, Szarek M, Pitt B, et al; SCORED Investigators. Sotagliflozin in patients with diabetes and chronic kidney disease. *N Engl J Med.* 2021;384(2):129-139.

48. Echt DS, Liebson PR, Mitchell LB, et al. Mortality and morbidity in patients receiving encainide, flecainide, or placebo. The Cardiac Arrhythmia Suppression Trial. *N Engl J Med.* 1991;324:781-788.

49. Roy D, Talajic M, Nattel S, et al. Rhythm control versus rate control for atrial fibrillation and heart failure. *N Engl J Med.* 2008;358:2667-2677.

50. Kober L, Torp-Pedersen C, McMurray JJ, et al. Increased mortality after dronedarone therapy for severe heart failure. *N Engl J Med.* 2008;358:2678-2687.

51. Marrouche NF, Brachmann J, Andresen D, et al. Catheter ablation for atrial fibrillation with heart failure. *N Engl J Med.* 2018;378:417-427.

52. Velazquez EJ, Lee KL, Deja MA, et al. Coronary-artery bypass surgery in patients with left ventricular dysfunction. *N Engl J Med.* 2011;364:1607-1616.

53. Velazquez EJ, Lee KL, Jones RH, et al. Coronary-artery bypass surgery in patients with ischemic cardiomyopathy. *N Engl J Med.* 2016;374:1511-1520.

54. Cleland JG, Daubert JC, Erdmann E, et al. The effect of cardiac resynchronization on morbidity and mortality in heart failure. *N Engl J Med.* 2005;352:1539-1549.

55. Tang AS, Wells GA, Talajic M, et al. Cardiac-resynchronization therapy for mild-to-moderate heart failure. *N Engl J Med.* 2010;363:2385-2395.

56. Hsu JC, Solomon SD, Bourgoun M, et al. Predictors of super-response to cardiac resynchronization therapy and associated improvement in clinical outcome: the MADIT-CRT (multicenter automatic defibrillator implantation trial with cardiac resynchronization therapy) study. *J Am Coll Cardiol.* 2012;59:2366-2373.

57. Abraham WT, Adamson PB, Bourge RC, et al. Wireless pulmonary artery haemodynamic monitoring in chronic heart failure: a randomised controlled trial. *Lancet.* 2011;377:658-666.

58. Stone GW, Lindenfeld J, Abraham WT, et al; COAPT Investigators. Transcatheter mitral-valve repair in patients with heart failure. *N Engl J Med.* 2018;379(24):2307-2318.

59. Rose EA, Gelijns AC, Moskowitz AJ, et al. Long-term use of a left ventricular assist device for end-stage heart failure. *N Engl J Med.* 2001;345:1435-1443.

60. Mehra MR, Naka Y, Uriel N, et al. A fully magnetically levitated circulatory pump for advanced heart failure. *N Engl J Med.* 2017;376:440-450.

61. Mehra MR, Goldstein DJ, Uriel N, et al. Two-year outcomes with a magnetically levitated cardiac pump in heart failure. *N Engl J Med.* 2018;378:1386-1395.

62. Mehra MR, Kobashigawa J, Starling R, et al. Listing criteria for heart transplantation: International Society for Heart and Lung Transplantation guidelines for the care of cardiac transplant candidates–2006. *J Heart Lung Transplant.* 2006;25:1024-1042.

63. Kaneko Y, Floras JS, Usui K, et al. Cardiovascular effects of continuous positive airway pressure in patients with heart failure and obstructive sleep apnea. *N Engl J Med.* 2003;348:1233-1241.

64. Cowie MR, Woehrle H, Wegscheider K, et al. Adaptive servo-ventilation for central sleep apnea in systolic heart failure. *N Engl J Med.* 2015;373:1095-1105.

65. Costanzo MR, Guglin ME, Saltzberg MT, et al. Ultrafiltration versus intravenous diuretics for patients hospitalized for acute decompensated heart failure. *J Am Coll Cardiol.* 2007;49:675-683.

66. Bart BA, Goldsmith SR, Lee KL, et al. Ultrafiltration in decompensated heart failure with cardiorenal syndrome. *N Engl J Med.* 2012;367:2296-2304.

67. Whellan DJ, Goodlin SJ, Dickinson MG, et al. End-of-life care in patients with heart failure. *J Card Fail.* 2014;20:121-134.

68. Masip J, Roque M, Sanchez B, et al. Noninvasive ventilation in acute cardiogenic pulmonary edema: systematic review and meta-analysis. *J Am Med Assoc.* 2005;294:3124-3130.

69. De Backer D, Biston P, Devriendt J, et al. Comparison of dopamine and norepinephrine in the treatment of shock. *N Engl J Med.* 2010;362:779-789.

70. Binanay C, Califf RM, Hasselblad V, et al. Evaluation study of congestive heart failure and pulmonary artery catheterization effectiveness: the ESCAPE trial. *J Am Med Assoc.* 2005;294:1625-1633.

71. Cheng JM, den Uil CA, Hoeks SE, et al. Percutaneous left ventricular assist devices vs. intra-aortic balloon pump counterpulsation for treatment of cardiogenic shock: a meta-analysis of controlled trials. *Eur Heart J.* 2009;30:2102-2108.

72. Hershberger RE, Hedges DJ, Morales A. Dilated cardiomyopathy: the complexity of a diverse genetic architecture. *Nat Rev Cardiol.* 2013;10:531-547.

73. Mason JW, O'Connell JB, Herskowitz A, et al. A clinical trial of immunosuppressive therapy for myocarditis. The Myocarditis Treatment Trial Investigators. *N Engl J Med.* 1995;333:269-275.

74. Elliott PM, Anastasakis A, Borger MA, et al. 2014 ESC guidelines on diagnosis and management of hypertrophic cardiomyopathy: the task force for the diagnosis and management of hypertrophic cardiomyopathy of the European Society of Cardiology (ESC). *Eur Heart J.* 2014;35:2733-2779.

75. Ommen SR, Mital S, Burke MA, et al. 2020 AHA/ACC guideline for the diagnosis and treatment of patients with hypertrophic cardiomyopathy. Executive summary: a report of the American College of Cardiology/American Heart Association Joint Committee on clinical practice guidelines. *J Am Coll Cardiol.* 2020;76(25):3022-3055.

76. Hershberger RE, Siegfried JD. Update 2011: clinical and genetic issues in familial dilated cardiomyopathy. *J Am Coll Cardiol.* 2011;57:1641-1649.

77. Bos JM, Towbin JA, Ackerman MJ. Diagnostic, prognostic, and therapeutic implications of genetic testing for hypertrophic cardiomyopathy. *J Am Coll Cardiol.* 2009;54:201-211.

78. Galve E, Sambola A, Saldana G, et al. Late benefits of dual-chamber pacing in obstructive hypertrophic cardiomyopathy: a 10-year follow-up study. *Heart.* 2010;96:352-356.

79. Ommen SR, Maron BJ, Olivotto I, et al. Long-term effects of surgical septal myectomy on survival in patients with obstructive hypertrophic cardiomyopathy. *J Am Coll Cardiol.* 2005;46:470-476.

80. Sorajja P, Valeti U, Nishimura RA, et al. Outcome of alcohol septal ablation for obstructive hypertrophic cardiomyopathy. *Circulation.* 2008;118:131-139.

81. Schatka I, Bengel FM. Advanced imaging of cardiac sarcoidosis. *J Nucl Med.* 2014;55:99-106.

82. Talreja DR, Nishimura RA, Oh JK, et al. Constrictive pericarditis in the modern era: novel criteria for diagnosis in the cardiac catheterization laboratory. *J Am Coll Cardiol.* 2008;51:315-319.

83. Maurer MS, Schwartz JH, Gundapaneni B, et al; ATTR-ACT Study Investigators. Tafamidis treatment for patients with transthyretin amyloid cardiomyopathy. *N Engl J Med.* 2018;379(11):1007-1016.

84. Gujja P, Rosing DR, Tripodi DJ, et al. Iron overload cardiomyopathy: better understanding of an increasing disorder. *J Am Coll Cardiol.* 2010;56:1001-1012.

85. Schiffmann R, Kopp JB, Austin HAIII, et al. Enzyme replacement therapy in Fabry disease: a randomized controlled trial. *J Am Med Assoc.* 2001;285:2743-2749.

CHAPTER 5

86. Eng CM, Guffon N, Wilcox WR, et al. Safety and efficacy of recombinant human alpha-galactosidase A replacement therapy in Fabry's disease. *N Engl J Med.* 2001;345:9-16.
87. Rubinow A, Skinner M, Cohen AS. Digoxin sensitivity in amyloid cardiomyopathy. *Circulation.* 1981;63:1285-1288.
88. Arany Z, Elkayam U. Peripartum cardiomyopathy. *Circulation.* 2016;133:1397-1409.
89. Davis MB, Arany Z, McNamara DM, Goland S, Elkayam U. Peripartum cardiomyopathy: JACC state-of-the-Art review. *J Am Coll Cardiol.* 2020;75(2):207-221.
90. Sliwa K, Fett J, Elkayam U. Peripartum cardiomyopathy. *Lancet.* 2006;368:687-693.
91. Hilfiker-Kleiner D, Kaminski K, Podewski E, et al. A cathepsin D-cleaved 16 kDa form of prolactin mediates postpartum cardiomyopathy. *Cell.* 2007;128:589-600.

6 Pericardial and Valvular Heart Disease

Phillip M. King and Nishath Quader

PERICARDIAL DISEASE

Acute Pericarditis

ETIOLOGY

Idiopathic, neoplastic (chemotherapy and radiation), autoimmune, viral, tuberculosis, bacterial (nontuberculous), uremia, post–cardiac surgery, trauma, post–myocardial infarction, drugs, dissecting aortic aneurysm, hypothyroidism.

Pathophysiology
- The pericardium is a fibrous sac surrounding the heart consisting of two layers: a thin visceral layer attached to the myocardium and a thicker parietal layer.
- The pericardial space is normally filled with 15–50 mL of fluid, and the two layers slide smoothly against each other, allowing for normal expansion and contraction of the heart.
- Pericarditis occurs when these layers are inflamed.

DIAGNOSIS

History
- The clinical presentation of acute pericarditis can vary depending on the underlying etiology.
- Chest pain: typically sudden onset, anterior chest, sharp and pleuritic; improved by sitting up and leaning forward, made worse by inspiration and lying flat, radiation to back, neck and shoulders, pain along the trapezius ridge.

Physical Examination
Pericardial friction rub: highly specific for acute pericarditis. Described as a "scratchy, grating, or squeaking sound," heard best with the diaphragm of the stethoscope.

Diagnostic Testing
- **Electrocardiogram (ECG):** diffuse ST-segment elevation (usually in more than one coronary artery distribution) and PR depression.
- **Transthoracic echocardiogram (TTE):** may observe an associated pericardial effusion.
- Other tests: complete blood count, C-reactive protein, erythrocyte sedimentation rate, blood cultures (if suspect infection), thyroid function, cytology (if suspecting neoplasm).

TREATMENT

- Treat the underlying cause whenever possible.
- **NSAIDs:** ibuprofen, aspirin, ketorolac.
- **Colchicine:** when added to conventional anti-inflammatory therapy, significantly reduces symptoms, recurrence rates, and hospitalizations (COPE trial).[1]
- **Glucocorticoids:** reserved for cases refractory to standard therapy or in the setting of uremia, connective tissue disease, or immune-mediated pericarditis. Increases risk of recurrence.

Constrictive Pericarditis

Constrictive pericarditis is often difficult to distinguish from restrictive cardiomyopathies. Multiple imaging modalities, invasive hemodynamic tests, history, and physical examination are often needed to confirm the diagnosis.

ETIOLOGY

Idiopathic, viral pericarditis (chronic or recurrent), postcardiotomy, chest irradiation, autoimmune connective tissue disorders, end-stage renal disease, uremia, malignancy (e.g., breast, lung, lymphoma), and tuberculosis (more common in endemic countries).

Pathophysiology

- In the setting of chronic inflammation, the pericardial layers become thickened, scarred, and calcified.
- The pericardial space is obliterated, and the pericardium becomes noncompliant. This impairs ventricular filling and leads to an equalization of pressures in all four chambers and subsequent heart failure symptoms.

DIAGNOSIS

History
The clinical presentation of constrictive pericarditis is insidious, with gradual development of fatigue, exercise intolerance, and venous congestion.

Physical Examination
- Features of right-sided heart failure: lower extremity edema, hepatomegaly, ascites, elevated jugular venous pressure (JVP).
- Other characteristic signs
  - **Kussmaul sign:** paradoxical increase in JVP with inspiration or lack of appropriate decrease in JVP with inspiration.
  - **Pericardial knock:** early, loud, high-pitched S_3.

Diagnostic Testing
- **TTE**
  - First-line diagnostic test.
  - Ventricular systolic function can be deceptively "normal."
  - Features suggestive of constrictive pericarditis include the following:
    - Increased pericardial thickness/tethering of the pericardium to the myocardium.
    - Dilated, incompressible inferior vena cava (IVC).
    - Septal bounce (exaggerated septal motion).

- Inspiratory variation in mitral flow velocity curves.
- Expiratory diastolic flow reversal in hepatic veins.
- Preserved (or increased) tissue Doppler velocities of the mitral annulus.
- Blunted superior vena cava flow.

- **Cardiac catheterization:** allows for simultaneous measurement of right ventricular and left ventricular pressures.
- **Cardiac CT and MRI**
  - Provide excellent visualization of pericardial anatomy (thickness and calcification).
  - An MRI and gated CT can show evidence of ventricular interdependence (septal bounce).
  - Can provide other anatomic information that may be helpful in making the diagnosis of constriction (i.e., engorgement of IVC and hepatic veins) and its etiology (i.e., lymph nodes, tumors).

TREATMENT

- Limited role for medical therapy: diuretics, low-sodium diet.
- Patients with constriction often have a resting sinus tachycardia. Because of limited stroke volume (SV), they are more dependent on heart rate for adequate cardiac output (CO). Avoid efforts to slow down the heart rate.
- **Surgical pericardiectomy is the only definitive treatment for constrictive pericarditis.** Operative mortality is 5%–15%; more advanced heart failure symptoms confer higher operative risk.

Cardiac Tamponade

Cardiac tamponade is a **clinical diagnosis** and is considered a medical emergency. Imaging is used to confirm the presence of a pericardial effusion; however, it should not be solely relied on to make the diagnosis of tamponade.

ETIOLOGY

Procedural complications, infection, neoplasms, or idiopathic pericarditis, postcardiotomy, autoimmune connective tissue disorders, uremia, trauma, radiation, myocardial infarction (subacute), drugs (hydralazine, procainamide, isoniazid, phenytoin, minoxidil), hypothyroidism

Pathophysiology

- Fluid accumulation in the pericardial space increases pericardial pressure. The pressure depends on the amount of fluid, the rate of accumulation, and the compliance of the pericardium.
- Tamponade develops when the pressure in the pericardial space is sufficiently high to interfere with adequate cardiac filling, resulting in a decrease in CO.

DIAGNOSIS

History

- The diagnosis of cardiac tamponade should be suspected in patients with **elevated JVP, hypotension, and distant heart sounds (Beck's triad).**
- Symptoms can include dyspnea, fatigue, anxiety, presyncope, chest discomfort, abdominal fullness, and lethargy.

Physical Examination

- **Pulsus paradoxus** refers to an abnormally large decrease in systolic blood pressure, SV, and pulse wave amplitude with inspiration.
- A normal fall in pressure is less than 10 mm Hg. **A decrease in systolic pressure >10 mm Hg is one of the physical examination findings in tamponade.**
- Patients are also frequently tachycardic and hypotensive.

Diagnostic Testing

- **Remember: Cardiac tamponade is a clinical diagnosis that can be made based on history, physical examination, and vital signs (blood pressure, pulse paradoxus) alone.**
- **ECG:** low voltage (more likely with larger pericardial effusions), sinus tachycardia, electrical alternans (specific but not sensitive).
- **TTE**
  - First-line diagnostic test to evaluate the hemodynamic significance of pericardial effusion.
  - Features suggestive of a hemodynamically significant pericardial effusion:
    - Dilated, incompressible IVC.
    - Significant respiratory variation of tricuspid and mitral inflow velocities (>25% mitral, >40% tricuspid).
    - Early diastolic collapse of the right ventricle and systolic collapse of the right atrium.

TREATMENT

- Limited role for medical therapy to treat cardiac tamponade. **Goal is to maintain adequate filling pressures** with IV fluids. Avoid diuretics, nitrates, and any other preload-reducing medications. Avoid efforts to slow down sinus tachycardia: it compensates for a reduced SV to try to maintain adequate CO.
- **Percutaneous pericardiocentesis** with echocardiographic guidance can be a relatively safe and effective way to drain the pericardial fluid; the approach should be guided by location of the fluid and is usually easiest when the effusion is in anterior location.
- Creation of a **pericardial window** is preferred for recurring effusions, loculated effusions, or those not safely accessible percutaneously.

VALVULAR HEART DISEASE

The 2020 American Heart Association/American College of Cardiology (AHA/ACC) Guidelines describe different stages in the progression of valvular heart disease (VHD).[2]
- **Stage A (at risk):** patients with risk factors for development of VHD.
- **Stage B (progressive):** patients with progressive VHD (mild to moderate severity and asymptomatic).
- **Stage C (asymptomatic severe):** asymptomatic patients who meet criteria for severe VHD.
  - C1: asymptomatic patients with a compensated left and right ventricle.
  - C2: asymptomatic patients with decompensation of the left or right ventricle.
- **Stage D (symptomatic severe):** patients who have developed symptoms as a result of VHD.

Mitral Stenosis

Mitral stenosis (MS) is characterized by incomplete opening of the mitral valve during diastole, which limits antegrade flow and yields a sustained diastolic pressure gradient between the left atrium (LA) and the left ventricle (LV).

ETIOLOGY

- **Rheumatic MS**
  - Because of the increased use of antibiotics, the incidence of rheumatic heart disease as a cause of MS has decreased.
  - Two-thirds of patients with rheumatic MS are female; may be associated with mitral regurgitation (MR).
  - Rheumatic fever can cause fibrosis, thickening, and calcification, leading to fusion of the commissures, leaflets, chordae, and/or papillary muscles.
- **Other causes of MS:** substantial mitral annular calcification (calcific MS), systemic lupus erythematosus (SLE), rheumatoid arthritis, congenital, oversewn or small mitral annuloplasty ring; "functional MS" may occur with obstruction of the LA outflow because of tumor (particularly myxoma), LA thrombus, or endocarditis with a large vegetation.

Pathophysiology

- Increased transvalvular flow or decreased diastolic filling time may lead to worsening symptoms of MS. This occurs with pregnancy, exercise, hyperthyroidism, atrial fibrillation (AF) with rapid ventricular response, and fever.
- MS causes increased pressure in the LA, which then dilates as a compensatory mechanism. This causes the LA to dilate and fibrose, which then leads to atrial arrhythmias and thrombus formation.
- A sustained increase in pulmonary venous pressures is transmitted backward to cause pulmonary hypertension (PH) and with time, increased pulmonary vascular resistance and right ventricular pressure overload and dysfunction.

DIAGNOSIS

History

After a prolonged asymptomatic period, patients may report any of the following: dyspnea, decreased functional capacity, orthopnea, paroxysmal nocturnal dyspnea, fatigue, palpitations, systemic embolism, hemoptysis, chest pain.

Physical Examination

- **Opening snap (OS)** caused by sudden tensing of the valve leaflets; the A_2-OS interval varies inversely with the severity of stenosis (shorter interval = more severe stenosis).
- **Mid-diastolic rumble:** low-pitched murmur heard best at the apex with the bell of the stethoscope; the severity of stenosis is related to the duration of the murmur, not intensity.
- Signs of right-sided heart failure and PH.

Diagnostic Testing

- **ECG:** left atrial enlargement (LAE), AF, right ventricular hypertrophy.
- **CXR:** enlarged chambers, calcification of the mitral valve and/or annulus.

- **TTE**
  - Assess valve leaflets and subvalvular apparatus.
  - Determine mitral valve area (MVA) and mean transmitral gradient (severe considered MVA ≤1.5 cm^2 or mean transmitral gradient of >5–10 mm Hg).
  - Estimate pulmonary artery systolic pressure (PASP) and evaluate right ventricular size and function.
- **Transesophageal echocardiogram (TEE):** Imaging modality of choice for evaluation of anatomy and functional significance. Also used to rule out left atrial thrombus.
- **Exercise stress testing:** indicated when symptoms are out of proportion to severity indicated by TTE.
- **Cardiac catheterization:** Rarely used. Useful in cases of discordant or inconclusive data by echocardiography. May provide clarification to the etiology of severe PH when out of proportion of the severity of MS. Typically performed in patients going for mitral valve replacement with risk factors for CAD.

TREATMENT

Medical Management

- Diuretics, β-blockers, and low-salt diet for heart failure symptoms.
- **AF** occurs in 30%–40% of patients with severe MS.
  - Therapy is mostly aimed at rate control and prevention of thromboembolism.
  - **Class I indication for anticoagulation** for prevention of systemic embolization in patients with MS regardless of CHADS2VASC score.[2]

Percutaneous Mitral Balloon Commissurotomy

- Balloon inflation separates the leaflets, yielding an increased valve area.
- Indicated only in rheumatic MS where there is thickening of the leaflets and annulus is mostly spared.
- Procedure of choice in experienced centers in patients without contraindications (such as moderate or severe MR and left atrial appendage thrombus).
- **Recommendations for percutaneous mitral balloon commissurotomy**[2]
  - Symptomatic patients with severe MS (valve area ≤1.5 cm^2) (stage D) and favorable valve anatomy in the absence of contraindications (i.e., LA clot or moderate to severe MR) (Class I)
  - Other indications: Asymptomatic patients with severe MS and pulmonary hypertension (PASP >50 mm Hg) or new onset AF (Class II)

Surgical Management

Recommendations for mitral valve surgery[2]: Severely symptomatic patients with severe MS who are not candidates for or failed previous percutaneous mitral balloon commissurotomy, or who are undergoing other cardiac procedures (Class I).

Aortic Stenosis

- **Aortic stenosis** (AS) is the most common cause of LV outflow tract obstruction.
- Other causes of obstruction occur above the valve (supravalvular) and below the valve (subvalvular), both fixed (i.e., subaortic membrane) and dynamic (i.e., hypertrophic cardiomyopathy with obstruction).

ETIOLOGY

- **Calcific/degenerative**
  - Most common cause in the US
  - Trileaflet calcific AS usually presents in the seventh to ninth decades of life
- **Bicuspid**
  - Occurs in 1%–2% of population (congenital lesion)
  - AS in this population occurs in much younger patients
  - Can be associated with aortopathies (i.e., dissection, aneurysm)
- **Rheumatic**
  - More common cause worldwide; much less common in the US
  - Almost always accompanied by MV disease
- **Radiation induced**

Pathophysiology

The pathophysiology for calcific AS involves both the valve and the ventricular adaptation to the stenosis (Figure 6-1).

DIAGNOSIS

History

- The classic triad of symptoms includes **angina, syncope, and heart failure.**
- Symptoms may be masked by a progressive decline in functional capacity as patients modify their activities to suit their symptoms.

Physical Examination

- **Harsh systolic crescendo–decrescendo murmur** heard best at the right upper sternal border and radiating to both carotids; time to peak intensity correlates with severity (later peak = more severe).
- Diminished or absent A_2 (soft S_2) suggests severe AS.
- **Pulsus parvus et tardus:** late-peaking and diminished carotid upstroke in severe AS.

Diagnostic Testing

- **ECG:** LAE, left ventricular hypertrophy (LVH).
- **CXR:** cardiomegaly, calcification of the aorta and/or aortic valve.
- **TTE**
  - Determine valve morphology (tricuspid vs. bicuspid), calculate valve area using continuity equation, and measure transvalvular mean and peak gradients.
  - **Severe AS:** peak jet velocity ≥4.0 m/s, mean gradient ≥40 mm Hg, valve area <1.0 cm^2.
- **TEE:** useful in select patients to better visualize valve morphology and determination of AS severity.
- **Dobutamine stress echocardiography**
  - Useful to assess the patient with a reduced SV (reduced or preserved ejection fraction [EF]) and small calculated valve area but a low (<30–40 mm Hg) mean transvalvular gradient.
  - Can help distinguish truly severe AS from pseudo–severe AS.
- **Cardiac catheterization**
  - Hemodynamic assessment of severity of AS in patients for whom noninvasive tests are inconclusive or when there is discrepancy between noninvasive tests and clinical findings regarding AS severity.

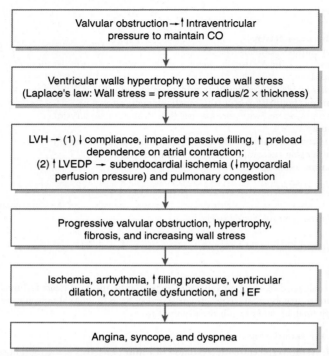

Figure 6-1. Pathophysiology of aortic stenosis. CO, cardiac output; EF, ejection fraction; LVEDP, left ventricular end-diastolic pressure; LVH, left ventricular hypertrophy.

- **Gorlin equation:** used to calculate aortic valve area during invasive hemodynamic assessment; based on principle that aortic valve area is equal to systolic flow across valve divided by systolic pressure gradient times a constant.

TREATMENT

- **Severe symptomatic AS requires surgery or percutaneous aortic valve replacement (AVR);** currently, there are no medical treatments proven to decrease mortality or to delay surgery.
- Hypertension should be addressed, and diuretics used for volume overload symptoms.
- Severe AS with decompensated HF or shock: Several options may help bridge the patient to definitive surgery or percutaneous procedure: intra-aortic balloon pump (IABP) (contraindicated in patients with moderate to severe aortic regurgitation [AR]), sodium nitroprusside, balloon aortic valvuloplasty.
- **AHA/ACC guideline indications for surgical or percutaneous AVR[2]**
  - Symptomatic patients with severe AS (Class I).
  - Asymptomatic patients with severe AS and an LVEF <50% (Stage C2) (Class I).
  - Asymptomatic patients with severe AS undergoing cardiac surgery for other indications (Class I).

○ Class IIB indications include: Asymptomatic patients with decreased exercise tolerance by stress testing, asymptomatic patients with very severe AS (aortic velocity >5 m/s), asymptomatic patients with elevated BNP, or increase in aortic velocity ≥0.3 m/s per year on serial examinations.

- **Decision for mechanical versus bioprosthetic AVR** involves shared decision-making with the patient regarding risks of anticoagulant therapy and expected longevity of new valve. In general, it is reasonable to recommend a mechanical prosthesis in patients <50 years of age who do not have a contraindication to anticoagulation due to the improved durability of this type of valve. Alternatively, it is reasonable to recommend a bioprosthetic valve over a mechanical valve in patients who are >65 years of age (Class IIa).[2]

- **Transcatheter aortic valve implantation (TAVI)** is an option for patients who are considering bioprosthetic AVR.
  ○ Requires evaluation by a team of cardiologists and cardiac surgeons. TAVI procedure uses fluoroscopic and echocardiographic guidance to place a stented bioprosthetic valve within the stenotic valve. This can be performed via a transfemoral, transaortic, subclavian, transcaval, or transapical approach.
  ○ To date, clinical trials have demonstrated that in patients at prohibitive risk for surgery, TAVI reduces mortality compared with medical therapy[3]; for high-risk patients and intermediate-risk patients, TAVI and surgical valve replacement have similar outcomes.[4-6]
  ○ **ACC/AHA guidelines for decision for surgical aortic valve replacement (SAVR) versus TAVI**[2]
    ▪ Class I indication for TAVI in patients who are at prohibitive risk for surgery if expected survival is >12 months with an acceptable quality of life.
    ▪ SAVR is recommended for patients with severe AS who are <65 years of age or have life expectancy of >20 years (Class I).
    ▪ In patients who are 65–80 years of age, either SAVR or transfemoral TAVI are options (Class I).
    ▪ For symptomatic patients with severe AS who are >80 years of age or for younger patients with a life expectancy <10 years, transfemoral TAVI is recommended in preference to SAVR (Class I).
  ○ Ongoing studies are assessing the role of TAVI in expanded patient populations.

PROGNOSIS

- AS is a progressive disease typically characterized by an asymptomatic phase until the valve area reaches a minimum threshold, generally <1.0 cm². In the absence of symptoms, patients with AS have a good prognosis with a risk of sudden death estimated to be approximately 1% per year.
- Once patients experience symptoms, their average survival is 2–3 years with a high risk of sudden death.

Mitral Regurgitation

- Prevention of MR is dependent on the integrated and proper function of the MV (annulus and leaflets), subvalvular apparatus (chordae tendineae and papillary muscles), LA, and LV; abnormal function or size of any one of these components can lead to MR.

- **Primary MR** refers to MR caused primarily by lesions to the valve leaflets and/or chordae tendineae (i.e., myxomatous degeneration, endocarditis, rheumatic).
- **Secondary MR,** or functional MR, refers to MR caused primarily by ventricular dysfunction usually with accompanying annular dilatation (i.e., dilated cardiomyopathy and ischemic MR).
- It is critical to define the mechanism of MR and the time course (acute vs. chronic) because these significantly impact clinical management.

ETIOLOGY

- **Primary MR**
  - **Degenerative** (overlap with MV prolapse syndrome)
    - Usually occurs as a primary condition (Barlow disease or fibroelastic deficiency) but has also been associated with heritable diseases affecting the connective tissue including Marfan syndrome, Ehlers–Danlos syndrome, osteogenesis imperfecta, etc.
    - Occurs in 1.0%–2.5% of the population in a female-to-male ratio of 2:1.
    - Myxomatous proliferation and cartilage formation can occur in the leaflets, chordae tendineae, and/or annulus.
  - **Rheumatic**
    - May be isolated MR or combined MR/MS.
    - Caused by thickening and/or calcification of the leaflets and chords.
  - **Infective endocarditis:** usually caused by destruction of the leaflet tissue (i.e., perforation).
- **Secondary MR**
  - **Dilated cardiomyopathy**
    - Annular dilatation from ventricular enlargement.
    - Papillary muscle displacement because of ventricular enlargement and remodeling prevents adequate leaflet coaptation.
  - **Ischemic**
    - Mechanism of MR usually involves one or both of the following: (1) annular dilatation from ventricular enlargement; (2) local LV remodeling with papillary muscle displacement (both the dilatation of the ventricle and the akinesis/dyskinesis of the wall to which the papillary muscle is attached can prevent adequate leaflet coaptation).
    - MR may develop acutely from papillary muscle rupture (see below).
- **Other causes of MR**
  Congenital, infiltrative diseases (i.e., amyloid), SLE (Libman–Sacks endocarditis), hypertrophic obstructive cardiomyopathy, mitral annular calcification, paravalvular prosthetic leak, drug toxicity (e.g., Fen-phen).
- **Acute causes of MR**
  - Ruptured papillary muscle or ruptured chordae tendineae, usually in setting of acute MI. The posteromedial papillary muscle is more likely to rupture than the anterolateral papillary muscle; the anterolateral muscle has dual blood supply from both the left anterior descending artery and left circumflex artery.
  - Infective endocarditis.

Pathophysiology

- Acute MR (Figure 6-2)
- Chronic MR (Figure 6-3)

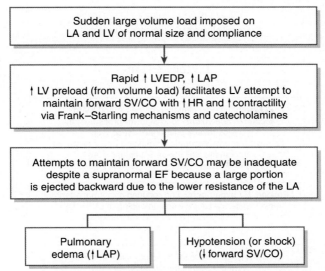

Figure 6-2. Acute mitral regurgitation. CO, cardiac output; EF, ejection fraction; HR, heart rate; LA, left atrium; LAP, left atrial pressure; LV, left ventricle; LVEDP, left ventricular end-diastolic pressure; SV, stroke volume.

DIAGNOSIS

History

- **Acute MR:** most prominent symptom is relatively rapid onset of significant shortness of breath, which may lead quickly to respiratory failure.
- **Chronic MR**
  - Symptoms will depend on the etiology of MR and timing of presentation.
  - In primary MR (usually degenerative MR) that has gradually progressed, the patient may be asymptomatic even when the MR is severe. As compensatory mechanisms fail, patients may note dyspnea on exertion (may be because of PH and/or pulmonary edema), palpitations (from an atrial arrhythmia), fatigue, and volume overload.

Physical Examination

- **Acute MR**
  - Tachypnea with respiratory distress, tachycardia, hypotension.
  - Systolic murmur, usually at the apex (may not be holosystolic and may be absent).
- **Chronic MR**
  - Apical holosystolic murmur that radiates to the axilla.
  - In MV prolapse, there is a midsystolic click heard before the murmur.
  - S_2 may be widely split because of an early A_2.
  - Other signs of heart failure (lower extremity edema, increased JVP, rales, etc.).

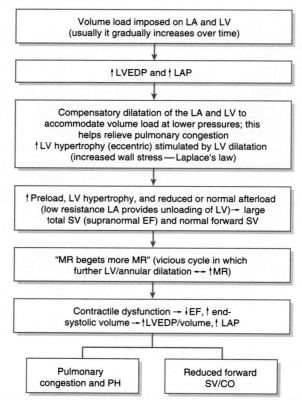

Figure 6-3. Chronic mitral regurgitation. CO, cardiac output; EF, ejection fraction; LA, left atrium; LAP, left atrial pressure; LV, left ventricle; LVEDP, left ventricular end-diastolic pressure; MR, mitral regurgitation; PH, pulmonary hypertension; SV, stroke volume.

Diagnostic Testing

- **ECG:** LAE, LVH, AF.
- **CXR:** enlarged LA, pulmonary edema, enlarged pulmonary arteries, and cardiomegaly.
- **TTE:** assess etiology of MR, LA size and LV dimensions (dilated in chronic severe MR), EF (LV dysfunction is present if EF ≤55%), qualitative and quantitative measures of MR severity.
- **TEE**
  - Provides better visualization of the valve to help define anatomy, presence of endocarditis (valvular vegetations), and feasibility of repair.
  - May help determine severity of MR when TTE is nondiagnostic, particularly in the setting of an eccentric jet.
- **Right heart catheterization**
  - Better characterize PH in patients with chronic severe MR and determine LA filling pressure in patients with unclear symptoms.
  - Giant "V" waves on pulmonary capillary wedge pressure tracing may suggest severe MR.

...ization
...erapeutic strategy in ischemic MR.

Left heart catheter...
○ May influenc...D in patients with risk factors undergoing MV surgery.

Evaluation...ing
○ ...tients with severe MR but with an inadequate assessment of EF by
...phy.

MRI/nu...
○ As ...itative measure of MR severity when echocardiography is
...c.

...essment may play a role in considering therapeutic strategy in isch-

...T

...Mitral Regurgitation

While awaiting surgery, aggressive afterload reduction with IV nitroprusside or an IABP can diminish the amount of MR and stabilize the patient by promoting forward flow and reducing pulmonary edema.

- These patients are usually tachycardic, but attempts to slow down their heart rate should be avoided because they are often heart rate dependent for an adequate forward CO.

Chronic Mitral Regurgitation

- **Chronic primary MR**
  ○ Medical therapy is reasonable in patients with chronic primary MR and LVEF less than 60% not undergoing surgery.
  ○ Angiotensin-converting enzyme (ACE) inhibitors and angiotensin receptor blockers have been shown to reduce the regurgitant fraction and aid with ventricular remodeling. β-Blockers have also been shown to reduce severity of MR in asymptomatic patients.
  ○ There is no benefit of vasodilator therapy in the asymptomatic patient with normal LV function and chronic severe MR.
- **Chronic secondary MR**
  ○ Treat symptoms related to LV dysfunction.
  ○ Guideline-directed medical therapy (GDMT) for LV systolic dysfunction, including ACE inhibitors and β-blockers, is indicated and has been shown to reduce mortality and the severity of MR.
  ○ Some patients may also qualify for cardiac resynchronization therapy, which can favorably remodel the LV and reduce the severity of MR.

Percutaneous Intervention[2]

- Transcatheter edge to edge repair (TEER) (i.e., MitraClip) pinches the leaflets together in an attempt to enhance coaptation (a percutaneous treatment analogous to the surgical Alfieri stitch), creating a double-orifice valve.
  ○ This procedure is performed via femoral venous access, and a transseptal puncture is used to position the delivery system in the LA.
  ○ Using fluoroscopy and TEE guidance, the clip is advanced and attempts are made to grasp the leaflet tips of the anterior and posterior MV leaflets and clip them together.
  ○ Indicated for chronic severe secondary MR with LVEF between 20% and 50% for patients with persistent symptoms despite GDMT and appropriate anatomy (Class IIa).

This recommendation comes from results of the COAPT~~ trial demonstrating~~ improvement in survival, symptoms, and quality of life in ~~patients with~~ moderate to severe secondary MR who underwent TEER as com~~medical~~ therapy alone.[7,8]

- ○ TEER is also an option for patients with severely symptomatic with ~~~~ MR at high or prohibitive surgical risk who have favorable anatomy (~~~~
- Transcatheter mitral valve replacement is an emerging structural interve~~~~ currently being investigated in a number of clinical trials. Currently, this te~~~~ is only reserved for degenerative MR.

Surgical Management
- **Primary MR**[2]
  - ○ Symptomatic with chronic severe primary MR (stage D) (Class I).
  - ○ Asymptomatic with chronic severe primary MR with EF ≤60% or LV end-systolic dimension ≥40 mm (stage C2; Class I).
  - ○ Chronic severe primary MR undergoing cardiac surgery for other indications (Class I).
  - ○ Repair is recommended over replacement (Class I).
  - ○ Asymptomatic patients with chronic severe primary MR (stage C1) in whom repair is highly likely (>95%) and operative mortality is low (<1%) (Class IIa).
- **Secondary MR**[2]
  - ○ Class IIa: chronic severe secondary MR undergoing cardiac surgery for other indications.
  - ○ Class IIb
    - Severely symptomatic patients despite GDMT (NYHA III/IV) with chronic severe secondary MR (stage D) and LVEF ≥50%.
    - Patients with persistent symptoms with chronic severe secondary MR (stage D) and LVEF <50% who do not have favorable anatomy for TEER.
  - ○ Note that the benefits of surgery are not well established for secondary MR.

Aortic Regurgitation

- AR may result from pathology of the aortic valve, the aortic root, or both; it is important that both the aortic valve and the aortic root are evaluated to determine the appropriate management and treatment.
- AR usually progresses insidiously with a long asymptomatic period; when it occurs acutely, patients are often very sick and must be managed aggressively.

ETIOLOGY

- **More common**
  Bicuspid aortic valve, rheumatic disease, calcific degeneration, infective endocarditis, idiopathic dilatation of the aorta, myxomatous degeneration, systemic hypertension, dissection of the ascending aorta, Marfan syndrome.
- **Less common**
  Traumatic injury to the aortic valve, collagen vascular diseases (ankylosing spondylitis, rheumatoid arthritis, reactive arthritis, giant cell aortitis, and Whipple disease), syphilitic aortitis, discrete subaortic stenosis, ventricular septal defect with prolapse of an aortic cusp.
- **Acute AR**
  Infective endocarditis, dissection of the ascending aorta, trauma.

Pathophysiology
- Acute AR (Figure 6-4)
- Chronic AR (Figure 6-5)

DIAGNOSIS

History
- **Acute AR:** patients with acute AR may present with **symptoms of cardiogenic shock and severe dyspnea.** Other presenting symptoms may be related to the cause of acute AR.
- **Chronic AR:** symptoms depend on the presence of LV dysfunction and whether the patient is in the **compensated versus decompensated stage.** Compensated patients are typically asymptomatic, whereas those in the decompensated stage may note decreased exercise tolerance, dyspnea, fatigue, and/or angina.

Physical Examination
- **Acute AR**
  - Widened pulse pressure may be present, but it is often not present because forward SV (and therefore systolic blood pressure) is reduced.
  - May hear brief soft diastolic murmur or systolic flow murmur.
  - Look for evidence of aortic dissection, infective endocarditis, and characteristics associated with Marfan disease.
- **Chronic AR**
  - LV heave; point of maximal impulse is laterally displaced.
  - Diastolic decrescendo murmur heard best at left sternal border leaning forward at end-expiration (**severity of AR correlates with duration, not intensity, of the murmur**).

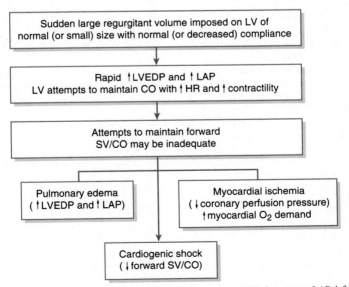

Figure 6-4. Acute aortic regurgitation. CO, cardiac output; HR, heart rate; LAP, left atrial pressure; LV, left ventricle; LVEDP, left ventricular end-diastolic pressure; SV, stroke volume.

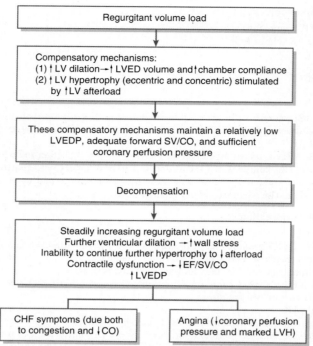

Figure 6-5. Chronic aortic regurgitation. CHF, congestive heart failure; CO, cardiac output; EF, ejection fraction; LV, left ventricle; LVED, left ventricular end-diastolic; LVEDP, left ventricular end-diastolic pressure; LVH, left ventricular hypertrophy; SV, stroke volume.

- ○ Systolic flow murmur (mostly because of volume overload; concomitant AS may also be present).
- ○ **Widened pulse pressure** (often >100 mm Hg) with a low diastolic pressure; there are numerous eponyms for the characteristic signs related to a wide pulse pressure.

Diagnostic Testing

- **ECG:** tachycardia, LVH, and LAE (more common in chronic AR).
- **CXR:** pulmonary edema, widened mediastinum, and cardiomegaly.
- **TTE**
  - ○ Assess LV systolic function, LV dimensions at end systole and diastole, leaflet number and morphology, assessment of the severity of AR.
  - ○ Look for evidence of endocarditis or aortic dissection, dimension of aortic root.
- **TEE**
  - ○ Clarify whether there is a bicuspid valve if unclear on TTE.
  - ○ Better sensitivity and specificity for aortic dissection than TTE.
  - ○ Clarify whether there is endocarditis with or without root abscess if unclear on TTE.
  - ○ Better visualization of aortic valve in patients with a prosthetic aortic valve.
- **Cardiac catheterization:** assessment of LV pressure, LV function, and severity of AR (via aortic root angiography) is indicated in symptomatic patients in whom the severity of AR is unclear on noninvasive imaging or discordant with clinical findings.

- **MRI/CT**
  - Either of these may be the imaging modality of choice for evaluating aortic dimensions and/or for evaluation of aortic dissection.
  - If echocardiography assessment of the severity of AR is inadequate, MRI is useful for assessing the severity of AR.

TREATMENT

- **The role of medical therapy in patients with AR is limited.**
- **Vasodilator therapy (i.e., nifedipine, ACE inhibitor, hydralazine)** is indicated to reduce systolic blood pressure in hypertensive patients with AR.
- When endocarditis is suspected or confirmed, appropriate antibiotic coverage is critical.

Surgical Management

- AHA/ACC recommendations for intervention[2]
  - Symptomatic patients with severe AR (stage D) regardless of LV systolic function (Class I).
  - Asymptomatic patients with chronic severe AR and LV systolic dysfunction (EF ≤55%) (stage C2; Class I).
  - Patients with severe AR (stage C or D) undergoing cardiac surgery for other indications (Class I).
  - Asymptomatic patients with severe AR and normal LV systolic function (EF >55%) but with severe LV dilation (LV end-systolic dimension >50 mm) (stage C2; Class IIa).
- **Acute, severe AR is almost universally symptomatic and is treated surgically.**
- If the aortic root is dilated, it may be repaired or replaced at the time of AVR. For patients with a bicuspid valve, Marfan syndrome, or a related genetically triggered aortopathy, surgery on the aorta should be considered at the time of AVR.

OUTCOME/PROGNOSIS

- Asymptomatic patients with normal LV systolic function (LVEF ≥55%): progression to symptoms and/or LV dysfunction approximately 6% per year.[9]
- Asymptomatic patients with LV dysfunction (LVEF <50%): progression to cardiac symptoms >25% per year.[9,10]
- Symptomatic patients: mortality rate approximately 9.4% per year.[9]

Prosthetic Heart Valves

- The choice of valve prosthesis depends on many factors including the patient, surgeon, cardiologist, and clinical scenario.
- With improvements in bioprosthetic valves, the recommendation for a mechanical valve in patients <65 years of age is no longer as firm, and bioprosthetic valve use has increased in younger patients.
- **Mechanical valves**
  - Ball-and-cage (Starr–Edwards): rarely, if ever, used today.
  - Bileaflet (i.e., St. Jude, Carbomedics): most commonly used.
  - Single tilting disk (i.e., Björk–Shiley, Medtronic Hall, Omnicarbon).
  - **Advantages of mechanical valve:** structurally stable, long-lasting, relatively hemodynamically efficient (particularly bileaflet).

- **Disadvantages of mechanical valve:** need for anticoagulation/risk of bleeding, risk of thrombosis/embolism despite anticoagulation, severe hemodynamic compromise if disk thrombosis or immobility occurs (single tilting disk), risk of endocarditis, anticoagulation issues in women of child-bearing age.
- **Bioprosthetic valves**
  - Porcine aortic valve tissue (i.e., Hancock, Carpentier-Edwards)
  - Bovine pericardial tissue (i.e., Carpentier-Edwards Perimount)
  - **Advantages of bioprosthetic valve:** no need for anticoagulation, low thromboembolism risk, low risk of catastrophic valve failure
  - **Disadvantages of bioprosthetic valve:** structural valve deterioration, risk of endocarditis, still a small risk (approximately 0.04%–0.34% per year in meta-analysis) of thromboembolism without anticoagulation[11]
  - **Homograft (cadaveric):** rarely used; most commonly used to replace the pulmonic valve

TREATMENT

- **Anticoagulation with a vitamin K antagonist (VKA) and international normalized ratio (INR) monitoring is recommended in patients with a mechanical prosthetic valve** (Class I).[2]
  - Goal INR of 2.5 is recommended in patients with a mechanical AVR and no risk factors for thromboembolism. Goal INR 3.0 in patients with a mechanical AVR and additional risk factors for thromboembolic events (AF, previous thromboembolism, LV dysfunction, or hypercoagulable conditions) or an older generation mechanical AVR (such as ball-in-cage) (Class I).
  - Goal INR 3.0 in patients with a mechanical MV replacement (Class I).
  - Aspirin in addition to VKA therapy for mechanical prosthetic valves is no longer routinely recommended in the absence of other indications for aspirin therapy.
  - Aspirin 75–100 mg daily is reasonable in all patients with a bioprosthetic aortic or mitral valve (Class IIa).
  - **Anticoagulant therapy with oral direct thrombin inhibitors or anti-Xa agents should not be used in patients with mechanical valve prostheses (Class III).**
- **Bridging therapy for prosthetic valves**[2]:
  - Continuation of VKA anticoagulation with a therapeutic INR is recommended in patients with mechanical heart valves undergoing minor procedures (i.e., dental extractions) where bleeding is easily controlled (Class I).
  - Temporary interruption of VKA anticoagulation, without bridging agents while the INR is subtherapeutic, is recommended in patients with bileaflet mechanical AVR and no other risk factors for thrombosis who are undergoing invasive or surgical procedures (Class I).
  - Bridging anticoagulation is reasonable for patients who are undergoing invasive procedures and have mechanical AVR with thromboembolic risk factors, an older generation mechanical AVR, or mechanical MVR (Class IIa).

Infective Endocarditis in Native or Prosthetic Valves

- Patients at risk or with suspected endocarditis should receive antibiotic therapy after two sets of blood cultures (Class I).[2]
- These patients should be evaluated for need and timing of surgery: early surgery is recommended (Class I) for those with valve dysfunction causing heart failure, resistant organisms (fungi, staphylococcus), heart block/abscess, persistent infection.

- Surgery is also recommended for relapsing prosthetic valve endocarditis (Class I).[2]
- Those with large mobile vegetations of the native valve and recurrent emboli can be evaluated for early surgery (Class II).[2]

Management of Pregnant Patients with Prosthetic Heart Valves (Figure 6-6)

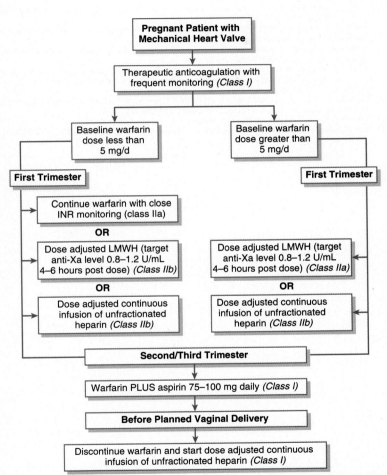

Figure 6-6. Anticoagulation management in pregnant patients with prosthetic valves. INR, international normalized ratio; LMWH, low molecular weight heparin. (Modified from Nishimura RA, Otto CM, Bonow RO, et al. 2014 AHA/ACC guideline for the management of patients with valvular heart disease: executive summary. A report of the American College of Cardiology/American Heart Association task force on practice guidelines. *J Am Coll Cardiol.* 2014;63:2438-2488. Copyright © 2014 American Heart Association, Inc., and the American College of Cardiology Foundation. With permission.)

REFERENCES

1. Imazio M, Bobbio M, Cecchi E, et al. Colchicine in addition to conventional therapy for acute pericarditis. *Circulation.* 2005;112:2012-2016.
2. Otto CM, Nishimura RA, Bonow RO, et al. 2020 ACC/AHA guideline for the management of patients with valvular heart disease: a report of the American College of Cardiology/American Heart Association Joint Committee on clinical practice guidelines. *Circulation.* 2021;143:e72-e227.
3. Leon MB, Smith CR, Mack M, et al. Transcatheter aortic-valve implantation for aortic stenosis in patients who Cannot undergo surgery. *N Engl J Med.* 2010;363:1597-1607.
4. Leon MB, Smith CR, Mack MJ, et al. Transcatheter or surgical aortic-valve replacement in intermediate-risk patients. *N Engl J Med.* 2016;374:1609-1620.
5. Smith CR, Leon MB, Mack MJ, et al. Transcatheter versus surgical aortic-valve replacement in high-risk patients. *N Engl J Med.* 2011;364:2187-2198.
6. Reardon MJ, Mieghem NMV, Popma JJ, et al. Surgical or transcatheter aortic-valve replacement in intermediate-risk patients. *N Engl J Med.* 2017;376:1321-1331.
7. Stone GW, Lindenfeld J, Abraham WT, et al. Transcatheter mitral-valve repair in patients with heart failure. *N Engl J Med.* 2018;379:2307-2318.
8. Mack MJ, Abraham WT, Lindenfeld J, et al. Cardiovascular outcomes assessment of the MitraClip in patients with heart failure and secondary mitral regurgitation: Design and rationale of the COAPT trial. *Am Heart J.* 2018;205:1-11.
9. Dujardin KS, Enriquez-Sarano M, Schaff HV, Bailey KR, Seward JB, Tajik AJ. Mortality and morbidity of aortic regurgitation in clinical practice. *Circulation.* 1999;99:1851-1857.
10. Maurer G. Aortic regurgitation. *Heart.* 2006;92:994.
11. Puri R, Auffret V, Rodés-Cabau J. Bioprosthetic valve thrombosis. *J Am Coll Cardiol.* 2017;69:2193-2211.

Cardiac Arrhythmias

Sandeep S. Sodhi, Daniel H. Cooper, and
Mitchell N. Faddis

TACHYARRHYTHMIAS

Approach to Tachyarrhythmias

GENERAL PRINCIPLES

- Tachyarrhythmias are encountered in both inpatient and outpatient settings.
- Recognition and stepwise analysis of these rhythms facilitate appropriate management.
- Clinical decision-making is guided by patient symptoms and signs of hemodynamic stability.

Definition
Cardiac rhythms whose ventricular rate exceeds **100 beats per minute** (bpm).

Classification
Broadly classified into the following based on the width of the QRS complex on the ECG:
- Narrow-complex tachyarrhythmia (QRS <120 ms): Arrhythmia originates within the atria (supraventricular tachycardia [SVT]) and rapidly activates the ventricles via His–Purkinje system.
- Wide-complex tachyarrhythmia (WCT) (QRS ≥120 ms): Arrhythmia originates within the ventricles and does not depend on the His–Purkinje system (ventricular tachycardia [VT]) or originates in the atria and travels to the ventricles either via an abnormal His–Purkinje system (SVT with aberrancy) or through an accessory pathway.

Etiology
Mechanism divided into disorders of **impulse conduction** and **impulse formation**
- **Disorders of impulse conduction:** Reentry is the most common mechanism of tachyarrhythmias. Reentrant mechanism can occur when differential refractory periods and conduction velocities allow for propagation of an activation wavefront in a unidirectional manner around a zone of scar or refractory cardiac tissue. Reentry of the activation wavefront around a myocardial circuit sustains the arrhythmia (e.g., VT).
- **Disorders of impulse formation: Enhanced automaticity** (e.g., accelerated junctional and accelerated idioventricular rhythm) **and triggered activity** (e.g., long QT syndrome [LQTS] and digitalis toxicity) are other, less common mechanisms of tachyarrhythmias.

DIAGNOSIS

Clinical Presentation

- Often produce symptoms that lead to patient presentation at outpatient or acute care settings.
- Can be associated with systemic illnesses in patients being evaluated in the emergency department or being treated in the inpatient setting.

History

- Symptoms generally guide clinical decision-making.
- **Dyspnea, angina, lightheadedness or syncope, and decreased level of consciousness** are severe symptoms that mandate urgent intervention.
- Symptoms that reflect **poor left ventricular (LV) function**, such as dyspnea on exertion, orthopnea, paroxysmal nocturnal dyspnea, and lower extremity swelling, are critical to identify.
- **Palpitations** are a common symptom of tachyarrhythmias. The pattern of onset and termination is useful to suggest the presence of a primary arrhythmia.
  - Sudden onset and termination of palpitations is highly suggestive of a reentrant tachyarrhythmia.
  - Termination with breath-holding or Valsalva maneuver is suggestive of SVT.
- History or presence of **structural heart disease** (i.e., ischemic, nonischemic, or valvular cardiomyopathy) or **endocrinopathy** (i.e., thyroid disease, pheochromocytoma) should be determined.
- History of **familial or congenital causes of arrhythmias** such as hypertrophic cardiomyopathy (HCM), LQTS, or other congenital cardiac conditions should be ascertained, as well.
  - **Hypertrophic obstructive cardiomyopathy** is associated with atrial arrhythmias (primarily atrial fibrillation [AF]) as well as malignant ventricular arrhythmias.
  - **Mitral valve prolapse** is associated with supraventricular and ventricular arrhythmias.
  - **Repaired congenital heart diseases,** such as surgically corrected tetralogy of Fallot and d-transposition of the great arteries with Mustard or Senning baffles, are substrates for ventricular tachyarrhythmia and SVTs, respectively.
- **Medication and ingestion history** (including over-the-counter drugs, herbal supplements, and illicit substances) should be taken to assess possible causal link.

Physical Examination

- If clinically stable, physical examination should focus on determining underlying cardiovascular abnormalities that may make certain rhythms more or less likely.
- Signs of **congestive heart failure (CHF)**, including elevated jugular venous pressure (JVP), pulmonary rales, peripheral edema, and S_3 gallop, make the diagnosis of malignant ventricular arrhythmias more likely.
- If an arrhythmia is sustained, special considerations during physical examination include the following:
  - **Palpation of the pulse** to assess for rate and regularity.
    - If the rhythm is irregular and the rate is approximately 150 bpm, suspect atrial flutter (AFL) with 2:1 block.
    - If the pulse is irregular with no pattern, suspect AF.
    - Irregular pulse with a discernible pattern (group beating) suggests the presence of second-degree heart block.

- o **Presence of "cannon" A waves:** Revealed on inspection of JVP; reflects atrial contraction against a closed tricuspid valve.
  - If irregular, may be suggestive of underlying atrioventricular (AV) dissociation and possible presence of VT.
  - If regular in a 1:1 ratio with peripheral pulse, then suggestive of an AV nodal reentrant tachycardia (AVNRT), AV reentrant tachycardia (AVRT), or a junctional tachycardia (JT), all leading to retrograde atrial activation occurring simultaneously with ventricular contraction.

Diagnostic Testing
Laboratories
Serum electrolytes, complete blood count (CBC), thyroid function tests, serum level of digoxin (if applicable), and urine toxicology screen should be considered for all patients.

Electrocardiography
- **Twelve-lead ECG, in the presence of the rhythm abnormality and in normal sinus rhythm (NSR),** is the most useful initial diagnostic test.
- If the patient is clinically stable, obtain 12-lead ECG and **continuous rhythm strip** with leads that best demonstrate atrial activation (e.g., V_1, II, III, aVF).
- Examine ECG for evidence of conduction abnormalities, such as preexcitation or bundle branch block, or signs of structural heart disease such as prior myocardial infarction (MI).
- Comparison of ECG obtained during arrhythmia with baseline can highlight subtle features of QRS deflection that indicate superposition of atrial and ventricular depolarization.
- Rhythm strip is useful to document response to interventions (e.g., vagal maneuvers, antiarrhythmic drug therapy, or electrical cardioversion).

Imaging
CXR and **transthoracic echocardiogram (TTE)** can help provide evidence of structural heart disease that may make ventricular arrhythmias more likely.

Other Diagnostic Testing
- Continuous ambulatory ECG monitoring
  - Aids in outpatient diagnosis of tachyarrhythmias.
  - A 24- or 48-hour Holter monitor; useful for documenting arrhythmias that occur with sufficient frequency.
  - Useful for assessment of patient's heart rate response to daily activities or antiarrhythmic drug treatment.
  - Correlation between patient-reported symptoms in a time-marked diary and heart rhythm recordings is key to determining if symptoms are attributable to arrhythmia.
- Event recorders
  - Weeks to months of ambulatory monitoring; useful for documenting symptomatic transient arrhythmias that occur infrequently.
  - Loop recorder—worn by the patient and continuously records the cardiac rhythm. When activated by the patient or via autodetection, a rhythm strip is saved with several minutes of preceding data.
  - **Implantable loop recorder (ILR)**—SC monitoring device used to provide an automated or patient-activated recording of significant arrhythmic events that occur very infrequently or for patients who are unable to activate external recorders.

CHAPTER 7

- Exercise ECG
  Useful for studying exercise-induced arrhythmias or assessing sinus node response to exercise.
- Inpatient telemetry monitoring
  Mainstay of surveillance monitoring during hospitalization for cardiac arrhythmia patients, especially those who are seriously ill or experiencing life-threatening arrhythmias.
- Electrophysiology study (EPS)
  ○ Invasive catheter-based procedure used to study susceptibility to arrhythmias or investigate the mechanism of a known arrhythmia.
  ○ EPS can be combined with catheter ablation for management of many arrhythmias.
  ○ Capability of EPS to induce and study arrhythmias is highest for reentrant mechanisms.

TREATMENT

Refer to treatment of individual tachyarrhythmias for hemodynamically unstable patients and advanced cardiac life support (ACLS) algorithm for tachycardias in Appendix C.

Supraventricular Tachyarrhythmias

GENERAL PRINCIPLES

- **SVTs**—often recurrent, rarely persistent, and can result in visits to emergency departments and primary care physician offices.
- Always begin with prompt assessment of hemodynamic stability and clinical status.
- Diagnostic and therapeutic discussion that follows is aimed at hemodynamically stable patients. If a patient is clinically unstable based on signs and symptoms, immediately proceed to cardioversion per ACLS guidelines.

Definition

- Tachyarrhythmias that require atrial or AV nodal tissue or both for their initiation and maintenance are termed SVT.
- The QRS complex in most SVTs is narrow (QRS <120 ms).
- SVTs can present as a wide-complex tachycardia (QRS ≥120 ms) if they are aberrantly conducted.

Classification

- Initially classified by ECG to help understand likely underlying arrhythmia mechanism.
- Diagnostic approach, based on the ECG, is summarized in Figure 7-1.
- Narrow QRS complex tachyarrhythmias can be divided into those requiring only atrial tissue for initiation and maintenance (atrial tachycardia [AT], AF, and AFL) versus those that require the AV junction for perpetuation (JT, AVNRT, and AVRT).
- **Paroxysmal SVT**—intermittent SVT other than AF, AFL, and multifocal AT (MAT).

Epidemiology

- The estimated prevalence of paroxysmal SVT is 2.25/1000, with an incidence of 35/100,000 person-years.[1]

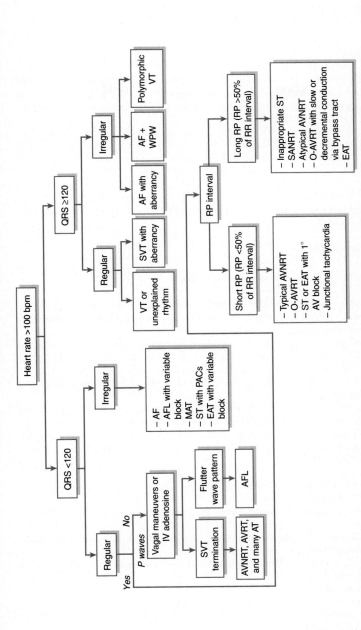

Figure 7-1. Diagnostic approach to tachyarrhythmias. AF, atrial fibrillation; AFL, atrial flutter; AT, atrial tachycardia; AV, atrioventricular; AVNRT, atrioventricular nodal reentrant tachycardia; AVRT, atrioventricular reentrant tachycardia; EAT, ectopic atrial tachycardia; MAT, multifocal atrial tachycardia; O-AVRT, orthodromic AVRT; PAC, premature atrial complex; SANRT, sinoatrial nodal reentrant tachycardia; ST, sinus tachycardia; SVT, supraventricular tachyarrhythmia; VT, ventricular tachycardia; WPW, Wolff–Parkinson–White.

CHAPTER 7

- In the absence of structural heart disease, SVT most commonly presents between ages 12 and 30 years.[1]
- Women are twice as likely to develop SVT as men.[1]

DIAGNOSIS

- **AF**—most common narrow-complex tachycardia seen in the inpatient setting. **AFL** can often accompany AF and is diagnosed one-tenth as often as AF, but first-time AFL is diagnosed twice as often as the paroxysmal SVTs. Remaining atrial tachyarrhythmias are far less common.[2]
- Mechanism of paroxysmal SVT is significantly influenced by gender and age. Irrespective of gender, AVRT tends to present at a younger age (most commonly in the first 2 decades of life), whereas AVNRT and AT tend to present more commonly later in life.[2]

Clinical Presentation
Clinical presentation for SVT is similar to tachyarrhythmias in general and has been previously outlined.

Differential Diagnosis
- **AF**
  Discussed as a separate topic later in this section.
- **AFL**
  - Adjusted for age, the incidence in men is more than 2.5 times that of women.[3]
  - AFL usually presents as a **regular rhythm** but can be **irregularly irregular** when associated with variable AV block.
  - **Mechanism:** Macroreentrant circuit usually within the right atrium around the perimeter of the tricuspid valve. This form of AFL is called "typical" AFL. Atrial rate is 250–350 bpm with conduction to ventricle that is usually not 1:1, but most often 2:1. **(SVT with regular ventricular rate of 150 bpm should raise suspicion for AFL.)**
  - Chronic AFL commonly coexists with AF and is associated with the same risk factors (obesity, hypertension [HTN], diabetes mellitus, and obstructive sleep apnea [OSA]).
  - **ECG:** In typical AFL, a "saw tooth" pattern best visualized in leads II, III, and aVF with negative deflections in those leads and either positive, negative, or biphasic atrial deflection in V_1.
- **MAT**
  - **Irregularly irregular** SVT generally seen in elderly hospitalized patients with multiple comorbidities.
  - Most often associated with chronic obstructive pulmonary disease (COPD) and CHF.
  - Also associated with glucose intolerance, hypokalemia, hypomagnesemia, drugs (e.g., theophylline), and chronic renal failure.
  - **ECG:** SVT with at least **three distinct P wave morphologies**, generally best visualized in leads II, III, aVF, and V_1.
- **Sinus tachycardia**
  - Most common mechanism of **long RP tachycardia.**
  - Usually, normal physiologic response to hyperadrenergic states (fever, pain, hypovolemia, anemia, hypoxia, etc.).

- Can be induced by illicit (cocaine, amphetamines, methamphetamine) and prescription (theophylline, atropine, β-adrenergic agonists) drugs.
  - **Inappropriate sinus tachycardia** refers to persistently elevated resting sinus rate (>100 bpm) in the absence of identifiable physical, pathologic, or pharmacologic influence.
- **Ectopic atrial tachycardia (EAT)**
  - EAT with variable block can present as an **irregularly irregular** rhythm and can be distinguished from AFL by an **atrial rate of 150–200 bpm.**
  - EAT with variable block is associated with **digoxin toxicity.**
  - Characterized by regular atrial activation pattern with P wave morphology originating outside the sinus node complex resulting in **long RP tachycardia.**
  - **Mechanism:** Enhanced automaticity, triggered activity, and possibly microreentry.
- **AVNRT**
  - Reentrant rhythm requiring functional dissociation of the AV node into two pathways with both antegrade and retrograde conduction through the AV node.
  - Not correlated with structural heart disease and can occur at any age, with a predilection for **middle age** and **female gender.**
  - **Typical AVNRT**—major cause of short RP tachycardia.
    - **ECG appearance has characteristic "absent P waves"** because atrial activation is coincident with the QRS complex. Commonly, atrial activation can occur at terminal portion of QRS to create a pseudo-r' (V_1) or pseudo-s' (II) compared with sinus rhythm (SR) QRS.
    - **Conduction occurs in an antegrade fashion down the slow AV nodal pathway with retrograde conduction occurring back up the fast pathway, manifesting in short RP tachycardia by ECG.**
  - **Atypical AVNRT**
    - Less common; antegrade conduction proceeds down a fast AV nodal pathway with retrograde conduction up a slow AV nodal pathway, leading to a **long RP tachycardia.**
    - **ECG:** Retrograde P wave inscribed well after QRS complex in second half of RR interval.
- **AVRT**
  - Reentrant tachycardia with circuit consisting of the normal AV conduction system and accessory pathway linking atrial and ventricular tissues.
  - **Orthodromic AVRT**—most common AVRT, accounting for about 95% of all AVRT.
    - Accessory pathway–mediated reentrant rhythm with antegrade conduction to the ventricle down the AV node and retrograde conduction to the atrium up an accessory or "bypass" tract, leading to **short RP tachycardia.**
    - **ECG:** Retrograde P waves frequently seen after the QRS complex and usually distinguishable from the QRS (i.e., separated by >70 ms).
    - Most common mechanism of SVT in patients with Wolff–Parkinson–White (WPW) syndrome who have preexcitation (defined by short PR and a delta wave on upstroke of QRS) present on SR ECG.
    - Can occur without preexcitation when conduction through bypass tract occurs only during tachycardia in retrograde fashion ("concealed pathway").
    - Less commonly, retrograde conduction through the accessory pathway to the atrium proceeds slowly enough for atrial activation to occur in the second half of the RR interval, leading to a **long RP tachycardia.**

CHAPTER 7

- **Antidromic AVRT (A-AVRT):** Occurs when conduction to the ventricle is down an accessory bypass tract with retrograde conduction through the AV node or second bypass tract.
  - **ECG:** QRS seems consistent with VT; however, the presence of preexcitation on the baseline QRS should be diagnostic for WPW syndrome.
  - A-AVRT is seen in <5% of patients with WPW syndrome.
- **JT**
  - Due to enhanced automaticity of AV junction. Electrical impulses conduct to the ventricle and atrium simultaneously, similar to typical AVNRT.
  - Retrograde P waves are frequently concealed within the QRS complex.
  - Uncommon in adults. Common in young children, particularly after cardiac surgery.
- **Sinoatrial (SA) nodal reentrant tachycardia**
  - Reentrant circuit localized at least partially within the SA node.
  - Abrupt onset and termination, triggered by premature atrial complex.
  - **ECG:** P wave morphology and axis identical to native sinus P wave during NSR.

TREATMENT

- Please refer to Table 7-1 for general therapeutic approach to common SVTs.
- Acute treatment of symptomatic SVT—follow **ACLS protocol** as outlined in Appendix C.
- Chronic treatment guided by severity of symptoms, as well as frequency and duration of recurrent events.[2]
- Many SVTs can be terminated by **AV nodal blocking agents or vagal techniques** (Table 7-2), whereas AF, AFL, and some ATs will persist despite a slowing of the ventricular rate because of partial AV nodal blockade.
- **Radiofrequency ablation (RFA):** Definitive cure with high success rates ranging from 80% to 100% for many SVTs including AVNRT, accessory bypass tract–mediated tachycardias, focal AT, and AFL.
- Complication risk generally <3% for ablation of common SVTs. Risks include major bleeding, cardiac perforation or tamponade, stroke, pulmonary embolism, and complete heart block requiring permanent pacemaker (PPM) implantation.[2]

Atrial Fibrillation

GENERAL PRINCIPLES

Definition

- Most common sustained cardiac arrhythmia encountered in clinical practice.
- Atrial tachyarrhythmia characterized by chaotic activation of the atria with loss of normal atrial mechanical function.
- Twelve-lead ECG characterized by the absence of consistent P waves. Rapid, low-amplitude oscillations or fibrillatory waves noted in baseline of leads that best demonstrate atrial activation (V_1, II, III, and aVF).
- Ventricular response to AF is characteristically irregular and, often, rapid in the presence of intact AV conduction.

TABLE 7-1	Treatment of Common Supraventricular Tachyarrhythmias
Treatment Strategies	
Atrial flutter (AFL)	Anticoagulation similar to AF; risk of thromboembolic complications is similar.
	Rate control with same agents as AF.
	If highly symptomatic or rate control difficult, electrical or chemical cardioversion is appropriate.
	If pacemaker present, overdrive atrial pacing can achieve cardioversion.
	Catheter ablation of typical right AFL with long-term success above 90% and rare complications.
Multifocal atrial tachycardia (MAT)	Therapy targeted at treatment of underlying pathophysiologic process.
	Antiarrhythmic, if symptomatic rapid ventricular response. Individualize β-adrenergic blockers versus calcium channel blocker therapy.
	DC cardioversion is not effective.
Sinus tachycardia (ST)	Therapy targeted at treatment of underlying pathophysiologic process.
Ectopic atrial tachycardia (EAT)	**Acute therapy:** Identify and treat precipitating factors like digoxin toxicity; if hemodynamically stable, then β-blockers and calcium channel blockers. In rare cases, amiodarone, flecainide, or sotalol.
	Chronic therapy: Rate control with β-adrenergic blockers and calcium channel blockers. If unsuccessful, options include catheter ablation (86% success rate), flecainide, propafenone, sotalol, or amiodarone.
AV nodal reentrant tachycardia (AVNRT)	Catheter ablation highly successful (96%) but has to be individualized to each patient.
	If medical therapy more desirable—β-adrenergic blockers, calcium channel blockers, and digoxin; then consider propafenone, flecainide, etc.
Orthodromic AV reentrant tachycardia (O-AVRT)	**Acute therapy:** Vagal maneuvers, adenosine, calcium channel blockers. If ineffective, then procainamide or β-blockers.
	Chronic suppressive therapy: Catheter ablation highly successful (95%) but has to be individualized to each patient. If medical therapy is more desirable for prevention, flecainide and procainamide are indicated.
Antidromic AV reentrant tachycardia (A-AVRT)	**Acute therapy:** Avoid adenosine or other AV node–specific blocking agents. Consider ibutilide, procainamide, or flecainide.
	Chronic suppressive therapy: Accessory pathway catheter ablation is preferred and successful (95%). If medical therapy desired, consider flecainide and propafenone.

AF, atrial fibrillation; AV, atrioventricular; DC, direct current.

CHAPTER 7

TABLE 7-2   Common Vagal Maneuvers and Adenosine

	Patient Preparation[a]	Mechanism	Dose/Duration/Details	Toxicity	Contraindication	Potentiators/ Antagonists	Common Side Effects
Valsalva	Describe the procedure.	Vagal stimulation during relaxation phase.	Exhale forcefully against a closed airway for several seconds followed by relaxation.	Well tolerated.	Patient unable to follow commands.	—	—
Carotid sinus massage	Check for carotid bruits and history of CVA; then place in recumbent position with neck extended.	Vagal stimulation.	First, apply enough pressure to simply feel carotid pulse with index and middle fingers. If no effect, then use rotating motion for 3–5 s.	Well tolerated. Risk of embolizing carotid plaque. **Never massage both carotids.**	Recent TIA or stroke or ipsilateral significant carotid artery stenosis or carotid artery bruit.	—	—
Adenosine	Explain the potential side effects to the patient.	AV nodal blocking agent. Short acting (serum half-life 4–8 min).	Initial: 6 mg IV rapid bolus via antecubital vein, followed by 10–30 mL saline flush. If desired or effect not achieved, can repeat 12 mg followed by 12 mg after 1- to 2-min intervals. Central venous line: 3 mg IV initial dose.	Precipitate prolonged asystole in patients with sick sinus syndrome or second- or third-degree AV block.	Significant bronchospasm.	Potentiators: Dipyridamole and carbamazepine. **Effect pronounced in heart transplant recipients.** Antagonists: Caffeine and theophylline.	Facial flushing, palpitations, chest pain, hypotension, and exacerbation of bronchospasm.

Atrioventricular nodal reentrant tachycardia, atrioventricular reentrant tachycardia, and many atrial tachycardias will terminate with vagal maneuvers or adenosine, and in atrial flutter, the appearance of flutter waveform will help diagnosis.

Water immersion, eyeball pressure, coughing, gagging, deep breathing, etc., are other alternative vagal maneuvers.

AV, atrioventricular; CVA, cerebrovascular accident; TIA, transient ischemic attack.

[a]Patients should be under continuous ECG monitoring for each of these procedures. To enhance diagnostic value of rhythm strip, use leads V_1 and II (atrial activity).

Classification

Five forms based on clinical presentation: first occurrence, paroxysmal, persistent, long-standing persistent, and permanent.

- **First occurrence** may be symptomatic or asymptomatic. Spontaneous conversion rate is high, measured at >60% in hospitalized patients.
- **Paroxysmal**—recurrent form of AF in which individual episodes are <7 days and usually <48 hours in duration.
- **Persistent**—recurrent form of AF in which individual episodes are >7 days in duration and may require electrical or chemical cardioversion to terminate.
- **Long-standing persistent**—AF for >1 year, still deemed manageable with cardioversion or RFA.
- **Permanent**—AF after failed attempts at electrical or chemical cardioversion, has been present for more than 1 year, or has been accepted due to contraindications for cardioversion or lack of symptoms.

Epidemiology

- Most common sustained tachyarrhythmia for which patients seek treatment and most likely etiology for irregularly irregular rhythm discovered on an inpatient ECG. Typically, a disease of the elderly, affecting >10% of those aged >75 years.
- Independent risk factors include advanced age, male gender, and comorbid presence of diabetes mellitus and cardiovascular diseases such as CHF, valvular heart disease, HTN, and previous MI.[4] Age <65 years, obesity, and OSA are important risk factors for new-onset AF.[5]
- Following cardiothoracic surgery, AF occurs in 20%–50% of patients.[6]

Pathophysiology

- Precise mechanisms giving rise to AF are not completely understood.
- Initiation due to rapid, repetitive firing of ectopic focus within the pulmonary veins with fibrillatory conduction to bodies of the atria.
- Maintenance likely requires multiple reentrant circuits varying in location and timing to explain the self-perpetuating characteristic of AF.
- Structural and electrical remodeling of the left atrium associated with cardiovascular disease promotes ectopic activity and heterogeneous conduction patterns that provide the substrate for AF. AF, when present, also promotes structural and electrical remodeling in the atria that stabilizes the rhythm.
- Inflammation and fibrosis may play major role in initiation and maintenance. Inflammatory markers, such as interleukin 6 and C-reactive protein (CRP), are increased in and correlate with duration of AF, success of cardioversion, and thrombogenesis.

Prevention

- Lack of prospective clinical data examining the value of risk factor modification in the prevention of non–postoperative AF.
- Some data suggest statins may reduce recurrent AF by 61%, independent of lipid-lowering effect.[7]
- Angiotensin-converting enzyme inhibitors (**ACE-I**) and angiotensin receptor blockers (**ARBs**) shown to prevent atrial remodeling in animals via suppression of the renin–angiotensin system. A meta-analysis of patients with CHF and HTN treated with either ACE-I or ARB has demonstrated reduction in new-onset AF by 20%–30%.[8]

• A number of pharmacologic and nonpharmacologic strategies have been evaluated to prevent postoperative AF. Perioperative continuation of **β-adrenergic antagonists (β-blockers)** has shown to reduce postoperative AF rates. **Amiodarone, sotalol, magnesium, and omega-3 fatty acids** used in perioperative period also demonstrated reduction in postoperative AF.[9]

DIAGNOSIS

• Diagnosed by 12-lead ECG with stereotypical pattern of irregularly fluctuating baseline with irregular, often rapid, ventricular rate (>100 bpm).
• Important to distinguish AF from other tachycardia mechanisms with an irregular ventricular response such as MAT and AFL with variable conduction.

Clinical Presentation

• Symptoms can range from nonexistent to nonspecific (fatigue) to severe (acute pulmonary edema, palpitations, angina, syncope).
• Symptoms usually secondary to rapid ventricular response (RVR) to AF rather than loss of atrial systole. However, patients with significant ventricular systolic or diastolic dysfunction can have symptoms directly attributable to loss of atrial systole.
• Prolonged tachycardia from AF may lead to **tachycardia-induced cardiomyopathy.**

TREATMENT

• Medical management is directed at three therapeutic goals: **(1) rate or (2) rhythm control and (3) prevention of thromboembolic events.**
• Previous studies have shown there is no mortality benefit to a strategy aimed at maintaining SR.[10] Therefore, rate control and management of thromboembolic risk are preferred strategy in asymptomatic and minimally symptomatic patients. Rhythm control is reserved for patients who remain symptomatic despite reasonable efforts at rate control.

Medications

• Medical management begins with consideration of appropriate antithrombotic therapy. Coumadin has shown to be superior to aspirin (ASA) or ASA in combination with clopidogrel for prevention of thromboembolic events in patients with nonvalvular-associated AF.
• Direct oral anticoagulants (DOAC) such as dabigatran, rivaroxaban, apixaban, and edoxaban have been directly compared with warfarin in randomized prospective trials and have been shown to be either noninferior or superior to coumadin in preventing stroke in AF patients.
• Rate control of AF is achieved with medications that limit conduction through the AV node such as **non-dihydropyridine calcium channel blockers** (verapamil, diltiazem, etc.), **β-adrenergic antagonists, and digoxin.**
• Rhythm control can be attempted with selected antiarrhythmic drugs. Pharmacologic control with antiarrhythmic drugs is more effective at preventing recurrence of AF than chemical cardioversion (Table 7-3).

First Line

• **Prevention of stroke and systemic emboli**—central tenet of AF management is guided by individual risk assessment. Systemic anticoagulation with coumadin or DOAC attenuates risk of stroke or systemic emboli associated with AF.

TABLE 7-3	Pharmacologic Agents Used for Heart Rate Control in Atrial Fibrillation				
Drug	Loading Dose	Onset of Action	Maintenance Dose	Major Side Effects	Recommendation
Without Evidence of Accessory Pathway					
Esmolol[a]	IV: 500 µg/kg over 1 min, followed by 50 µg/kg for 4 min	IV: 2–10 min	IV: Up to 200 µg/kg/min continuous infusion	↓BP, ↓HR, HB, HF, bronchospasm	I
Metoprolol[a]	IV: 2.5–5 mg over 2 min, repeat doses every 5 min as needed up to 15 mg	IV: 20 min	–	↓BP, ↓HR, HB, HF, bronchospasm	I
	PO: 50–100 mg (in single or divided doses depending upon formulation)	PO: Within 1 h	PO: Up to 400 mg daily	–	–
Propranolol[a]	IV: 1 mg over 1 min, repeat every 2 min as needed up to 3 doses	–	–	↓BP, ↓HR, HB, HF, bronchospasm	I
	PO: 10–30 mg every 6–8 h	PO: 1–2 h	PO: 10–40 mg tid or qid	–	–
Diltiazem	IV: 0.25 mg/kg over 2 min, followed by 0.35 mg/kg over 2 min if needed	IV: 3 min	IV: 5–10 mg/h, up to 15 mg/h	↓BP, HB, HF	I
	PO: 120 mg daily (in single or divided doses depending upon formulation)	PO: 30–60 min (for immediate release formulation)	PO: 120–360 mg daily	–	–
Verapamil	IV: 0.075–0.15 mg/kg over 2 min, followed by 10 mg bolus after 15–30 min if needed	IV: 3–5 min	IV: 5 mg/h	↓BP, HB, HF	I
	PO: 180–480 mg daily (in single or divided doses depending upon formulation)	PO: 1–2 h (for immediate release formulation)	PO: Up to 480 mg daily	–	–

(continued)

CHAPTER 7

TABLE 7-3	Pharmacologic Agents Used for Heart Rate Control in Atrial Fibrillation *(continued)*				
Drug	Loading Dose	Onset of Action	Maintenance Dose	Major Side Effects	Recommendation
Amiodarone	IV: 150 mg over 10 min, followed by 1 mg/min for 6 h, followed by 0.5 mg/min for 18 h PO: 600–800 mg daily in divided doses for total load of 10 g over 2–4 wk	2 d–3 wk for anti-arrhythmic effects of IV and PO	PO: 200 mg once daily, can be decreased to 100 mg in elderly and patients with low BMI	↓BP, HB, ↓HR, warfarin interaction; see text for description of dermatologic, thyroid, pulmonary, corneal, and liver side effects	Acute setting: IIa (IV) Nonacute/chronic: IIb (PO)
With Evidence of Accessory Pathway[c]					
Amiodarone	IV: 150 mg over 10 min, followed by 1 mg/min for 6 h, followed by 0.5 mg/min for 18 h	2 d–3 wk	PO: 200 mg once daily	See above	IIa
With Heart Failure and Without Accessory Pathway					
Digoxin	IV: 0.25–0.5 mg over several min, repeat 0.25 mg doses every 6 h to maximum dose of 1.5 mg in 24 h; dose may need to be reduced by 50% in patients with CKD/ESRD	IV: 5–60 min PO: 1–2 h	PO: 0.125–0.25 mg once daily; 0.0625 mg once daily for GFR of 10–50 mL/min; 0.0625 mg once every 48 h for GFR <10 mL/min	Digoxin toxicity, HB, ↓HR	I

BMI, body mass index; ↓BP, hypotension; CKD, chronic kidney disease; ESRD, end-stage renal disease; GFR, glomerular filtration rate; HB, heart block; HF, heart failure; ↓HR, bradycardia; NA, not applicable.

[a]Only representative β-blockers are included in the table, but other similar agents could be used for this indication in appropriate doses.

[b]Onset is variable, and some effects occur earlier.

[c]Conversion to sinus rhythm and catheter ablation of the accessory pathway are generally recommended; pharmacologic therapy for rate control may be appropriate therapy in certain patients. See text for discussion of atrial fibrillation in setting of preexcitation/Wolff–Parkinson–White syndrome.

[d]Amiodarone can be useful to control the heart rate in patients with atrial fibrillation when other measures are unsuccessful or contraindicated.

- Use of oral anticoagulants requires careful risk–benefit analysis to identify patients who are at sufficient risk for thromboembolic events without significant risk of hemorrhagic complications.
  - **CHA_2DS_2-VASc score**—validated risk stratification tool used in nonvalvular AF to predict stroke or systemic embolus risk based on the presence of following risk factors: CHF, HTN, **a**ge >65 or >75 years, **d**iabetes mellitus, female gender, prior **s**troke or transient ischemic attack (TIA), and history of **v**ascular disease (Table 7-4).[11]
  - Antithrombotic therapy can be omitted in patients with a **CHA_2DS_2-VASc score = 0.**
  - In patients with a **CHA_2DS_2-VASc score of 1, no antithrombotic therapy or treatment with an oral anticoagulant or ASA may be considered.**
  - Systemic anticoagulation with coumadin or DOAC is recommended for male patients with a CHA_2DS_2-VASc risk of ≥2 and female patients with a CHA_2DS_2-VASc risk of ≥3 in women who have no contraindications for anticoagulation.
  - DOACs are recommended over coumadin for DOAC-eligible patients.
  - Measurement of renal function is critical to assess safety and dosing of certain DOACs in patients with **CHA_2DS_2-VASc score of ≥2 and chronic kidney disease.**
  - For AF patients at risk for thromboembolism but unable to tolerate long-term anticoagulation, consideration can be given to percutaneous occlusion or surgical ligation of left atrial appendage (LAA).
  - Role of antithrombotic therapy leading up to and after restoration of SR discussed in the context of cardioversion.
- **Pharmacologic rate control** of AF is achieved with drugs that prolong conduction through the AV node. Principally, these include the non-dihydropyridine calcium channel blockers (diltiazem, verapamil), β-adrenergic blockers, and digoxin. Refer to Table 7-3 for loading and dosing recommendations.
  Digoxin can be useful in controlling the resting ventricular rate in AF in the setting of LV dysfunction and CHF when other agents fail. Utility in other clinical settings

TABLE 7-4	Annual Stroke Risk in Patients With Nonvalvular Atrial Fibrillation Not Treated With Anticoagulation According to the CHA_2DS_2-VASc Score
CHA_2DS_2-VASc Score	**Stroke Risk (%)[a]**
0	0
1	1.3
2	2.2
3	3.2
4	4.0
5	6.7
6	9.8
7	9.6
8	12.5
9	15.2

CHA_2DS_2-VASc, cardiac failure, hypertension, age 65–74 years or age >74 years (doubled), diabetes, female sex, stroke (doubled), and a history of vascular disease.
[a]The adjusted stroke rate was derived from multivariate analysis assuming no aspirin usage.

is limited by reduced efficacy of rate control during exertion and significant concerns of toxicity.

- ○ **Digitalis toxicity** is characterized by **nausea, abdominal pain, vision changes, confusion, and delirium.** Patients with renal dysfunction are at risk for digitalis toxicity as are patients on agents known to increase digoxin levels (e.g., verapamil, diltiazem, erythromycin, cyclosporine).
- ○ **Paroxysmal AT with varying degrees of AV block and bidirectional VT**—most commonly seen arrhythmias in association with digitalis toxicity. Treatment is supportive (i.e., withholding drug, inserting temporary pacemaker for prolonged AV block, administering **IV phenytoin for bidirectional VT**).
- • **Nonpharmacologic rate control**—accomplished by AV nodal ablation in association with PPM implantation. Strategy reserved for patients deemed to be in permanent AF, who have failed pharmacologic rate control, and in whom rhythm control is either ineffective or contraindicated.

Second Line

Pharmacologic rhythm control of AF accomplished with antiarrhythmic drugs that modify impulse formation or propagation to prevent initiation of AF. **Risk of thromboembolism associated with pharmacologic cardioversion should be considered before beginning antiarrhythmic drug therapy.**

- • **Pharmacologic cardioversion** should be performed in hospital setting with continuous ECG monitoring due to small risk of life-threatening tachy- or bradyarrhythmias.
  - ○ **Ibutilide**—only drug approved by US Food and Drug Administration for pharmacologic cardioversion. Clinical trials have shown a 45% conversion rate for AF and a 60% conversion rate for AFL.
  - ○ Ibutilide is associated with 4%–8% risk for torsades de pointes (TdP), especially in first 2–4 hours after administration. Because of this risk, patients must be monitored on telemetry with an external defibrillator immediately available during ibutilide infusion and for at least 4 hours after infusion. The risk for TdP is higher in patients with cardiomyopathy and CHF.
  - ○ Ibutilide is administered intravenously, at dosage of 1 mg (0.01 mg/kg if patient is <60 kg), **infused slowly over 10 minutes.** Faster administration can promote TdP.
  - ○ Efficacy of antiarrhythmics to achieve pharmacologic conversion drops sharply when AF is >7 days in duration. For shorter duration episodes, dofetilide, sotalol, flecainide, and propafenone have some efficacy; amiodarone has limited efficacy to achieve pharmacologic cardioversion.
- • **Maintenance of** NSR with antiarrhythmic agents is associated with small risk for life-threatening proarrhythmia. As a result, antiarrhythmic therapy should be reserved for patients who have symptomatic AF with or without adequate rate control. Commonly used antiarrhythmic agents, their major route of elimination, and dosing regimens are listed in Table 7-5. Most effective agents for maintenance of SR are flecainide, propafenone, sotalol, dofetilide, amiodarone, and dronedarone.
  - ○ **Flecainide and propafenone**
    - ▪ For maintenance of NSR in patients with **structurally normal hearts.**
    - ▪ Associated with increased mortality rate in patients with structural heart disease.[12]
    - ▪ Potent negative inotropes that can provoke or exacerbate heart failure.
    - ▪ Prolong QRS duration as early manifestation of toxicity.
      - □ Toxicity increases with heart rate because of preferential blockade of active sodium channels. Property is described as **positive-use dependence.**

TABLE 7-5	Commonly Used Antiarrhythmic Drugs			
Class	Drug	Route of Administration (Elimination)	Initial/Loading Dose	Maintenance Dose	Major Adverse Effects[a]/ Comments

Class	Drug	Route of Administration (Elimination)	Initial/Loading Dose	Maintenance Dose	Major Adverse Effects[a]/ Comments
Ia	Procainamide	IV (R, H) PO (R, H)	15–18 mg/kg at 20 mg/min 50 mg/kg/24 h, max: 5 g/24 h	1–4 mg/min IR: 250–500 mg q3–6h SR: 500 mg q6h Procanbid: 1000–2500 mg q12h	GI, CNS, +ANA/SLE-like syndrome, fever, hematologic, anticholinergic. Follow QT_c, serum procainamide (4–8 mg/L) and NAPA levels (<20 mg/mL)
	Quinidine	PO (H)	Sulfate, 200–400 mg q6h; gluconate, 324–972 mg q8–12h	NA	↑QT, TdP, ↓BP, thrombocytopenia, cinchonism, GI upset
	Disopyramide	PO (H, R)	300–400 mg	IR: 100–200 mg q6h SR: 200–400 mg q12h	Anticholinergic, HF
Ib	Lidocaine	IV (H)	1 mg/kg over 2 min (may repeat × 2 up to 3 mg/kg total)	1–4 mg/min	↓HR, CNS, GI; adjust dose in patients with hepatic failure, AMI, HF, or shock
	Mexiletine	PO (H)	400 mg one-time dose	200–300 mg q8h	GI, CNS
Ic	Flecainide	PO (H, R)	50 mg q12h	Increase by 50–100 mg/d every 4 d to max 400 mg/d	HF, GI, CNS, blurred vision
	Propafenone	PO (H)	IR: 150 mg q8h ER: 225 mg q12h	IR: Increase at 3- to 4-day intervals up to 300 mg q8h ER: May increase at 5-day intervals, up to 425 mg q12h	GI, dizziness

(continued)

TABLE 7-5	Commonly Used Antiarrhythmic Drugs *(continued)*			
Class	Drug	Route of Administration (Elimination)	Initial/Loading Dose	Maintenance Dose	Major Adverse Effects[a]/ Comments
III	Sotalol	PO (R)	80 mg q12h	May increase every 3 d up to 240–320 mg/d in two to three divided doses	↓HR, ↓BP, CHF, CNS Limit QT$_c$ prolongation to <550 ms
	Dofetilide	PO (R, H)	CrCl (mL/min): Dose (µg bid): >60: 500 40–60: 250 20–39: 125 <20: Contraindicated	Dose adjusted based on QT$_c$ 2–3 h after inpatient doses 1 through 5 Chronic therapy requires calculation of QT$_c$ and CrCl every 3 mo with adjustment as necessary	↑QT, VT/TdP, HA, dizziness; see text for further details on initiating and monitoring treatment
	Ibutilide	IV (H)	1 mg (0.01 mg/kg if patient <60 kg) over 10 min; can repeat if no response 10 min after initial infusion	NA	↑QT, TdP, AV block, GI, HA
	Amiodarone	IV (H) PO (H)	IV: 150 mg over 10 min PO: 800 mg/d for 1 wk, then 600 mg/d for 1 wk, then 400 mg/d for 1 wk	1 mg/min × 6 h, then 0.5 mg/min 100–400 mg PO daily	↓BP, HB, ↓HR, warfarin interaction; see text for description of dermatologic, thyroid, pulmonary, corneal, and liver effects

AMI, acute myocardial infarction; ANA, antinuclear antibodies; ↓BP, hypotension; CNS, central nervous system; CHF, congestive heart failure; CrCl, creatinine clearance; ER, extended release; GI, gastrointestinal; H, hepatic; HA, headache; HB, heart block; HF, heart failure; ↓HR, bradycardia; IR, immediate release; NA, not applicable; NAPA, N-acetylprocainamide; R, renal; SLE, systemic lupus erythematosus; SR, sustained release; TdP, torsades de pointes; VT, ventricular tachycardia.

[a]Either common or life-threatening adverse effects of these medications are listed. This is not a comprehensive list of all possible adverse effects.

- □ Exercise ECG used to give additional information about dose safety at higher heart rates.
- □ Flecainide should be used cautiously without concomitant dosing with AV nodal blocker because paradoxical increase in the ventricular rate may occur from drug-induced conversion of AF to AFL. Propafenone is less prone to this because of intrinsic β-adrenergic antagonism.

○ **Sotalol**—mixture of stereoisomers (DL-)
- D-sotalol is a potassium channel blocker, whereas L-sotalol is a β-antagonist. Side effects of the drug reflect both mechanisms of action.
- DL-sotalol may result in QT interval prolongation leading to TdP as well as sinus bradycardia or AV conduction abnormalities.
- Should not be used in patients with decompensated CHF (because of negative inotropic effect) or with a prolonged QT interval.
- Initiation should be performed in an inpatient monitored setting.
- Renal adjustment is necessary as sotalol is excreted by the kidneys.

○ **Dofetilide**—pure potassium channel blocker.
- Initiation of dofetilide should be done in an inpatient monitored setting due to increased risk of QT interval prolongation leading to TdP.
- QT prolongation with sotalol or dofetilide is intensified by bradycardia, known as "**reverse-use dependence.**"
- Contraindicated in patients with baseline corrected QT interval (QT_c) >440 ms (or >500 ms with baseline bundle branch block).
- Dosing is based on the creatinine clearance. A 12-lead ECG should be obtained before the first dose and 1–2 hours after each dose, thereafter. If QT_c prolongs by 15% of baseline or exceeds 500 ms, 50% dosage reduction is indicated. If the QT_c exceeds 500 ms after the second dose, dofetilide must be discontinued.
- Several medications block renal secretion of dofetilide (verapamil, cimetidine, prochlorperazine, trimethoprim, megestrol, ketoconazole) and are contraindicated with the use of dofetilide.
- Not associated with increased mortality in patients with LV dysfunction and does not cause conduction disturbances.

○ **Dronedarone**—newest antiarrhythmic agent approved for management of AF.
- Shares properties with Vaughan Williams classes I–IV antiarrhythmic drugs.
- More effective than placebo but less effective than amiodarone at maintaining SR after cardioversion.
- Incidence of proarrhythmia and organ toxicity low with dronedarone.
- Trend toward increased mortality has been shown in patients with advanced heart failure symptoms; as such, it is contraindicated in this patient group.
- Metabolized by the liver and should not be used in patients with significant hepatic dysfunction.
- Can be used in patients with significant renal dysfunction.

○ **Amiodarone**—most effective antiarrhythmic agent for maintenance of SR.
- **Because of extensive toxicity profile, should not be considered first-line agent for rhythm control of AF in patients in whom alternative antiarrhythmic can be safely used.**
- Low efficacy for acute conversion of AF, although conversion after several days of IV has been observed. Adverse effects of oral amiodarone are partially dose dependent and may occur in up to 75% of patients treated at high doses for 5 years. At lower doses (200–300 mg/d), adverse effects that require discontinuation occur in approximately 5%–10% of patients per year.

- **Pulmonary toxicity** in 1%–15% of treated patients but appears less likely in those who receive <300 mg/d.[13]
    - Dry cough and dyspnea associated with pulmonary infiltrates and rales.
    - Process reversible if detected early, but undetected cases may result in mortality rate of up to 10%.
    - CXR and pulmonary function tests should be obtained at baseline and every 12 months or when patients report symptoms of dyspnea. The presence of interstitial infiltrates on CXR and decreased diffusion capacity raise concern for amiodarone-induced pulmonary toxicity.
  - **Photosensitivity**—common adverse reaction. Violaceous skin discoloration can develop in sun-exposed areas; blue-gray discoloration may not resolve completely with discontinuation of therapy.
  - **Thyroid dysfunction**—common adverse effect. Both hypothyroidism and hyperthyroidism are reported, with an incidence of 2%–5% per year. Thyroid-stimulating hormone should be obtained at baseline and monitored every 6 months. If hypothyroidism develops, concurrent treatment with levothyroxine may allow continued amiodarone use.
  - **Corneal microdeposits**—detectable on slit-lamp examination, develop in virtually all patients. Deposits rarely interfere with vision and not an indication for discontinuation of drug. Optic neuritis, leading to blindness, is rare but has been reported in association with amiodarone.
  - Most common **ECG changes** are lengthened PR interval and bradycardia; however, high-grade AV block may occur in patients who have preexisting conduction abnormalities. May prolong QT intervals, although usually not extensively, and **TdP is rare.** Other QT-prolonging agents should be avoided in patients taking amiodarone.
  - **Liver dysfunction** usually manifests in asymptomatic and transient rise in hepatic transaminases. If increase exceeds three times normal or doubles in patient with an elevated baseline level, amiodarone should be discontinued or dose should be reduced. Aspartate transaminase and alanine transaminase should be monitored every 6 months.
  - **Drug interactions**—amiodarone may raise blood levels of warfarin and digoxin; these drugs should be reduced routinely by one-half when amiodarone is initiated, and levels followed closely.

Nonpharmacologic Therapies

- Nonpharmacologic methods of rhythm control include electrical cardioversion, catheter ablation, or surgical techniques that block initiation and maintenance of AF.
- **Direct current cardioversion (DCCV)**—safest and most effective method of acutely restoring SR. Prior to cardioversion:
  - Consideration of anticoagulation is critical, to minimize thromboembolic events triggered by the cardioversion process.
  - AF with RVR in setting of ongoing myocardial ischemia, MI, hypotension, or respiratory distress should receive prompt cardioversion regardless of the anticoagulation status.
  - If duration of AF is **<48 hours**, cardioversion may proceed without anticoagulation. If AF has persisted for **>48 hours** (or for unknown duration), patients should be therapeutically anticoagulated for at least 3 weeks before cardioversion (elective situation), and anticoagulation should be continued following successful cardioversion for a minimum of 4 weeks.

- ○ Alternative to anticoagulation for 3 weeks prior to cardioversion is to perform **transesophageal echocardiogram** to rule out LAA thrombus before cardioversion. This method is safe and has advantage of shorter time to cardioversion. Therapeutic anticoagulation is indicated after cardioversion for minimum of 4 weeks.[14]
- ○ When practical, periprocedural sedation is accomplished with midazolam (1–2 mg IV q2min to a maximum of 5 mg), methohexital (25–75 mg IV), etomidate (0.2–0.6 mg/kg IV), or propofol (initial dose, 5 mg/kg/h IV).
- ○ Proper synchronization of DC shock to the QRS is critical to avoid induction of VT by shock delivered during vulnerable period of the ventricle.
- ○ For cardioversion of atrial arrhythmias, anterior patch electrode should be positioned just right of the sternum at the level of third or fourth intercostal space, with second electrode positioned just below left scapula posteriorly. **Care should be taken to position patch electrodes at least 6 cm from PPM or implantable cardioverter–defibrillator (ICD) generators.** If electrode paddles are used, firm pressure and conductive gel should be applied to minimize contact impedance. Direct contact with the patient or the bed should be avoided. Atropine (1 mg IV) should be readily available to treat prolonged pauses. Reports of serious arrhythmias, such as VT, ventricular fibrillation (VF), or asystole are rare and more likely in setting of improperly synchronized cardioversions, digitalis toxicity, or concomitant antiarrhythmic drug therapy.
- **Catheter ablation of AF**—highly effective in younger patients with structurally normal hearts and paroxysmal pattern of AF.[6]
- ○ Success rates in this cohort are in the range of 70%–80% over 12–18 months follow-up period.
- ○ Success rates are diminished in patients with structural heart disease, advanced age, and persistent AF. A significant fraction of patients require more than one ablation procedure to achieve long-term successful elimination of AF.
- ○ Goal of catheter ablation in paroxysmal AF patients is to achieve electrical isolation of the pulmonary veins. In patients with persistent AF, this goal is frequently combined with substrate modification strategies whereby regions of the atria are targeted for ablation to block reentry or the presence of focal drivers of AF.

Surgical Management

Surgical techniques for cure of AF have been evaluated since the 1980s. Among these, the Cox maze procedure has highest demonstrated efficacy and most robust follow-up data documenting sustained efficacy. Including patients with persistent AF and structural heart disease, success rates approach 90%. Because of its invasive nature, surgical treatment is usually reserved for those who have failed catheter ablation or who have planned concomitant cardiac surgery.[6]

Ventricular Tachyarrhythmias

GENERAL PRINCIPLES

- Ventricular tachyarrhythmias should be initially approached with assumption that they will have malignant course, until proven otherwise.
- Characterization of the arrhythmia involves consideration of hemodynamic stability, duration and ECG morphology of tachycardia, and the presence or lack of underlying structural heart disease.
- Characterization will aid in determining the patient's risk for **sudden cardiac arrest (SCA)** and need for therapeutic intervention and/or device implantation.

CHAPTER 7

Definition

- **Nonsustained ventricular tachycardia (NSVT):** Three or more consecutive ventricular complexes (>100 bpm) that terminate spontaneously within 30 seconds.
- **Sustained monomorphic ventricular tachycardia (SMVT):** Tachycardia of ventricular origin with single QRS morphology lasting longer than 30 seconds or requiring cardioversion due to hemodynamic compromise.
- **Polymorphic ventricular tachycardia (PMVT):** VT is characterized by evolving QRS morphology. **TdP** is a variant of PMVT typically preceded by prolonged QT interval in SR. PMVT is associated with hemodynamic collapse or instability.
- **VF:** Associated with disorganized mechanical contraction of ventricles, hemodynamic collapse, and sudden death. ECG reveals irregular and rapid oscillations (250–400 bpm) of highly variable amplitude without clearly identifiable QRS complexes or T waves.
- Ventricular arrhythmias—major cause of **sudden cardiac death (SCD).**
  - **SCD**—unexpected death that generally occurs within 1 hour of onset of symptoms in person without prior condition that would appear fatal. In the US, approximately 350,000 cases of SCD occur annually.
    - Among patients with aborted SCD, ischemic heart disease is most commonly associated cardiac structural abnormality. Most cardiac arrest survivors do not have evidence of acute MI; however, >75% have evidence of previous infarcts.
    - Nonischemic cardiomyopathy (NICM) is also associated with an elevated risk for SCD.[15]

Etiology

- **VT associated with structural heart disease**
  - Most ventricular arrhythmias are associated with structural heart disease, typically related to active ischemia or prior infarct.
    - Scar and the peri-infarct area provide substrate for reentry that produces SMVT.
    - PMVT and VF—commonly associated with ischemia and are presumed cause of most out-of-hospital SCD.
  - NICM typically involves progressive dilation and fibrosis of ventricular myocardium, providing arrhythmogenic substrate.
  - Infiltrative cardiomyopathies (secondary to sarcoidosis, hemochromatosis, amyloidosis, etc.) affect smaller patient population that is at significant risk for ventricular arrhythmias and whose management is less clearly defined.
  - Adults with prior repair of congenital heart disease are commonly afflicted with both VT and SVT.
  - Arrhythmogenic right ventricular dysplasia (ARVD) or cardiomyopathy—marked by fibrofatty replacement of the RV (and sometimes LV) myocardium giving rise to left bundle branch block (LBBB) morphology VT and is associated with sudden death, particularly in young athletes.
  - Bundle branch reentry VT—form of ventricular tachyarrhythmia that uses His–Purkinje system in a reentrant circuit and is typically associated with cardiomyopathy and abnormal conduction system.
- **VT in the absence of structural heart disease**
  - Inherited ion channelopathies, such as those seen in Brugada syndrome and LQTS, can lead to PMVT and sudden death in patients without evidence of structural heart disease.
  - Catecholaminergic PMVT involves inherited, exercise-induced VT related to irregular calcium processing.

- ○ **Idiopathic VT**—diagnosis of exclusion that requires documented absence of structural heart disease, genetic disorders, and reversible etiologies (i.e., ischemia, metabolic abnormalities).
  - ▪ Most originate from RV outflow tract (RVOT) and are amenable to ablation.
  - ▪ LV outflow tract (LVOT) VTs, arising from near the coronary cusps or aortomitral continuity, or fascicular VTs (using anterior and posterior divisions of the left bundle branch) are less common forms of idiopathic VT.
  - ▪ Tachycardia-mediated cardiomyopathy can result if left untreated.

DIAGNOSIS

Clinical Presentation

- Evaluation of WCTs should always begin with prompt assessment of vital signs and symptoms. If arrhythmia is poorly tolerated, postpone further evaluation and proceed to acute management per ACLS guidelines. If patient is clinically stable, rhythm should be carefully analyzed to distinguish VT from SVT. A common mistake is the assumption that hemodynamic stability supports the diagnosis of SVT over VT.
- VT represents the majority of WCT seen in the inpatient setting with reported prevalence of ~80%. Eliciting historical points of emphasis and closely assessing ECG properties can help delineate mechanism of underlying rhythm disturbance. Begin with the following questions:
  - ○ Does patient have history of structural heart disease?
    - ▪ Patients with structural heart disease are much more likely to have VT than SVT as etiology of WCT. In one analysis, 98% of patients with WCT on ECG who had prior MI proved to have VT.[16]
  - ○ Does patient have implanted device (PPM or ICD) or wide QRS at baseline?
    - ▪ Presence of either pacemaker or ICD should raise suspicion for device-mediated WCT.
    - ▪ **Device-mediated WCT** can occur from ventricular pacing at rapid rate either caused by tracking of an atrial tachyarrhythmia or alternatively by "endless loop tachycardia" from tracking of retrograde atrial impulses created by preceding ventricular paced beat. In either case, tachycardia rate is a clue to mechanism because it is typically equal to programmed upper rate limit (URL) of the device. A commonly programmed URL is 120 bpm. Tachycardia rate above URL effectively excludes device-mediated WCT.
    - ▪ Presence of an implantable device can be confirmed by inspection of the chest wall (usually left chest for right-handed patients), CXR, or appearance of pacing spikes on ECG or telemetry.
    - ▪ Patients with known right bundle branch block (RBBB), LBBB, or intraventricular conduction delay (IVCD) at baseline presenting with WCT will have QRS morphology identical to baseline in the presence of SVT. In contrast, some patients with narrow QRS at baseline will manifest WCT due to SVT when a rate-related bundle branch block is present (SVT with aberrancy).
  - ○ What are patient's home medications?
    - ▪ Home medication list should be carefully reviewed for any drugs with proarrhythmic side effects, especially those that can prolong the baseline QT interval—including many class I and III antiarrhythmics, certain antibiotics, and antipsychotics.
    - ▪ Medications that can lead to electrolyte derangements, such as loop and potassium-sparing diuretics, ACE-I, ARB, and digoxin toxicity, if applicable, should be considered in setting of any arrhythmia.

CHAPTER 7

Differential Diagnosis

- WCT is secondary to either SVT with aberrant conduction or VT. Differentiation between these rhythm abnormalities is of utmost importance. **The pharmacologic agents used in the management of SVT (i.e., adenosine, β-blockers, calcium channel blockers) may cause hemodynamic instability if used in the setting of VT.** Therefore, all WCTs are considered ventricular in origin until proven otherwise.
- Other less common mechanisms of WCT include **A-AVRT, hyperkalemia-induced arrhythmia, or pacemaker-induced tachycardia.**
- **Telemetry artifact** from poor lead contact or repetitive patient motion (tremor, shivering, brushing teeth, chest physical therapy, etc.) can mimic VT or VF.

Diagnostic Testing

Laboratories
- Basic studies should include CBC, complete metabolic panel, magnesium level, and serial troponins.
- Additional labs based on clinical suspicion should also be obtained during initial workup.

Electrocardiography
- **Differentiation of SVT with aberrancy from VT** based on ECG analysis is critical for determination of appropriate therapy. Features diagnostic of VT: **AV dissociation**, **capture or fusion beats**, an absence of RS morphology in all precordial leads (V_1–V_6), and **LBBB morphology with right axis deviation.** In absence of these features, examination of an RS complex in a precordial lead for an RS interval >100 ms is consistent with VT. In addition, characteristic QRS morphologies that are suggestive of VT may be sought, as shown in Figure 7-2.
- **ECG pearls**
  - **Brugada syndrome ECG patterns**
    - Type 1: characterized by ST segment elevation of at least 2 mm with a coved morphology in leads V_1 and V_2, associated with an incomplete or complete RBBB, and followed by descending T wave.
    - Type 2 (also referred to as "saddleback" pattern): characterized by ST segment elevation of 2 mm followed by a trough within the ST segment with continued ST elevation of ≥1 mm and positive or biphasic T wave.
    - Patterns may be observed spontaneously or unmasked after fever, drug administration, stress, etc.
    - Only type 1 pattern is diagnostic of Brugada syndrome, while type 2 is suggestive but not specific.
  - **ARVD**
    - NSR ECG at baseline with the presence of an epsilon wave (late potential just after QRS) and/or T wave inversions in the right precordial leads is a diagnostic criterion for ARVD.
    - VT in ARVD generally arises from an RV origin and is therefore likely to have LBBB configuration; patients may present with NSVT or PMVT.
  - **Bundle branch reentrant VT**
    - Baseline ECG often shows IVCD.
    - In VT, ECG typically presents with LBBB morphology with electrical impulse traveling "down" the right bundle and "up" the left bundle.
  - **Fascicular VT**
    ECG in VT shows RBBB morphology with superior axis.

○ **LQTS**
- Abnormal prolongation of QT interval on ECG at baseline (ideally measured in leads II and V_5 or V_6).
- QT_c ≥450 ms in men and 460 ms in women.
- ECG in VT often shows TdP degenerating into VF.

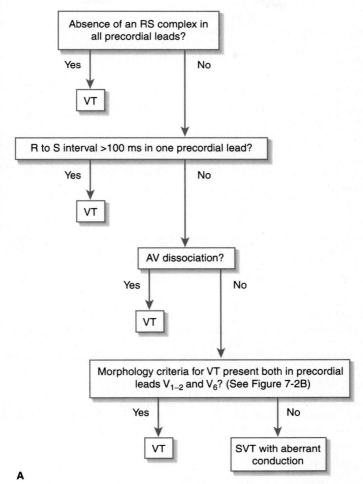

A

Figure 7-2. A and B, Brugada criteria for distinguishing ventricular tachycardia from supra-ventricular tachycardia with aberrancy in wide-complex tachycardias. LBBB, left bundle branch block; RBBB, right bundle branch block; SVT, supraventricular tachyarrhythmia; VT, ventricular tachycardia. (Reprinted with permission from Sharma S, Smith T. Advanced electrocardiography. In: Cuculich PS, Kates AM, eds. *The Washington Manual of Cardiology Subspecialty Consult.* 3rd ed. Lippincott, Williams & Wilkins; 2014.)

	LBBB		RBBB	
	VT	**SVT**	**VT**	**SVT**
Lead V1	In V1, V2 any of: (a) r ≥0.04 s (b) Notched S downstroke (c) Delayed S nadir >0.06 s	In V1, V2 absence of: (a) r ≥0.04 s (b) Notched S downstroke (c) Delayed S nadir >0.06 s	Taller left peak Biphasic RS or QR	Triphasic rsR' or rR'
	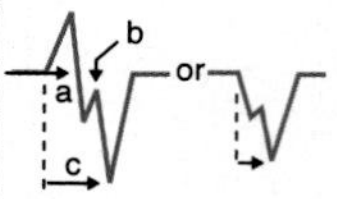	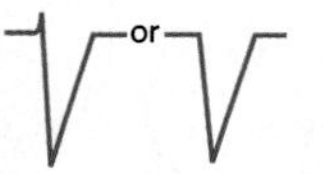	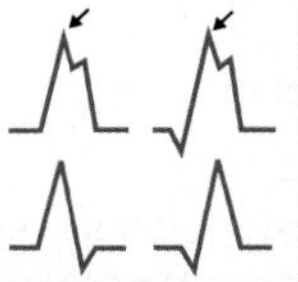	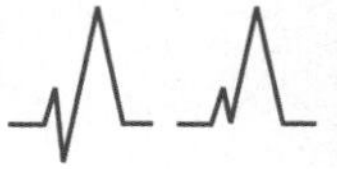
Lead V6	Monophasic QS 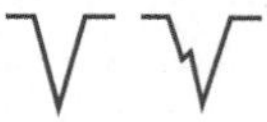		Biphasic rS 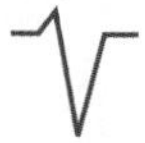	Triphasic qRs 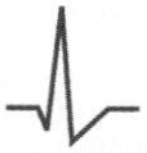

B

Figure 7-2. Cont'd

- ○ **Outflow tract VT**
  - ▪ ECG characteristically has inferior axis with LBBB morphology.
  - ▪ R/S transition in precordial leads can aid in localization: early transition (V₁ or V₂) suggests an LVOT origin, whereas later transition (V₄ or after) is suggestive of an RVOT origin.

Imaging
- Presence or absence of structural heart disease should be initially evaluated by TTE.
- Further imaging (cardiac MRI, noninvasive stress test, coronary angiogram, etc.) should be obtained based on suspected etiology.

TREATMENT

- **Differentiation of SVT with aberrancy from VT** based on analysis of surface ECG is critical in the determination of appropriate treatment.
  For acute therapy of SVT, IV medications such as adenosine, calcium channel blockers, or β-blockers are used (see "Treatment" of "Supraventricular Tachyarrhythmias" earlier in this chapter). However, calcium channel blockers and β-blockers can produce hemodynamic instability in patients with VT.
- Immediate unsynchronized DCCV is the primary therapy for pulseless VT and VF.

Nonpharmacologic Therapies

- **ICDs** provide automatic recognition and treatment of ventricular arrhythmias. ICD implantation improves survival in patients resuscitated from ventricular arrhythmias (secondary prevention of SCD) and in individuals without prior symptoms who are at high risk for SCD (primary prevention of SCD).
  - ○ Idiopathic VT is thought to be benign in the absence of structural heart disease. Therefore, ICD implantation is not appropriate.
  - ○ **Secondary prevention of SCD** with ICD implantation is indicated for most patients who survive SCD outside of the peri-MI setting. The superiority of ICD therapy to chronic antiarrhythmic drug therapy has been demonstrated.[17]
  - ○ **Primary prevention of SCD** with ICD implantation is indicated for patients who are at high risk of SCD. The efficacy of ICD implantation for primary prevention of SCD in the setting of cardiomyopathy has been established in multiple prospective clinical trials.[18-20] Most patients with LV ejection fraction of <35% for more than 3 months on optimal medical therapy for cardiomyopathy meet indications for prophylactic ICD implantation.
  - ○ **Alternative indications for ICD placement**
    - Phenotypes associated with **HCM, ARVD, cardiac sarcoid, congenital LQTS, or Brugada syndrome have higher risk of SCD.** ICD implantation indicated if patients with one of these syndromes have had resuscitated cardiac arrest or documented ventricular arrhythmia. Prophylactic ICD implantation is based on disease-specific risk factors.
    - Patients awaiting cardiac transplantation are at high risk for SCD, especially if they are receiving an IV inotrope. Prophylactic ICD implantation is reasonable to protect against SCD prior to transplantation.
    - ICDs are **contraindicated** in patients who have incessant VT, recent MI <40 days or revascularization <3 months in the case of primary prevention, significant psychiatric illnesses, or life expectancy of <12–24 months.
- **RFA of VT**—most successfully performed in patients with hemodynamically stable forms of idiopathic VT not associated with structural heart disease. Long-term cure rates are similar to those for catheter ablation of SVT. In structural heart disease, catheter ablation has a lower efficacy and higher morbidity but is an important treatment option, particularly in drug refractory VT leading to ICD therapy.
  - ○ **Idiopathic VT** is amenable to treatment with RFA or drug therapy.
  - ○ **VT associated with ischemic heart disease** can also be treated by catheter ablation targeting scar-based substrate. Emergent catheter ablation in setting of frequent hemodynamically unstable VT requiring defibrillation (VT storm) can be life-saving. Ablation has been shown to reduce ICD therapy and to improve quality of life.
  - ○ **Ablation of VT** in NICM—reasonable option, particularly in drug refractory patients. However, VT circuits may be intramyocardial or epicardial. As a result, success rates are typically lower than with ischemic VT. Referral to a center that routinely performs both endocardial and epicardial ablations should be considered.

Medications

- **Outflow tract VT** can be responsive to β-adrenergic blockers, diltiazem, verapamil, and/or adenosine.
- VT or VF resistant to external defibrillation requires addition of IV antiarrhythmic agents.
  - ○ IV lidocaine is frequently used; however, IV amiodarone appears to be more effective in increasing survival of VF when used in conjunction with defibrillation.[21]
  - ○ After successful defibrillation, continuous IV infusion of effective antiarrhythmic therapy should be maintained until reversible causes have been corrected.

CHAPTER 7

- Chronic antiarrhythmic drug therapy is indicated for treatment of recurrent symptomatic ventricular tachyarrhythmias. In setting of hemodynamically unstable ventricular arrhythmias treated with an ICD, antiarrhythmic drug therapy is often necessary to prevent frequent shocks.

Acute Drug Therapy
- **Amiodarone**—safe and well-tolerated for acute management of ventricular arrhythmias. Amiodarone has complex pharmacokinetics and is associated with significant toxicities arising from chronic therapy.
  After loading, amiodarone prevents recurrence of sustained VT or VF in up to 60% of patients. Therapeutic latency of more than 5 days exists before beneficial antiarrhythmic effects are observed with oral dosing, and full suppression of arrhythmias may not occur for 4–6 weeks after therapy is initiated. Unfortunately, recurrence of ventricular arrhythmias during long-term follow-up is common.
- **Lidocaine—class Ib** agent available only in IV form with efficacy in management of sustained and recurrent VT/VF. Prophylactic use for suppression of premature ventricular contractions and NSVT in otherwise uncomplicated post-MI setting should be avoided.
  ○ Toxicities can include central nervous system (CNS) effects (convulsions, confusion, stupor, and, rarely, respiratory arrest), all of which resolve with discontinuation of therapy.
  ○ Serum levels should be monitored during prolonged use.
- **Class II** agents, β-adrenergic antagonists, are the only class of antiarrhythmic agents to have consistently shown improved survival in post-MI patients.
  ○ β-adrenergic blockers reduce postinfarction total mortality by 25%–40% and SCD by 32%–50%.[22-25]
  ○ After acute therapy of VT/VF and stabilization, β-adrenergic blockers should be initiated and titrated as blood pressure and heart rate allow.

Chronic Drug Therapy
- **Sotalol—class III** agent indicated for chronic treatment of VT/VF. Sotalol prevents recurrence of sustained VT and VF in 70% of patients but must be used with caution in individuals with CHF.
- **Class I** agents have not been shown to reduce mortality in patients with VT/VF. In fact, class Ic agents, **flecainide** and **propafenone**, are associated with increased mortality in patients with ventricular arrhythmias after MI.[12] **Mexiletine** is similar to lidocaine (also an Ib agent) but is available in oral form. **Mexiletine is most often used in combination with either amiodarone or sotalol for chronic treatment of refractory ventricular arrhythmias.** CNS toxicity includes tremor, dizziness, and blurred vision. Higher levels may result in dysarthria, diplopia, nystagmus, and an impaired level of consciousness. Nausea and vomiting are common.
- **Phenytoin** can be used in the treatment of **digitalis-induced ventricular arrhythmias.** It may have limited role in treatment of ventricular arrhythmias associated with congenital LQTS and those with structural heart disease.

SPECIAL CONSIDERATIONS

- **Class IV** agents have no role in chronic management of VT associated with structural heart disease.
- Primary therapy for VF that occurs secondary to ischemia in the setting of an MI is complete revascularization. In the absence of complete revascularization, patients remain at high risk for recurrent VT/VF.

- In **TdP associated with LQTS**, acute therapy is immediate defibrillation.
- Bolus administration of magnesium sulfate in 1- to 2-g increments up to 4–6 g IV is effective.
- In cases of acquired long QT, identification and treatment of underlying condition should be performed, if possible.
- Elimination of long–short triggering sequences and shortening of the QT interval can be achieved by increasing the heart rate to the range of 90–120 bpm by either IV isoproterenol infusion (initial rate at 1–2 μg/min) or temporary transvenous pacing (TVP).

ALTERNATIVE THERAPIES

- For patients with ventricular arrhythmias that persist despite antiarrhythmic drug therapy and/or catheter ablation, consideration can be given to cervical sympathectomy or targeted stereotactic body radiation therapy (SBRT) at capable centers.
- Cervical sympathectomy is performed either unilaterally (on the left) or bilaterally for the purposes of reducing ICD shocks. Sympathectomy is generally preceded by stellate ganglion block to evaluate the short-term response to neuromodulation.[26]
- SBRT for the management of refractory VT is a relatively novel modality that has been shown to reduce both the burden of VT and ICD shocks in treated patients.[27]

BRADYARRHYTHMIAS

GENERAL PRINCIPLES

- Bradyarrhythmias can be encountered in both the inpatient and outpatient settings.
- Clinical decision-making is guided by patient symptoms and signs of hemodynamic stability.

Definition
Cardiac rhythms whose ventricular rate is below **60 bpm**.
- **Anatomy of the conduction system**
  - **The SA node**—collection of specialized pacemaker cells located in high right atrium. Under normal conditions, a wave of depolarization spreads inferiorly and leftward via atrial myocardium and intranodal tracts, producing atrial systole.
  - Wave of depolarization then reaches another group of specialized cells, the **AV node**, located in the lower right atrial side of the interatrial septum. Normally, AV node should serve as lone electrical connection between the atria and ventricles.
  - From the AV node, wave of depolarization travels down the **His bundle**, located in the membranous septum, and into **right and left bundle branches** before reaching the **Purkinje fibers** that depolarize the remaining ventricular myocardium.

Etiology
Common causes of bradycardia are listed in Table 7-6.

DIAGNOSIS

Clinical Presentation
- When evaluating suspected bradyarrhythmia, history, physical examination, and available data should be used to address stability, symptoms, reversibility, site of dysfunction, and the need for temporary as well as permanent pacing.

CHAPTER 7

TABLE 7-6	Causes of Bradycardia

Intrinsic

Congenital disease (may present later in life)

Idiopathic degeneration (aging)

Infarction or ischemia

Cardiomyopathy

Infiltrative disease: sarcoidosis, amyloidosis, hemochromatosis

Collagen vascular diseases: systemic lupus erythematosus, rheumatoid arthritis, scleroderma

Surgical trauma: valve surgery, transplantation

Infectious disease: endocarditis, Lyme disease, Chagas disease

Extrinsic

Autonomically mediated

Neurocardiogenic syncope

Carotid sinus hypersensitivity

Increased vagal tone: coughing, vomiting, micturition, defecation, intubation

Drugs: β-blockers, calcium channel blockers, digoxin, antiarrhythmic agents

Hypothyroidism

Hypothermia

Neurologic disorders: increased intracranial pressure

Electrolyte imbalances: hyperkalemia, hypermagnesemia

Hypercarbia/obstructive sleep apnea

Sepsis

- If patient demonstrates signs of poor perfusion (hypotension, confusion, decreased consciousness, cyanosis, etc.), immediate management per ACLS protocol should be initiated. Clinical manifestations of bradyarrhythmias are variable, ranging from asymptomatic to nonspecific (lightheadedness, fatigue, weakness, exercise intolerance) to overt (syncope).
- Emphasis should be placed on determining **if presenting symptoms have a direct temporal relationship to underlying bradycardia.** Other historical points of emphasis include the following:
  - Ischemic heart disease, particularly involving right coronary circulation, can precipitate a number of bradyarrhythmias. Therefore, signs and symptoms of acute coronary syndrome should be thoroughly investigated.
  - **Precipitating circumstances** (micturition, coughing, defecation, noxious smells) surrounding episodes may help identify neurocardiogenic etiology of bradycardia.
  - Tachyarrhythmias, particularly in patients with underlying sinus node dysfunction, can be followed by long pauses **(conversion pauses)** because of sinus node suppression during tachycardia.
  - History of structural heart disease, hypothyroidism, OSA, collagen vascular disease, infections (bacteremia, endocarditis, Lyme, Chagas), infiltrative diseases

(amyloid, hemochromatosis, and sarcoid), neuromuscular diseases, and prior cardiac surgery (valve replacement, congenital repair) should be elicited.
  ○ **Medications** should be reviewed with emphasis on those that affect the SA and AV nodes (i.e., calcium channel blockers, β-adrenergic blockers, digoxin).
• After hemodynamic stability is confirmed, a more thorough examination with emphasis on the cardiovascular system and any findings consistent with the above comorbidities is appropriate (Figure 7-3).

Diagnostic Testing
Laboratories
The laboratory testing should include serum electrolytes and thyroid function tests in most patients. Digoxin levels and serial troponins should be drawn when clinically appropriate.

Electrocardiography
• A **12-lead ECG** is the cornerstone for diagnosis in any workup where arrhythmia is suspected.
• Rhythm strips from leads that provide best view of atrial activity (II, III, aVF, or V_1) should be examined closely.
• Emphasis should be placed on identifying evidence of **SA node dysfunction** (P wave intervals) or **AV conduction abnormalities** (PR interval).

Special Considerations
• Episodes of bradycardia are often transient and episodic; therefore, a baseline ECG may not be sufficient to capture bradycardia. Some form of continuous monitoring can be required.
  ○ In inpatient setting, **continuous central telemetry monitoring** can be used.
  ○ If further workup is done as an outpatient, **short-term Holter monitoring** can be used if the episodes occur somewhat frequently. If infrequent, **an event recorder** or **ILR** should be considered.
  ○ Vital to correlate symptoms with rhythm disturbances discovered via continuous monitoring. Importance of accurate symptom diaries in ambulatory setting should be emphasized to patients.
• To evaluate sinus node response to exertion (chronotropic competence), walking the patient under supervision is easy and inexpensive. Formal **exercise ECG** can be ordered, if necessary.
• **EPS** can be used to assess sinus node function and AV conduction but is rarely necessary if rhythm is already diagnosed by noninvasive modalities.

Differential Diagnosis
• **Sinus node dysfunction,** or sick sinus syndrome (SSS), represents most common reason for pacemaker implantation in the US. Manifestations of SSS include the following (Figure 7-4):
  ○ **Sinus bradycardia**—regular rhythm with QRS complexes preceded by "-sinus" P waves (upright in II, III, aVF) at a rate of <60 bpm. Young patients and athletes often have resting sinus bradycardia that is well tolerated. Nocturnal heart rates are lower in all patients, but elderly tend to have higher resting heart rates and sinus bradycardia is less common normal variant.
  ○ **Sinus arrest** and **sinus pauses**—failure of sinus node to depolarize; manifests as periods of atrial asystole (no P waves). May be accompanied by ventricular asystole or escape beats from junctional tissue or ventricular myocardium. Pauses of 2–3

CHAPTER 7

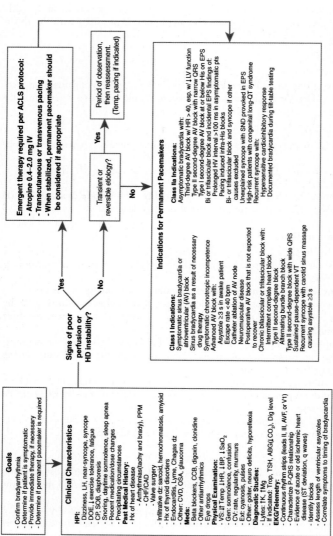

Goals
- Confirm bradyarrhythmia
- Determine if patient is symptomatic
- Provide immediate therapy, if necessary
- Determine if permanent pacemaker is required

Clinical Characteristics

HPI:
- Dizziness, LH, near-syncope, syncope
- DOE, ↓ exercise tolerance, fatigue
- CP, SOB, diaphoresis
- Snoring, daytime somnolence, sleep apnea
- Recent medication/dose changes
- Precipitating circumstances

Past Medical History:
- Hx of heart disease
  - Arrhythmias(tachy and brady), PPM
  - CHF/CAD
  - Valve surgery
- Infiltrative dz: sarcoid, hemochromatosis, amyloid
- Hx of thyroid disorders
- Endocarditis, Lyme, Chagas dz
- Other: CVD, OSA, glaucoma

Meds:
- Beta blockers, CCB, digoxin, clonidine
- Other antiarrhythmics
- Eye drops

Physical Examination:
- VS: ↓↑ Temp ↓HR ↓BP, ↓SaO₂
- Gen: somnolence, confusion
- CV: rate, regularity, murmurs
- Ext: cyanosis, pulses
- Other: goiter, neuro deficits, hyporeflexia

Diagnostic Studies:
- Lytes: ↑K, ↑Mg
- If indicated: Trop, TSH, ABG(↓CO₂), Dig level

EKG/Telemetry:
- Continuous rhythm strips (leads II, III, AVF, or V1)
- Characterize P-QRS relationship
- Evidence of acute or old ischemic heart disease (ST deviation, q waves)
- Identify blocks
- Assess length of ventricular asystoles
- Correlate symptoms to timing of bradycardia

Signs of poor perfusion or HD instability?

Emergent therapy required per ACLS protocol:
- Atropine 0.4–2.0 mg IV
- Transcutaneous or transvenous pacing
- When stabilized, permanent pacemaker should be considered if appropriate

Transient or reversible etiology?

Period of observation, then reassessment.
(Temp: pacing if indicated)

Indications for Permanent Pacemakers

Class I Indications:
Symptomatic sinus bradycardia or atrioventricular (AV) block
Sinus bradycardia as a result of necessary drug therapy
Symptomatic chronotropic incompetence
Advanced AV block with:
  Asystole ≥3 s in awake patient
  Escape rate <40 bpm
  Catheter ablation of AV node
  Neuromuscular disease
  Postoperative AV block that is not expected to recover
Chronic bifascicular or trifascicular block with:
  Intermittent complete heart block
  Type II second-degree block
  Alternating bundle branch block
Type II second-degree block with wide QRS
Sustained pause-dependent VT
Recurrent syncope with carotid sinus massage causing asystole ≥3 s

Class IIa Indications:
Asymptomatic bradycardia with:
  Third-degree AV block w/ HR >40, esp. w/ LV function
  Type II second-degree AV block with narrow QRS
  Type I second-degree AV block at or below His on EPS
Bi or trifascicular block and incidental EPS findings of:
  Prolonged HV interval >100 ms in asymptomatic pts
  Pacing induced infra-His block
Bi- or trifascicular block and syncope if other causes excluded
Unexplained syncope with SND provoked on EPS
High-risk patients with congenital long-QT syndrome
Recurrent syncope with:
  Hypersensitive cardioinhibitory response
  Documented bradycardia during tilt-table testing

Figure 7-3. Approach to bradyarrhythmias. ABG, arterial blood gas; ACLS, advanced cardiac life support; ↓BP, hypotension; CAD, coronary artery disease; CCB, calcium channel blocker; CHF, congestive heart failure; CP, chest pain; CVD, cerebrovascular disease; DOE, dyspnea on exertion; dz, disease; EPS, electrophysiologic study; HD, hemodynamic; HPI, history of present illness; ↓HR, bradycardia; Hx, history; ↑K, hyperkalemia; LH, lightheadedness; ↑Mg, hypermagnesemia; OSA, obstructive sleep apnea; PPM, permanent pacemaker; ↓SaO₂, hypoxia; SND, sinus node dysfunction; SOB, shortness of breath; TSH, thyroid-stimulating hormone; VS, vital signs; VT, ventricular tachycardia. (Reprinted with permission from Fansler D, Chen J. Bradyarrhythmias and permanent pacemakers. In: Cuculich PS, Kates AM, eds. *The Washington Manual Cardiology Subspecialty Consult.* 3rd ed. Lippincott, Williams & Wilkins; 2014.)

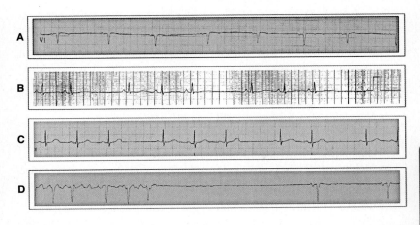

Figure 7-4. Examples of sinus node dysfunction. A, Sinus bradycardia. The sinus rate is approximately 45 bpm. B, Sinoatrial node exit block. Note that the PP interval in which the pause occurs is exactly twice that of the nonpaused PP interval. C, Blocked premature atrial complexes. This rhythm is often confused for sinus node dysfunction or atrioventricular block. Note the premature, nonconducted P waves inscribed in the T wave that resets the sinus node leading to the observed pauses. D, Tachy–brady syndrome. Note the termination of the irregular tachyarrhythmia followed by a prolonged 4.5-second pause prior to the first sinus beat. (Reprinted with permission from Fansler D, Chen J. Bradyarrhythmias and permanent pacemakers. In: Cuculich PS, Kates AM, eds. *The Washington Manual Cardiology Subspecialty Consult.* 3rd ed. Lippincott, Williams & Wilkins; 2014.)

seconds can be found in healthy, asymptomatic people, especially during sleep. Pauses >3 seconds, particularly during daytime hours, raise concern for sinus node dysfunction.
- ◦ **Sinus exit block**—appropriate firing of sinus node, but wave of depolarization fails to traverse past perinodal tissue. Indistinguishable from sinus arrest on surface ECGs except that the RR interval will be a multiple of RR preceding the bradycardia.
- ◦ **Tachy–brady syndrome**—when tachyarrhythmias alternate with bradyarrhythmias. Can be seen in conjunction with a number of types of SVT but is most commonly noted in patients with paroxysmal AF.
- ◦ **Chronotropic incompetence**—inability to increase the heart rate appropriately in response to metabolic need. Usually determined by exercising patients.
- **AV conduction disturbances**
- ◦ AV conduction can be **diverted** (fascicular or bundle branch blocks); **delayed** (first-degree AV block); **occasionally interrupted** (second-degree AV block); **frequently, but not always, interrupted** (advanced or high-degree AV block); or **completely absent** (third-degree AV block). Assignment of the bradyarrhythmia under investigation to one of these categories determines prognosis and guides therapy.
- ◦ **First-degree AV block**—conduction delay that results in PR interval >200 ms on surface ECG.

- ○ **Second-degree AV block**—periodic interruptions (i.e., "dropped beats") in AV conduction. Distinction between Mobitz I and II is important because entities possess differing natural rates of progression to complete heart block.
  - **Mobitz type I block (Wenckebach)**—progressive delay in AV conduction with successive atrial impulses until an impulse fails to conduct. On ECG, classic Wenckebach block manifests as follows:
    - □ Progressive prolongation of PR interval of each successive beat before dropped beat.
    - □ Shortening of each subsequent RR interval before dropped beat.
    - □ A regularly irregular grouping of QRS complexes (group beating).
    - □ Type I block usually within the AV node and portends more benign history with progression to complete heart block unlikely.
    - □ **Mobitz type II block** carries less favorable long-term prognosis and is characterized by abrupt AV conduction block without evidence of progressive conduction delay.
    - □ On ECG, PR intervals remain unchanged preceding nonconducted P wave.
    - □ Presence of type II block, particularly if bundle branch block is present, often antedates progression to complete heart block.
  - Presence of **2:1 AV block** makes differentiation between Mobitz type I and II mechanisms difficult. Diagnostic clues to the site of block include the following:
    - □ Concomitant first-degree AV block, periodic AV Wenckebach, or improved conduction (1:1) with enhanced sinus rates or sympathetic input suggests more proximal interruption of conduction (i.e., Mobitz type I mechanism).
    - □ Concomitant bundle branch block, fascicular block, or worsened conduction (3:1, 4:1, etc.) with enhanced sympathetic input localizes site of block more distally (Mobitz type II mechanism).
- ○ **Third-degree (complete) AV block**—all atrial impulses fail to conduct to ventricles. Complete dissociation between the atria and ventricles ("A > V" rates). Should be distinguished from dissociation with competition at AV node ("V > A" rates).
- ○ **Advanced or high-degree AV block**—more than one consecutive atrial depolarization fails to conduct to the ventricles (i.e., 3:1 block or greater). On ECG, consecutive P waves seen without associated QRS complexes. However, there will be demonstrable P:QRS conduction somewhere on the record to avoid a "third-degree" designation (Figure 7-5).

Imaging
- Presence or absence of structural heart disease should be initially evaluated by TTE.
- Further imaging should be obtained based on suspected etiology.

TREATMENT

Pharmacologic Therapy
- Bradyarrhythmias leading to significant symptoms and hemodynamic instability should be managed emergently as outlined in ACLS guidelines (see Appendix C).
- **Atropine**, an anticholinergic agent given in doses of 0.5–2.0 mg IV, is cornerstone pharmacologic agent for emergent bradycardia treatment.
  - ○ Dysfunction localized more proximally in conduction system (i.e., symptomatic sinus bradycardia, first-degree AV block, Mobitz I second-degree AV block) tends to be responsive to atropine.
  - ○ Distal disease is not responsive and can be worsened by atropine.

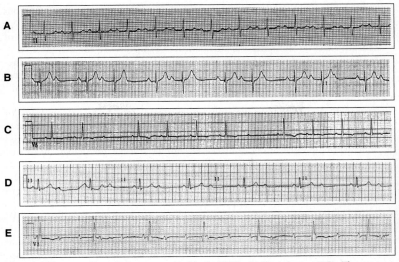

Figure 7-5. Examples of atrioventricular block (AVB). A, First-degree AVB. There are no dropped beats, and the PR interval is >200 ms. B, 3:2 second-degree AVB—Mobitz I. Note the "group beating" and the prolonging PR interval prior to the dropped beat. The third P wave in the sequence is subtly inscribed in the T wave of the preceding beat. C, Second-degree AVB—Mobitz II. Note the abrupt atrioventricular conduction block without evidence of progressive conduction delay. D, 2:1 AVB. This pattern makes it difficult to distinguish between Mobitz I versus II type mechanisms of block. Note the narrow QRS complex, which supports a more proximal origin of block (type I mechanism). A wider QRS (concomitant bundle branch or fascicular block) would suggest a type II mechanism. E, Complete heart block. Note the independent regularity of both the atrial and ventricular rhythms (junctional escape) with no clear association with each other throughout the rhythm strip. (Reprinted with permission from Fansler D, Chen J. Bradyarrhythmias and permanent pacemakers. In: Cuculich PS, Kates AM, eds. *The Washington Manual Cardiology Subspecialty Consult*. 3rd ed. Lippincott, Williams & Wilkins; 2014.)

- ○ Reversible causes of bradyarrhythmias should be identified, and any agents (digoxin, calcium channel blockers, β-adrenergic blockers) that caused or exacerbated the underlying dysrhythmia should be withheld.

Nonpharmacologic Therapies

- For bradyarrhythmias that have irreversible etiologies or that are secondary to medically necessary pharmacologic therapy, pacemaker therapy should be considered.
  - ○ Temporary pacing indicated for symptomatic second- or third-degree heart block caused by transient drug intoxication or electrolyte imbalance and complete heart block or Mobitz II second-degree AV block in the setting of an acute MI.
  - ○ Sinus bradycardia, AF with a slow ventricular response, or Mobitz I second-degree AV block should be treated with temporary pacing only if significant symptoms or hemodynamic instability is present.
  - ○ Temporary pacing is achieved preferably via insertion of a TVP. Transthoracic external pacing can be used, although the lack of reliability of capture and patient discomfort make this a second-line modality.

- Once hemodynamic stability has been established, attention turns to the indications for PPM placement.
  - In symptomatic patients, key determinants include **potential reversibility of causative factors** and **temporal correlation of symptoms to the arrhythmia.**
  - In asymptomatic patients, key determinant based on whether **discovered conduction abnormality has natural history of progression to higher degrees of heart block** that portends poor prognosis.
- **Permanent pacing**
  - Permanent pacing involves placement of anchored, intracardiac pacing leads for the purpose of maintaining heart rate sufficient to avoid symptoms and hemodynamic instability. Current devices, through maintenance of AV synchrony and rate-adaptive programming, more closely mimic normal physiologic heart rate behavior.
    - Class I and IIa indications for permanent pacing are listed in Figure 7-3.
    - Pacemakers are designed to provide an electrical stimulus to the heart whenever the rate drops below a preprogrammed **lower rate limit.** Therefore, the ECG appearance of a PPM varies depending on the heart rate and state of AV conduction.
    - Pacing spikes produced by modern pacemakers are low amplitude, sharp, and immediately preceding the generated P wave or QRS complex indicating capture of the chamber. Figure 7-6 illustrates some common ECG appearances of normally and abnormally functioning pacemakers.
  - Pacemaker generator is commonly placed subcutaneously in pectoral region on the side of the nondominant arm. The electronic lead(s) is/are placed in the cardiac chamber(s) via central veins. Complications of placement include **pneumothorax, device infection, bleeding, and, rarely, cardiac perforation with tamponade.**
    - Before implantation, patient must be free of any active infections, and anticoagulation issues must be carefully considered. Hematomas in the pacemaker pocket develop most commonly in patients who are receiving IV heparin or SC low-molecular-weight heparin.
    - Following implant, **posteroanterior and lateral CXR** are obtained to confirm appropriate lead placement. Pacemaker is interrogated at appropriate intervals—typically, before discharge, 2–6 weeks following implantation, and every 6–12 months thereafter.
  - **Pacing modes**—classified by sequence of three to five letters. Most pacemakers are referred to by the three-letter code alone.
    - **Position I denotes the chamber that is paced:** A for atria, V for ventricle, or D for dual (A + V).
    - **Position II refers to the chamber that is sensed:** A for atria, V for ventricle, D for dual (A + V), or O for none.
    - **Position III denotes the type of response the pacemaker will have to a sensed signal:** I for inhibition, T for triggering, D for dual (I + T), or O for none.
    - **Position IV is used to signify the presence of rate-adaptive pacing (R)** in response to increased metabolic need.
  - The most common pacing systems used today include VVI, DDD, or AAI.
    - AAI systems used only for sinus node dysfunction in the absence of any AV conduction abnormalities.
    - Presence of AV nodal or His–Purkinje disease makes a dual-chamber device (i.e., DDD) more appropriate.
    - Patients in permanent AF warrant a single ventricular lead with VVI programming.

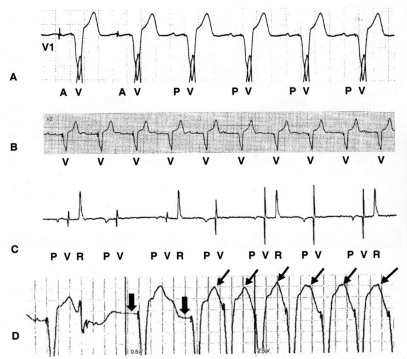

Figure 7-6. Pacemaker rhythms. A, Normal dual-chamber device (DDD) pacing. First two complexes are atrioventricular (AV) sequential pacing, followed by sinus with atrial sensing and ventricular pacing. B, Normal single-chamber (VVI) pacing. The underlying rhythm is atrial fibrillation (no distinct P waves), with ventricular pacing at 60 bpm. C, Pacemaker malfunction. The underlying rhythm is sinus (P) at 80 bpm with 2:1 heart block and first-degree AV block (long PR). Ventricular pacing spikes are seen (V) after each P wave, demonstrating appropriate sensing and tracking of the P waves; however, there is failure to capture. D, Pacemaker-mediated tachycardia. A, paced atrial events; P, sensed atrial events; R, sensed ventricular events; V, paced ventricular events. (Reprinted with permission from Fansler D, Chen J. Bradyarrhythmias and permanent pacemakers. In: Cuculich PS, Kates AM, eds. *The Washington Manual Cardiology Subspecialty Consult.* 3rd ed. Lippincott, Williams & Wilkins; 2014.)

- ○ Modern-day pacemakers also have the capability of **mode switching.**
  - ■ Useful in patients with DDD pacers who have concurrent paroxysmal atrial tachyarrhythmias. When an atrial arrhythmia faster than a programmed mode switch rate develops, the device will change to a mode (i.e., VVI) that does not track atrial signals. It will return to DDD when the tachyarrhythmia resolves.
  - ■ Another common mode switch setting is used in patients with low-grade or intermittent high-grade AV conduction disease to minimize ventricular pacing. The device will attempt to stay in AAI and switch to DDD only when conduction through the AV node fails. This allows for preferential conduction to the ventricles through the native conduction system as much as possible and reduces the chance for pacemaker-mediated cardiomyopathy.

○ Although infrequent, **pacemaker malfunction** is potentially life-threatening, particularly for patients who are pacemaker dependent. The workup of suspected malfunction should begin with a 12-lead ECG.

■ If no pacing activity is seen, place a magnet over the pacemaker to assess for output failure and ability to capture. **Application of the magnet switches the pacemaker to an asynchronous pacing mode.** For example, VVI mode becomes VOO (ventricular asynchronous pacing) and DDD mode becomes DOO (asynchronous AV pacing).

■ If malfunction is obvious or if the ECG is unrevealing and malfunction is still suspected, then formal interrogation of the device should be performed. **Patients are given a card on implantation that will identify the make and model of the device to facilitate this evaluation.**

■ **Two view CXR** should also be obtained to assess for evidence of overt lead abnormalities (dislodgement, fracture, migration, etc.).

○ General categories of pacemaker malfunction include failure to pace (output failure), failure to capture, failure to sense (undersensing), and pacemaker-mediated dysrhythmias.

Syncope

GENERAL PRINCIPLES

Syncope is a common clinical problem. Primary goal of evaluation is to determine whether the patient is at increased risk of SCD.

Definition

Sudden, self-limited loss of consciousness and postural tone caused by transient global cerebral hypoperfusion, followed by spontaneous, complete, and prompt recovery.

Classification

Four major categories based on etiology[28]
- **Neurocardiogenic** (most common): vasovagal, carotid sinus hypersensitivity, and situational.
- **Orthostatic hypotension:** hypovolemia, medication-induced (iatrogenic), and autonomic dysfunction.
- **Cardiovascular**
  ○ **Arrhythmogenic:** sinus node dysfunction, AV block, pacemaker malfunction, VT/VF, SVT (rare).
  ○ **Mechanical:** HCM, valvular stenosis, aortic dissection, myxomas, pulmonary embolism, pulmonary HTN, acute MI, subclavian steal, etc.
- **Miscellaneous** (not true syncope): seizures, stroke/TIA, hypoglycemia, hypoxia, psychogenic, etc.
  Atherosclerotic cerebral artery disease is a rare cause of true syncope; the exception is severe obstructive four-vessel cerebrovascular disease (expect focal neurologic findings prior to syncope).

Epidemiology

- Common in general population: 6% of medical admissions and 3% of emergency room visits.[29]
- Incidence is similar among men and women; one of the largest epidemiologic studies revealed an 11% incidence during an average follow-up of 17 years, with sharp rise after age 70 years.[29]

Pathophysiology

- Two components of **neurocardiogenic syncope** are described as **cardioinhibitory**, in which bradycardia or asystole results from increased vagal outflow to the heart, and **vasodepression**, where peripheral vasodilation results from sympathetic withdrawal to peripheral arteries. Most patients have a combination of both components as mechanism.
- Specific stimuli (e.g., micturition, defecation, coughing, swallowing) may evoke a neurocardiogenic mechanism, leading to **situational syncope.**

Risk Factors

- **Cardiovascular disease**, history of **stroke or TIA**, and **HTN have been shown to predispose patients to syncope.**[30]
- Low body mass index (BMI), increased alcohol intake, and diabetes are also associated with syncope.[30]

DIAGNOSIS

Clinical Presentation

History

- Meticulous history and physical examination are vital to accurate diagnosis of etiology of syncope. In 40% of episodes, the mechanism of syncope remains unexplained.[31,32]
- Special attention should be focused on **symptoms** that **precede and follow** syncopal episode, **eyewitness** accounts during the event, **time course** of loss and resumption of consciousness (abrupt vs. gradual), and patient's **medical history.**
- Characteristic prodrome of nausea, diaphoresis, visual changes, or flushing suggests neurocardiogenic syncope.
  ○ Identification of emotional or situational trigger and post-episode fatigue are also clues to neurocardiogenic/situational cause of syncope.
- Alternatively, unusual sensory prodrome, incontinence, or a decreased level of consciousness that gradually clears suggests a seizure as a likely diagnosis.
- With transient ventricular arrhythmias, abrupt loss of consciousness with rapid recovery may occur.
- Syncope with exertion concerning for structural heart disease, pulmonary HTN, and/or CAD.

Physical Examination

- **Cardiovascular** and **neurologic** examinations are primary focus of initial evaluation.
- Orthostatic vital signs aid in the diagnosis of orthostatic hypotension. Patients should have blood pressure checked in both arms.
- Cardiac examination findings may detect valvular heart disease, LV dysfunction, pulmonary HTN, etc.
- Neurologic findings are often absent but, if present, may point to a neurologic etiology.
- Carotid sinus massage for 5–10 seconds with reproduction of symptoms and consequent ventricular pause >3 seconds is considered positive for carotid sinus hypersensitivity. Take proper precautions of telemetry monitoring, availability of bradycardia treatments, and avoidance of the maneuver in patients with known or suspected carotid disease.

CHAPTER 7

Diagnostic Testing

- Presence of known **structural heart disease, abnormal ECG, age >65 years, focal neurologic findings, and severe orthostatic hypotension** suggest more ominous etiology of a syncopal event. These patients should be admitted for further workup to avoid delay and adverse outcomes.
- After history and physical examination, ECG is the most important diagnostic tool in the evaluation of syncope. It will be abnormal in 50% of cases but alone will yield a diagnosis in only 5% of these patients.
- If no history of heart disease or baseline or ECG abnormalities, **tilt table testing** has been used to evaluate hemodynamic response during transition from supine to an upright state to precipitate a neurocardiogenic response. In an unselected population, the predictive value of this test is low.
- Refer to Figure 7-7 for the diagnostic approach to syncope.

TREATMENT

- Therapy is tailored to the underlying etiology of syncope with goals of preventing recurrence and reducing risk of injury or death.
- **Neurocardiogenic syncope**
  - **Counsel** patients to take steps to avoid injury by being aware of prodromal symptoms and maintaining a **horizontal position** at those times.

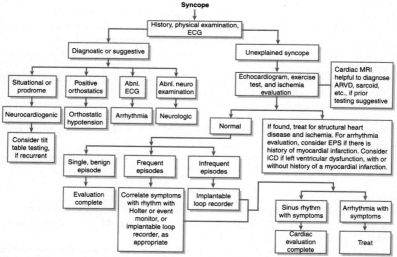

Figure 7-7. Algorithm for the evaluation of syncope. ARVD, arrhythmogenic right ventricular dysplasia; EPS, electrophysiology study; ICD, implantable cardioverter–defibrillator. (Modified from Strickberger SA, Benson DW, Biaggioni I, et al. AHA/ACCF scientific statement on the evaluation of syncope from the American Heart Association Councils on Clinical Cardiology, Cardiovascular Nursing, Cardiovascular Disease in the Young, and Stroke, and the Quality of Care and Outcomes Research Interdisciplinary Working Group; and the American College of Cardiology Foundation in Collaboration with the Heart Rhythm Society. *J Am Coll Cardiol.* 2006;47(2):473-484. Copyright © 2006 American College of Cardiology Foundation. With permission.)

- ○ Avoid known precipitants and maintain adequate **hydration.**
- ○ Employ **isometric muscle contraction** during prodrome to abort a syncopal episode.
- ○ Evidence suggests that β-adrenergic blockers are probably unhelpful; **selective serotonin reuptake inhibitor antidepressants** and **fludrocortisone** have debatable effect; **midodrine** (initiated at 5 mg PO tid and can be increased to 15 mg tid) is probably helpful in treatment of neurocardiogenic syncope.[33-35]
- ○ In general, **PPMs** have no proven benefit in the management of neurocardiogenic syncope. However, permanent dual-chamber pacemakers with hysteresis function (high-rate pacing in response to a detected sudden drop in heart rate) have been shown to be useful in highly selected patients with recurrent neurocardiogenic syncope with a prominent cardioinhibitory component.[36]
- ○ **Cardiac pacing** for **carotid sinus hypersensitivity** is appropriate in syncopal patients.
- ○ In general, neurocardiogenic syncope is not associated with increased risk of mortality.
- • **Orthostatic hypotension**
  - ○ **Adequate hydration** and elimination of offending drugs.
  - ○ Salt supplementation, compressive stockings, and counseling on gradual position changes.
  - ○ Midodrine and fludrocortisone can help by increasing systolic BP and expanding plasma volume, respectively.
- • **Cardiovascular (arrhythmia or mechanical)**
  - ○ Treatment of **underlying disorder** (valve replacement, antiarrhythmic agent, coronary revascularization, etc.)
  - ○ **Cardiac pacing** for sinus node dysfunction or high-degree AV block
  - ○ Discontinuation of QT-prolonging drugs
  - ○ Catheter **ablation** procedures in select patients with syncope associated with SVT
  - ○ **ICD** for documented VT without correctable cause and for syncope in the presence of significant LV dysfunction even in the absence of documented arrhythmia

REFERENCES

1. Porter MJ, Morton JB, Denman R, et al. Influence of age and gender on the mechanism of supraventricular tachycardia. *Heart Rhythm.* 2004;1:393-396.
2. Page RL, Joglar JA, Caldwell MA, et al. 2015 ACC/AHA/HRS guideline for the management of adult patients with supraventricular tachycardia: a report of the American College of Cardiology/American Heart Association task force on clinical practice guidelines and the Heart Rhythm Society. *J Am Coll Cardiol.* 2016;67:e27-e115.
3. Granada J, Uribe W, Chyou PH, et al. Incidence and predictors of atrial flutter in the general population. *J Am Coll Cardiol.* 2000;36:2242-2246.
4. Benjamin EJ, Levy D, Vaziri SM, et al. Independent risk factors for atrial fibrillation in a population-based cohort. The Framingham Heart Study. *J Am Med Assoc.* 1994;271:840-844.
5. Gami AS, Hodge DO, Herges RM, et al. Obstructive sleep apnea, obesity, and the risk of incident atrial fibrillation. *J Am Coll Cardiol.* 2007;49:565-571.
6. January CT, Wann LS, Alpert JS, et al. 2014 AHA/ACC/HRS guideline for the management of patients with atrial fibrillation: a report of the American College of Cardiology/American Heart Association task force on practice guidelines and the Heart Rhythm Society. *J Am Coll Cardiol.* 2014;64:e1-e76.
7. Fauchier L, Pierre B, de Labriolle A, et al. Antiarrhythmic effect of statin therapy and atrial fibrillation a meta-analysis of randomized controlled trials. *J Am Coll Cardiol.* 2008;51:828-835.
8. Healey JS, Baranchuk A, Crystal E, et al. Prevention of atrial fibrillation with angiotensin-converting enzyme inhibitors and angiotensin receptor blockers: a meta-analysis. *J Am Coll Cardiol.* 2005;45:1832-1839.
9. Baker WL, White CM. Post-cardiothoracic surgery atrial fibrillation: a review of preventive strategies. *Ann Pharmacother.* 2007;41:587-598.
10. Van Gelder IC, Hagens VE, Bosker HA, et al. A comparison of rate control and rhythm control in patients with recurrent persistent atrial fibrillation. *N Engl J Med.* 2002;347:1834-1840.

11. Lip GY, Nieuwlaat R, Pisters R, et al. Refining clinical risk stratification for predicting stroke and thromboembolism in atrial fibrillation using a novel risk factor-based approach: the euro heart survey on atrial fibrillation. *Chest.* 2010;137:263-272.
12. Echt DS, Liebson PR, Mitchell LB, et al. Mortality and morbidity in patients receiving encainide, flecainide, or placebo. The Cardiac Arrhythmia Suppression Trial. *N Engl J Med.* 1991;324:781-788.
13. Dusman RE, Stanton MS, Miles WM, et al. Clinical features of amiodarone-induced pulmonary toxicity. *Circulation.* 1990;82:51-59.
14. Berger M, Schweitzer P. Timing of thromboembolic events after electrical cardioversion of atrial fibrillation or flutter: a retrospective analysis. *Am J Cardiol.* 1998;82:1545-1547, A8.
15. Al-Khatib SM, Stevenson WG, Ackerman MJ, et al. 2017 AHA/ACC/HRS guideline for management of patients with ventricular arrhythmias and the prevention of sudden cardiac death: executive summary. A report of the American College of Cardiology/American Heart Association task force on clinical practice guidelines and the Heart Rhythm Society. *Heart Rhythm.* 2018;15:e190-e252.
16. Tchou P, Young P, Mahmud R, et al. Useful clinical criteria for the diagnosis of ventricular tachycardia. *Am J Med.* 1988;84:53-56.
17. Antiarrhythmics Versus Implantable Defibrillators (AVID) Investigators. A comparison of antiarrhythmic-drug therapy with implantable defibrillators in patients resuscitated from near-fatal ventricular arrhythmias. *N Engl J Med.* 1997;337:1576-1583.
18. Moss AJ, Hall WJ, Cannom DS, et al. Improved survival with an implanted defibrillator in patients with coronary disease at high risk for ventricular arrhythmia. Multicenter Automatic Defibrillator Implantation Trial (MADIT) Investigators. *N Engl J Med.* 1996;335:1933-1940.
19. Buxton AE, Lee KL, Fisher JD, et al. A randomized study of the prevention of sudden death in patients with coronary artery disease. Multicenter Unsustained Tachycardia Trial Investigators. *N Engl J Med.* 1999;341:1882-1890.
20. Moss AJ, Zareba W, Hall WJ, et al. Prophylactic implantation of a defibrillator in patients with myocardial infarction and reduced ejection fraction. *N Engl J Med.* 2002;346:877-883.
21. Dorian P, Cass D, Schwartz B, et al. Amiodarone as compared with lidocaine for shock-resistant ventricular fibrillation. *N Engl J Med.* 2002;346:884-890.
22. Hjalmarson A, Elmfeldt D, Herlitz J, et al. Effect on mortality of metoprolol in acute myocardial infarction. A double-blind randomised trial. *Lancet.* 1981;2:823-827.
23. CIBIS-II Investigators and Committees. The Cardiac Insufficiency Bisoprolol Study II (CIBIS-II): a randomised trial. *Lancet.* 1999;353:9-13.
24. MERIT-HF Study Group. Effect of metoprolol CR/XL in chronic heart failure: Metoprolol CR/XL Randomised Intervention Trial in Congestive Heart Failure (MERIT-HF). *Lancet.* 1999;353:2001-2007.
25. Dargie HJ. Effect of carvedilol on outcome after myocardial infarction in patients with left-ventricular dysfunction: the CAPRICORN randomised trial. *Lancet.* 2001;357:1385-1390.
26. Ajijola OA, Lellouche N, Bourke T, et al. Bilateral cardiac sympathetic denervation for the management of electrical storm. *J Am Coll Cardiol.* 2012;59(1):91-92.
27. Cuculich PS, Schill MR, Kashani R, et al. Noninvasive cardiac radiation for ablation of ventricular tachycardia. *N Engl J Med.* 2017;377:2325-2336.
28. Strickberger SA, Benson DW, Biaggioni I, et al. AHA/ACCF scientific statement on the evaluation of syncope from the American Heart Association Councils on Clinical Cardiology, Cardiovascular Nursing, Cardiovascular Disease in the Young, and Stroke, and the Quality of Care and Outcomes Research Interdisciplinary Working Group; and the American College of Cardiology Foundation: in collaboration with the Heart Rhythm Society. *Circulation.* 2006;113:316-327.
29. Soteriades ES, Evans JC, Larson MG, et al. Incidence and prognosis of syncope. *N Engl J Med.* 2002;347:878-885.
30. Chen L, Chen MH, Larson MG, et al. Risk factors for syncope in a community-based sample (the Framingham Heart Study). *Am J Cardiol.* 2000;85:1189-1193.
31. Linzer M, Yang EH, Estes NAIII, et al. Diagnosing syncope. Part 1: value of history, physical examination, and electrocardiography. Clinical efficacy assessment project of the American College of Physicians. *Ann Intern Med.* 1997;126:989-996.
32. Linzer M, Yang EH, Estes NAIII, et al. Diagnosing syncope. Part 2: unexplained syncope. Clinical efficacy assessment project of the American College of Physicians. *Ann Intern Med.* 1997;127:76-86.
33. Sheldon R, Connolly S, Rose S, et al. Prevention of Syncope Trial (POST): a randomized, placebo-controlled study of metoprolol in the prevention of vasovagal syncope. *Circulation.* 2006;113:1164-1170.
34. Samniah N, Sakaguchi S, Lurie KG, et al. Efficacy and safety of midodrine hydrochloride in patients with refractory vasovagal syncope. *Am J Cardiol.* 2001;88:A7, 80-83.
35. Kuriachan V, Sheldon RS, Platonov M. Evidence-based treatment for vasovagal syncope. *Heart Rhythm.* 2008;5:1609-1614.
36. Connolly SJ, Sheldon R, Thorpe KE, et al. Pacemaker therapy for prevention of syncope in patients with recurrent severe vasovagal syncopesecond Vasovagal Pacemaker Study (VPS II): a randomized trial. *J Am Med Assoc.* 2003;289:2224-2229.

Critical Care

David B. Rose and Marin H. Kollef

Respiratory Failure

GENERAL PRINCIPLES

Definitions

- **Hypoxemic (type 1) respiratory failure:** Occurs when normal gas exchange is seriously impaired, causing hypoxemia (arterial oxygen tension [PaO_2] <60 mm Hg or arterial oxygen saturation [SaO_2] <90%). Usually associated with tachypnea and hypocapnia; however, progression can lead to hypercapnia as well. **Acute respiratory distress syndrome (ARDS)** is an important form of hypoxemic respiratory failure caused by acute lung injury. The common end result is disruption of the alveolocapillary membrane, leading to increased vascular permeability and accumulation of inflammatory cells and protein-rich fluid within the alveolar space.
  - The ARDS Definition Task Force defined ARDS as follows[1]:
    - Onset within 1 week of a known clinical insult or new or worsening respiratory symptoms;
    - Bilateral opacities not fully explained by effusions, lobar/lung collapse, or nodules;
    - Respiratory failure not fully explained by cardiac failure or volume overload; and
    - Impaired oxygenation with low PaO_2 to fraction of inspired oxygen (FIO_2) ratio (PaO_2/FIO_2 ≤300 mm Hg).
  - The severity of ARDS is stratified based on PaO_2/FIO_2.
    - Mild: 200 <PaO_2/FIO_2 ≤300 mm Hg with positive end-expiratory pressure (PEEP) or continuous positive airway pressure (CPAP) ≥5 cm H_2O
    - Moderate: 100 <PaO_2/FIO_2 ≤200 mm Hg with PEEP ≥5 cm H_2O
    - Severe: PaO_2/FIO_2 ≤100 mm Hg with PEEP ≥5 cm H_2O
- **Hypercapnic (type 2) respiratory failure:** Occurs with acute elevation of carbon dioxide (arterial carbon dioxide tension [$PaCO_2$] >45 mm Hg), producing a respiratory acidosis (pH <7.35).
- **Postoperative (type 3) respiratory failure:** Occurs when patients develop atelectasis from pain or the use of sedatives postoperatively. In reality, this is a subset of type 1 or 2 respiratory failure; however, as this is so common, it is often classified as its own type of respiratory failure.
- **Respiratory failure from shock (type 4):** Respiratory failure where the metabolic demands of the patient are too high for the respiratory system to compensate for (e.g., from sepsis or fever). Patients are often intubated in the process of resuscitation to off-load the respiratory system and decrease oxygen consumption.
- **Mixed respiratory failure:** Most commonly, respiratory failure is due to multiple pathophysiologic processes that can lead to both hypercarbia and hypoxemia.

Pathophysiology

- **Hypoxemic respiratory failure (type 1):** Usually is the result of the lung's reduced ability to deliver oxygen across the alveolocapillary membrane. The severity of gas exchange impairment is determined by calculating the $P(A–a)\ O_2$ gradient (A-a gradient) using the alveolar gas equation:

$$PAO_2 = FIO_2\left(P_{ATM} - P_{H_2O}\right) - \frac{PACO_2}{R}$$

where FIO_2 = the fraction of inspired oxygen, P_{ATM} = atmospheric pressure, P_{H_2O} = water vapor pressure, and R = the respiratory quotient. Hypoxemia is caused by one of the following five mechanisms:

○ **Ventilation–perfusion (V/Q) mismatch:** Occurs when perfusion does not compensate for a change in ventilation or vice versa (e.g., emphysema, pneumonia, pulmonary edema, pulmonary embolism). V/Q mismatch leads to an elevated A-a gradient. Administration of supplemental oxygen increases PaO_2 (of note, supplemental oxygen paradoxically worsens V/Q mismatching in emphysema via reversing hypoxic vasoconstriction of pulmonary capillaries supplying poorly ventilated alveoli).

○ **Shunt:** Occurs when mixed venous blood bypasses lung units and enters systemic arterial circulation without receiving oxygenation. Shunts can be congenital (e.g., intracardiac shunt) or acquired (atelectasis, hepatopulmonary syndrome). Shunt leads to an elevated A-a gradient. In pure shunt, administration of supplemental oxygen does not increase PaO_2. See Table 8-1 for different causes of shunt.

○ **Diffusion abnormality:** Occurs owing to abnormalities of the interstitium wherein the time it takes for gas equilibration is longer than the red blood cell transit time through the pulmonary capillaries (e.g., pulmonary fibrosis, pulmonary hypertension). Diffusion abnormalities lead to an elevated A-a gradient. Administration of supplemental oxygen increases PaO_2.

○ **Hypoventilation:** Occurs owing to a decrease in minute ventilation that results in an increase in $PaCO_2$ (see the causes of hypercapnia under "Hypercapnic respiratory failure [type 2]") and displacement of oxygen. The A-a gradient is normal. Primary treatment is directed at correcting the cause of hypoventilation. Administration of supplemental oxygen increases PaO_2.

○ **Low inspired oxygen:** Occurs owing to a low partial pressure of inspired oxygen (e.g., high-altitude travel). A-a gradient is normal. Administration of supplemental oxygen increases PaO_2.

• **Hypercapnic respiratory failure (type 2):** Primarily occurs owing to ventilatory failure, resulting in an elevated $PaCO_2$ >45 mm Hg:

$$PaCO_2 = \frac{\dot{V}CO_2}{\dot{V}_A} = \frac{\dot{V}CO_2}{\dot{V}_E - \dot{V}_D}$$

where CO_2 = CO_2 production, V_A = alveolar ventilation, V_E = expired total ventilation, and V_D = dead space ventilation. The cause of hypercapnia is generally failure of one of the following components of the respiratory system:

○ Disorders of the central nervous system: An impaired respiratory drive causes a decreased respiratory rate ("won't breathe"); e.g., opiate overdose, central apnea/hypoventilation, metabolic alkalosis, central nervous system (CNS) infection.

○ Disorders of anterior horn cells, peripheral nervous system, or muscles: Neuromuscular failure or muscle weakness causes decreased tidal volume ("can't breathe"); e.g., Guillain–Barré syndrome, myasthenia gravis, amyotrophic lateral sclerosis, muscular dystrophies, myopathies.

○ Disorders of the thoracic cavity: Anatomic abnormality causes decreased tidal volume; e.g., kyphoscoliosis, morbid obesity, pleural effusions, abdominal distention, diaphragmatic injury.

TABLE 8-1	Causes of Shunt
Cause	Examples
Pulmonary Shunts	
Pus	Pneumonia
Water	Cardiogenic pulmonary edema
	Acute myocardial infarction
	Systolic or diastolic left ventricular failure
	Mitral regurgitation or stenosis
	Noncardiogenic pulmonary edema
	Primary acute respiratory distress syndrome
	Aspiration
	Inhalational injury
	Near drowning
	Secondary acute respiratory distress syndrome
	Sepsis
	Pancreatitis
	Reperfusion injury
	Upper airway obstruction pulmonary edema
	Neurogenic pulmonary edema
	High-altitude pulmonary edema
Blood	Diffuse alveolar hemorrhage
Atelectasis	Pleural effusion with atelectasis
	Mucous plugging with lobar collapse
Cardiac shunts	Patent foramen ovale
	Atrial septal defect
	Ventricular septal defect
Vascular shunts	Arteriovenous malformation

- Disorders of the airway or lung parenchyma: Lung pathology causes increased dead space; e.g., asthma, chronic obstructive pulmonary disease (COPD), severe ARDS.
- Hypermetabolic states can cause increased CO_2 production and lead to hypercapnia; e.g., sepsis, seizure, thyrotoxicosis, serotonin syndrome.

Noninvasive Oxygen Therapy

GENERAL PRINCIPLES

- **Nasal cannulas:** Most commonly used, but the exact FIO_2 delivered is unknown because it is influenced by peak inspiratory flow demand. Each additional liter of flow increases FIO_2 by approximately 4% (e.g., 2 L/min delivers ~28%). Flow rates should generally be limited to ≤6 L/min. An oxygen reservoir device can increase oxygen delivery.

- **Simple facemask:** Delivers oxygen at FIO_2 of 35%–55% using flows of 5–12 L/min (lower flow rates should be avoided to prevent breathing in expired CO_2).
- **Venturi masks:** Allow the precise administration of oxygen via a facemask by delivering a mix of ambient air with oxygen. Usual FIO_2 values delivered are 24%, 28%, 31%, 35%, 40%, and 50%. As FIO_2 increases, total flow decreases.
- **Nonrebreathing masks:** Use a reservoir bag to achieve higher oxygen concentrations (up to 80%). Flow rates are generally at least 8–15 L/min. A one-way valve prevents exhaled gases from entering the reservoir bag, maximizing the FIO_2 that is inspired.
- **Heated humidified high-flow nasal cannula (HFNC):** Delivers heated and humidified oxygen at high flows and concentrations such that it flushes out a significant amount of nonoxygenated air from the upper airway. The system can be titrated up to 60 L/min and 100% FIO_2 and may provide a small amount of PEEP at high flow rates.
  - The use of HFNC devices has increased recently with some studies showing encouraging benefits. In one open-label trial, patients with hypoxemic non-hypercapnic respiratory failure were randomly assigned to HFNC versus standard oxygen therapy or noninvasive positive-pressure ventilation (NPPV). Intubation rates were similar between groups; however, there was a significant improvement in 90-day mortality in patients who received HFNC as compared with other modalities.[2]
  - In a meta-analysis of nine trials comparing HFNC to low-flow oxygen in patients with hypoxemic respiratory failure, HFNC decreased the need for both intubation and escalation of oxygen therapy.[3]
  - The role of HFNC following extubation is discussed in "Mechanical Ventilation."
- **NPPV:** Delivers respiratory support with positive airway pressure via a sealed facemask, nasal mask, or helmet device. NPPV most commonly refers to continuous positive airway pressure (CPAP) and bilevel positive airway pressure (BiPAP) ventilation. NPPV can be delivered by home devices or ventilators.
  - CPAP: Delivers continuous positive airway pressure throughout the respiratory cycle and prevents alveolar collapse during expiration. CPAP is often used in the treatment of obstructive sleep apnea and pulmonary edema. Initially, 5 cm H_2O of pressure should be applied, and if hypoxemia persists, the level should be increased by 3–5 cm H_2O up to a level of 10–15 cm H_2O.
  - BiPAP: Delivers two different airway pressures during inspiration and expiration to decrease the work of breathing. BiPAP is often used for COPD exacerbations, weaning, and neuromuscular weakness. An inspiratory pressure support of 5–10 cm H_2O and an expiratory pressure of 5 cm H_2O are reasonable starting points. Ventilation is determined by the difference between inspiratory and expiratory pressures (i.e., "drive pressure"), and inspiratory pressures can be uptitrated to achieve adequate tidal volumes and minute ventilation.
  - Benefits of NPPV: NPPV decreases the need for mechanical ventilation in appropriately selected patients.[4] The benefits of NPPV are particularly strong in patients with neuromuscular disease, COPD, pulmonary edema, and postoperative respiratory insufficiency.[5] A 2016 single-center trial found that NPPV delivered via a transparent helmet device covering the entire head reduced the need for intubation and improved survival in patients with ARDS.[6]
  - There has been conflicting evidence over the years regarding the use of NPPV in severe acute exacerbations of asthma. A recent retrospective analysis of >50,000 patients found that the use of NPPV was associated with lower odds of receiving invasive mechanical ventilation and in-hospital mortality.[7]

○ **Potential harms of NPPV:** NPPV is generally safe but can cause skin damage, eye irritation, claustrophobia, and aerophagia and can be difficult to tolerate for some patients. Use should be limited to patients who are conscious, cooperative, able to protect their airway, and hemodynamically stable.[8] **NPPV use should be limited to those with an anticipated short duration of respiratory failure. Close monitoring is required during its use.**

Airway Management and Endotracheal Intubation

GENERAL PRINCIPLES

Airway Management Before Intubation

- **Head and jaw positioning:** First, the oropharynx should be inspected, and all foreign bodies should be removed. If the patient is unresponsive, the head tilt–chin lift maneuver should be performed. If neck immobilization is required, jaw thrust should be performed.
- **Oral and nasopharyngeal airways:** Airway adjunct devices can be used to maintain a patent airway. Initially inserted with the concave curve of the airway facing toward the roof of the mouth. The oral airway then is turned 180 degrees as it is inserted so that the concave curve of the airway follows the natural curve of the tongue. Careful monitoring of airway patency is required, as malpositioning can push the tongue posteriorly and result in oropharyngeal obstruction. Nasopharyngeal airways are made of soft plastic and passed easily down one of the nasal passages to the posterior pharynx after topical nasal lubrication and anesthesia with viscous lidocaine jelly.
- **Bag-valve-mask ventilation:** Ineffective respiratory efforts can be augmented with simple bag-valve-mask ventilation. Proper fitting and positioning of the mask using the "EC" hand position—thumb and index finger forming a "C" around the mask, and the remaining fingers forming an "E" to support the jaw—ensure a tight seal around the mouth and nose. This maneuver should be used in conjunction with proper positioning and airway adjuncts (e.g., an oral airway). If possible, two hands should be used to optimize seal while a second clinician ventilates the patient. Bag-valve-mask ventilation is a critical skill in airway management and is frequently incorrectly performed.
- **Laryngeal mask airway (LMA):** The LMA is a supraglottic airway device shaped like an endotracheal tube connected to an elliptical mask. It is designed to be inserted over the tongue and seated in the hypopharynx, covering the supraglottic structures and relatively isolating the trachea. It is a temporary airway and should not be used for prolonged ventilatory support. LMAs can be lifesaving in establishing an airway when endotracheal intubation cannot be easily achieved.

Endotracheal Intubation

- **Indications:** Refractory hypoxemic respiratory failure, hypercapnic respiratory failure, airway protection (e.g., intoxication, head trauma, severe upper GI bleeding with hematemesis), upper airway obstruction (e.g., angioedema, tumor), severe metabolic acidosis or shock (e.g., type 4 respiratory failure, severe diabetic ketoacidosis), and need for hyperventilation as a treatment for increased intracranial pressure.

CHAPTER 8

- **Before endotracheal tube intubation** is attempted:
  - Ensure that monitoring equipment is working (including pulse oximetry, telemetry, and blood pressure monitoring) and that the patient has adequate working intravenous (IV) access.
  - Ensure that all necessary equipment is at the bedside including working suction equipment, endotracheal tube (with stylet, lubricant, and balloon tested), 10 mL syringe to fill endotracheal tube balloon, oral or nasopharyngeal airway, bag-valve-mask connected to 15 L/min oxygen, direct or video laryngoscope, end-tidal CO_2 monitor, medications for intubation, and tape or endotracheal holder.
  - Have the plan articulated and the equipment at the bedside (e.g., tracheal tube introducer and supraglottic device) in case of a difficult airway.
  - Evaluate head and neck positioning: Oral, pharyngeal, and tracheal axes should be aligned by flexing the neck and extending the head, achieving the "sniffing" position. Obese patients may require a shoulder roll or ramp.
  - The selected agents for intubation including neuromuscular blocking agents, opiates, and anxiolytics should be chosen based on their respective advantages and disadvantages in the given clinical situation. Commonly used agents for intubation are listed in Table 8-2.
  - If patient not in extremis/cardiac arrest, a verbal time-out should be performed.
- Techniques
  - Direct laryngoscopic orotracheal intubation: Most commonly used, requiring only a direct laryngoscope and light source. Procedure available in Table 8-3.
  - Video laryngoscopic orotracheal intubation: Allows for direct visual confirmation of intubation by a second observer via video monitoring and is particularly beneficial in more difficult airways.
  - Advanced techniques for specialists include blind nasotracheal intubation and flexible fiber optically guided orotracheal or nasotracheal intubation.
- Verification of correct endotracheal tube location and positioning: Proper tube location must be ensured by:
  - Fiber optic inspection of the airways through the endotracheal tube; *or*
  - Direct visualization of the endotracheal tube passing through the vocal cords; *and*
  - Use of an end-tidal CO_2 monitor; *and*
  - CXR.
  - Clinical evaluation of the patient (i.e., listening for bilateral breath sounds over the chest and the absence of ventilation over the stomach) and radiographic evaluation alone are unreliable for establishing correct endotracheal tube location.
  - The tip of the endotracheal tube should be 3–5 cm above the carina, depending on head and neck position.
- After successful intubation:
  - Tracheal tube cuff pressures: Should be monitored at regular intervals and maintained below capillary filling pressure (25 mm Hg) to prevent ischemic mucosal injury.
  - Sedation: Anxiolytics and opiates are frequently used to facilitate endotracheal intubation and mechanical ventilation. Commonly used agents are listed in Table 8-4.
- **Complications:** Improper endotracheal tube location or positioning is the most important immediate complication to be recognized and corrected.
  - Esophageal intubation should be suspected if no end-tidal CO_2 is detected after three to five breaths, hypoxemia persists or develops, there is a lack of breath sounds, or abdominal distention or regurgitation of stomach contents occurs.
  - Mainstem intubation should be suspected if peak airway pressures are elevated or there are unilateral breath sounds.
  - Other complications include dislodgment of teeth and upper airway trauma.

TABLE 8-2	Drugs to Facilitate Endotracheal Intubation				
Drug	Action	Dose (IV)	Onset (s)	Duration (min)	Comment
Propofol	Sedation, amnesia	Unstable: 0.5 mg/kg Stable 1–1.5 mg/kg	30–60	5–10	Causes hypotension and bradycardia; beneficial in seizures
Midazolam	Sedation, amnesia	0.02–0.08 mg/kg (generally 1–5 mg in adult)	30–60	15–30	Causes hypotension; beneficial in seizures
Fentanyl	Analgesia	~2 µg/kg	15	30–60	Causes hypotension; used at lower doses as an adjunctive agent
Etomidate	Sedation	Unstable: 0.15 mg/kg Stable 0.3 mg/kg	15–45	3–12	Hemodynamically neutral; inhibits cortisol synthesis; decreases seizure threshold
Ketamine	Sedation, amnesia, analgesia	1–3 mg/kg	30	5–10	Increases HR and BP; bronchodilator; may elevate ICP
Succinylcholine	Paralytic	1–1.5 mg/kg	30–60	5–15	Contraindicated in hyperkalemia, history of malignant hyperthermia, myopathy
Rocuronium	Paralytic	1 mg/kg	45–60	30–45	Caution if difficult intubation or bag-valve-mask ventilation anticipated

BP, blood pressure; HR, heart rate; ICP, intracranial pressure.

TABLE 8-3	Procedure for Endotracheal Intubation, Needle Cricothyrotomy, and Cricothyrotomy

Endotracheal Intubation Using Direct Laryngoscopy

Equipment		Oxygen tubing, bag-valve-mask device, suction and tubing, oral airway, laryngoscope, laryngoscope blades, endotracheal tube with stylet, syringe, end-tidal carbon dioxide colorimeter
Technique	Step 1	Place the patient in the "sniffing" position, with neck flexed and head extended; obese patients will require shoulder roll or ramp.
	Step 2	Preoxygenate the patient with 100% oxygen through the bag-valve-mask device until saturations are maintained at >95% for 3–5 min and suction oral secretions as necessary.
	Step 3	During preoxygenation, ensure that all equipment necessary is present and functional: check the endotracheal tube cuff with inflation and deflation and that the light of the laryngoscope is functional.
	Step 4	Administer intravenous (IV) sedation; once the patient is appropriately sedated, open the mouth with the right hand and insert the laryngoscope blade into the right side of mouth with the left hand, sweeping the tongue to the left.
	Step 5	Advance the blade to the base of the tongue and then lift vertically to visualize the vocal cords; **do not tilt the laryngoscope**.
	Step 6	If vocal cords are visible, insert the endotracheal tube with the stylet with the right hand; once the cuff is past the vocal cords, remove stylet. **Do not attempt intubation if the vocal cords are not visible**.
	Step 7	Advance the endotracheal tube until it is at 21 cm at the gum/teeth for women and 22 cm for men and inflate the cuff.
	Step 8	**Check tube location** with end-tidal carbon dioxide colorimeter, auscultation over the chest and abdomen, AND chest radiograph.

Needle Cricothyrotomy

Equipment		Large-bore IV catheter with needle stylet, 3-mL Luer lock syringe with plunger removed, 7-mm inner diameter endotracheal tube adapter
Technique	Step 1	Extend the neck and identify the cricothyroid membrane, located inferior to the thyroid cartilage and superior to the thyroid gland.
	Step 2	Stabilize the thyroid cartilage with the nondominant hand and, using the dominant hand, introduce the IV catheter with the needle stylet at a 45-degree angle through the cricothyroid membrane into the trachea, aspirating air to confirm location.

TABLE 8-3	Procedure for Endotracheal Intubation, Needle Cricothyrotomy, and Cricothyrotomy (*continued*)
	Step 3	Advance the catheter to the hub, and remove the needle stylet.
	Step 4	Attach the Luer lock syringe to the catheter and then the endotracheal tube adapter to the syringe to allow for bag-valve ventilation.

Cricothyrotomy

Equipment	Scalpel, Kelly forceps, 6-mm inner diameter or smaller endotracheal tube	
Technique	Step 1	Extend the neck and identify the cricothyroid membrane, located inferior to the thyroid cartilage and superior to the thyroid gland.
	Step 2	Stabilize the thyroid cartilage with the nondominant hand and, using the dominant hand, make a 1-cm horizontal incision just above the superior border of the cricoid.
	Step 3	Using the Kelly forceps, dissect until the cricothyroid membrane is visualized and then make a vertical incision through the midline of the membrane, being careful to not pass the blade too deeply.
	Step 4	Widen the incision with Kelly forceps until the endotracheal tube can be inserted and then inflate the cuff.

CHAPTER 8

TABLE 8-4	Commonly Used Sedation Medications in the Intensive Care Unit		
Drug	Dose (IV)	Time to Arousal	Comment
Propofol	20–100 µg/kg/min	10–15 min	Causes hypotension, may cause hypertriglyceridemia or propofol-related infusion syndrome, beneficial in bronchospasm
Midazolam	1–10 mg/h	1–2 h	Arousal time can be prolonged; active metabolite accumulates in renal failure; associated with delirium
Fentanyl	25–200 µg/h	15 s	Can cause chest wall rigidity and serotonin syndrome at higher doses
Ketamine	0.5–3 mg/kg/h	5–10 min	May cause hypertension and tachycardia; may experience reemergence hallucinations, beneficial in bronchospasm.
Dexmedetomidine	0.1–1.5 mg/kg/h	6–10 min	Does not cause respiratory depression, can cause hypotension and bradycardia

Surgical Airways

- **Indications** for surgical airways in critical care
  - Life-threatening upper airway obstruction (e.g., epiglottitis, angioedema, facial burns, laryngeal/vocal cord edema) preventing bag-valve-mask ventilation and endotracheal intubation.
  - Need for prolonged respiratory support.
- **Needle cricothyrotomy:** Indicated in emergency settings when the patient cannot be ventilated noninvasively, standard endotracheal intubation is unsuccessful, and a surgical airway cannot be immediately performed. The steps of the procedure are listed in Table 8-3.
- **Cricothyrotomy:** Indicated in emergency settings when the patient cannot be ventilated noninvasively and standard endotracheal intubation is unsuccessful. The steps of the procedure are listed in Table 8-3.
- **Tracheostomy:** Predominantly performed owing to need for prolonged respiratory support.
  - The optimal time to perform a tracheostomy in a patient requiring prolonged respiratory support is somewhat controversial. A 2010 randomized controlled trial (RCT) did not demonstrate any benefit in regard to occurrence of ventilator-associated pneumonia (VAP) or long-term outcomes for those who received an early tracheostomy (after 6–8 days of intubation) compared with late tracheostomy (after 12–14 days of intubation).[9] A 2013 multicenter RCT from the United Kingdom comparing early (within 4 days of intubation) vs late (after 10 days) tracheostomy found no difference in 30-day mortality, ICU length of stay (LOS), or hospital LOS between the two groups.[10] **Generally, tracheostomy should be considered if prolonged ventilatory support is anticipated after 10–14 days of endotracheal intubation.**
  - **Complications:** Tracheostomy sites require at least 72 hours to mature, and tube dislodgment before maturation can lead to serious and life-threatening complications.
    - A tracheostomy tube that has been dislodged before stoma maturation **should not be reinserted** owing to the risk of creating a false tract.
    - **Standard endotracheal intubation** should be performed if a tracheostomy tube is dislodged before stoma maturation.
    - **Tracheoinnominate artery fistulas** are an uncommon but life-threatening complication of a tracheostomy that occurs when an abnormal tract develops between the innominate artery and trachea, leading to hemorrhage. This complication most commonly occurs 7–14 days after the tracheostomy but can occur up to 6 weeks after the procedure. Immediate management includes overinflation of the tracheostomy tube cuff, digital compression of the stoma, and surgical exploration.[11]

Mechanical Ventilation

GENERAL PRINCIPLES

Basic modes of ventilation: One can determine how the ventilator initiates a breath (triggering), how the breath is delivered, how patient-initiated breaths are supported, and when to terminate the breath to allow expiration (cycling).

- **Initiation of a breath:** Triggering of a ventilator occurs after a period of time has elapsed (time triggered) or when the patient has generated sufficient negative airway pressure or inspiratory flow exceeding a predetermined threshold (patient triggered).

- **Modes of ventilation**
  - **Assist-control (AC) ventilation:** Ventilator delivers a fully supported breath whether time or patient triggered. Primary mode of ventilation used in respiratory failure.
  - **Synchronized intermittent mandatory ventilation (SIMV):** Ventilator delivers a fully supported breath when time triggered. However, when the breath is patient triggered, the ventilator delivers a pressure-supported breath (at a level set by the clinician). The size of the patient-triggered breath depends on lung compliance and patient's effort. This mode is commonly used in surgical patients.
  - **Pressure support ventilation (PSV):** Spontaneous mode of ventilation without a set respiratory rate. Delivers a clinician-determined inspiratory pressure during patient-triggered breathing. **No respiratory rate is set, so there is no guaranteed minute ventilation.**
- **Type of breath delivered**
  - **Volume control (VC):** Ventilator delivers a clinician-determined tidal volume (V_T) for each breath regardless of whether the breath was time or patient triggered. When predetermined V_T is delivered, airflow is terminated and exhalation occurs.
  - **Pressure control (PC):** Delivers a practitioner-determined inspiratory pressure for each breath. When inspiratory time has elapsed, inspiratory pressure is terminated and exhalation occurs. The tidal volume varies based on lung compliance. **PC ventilation does not deliver a guaranteed V_T or minute ventilation and may lead to hypoventilation.** However, PC may improve patient synchrony and comfort while on the ventilator.
- **Basic ventilator terminology and management:** Flow-time and pressure-time tracings are demonstrated in Figure 8-1.
  - **Minute ventilation:** Defined as the product of V_T and respiratory rate ($V_T \times RR$). Normally between 5 and 10 L/min in resting adults, but may be much higher in high metabolic states, e.g., septic shock.
  - **Peak airway pressure:** Composed of pressures necessary to overcome inspiratory airflow resistance, chest wall recoil resistance, and alveolar opening resistance. Does not reflect alveolar pressure.
  - **Mean airway pressure:** Mean pressures applied during the inspiratory cycle. Approximates alveolar pressure until overdistention occurs.
  - **Plateau pressure (P_{plat}):** Reflects alveolar pressure. Checked by performing an end-inspiratory hold maneuver to allow pressures through the tracheobronchial tree to equilibrate.

Ventilator Settings

Initial ventilator settings: One must decide on a ventilator mode (AC vs. SIMV), control (VC vs. PC), respiratory rate, FIO_2, and PEEP. AC/VC is the most commonly used mode.
- For VC, the following must be entered:
  - **V_T:** Generally, begin at 6–8 mL/kg ideal body weight (IBW) to prevent barotrauma. There is growing evidence that low tidal volume ventilation may be beneficial in patients whether or not they have acute ARDS and should be routinely used whenever possible.[12] IBW can be calculated as follows: Male IBW = 50 kg + 2.3 kg/in. × (Height in inches − 60) (imperial), 50 kg + 1.1 kg/cm × (Height in cm − 152.4) (metric); Female IBW = 45.5 kg + 2.3 kg/in. × (Height in inches − 60) (imperial), 45.5 kg + 1.1 kg/cm × (Height in cm − 152.4) (metric).

CHAPTER 8

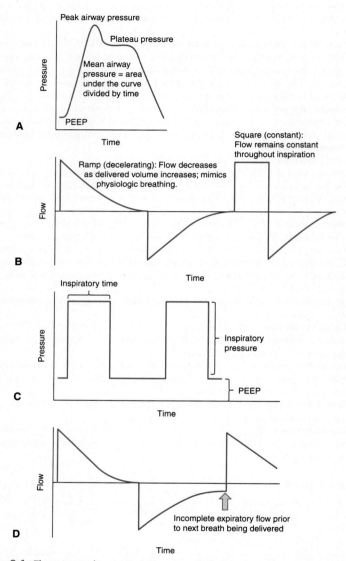

Figure 8-1. Flow–time and pressure–time tracings. A, Pressure–time curve for one breath. B, Flow–time curve for volume control ventilation. Pressure varies throughout inspiratory time, depending on lung compliance. C, Pressure–time curve for pressure control ventilation. Flow varies throughout inspiratory time, depending on lung compliance. D, Flow–time curve demonstrating auto–positive end-expiratory pressure (auto-PEEP).

- ○ **Inspiratory flow rate:** May be constant (square wave) or ramp (decelerating). Recommend 60 L/min or greater. Higher flow rates increase expiration time, which may be important in obstructive lung disease to prevent auto-PEEP (ventilator delivers a breath before the patient has been able to fully expire).
- **FIO$_2$:** It is reasonable to start at 100%, but FIO$_2$ should be weaned down quickly to maintain SaO$_2$ >87% or PaO$_2$ >55 mm Hg. There is growing evidence that tolerating hyperoxia after intubation may actually worsen patient survival.[13] FIO$_2$ can generally be quickly titrated down based on pulse oximetry alone.
- **PEEP:** It is generally reasonable to start at 5–10; however, higher values are frequently used in the treatment of ARDS.
  - ○ ARDSNet publishes recommended strategies for PEEP and FIO$_2$ levels, which are available on their website (http://www.ardsnet.org).
  - ○ Morbidly obese patients may also require higher PEEP.

Advanced Modes of Ventilation

Advanced modes should generally only be used after discussion with higher level practitioners.
- **Pressure-regulated VC ventilation:** Ventilator determines, after each breath, if inspiratory pressure was sufficient to achieve targeted V$_T$; if insufficient or excessive, then ventilator will adjust inspiratory pressure to achieve desired V$_T$. PRVC applies a constant pressure throughout inspiration, resulting in a decelerating and variable flow pattern that is more comfortable for some patients.
- **Inverse-ratio ventilation (IRV):** A pressure-controlled method of ventilation most commonly used in ARDS. Inspiratory time exceeds expiratory time to improve oxygenation at the expense of ventilation; patients are permitted to become hypercapnic to pH 7.20. If obstructive lung disease is present, can cause auto-PEEP and excessive hypercapnia.
- **Airway pressure release ventilation (APRV):** An extreme version of IRV; inspiratory pressure (P$_{high}$) applied for a prolonged period of time (T$_{high}$) with a short expiratory time (T$_{low}$, or release time)—usually <1 second—to allow for ventilation. Like IRV, patients are permitted to be hypercapnic to pH 7.20.
- **High-frequency oscillatory ventilation (HFOV):** A pressure control form of ventilation that delivers very small, rapid (as many as several per second) breaths superimposed on a mean airway pressure. The pressure is set at a level that was previously required to maintain oxygenation, whereas the small breaths facilitate CO$_2$ clearance. HFOV was previously thought to improve outcomes in ARDS,[14] though subsequent prospective RCTs demonstrated no reduction[15] and possibly an increase in mortality.[16]

Mechanical Ventilation Principles for Patients With ARDS

Owing to severe hypoxia associated with ARDS, oxygenation and prevention of barotrauma may have to be prioritized over ventilation, resulting in hypercapnia.
- Hypercapnia resulting in a pH of 7.20–7.35 often is tolerated to sufficiently oxygenate the patient ("**permissive hypercapnia**").
- The plateau pressure should be checked and the tidal volume should be decreased down to 4 mL/kg of IBW as pH allows to achieve a plateau pressure ≤30 cm H$_2$O.
- There is growing evidence that driving pressure (ratio of V$_T$/respiratory system compliance, or P$_{plat}$ − PEEP) is an important predictor of mortality in patients with ARDS. While there is no standard target value, data suggest that driving pressures below 14 cm H$_2$O are associated with better outcomes.[17,18] Practically, driving pressure can be used to identify patients with recruitable lung units who may benefit from higher PEEP strategies.

CHAPTER 8

ADJUNCTS TO MECHANICAL VENTILATION

- **Nitric oxide (NO):** Improves oxygenation by preferential vasodilation of capillary beds of ventilated lung.
  - NO may have some benefit in patients with pulmonary hypertension who are severely hypoxemic.
  - The use of NO in patients without pulmonary hypertension is limited. Studies have suggested that its usage does not improve mortality in patients with ARDS regardless of the degree of hypoxia[19] and increases the risk for renal dysfunction.[20]
- **Inhaled prostacyclins:** Similar to NO, theoretically, inhalation of prostacyclins—a class of vasodilators—improves oxygenation by preferential vasodilation of the capillary beds of ventilated lung.
  - Studies have shown that inhaled prostaglandins improve oxygenation and pulmonary artery pressure in patients with ARDS.[21] However, no studies have been performed to investigate whether mortality benefit exists.
  - Have antiplatelet effects, so theoretical concern for worsening diffuse alveolar hemorrhage.
- **Helium–oxygen mixture (Heliox):** Used in asthma and severe bronchospasm. Usually, a mixture of 70%–80% helium and 20%–30% oxygen. Theoretically decreases airway resistance owing to its low density, leading to improvement in the ratio of laminar to turbulent flow, thereby decreasing the work of breathing. Studies have suggested some benefit in patients with severe asthma exacerbations.[22]

CONSIDERATIONS IN ACUTE RESPIRATORY DISTRESS SYNDROME

- **Fluids:** Conservative fluid management (pulmonary capillary wedge pressure <8, central venous pressure [CVP] <4) in an ARDS patient is associated with shorter mechanical ventilation time.[23]
- **Steroids:** The use of glucocorticoids later in the course of ARDS (≥14 days) is not beneficial and may be harmful. The use of glucocorticoids earlier in the course of ARDS is less clear, but, generally speaking, there is no good evidence of benefit. Steroids are often avoided owing to their detrimental side effects, particularly when used together with paralytics.[24]
  One notable exception involves patients with severe COVID-19. In a meta-analysis of seven trials that included 1703 critically ill patients with COVID-19, glucocorticoids reduced 28-day mortality compared with standard care or placebo. They were not associated with an increased risk of severe adverse events.[25]
- **Paralysis:** Decreases oxygen consumption from accessory inspiratory muscle use and is frequently used in ARDS. Data regarding their benefit are conflicting.
  - A randomized controlled multicenter trial showed that early neuromuscular blockade with cisatracurium was associated with an improvement in 90-day mortality and fewer ventilator days in patients with PaO_2/FIO_2 <120 mm Hg.[26]
  - However, a second RCT from 2019 with cisatracurium done in patients with P:F <150 mm Hg did not result in lower in-hospital mortality, ventilator-free days, or rates of baurotrauma when compared with patients receiving light sedation.[27]
- **Prone positioning:** Improves oxygenation in patients with ARDS by reducing V/Q mismatching and improving shunting by decreasing the amount of atelectatic lung.
  - Early application of prone positioning is associated with improved mortality in patients with ARDS with a PaO_2/FIO_2 <150 mm Hg ARDS.[28]
  - Patients should receive neuromuscular blockade to tolerate proning.
  - Absolute contraindications to proning include spinal instability or unstable fractures. Use of vasopressors, renal replacement therapy, and obesity are not contraindications to proning, but obesity can make proning challenging.

○ Patients should remain proned for at least 16 consecutive hours at a time for benefit and to limit the frequency of turns.
- **Extracorporeal membrane oxygenation (ECMO):** Veno-venous ECMO provides gas exchange in patients with ARDS regardless of the extent of their lung pathology. One study found that referral to a hospital that provides ECMO was associated with improved survival in patients with ARDS from H1N1 influenza.[29] However, this study was limited by the fact that care likely differed between hospitals that provide ECMO and those that do not. A recent study found that mortality did not differ between patients with severe ARDS who received early ECMO as compared with patients who received conventional therapy with ECMO used as a rescue therapy.[30] ECMO remains an important option for carefully selected patients with severe ARDS who are failing conventional therapy.

COMMON COMPLICATIONS OF MECHANICAL VENTILATION

- **Airway malpositioning and occlusion:** See "Airway Management and Endotracheal Intubation."
- **Troubleshooting ventilator alarms:** See Figure 8-2.
- **Auto-PEEP:** Occurs when inspiration is initiated before complete exhalation is complete. May be detected on physical examination by wheezing that does not terminate before the next breath. Demonstrated on ventilator flow-time loop by flow not returning to baseline before delivery of next breath (Figure 8-1). Excessive auto-PEEP can lead to cardiac decompensation owing to tension pneumothorax–like physiology. Treated by adjusting ventilator settings to prolong the expiratory time (either by increasing the flow or decreasing the respiratory rate) and treating any reversible airway obstruction. In the acute setting, the patient may need to be disconnected from the ventilator to allow for full exhalation.
- **Barotrauma/volutrauma:** Occurs when excessive PEEP, inspiratory pressures, or tidal volumes are applied, resulting in alveolar rupture and dissection of air along interstitial tissues causing pneumothorax, pneumomediastinum, pneumopericardium, or pneumoperitoneum. If undetected, can result in life-threatening cardiac decompensation.
- **Ventilator-associated pneumonia (VAP):** Defined as pneumonia in a patient who has been intubated for >48 hours.
  ○ VAP is generally identified by a new infiltrate on CXR in addition to ≥2 of the following criteria: fever, leukocytosis, worsening oxygenation, and purulent secretions.
  ○ When VAP is suspected, microbiologic specimens should be obtained via tracheal aspirate or bronchoscopy with bronchoalveolar lavage.
  ○ Treatment with broad-spectrum empiric antibiotics based on the local prevalence of pathogens and antibiotic sensitivities should be initiated if there is high clinical suspicion for VAP. If an organism has been identified, the antibiotic choice should be tailored to the specific pathogen. Generally, the two most common causes of VAP are *Staphylococcus aureus* and *Pseudomonas aeruginosa*.
  ○ The antibiotic duration for VAP is generally 7 days, as longer durations are not more effective and may increase the risk of antibiotic resistance.[31,32]
- **Stress-induced peptic ulcer disease:** Critically ill patients are at an increased risk of developing upper gastrointestinal (GI) bleeding, which can be prevented by appropriate use of pharmacologic prophylaxis.
  ○ The primary indications for stress ulcer prophylaxis are the presence of a significant coagulopathy (platelets <50k, international normalized ratio >1.5, or partial thromboplastin time >2 upper limits of normal) or the use of mechanical ventilation >48 hours. The other indications for prophylaxis include a history of an upper GI bleed in the last year, presence of brain or spinal cord injury, or any two

CHAPTER 8

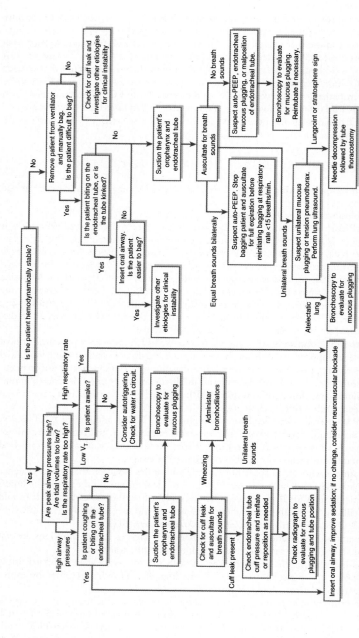

Figure 8-2. Troubleshooting ventilator alarms: what to do when the patient is hypoxic. *Auto-PEEP*, auto–positive end-expiratory pressure.

of the following: occult bleeding for ≥6 days, use of high-dose steroids (>250 mg of hydrocortisone), sepsis, or an intensive care unit (ICU) stay >1 week.

○ A histamine-2 receptor antagonist or proton pump inhibitor can be used for prophylaxis with some controversy on what agent is preferred.

○ The use of ulcer prophylaxis may increase the risk of nosocomial infections, but benefits are likely greater than risks in the above patients.

• **Oxygen toxicity:** Breathing high FIO_2 can lead to excessive free radical generation and result in lung injury.

○ Reducing FIO_2 to the lowest tolerable oxygen saturation (O_2 saturation of 90% or PaO_2 of 65 mm Hg) is advisable. There is evidence that tolerating hyperoxia after intubation may worsen patient survival.[13]

LIBERATION FROM MECHANICAL VENTILATION

• **Parameters demonstrating readiness to wean:** Daily assessment of readiness for extubation should be done once the underlying disease process begins to resolve and minimal ventilator support is required. The following criteria should generally be met before extubation:

○ Minimal ventilator support: FIO_2 ≤40%, PEEP 5 cm H_2O to maintain SpO_2 >90%.

○ Arterial blood gas: pH and $PaCO_2$ should be at the patient's baseline; particularly important for patients with chronic CO_2 retention.

○ Ventilation requirement: Minute ventilation should be <10 L/min and respiratory rate <30 breaths/min.

○ Mental status: Patient should be awake, alert, and cooperative.

○ Secretions: Secretions should be thin, scant in amount, and easily suctioned; patient should not require suctioning more frequently than every 4 hours before extubation.

○ Strength: Patient should have strong cough and be able to lift head off the bed and hold it in flexion for >5 seconds.

○ Breathing trial: Patient should be able to generate spontaneous V_T >5 mL/kg IBW.

○ **Rapid shallow breathing index (RSBI): RSBI should be ≤105.** Defined as ratio of respiratory rate to V_T in liters (f/V_T). RSBI >105 accurately predicts weaning failure, but RSBI ≤105 is less accurate at predicting weaning success.[33]

○ **Patency of airway:** In patients with concern for laryngeal edema (e.g., angioedema, traumatic intubation), cuff leak should be checked before extubation. **Absence of cuff leak should generally preclude extubation**, and patients should be treated with IV corticosteroids for 12–24 hours before extubation.[34]

○ Some patients felt to be ready to extubate based on all objective criteria will still fail extubation. Failure rates as high as 23.5% have been reported.[35]

• **Weaning strategies: Sedation interruption and breathing trials for 30–120 minutes should be done daily** and is the most important predictor of timely liberation from mechanical ventilation.[36] Weaning strategies include the following:

○ **PSV:** No time-triggered breaths, but patient remains connected to the ventilator. PEEP is usually at 5 cm H_2O, with low levels of pressure support (5–10 cm H_2O) during spontaneous breathing.

○ **T-piece/spontaneous breathing trial:** Patient is removed from the ventilator but remains intubated. Endotracheal tube is connected to a heated, humidified circuit with minimal or no supplemental oxygen. End-tidal CO_2 monitoring may be used for additional safety.

○ **SIMV:** Used most frequently in surgical and neurosurgical patients. Set respiratory rate is gradually decreased over hours to days until patient is primarily breathing spontaneously.

○ SIMV has the poorest weaning outcomes of all techniques. However, neither T-piece nor PSV has proven to be more predictive of successful extubation.[37]

- **Management following extubation:** Patients need to be closely monitored following extubation. Good airway clearance and oxygenation decrease the risk of reintubation.
  - **Extubation to NPPV:** In patients with COPD who are intubated for acute respiratory failure, extubation to NPPV is associated with a reduction in mortality and health care–associated pneumonia.[38] More generally, in patients with chronic hypercapnic respiratory failure, two trials have found that the use of NPPV reduces rates of reintubation following extubation.[39,40] Similar benefit of NPPV has not been demonstrated in other etiologies of respiratory failure.
  - **Extubation to HFNC:** The use of HFNC may also have a beneficial role in the prevention of postextubation respiratory failure in select low-risk patients. When patients were randomly assigned to HFNC versus conventional oxygen therapy after extubation, patients who received HFNC were less likely to be intubated within 48–72 hours.[41,42] Other studies have shown HFNC to be noninferior when compared with NPPV in preventing reintubation.[43]
- **Failure to wean:** Defined as inability to liberate from mechanical ventilation 48–72 hours after resolution of underlying disease process. Factors that should be considered include the following:
  - Endotracheal tubes with smaller inner diameter increase airway resistance and may make breathing trials more difficult.
  - Use of neuromuscular blockade is associated with prolonged weakness, particularly when used with corticosteroids.[44]
  - Critical illness myopathy and polyneuropathy places the patient at risk for recurrent respiratory failure.
  - Psychiatric illnesses (delirium, anxiety, PTSD, etc.) may interfere with SBTs and other standard weaning protocols.
  - Acid–base disturbances may make liberation from mechanical ventilation difficult.
    - Non–anion gap metabolic acidosis causes compensatory increase in minute ventilation (respiratory alkalosis) to normalize pH, which can lead to tachypnea and respiratory fatigue upon extubation.
    - Metabolic alkalosis causes blunting of ventilatory drive and decrease in minute ventilation (respiratory acidosis) to maintain normal pH, which can lead to hypercapnia upon extubation.

Shock

GENERAL PRINCIPLES

- A process in which blood flow and oxygen delivery to tissues are deranged, leading to tissue hypoxia and resultant compromise of cellular metabolic activity and organ function.
- Main goal of therapy is rapid cardiovascular resuscitation to reestablish tissue perfusion.
- Definitive treatment requires reversal of underlying processes.

Classifications of Shock

Hemodynamic patterns associated with the different shock states are listed in Table 8-5.

- **Distributive:** Shock caused by massive vasodilation and impaired distribution of blood flow, resulting in tissue hypoxia. Usually associated with hyperdynamic cardiac function, unless cardiac function is somehow impaired (see later discussion of cardiogenic shock).

TABLE 8-5	Hemodynamic Patterns Associated With Specific Shock States							
Type of Shock	CI	SVR	PVR	SvO₂	RAP	RVP	PAP	PAOP
Cardiogenic	↓	↑	N	↓	↑	↑	↑	↑
Hypovolemic	↓	↑	N	↓	↓	↓	↓	↓
Distributive	N–↑	↓	N	N–↑	N–↓	N–↓	N–↓	N–↓
Obstructive[a]	↓	↑–N	↑	N–↓	↑	↑	↑	N–↓

[a]Equalization of RAP, PAOP, diastolic PAP, and diastolic RVP establishes a diagnosis of cardiac tamponade.
CI, cardiac index; N, normal; PAOP, pulmonary artery occlusion pressure; PAP, pulmonary artery pressure; PVR, pulmonary vascular resistance; RAP, right atrial pressure; RVP, right ventricular pressure; SvO_2, mixed venous oxygen saturation; SVR, systemic vascular resistance.

- ○ **Primary etiologies** are septic shock and anaphylactic shock. Septic shock is most commonly seen in medical ICUs and will be further discussed in the next section. Anaphylaxis is discussed in Chapter 11, Allergy and Immunology. Other less common types include neurogenic shock and adrenal shock.
- ○ **Hemodynamic parameters** will generally demonstrate increased cardiac output (CO), decreased systemic vascular resistance (SVR) due to vasodilation, and elevated central venous oxygen saturation ($ScvO_2$) due to ineffective oxygen extraction by tissue.
- ○ Primary goals of therapy
  - ▪ Volume resuscitation: Owing to massive peripheral vasodilation, patients have a functionally decreased oxygen-carrying capacity, requiring volume resuscitation. IV crystalloid fluids are primarily used.
  - ▪ Treatment of underlying infection: Inadequate initial antimicrobial therapy is an independent risk factor for in-hospital mortality in patients with septic shock, so timely, effective antimicrobial therapy is a cornerstone of treatment.
  - ▪ Removal of the offending agent in anaphylactic shock.
  - ▪ Cardiovascular support with vasoactive agents (e.g., norepinephrine). Vasoactive agents will be discussed in more detail in a later section.
- • **Hypovolemic:** Shock caused by a decrease in effective intravascular volume and decreased oxygen-carrying capacity.
  - ○ **Primary etiologies** are hemorrhagic (e.g., trauma, gastrointestinal bleeding) or fluid depletion (e.g., diarrhea, vomiting).
  - ○ **Hemodynamic parameters** will generally demonstrate a decreased CO, increased SVR, and decreased $ScvO_2$ due to increased oxygen extraction by peripheral tissue.
  - ○ Primary goals of therapy
    - ▪ Volume resuscitation: IV blood product and crystalloid are used for resuscitation of hemorrhagic and fluid depletion shock, respectively, with goal mean arterial pressure (MAP) of 60–65 mm Hg. Overresuscitation may be detrimental in hemorrhagic shock and patients without significant comorbidities may tolerate lower hemoglobin levels (7 g/dL) than previously believed.
    - ▪ Definitive treatment of underlying etiology of volume loss: For hemorrhagic shock, surgical intervention may be necessary.
- • **Obstructive:** Shock caused by obstruction of the heart or great vessels, resulting in decreased left ventricular filling and cardiovascular collapse.
  - ○ **Primary etiologies** are pulmonary embolism, cardiac tamponade, and tension pneumothorax.
  - ○ **Hemodynamic parameters** will generally demonstrate decreased CO, normal to increased SVR, and normal to decreased $ScvO_2$.

○ Primary goals of therapy
  ▪ Supportive: Although patients are preload dependent, excessive fluid administration can lead to right ventricular overload and impairment of LV filling, thereby worsening shock.
  ▪ Definitive therapy involves relieving the obstruction (e.g., thoracostomy in the case of a pneumothorax, and pericardiocentesis in tamponade).
  ▪ In a carefully selected group of patients, thrombolytic therapy may be beneficial in patients with pulmonary emboli.
• **Cardiogenic:** Shock caused by left ventricular systolic failure, resulting in decreased CO and subsequent insufficient oxygen distribution.
  ○ **Primary etiologies** are myocardial infarction, acute mitral regurgitation, and myocarditis.
  ○ **Hemodynamic parameters** will demonstrate decreased CO, increased SVR, and decreased $ScvO_2$.
  ○ Primary goals of therapy
    ▪ Mitigation of pulmonary edema: NPPV or endotracheal intubation with mechanical ventilation reduces afterload, thereby encouraging forward flow, as well as preload. Additionally, the application of positive pressure to the alveolar space causes pulmonary edema fluid to move to the interstitial space.
    ▪ Careful fluid management: Adequate preload to optimize ventricular function is important, but volume overload will worsen respiratory status, so careful fluid management is necessary. Volume removal (whether via diuresis or hemodialysis) is often a critical component of early management.
    ▪ Definitive therapy for underlying cardiac disease: In the event of myocardial infarction, percutaneous revascularization should be performed in a timely fashion.
    ▪ Supportive: Inotropic agents such as dobutamine may be used to augment CO. Other inotropes are discussed in "Pharmacologic Therapies." Mechanical circulatory assist devices, including left ventricular assist devices and intra-aortic balloon pumps, may be necessary in patients who do not respond to medical therapy.

Septic Shock

• **Definition of sepsis:** Sepsis is defined as a life-threatening organ dysfunction caused by dysregulation of the host response to an infection.
  ○ Sepsis was previously identified based on the presence of at least two systemic inflammatory response syndrome (SIRS) criteria:
    ▪ Tachypnea: Respiratory rate >20 breaths/min or $PaCO_2$ <32 mm Hg
    ▪ White blood cell count <4000 cells/μL or >12,000 cells/μL
    ▪ Tachycardia: Pulse >90 bpm
    ▪ Hypo- or hyperthermia: Temperature >38°C or <36°C
  ○ The new sepsis guidelines now identify organ dysregulation in sepsis as an increase in the Sequential Organ Failure Assessment (SOFA) score of ≥2.[45]
  ○ Septic shock is a subset of sepsis identified by persistent hypotension requiring vasopressors to maintain a mean arterial blood pressure ≥65 mm after adequate volume resuscitation. Mortality in these patients is ~40%.
• **Management of septic shock:** Management of septic shock involves early aggressive volume resuscitation and attempting to achieve hemodynamic stability quickly.[46]
  ○ **Volume resuscitation:** Patients should begin to receive **at least 30 mL/kg IBW IV crystalloid fluid** within the first hour of presentation.[47] Smaller amounts of fluid may be needed if there is concomitant heart failure or pulmonary edema, whereas additional volume may be required if the patient remains volume responsive after the initial 30 mL/kg bolus. Parameters to determine volume responsiveness

(discussed in "Hemodynamic Measurements") should be closely monitored during volume resuscitation to prevent volume overload.

- A recent RCT found that balanced crystalloids (i.e., lactated Ringer solution) may be associated with lower rates of renal dysfunction and even improved mortality when used as compared with normal saline.[48]
- Several trials have not found significant benefit in albumin administration when compared with crystalloid in septic patients.[49]
  ○ **Cardiovascular support:** Vasoactive medications may be necessary if volume resuscitation is insufficient to maintain MAP ≥65 mm Hg. **Norepinephrine has become the first-line agent** after it was demonstrated that dopamine had more adverse events.[50] Vasopressin is frequently used as a second-line agent. Mechanisms of action and other agents are discussed in "Pharmacologic Therapies."
  ○ **Timely, effective antimicrobial administration:** Delays in starting appropriate antimicrobials are associated with increased mortality.[51] The Surviving Sepsis Guidelines recommend starting antibiotics immediately after obtaining blood cultures, if possible.[47]
  ○ **Source control:** If a specific anatomical source of infection is identified (e.g., necrotizing soft tissue infection), intervention for source control should be performed as soon as reasonably possible.[52]
  ○ **Early goal-directed therapy:** Protocol for management of the **first 6 hours** of sepsis proposed by Rivers et al. in 2001.[46] Widely adapted in practice before recent multicenter, prospective, RCTs called its effectiveness into question.[53,54] However, these studies were limited by practice changes in control group (Figure 8-3).
  ○ **Lactate clearance:** Lactate clearance is associated with improved mortality in septic patients.[55] The most recent Surviving Sepsis Guidelines recommend targeting resuscitation to normalize lactate in patients with elevated lactate levels.[47]
  ○ **Procalcitonin (PCT):** PCT is a biomarker that may aid in diagnosing sepsis, assessing treatment response, and determining antibiotic duration. An elevated PCT >0.5 ng/mL is suggestive of a bacterial infection while a PCT <0.1 ng/mL makes bacterial infection less likely.[56] Some studies have shown that use of PCT may reduce the unnecessary usage of antibiotics.[57] However, caution must be used, as a low PCT does not exclude the possibility of a severe bacterial infection.

Pharmacologic Therapies
Vasoconstrictive and Inotropic Agents
- **Norepinephrine:** Causes potent vasoconstriction via α_1- and β_1-adrenergic activity. Preferred agent in septic shock.
- **Vasopressin:** Causes vasoconstriction via three different G-peptide receptors. Primarily used as an adjunct to norepinephrine. Weak evidence that it may have mortality benefit over norepinephrine in less severe septic shock (defined as requiring treatment with norepinephrine 5–14 μg/min to maintain MAP ≥65 mm Hg).[58]
- **Epinephrine:** Has inotropic and vasoconstrictive properties in a dose-dependent fashion owing to α_1- and β-adrenergic activity. At low doses (≤0.05 μg/kg/min), it increases CO and slightly reduces SVR owing to predominant β activity. At higher doses (>0.05 μg/kg/min), vasoconstriction predominates owing to increased α_1 activity. Preferred agent for anaphylactic shock, and is also frequently used in cardiogenic shock.
- **Phenylephrine:** Selective α_1-receptor agonist causing vasoconstriction of larger arterioles. Few studies supporting its use in septic shock.
- **Angiotensin II:** Recent studies have investigated angiotensin II which engages the renin–angiotensin–aldosterone system. These studies showed that angiotensin II increased blood pressure in patients with vasodilatory shock.[59]

CHAPTER 8

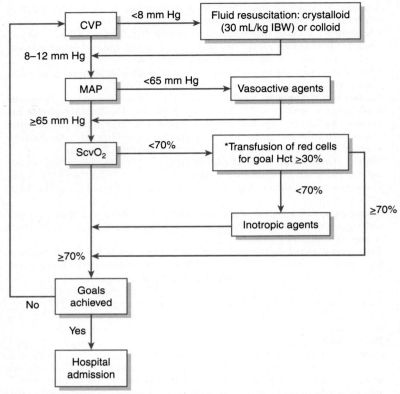

Figure 8-3. Early goal-directed therapy protocol. (Adapted from Rivers E, Nguyen B, Havstad S, et al. Early goal-directed therapy in the treatment of severe sepsis and septic shock. *N Engl J Med.* 2001;345:1368-1377.)

*Although included in the original early goal-directed therapy protocol, more recent trials have demonstrated a trend toward increased harm in patients who receive more transfusions; current Surviving Sepsis Guidelines do not recommend transfusing to achieve Hct of 30%. CVP, central venous pressure; Hct, hematocrit; IBW, ideal body weight; MAP, mean arterial pressure; $ScvO_2$, central venous oxygen saturation.

- **Dobutamine:** Inotropic agent that reduces afterload and increases stroke volume and heart rate via β_1-agonist activity. Good agent for cardiogenic shock but increases risk of cardiac arrhythmias.
- **Dopamine:** Has inotropic, vasodilatory, and vasoconstrictive properties in a dose-dependent fashion due to action on peripheral α_1-receptors, cardiac β_1-receptors, and renal and splanchnic dopaminergic receptors. At doses <5 µg/kg/min, primarily behaves as a vasodilator, increasing renal blood flow. At doses of 5–10 µg/kg/min, behaves as an inotrope. At doses >10 µg/kg/min, behaves as a vasopressor. Is associated with a higher rate of cardiac arrhythmias than norepinephrine.[50]
- **Milrinone:** Phosphodiesterase III inhibitor that has positive inotropic effect, causing increase in CO. Also causes systemic vasodilation, which decreases afterload, making it an alternative option for cardiogenic shock.

- Regarding **venous access**, low-dose norepinephrine, phenylephrine, and epinephrine may be infused peripherally for a limited period of time. However, central access is preferred as medication extravasation can lead to local ischemia.
  - If extravasation occurs, phentolamine (an α-antagonist) can be injected into the area of extravasation to reduce ischemic injury.
  - Peripheral administration of vasopressin and angiotensin II is not recommended.

Adjunctive Therapies
- **Corticosteroids:** Relative adrenal insufficiency may contribute to refractory hypotension during septic shock. Data do not support the use of corticosteroids in mild septic shock. However, corticosteroids should be considered on an individual basis in patients with more severe shock, particularly in patients chronically on steroids. Generally, hydrocortisone 200–300 mg daily divided on a q6–8h basis is given. Previous trials have shown faster resolution of shock when administering hydrocortisone, but no difference in mortality.[60,61] Another recent trial showed a benefit in 90-day mortality when hydrocortisone (50 mg every 6 hours) and fludricortisone (50 μg daily) were administered in conjunction.[62]
- **Sodium bicarbonate:** No evidence supports the use of bicarbonate therapy in lactic acidemia from sepsis with a pH ≥7.15. Effect of bicarbonate on hemodynamics and vasopressor requirements with more severe acidemia is unknown, but bicarbonate is often recommended in patients with severe lactic acidemia (pH <7.1) who are hemodynamically unstable.
- **Methylene blue:** Selective guanylate cyclase inhibitor, thereby mitigating nitric oxide–mediated vasodilation. Observational studies have demonstrated beneficial effects on hemodynamic parameters, but effects on morbidity and mortality are unknown.[63]

Hemodynamic Measurements

Although CVP, MAP, and SvO_2/$ScvO_2$ are used as therapeutic end points in treating shock, there is evidence that these parameters do not reflect intravascular volume. There is a growing body of evidence that dynamic parameters, including pulse pressure variation and inferior vena cava (IVC) diameters, may better reflect intravascular volume, but it is unclear that the use of these leads to improved outcomes.
- **Static parameters**
  - **CVP:** An approximation of right atrial pressure and, therefore, preload. Should be measured from an internal jugular or subclavian venous catheter because readings from femoral catheters are influenced by intra-abdominal pressures and thus inaccurate. There is a poor relationship between CVP and blood volume,[64] but low values (<4 mm Hg) should generally lead to fluid resuscitation with careful monitoring.[65]
  - **$ScvO_2$/SvO_2:** $ScvO_2$ is a surrogate that is often used to reflect SvO_2, which is the percentage of oxygen bound to hemoglobin in blood returning to the right side of the heart. $ScvO_2$ is measured from an internal jugular or subclavian venous catheter, while a true SvO_2 must be measured with a pulmonary artery catheter (PAC). Normal values are 65%–75%. A high value often represents decreased oxygen consumption (commonly seen in mitochondrial dysfunction with sepsis), whereas low values indicate inadequate oxygen delivery (often due to low CO states such as cardiogenic shock). Previous guidelines recommended targeting an $ScvO_2$ >70% with dobutamine administration if needed, though more recent trials have shown that using lactate clearance as a resuscitation goal is noninferior.[66]
  - **PACs:** A PAC catheter provides direct measurements of pressures in the right atrium, right ventricle, and pulmonary artery, as well as a pulmonary capillary wedge pressure. Previously commonly used in the management of septic shock and ARDS but did not affect mortality or morbidity.[67]

CHAPTER 8

- **Dynamic parameters**
  - **Esophageal Doppler:** A Doppler probe is placed into the esophagus and rotated to measure blood flow through the descending aorta. System can be used to calculate CO and stroke volume, and correlates well with CO as measured by PAC.[68] Predicts volume responsiveness in critically ill ventilated patients without spontaneous breathing.[69]
  - **Pulse pressure variation (ΔPp):** Requires arterial line placement. Calculated as the difference between maximal and minimal systolic blood pressures measured over one respiratory cycle divided by the mean of those values. ΔPp of 13% was an accurate predictor of fluid responsiveness in mechanically ventilated patients without spontaneous breathing.[70]
  - **IVC distensibility index (dIVC):** Calculated as the difference between maximal and minimal IVC diameter measured over one respiratory cycle divided by the minimal IVC diameter. dIVC of 18% discriminated between volume responders and nonresponders with 90% sensitivity and specificity in mechanically ventilated patients without spontaneous breathing in one study,[71] but more recent studies have shown this method to be a poor predictor of fluid responsiveness.[72]
  - **Thoracic bioreactance:** A noninvasive device is applied to the chest and measures bioreactance across the thorax using sensor pads placed on a patient's thorax surrounding their heart. Blood flow (which is predominately in the aorta in the thorax) causes phase shifts in impedance, which is detected by the sensors. From these measurements, stroke volume and CO can be estimated. There are conflicting data on the ability of thoracic bioreactance devices to reliably determine fluid responsiveness.[73,74]

Critical Care Ultrasound

The use of bedside ultrasonography has greatly expanded recently and is rapidly becoming standard of care in ICUs. Courses in critical care ultrasonography are becoming more readily available and are necessary for complete proficiency. This section is intended to serve as an overview of basic concepts only. Critical care ultrasound should be used as an adjunct to other clinical data.

- **Basic concepts:** Air and calcified structures transmit sound waves poorly. Free-flowing fluids transmit sound waves well.
- **Basic definitions**
  - Echogenicity: The ability of an object to reflect sound waves.
  - Hyperechoic: Structures that reflect sound waves well; shows as white on ultrasound (e.g., bone, pleura, lung).
  - Hypoechoic: Structures that reflect sound waves poorly; shows as gray on ultrasound. Deeper structures are also more hypoechoic owing to attenuation with distance (e.g., lymph nodes, adipose tissue, muscle).
  - Anechoic: Containing structures that allow sound waves to pass through freely; shows as black on ultrasound (e.g., blood vessels, transudative pleural effusion).
- **Ultrasound to facilitate vascular access:** More detailed instructions are available in the **Washington Manual of Critical Care**, Section XIX. Use of ultrasound to guide central venous access results in increased success and reduced complication rates.
  - Location: Ultrasound guidance is most commonly used for internal jugular and femoral venous access.
  - Before starting the procedure: Both internal jugular and femoral veins should be scanned to evaluate for aberrant anatomy or venous thrombosis.
  - After applying the sterile field: The probe is positioned so that the needle is visualized for the entire duration of accessing the vessel.
  - During the procedure: Following insertion of the guidewire, the length of the vessel is scanned to ensure that the guidewire did not inadvertently enter any adjacent arteries.
  - After the procedure: Lung ultrasound can be used to rule out a pneumothorax.

- **Cardiac ultrasound:** Includes five standard views, reviewed below. Uses body transducer. Intended to facilitate assessment of volume responsiveness, global left and right ventricular systolic function, and valvular function.
  - ○ Parasternal long-axis view: Probe is placed adjacent to the sternum in the left third to fifth intercostal space with the orientation marker pointing toward the patient's right shoulder. The right ventricular outflow tract, left ventricular cavity, ascending aorta, mitral valve, and left atrium should be visualized. Assesses for pericardial effusion, left and right ventricular dysfunction, and valvular pathologies.
  - ○ Parasternal short-axis view: Probe remains adjacent to the sternum in the left third to fifth intercostal space, but orientation marker is rotated 90 degrees clockwise to point at the patient's left shoulder. Cross-sectional view of the left and right ventricles at the level of the papillary muscles should be visualized. Assesses for pericardial effusion and left and right ventricular dysfunction.
  - ○ Apical four-chamber view: Probe is placed between the midclavicular and midaxillary lines of the left lateral chest between the fifth and seventh intercostal spaces, underneath the left nipple, with the orientation marker pointed at 3 o'clock. The left and right ventricles and atria, as well as the tricuspid and mitral valves, should be visualized. Assesses left and right ventricular size and function. See Figure 8-4.
  - ○ Subcostal long-axis view: Probe is placed below the xiphoid process with the orientation marker pointed at 3 o'clock. The left and right ventricles and atria should be visualized. Assesses for pericardial effusion and left and right ventricular dysfunction. May be used for rapid assessment of cardiac function during performance of cardiopulmonary resuscitation.
  - ○ IVC longitudinal view: Probe remains below the xiphoid process, but orientation marker is rotated 90 degrees counterclockwise to point at 12 o'clock. IVC in the longitudinal axis should be visualized. Assesses IVC diameter during the respiratory cycle to determine volume responsiveness.
- **Thoracic ultrasound:** Includes four standard positions, performed bilaterally. Uses the body transducer on the abdominal setting to examine lung parenchyma; vascular transducer may be used for detailed examination of the pleura. Intended to facilitate the diagnosis of pleural effusion, pulmonary edema, pulmonary consolidation, and pneumothorax. Also used to guide a safe thoracentesis.
  - ○ **Probe placement:** Bedside lung ultrasound in emergency (BLUE)s protocol, intended for immediate diagnosis of acute respiratory failure, defines four areas for investigation.[75] The orientation marker should be pointed toward the patient's head.
    - ▪ Upper BLUE point: Midclavicular line, second intercostal space

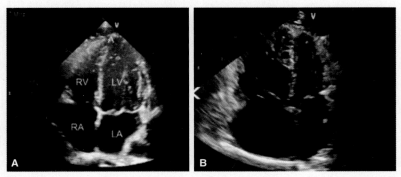

Figure 8-4. Cardiac ultrasound. Left (A): normal apical four-chamber view. A, apex; RV, right ventricle; RA, right atrium; LV, left ventricle; LA, left atrium. Right (B): demonstrates same view in a patient with right ventricular hypertrophy and dilation.

CHAPTER 8

- Lower BLUE point: Anterior axillary line, fourth or fifth intercostal space
- Phrenic point: Midaxillary line, sixth or seventh intercostal space; location of the diaphragm
- Posterolateral alveolar and/or pleural syndrome point: Posterior to the posterior axillary line, fourth or fifth intercostal space
  ○ **Anatomic landmarks and ultrasound appearance:** Knowledge of the normal sonographic appearance of thoracic anatomy is paramount to identifying key structures.
- Chest wall: Hypoechoic, linear shadows of soft tissue density.
- Ribs: Hyperechoic, curvilinear structures with a deep, hypoechoic, posterior acoustic shadow.
- Pleura: Bright, hyperechoic, roughly horizontal line located approximately 0.5 cm below rib shadows.
- Diaphragm: Curvilinear, hyperechoic line that moves caudally with inspiration. In a seated patient, it is located caudad to the ninth rib.
- Splenorenal and hepatorenal recesses: Should be confirmed before any procedure because its curvilinear appearance is similar to that of the diaphragm. Identified by visualization of the liver or spleen and the kidney caudally.
- Lung: Air-filled lung appears hyperechoic due to the poor echogenicity of air. Atelectatic or consolidated lung appears hypoechoic relative to normal lung.
  ○ **Sonographic artifacts and terminology:** A number of sonographic artifacts are caused by air–tissue interfaces, and presence or absence of these artifacts is indicative of disease.[76]
- Pleural line: Brightly echogenic, roughly horizontal line; caused by parietopulmonary interface and indicating the lung surface.
- A-lines: Brightly echogenic horizontal lines roughly parallel to the chest wall; caused by reverberations of the pleural line.
- B-lines: Also called "comet tails"; a grouping within one intercostal space is called "lung rockets." Hyperechoic line arising perpendicularly from the pleural line that extends across the whole screen without fading, erasing A-lines; moves with lung slide. Caused by thickened interlobular septa or ground-glass areas; isolated B-lines are a normal variant. See Figure 8-5.

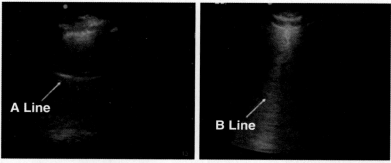

Figure 8-5. Lung ultrasound. A-lines demonstrated on left are equidistant horizontal lines created by reflections of the pleural line. B-lines demonstrated on the right are bright vertical lines that move with the pleura and extend to the bottom of the screen representing thickened fluid-filled interlobular septae.

- **Lung slide:** "Twinkling" movement of the pleural line that occurs with the respiratory cycle; caused by movement of the lung along the craniocaudal axis during respiration. In M-mode, lung slide is visualized as the "seashore sign," with the chest wall generating the "waves," the aerated lung forming the "sand," and the pleural line as the interface.
- **Lung pulse:** Pulsation of the pleural line due to transmission of the heartbeat through noninflated lung.
- **Ultrasonography of lung pathology**
  - **Pleural effusion:** A fluid collection bordered by the diaphragm, chest wall, and lung surface. Transudative effusions are typically anechoic; exudative effusions may have some echogenicity. If the effusion is loculated, septations—visualized as hyperechoic, weblike structures—may be seen. Atelectatic lung may be seen in the effusion.
  - **Pneumothorax:** Owing to air's poor echogenicity, diagnosis of pneumothorax on ultrasound is made by artifact analysis.
    - The presence of lung slide or lung pulse effectively rules out pneumothorax in the location being investigated.
    - Abolishment of lung slide has a characteristic stratosphere sign in M-mode, with loss of the "sand," but is neither sufficient nor specific for diagnosis of pneumothorax.
    - Lung point is pathognomonic for pneumothorax but has poor sensitivity. Occurs at the interface of the pneumothorax and aerated lung. Characterized by alternation between absent lung slide and present lung slide or B-lines in one location with respirations. In M-mode, will transition between seashore sign and stratosphere sign.
  - **Pneumonia:** Can only be visualized when the consolidation abuts the pleura. A heterogeneous, hypoechoic area with irregular margins where aerated lung abuts the consolidated area. Air bronchograms should be seen to make the diagnosis of pneumonia.
  - **Pulmonary edema:** Presence of multiple B-lines within one intercostal space ("lung rockets") may indicate cardiogenic or noncardiogenic pulmonary edema. Corresponds to the Kerley B-lines seen on chest radiograph. Isolated B-lines are a normal variant.
- **Abdominal ultrasound:** Abdominal ultrasound in critical care is limited and intended to evaluate for intra-abdominal fluid and assess the urinary tract and abdominal aorta.
  - Evaluating for intra-abdominal fluid: Standard evaluation of the trauma patient who may have intra-abdominal bleeding includes the focused assessment with sonography for trauma (FAST) examination. The patient is in the supine position, and four views are obtained:
    - **Hepatorenal space:** The probe is placed on the right in the 10th or 11th intercostal space at the posterior axillary line with the orientation mark pointed cephalad.
    - **Pelvis:** The probe is placed in the suprapubic area with the orientation mark in the 3-o'clock position.
    - **Perisplenic space:** The probe is placed on the left in the 10th or 11th space at or slightly posterior to the posterior axillary line with the orientation mark pointed cephalad.
    - **Pericardial space:** The probe is placed in the subxiphoid position with the orientation marker in the 3-o'clock position.

- Paracentesis: Paracentesis should be performed under ultrasound guidance because there is evidence supporting a decrease in complications. More details can be found in the *Washington Manual for Critical Care*, Section XIX.
- Assessment of the urinary tract: Bedside ultrasonography can identify bladder distention or hydronephrosis.
  - Bladder distention: The probe is placed in the suprapubic position with the orientation marker pointed cephalad for longitudinal dimensions and in the 3-o'clock position for transverse dimensions.
  - Hydronephrosis: The probe should be placed slightly caudad to the locations used for examination of the hepatorenal and perisplenic spaces in the FAST examination. Hydronephrosis is characterized by thinning of the renal cortex as the collecting system dilates.
- Assessment of the abdominal aorta: The goal is to visualize the entire abdominal aorta to ensure that its diameter from outer wall to outer wall is <3 cm. The examination begins caudad to the xiphoid process, with the probe perpendicular to the abdominal wall and the orientation marker in the 3-o'clock position.
- **Vascular diagnostic ultrasound:** Bedside ultrasonography may be performed to evaluate for deep vein thrombosis when clinically indicated. The target vein is visualized in the transverse plane. A vessel with normal blood flow should appear internally anechoic and should be easily compressible. Organized thrombus appears as a discrete, echogenic structure within the venous lumen. A very recently formed thrombus may be anechoic, but the vessel will be incompressible.

REFERENCES

1. Force ADT, Ranieri VM, Rubenfeld GD, et al. Acute respiratory distress syndrome: the Berlin definition. *J Am Med Assoc.* 2012;307:2526-2533.
2. Frat JP, Thille AW, Mercat A, et al. High-flow oxygen through nasal cannula in acute hypoxemic respiratory failure. *N Engl J Med.* 2015;372:2185-2196.
3. Rochwerg B, Granton D, Wang DX, et al. High flow nasal cannula compared with conventional oxygen therapy for acute hypoxemic respiratory failure: a systematic review and meta-analysis. *Intensive Care Med.* 2019;45(5):563.
4. Peter JV, Moran JL, Phillips-Hughes J, et al. Effect of non-invasive positive pressure ventilation (NIPPV) on mortality in patients with acute cardiogenic pulmonary oedema: a meta-analysis. *Lancet.* 2006;367:1155-1163.
5. Barreiro TJ, Gemmel DJ. Noninvasive ventilation. *Crit Care Clin.* 2007;23:201-222, ix.
6. Patel BK, Wolfe KS, Pohlman AS, et al. Effect of noninvasive ventilation delivered by helmet vs face mask on the rate of endotracheal intubation in patients with acute respiratory distress syndrome: a randomized clinical trial. *J Am Med Assoc.* 2016;315:2435-2441.
7. Althoff MD, Holguin F, Yang F, et al. Noninvasive ventilation use in critically ill patients with acute asthma exacerbations. *Am J Respir Crit Care Med.* 2020;202(11):1491-1493.
8. Antonelli M, Conti G, Rocco M, et al. A comparison of noninvasive positive-pressure ventilation and conventional mechanical ventilation in patients with acute respiratory failure. *N Engl J Med.* 1998;339:429-435.
9. Terragni PP, Antonelli M, Fumagalli R, et al. Early vs late tracheotomy for prevention of pneumonia in mechanically ventilated adult ICU patients: a randomized controlled trial. *J Am Med Assoc.* 2010;303:1483-1489.
10. Young D, Harrison DA, Cuthbertson BH, Rowan K; TracMan Collaborators. Effect of early vs late tracheostomy placement on survival in patients receiving mechanical ventilation: the TracMan randomized trial. *J Am Med Assoc.* 2013;309(20):2121-2129.
11. Grant CA, Dempsey G, Harrison J, Jones T. Tracheo-innominate artery fistula after percutaneous tracheostomy: three case reports and a clinical review. *Br J Anaesth.* 2006;96:127-131.
12. Futier E, Constantin JM, Paugam-Burtz C, et al. A trial of intraoperative low-tidal-volume ventilation in abdominal surgery. *N Engl J Med.* 2013;369:428-437.
13. Page D, Ablordeppey E, Wessman BT, et al. Emergency department hyperoxia is associated with increased mortality in mechanically ventilated patients: a cohort study. *Crit Care.* 2018;22:9.
14. Sud S, Sud M, Friefrich JO, et al. High frequency oscillation in patients with acute lung injury and acute respiratory distress syndrome (ARDS): systematic review and meta-analysis. *Br Med J.* 2010;340:c2327.

15. Yung D, Lamb SE, Shah S, et al. High-frequency oscillation for acute respiratory distress syndrome. *N Engl J Med*. 2013;368:806.
16. Ferguson ND, Cook DJ, Guyatt GH, et al. High-frequency oscillation in early acute respiratory distress syndrome. *N Engl J Med*. 2013;368:795.
17. Grieco DL, Chen L, Dres M, Brochard L. Should we use driving pressure to set tidal volume? *Curr Opin Crit Care*. 2017;23:38-44.
18. Amato MB, Meade MO, Slutsky AS, et al. Driving pressure and survival in the acute respiratory distress syndrome. *N Engl J Med*. 2015;372:747-755.
19. Adhikari NK, Dellinger RP, Lundin S, et al. Inhaled nitric oxide does not reduce mortality in patients with acute respiratory distress syndrome regardless of severity: systematic review and meta-analysis. *Crit Care Med*. 2014;42:404-412.
20. Ruan SY, Wu HY, Kun HH, et al. Inhaled nitric oxide and the risk of renal dysfunction in patients with acute respiratory distress syndrome: a propensity-matched cohort study. *Crit Care*. 2016;20:389.
21. Fuller BM, Mohr NM, Skrupky L, et al. The use of inhaled prostaglandins in patients with ARDS: a systematic review and meta-analysis. *Chest*. 2015;147:1510-1522.
22. Rodrigo GJ, Castro-Rodriguez JA. Heliox-driven β2-agonists nebulization for children and adults with acute asthma: a systematic review with meta-analysis. *Ann Allergy Asthma Immunol*. 2014;112:29-34.
23. National Heart Lung, and Blood Institute Acute Respiratory Distress Syndrome Clinical Trials Network; Wiedemann HP, Wheeler AP, Bernard GR, et al. Comparison of two fluid-management strategies in acute lung injury. *N Engl J Med*. 2006;354:2564-2575.
24. Steinberg KP, Hudson LD, Goodman RB, et al. Efficacy and safety of corticosteroids for persistent acute respiratory distress syndrome. *N Engl J Med*. 2006;354:1671-1684.
25. WHO Rapid Evidence Appraisal for COVID-19 Therapies (REACT) Working Group; Sterne JAC, Murthy S, Diaz JV, et al. Association between administration of systemic corticosteroids and mortality among critically ill patients with COVID-19: a meta-analysis. *J Am Med Assoc*. 2020;324(13):1330.
26. Papazian L, Forel JM, Gacouin A, et al. Neuromuscular blockers in early acute respiratory distress syndrome. *N Engl J Med*. 2010;363:1107-1116.
27. National Heart, Lung, and Blood Institute PETAL Clinical Trials Network; Moss M, Huang DT, Brower RG, et al. Early neuromuscular blockade in the acute respiratory distress syndrome. *N Engl J Med*. 2019;380(21):1997.
28. Guerin C, Reignier J, Richard JC, et al. Prone positioning in severe acute respiratory distress syndrome. *N Engl J Med*. 2013;368:2159-2168.
29. Noah MA, Peek GJ, Finney SJ, et al. Referral to an extracorporeal membrane oxygenation center and mortality among patients with severe 2009 influenza A(H1N1). *J Am Med Assoc*. 2011;306:1659-1668.
30. Combes A, Hajage D, Capellier G, et al. Extracorporeal membrane oxygenation for severe acute respiratory distress syndrome. *N Engl J Med*. 2018;378:1965-1975.
31. Kollef MH. Health care-associated pneumonia: perception versus reality. *Clin Infect Dis*. 2009;49:1875-1877.
32. Kalil AC, Metersky ML, Klompas M, et al. Management of adults with hospital-acquired and ventilator-associated pneumonia: 2016 clinical practice guidelines by the Infectious Diseases Society of America and the American Thoracic Society. *Clin Infect Dis*. 2016;63:e61-e111.
33. Yang KL, Tobin MJ. A prospective study of indexes predicting the outcome of trials of weaning from mechanical ventilation. *N Engl J Med*. 1991;324:1445-1450.
34. Khemani RG, Randolph A, Markovitz B. Corticosteroids for the prevention and treatment of post-extubation stridor in neonates, children and adults. *Cochrane Database Syst Rev*. 2009;(3):CD001000.
35. Boles JM, Bion J, Connors A, et al. Weaning from mechanical ventilation. *Eur Respir J*. 2007;29:1033-1056.
36. Blackwood B, Burns KE, Cardwell CR, O'Halloran P. Protocolized versus non-protocolized weaning for reducing the duration of mechanical ventilation in critically ill adult patients. *Cochrane Database Syst Rev*. 2014;(11):CD006904.
37. Hess D. Ventilator modes used in weaning. *Chest*. 2001;120:474S-476S.
38. Burns KE, Meade MO, Premji A, Adhikari NK. Noninvasive positive-pressure ventilation as a weaning strategy for intubated adults with respiratory failure. *Cochrane Database Syst Rev*. 2013;(12):CD004127.
39. Nava S, Gregoretti C, Fanfulla F, et al. Noninvasive ventilation to prevent respiratory failure after extubation in high-risk patients. *Crit Care Med*. 2005;33:2465-2470.
40. Ferrer M, Sellares J, Valencia M, et al. Non-invasive ventilation after extubation in hypercapnic patients with chronic respiratory disorders: randomised controlled trial. *Lancet*. 2009;374:1082-1088.
41. Hernandez G, Vaquero C, Gonzalez P, et al. Effect of postextubation high-flow nasal cannula vs conventional oxygen therapy on reintubation in low-risk patients: a randomized clinical trial. *J Am Med Assoc*. 2016;315:1354-1361.
42. Maggiore SM, Idone FA, Vaschetto R, et al. Nasal high-flow versus Venturi mask oxygen therapy after extubation. Effects on oxygenation, comfort, and clinical outcome. *Am J Respir Crit Care Med*. 2014;190(3):282-288.
43. Hernandez G, Vaquero C, Colinas L, et al. Effect of postextubation high-flow nasal cannula vs noninvasive ventilation on reintubation and postextubation respiratory failure in high-risk patients: a randomized clinical trial. *J Am Med Assoc*. 2016;316:1565-1574.

CHAPTER 8

44. De Jonghe B, Sharshar T, Hopkinson N, Outin H. Paresis following mechanical ventilation. *Curr Opin Criti Care*. 2004;10:47-52.
45. Singer M, Deutschman CS, Seymour CW, et al. The third international consensus definitions for sepsis and septic shock (Sepsis-3). *J Am Med Assoc*. 2016;315:801-810.
46. Rivers E, Nguyen B, Havstad S, et al. Early goal-directed therapy in the treatment of severe sepsis and septic shock. *N Engl J Med*. 2001;345:1368-1377.
47. Levy MM, Evans LE, Rhodes A. The surviving sepsis campaign bundle: 2018 update. *Crit Care Med*. 2018;46:997-1000
48. Semler MW, Self WH, Wanderer JP, et al. Balanced crystalloids versus saline in critically ill adults. *N Engl J Med*. 2018;378:829-839.
49. Finfer S, Bellomo R, Boyce N, et al. A comparison of albumin and saline for fluid resuscitation in the intensive care unit. *N Engl J Med*. 2004;350(22):2247.
50. De Backer D, Biston P, Devriendt J, et al. Comparison of dopamine and norepinephrine in the treatment of shock. *N Engl J Med*. 2010;362:779-789.
51. Liu VX, Fielding-Singh V, Greene JD, et al. The timing of early antibiotics and hospital mortality in sepsis. *Am J Respir Crit Care Med*. 2017;196:856-863.
52. Marshall JC, Maier RV, Jimenez M, Dellinger EP. Source control in the management of severe sepsis and septic shock: an evidence-based review. *Crit Care Med*. 2004;32:S513-S526.
53. Pro CI, Yealy DM, Kellum JA, et al. A randomized trial of protocol-based care for early septic shock. *N Engl J Med*. 2014;370:1683-1693.
54. ARISE Investigators; ANZICS Clinical Trials Group; Peake SL, Delaney A, Bailey M, et al. Goal-directed resuscitation for patients with early septic shock. *N Engl J Med*. 2014;371:1496-1506.
55. Marty P, Roquilly A, Vallee F, et al. Lactate clearance for death prediction in severe sepsis or septic shock patients during the first 24 hours in Intensive Care Unit: an observational study. *Ann Intensive Care*. 2013;3:3.
56. Wacker C, Prkno A, Brunkhorst FM, Schlattmann P. Procalcitonin as a diagnostic marker for sepsis: a systematic review and meta-analysis. *Lancet Infect Dis*. 2013;13:426-435.
57. Schuetz P, Wirz Y, Sager R, et al. Procalcitonin to initiate or discontinue antibiotics in acute respiratory tract infections. *Cochrane Database Syst Rev*. 2017;(10):CD007498. doi:10.1002/14651858. CD007498.pub3
58. Russell JA, Walley KR, Singer J, et al. Vasopressin versus norepinephrine infusion in patients with septic shock. *N Engl J Med*. 2008;358:877-887.
59. Khanna A, English SW, Wang XS, et al. Angiotensin II for the treatment of vasodilatory shock. *N Engl J Med*. 2017;377:419-430.
60. Sprung CL, Annane D, Keh D, et al. Hydrocortisone therapy for patients with septic shock. *N Engl J Med*. 2008;358:111-124.
61. Venkatesh B, Finfer S, Cohen J, et al. Adjunctive glucocorticoid therapy in patients with septic shock. *N Engl J Med*. 2018;378:797-808.
62. Annane D, Renault A, Brun-Buisson, et al. Hydrocortisone plus fludrocortisone for adults with septic shock. *N Engl J Med*. 2018;378:809-818.
63. Paciullo CA, McMahon Horner D, Hatton KW, Flynn JD. Methylene blue for the treatment of septic shock. *Pharmacotherapy*. 2010;30:702-715.
64. Marik PE, Baram M, Vahid B. Does central venous pressure predict fluid responsiveness? A systematic review of the literature and the tale of seven mares. *Chest*. 2008;134:172-178.
65. Antonelli M, Levy M, Andrews PJ, et al. Hemodynamic monitoring in shock and implications for management. International Consensus Conference, Paris, France, 27–28 April 2006. *Intensive Care Med*. 2007;33:575-590.
66. Jones AE, Shapiro NI, Trzeciak S, et al.; Emergency Medicine Shock Research Network (EMShockNet) Investigators. Lactate clearance vs central venous oxygen saturation as goals of early sepsis therapy: a randomized clinical trial. *J Am Med Assoc*. 2010;303(8):739-746.
67. Richard C, Warszawski J, Anguel N, et al. Early use of the pulmonary artery catheter and outcomes in patients with shock and acute respiratory distress syndrome: a randomized controlled trial. *J Am Med Assoc*. 2003;290:2713-2720.
68. Dark PM, Singer M. The validity of trans-esophageal Doppler ultrasonography as a measure of cardiac output in critically ill adults. *Intensive Care Med*. 2004;30:2060-2066.
69. Monnet X, Rienzo M, Osman D, et al. Esophageal Doppler monitoring predicts fluid responsiveness in critically ill ventilated patients. *Intensive Care Med*. 2005;31:1195-1201.
70. Michard F, Boussat S, Chemla D, et al. Relation between respiratory changes in arterial pulse pressure and fluid responsiveness in septic patients with acute circulatory failure. *Am J Respir Crit Care Med*. 2000;162:134-138.
71. Barbier C, Loubieres Y, Schmit C, et al. Respiratory changes in inferior vena cava diameter are helpful in predicting fluid responsiveness in ventilated septic patients. *Intensive Care Med*. 2004;30:1740-1746.

72. Corl K, Napoli AM, Gardiner F. Bedside sonographic measurement of the inferior vena cava caval index is a poor predictor of fluid responsiveness in emergency department patients. *Emerg Med Australas.* 2012;24:534-539.
73. Kupersztych-Hagege E, Teboul JL, Artigas A, et al. Bioreactance is not reliable for estimating cardiac output and the effects of passive leg raising in critically ill patients. *Br J Anaesth.* 2013;111:961-966.
74. Benomar B, Ouattara A, Estagnasie P, et al. Fluid responsiveness predicted by noninvasive bioreactance-based passive leg raise test. *Intensive Care Med.* 2010;36:1875-1881.
75. Lichtenstein DA. Lung ultrasound in the critically ill. *Ann Intensive Care.* 2014;4:1.
76. Lichtenstein DA. Ultrasound in the management of thoracic disease. *Crit Care Med.* 2007;35:S250-S261.

9 Obstructive Lung Disease

James G. Krings, Laura Halverson,
Rodrigo Vazquez Guillamet, and Kaharu Sumino

Chronic Obstructive Pulmonary Disease

GENERAL PRINCIPLES

Definition

- Chronic obstructive pulmonary disease (COPD) is defined by the Global Initiative for Chronic Obstructive Lung Disease (GOLD) as a mostly preventable and treatable disorder characterized by an expiratory airflow limitation that is not fully reversible. Exposure to noxious particles and gases, as well as abnormalities in lung development, predisposes individuals to the development of COPD. The trajectory of the disease is variable and not necessarily progressive.
- Recently, there has been a suggestion to expand the diagnostic criteria of COPD from a single measure of lung function (expiratory airflow limitation) to include environmental exposure, symptoms, and abnormal findings on CT scans. There is now recognition that a COPD definition that solely relies on lung function misses patients in the early stages of the disease.
- **The airflow obstruction in COPD is caused by emphysema and airway disease.**
  - Emphysema is defined pathologically as permanent enlargement of air spaces distal to the terminal bronchiole accompanied by destruction of the alveolar walls and the absence of associated fibrosis. However, fibrosis can coexist with emphysema in a syndrome called combined pulmonary fibrosis and emphysema (CPFE).
  - The airway disease in COPD occurs primarily in small airways (i.e., those with an internal diameter of <2 mm). Chronic bronchitis is a common feature of COPD and is defined clinically as a productive cough, on most days, for at least 3 consecutive months per year and for at least 2 consecutive years, and in the absence of other lung diseases that could account for this symptom.
  - Emphysema and chronic bronchitis can be insidious and present in the absence of airflow obstruction. Even in the absence of airflow obstruction, COPD is still associated with adverse health outcomes.

Epidemiology

- Although the true prevalence of COPD is difficult to determine, COPD is estimated to affect approximately 15 million people in the US.
- Prior to the COVID-19 pandemic, COPD and other chronic lower respiratory diseases represented the third leading cause of death in the US.[1] In 2020, COVID-19 was the third leading underlying cause of death after heart disease and cancer, with COPD and chronic lower respiratory disease ranking sixth. The mortality rate for COPD has steadily increased since 2012, and globally the burden

remains high. The World Health Organization estimated that approximately 3.2 million deaths were caused by COPD in 2015, accounting for 5% of all worldwide deaths that year.

- COPD is protracted in time and is responsible for more years lived with disability (3.6%) than all other respiratory diseases combined.[1]

Etiology

- Most cases of COPD are attributable to **cigarette smoking** in the US.
- **Environmental and occupational dusts** (e.g., wood-burning stoves, fumes, gases, and chemicals) are other common causes of COPD worldwide. Household indoor air pollution is a major cause of fatal COPD, particularly in developing countries and rural areas.[2]
- **α1-Antitrypsin (A1AT) deficiency** is found in 1%–2% of COPD patients. Clinical characteristics of affected patients may include a minimal or nonexistent smoking history, early-onset COPD (e.g., younger than 45 years), a family history of lung disease, or lower lobe–predominant panacinar emphysema.

Pathophysiology

- The pathogenesis of COPD involves inflammation, immune reactions, imbalance of proteinases and antiproteinases, turnover of the extracellular matrix, oxidative stress, and apoptosis.
- Pathologic features include destruction of alveolar tissue and small airways, airway wall inflammation, edema and fibrosis, and intraluminal mucus.
- Pulmonary function changes include decreased maximal expiratory airflow, hyperinflation, air trapping, and alveolar gas exchange abnormalities.
- An increased incidence of osteoporosis, skeletal muscle dysfunction, and coronary artery disease occur in COPD, perhaps indicating a systemic component of inflammation.[3]

Prevention

- **In Western countries, abstinence from smoking is the most effective measure for preventing COPD.**
- Domestic biomass fuel smoke inhalation is responsible for COPD in nonsmoking patients in rural settings and developing countries, who sometimes have comparatively low cigarette smoking rates. Strategies aimed at improving access to cookstoves and cleaner fuel sources along with increased ventilation are essential in these populations (e.g., the Global Alliance for Clean Cookstoves has been established for this purpose).
- In patients with COPD, smoking cessation may result in a reduction in the rate of lung function decline and improved survival.[4,5]
- Tobacco cessation attempts warrant repeating until the patient stops smoking. Most smokers fail initial attempts at smoking cessation, and relapse reflects the nature of the nicotine dependence and not the failure of the patient or the physician.
- A multimodality approach is recommended to optimize smoking cessation.
  - Counseling on the preventable health risks of smoking, providing advice to stop smoking, and encouraging further attempts to stop smoking even after previous failures.
  - Providing smoking cessation materials to patients.
  - Prescribing pharmacotherapy (Table 9-1); providers should take every advantage to counsel and provide pharmacotherapy.
  - The US Department of Health and Human Services has developed a telephone-based support system (1-800-QUIT-NOW) with an Internet analog (smokefree.gov).

CHAPTER 9

TABLE 9-1	Pharmacotherapy for Smoking Cessation	
Product	Dosing	Side Effects/Precautions
Nicotine Replacement Therapy[a]		
Transdermal patch[b]	7, 14, or 21 mg/24 h Usual regimen = 21 mg/d = 6 wk, 14 mg/d × 2 wk, 7 mg/d × 2 wk	Headache, insomnia, night-mares, nausea, dizziness, blurred vision (applies to all nicotine products)
Chewing gum, lozenges	2–4 mg q1–8h Gradually taper use	
Inhaler	10 mg/cartridge (4 mg delivered dose) 6–16 cartridges/d	
Nasal spray	0.5 mg/spray 1–2 sprays in each nostril q1h	
Nonnicotine Pharmacotherapy		
Bupropion ER (*Zyban*)	150 mg/d × 3 d, then bid × 7–12 wk Start 1 wk before quit date	Dizziness, headache, insomnia, nausea, xerostomia, hypertension, seizure Avoid monoamine oxidase inhibitors
Varenicline (*Chantix*)	0.5 mg/d × 3 d, bid × 4 days, then 1 mg bid × 12–24 wk Start 1 wk before quit date	Nausea, vomiting, headache, insomnia, abnormal dreams Worsening of underlying psychiatric illness

[a]Combination therapy is often used. A long-acting product (e.g., patch) is used for basal nicotine replacement, with a short-acting product (e.g., inhaler or gum) used for breakthrough cravings.

[b]If patient smokes less than a half pack per day, start at 14-mg dose.

See also FioreMC, BakerTB. Clinical practice. Treating smokers in the health care setting. *N Engl J Med*. 2011;365:1222-1231 for strategies and approach.

DIAGNOSIS

Clinical Presentation

History

- Patients are usually older than 40 years at diagnosis.
- Clinicians should obtain a smoking history and quantify exposure to environmental and occupational risk factors. A family history of COPD, maternal tobacco use during pregnancy, and secondhand tobacco exposure also increase the risk of developing COPD.
- Common symptoms are dyspnea on exertion, cough, sputum production, and wheezing. Typically, dyspnea on exertion progresses gradually over years.
- Symptom presence and severity of COPD can be collected using standardized questionnaires like the COPD Assessment Test (CAT) (Table 9-2).
- Overlap with asthma, obstructive sleep apnea (OSA), bronchiectasis, and interstitial lung disease (ILD) exists.

TABLE 9-2	Chronic Obstructive Pulmonary Disease Assessment Tool (CAT)					
I never cough.	1	2	3	4	5	I cough all the time.
I have no phlegm or mucus in my chest.	1	2	3	4	5	My chest is completely full of mucus or phlegm.
My chest does not feel tight.	1	2	3	4	5	My chest feels tight.
When I walk up a hill or one flight of stairs, I am not breathless.	1	2	3	4	5	When I walk up a hill or one flight of stairs, I am very breathless.
I am not limited doing any activities at home.	1	2	3	4	5	I am limited doing activities at home.
I am confident leaving my home despite my lung condition.	1	2	3	4	5	I am not at all confident leaving my home because of my lung condition.
I sleep soundly.	1	2	3	4	5	I do not sleep soundly because of my lung condition.
I have lots of energy.	1	2	3	4	5	I have no energy at all.

Total score is sum of scores from individual question scales.
From Jones PW, Harding G, Berry P, et al. Development and first validation of the COPD Assessment Test. *Eur Respir J.* 2009;34:648-654. Reproduced with permission from GlaxoSmithKline. GlaxoSmithKline is the copyright owner of the COPD Assessment Test (CAT). However, third parties will be allowed to use the CAT free of charge. The CAT must always be used in its entirety. Except for limited reformatting the CAT may not be modified or combined with other instruments without prior written approval. The eight questions of the CAT must appear verbatim, in order, and together as they are presented and not divided on separate pages. All trademark and copyright information must be maintained as they appear on the bottom of the CAT and on all copies. The final layout of the final authorised CAT questionnaire may differ slightly but the item wording will not change. The CAT score is calculated as the sum of the responses present. If more than two responses are missing, a score cannot be calculated; when one or two items are missing their scores can be set to the average of the non-missing item scores.

- Beyond coexistence with other respiratory disease, patients with COPD frequently have comorbidities that impact quality of life and prognosis. Osteoporosis, anxiety, depression, cardiovascular disease, tobacco related malignancies, malnutrition, and diabetes are all more common than expected among patients with COPD. Symptoms related to comorbidities should be investigated.[3]
- As the disease advances, cause-specific mortality for patients with COPD shifts from cardiovascular disease and malignancies in the early stages to respiratory failure. Both severe airflow obstruction and a high frequency of exacerbations increase the likelihood of a respiratory death.[6]
- Disease severity should be established using multidimensional tools such as the **B**ody mass index, airflow **O**bstruction, **D**yspnea, and **E**xercise capacity (BODE) index (Table 9-3). The BODE index has been validated as a more accurate predictor of COPD mortality than forced expiratory volume in 1 second (FEV_1) alone.[7,8]
- A novel definition of COPD is currently being examined as introduced through the COPDGene Study.[9] The use of environmental exposures (e.g., smoking), symptoms (e.g., shortness of breath, chronic cough, and phlegm production), structural abnormalities on CT scans (e.g., emphysema, gas trapping, and airway wall thickness),

TABLE 9-3	Body Mass Index, Airflow Obstruction, Dyspnea, and Exercise Capacity Index			
	Points			
	0	1	2	3
FEV$_1$% predicted	≥65	50–64	36–49	≤35
6MWT (m)	250	250–349	150–249	≤149
mMRC dyspnea scale	0–1	2	3	4
BMI (kg/m^2)	≥21	<21		

A total score is calculated by adding all the variables. The result provides estimates of 4-year survival: 1 point = 80%, 4 points = 67%, 7 points = 18%. 6MWT, 6-minute walk test; BMI, body mass index; FEV$_1$%, forced expiratory volume in the first second percent predicted; mMRC, modified Medical Research Council. In the absence of a 6MWT, the BODEX index can be calculated substituting 6MWT for number of exacerbations with similar predictive value up to a score of 5.

and lung function or spirometry (e.g., FEV$_1$, forced vital capacity [FVC]) are used in combination to identify those with possible, probable, or definite COPD. In this study, smokers diagnosed with COPD, but who would not have previously met the definition of COPD based on spirometry alone, were more likely to experience lung function decline and death within 5 years.

Physical Examination
• By the time physical examination findings of COPD are present, the disease is usually at an advanced stage (e.g., FEV$_1$ < 50% predicted).
• On inspection, pursed lip breathing, barrel chest secondary to hyperinflation, use of accessory muscles of respiration, and central and peripheral cyanosis can be present.
• Palpation should focus on supraclavicular and axillary lymphadenopathies, the presence of abdominal hernias, abdominal aortic aneurysms, and the presence and quality of peripheral pulses.
• Percussion is hyperresonant in advanced emphysema. Diaphragmatic excursion can be reduced due to hyperinflation.
• Auscultation in severe COPD may expose prolonged (i.e., >6 seconds) breath sounds on a maximal forced exhalation and decreased breath sounds. Expiratory wheezing and rhonchi may or may not be present.
• Signs of pulmonary hypertension and right-sided heart failure may be present, and heart sounds may be muffled from the interposed hyperinflated lungs.
• **Clubbing is not a feature of COPD** alone, so its presence should prompt an evaluation for other conditions, especially lung cancer.
• Given the high incidence of cardiovascular comorbidities, an evaluation for signs of arrhythmias and decompensated heart failure is also paramount. Abnormalities of cardiac auscultation or significant lower extremity edema should trigger further investigation.

Differential Diagnosis
• Obesity hypoventilation syndrome is commonly misdiagnosed as COPD in patients admitted to the hospital with acute hypercapnic respiratory syndrome.
• Debut presentation to the hospital with acute hypercapnic respiratory failure is common. In this scenario, pulmonary function tests (PFTs) are often not available and

a careful evaluation of the clinical history, physical examination including bedside ultrasound, CT, and physiologic measurements while on mechanical ventilation (e.g., airway resistance, auto-PEEP [positive end-expiratory pressure]) can help narrow the differential diagnosis.[9-11] On discharge, all such patients should be referred for PFTs.

Diagnostic Testing

Consider the diagnosis of COPD in any patient with chronic cough, dyspnea, or sputum production and a history of exposure to COPD risk factors, especially cigarette smoking.

Pulmonary Function Testing

- A definitive diagnosis of COPD requires the presence of expiratory airflow limitation on postbronchodilator spirometry, measured using the FEV_1/FVC ratio, after 400 μg of albuterol is administered. Although a ratio of 0.7 is taken as the lower limit of normal for all adults, with advancing age, the ratio may decrease below 0.7 in individuals who are asymptomatic and have never smoked. Therefore, a reduced ratio should not be interpreted automatically as diagnostic of COPD.
- The postbronchodilator FEV_1 relative to the predicted normal defines the severity of expiratory airflow obstruction (Table 9-4) and is an independent predictor of COPD-associated mortality.
- The total lung capacity, functional residual capacity, and residual volume often increase to supranormal values in patients with COPD, indicating lung hyperinflation and air trapping.
- The diffusing capacity for carbon monoxide (DLCO) may be reduced in patients with emphysema.
- The 6-minute walk test is a submaximal exercise test. The distance covered by the patient is one of the components of many multidimensional mortality prediction tools. It can also unmask exercise-induced hypoxemia and muscle dysfunction. Healthy individuals will generally cover >450 m.

Laboratory Studies

- A baseline arterial blood gas (ABG) is recommended for patients with severe COPD to assess for the presence and severity of hypoxemia and hypercapnia. Annual monitoring may be considered.
- Elevated venous bicarbonate may signify chronic hypercapnia.

TABLE 9-4	Classification of Severity of Airflow Limitation in Chronic Obstructive Pulmonary Disease (Based on Postbronchodilator FEV_1)	
In Patients With FEV_1/FVC <0.70:		
GOLD 1	Mild	$FEV_1 \geq 80\%$ predicted
GOLD 2	Moderate	$50\% \leq FEV_1 < 80\%$ predicted
GOLD 3	Severe	$30\% \leq FEV_1 < 50\%$ predicted
GOLD 4	Very severe	$FEV_1 < 30\%$ predicted

Reprinted from the *Global Strategy for Diagnosis, Management, and Prevention of COPD*; 2021. © Global Initiative for Chronic Obstructive Lung Disease (GOLD), all rights reserved. Available from http://www.goldcopd.com
FEV_1, forced expiratory volume in 1 second; FVC, forced vital capacity; GOLD, Global Initiative for Chronic Obstructive Lung Disease.

- Polycythemia may reflect a physiologic response to chronic hypoxemia and inadequate supplemental oxygen use.
- Peripheral eosinophils >300 cells/μL support the initial use of an inhaled corticosteroid (ICS).
- A1AT levels: Because of its prognostic implications, unique set of comorbidities (e.g., liver disease), and the availability of A1AT replacement therapy, all COPD patients should be screened at least once for A1AT deficiency.[12]

Imaging
- CXRs are not sensitive for determining the presence of COPD, but they are useful for evaluating alternative diagnoses and to establish a baseline.
- Chest CT without contrast can detect emphysema, changes in airway wall thickness, air trapping, and other conditions associated with tobacco smoking and COPD, such as lung cancer or atherosclerosis (see "Treatment" section). Symptomatic smokers with normal spirometry will often have CT abnormalities as listed above to explain their symptoms.
- With increasing severity of COPD, patients often develop radiographic signs of thoracic hyperinflation, including flattening of the diaphragm, increased retrosternal/retrocardiac air spaces, and lung hyperlucency with diminished vascular markings. Bullae may be visible. In severe disease, chest CT is used to determine candidacy for lung volume reduction surgery (LVRS) (see "Maximizing lung function" in "Treatment" section).

TREATMENT

- Long-term management of patients with COPD aims to improve quality of life, decrease the frequency and severity of acute exacerbations, slow the progression of disease, and prolong survival. These goals are pursued by decreasing exposures to noxious agents; maximizing lung function; maximizing/supplementing compensatory mechanisms; diagnosing and managing comorbidities; and implementing exacerbation prevention strategies.
- **Decreasing exposure to noxious agents**
  - Smoking cessation as detailed above (prevention).
  - Avoidance of biomass fuels at home and at work (e.g., avoiding the use of coal and wood to heat and cook).
  - Using personal protective equipment during activities that produce dust and fumes.
  - Improving ventilation and avoiding the use of caustic chemicals in home cleaning, hobbies, etc.
- **Maximizing lung function**
  - Bronchodilators
    - The inhaled route maximizes drug levels in the airways and helps reduce systemic toxicities.
    - Inhaled bronchodilators work primarily by relaxing airway smooth muscle tone. This results in a reduction in expiratory airflow obstruction. Inhaled bronchodilators can be long-acting (e.g., muscarinic antagonists [LAMAs], β$_2$-agonists [LABAs]) or short-acting (e.g., muscarinic antagonists and β$_2$-agonists [SABAs]).
    - LAMAs and LABAs alone and in combination result in improvements in lung function, reductions in COPD exacerbations, and improvements in quality of life.[13,14] However, they do not slow the rate of lung function decline and do not improve survival.

- ○ ICS
  - ICS are not recommended as monotherapy in COPD. Initial combination therapy with ICS/LABA can be considered in patients with peripheral eosinophil counts >300 cells/μL.[15]
  - ICS can be used in patients already on LAMA/LABA who have continued frequent COPD exacerbations, blood eosinophil counts >300 cells/μL, or a history of asthma.
  - ICS withdrawal should be considered in patients with a history of <2 exacerbations in a year, no COPD-related hospitalizations, and an eosinophil count < 300 cells/μL.[16]
- ○ Initial inhaled therapy
  - In the latest GOLD statement, initial inhaled therapy is based on symptoms and history of exacerbations and *not* on the severity of airflow obstruction. Four groups, A, B, C, and D, are defined as outlined in Table 9-5.
  - Recommended initial therapy: Group A, a bronchodilator; Group B, a LABA or LAMA; Group C, a LAMA; and Group D, a LAMA. For Group D with CAT > 20, combination LABA and LAMA is recommended. If group D and eosinophils >300 cells/μL, consider ICS plus LABA.
  - Table 9-6 lists commonly available inhaled bronchodilators.
  - Providers should routinely assess a patient's inhaler technique and provide teaching.
- ○ Bronchoscopic and LVRS
  - In selected patients, LVRS or bronchoscopic lung volume reduction (such as using a one-way endobronchial valve) can improve FEV_1, oxygenation, and functional outcomes. With these procedures, total thoracic lung volume is reduced, heathier lung is preferentially ventilated and perfused, and respiratory muscles may become more effective at ventilation. In a very carefully selected group of patients, LVRS may be associated with a survival benefit.[17]

TABLE 9-5	Refined ABCD Assessment Tool for Chronic Obstructive Lung Disease
Group	Description
A	0–1 exacerbations, no hospitalizations, minimal symptoms: mMRC 0–1 or CAT <10
B	0–1 exacerbations, no hospitalizations, moderate to severe symptoms: mMRC ≥2 or CAT ≥10
C	>2 exacerbations or >1 hospitalization, minimal symptoms: mMRC 0–1 or CAT <10
D	>2 exacerbations or >1 hospitalization, moderate to severe symptoms: mMRC ≥2 or CAT ≥10

Data from the *Global Strategy for Diagnosis, Management, and Prevention of COPD*; 2021. © Global Initiative for Chronic Obstructive Lung Disease (GOLD).
CAT, COPD Assessment Test; mMRC, modified Medical Research Council Dyspnea Scale.
Initiative for chronic obstructive lung disease. Recommended initial therapy: Group A, a bronchodilator; Group B, a long-acting β₂-agonist or long-acting muscarinic antagonist; Group C, a long-acting muscarinic antagonist; and Group D, a long-acting muscarinic antagonist. For Group D with CAT >20, combination long-acting β₂-agonist and long-acting muscarinic antagonist. If group D and eosinophils >300 cells/μL, consider inhaled corticosteroid plus long-acting β₂-agonist.

CHAPTER 9

TABLE 9-6	Inhaler Pharmacotherapy for Chronic Asthma and Chronic Obstructive Pulmonary Disease[a]	
Name	**Dose**	**Side Effects[b]**
Short-Acting β_2-Agonists and Muscarinic Antagonists (SABA and SAMA)		
Albuterol (*ProAir, Ventolin, Proventil*)	MDI: 2 inh q4–6h Nebulizer: 2.5 mg q6–8h	Palpitations, tremor, anxiety, nausea/vomiting, throat irritation, dyspepsia, tachycardia, arrhythmia, hypertension
Levalbuterol (*Xopenex*)	MDI: 2 inh q4–6h Nebulizer: 0.63–1.25 mg q6–8h	Cardiovascular effects may be less common with levalbuterol
Ipratropium[c] (*Atrovent*)	MDI: 2 inh q4–6h Nebulizer: 0.5 mg q6–8h	Xerostomia, cough, nausea/vomiting, diarrhea, urinary retention
Albuterol/ipratropium (*Combivent Respimat, DuoNeb*)	SMI: 1–2 inh q6h Nebulizer: 1 vial (3 mL) qid	As above for each individual medication
Long-Acting β_2-Agonists (LABA)		
Salmeterol (*Serevent Diskus*)	DPI: 1 inh bid	Headache, upper respiratory tract infection, cough, palpitations, fatigue, diarrhea
Olodaterol (*Striverdi*)	2 inh q24h	
Long-Acting Muscarinic Antagonists (LAMA)		
Umeclidinium (*Incruse*)	DPI: 1 inh q24h	Xerostomia, cough, nausea/vomiting, diarrhea, urinary retention
Tiotropium (*Spiriva*)	DPI: 1 inh q24h	
Combination Inhaled Corticosteroid (ICS)/LABA		
Fluticasone/salmeterol (*Advair Diskus, Advair HFA, Wixela Inhub, AirDuo*)	Advair DPI: 1 inh bid Advair HFA: 1 inh bid Wixela: 1 inh bid AirDuo: 1 inh bid	As above, plus lower respiratory tract infection (pneumonia) and oral candidiasis
Budesonide/formoterol (*Symbicort*)	DPI: 2 inh bid	
Mometasone/formoterol (*Dulera*)	HFA: 2 inh bid	
Fluticasone/vilanterol (*Breo*)	DPI: 1 inh q24h	
Combination LABA/LAMA		
Umeclidinium/vilanterol (*Anoro*)	DPI: 1 inh q24h	As above for each individual medication class
Tiotropium/olodaterol (*Stiolto*)	SMI: 2 inh q24h	

TABLE 9-6	Inhaler Pharmacotherapy for Chronic Asthma and Chronic Obstructive Pulmonary Disease[a] *(continued)*	
Name	Dose	Side Effects[b]
Triple Combination (ICS–LAMA–LABA)		
Fluticasone/umeclidinium/vilanterol (*Trelegy Ellipta*	DPI: 1 inh q24h	As above for each individual medication class
Budesonide/glycopyrrolate/formoterol (*Breztri*)	MDI: 2 inh bid	

DPI, dry powder inhaler; inh, inhalation(s); MDI, metered-dose inhaler; SMI, soft mist inhaler.
[a]Table is not exhaustive and only lists some commonly prescribed inhalers. Inhaled corticosteroid (ICS) monotherapy inhalers are listed in the "Asthma" section in Table 9-14.
[b]Only the most common side effects are listed.
[c]Short-acting anticholinergic therapy (e.g., ipratropium) is usually discontinued with initiation of long-acting anticholinergic therapy (e.g., tiotropium), because minimal additional benefit is expected, side effects may increase, and use of two inhaled anticholinergic agents has had limited evaluation.

- Lung transplantation
  - Lung transplantation in COPD is reserved for patients with advanced disease (BODE >7) and nonfatal comorbidities. Single and double lung transplant procedures can be performed in COPD with better long-term survival for double-lung transplantation.[18] Transplantation is rare in patients older than 75 years.
  - Quality of life improves significantly for the vast majority of appropriately selected patients.[19]
  - Median survival after transplantation is approximately 6 years. Importantly, survival is improved for some but not all patients with COPD after lung transplantation.[20]
- **Maximizing/supplementing compensatory mechanisms**
  - Exercise training
    - When possible, exercise should be performed in the setting of a **pulmonary rehabilitation** program.
    - All patients being discharged from the hospital for a COPD exacerbation, at initial diagnosis, and prior to LVRS or lung transplantation should be referred to a pulmonary rehabilitation program.
    - Exercise training consists of aerobic exercise at 60%–80% of maximal exercise capacity. High intensity interval training can help achieve similar workloads in patients with limited mobility and exercise tolerance. Upper extremity strength training helps improve upper extremity specific task performance (e.g., laundry, doing dishes).[21]
  - Supplemental oxygen
    - Oxygen supplementation improves survival and quality of life and reduces exacerbations.
    - The current **indications for oxygen therapy** in COPD are as follows:
      - PaO_2 ≤55 mm Hg or SpO_2 ≤88% at rest.
      - PaO_2 56–59 mm Hg or SpO_2 <89% if there is right heart failure, cor pulmonale, or erythrocytosis with a hematocrit >55%.

CHAPTER 9

- In patients with moderate resting desaturation (i.e., SpO_2 89%–93%) or exercise-induced desaturation (i.e., $SpO_2 \geq 80\%$ for ≥5 minutes and <90% for ≥10 seconds), oxygen therapy did not improve mortality in a recent clinical trial.[22]
- In patients with nocturnal desaturations but without sleep-disordered breathing or severe daytime hypoxemia, nocturnal oxygen therapy does not improve survival.[23]

○ Noninvasive positive pressure ventilation

The use of nocturnal noninvasive positive pressure ventilation in patients with a resting $paCO_2 \geq 52$ mm Hg improves dyspnea, exercise capacity, time to hospital readmission, and possibly survival in small randomized controlled trials and uncontrolled case series.[24,25]

○ Nutritional supplementation

- Malnutrition, usually measured by the body mass index (BMI), is associated with increased mortality. Nutritional advice can be obtained as a part of most **pulmonary rehabilitation** programs.
- Small frequent meals and resting before eating can alleviate meal-induced dyspnea.
- Supplementation with 120 mL of dietary supplements three times daily can improve BMI, exercise tolerance, and quality of life in advanced COPD.[26]

- **Management of comorbidities**
  ○ Population-based studies reveal a diagnosis of COPD as a major event in a patient's trajectory, that is often followed by the occurrence of multiple complications and the diagnosis of many comorbidities.
  ○ Providers should screen for and manage frequently encountered comorbidities following general guidelines without significant deviation.
  ○ β-Blockers, used in the management of heart failure and coronary artery disease among others, are not contraindicated in patients with COPD.
  ○ The presence of atrial arrhythmias should not generally alter inhaler selection with the exception of avoiding high-dose SABA and systemic theophylline.
  ○ Intermittent claudication secondary to peripheral vascular disease is a common contributor to low exercise capacity.
  ○ Coronary artery disease and heart failure can mimic COPD exacerbations.
  ○ **Lung cancer screening**
    - Updated US Preventive Services Task Force guidelines in 2021 recommend current smokers or those who quit during the past 15 years, have a cumulative smoking history of ≥20 pack-years, and are also between the ages of 50 and 80 years undergo low-dose CT lung cancer screening as it has been associated with improved survival.[27]
    - Screening CTs should be discontinued once a person has not smoked for 15 years or if they develop a health problem that limits life expectancy or the ability to tolerate treatment targeted at a diagnosed lung cancer.
  ○ Overlap with other respiratory diseases:
    - Patients with clinical, historical, and spirometric evidence of an asthma overlap (e.g., bronchodilator response >15% or 400 mL for FEV_1, personal history of asthma, peripheral eosinophilia) may be considered to have asthma–COPD overlap (ACO) and should have treatment that addresses the predominant disease entity (e.g., if they have predominant asthma, treat as asthma; if predominant COPD, treat as COPD; and if features of both, start treatment as asthma pending further investigation).[28]

- In patients with ILD overlap, the prognosis is usually determined by the underlying ILD.
- Overlap with bronchiectasis may benefit from therapies aimed at improving airway clearance and avoidance of ICSs.
- **Exacerbation prevention strategies**
  - Consistent use of inhaled therapies, avoidance of noxious exposures, diagnosis and management of comorbidities, exercise training, nutritional support, oxygen and ventilatory support are necessary to prevent exacerbations and their complications.
  - **Vaccinations**
    - All patients with COPD should receive influenza vaccination yearly preferably with killed or live inactivated viruses.
    - One dose of pneumococcal vaccine (PPSV23) should be administered before the age of 65 years and a second dose after the age of 65 years (and at least 5 years after the first dose).
    - Pneumococcal vaccines (PCV13) are recommended for all patients older than 65 years or in younger patients in the presence of immunocompromising conditions or immunosuppression.[29]
    - PCV13 and PPSV23 should not be administered during the same visit.
    - If both PCV13 and PPSV23 are to be administered, PCV13 should be administered first.
    - PCV13 and PPSV23 should be administered at least 1 year apart unless they are being administered to an immunocompromised patient in which case they can be administered 8 weeks apart.[30]
    - COVID-19 vaccination is recommended to all patients with COPD.[31]
  - **Macrolide antibiotics** (e.g., azithromycin 250 mg daily)
    - It may function as an anti-infective or direct anti-inflammatory in COPD.
    - In patients with previous exacerbations, the frequency of subsequent exacerbations is decreased by 19%; however, improvement in clinical symptoms was modest.[32]
    - The benefit may be absent in current smokers and greater in older individuals (>65 years) and those with milder disease (FEV_1 >50%).
    - Hearing loss in the absence of tinnitus was reported, suggesting routine monitoring with audiometry should be considered with chronic therapy.
  - **Phosphodiesterase-4 inhibitors** (e.g., roflumilast 500 μg daily)
    - The US Food and Drug Administration (FDA) approved for a relatively narrow indication of severe COPD (FEV_1 <50%) and chronic bronchitis with frequent exacerbations, demonstrating a 17% reduction in exacerbations.[33]
    - It appears to be safe when used as additional therapy to chronic bronchodilators.
    - It did not result in improvements in clinical symptoms possibly due to a higher frequency of side effects, particularly gastrointestinal, which limit the dose tolerated.
    - Limited long-term data and the possibility of weight loss and increased psychiatric symptoms suggest that close monitoring is indicated.
  - **Theophylline** (200–300 mg twice daily in sustained release tablets)
    - Theophylline is a xanthine derivative with bronchodilator properties. High-risk patients not responding adequately to dual inhaled bronchodilator therapy may benefit from the addition of theophylline.
    - Theophylline is generally not recommended due to limited efficacy, a narrow therapeutic margin, and multiple drug interactions.
    - Patients with severe COPD may experience clinical deterioration with discontinuation of theophylline.

- Theophylline clearance is increased in current smokers and reduced in the elderly and patients with liver disease or congestive heart failure.
  - **Systemic corticosteroids** are not recommended for the long-term management of COPD owing to an unfavorable side effect profile and limited efficacy. However, they are sometimes used in patients with severe disease who are not responding to other therapies. If used, chronic oral steroid therapy should be administered at the minimum effective dose and discontinued as soon as is feasible. Routine bone mineral density assessment to prevent complications of osteoporosis should be incorporated.
  - IV A1AT augmentation therapy may benefit select patients with severe A1AT deficiency and COPD.[34] Weekly infusion of 60 mg/kg is the standard treatment.

SPECIAL CONSIDERATIONS

Acute Exacerbation of COPD

- A COPD exacerbation is defined as increased dyspnea, often accompanied by increased cough, sputum production, sputum purulence, wheezing, chest tightness, or other symptoms (and signs) of acutely worsened respiratory status, in the absence of an alternative explanation.[35]
- Respiratory infections (viral and bacterial) and air pollution cause most exacerbations.
- The differential diagnosis includes pneumothorax, pneumonia, pleural effusion, congestive heart failure, cardiac ischemia, and pulmonary embolism.
- In addition to the history and physical examination, assessment of a patient with a suspected COPD exacerbation should include oxyhemoglobin saturation, ABG, ECG, and CXR.
- Criteria for hospital admission include a significant increase in symptom severity, severe underlying COPD, significant comorbidities, failure to respond to initial medical management, diagnostic uncertainty, and insufficient home support.
- Criteria for admission to an intensive care unit include the need for invasive mechanical ventilation, hemodynamic instability, severe dyspnea that does not adequately respond to therapy, mental status changes, and persistent or worsening hypoxemia, hypercapnia, or respiratory acidosis despite supplemental oxygen and noninvasive ventilation (NIV).
- **Pharmacotherapy** (Table 9-7)
  - **SABAs are the first-line therapy for COPD exacerbations.** Short-acting anticholinergic agents can be added in the event of inadequate response to SABAs.
  - Many patients experiencing an acute exacerbation of COPD have difficulty performing optimal metered-dose inhaler (MDI) technique. Therefore, numerous clinicians opt to deliver bronchodilators via nebulization.
  - Long-acting bronchodilators should be considered once stable.
  - Owing to the risk of serious side effects, clinicians typically avoid using methylxanthines (e.g., theophylline) for acute exacerbations. However, if a patient uses methylxanthines chronically, discontinuation during an exacerbation is discouraged because of the risk of decompensation.
  - **Systemic corticosteroids** produce improvement in hospital length of stay, lung function, and the incidence of relapse. They are recommended for all inpatients and most outpatients experiencing an exacerbation of COPD. A prednisone dose of 40 mg for 5 days is recommended over longer regimens.[36]

TABLE 9-7	Pharmacotherapy for Acute Exacerbations of Chronic Obstructive Pulmonary Disease	
Medication Name	**Dose**	
Albuterol	MDI: two to four puffs q1–4h Nebulizer: 2.5 mg q1–4h	
Ipratropium	MDI: two puffs q4h Nebulizer: 0.5 mg q4h	
Prednisone	40 mg/d × 5 d	
Antibiotics[a]		
Patient Characteristics	Pathogens to Consider	Antibiotic[b] (One of the Following)
No risk factors for poor outcome or drug-resistant pathogen[c]	*Haemophilus influenzae* *Streptococcus pneumoniae* *Moraxella catarrhalis*	Macrolide, second- or third-generation cephalosporin, doxycycline, trimethoprim/sulfamethoxazole
Risk factors present	As above, plus gram-negative rods, including *Pseudomonas*	Antipseudomonal fluoroquinolone or β-lactam

MDI, metered-dose inhaler.

[a]Reprinted from the Global Strategy for Diagnosis, Management, and Prevention of COPD; 2021. © Global Initiative for Chronic Obstructive Lung Disease (GOLD), all rights reserved. Available from http://www.goldcopd.com.[1]

[b]Treat for 3–7 days. If recent antibiotic exposure, select an agent from an alternative class. Take local resistance patterns into account.

[c]Risk factors: age >65 years, comorbid conditions (especially cardiac disease), forced expiratory volume in 1 second (FEV_1) <50%, more than three exacerbations/year, and antibiotic therapy within the past 3 months.

- **Antibiotic therapy** is routinely administered but most often benefits patients with sputum purulence as well as patients with a need for mechanical ventilation. Duration of therapy should be 5–7 days. Antibiotic choice should be guided by local resistance patterns, previous patient exposures, and severity of COPD.
- **Supplemental oxygen** should be administered with a target oxygen saturation of 88%–92%.
- **Thromboprophylactic measures** should be used given the increased risk of deep venous thrombosis in patients hospitalized for COPD exacerbations.[37]
- **NIV** (Table 9-8) should be considered the first mode of ventilator support as it reduces intubation rate, improves respiratory acidosis, decreases respiratory rate, and decreases hospital length of stay.
- **Endotracheal intubation** and invasive mechanical ventilation are required in some patients (Table 9-9).
- Discharge criteria for patients with acute exacerbations of COPD include the need for inhaled bronchodilators less frequently than every 4 hours; clinical and ABG stability for at least 12–24 hours; the ability to eat, sleep, and ambulate fairly comfortably; adequate patient understanding of home therapy; and adequate home arrangements. Before discharging from the hospital, chronic therapy issues should be readdressed, including supplemental oxygen requirements, vaccinations, smoking cessation, assessment of inhaler technique, and referral to pulmonary rehabilitation.

CHAPTER 9

TABLE 9-8	Indications and Contraindications for Noninvasive Ventilation in Acute Exacerbations of Chronic Obstructive Pulmonary Disease
Indications	**Contraindications**
Moderate to severe dyspnea with evidence of increased work of breathing	Respiratory arrest
	Hemodynamic instability
	Altered mental status, inability to cooperate
Acute respiratory acidosis with pH ≤7.35 and/or $PaCO_2$ >45 mm Hg (6 kPa)	High risk of aspiration
	Viscous or copious secretions
	Recent facial or gastroesophageal surgery
Respiratory rate >25/min	Craniofacial trauma
	Fixed nasopharyngeal abnormalities
	Burns
	Extreme obesity

Data from the *Global Strategy for Diagnosis, Management, and Prevention of COPD*; 2021. © Global Initiative for Chronic Obstructive Lung Disease (GOLD).

TABLE 9-9	Indications for Invasive Mechanical Ventilation in Acute Exacerbations of Chronic Obstructive Pulmonary Disease
Failure to improve with or not a candidate for noninvasive ventilation (see Table 9-8)	
Severe dyspnea with evidence of increased work of breathing	
Acute respiratory acidosis with pH <7.25 and/or $PaCO_2$ >60 mm Hg (8 kPa)	
PaO_2 <40 mm Hg (5.3 kPa)	
Respiratory rate >35/min	
Coexisting conditions such as cardiovascular disease, metabolic abnormalities, sepsis, pneumonia, pulmonary embolism, pneumothorax, and large pleural effusion	

Data from the *Global Strategy for Diagnosis, Management, and Prevention of COPD*; 2021. © Global Initiative for Chronic Obstructive Lung Disease (GOLD).

Asthma

GENERAL PRINCIPLES

Definition

- Asthma is a common airway disease characterized by chronic airway inflammation and variable obstruction wherein patients frequently have paroxysms of cough, dyspnea, chest tightness, and wheezing.
- **Patients with asthma frequently have episodic acute exacerbations that are interspersed with periods of symptomatic variability.** Exacerbations are characterized by a progressive increase in asthma symptoms that can last minutes to hours and are frequently associated with viral infections, allergens, and occupational exposures.

Classification

- When treating asthma, severity should be carefully classified by the clinician based on both level of impairment (symptoms, lung function, daily activities, and rescue medication use) and risk (exacerbations, lung function decline, and medication side effects).
- At the initial clinical evaluation, a clinician should determine a patient's asthma severity level. If the patient is not already on controller medications, severity is determined based on the most severe category in which any feature appears (Table 9-10). On subsequent visits, or if the patient is already on a controller medication at the initial encounter, severity is based on the lowest step of therapy required to maintain clinical control (Table 9-11).
- The severity of an asthma exacerbation should be classified based on symptoms, signs, and objective measures of lung function (Table 9-12).
- While the majority of patients with asthma can achieve disease control with controller therapy, approximately 5% of patients with asthma have severe persistent disease that remains inadequately controlled despite adherence to standard treatments. These patients carry a significant amount of the morbidity, mortality, and healthcare utilization that is associated with asthma.

Epidemiology

In the US
- Asthma is highly prevalent affecting more than 300 million people worldwide and approximately 8% of the American population.[38]
- The prevalence of asthma is highest among African-Americans, is inversely associated with socioeconomic status, and is a well-recognized health inequity in the US.[39]

Etiology

Possible factors associated with asthma development can be broadly divided into host, genetic, and environmental factors.
- There have been multiple genes, chromosomal regions, and epigenetic changes associated with the development of asthma. Racial and ethnic differences have also been reported in asthma and are likely the result of a complex interaction between genetic, socioeconomic, and environmental factors.
- There are multiple environmental factors that contribute to the development and persistence of asthma. Severe viral infections early in life, particularly respiratory syncytial virus and rhinovirus, are associated with the development of asthma in childhood and play a role in its pathogenesis.
- Childhood exposure and sensitization to a variety of aeroallergens and irritants (e.g., cigarette smoke, mold, pet dander, dust mites, cockroaches) may play a role in the development of asthma, but the exact nature of this relationship is not yet fully elucidated. By contrast, early-life exposure to indoor allergens together with certain bacteria (microbiota) may be protective for urban children. The prevalence of asthma in children raised in a rural setting is reduced, although the reason for this is not fully known.

Pathophysiology

Asthma is characterized by variable airflow obstruction, hyperinflation, and airflow limitation resulting from multiple processes including the following:
- Acute and chronic airway inflammation characterized by infiltration of the airway wall, mucosa, and lumen by activated eosinophils, mast cells, macrophages, and T lymphocytes. Components of innate immunity including natural killer T cells, neutrophils, and innate lymphoid lymphocytes are also implicated.

CHAPTER 9

TABLE 9-10   Classification of Asthma Severity on Initial Assessment

	Intermittent	Mild Persistent	Moderate Persistent	Severe Persistent
Daytime symptoms	≤2 d/wk	≥2 d/wk but not daily	Daily	Throughout the day
Nighttime symptoms	≤2x/mo	3–4x/mo	≥1x/wk but not nightly	Nightly
Activity limitations	None	Minor	Some	Extreme
Reliever medicine use	≤2 d/wk	≥2 d/wk but not daily	Daily	Several times per day
FEV$_1$	≥80%	≥80%	60%–80%	<60%
Exacerbations	0–1x/y	≥2x/y	≥2x/y	≥2x/y
Management	Step 1	Step 2	Step 3	Step 4	Step 5
Preferred	SABA as needed or low-dose ICS + rapid onset LABA as needed	Low-dose ICS + SABA as needed or low-dose ICS + rapid onset LABA as needed	Low-dose ICS-LABA or medium-dose ICS with SABA as needed	Medium- or high-dose ICS + LABA	Add-on therapy: i.e., anti-IL-5/α, anti-IL-4α, omalizumab
Alternative	Low-dose ICS + SABA as needed	Low-dose ICS + SABA as needed or daily LTRA	Low-dose ICS with LTRA	High-dose ICS + LTRA or theophylline	Consider LAMA, short-course OCS, chronic macrolide, bronchial thermoplasty

In 2–6 wk, evaluate level of asthma control and adjust therapy accordingly.

Data from the 2020 GINA Report: Global Strategy for Asthma Management and Prevention. Global Initiative for Asthma – GINA. Updated 2020. Accessed February 24, 2021. https://ginasthma.org/gina-reports/ and NAEPP Third Expert Panel on the Diagnosis and Management of Asthma. https://www.jacionline.org/action/showPdf?pii=S0091-6749%2820%2931404-4. Accessed February 24, 2021.

FEV$_1$, forced expiratory volume in 1 second; ICS, inhaled corticosteroid; IL, interleukin; LABA, long-acting β$_2$-agonist; LAMA, long-acting muscarinic antagonist; LTRA, leukotriene receptor antagonist; OCS, oral corticosteroid; SABA, short-acting β$_2$-agonist.

TABLE 9-11	Assessment of Asthma Control		
	Well Controlled	Not Well Controlled	Very Poorly Controlled
Daytime symptoms	≤2 d/wk	>2 d/wk	Throughout the day
Nighttime symptoms	None	1–3×/wk	≥4×/wk
Activity limitations	None	Some	Extreme
Reliever medicine use	≤2×/wk	>2×/wk	Frequent
FEV_1 or PEF	≥80%	60%–80%	<60%
Validated questionnaire	ACT ≥ 20 ACQ < 0.75	ACT 16–19 ACQ > 1.5	ACT ≤ 15
Exacerbations	0–1/y	≥2×/y	≥2×/y
Management	Maintain at lowest step possible Consider step down if well controlled for ≥3 mo	Step up one step	Step up one to two steps and consider short-course OCS
Follow-up	1–6 mo	2–6 wk	2 wk

Data from the *2020 GINA Report: Global Strategy for Asthma Management and Prevention. Global Initiative for Asthma – GINA. Updated 2020. Accessed February 24, 2021. https://ginasthma.org/gina-reports/* and NAEPP Third Expert Panel on the Diagnosis and Management of Asthma. Accessed February 24, 2021, https://www.jacionline.org/action/showPdf?pii=S0091-6749%2820%2931404-4
ACQ, Asthma Control Questionnaire; ACT, Asthma Control Test; FEV_1, forced expiratory volume in 1 second; OCS, oral corticosteroids; PEF, peak expiratory flow.

- Bronchial smooth muscle contraction resulting from mediators released by a variety of cell types including inflammatory, local neural, and epithelial cells.
- Epithelial damage manifested by denudation and desquamation of the epithelium leading to mucus plugs that obstruct the airway.
- Airway remodeling characterized by the following findings:
  - Subepithelial fibrosis, specifically thickening of the lamina reticularis from collagen deposition.
  - Smooth muscle hypertrophy and hyperplasia.
  - Goblet cell and submucosal gland hypertrophy and hyperplasia resulting in mucus hypersecretion.
  - Airway angiogenesis.
  - Airway wall thickening due to edema and cellular infiltration.

Risk Factors

A number of factors increase airway hyperresponsiveness and can cause an acute and chronic increase in the severity of asthma:
- Allergens such as dust mites, cockroaches, pollens, molds, and pet dander in susceptible patients.
- Viral upper respiratory tract infections.

CHAPTER 9

TABLE 9-12	Classification of Asthma Exacerbation Severity		
	Moderate	Severe	Impending Respiratory Arrest
FEV$_1$ or PEF predicted or personal best	40%–69%	<40%	<25% or unable to measure
Symptoms	DOE or SOB with talking	SOB at rest	Severe SOB
Examination	Expiratory wheeze	Inspiratory and expiratory wheeze	Wheeze may become absent
	Some accessory muscle use	Increased accessory muscle use	Accessory muscle use with paradoxical thoracoabdominal movement
		Chest retraction	
		Agitation or confusion	Depressed mental status
Vitals	RR <28/min	RR >28/min	Same as severe but could develop respiratory depression and/or bradycardia
	HR <110 bpm	HR >110 bpm	
	O$_2$sat >91% RA	O$_2$sat <91% RA	
	No pulsus paradoxus	Pulsus paradoxus >25 mm Hg	
PaCO$_2$	Normal to hypocapnia	>42 mm Hg	Hypercapnia is a late sign

Data from the *2020 GINA Report: Global Strategy for Asthma Management and Prevention. Global Initiative for Asthma – GINA.* Updated 2020. Accessed February 24, 2021. https://ginasthma.org/gina-reports/ and NAEPP Third Expert Panel on the Diagnosis and Management of Asthma. Accessed February 24, 2021. https://www.jacionline.org/action/showPdf?pii=S0091-6749%2820%2931404-4

DOE, dyspnea on exertion; FEV$_1$, forced expiratory volume in 1 second; HR, heart rate; O$_2$sat, oxygen saturation; PEF, peak expiratory flow; RA, room air; RR, respiratory rate; SOB, shortness of breath.

- Many occupational allergens and irritants such as perfumes, cleaners, or detergents, even in small doses.
- Changes in weather (i.e., from warm to cold), strong emotional stimuli, and exercise.
- Indoor and outdoor pollutants, such as nitrogen dioxide (NO_2) and tobacco and wood smoke.
- Obesity.
- Medications such as β-blockers (including ophthalmic preparations), aspirin, and NSAIDs can cause the sudden onset of severe airway obstruction.

Prevention

- Rigorous treatment adherence and appropriate follow-up can help prevent worsening of asthma control.
- Identification and avoidance of risk factors (allergens, irritants) that exacerbate symptoms play a key role in prevention.
- Recognition and management of comorbidities such as obesity, sinonasal diseases, gastroesophageal reflux disease (GERD), and psychiatric disorders is important.

Associated Conditions

- Rhinosinusitis, with or without nasal polyps, is frequently present and should be treated with intranasal or oral corticosteroids, saline rinses, and/or antihistamines. Antibiotics should be reserved for superimposed bacterial infections.
- **Vocal cord dysfunction (VCD) or paradoxical vocal fold movement** can coexist with or masquerade severe, uncontrolled asthma. Diagnosis often requires provocation testing with laryngoscopy by otolaryngology specialists. Treatment consists of speech and, if needed, behavioral therapy.
- Symptomatic GERD can cause worsening asthma control and treatment with H_2 blockers or proton pump inhibitors is recommended in these cases. However, empiric treatment of GERD in asymptomatic patients with uncontrolled asthma is not an effective strategy.
- Obesity is increasingly recognized as an important comorbid condition and its presence is inversely correlated with asthma control. This association may be related to altered lung mechanics, altered respiratory patterns, or an increase in systemic inflammation. Healthy weight loss should be an integral part of a comprehensive asthma treatment plan.
- Smoking prevalence in patients with asthma is the same as the general population. Although no convincing evidence links tobacco use with developing asthma, it may make patients less responsive to ICS and more difficult to control. Tobacco cessation should be encouraged in all patients.
- OSA may make asthma more difficult to control and should be addressed with an overnight polysomnogram if suspected.

DIAGNOSIS

Clinical Presentation

History
- Recurring episodes of cough, dyspnea, chest tightness, and wheezing are suggestive of asthma. Symptoms are often worse at night or early morning, in the presence of potential triggers, and/or in a seasonal pattern.
- A personal or family history of atopy increases the likelihood of an asthma diagnosis.
- Patients older than 50 years presenting for the first time, patients with >20 pack-years of smoking, and patients with a lack of response to asthma therapy are features that make asthma less likely as the sole cause of respiratory symptoms. Alternative diagnoses including COPD, ACO, and others should be carefully considered in these patients.

Physical Examination
- Chronic asthma
  - Auscultation of wheezing and a prolonged expiratory phase can be present on examination, but a normal chest examination does not exclude asthma.
  - Signs of atopy, such as eczema, rhinitis, or nasal polyps, often coexist with asthma. The presence of nasal polyps should prompt questioning regarding the possibility of aspirin-exacerbated respiratory disease (AERD).
- Asthma exacerbation
  - During a suspected asthma exacerbation, a rapid assessment should be performed to identify patients who require immediate intervention (Table 9-12).
  - The presence or intensity of wheezing is an unreliable indicator of the severity of an attack.

Diagnostic Criteria

- In general, the diagnosis is supported by the presence of symptoms consistent with asthma combined with demonstration of variable expiratory airflow obstruction.
- Adequate response to asthma treatment assists with making the diagnosis.
- Methacholine challenge test can be considered when the diagnosis is in question. Note that airway hyperresponsiveness can be seen in diseases other than asthma (e.g., COPD, sarcoidosis) and effective asthma controller medications (such as ICS) can normalize the result (see "Diagnostic Testing" below).

Differential Diagnosis

Other conditions may present with wheezing and must be considered, especially in patients who are not responsive to therapy (Table 9-13).

Diagnostic Testing

Laboratory Studies

- Chronic asthma
  - Although laboratory analysis is not necessary for a diagnosis, a complete blood count with cellular differential should be obtained to assist with clinical phenotyping (i.e., to identify those with predominant eosinophilia—absolute peripheral blood eosinophil level of $0.3 \times 10^9/mm^3$ or greater).
  - A diagnosis of allergic bronchopulmonary aspergillosis (ABPA), which is due to a hypersensitivity reaction to *Aspergillus fumigatus*, should be carefully considered in each patient and is present in 1%–2% of asthma patients with persistent disease. Serum IgE levels, precipitating antibodies to *A. fumigatus*, or elevated *A. fumigatus*–specific antibodies should be tested to aid in the diagnosis.
  - Allergy skin tests or immunoassays for allergen-specific IgE are helpful to identify sensitization to specific inhalant allergens when allergen exposures are being concerned as a trigger. Results of allergy tests must correlate with history and clinical presentation.
  - Fractional concentration of exhaled nitric oxide (FeNO) may be used as a marker of eosinophilic airway inflammation in asthma. An FeNO level >50 parts per billion (ppb) is associated with a good response to ICS therapy.
- Asthma exacerbation
  - During an exacerbation, monitor oxygen saturation. ABG measurement should be considered in patients in severe distress or with an FEV_1 of <40% of predicted values after initial treatment.
  - A PaO_2 <60 mm Hg is a sign of severe bronchoconstriction or of a complicating condition, such as pulmonary edema, pulmonary embolism, or pneumonia.
  - Initially, during an exacerbation, the $PaCO_2$ is low due to an increase in respiratory rate. With a prolonged attack, the $PaCO_2$ may rise as a result of severe airway obstruction, increased dead space ventilation, and respiratory muscle fatigue. **A normal or increased $PaCO_2$ is a sign of impending respiratory failure and necessitates hospitalization and close monitoring.**

Imaging

- Although not necessary for the diagnosis of asthma, CXRs may be helpful to examine for alternative diagnoses that are associated with wheezing such as emphysema, pulmonary edema, or tracheobronchial obstruction. CXRs are often normal in patients with asthma.
- CTs of the chest can be considered in patients with severe disease wherein the diagnosis is not entirely clear or alternative diagnoses are being seriously considered. Patients with asthma may have mucus plugging, air trapping, bronchial wall thickening, and luminal narrowing on CT.

Diagnostic Procedures

- **PFTs** are essential to the diagnosis of asthma. In patients with asthma, PFTs often, but not always, demonstrate an obstructive pattern—the hallmark of which is a decrease in expiratory flow rates.
  - A reduction in FEV_1 and a proportionally smaller reduction in the FVC occur. This produces a decreased FEV_1/FVC ratio (generally <0.7 or the lower limit of normal value). With mild obstructive disease that involves only the small airways, the FEV_1/FVC ratio may be normal, with the only abnormality being a decrease in airflow at midlung volumes (forced expiratory flow 25%–75%).
  - The clinical diagnosis of asthma is supported by an obstructive pattern that improves after bronchodilator therapy. **Improvement is defined as an increase in FEV_1 of >12% and 200 mL after two to four puffs of a short-acting bronchodilator.** Bronchodilator response is helpful in the diagnosis of asthma, but absence will not exclude the diagnosis as some patients may need repeat testing to demonstrate reversibility.
  - In patients with chronic, severe asthma, the airflow obstruction may no longer be completely reversible. In these patients, the most effective way to establish the maximal degree of airway reversibility is to repeat PFTs after a course of oral corticosteroids (usually 40 mg/day for 10–14 days) and to use the same criteria as above for reversibility. The lack of demonstrable airway obstruction or reactivity does not rule out a diagnosis of asthma.
  - In cases in which spirometry is normal, the diagnosis can be made by showing heightened airway responsiveness to a **methacholine challenge.** A methacholine challenge is considered positive when a provocative concentration of 8 mg/mL or less causes a drop in FEV_1 of 20% (PC_{20}). If the patient is on an ICS, a PC_{20} of 8–16 mg/mL is considered borderline positive. A PC_{20} >16 mg/mL is considered a negative test. Repeat testing with the patient off of their ICS may be necessary.
- An objective measurement of airflow obstruction is essential to the evaluation of an exacerbation. The severity of the exacerbation should be classified as follows:
  - Mild (peak expiratory flow [PEF] or FEV_1 >70% of predicted or personal best)
  - Moderate (PEF or FEV_1 40%–69%)
  - Severe (PEF or FEV_1 <40%)
  - Life-threatening/impending respiratory arrest (PEF or FEV_1 <25%).

PRINCIPLES OF MANAGEMENT OF CHRONIC ASTHMA

Medical management involves chronic management and a plan for acute exacerbations, otherwise known as an **asthma action plan.** Most often, management includes the daily use of an anti-inflammatory, disease-modifying medication (long-term control medications) and as-needed use of a short-acting bronchodilator (quick-relief medications).

- The goals of daily management are to **avoid impairment** (lack of symptoms while maintaining normal activity and pulmonary function) and to **minimize risk** (preventing exacerbations, loss of lung function, and medication side effects). Successful management requires patient education, objective measurement of airflow obstruction, and a medication plan for daily use and for exacerbations.
- When initiating therapy for a patient not already on a controller medicine, one should assess the patient's severity and assign the patient to the highest level in which any one feature has occurred over the previous 2–4 weeks (see Table 9-10).
- Assessment of control on subsequent visits is used to modify therapy when following patients already on controller medication (see Table 9-11).

- A clinician should address the following issues before stepping up therapy when there is a poor response to a controller:
  - **Nonadherence to medications**: Specifically, poor adherence to ICS therapy is associated with an increased frequency of asthma exacerbations, accelerated longitudinal lung function decline, a greater number of missed school and workdays, asthma-related hospitalizations, and asthma-related death
  - Incorrect inhaler technique
  - Ongoing exposure to allergens and/or irritants
  - Comorbidities: Obesity, sinonasal diseases, GERD, OSA, and depression
  - Alternative diagnoses (see Table 9-13)
- The goal of the stepwise approach is to gain control of symptoms as quickly as possible. At the same time, level of control varies over time and, consequently, medication requirements may vary over time as well. Therapy should be reviewed regularly to check whether stepwise reduction is possible (Figure 9-1).

TABLE 9-13	Conditions That Can Present as Refractory Asthma

Upper Airway Obstruction
Tumor
Epiglottitis
Vocal cord dysfunction
Obstructive sleep apnea

Lower Airway Disease
Allergic bronchopulmonary aspergillosis
Chronic obstructive pulmonary disease
Cystic fibrosis
$\alpha 1$-Antitrypsin deficiency
Bronchiectasis
Bronchiolitis obliterans
Tracheomalacia
Endobronchial lesion
Foreign body
Herpetic tracheobronchitis

Adverse Drug Reaction
Aspirin
β-Adrenergic antagonist
Angiotensin-converting enzyme inhibitors
Inhaled pentamidine
Congestive heart failure
Gastroesophageal reflux
Sinusitis
Hypersensitivity pneumonitis
Eosinophilic granulomatosis with polyangiitis (Churg–Strauss)
Eosinophilic pneumonia
Hyperventilation with panic attacks
Dysfunctional breathlessness

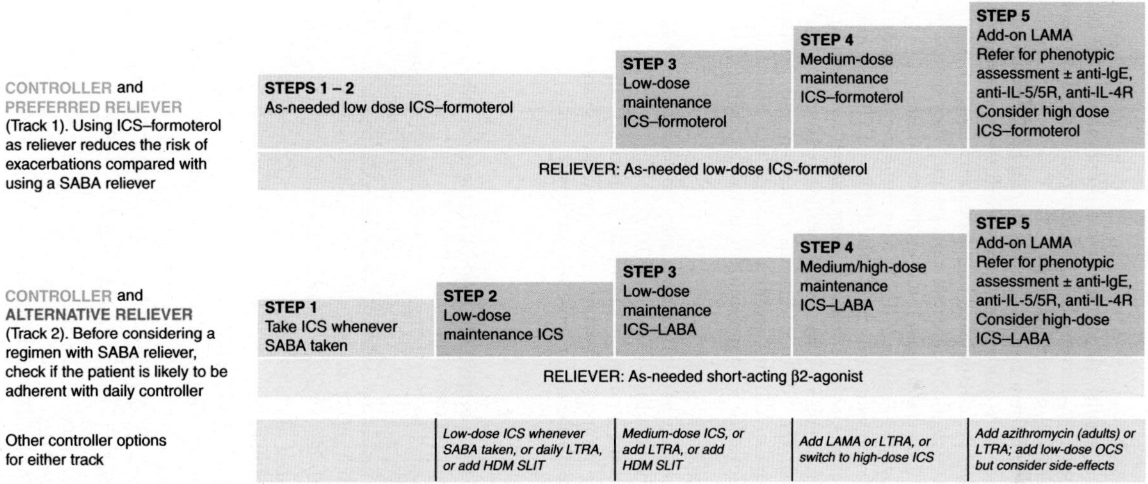

Figure 9-1. Management algorithm based on level of control. ICS, inhaled corticosteroids; IL, interleukin; LABA, long-acting β₂-agonist; LAMA, long-acting muscarinic antagonist; LTRA, leukotriene receptor antagonist; SABA, short-acting β₂-agonist. *Figure reflects recommendations for adults and adolescents aged 12+ years. (Copyright © 2022 Global Initiative for Asthma, used with express permission, www.ginasthma.org)

Pharmacologic Therapies

When choosing a treatment regimen, the patient's asthma severity should be classified as described above.

Short-Acting β_2-Agonists

* Regardless of asthma severity, all patients with asthma should have access to quick-relief medications used on an as-needed basis for treatment of symptoms and exacerbations (via either MDI or nebulization).
* Traditionally, for intermittent asthma, SABAs should be used on an as-needed basis (e.g., albuterol, two puffs q6h). Additionally, SABAs are considered the drug of choice for preventing exercise-induced bronchoconstriction.
* All SABAs now use hydrofluoroalkane as a propellant. They should be primed with four puffs when first used and again if not used over 2 weeks.
* The Global Initiative for Asthma (GINA) now recommends against using SABA-only treatment for mild asthma in the GINA 2019 and 2020 strategy report. This is based on data that serious adverse events from asthma can occur in those patients with infrequent symptoms and that SABA overuse is associated with risk of poor outcomes. However, the National Asthma Education and Prevention Program (NAEPP) EPR-4 update did not specifically address this issue and SABAs remain the treatment of choice for mild intermittent asthma according to the NAEPP.[40]

Inhaled Corticosteroids

* ICS inhalers are generally administered via a dry powder inhaler, MDI with a spacing device, or can be nebulized (Table 9-14).
* Systemic corticosteroid absorption can occur in patients who use high doses of ICS. Consequently, prolonged therapy with high-dose ICS should be reserved for patients with severe disease or for those who otherwise require oral corticosteroids.

TABLE 9-14	Comparative Daily Adult Dosages for Inhaled Corticosteroids		
Drug	Low Dose (µg)	Medium Dose (µg)	High Dose (µg)
Beclomethasone HFA (40 or 80 µg/puff)	80–240	>240–480	>480
Budesonide DPI (90, 180, or 200 µg/dose)	180–600	>600–1200	>1200
Budesonide nebulized respules (250, 500, or 1000 µg/respules)	250–500	>500–1000	>1000
Ciclesonide HFA (80 or 160 µg/puff)	160–320	>320–640	>640
Fluticasone propionate HFA (44, 110, or 220 µg/puff)	88–264	>264–440	>440
Fluticasone furoate (100, 220 µg/puff)	100–300	>300–500	>500
Mometasone furoate DPI (110 or 220 µg/ puff)	220	440	>440

Data from the *2020 GINA Report: Global Strategy for Asthma Management and Prevention. Global Initiative for Asthma – GINA. Updated 2020. Accessed February 24, 2021. https://ginasthma.org/gina-reports/* and NAEPP Third Expert Panel on the Diagnosis and Management of Asthma. Accessed February 24, 2021. https://www.jacionline.org/action/showPdf?pii=S0091-6749%2820%2931404-4
DPI, dry powder inhaler; HFA, hydrofluoroalkane; MDI, metered-dose inhaler.

- Pharmacological inhibitors of cytochrome P450 may reduce steroid elimination in patients on ICS, thus increasing steroid side effects.
- Attempts should be made to decrease the dose of ICS every 2–3 months to the lowest possible dose to maintain control.
- Traditionally, patients with mild persistent asthma are treated with a daily maintenance low-dose ICSs that are to be taken as prescribed regardless of symptoms. Patients are further instructed to take a SABA with symptoms.

Combination Therapy
- Alternative regimens in moderate persistent asthma include a maintenance low-dose ICS/LABA (or medium-dose ICS) taken as a maintenance inhaler with a SABA used as needed.
- In addition, the treatment of moderate persistent asthma can include a low-dose ICS/LAMA. At the moment tiotropium (Spiriva) is the only FDA-approved stand-alone muscarinic antagonist for asthma specifically.
- A low-dose ICS plus a leukotriene modifier (LTM) or theophylline can be considered but is generally less preferred.

Regimen Using ICS/Formoterol
- Formoterol is a LABA, but it can provide relief of symptoms quickly (similar to SABAs) due to formoterol's rapid onset of action as compared to other LABAs. Using this characteristic, several as-needed options for ICS/formoterol have been studied and shown efficacy.[41] However, at the moment, these treatment methods are still off-label in the US.
- Low-dose ICS in combination with formoterol used as needed can be an option for treatment of mild asthma rather than a maintenance ICS and as-needed SABA.
- Single maintenance and reliever therapy (SMART) uses a low- or medium-dose ICS combined with formoterol on a maintenance basis and as needed for relief of asthma symptoms. SMART has been shown to reduce exacerbations and is a preferred treatment for mild or mild to moderate persistent asthma.

Leukotriene Agents
- Leukotrienes are mediators in the inflammatory cascade.
- **LTMs include montelukast** and **zafirlukast**, which are oral leukotriene receptor antagonists (LTRA), and **zileuton**, which is an oral 5-lipoxygenase inhibitor.
- These medications can be considered as an alternative first-line medication for mild persistent asthma and as an add-on to ICS for more severe forms of asthma.
- In particular, these medications should be considered for patients with aspirin-sensitive asthma, exercise-induced bronchoconstriction, concurrent allergic rhinitis, or in individuals who cannot master the use of an inhaler.

Pharmacologic Therapies in Severe Persistent Asthma

- Optimal treatment of severe persistent asthma is of the utmost importance given the high degree of morbidity and mortality in this group and deserves particular attention.
- Treatment of severe persistent asthma generally involves the use of a medium-dose or high-dose ICS/LABA as a maintenance inhaler. However, use of a LAMA in the place of a LABA can be considered.
- In patients not controlled on high-dose ICS/LABA therapy, consideration should be given to add-on therapy with tiotropium or an LTM.
- Selected patients who have uncontrolled asthma despite the use of high-dose ICS/LABA therapy and in whom medication adherence is not an issue should be carefully considered for biologic therapy.

- Biologic therapy with monoclonal antibodies against IgE and interleukin (IL)-4, IL-5, and IL-13 has been shown to be highly effective in certain patients with severe persistent asthma not controlled on high doses of ICS plus long-acting bronchodilators (see Table 9-15).
  - **Omalizumab** is a monoclonal antibody against IgE that has been shown to reduce exacerbation rates, decrease emergency healthcare utilization, and improve asthma-related quality of life in patients with moderate to severe persistent allergic asthma with a demonstrable sensitivity to a perennial allergen and incomplete symptom control with ICS.[42]
  - **Mepolizumab and reslizumab** are humanized monoclonal antibodies against IL-5, which reduce eosinophilic inflammation and have been shown to significantly reduce the frequency of exacerbations and hospitalizations in patients

TABLE 9-15	FDA-Approved Biologics for Asthma		
Biologic Medication	Mechanism of Action	Indication	Dosing and Administration
Omalizumab	Binds free IgE	≥6 y old with moderate to severe persistent asthma, an IgE level of 30–700 IU/mL (US ≥12 y) and 30–1300 IU/mL (US 6–11 y), and positive IgE specific tests or skin testing to a perennial allergen.	150–375 mg SC q2-4 weeks depending on IgE level
Mepolizumab	Binds to IL-5 ligand	≥12 y old (US) or ≥6 y old (EU) with severe eosinophilic asthma unresponsive to GINA Step 4–5 therapy. Serum AEC ≥150–300 cells/µL.	100 mg SC q4wk
Reslizumab	Binds to IL-5 ligand	≥18 y old with severe eosinophilic asthma unresponsive to GINA Step 4–5 therapy. Serum AEC ≥400 cells/µL.	3 mg/kg IV q4wk
Benralizumab	Binds to IL-5 receptor α	≥12 y old with severe eosinophilic asthma unresponsive to GINA Step 4–5 therapy. Serum AEC ≥300 cells/µL.	30 mg SC q4wk for first three doses followed by 30 mg q8wk
Dupilumab	Binds to IL-4 receptor α; blocks signaling of IL-4 and IL-13	≥12 y old with severe eosinophilic asthma unresponsive to GINA Step 4–5 therapy. Serum AEC ≥150 cells/µL or FeNO ≥25 ppb.	400–600 mg SC loading dose initially followed by 200–300 mg SC q2wk

AEC, absolute eosinophil count; FeNO, fractional nitric oxide concentration in exhaled breath; GINA, Global Initiative for Asthma; IL, interleukin; IU, international unit.

with severe asthma. Mepolizumab is delivered subcutaneously (and can now be self-administered at home), while reslizumab is delivered based on weight dosing intravenously.[43,44]

○ **Benralizumab** is a monoclonal antibody directed against the α receptor of IL-5 that has been shown to significantly decrease exacerbations, improve lung function, and reduce systemic corticosteroid exposure in patients with severe, steroid-dependent asthma. Benralizumab can be self-administered at home and carries the benefit of every 8 week dosing (after the first three doses).[45]

○ **Dupilumab** is a human monoclonal antibody against the α receptor of IL-4 that blocks signaling for IL-4 and IL-13. Among patients with uncontrolled severe asthma, dupilumab was shown to decrease the rate of severe exacerbation, improve lung function, and improve asthma control. This effect was most pronounced in patients with an eosinophil count >300 cells/mm^3 or FeNO ≥25 ppb. Dupilumab can be self-administered at home and should be administered every 2 weeks.[46]

Management of Asthma Exacerbations

• Management of an exacerbation requiring hospital-based care should follow a treatment algorithm to triage patients based on response to treatment.

○ The response to initial treatment (three treatments with a short-acting bronchodilator every 20 minutes for 60–90 minutes) can be a better predictor of the need for hospitalization than the severity of an exacerbation.

○ Patients at high risk of asthma-related death should be advised to seek medical attention early in the course of an exacerbation.

○ A low threshold for admission is appropriate for patients with recent hospitalization, a failure of aggressive outpatient management (with oral corticosteroids), or a previous life-threatening attack.

○ During an exacerbation, reversal of airflow obstruction is achieved most effectively by frequent administration of an inhaled SABA.

  ▪ For a **mild to moderate exacerbation**, initial treatment starts with two to six puffs of albuterol via MDI with a spacer or 2.5 mg via nebulizer and is repeated q20min until improvement is obtained or toxicity is noted.

  ▪ For a **severe exacerbation**, albuterol 2.5–5 mg q20min with ipratropium bromide 0.5 mg q20min should be administered via nebulizer. Alternatively, albuterol 10–15 mg, administered continuously over an hour, may be more effective in severely obstructed adults. If used, telemetry monitoring is necessary.

  ▪ Levalbuterol four to eight puffs or nebulized 1.25–2.5 mg q20min can be substituted for albuterol but has not been associated with fewer side effects in adults.

○ **During an exacerbation, systemic corticosteroids speed the resolution of exacerbations of asthma and should be administered promptly to all patients.**

  ▪ The ideal dose of corticosteroid needed to speed recovery and limit symptoms is not well defined. A single or divided daily dose equivalent to prednisone 40–60 mg is usually adequate. Oral corticosteroid administration seems to be as effective as IV administration if given in equivalent doses.

  ▪ For maximal therapeutic response, tapering of high-dose corticosteroids should not take place until objective evidence of clinical improvement is observed (usually 36–48 hours or when PEF >70%). Initially, patients are given a daily dose of oral prednisone, which is then reduced slowly.

  ▪ A 7- to 14-day tapering dose of prednisone is usually successful in combination with an ICS instituted at the beginning of the tapering schedule. In patients with severe disease or with a history of respiratory failure, a slower dose reduction is appropriate.

- Patients discharged from the ED should receive oral corticosteroids. A dose of prednisone, 40 mg/day for 5–7 days, can be substituted for a tapering schedule in selected patients. Either regimen should be accompanied by the initiation of an ICS or an increase in the previous dose of ICS.
- For selected patients having a mild or moderate exacerbation, an alternative to oral corticosteroids is a recommendation that patients having an exacerbation quadruple their ICS.

Other Asthma Therapies

- **Methylxanthines:** Theophylline has historical utility in the management of asthma but should be a last-line option given the wide variety of options with less toxicity.
- **IV magnesium sulfate:** During a severe exacerbation refractory to standard treatment over 1 hour, one dose of 2 g IV over 20 minutes in the ED should be considered. It has been shown to acutely improve lung function especially in those with severe, life-threatening exacerbations.
- **Inhaled heliox:** During a severe exacerbation refractory to standard treatment over 1 hour, heliox-driven albuterol nebulization in a mixture with oxygen (70:30) should be considered. It has been shown to acutely improve lung function, especially in those with severe, life-threatening exacerbations.[47]
- **Macrolides:** Antibiotics have not been shown to have any benefit when used to treat asthma exacerbations. Although results are conflicting across trials, chronic azithromycin therapy can be considered in patients with severe persistent asthma who are poorly controlled despite maximal therapy.
- **SC allergen immunotherapy (SCIT)** can be considered in allergic patients with mild to moderate disease with persistent symptoms despite adherence to allergen avoidance and medications. SCIT is relatively contraindicated in patients with severe or unstable asthma (chronic oral corticosteroid use or severe exacerbations requiring hospitalization or intubation in the previous 6 months).
- **Bronchial thermoplasty:** Bronchial thermoplasty is a novel therapy for severe asthma in which a specialized radiofrequency catheter is introduced through a bronchoscope to deliver thermal energy to smaller airways to reduce smooth muscle mass surrounding the airways. Bronchial thermoplasty should be only performed in very selected patients by experienced bronchoscopists in conjunction with an asthma specialist, and ideally as part of a clinical registry.

Oxygenation and Mechanical Ventilation

- **Supplemental oxygen** should be administered to the patient who is awaiting an assessment of arterial oxygen tension and should be continued to maintain an oxygen saturation >92% (95% in patients with coexisting cardiac disease or pregnancy).
- **Mechanical ventilation** may be required for respiratory failure.
  - General principles include use of a **large endotracheal tube (≥7.5 mm), prolonged expiratory time with high inspiratory flows, and low respiratory rate. PEEP should be patient targeted and may need to be upwardly adjusted in some cases to avoid development of intrinsic PEEP.**
  - Ketamine and propofol may provide modest bronchodilatory effects in addition to sedation. After deep sedation, paralytics may have an advantage in decreasing muscular tone and minimizing patient–ventilator dyssynchrony.

- ○ Recent trials have shown that NIV may be carefully used in patients with acute asthma exacerbations and decreases the risk of endotracheal intubation.[48] Data on a survival benefit in using NIV in this group are conflicting.
- ○ Although prospective data are lacking, extracorporeal life support may be beneficial in cases of severe ventilatory failure associated with asthma exacerbations in patients who are deteriorating on mechanical ventilation.

Lifestyle/Risk Modification

Diet

There is no general diet that is known to improve asthma control. However, a small percentage of patients may have reproducible deterioration after exposure to dietary sulfites used to prevent discoloration in foods such as beer, wine, processed potatoes, and dried fruit. These foods should be avoided in patients if they have had prior reactions to them.

Activity

Patients should be encouraged to lead an active lifestyle. If asthma is well controlled, patients should expect to be as physically active as they desire. If exercise is a trigger, patients should be advised to continue physical activity after prophylactic use of an LTM (montelukast 10 mg 2 hours before exercise) or an inhaled β_2-agonist (two to four puffs 15–20 minutes before exposure).

SPECIAL CONSIDERATIONS

During pregnancy, patients should have more frequent follow-up because the severity of asthma often changes and requires medication adjustment. **There is more potential risk to the fetus with poorly controlled asthma than with exposure to asthma medications, most of which are generally considered safe.**

- Occupational asthma requires a detailed history of occupational exposure to a sensitizing agent, lack of asthma symptoms before exposure, and a documented relationship with symptoms and the workplace. Beyond standard asthma medical treatment, exposure avoidance is crucial.
- AERD: Patients with aspirin sensitivity and chronic rhinosinusitis with nasal polyps typically have onset of asthma in the third or fourth decade of life. Aspirin desensitization may be considered in patients with corticosteroid-dependent asthma or those requiring daily aspirin/NSAID therapy for other medical conditions.

COMPLICATIONS

Medication Side Effects

- **SABA:** Sympathomimetic symptoms (tremor, anxiety, tachycardia), decrease in serum potassium and magnesium, mild lactic acidosis, prolonged QTc.
- **ICS**
  - ○ Increased risk for systemic effects at high doses (equivalent >1000 µg/day of beclomethasone) including skin bruising, cataracts, elevated intraocular pressure, and accelerated loss of bone mass.
  - ○ Pharyngeal and laryngeal effects are common, such as sore throat, hoarse voice, and oral candidiasis. **Patients should be instructed to rinse their mouth after each administration to reduce the possibility of thrush.** A change in the delivery method and/or use of a valved holding chamber/spacer may alleviate the other side effects.

CHAPTER 9

- **LABA**
  - Fewer sympathomimetic-type side effects.
  - Associated with an increased risk of severe asthma exacerbations and asthma-related death when used without ICS based on the Salmeterol Multicenter Asthma Research Trial, which showed a very low but significant increase in asthma-related deaths in patients receiving salmeterol (0.01%–0.04%).[49]
  - Should only be used in combination with ICS. FDA recommends discontinuation of LABA once asthma control is achieved and maintained.
- **LTM**
  - Cases of newly diagnosed eosinophilic granulomatosis with polyangiitis (Churg-Strauss) after exposure to LTRA have been described, but it is unclear whether they are related to unmasking of a preexisting case with concurrent corticosteroid tapering or whether there is a causal relationship.
  - Zileuton can cause a reversible hepatitis, so it is recommended that hepatic function be monitored at initiation once a month during the first 3 months, every 3 months for the first year, and then periodically.
- **Biologic therapy:** All biologic therapies pose the risk of immunogenicity, hypersensitivity, or, rarely, anaphylaxis. Today most biologic therapies can safely be administered at home.
- **Methylxanthines**
  - Theophylline has a narrow therapeutic range with significant toxicities, such as arrhythmias and seizures, as well as many potential drug interactions, especially with antibiotics.
  - Serum concentrations of theophylline should be monitored on a regular basis, aiming for a peak level of 5–10 µg/mL; however, at the lower doses used for asthma, toxicity is much less likely.

REFERRAL

Referral to a specialist should be considered in the following situations:
- Patients who require step 4 (see Figure 9-1) or higher treatment, or patients who have had a life-threatening asthma exacerbation.
- Patients being considered for biologic therapy, bronchial thermoplasty, or other alternative treatments.
- Patients with atypical signs or symptoms that make the diagnosis uncertain.
- Patients with comorbidities such as chronic sinusitis, nasal polyposis, ABPA, VCD, severe GERD, severe rhinitis, or significant psychiatric or psychosocial difficulties interfering with treatment.
- Patients requiring additional diagnostic testing, such as rhinoscopy or bronchoscopy, bronchoprovocation testing, or allergy skin testing.
- Patients who need to be evaluated for allergen immunotherapy.

REFERENCES

1. Institute for Health Metrics and Evaluation. *GBD Compare.* IHME, University of Washington; 2015.
2. Martin WJ, Glass RI, Balbus JM, Collins FS. A major environmental cause of death. *Science.* 2011;334:180-181.
3. Divo M, Cote C, de Torres JP, et al. Comorbidities and risk of mortality in patients with chronic obstructive pulmonary disease. *Am J Respir Crit Care Med.* 2012;186:155-161.
4. Anthonisen NR, Connett JE, Murray RP. Smoking and lung function of Lung Health Study participants after 11 years. *Am J Respir Crit Care Med.* 2002;166:675-679.
5. Anthonisen NR. The effects of a smoking cessation intervention on 14.5-year mortality: a randomized clinical trial. *Ann Intern Med.* 2005;142:233.

6. Abukhalaf J, Davidson R, Villalobos N, et al. Chronic obstructive pulmonary disease mortality, a competing risk analysis. *Clin Respir J.* 2018;12:2598-2605.
7. Celli BR, Cote CG, Marin JM, et al. The body-mass index, airflow obstruction, dyspnea, and exercise capacity index in chronic obstructive pulmonary disease. *N Engl J Med.* 2004;350:1005-1012.
8. Espantoso-Romero M, Román Rodríguez M, Duarte-Pérez A, et al. External validation of multidimensional prognostic indices (ADO, BODEx and DOSE) in a primary care international cohort (PROEPOC/COPD cohort). *BMC Pulm Med.* 2016;16:143.
9. Lowe KE, Regan EA, Anzueto A, et al. COPDGene® 2019: redefining the diagnosis of chronic obstructive pulmonary disease. *Chronic Obstr Pulm Dis.* 2019;6:384-399.
10. Lichtenstein DA, Mezière GA. The BLUE-points: three standardized points used in the BLUE-protocol for ultrasound assessment of the lung in acute respiratory failure. *Crit Ultrasound J.* 2011;3:109-110.
11. Hall JB, Kress J, Schmidt GA. *Principles of Critical Care.* 4th ed. McGraw-Hill Education; 2015.
12. Chapman KR, Burdon JGW, Piitulainen E, et al. Intravenous augmentation treatment and lung density in severe α1 antitrypsin deficiency (RAPID): a randomised, double-blind, placebo-controlled trial. *Lancet.* 2015;386:360-368.
13. Tashkin DP, Celli B, Senn S, et al. A 4-year trial of tiotropium in chronic obstructive pulmonary disease. *N Engl J Med.* 2008;359:1543-1554.
14. Lasserson TJ, Ferrara G, Casali L. Combination fluticasone and salmeterol versus fixed dose combination budesonide and formoterol for chronic asthma in adults and children. *Cochrane Database Syst Rev.* 2011;(12):CD004106.
15. Lipson DA, Barnhart F, Brealey N, et al. Once-daily single-inhaler triple versus dual therapy in patients with COPD. *N Engl J Med.* 2018;378:1671-1680.
16. Chalmers JD, Laska IF, Franssen FME, et al. Withdrawal of inhaled corticosteroids in COPD: a European Respiratory Society guideline. *Eur Respir J* 2020;55:2000351.
17. Criner GJ, Cordova F, Sternberg AL, Martinez FJ. The National Emphysema Treatment Trial (NETT): part I – lessons learned about emphysema. *Am J Respir Crit Care Med.* 2011;184:763-770.
18. Weill D, Benden C, Corris PA, et al. A consensus document for the selection of lung transplant candidates: 2014—an update from the Pulmonary Transplantation Council of the International Society for heart and lung transplantation. *J Heart Lung Transplant.* 2015;34:1-15.
19. Eskander A, Waddell TK, Faughnan ME, Chowdhury N, Singer LG. BODE index and quality of life in advanced chronic obstructive pulmonary disease before and after lung transplantation. *J Heart Lung Transplant* 2011;30:1334-1341.
20. Valapour M, Lehr CJ, Skeans MA, et al. OPTN/SRTR 2018 annual data report: lung. *Am J Transplant.* 2020;20:427-508.
21. Casaburi R, ZuWallack R. Pulmonary rehabilitation for management of chronic obstructive pulmonary disease. *N Engl Journal Med.* 2009;360:1329-1335.
22. Group TL-TOTTR. A randomized trial of long-term oxygen for COPD with moderate desaturation. *N Engl J Med.* 2016;375:1617-1627.
23. Lacasse Y, Series F, Corbeil F, et al. Randomized trial of nocturnal oxygen in chronic obstructive pulmonary disease. *N Engl J Med.* 2020;383:1129-1138.
24. Murphy PB, Rehal S, Arbane G, et al. Effect of home noninvasive ventilation with oxygen therapy vs oxygen therapy alone on hospital readmission or death after an acute COPD exacerbation: a randomized clinical trial. *JAMA.* 2017;317:2177-2186.
25. Köhnlein T, Windisch W, Köhler D, et al. Non-invasive positive pressure ventilation for the treatment of severe stable chronic obstructive pulmonary disease: a prospective, multicentre, randomised, controlled clinical trial. *Lancet Respir Med.* 2014;2:698-705.
26. Pison CM, Cano NJ, Chérion C, et al. Multimodal nutritional rehabilitation improves clinical outcomes of malnourished patients with chronic respiratory failure: a randomised controlled trial. *Thorax.* 2011;66:953-960.
27. Aberle DR, Adams AM; National Lung Screening Trial Research Team, et al. Reduced lung-cancer mortality with low-dose computed tomographic screening. *N Engl J Med.* 2011;365:395-409.
28. Cosentino J, Zhao H, Hardin M, et al. Analysis of asthma-chronic obstructive pulmonary disease overlap syndrome defined on the basis of bronchodilator response and degree of emphysema. *Ann Am Thorac Soc.* 2016;13:1483-1489.
29. Walters JA, Tang JNQ, Poole P, Wood-Baker R. Pneumococcal vaccines for preventing pneumonia in chronic obstructive pulmonary disease. *Cochrane Database Syst Rev.* 2017;1:CD001390.
30. Centers for Disease Control and Prevention. *Recommended Adult Immunization Schedule for ages 19 years or older 2021.* Accessed May 9, 2021. Available at https://www.cdc.gov/vaccines/schedules/downloads/adult/adult-combined-schedule.pdf.
31. Lee SC, Son KJ, Han CH, Park SC, Jung JY. Impact of COPD on COVID-19 prognosis: a nationwide population-based study in South Korea. *Sci Rep.* 2021;11:3735.
32. Albert RK, Connett J, Bailey WC, et al. Azithromycin for prevention of exacerbations of COPD. *N Engl J Med.* 2011;365:689-698.

33. Martinez FJ, Calverley PMA, Goehring UM, Brose M, Fabbri LM, Rabe KF. Effect of roflumilast on exacerbations in patients with severe chronic obstructive pulmonary disease uncontrolled by combination therapy (REACT): a multicentre randomised controlled trial. *Lancet*. 2015;385:857-866.

34. Stoller JK, Aboussouan LS. A review of α1-antitrypsin deficiency. *Am J Respir Crit Care Med*. 2012;185:246-259.

35. Aaron SD, Fergusson D, Marks GB, et al. Counting, analysing and reporting exacerbations of COPD in randomised trials. *Thorax*. 2008;63:122-128.

36. Leuppi JD, Schuetz P, Bingisser R, et al. Short-term vs conventional glucocorticoid therapy in acute exacerbations of chronic obstructive pulmonary disease: the REDUCE randomized clinical trial. *JAMA*. 2013;309:2223-2231.

37. Rizkallah J, Man SFP, Sin DD. Prevalence of pulmonary embolism in acute exacerbations of COPD: a systematic review and metaanalysis. *Chest*. 2009;135:786-793.

38. Braman SS. The global burden of asthma. *Chest*. 2006;130:4S-12S.

39. Shanawani H. Health disparities and differences in asthma: concepts and controversies. *Clin Chest Med*. 2006;27:17-28, v.

40. Cloutier MM, Baptist AP; Expert Panel Working Group of the National Heart, Lung, and Blood Institute(NHLBI) administered and coordinated National Asthma Education and Prevention Program Coordinating Committee (NAEPPCC), et al. 2020 Focused updates to the asthma management guidelines: a report from the National asthma education and prevention program coordinating committee expert panel working group. *J Allergy Clin Immunol* 2020;146:1217-1270.

41. O'Byrne PM, FitzGerald JM, Bateman ED, et al. Inhaled combined budesonide-formoterol as needed in mild asthma. *N Engl J Med*. 2018;378:1865-1876.

42. Normansell R, Walker S, Milan SJ, Walters EH, Nair P. Omalizumab for asthma in adults and children. *Cochrane Database Syst Rev*. 2014;(1):CD003559.

43. Castro M, Zangrilli J, Wechsler ME, et al. Reslizumab for inadequately controlled asthma with elevated blood eosinophil counts: results from two multicentre, parallel, double-blind, randomised, placebo-controlled, phase 3 trials. *Lancet Respir Med*. 2015;3:355-366.

44. Ortega HG, Liu MC, Pavord ID, et al. Mepolizumab treatment in patients with severe eosinophilic asthma. *N Engl J Med*. 2014;371:1198-1207.

45. Nair P, Wenzel S, Rabe KF, et al. Oral glucocorticoid-sparing effect of Benralizumab in severe asthma. *N Engl J Med*. 2017;376:2448-2458.

46. Castro M, Corren J, Pavord ID, et al. Dupilumab efficacy and safety in moderate-to-severe uncontrolled asthma. *N Engl J Med*. 2018;378:2486-2496.

47. Valli G, Paoletti P, Savi D, Martolini D, Palange P. Clinical use of Heliox in asthma and COPD. *Monaldi Arch Chest Dis*. 2007;67:159-164.

48. Althoff MD, Holguin F, Yang F, et al. Noninvasive ventilation use in critically ill patients with acute asthma exacerbations. *Am J Respir Crit Care Med*. 2020;202:1520-1530.

49. Nelson HS, Weiss ST, Bleecker ER, et al. The salmeterol multicenter asthma research trial: a comparison of usual pharmacotherapy for asthma or usual pharmacotherapy plus salmeterol. *Chest*. 2006;129(1):15-26.

10 Pulmonary Diseases

Adrian Shifren, Murali Chakinala, Alexander Chen,
Gabriel Schroeder, Katherine Dittman, Paul Kannarkat,
Nathaniel Moulton, Praveen Chenna, James G. Krings,
and Tonya D. Russell

Pulmonary Hypertension

GENERAL PRINCIPLES

Definition

Pulmonary hypertension (PH) is defined by sustained elevation of the mean pulmonary artery pressure (mPAP) to >20 mm Hg (at rest).[1]

Classification

- PH is subcategorized into five major groups (Table 10-1):
  - Group I—**Pulmonary arterial hypertension (PAH)**
  - Group II—**PH due to left heart disease**
  - Group III—**PH due to lung diseases and/or hypoxia**
  - Group IV—**PH due to pulmonary artery obstructions**
  - Group V—**PH with unclear multifactorial mechanisms**
- **PAH is a specific group of disorders with similar pathologies and clinical presentation, and a high propensity for right heart failure in the absence of elevated left-sided pressures.**
  - Hemodynamic definition = **mPAP > 20 mm Hg, pulmonary artery wedge pressure (PAWP) ≤ 15 mm Hg, and pulmonary vascular resistance (PVR) ≥ 3 Wood units**[1]

Epidemiology

- PH is most often due to left heart disease (Group II) or parenchymal lung disease (Group III).
- Prevalence of **idiopathic PAH (IPAH)** (Group I) is 6–9 cases per million compared with overall PAH prevalence of 15–26 cases per million.[2,3]
  - Average age of PAH patients is ~50 years.[2–4] IPAH patients tend to be even younger, with a mean age of ~35 years.[5]
- IPAH and PAH associated with connective tissue diseases (CTD) are the most common subtypes.[4,6]
- Incidence of chronic thromboembolic pulmonary hypertension (**CTEPH**) (Group IV) may be as high as 4% among survivors of acute pulmonary embolism.[7]

Pathophysiology

- PAH is suspected to develop in susceptible individuals who develop a comorbid condition (e.g., systemic sclerosis or portal hypertension), contract an infection (e.g., HIV), or get exposed to a culpable drug/toxin (e.g., fenfluramine, methamphetamines, or dasatinib).

TABLE 10-1	**Clinical Classification of Pulmonary Hypertension: Dana Point (2008) Classification System of Pulmonary Hypertension**

Group I: Pulmonary arterial hypertension (PAH)

Idiopathic (IPAH)

Heritable (HPAH)

Drugs and toxin-induced: methamphetamines, fenfluramine, dasatinib

Associated (APAH)

- Connective tissue diseases
- HIV infection
- Portal hypertension
- Congenital heart disease (systemic-to-pulmonary shunt)
- Schistosomiasis

PAH long-term responders to calcium channel blockers

PAH with overt features of venous/capillaries (PVOD/PCH) involvement

Group II: Pulmonary hypertension (PH) due to left heart disease

PH due to heart failure with preserved LVEF

PH due to heart failure with reduced LVEF

Valvular disease

Group III: PH due to lung disease and/or hypoxia

Obstructive lung disease

Restrictive lung disease

Other pulmonary diseases with mixed restrictive and obstructive pattern

Hypoxia without lung disease

Developmental lung disorders

Group IV: PH due to pulmonary artery obstructions

Chronic thromboembolic PH

Other pulmonary artery obstructions

Group V: PH with unclear and/or multifactorial mechanisms

Hematologic disorders: myeloproliferative disorders, hemoglobinopathies

Systemic and metabolic disorders: sarcoidosis, PLCH, LAM, neurofibromatosis, glycogen storage disease, Gaucher disease

Others: tumoral obstruction, fibrosing mediastinitis, chronic renal failure on dialysis

Complex congenital heart disease

LAM, lymphangioleiomyomatosis; LVEF, left ventricular ejection fraction; PCH, pulmonary capillary hemangiomatosis; PLCH, pulmonary Langerhans cell histiocytosis; PVOD, pulmonary veno-occlusive disease.

○ Mutations in bone morphogenetic protein receptor II (*BMPR-II*) gene account for ~70% of heritable PAH (HPAH).[8]

○ Mutations in the eukaryotic translation initiation factor 2 alpha kinase 4 (*EIF2AK4*) gene cause PAH with significant venous/capillary involvement (formerly known as pulmonary veno-occlusive disease).[9]

- Other susceptibility factors are speculated to exist but have not been identified.
- Comprehensive gene panels are commercially available.
- PAH involves a complex interplay of factors resulting in progressive vascular remodeling with endothelial cell and smooth muscle proliferation, vasoconstriction, and in situ thrombosis at an arteriolar level. Vessel wall changes and luminal narrowing restrict the flow of blood and lead to higher-than-normal pressure as blood flows through the vessels, which is quantifiable by an elevated PVR.[10]
  - Elevated PVR results in increased afterload for the right ventricle (RV), which increases RV wall tension and work, leading to reduced RV contractility, decreasing cardiac output and progressive exercise intolerance.
  - The RV has limited ability to hypertrophy and tolerates high afterload poorly, causing "vascular–ventricular uncoupling" and eventual RV failure and death.
- Mechanisms of PH in Groups II–V vary and include high postcapillary pressures, hypoxemia-mediated vasoconstriction, vascular remodeling, parenchymal destruction, thromboembolic narrowing or occlusion of large arteries, compression of proximal vasculature, and hyperdynamic states leading to increased circulatory flow.
- **Combined pre- and postcapillary PH** describes situations when multiple conditions lead to elevated pressures in the left-sided heart chambers (postcapillary) and simultaneous abnormalities in the pulmonary arterial side (precapillary).
  - **Hemodynamic definition = mean PAP > 20 mm Hg, PAWP > 15 mm Hg, and PVR ≥ 3 Wood units**[1]

Prevention

Yearly screening transthoracic echocardiogram (TTE) is indicated for high-risk groups including individuals with known *BMPR-II* mutation, scleroderma, portal hypertension undergoing liver transplantation evaluation, and congenital systemic-to-pulmonary shunts (e.g., ventricular septal defects, patent ductus arteriosus).
- More formal screening algorithm for early detection of PAH in scleroderma is available.[11]

DIAGNOSIS

Clinical Presentation

- **Symptoms** include **dyspnea** (most common), fatigue, palpitations, exertional dizziness, **syncope**, chest pain, lower extremity swelling, and increased abdominal girth (ascites).
- Explore underlying exposures (i.e., methamphetamines, chemotherapeutic agents)[1] or associated conditions (e.g., CTDs, left-sided cardiac disease, parenchymal lung diseases, obstructive sleep apnea syndrome [OSAS], and venous thromboembolism).
- Auscultatory signs of PH include **prominent second heart sound** (loud S2) with loud P2 component, RV S3, tricuspid regurgitation, and pulmonary insufficiency murmurs.
- **Signs of right heart failure are** jugular venous distention, pedal edema, hepatomegaly, pulsatile liver, and ascites.
- Examination findings of underlying conditions linked to PH include skin changes of scleroderma, stigmata of liver disease, clubbing (congenital heart disease), aortic/mitral murmurs, and abnormal breath sounds (parenchymal lung disease).

Diagnostic Testing

- **Confirm clinical suspicion and determine etiology of PH, while gauging the severity of the condition.**

- Acute illnesses can cause mild elevations of pulmonary artery systolic pressure (PASP) (<50 mm Hg).
- Evaluation of **chronic PH** is necessary if pressures remain elevated after resolution of acute conditions.
- **TTE is the initial test** when chronic PH is suspected or if screening a vulnerable population.

TTE With Doppler and Agitated Saline Injection
- **Estimate PASP** by Doppler interrogation of tricuspid valve regurgitant jet.
  - Sensitivity for PH is 80%–100%, and correlation coefficient with invasive measurement is 0.6–0.9.[12]
  - Absence of tricuspid regurgitation does not exclude elevated pressures or PH.
- **RV findings of significance:**
  - RV hypertrophy and dilation, depressed systolic function (reduced tricuspid annular systolic excursion [<1.8 cm associated with worse survival[13]], systolic velocity of the tricuspid valve annulus, and free wall strain), intraventricular septal displacement and paradoxical motion leading to left ventricular (LV) compression, and pericardial effusion.
- **Identify causes of PH** (e.g., LV systolic or **diastolic dysfunction**, left-sided valvular disease, left atrial structural anomalies, and congenital systemic-to-pulmonary shunts).
  - Left atrial enlargement is an important clue for diastolic dysfunction that frequently leads to PH, especially in the elderly.[14]
- Transesophageal echocardiogram (TEE) is indicated to exclude intracardiac shunts suspected by TTE; patent foramen ovale is most common shunt and does not require further evaluation.
- Additional studies outlined in the following text and Figure 10-1 should be completed if PH is unexplained by TTE, if lung disease is suspected, or if PAH is still a consideration.[12,15]

Laboratories
- Evaluate for associated conditions and gauge degree of cardiac impairment.
  - Complete blood counts (CBCs), blood urea nitrogen, serum creatinine, hepatic function tests, natriuretic peptides, HIV serology, CTD serologies (antinuclear, antitopoisomerase antibody, and anticentromere antibodies; extractable nuclear antigen [ENA]; and other potential serologies based on clinical presentation).
- Other contingent laboratories include thyroid function studies, hepatitis B and C serologies, hemoglobin electrophoresis, antiphospholipid antibody, and lupus anticoagulant.

Electrocardiography
Signs of **right heart enlargement** are RV hypertrophy, right atrial enlargement, right bundle branch block, and RV strain pattern (S wave in lead I with Q wave and inverted T wave in lead III), but these findings have low sensitivity in milder PH.

Pulmonary Function Testing
- **Spirometry and lung volumes** to look for obstructive (e.g., **chronic obstructive lung disease**) or restrictive (e.g., interstitial lung disease [ILD]) ventilatory abnormalities.
- **Diffusing capacity for carbon monoxide (DLCO)** is mildly reduced in PAH; but more severe reduction in DLCO (i.e., <40% predicted) is a clue for parenchymal lung disease or PAH associated with significant venous/capillary involvement.

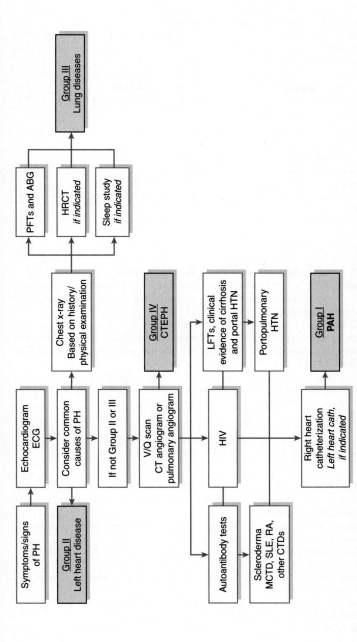

Figure 10-1. Algorithm for diagnostic workup of pulmonary hypertension. ABG, arterial blood gas; CTD, connective tissue disease; CTEPH, chronic thromboembolic pulmonary hypertension; HRCT, high-resolution CT; HTN, hypertension; LFT, liver function test; MCTD, mixed connective tissue disease; PAH, pulmonary arterial hypertension; PFT, pulmonary function test; PH, pulmonary hypertension; RA, rheumatoid arthritis; SLE, systemic lupus erythematosus; V/Q, ventilation–perfusion.

CHAPTER 10

- **Arterial blood gas (ABG):** Elevated arterial partial pressure of carbon dioxide ($PaCO_2$) suggests hypoventilation syndrome or severe obstructive ventilatory defect.
- **Six-minute walk (6MW) or simple exercise test:**
  ○ Distance walked correlates with the World Health Organization functional classification and overall prognosis.[16]
- **Nocturnal oximetry:** Desaturations could indicate OSAS.
  ○ Nocturnal desaturations are common in PAH, even in absence of OSAS, and should be treated with nocturnal supplemental oxygen.[17]
- Symptoms of sleep-disordered breathing and daytime hypercarbia should be evaluated with polysomnography (PSG).

Imaging
- **CXR:**
  ○ Central pulmonary arteries and RV enlargement
  ○ Clues to specific PH diagnosis include the following:
    ▪ Decreased peripheral vascular markings or pruning (PAH)
    ▪ Large pulmonary vasculature throughout lung fields (congenital-to-systemic shunt)
    ▪ Regional oligemia of pulmonary vasculature (chronic thromboembolic disease)
    ▪ Interstitial infiltrates (ILD)
    ▪ Hyperinflated lungs (chronic obstructive lung disease)
- **Ventilation–perfusion (V/Q) lung scan:**
  ○ **Critical for excluding chronic thromboembolic disease** but could also be abnormal in PAH with venous/capillary involvement and fibrosing mediastinitis.
  ○ Presence of one or more segmental mismatches should warrant CT angiography or pulmonary angiography.[15]
- **Chest CT scan:**
  ○ Angiogram can confirm CTEPH, if initial screening V/Q scan is suspicious, and also helps determine surgical feasibility; **CT should generally not be used to screen for CTEPH.**
  ○ High-resolution images to assess for interstitial or bronchiolar disease.
- **Pulmonary angiography** can be done safely in severe PH and confirms CTEPH and determines surgical feasibility.
- **Cardiac MRI:**
  ○ Provides RV anatomic and functional information, including ventricular volumes, ejection fraction, and stroke volume index, which have prognostic value.[18]
  ○ Identifies cardiac anomalies associated with PAH (if TEE contraindicated).

Diagnostic Procedures
- **Lung biopsy** is usually prohibited by severe PH or RV dysfunction if present; rarely performed when suspecting PAH associated with venous/capillary involvement.
- **Right heart catheterization:**
  ○ **Essential when PAH suspected and pulmonary vasodilators being considered.**
  ○ **Confirms PH** because TTE can be inaccurate.[19]
  ○ **Excludes left heart disease** by measuring end-expiratory PAWP and systemic-to-pulmonary shunts (by noting "step-up" in oxygen saturations).
    ▪ **Measure direct LV end-diastolic pressure** if PAWP not reliable, especially in patients older than 65 years.
  ○ **Reduced cardiac output and elevated mean right atrial pressure (RAP) are important predictors of mortality.**[5]
  ○ **Acute fluid challenge** (7 mL/kg over 5 minutes) can unmask LV dysfunction that could be etiology of mild PH.[20]

- **Acute vasodilator testing** recommended when IPAH, HPAH, or drug/toxin-induced PAH suspected, unless extreme right heart failure present (mean RAP > 20 mm Hg).
  - Use short-acting vasodilator, such as IV adenosine or inhaled nitric oxide.[21]
  - **Significant response is acute drop in mPAP ≥ 10 mm Hg *and* concluding mPAP < 40 mm Hg with stable or improved cardiac output.**[21]
  - **Only acute responders should receive long-term CCBs** (see "Treatment" section).

TREATMENT

- **Supplemental oxygen** to keep arterial saturations (>89%) to avoid hypoxic vasoconstriction. Normoxemia may not be possible with significant right-to-left intracardiac shunting.
- **In-line IV filters** to prevent paradoxical air emboli in patients with large right-to-left shunts.
- **Deep Valsalva** maneuvers raise intrathoracic pressure and reduce central venous return (e.g., vigorous exercise, severe coughing, straining during defecation, or micturition) and **high altitudes** (>5000 ft) because of low inspired concentration of oxygen.
- Avoid **pregnancy** because of hemodynamic alterations that further strain the RV.
- Pulmonary rehabilitation is recommended for treated PAH patients who remain limited due to physical deconditioning.
- **Management of PH depends on the specific category of PH.**
  - Group II PH should receive appropriate therapy for underlying causative condition with the goal of **minimizing postcapillary pressures.**
  - Group III PH should receive treatment for specific condition, for example, bronchodilators for obstructive lung disease, immunomodulators, or antifibrotics for ILD, noninvasive ventilation for OSAS or obesity hypoventilation syndrome, and supplemental oxygen.
    - Select PH–ILD patients can benefit from the inhaled pulmonary vasodilator, treprostinil.
  - CTEPH is usually treated by **pulmonary thromboendarterectomy or percutaneous balloon angioplasty** at specialized centers and requires careful evaluation to determine best intervention.[22,23] Inoperable or persistent CTEPH (after intervention) benefit from medical therapy.

Medications

- **PAH patients are candidates for vasomodulator/vasodilator** therapy (see Table 10-2).
  - Four categories of PAH-specific therapies with unique mechanisms of action:
    - **Endothelin receptor antagonists** block endothelin-1's effect on pulmonary artery smooth muscle cells, thus abrogating vasoconstriction and cellular growth.
    - **Phosphodiesterase 5 inhibitors** block enzyme that shuts down nitric oxide–mediated vasodilation.
    - **Soluble guanylate cyclase stimulator** activates the downstream signal of nitric oxide and induces vasodilation.
    - **Prostacyclin pathway activators, including prostacyclin analogues and prostacyclin receptor agonists,** induce vasodilation, inhibit cellular growth, and inhibit platelet aggregation.

TABLE 10-2	Vasomodulator/Vasodilatory Therapy for Pulmonary Arterial Hypertension				
Drug	Therapeutic Class	Route of Delivery	Dosing Range	Adverse Effects	Cautions
Nifedipine, amlodipine, diltiazem	Calcium channel blockers	PO	Varies by patient tolerance	Peripheral edema, hypotension, fatigue	**Use only in patients who are vasoresponsive during acute vasodilator challenge;** avoid if low cardiac output or decompensated right heart failure
Sildenafil Tadalafil	Phosphodiesterase type 5 inhibitor	PO	20 mg TID 40 mg/d	Headache, hypotension, dyspepsia, myalgias, visual disturbances	Avoid using with **nitrates or protease inhibitors**
Riociguat	Soluble guanylate cyclase stimulator	PO	2.5 mg TID	Hypotension	Avoid using with nitrates; **approved for PAH and CTEPH,** i.e., **inoperable or** persistent after endarterectomy
Bosentan	Endothelin receptor antagonist	PO	125 mg BID	Hepatotoxic, teratogen, peripheral edema	**Monthly liver function monitoring;** avoid using with glyburide and glipizide
Ambrisentan	Endothelin receptor antagonist	PO	5–10 mg/d	Teratogen, peripheral edema	Fluid retention, particularly in older patients
Macitentan	Endothelin receptor antagonist	PO	10 mg/d	Teratogen, peripheral edema	Monitor for anemia
Iloprost Treprostinil	Prostacyclin analogue	IH	2.5–5 µg 6–8/d ≥9 breaths QID	Cough, flushing, headache, trismus	**Suboptimal adherence due to dosing frequency;** overnight drug holiday
Selexipag	Prostacyclin receptor agonist	PO	200–1600 µg BID	Headache, jaw pain, diarrhea, extremity pain	Hyperthyroidism
Treprostinil	Prostacyclin analogue	SC, IV, or PO	Varies by patient tolerance	Headache, jaw pain, diarrhea, extremity pain	**With continuous parenteral use,** catheter-related complications (IV); **site pain/reaction (SC);** GI distress with PO use
Epoprostenol	Prostacyclin analogue	IV	Varies by patient tolerance	Headache, jaw pain, diarrhea, extremity pain	**Continuous parenteral agent; very short half-life;** catheter-related complications (IV); **high-output state at higher doses**

CTEPH, chronic thromboembolic pulmonary hypertension; GI, gastrointestinal; IH, inhaled; PAH, pulmonary arterial hypertension; PO, oral.

- ○ Choice of PAH-specific therapy should be individualized by severity of condition based on established risk assessment tools that are available online (see Figure 10-2 and Table 10-3).
  - **REVEAL 2.0 and REVEAL Lite** calculate a weighted score based on multiple variables (such as PAH subtype, demographics, New York Heart Association [NYHA] functional class, 6MW distance, natriuretic peptides, hemodynamics, vital signs) and determine low, intermediate, or high risk for death.[24,25]
  - **French Registry** method tallies the number of low-risk characteristics (including NYHA function class I or II, 6MW distance > 440 m, RAP < 8 mm Hg, cardiac index > 2.5 L/min/m²); ≥3 criteria signifies low-risk category and predicts improved survival.[26]

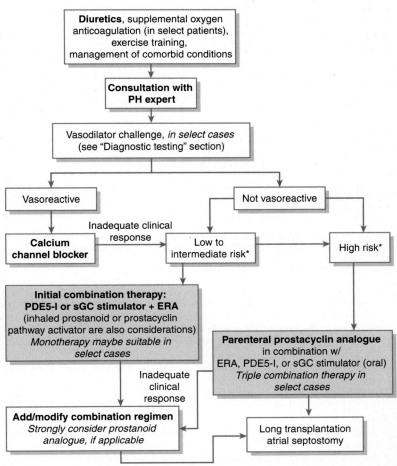

Figure 10-2. Algorithm for management of pulmonary arterial hypertension. ERA, endothelin receptor antagonist; PDE5-I, phosphodiesterase type 5 inhibitor; PH, pulmonary hypertension; sGC, soluble guanylate cyclase. *Risk determined by composite assesment of predictors of survival (see "Treatment" section).

CHAPTER 10

TABLE 10-3	Validated Risk Assessment Tools in PAH	
French Pulmonary Hypertension Registry	**REVEAL 2.0**	**REVEAL Lite**
Low-risk criteria:	*Poor predictors:*	*Poor predictors:*
Functional class I or II 6MWD > 440 m RAP < 8 mm Hg Cardiac index ≥ 2.5 L/min/m²	Connective tissue disease Heritable PAH Portopulmonary HTN Males > 60 y eGFR < 60 mL/min	eGFR < 60 mL/min Functional class III or IV Systolic BP < 110 mm Hg Pulse > 92 beats/min 6MWD < 165 m BNP > 180 pg/mL
Meeting ≥ 3 criteria associated with favorable 5-y prognosis	Functional class III or IV Systolic BP < 110 mm Hg Pulse > 92 beats/min Hospitalization within 6 mo. 6MWD < 165 m BNP > 200 pg/mL NT-proBNP > 1100 pg/mL Pericardial effusion DLCO < 40% predicted RAP > 20 mm Hg	*Favorable predictors:* Functional class I 6MWD > 440 m BNP < 50 pg/mL **Risk category based on weighted aggregate score**
	Favorable predictors: Functional class I 6MWD > 320 m BNP < 50 pg/mL or NT-proBNP < 300 pg/mL PVR < 5 Wood Units **Risk Category based on weighted aggregate score**	

6MWD, six-minute walk distance; BNP, brain natriuretic peptide; BP, blood pressure; DLCO, diffusing capacity for carbon monoxide; eGFR, estimated glomerular filtration rate; HTN, hypertension; NT-proBNP, N-terminal pro b-type natriuretic peptide; PAH, pulmonary arterial hypertension; PVR, pulmonary vascular resistance; RAP, right atrial pressure.

- ○ Combination therapy regimens with medications from more than one class of therapy are the preferred approach, even for newly diagnosed patients.[27]
  - ■ **Because of the complexity of some therapies, an individual's comorbid conditions, cognitive abilities, and psychosocial factors must also be considered.**
  - ○ Close monitoring and regular risk assessment is needed as deterioration often occurs, requiring alternative/additional medical and possibly surgical intervention.
- **Diuretics,** often in combination (e.g., loop diuretic + aldosterone antagonist), lessen **right heart failure** and symptoms.
- **Anticoagulation:**
  - ○ Chronic anticoagulation may improve survival in IPAH, while benefits in other PAH subtypes are unclear.[28,29]
  - ○ Warfarin is dosed to **target international normalized ratio of 1.5–2.5.**[21]
  - ○ Anticoagulant therapy is not urgent and bridging therapy is unnecessary.
- **Inotropes,** such as dobutamine and milrinone, are used in extremely decompensated states.

Surgical Management

- **Lung transplantation or heart–lung transplantation:**
  - For PAH patients who **remain in advanced functional class III–IV despite maximal medical therapy, which usually includes a parenteral prostanoid.**
  - Group III PH also impacts timing of transplant in parenchymal lung diseases.
  - Because the RV recovers after isolated lung transplantation, heart–lung transplantation is usually reserved for complex congenital heart defects that cannot be repaired.
- **Atrial septostomy:**
  - Palliative right-to-left intracardiac shunt created percutaneously in cases of severe right heart failure (i.e., syncope, hepatic congestion, prerenal azotemia) refractory to medical therapy.
  - Despite arterial oxyhemoglobin desaturation and hypoxemia, oxygen delivery increases from improved LV filling and cardiac output.
- **Septal defect closure:**
  - Intracardiac defects with significant net left-to-right shunting can be closed percutaneously or surgically.
  - Criteria for closure are evolving and some patients may be candidates after a period of treatment with pulmonary vasodilator therapy.[30]

PROGNOSIS

The 1-, 3-, and 5-year survival rates in PAH are 85%, 70%, and 55%, respectively.[31,32]

Obstructive Sleep Apnea–Hypopnea Syndrome

GENERAL PRINCIPLES

Definition

Obstructive sleep apnea (OSA) is a disorder in which patients experience apneas or hypopneas because of upper airway narrowing. When it is associated with excessive daytime somnolence, it is referred to as obstructive sleep apnea–hypopnea syndrome (OSAHS).[33]

Classification

- **Apneas** represent complete cessation of airflow.
  - Obstructive events are associated with continued respiratory effort.
  - Central events are associated with no respiratory effort.
- **Hypopneas** represent diminished airflow associated with at least a 3%–4% oxygen desaturation.
- **Respiratory effort–related arousals (RERAs)** represent changes in airflow that lead to an arousal, but do not meet criteria for an apnea or hypopnea.
- **All respiratory events** must last **at least 10 seconds** to be counted.
- **Apnea–hypopnea index (AHI)** is the number of apneas and hypopneas per hour of sleep.
- **Respiratory disturbance index (RDI)** is the number of apneas, hypopneas, and RERAs per hour of sleep.

Epidemiology

- The prevalence of OSAHS in the general population is estimated to be about 4%, with men being twice as likely as women to be affected.[34]
- Obesity is a significant risk factor for OSA.[34]

- Given the significant increase in the prevalence of obesity since the original epidemiological studies on OSA were performed, it is estimated that the current prevalence of moderate OSA as defined by an AHI > 15 is 13% in men and 6% in women.[35]

Etiology

- **OSA:** Narrowing of the upper airway because of excessive soft-tissue or structural abnormalities.
- **Central sleep apnea:** Disturbance of central control of respiration during sleep.

Pathophysiology

OSA occurs because of narrowing of the upper airway, which results in diminished airflow or cessation of airflow leading to arousals that fragment sleep.

Risk Factors

Risk factors for OSA include obesity (body mass index [BMI] > 30 kg/m^2), large neck circumference (>17 in for men and >16 in for women), increased soft tissue of the posterior oropharynx (enlarged tonsils, macroglossia, or elongated uvula), and abnormal jaw structure (micrognathia or retrognathia). Patients with comorbid conditions such as congestive heart failure, coronary artery disease, atrial fibrillation (AFib), difficult-to-control hypertension, and diabetes are also more likely to have OSA.[32]

Prevention

- Weight loss
- Avoiding sedatives such as hypnotic medications or alcohol

Associated Conditions

- **Cardiovascular disease**, including systemic hypertension, heart failure, arrhythmia, myocardial infarction, and stroke.[36] OSA has been established as an independent risk factor for hypertension.[37]
- **Increased risk of death in moderate-to-severe OSA**, mainly because of cardiovascular events.[38,39]
- Increased prevalence of **diabetes** has been noted in patients with OSAHS, independent of the effect of obesity.[40]
- There is approximately a 2.5-fold increased risk of **motor vehicle accidents** (MVA) in patients with OSA when compared with those without OSA. However, compliance with continuous positive airway pressure (CPAP) treatment can significantly reduce the risk of MVA in patients with OSA.[41]

DIAGNOSIS

Clinical Presentation

History

- **Habitual loud snoring** is the most common symptom of OSA, although not all people who snore have this syndrome. Patients with OSA may experience snore arousals along with a sensation of gasping or choking.
- Excessive daytime sleepiness (**hypersomnolence**) is a classic symptom of OSAHS (Table 10-4). Patients may describe falling asleep while driving or having difficulty concentrating at work.
- Patients may also complain of personality changes, intellectual deterioration, morning headaches, nocturnal angina, loss of libido, and chronic fatigue.

TABLE 10-4	Symptoms Associated With Obstructive Sleep Apnea–Hypopnea Syndrome

Excessive daytime sleepiness

Snoring

Nocturnal arousals

Nocturnal apneas

Nocturnal gasping, grunting, and choking

Nocturia

Enuresis

Awakening without feeling refreshed

Morning headaches

Impaired memory and concentration

Irritability and depression

Impotence

TABLE 10-5	Mallampati Airway Classification	
Class	Visible Structures With Mouth Maximally Opened and Tongue Protruded	
I	Hard palate, soft palate, uvula, tonsillar pillars	
II	Hard palate, soft palate, uvula	
III	Hard palate, soft palate, base of uvula	
IV	Hard palate	

Adapted from Mallampati SR, Gatt SP, Gugino LD, et al. A clinical sign to predict difficult tracheal intubation: a prospective study. *Can Anaesth Soc J*. 1985;32:429-434.

Physical Examination
- All patients should have a thorough nose and throat examination to detect sources of upper airway obstruction.
- Increased severity of OSA has been associated with a higher **Mallampati class** (Table 10-5).[42]

Diagnostic Criteria
A polysomnogram (**PSG**) demonstrating obstructive events with an AHI or RDI > 5 is diagnostic of OSA. If the RDI is between 5 and 15, a patient will qualify for positive airway pressure (PAP) if there is a comorbid condition such as hypertension, coronary artery disease, depression, or hypersomnolence. If there are no comorbid conditions, then the patient will qualify for PAP if the RDI is >15.

Differential Diagnosis
- In addition to OSAHS and sleep-related hypoventilation, the differential diagnosis for daytime sleepiness includes sleep deprivation, periodic limb movement disorder, narcolepsy, and medication side effects.
- Patients should also be evaluated for other medical conditions that may cause nighttime awakenings and dyspnea and thus mimic OSA, such as chronic lung disease, congestive heart failure, and gastroesophageal reflux disease (GERD).

CHAPTER 10

Diagnostic Testing

- The gold standard for the diagnosis of OSA is overnight PSG with direct observation by a qualified technician.[43] Sleep studies are typically performed in the outpatient setting.
- Typical indications for a sleep study include snoring with excessive daytime sleepiness, titration of optimal PAP therapy, and assessment of objective response to therapeutic interventions.
- PSG involves determination of sleep stages using electroencephalography, electromyography, and electrooculography and assessment of respiratory airflow and effort, oxyhemoglobin saturation, cardiac electrical activity (e.g., ECG), and body position. Transcutaneous CO_2 can be monitored to assess for hypoventilation in the appropriate clinical setting.
- Data are analyzed for sleep staging, the frequency of respiratory events, limb movements, and abnormal behaviors. Respiratory events are categorized as obstructive or central.
- Most sleep studies are performed as "split studies," where the first few hours of the study are diagnostic and the latter part of the study is used for PAP titration. Per the American Academy of Sleep Medicine guidelines, PAP should be started if the AHI/RDI during the diagnostic portion of the night is ≥40, but the threshold for starting PAP can be lowered to an AHI/RDI of ≥20 if there are significant comorbid conditions.
- Some patients only have significant events when lying in certain positions (usually supine) or during rapid eye movement sleep. These patients may require a complete overnight study for diagnosis and a second study for initiation of therapy.
- The American Academy of Sleep Medicine supports the use of unattended portable monitoring as an alternative to PSG for patients with a high pretest probability of moderate to severe OSA without significant comorbid medical conditions or other suspected sleep disorders.
  - The portable device must record airflow, respiratory effort, and blood oxygenation. A sleep specialist should review the results.
  - Portable devices can underestimate the severity of OSA because the number of events per hour is calculated using total recording time rather than total sleep time. If the portable sleep study is inconclusive, strong consideration should be given to performing an in-lab PSG.[43]

TREATMENT

The therapeutic approach to OSA depends on the severity of the disease, comorbid medical conditions, patient preference, and expected compliance. Treatment must be highly individualized, with special attention paid to correcting potentially reversible exacerbating factors.

Medications

- No pharmacologic agent has sufficient efficacy to warrant replacement of PAP as the primary therapeutic modality for OSAHS.
- Stimulant pharmacotherapy with **modafinil** or **armodafinil** may improve objective and subjective daytime sleepiness in patients with persistent symptoms despite adequate PAP use.[44]
- Medical treatment of conditions that may contribute to muscle hypotonia or weight gain, such as hypothyroidism, is of benefit.

Nonpharmacologic Therapies
- **PAP:**
  - **CPAP** delivers air via a face mask at a constant pressure throughout the respiratory cycle with the goal of pneumatically splinting open the upper airway, thus preventing collapse and airflow obstruction.
  - The PAP titration determines the PAP (expressed in cm H_2O) required to optimize airflow. The pressure setting is gradually increased until obstructive events, snoring, and oxygen desaturations are minimized.
  - The benefits of PAP include consolidated sleep and decreased daytime sleepiness. Hypertension, nocturia, peripheral edema, polycythemia, and PH may also improve.
  - CPAP is a highly cost-effective intervention.[45] The impact of CPAP treatment on associated cardiovascular comorbidities is variable with some studies showing improvement[46] and others showing no improvement.[47] Treatment of OSA results in a higher AFib-free survival rate after pulmonary vein isolation.[48]
  - **Nasal CPAP (nCPAP) is the current treatment of choice for most patients with OSAHS.**
    - The compliance rate with nCPAP is approximately 50%.
    - Compliance can be improved with education, instruction, follow-up, adjustment of the mask for fit and comfort, humidification of the air to decrease dryness, and treatment of nasal or sinus symptoms.
    - Use of a full-face mask (oronasal) has not been shown to improve compliance compared with the use of nCPAP.[49] However, full-face masks are frequently used in patients who "mouth breathe" or patients who require higher CPAP pressures because they will often experience air leak through the mouth when using nCPAP.
  - Autotitrating positive airway pressure (**APAP**) machines use flow and pressure transducers to sense airflow patterns and then automatically adjust the pressure setting in response. Small studies have shown that APAP may be as effective as traditional CPAP and appears to be preferred by patients.[50,51]
  - **Bilevel PAP** is typically used to treat OSA in the following settings: pressures >15–20 cm and H_2O are required, intolerance of CPAP, or concern for concomitant hypoventilation.
  - All positive pressure devices may induce dryness of the airway, nasal congestion, rhinorrhea, epistaxis, skin reactions to the mask, nasal bridge abrasions, and aerophagia. Some of these nasal symptoms may be treated with nasal saline, decongestants, and use of a humidifier.
  - Some patients, such as those with coexisting chronic obstructive pulmonary disease, require supplemental oxygen to maintain adequate nocturnal oxygen saturations ($SaO_2 \geq 90\%$).
- **Oral appliances:**
  - Used for mild OSAHS, with the aim to increase airway size to improve airflow. These devices, such as the mandibular advancement device, can be fixed or adjustable, and most require customized fitting. Many devices have not been well studied.
  - Contraindications include temporomandibular joint disease, bruxism, full dentures, and inability to protrude the mandible.
- **Upper airway stimulation device:**
  - A hypoglossal nerve stimulator to improve tongue protrusion is approved for use in patients with moderate to severe OSA who cannot tolerate CPAP. Use of the stimulator is limited to patients with a BMI < 32 kg/m^2.[52]
  - Although AHI and daytime sleepiness improved with this device, there was residual mild OSA.[53]

CHAPTER 10

Surgical Management

* **Tracheostomy:**
  ○ Tracheostomy is very effective in treating OSAHS but is rarely used since the advent of PAP therapy.
  ○ Tracheostomy should be reserved for patients with life-threatening disease (cor pulmonale, arrhythmias, or severe hypoxemia) or significant alveolar hypoventilation that cannot be controlled with other measures.
* **Uvulopalatopharyngoplasty (UPPP):**
  ○ UPPP is the most common surgical treatment of mild to moderate OSAHS in patients who do not respond to medical therapy.
  ○ UPPP enlarges the airway by removing tissue from the tonsils, tonsillar pillars, uvula, and posterior palate. UPPP may be complicated by change in voice, nasopharyngeal stenosis, foreign body sensation, velopharyngeal insufficiency with associated nasal regurgitation during swallowing, and PAP tolerance problems.
  ○ The success rate of UPPP for the treatment of OSAHS is only approximately 50%, when defined as a 50% reduction of the AHI, and improvements related to UPPP may diminish over time.[54] Thus, UPPP is considered a second-line treatment for patients with mild to moderate OSAHS who cannot successfully use PAP and who have retropalatal obstruction.
* **Staged procedures:**
  ○ In experienced centers, other staged procedures for OSA can be performed, including mandibular osteotomy with genioglossus advancement, hyoid myotomy with suspension, and maxillomandibular advancement (MMA).[53] Significant reductions in AHI have been reported with MMA, but more research is needed.[55]

Lifestyle/Risk Modification

* Weight loss, both surgical and through reduced caloric intake, has been shown to reduce the severity of OSA by reduction in AHI.[56,57]
* OSAHS patients should avoid use of alcohol, tobacco, and sedatives.
* Clinicians should counsel patients with OSAHS regarding the increased risk of driving and operating dangerous equipment.

SPECIAL CONSIDERATIONS

Patients with a BMI > 40 kg/m^2 are at increased risk for concomitant sleep-related hypoventilation because of morbid obesity.

COMPLICATIONS

* Patients with OSAHS are at greater risk for perioperative complications because of intubation difficulty and/or impaired arousal secondary to the effects of anesthetics, narcotics, and sedatives.[58]
* The risk of death, hypertension, and poor neuropsychological functioning rises with increasing severity of OSA.

REFERRAL

Patients with risk factors and symptoms or sequelae of OSAHS should be referred to a sleep specialist and sleep laboratory for further evaluation.

Interstitial Lung Disease

GENERAL PRINCIPLES

Definition

ILDs are a heterogeneous group of >200 disorders characterized by infiltration of the lung interstitium by cells, fluid, and/or connective tissue.

ILDs can present acutely or chronically, and they are often diagnosed using a multidisciplinary approach employing pulmonary clinicians, radiologists, and pathologists.

Classification

- ILDs can be broadly classified into those with known causes and those without (idiopathic).
  - Idiopathic interstitial pneumonias:[59]
    - Idiopathic pulmonary fibrosis (IPF) (idiopathic usual interstitial pneumonia [UIP])
    - Idiopathic nonspecific interstitial pneumonia (NSIP)
    - Desquamative interstitial pneumonia (DIP)
    - Respiratory bronchiolitis–associated interstitial lung disease (RB-ILD)
    - Cryptogenic organizing pneumonia (COP) (idiopathic OP)
    - Acute interstitial pneumonia (AIP)
    - Lymphoid interstitial pneumonia (LIP) (rare)
    - Idiopathic pleuroparenchymal fibroelastosis (rare)
  - Medication/therapy induced:
    - Bleomycin
    - Amiodarone
    - Nitrofurantoin
    - Checkpoint inhibitors
    - NSAIDs
    - Thalidomide
    - Rituximab
    - Azathioprine
    - Methotrexate
    - Radiation therapy
  - CTD-ILD:
    - Rheumatoid arthritis
    - Scleroderma
    - Sjögren syndrome
    - Antisynthetase syndrome
    - Mixed CTD
    - Systemic lupus erythematosus
  - Vasculitides:
    - Granulomatosis with polyangiitis
    - Eosinophilic granulomatosis with polyangiitis
    - Microscopic polyangiitis
    - Goodpasture syndrome
  - Pneumoconiosis (diseases of the lung due to dust inhalation):
    - Coal miners' pneumoconiosis
    - Asbestosis
    - Silicosis

- Siderosis
- Stannosis
- Mixed dust pneumoconiosis
○ Granulomatous ILD:
  - Sarcoidosis
  - Berylliosis
  - Hypersensitivity pneumonitis (HP)
  - Granulomatous–lymphocytic interstitial lung disease
  - Bronchocentric granulomatosis
○ Cystic lung diseases:
  - Lymphangioleiomyomatosis (LAM)
  - Pulmonary Langerhans cell histiocytosis (PLCH)
  - Birt–Hogg–Dubé (BHD) syndrome
  - Pulmonary amyloidosis
  - Light chain deposition disease
  - Postinfectious
○ Miscellaneous:
  - Erdheim–Chester disease
  - Pulmonary alveolar proteinosis
  - Lipoid pneumonia
  - Pulmonary alveolar microlithiasis
  - Acute eosinophilic pneumonia
  - Chronic eosinophilic pneumonia

Clinical Presentation

History

- Obtaining a thorough history is of paramount importance in patients presenting with ILD and is often crucial in making a diagnosis.
- Patients most often present with progressive dyspnea and persistent dry cough.
- Duration of symptoms may help in differentiating ILDs. While many ILDs present with years of progressive dyspnea and cough, a subset of ILD patients present with acute or subacute onset of symptoms (AIP, acute eosinophilic pneumonia, OP), which may mimic infectious pneumonias with atypical organisms.
- Past medical history is very important, not only for underlying diseases but also to identify ILDs related to disease management. Examples include CTDs and immunosuppressive agents; cancers along with chemo-, immuno-, and radiotherapies; and other systemic diseases that can potentially affect the lungs such as inflammatory bowel disease. It is important not to forget the use of over-the-counter medications.
- Documenting a smoking history is essential. Some ILDs manifest almost exclusively in smokers (Langerhans cell histiocytosis, DIP, and RB-ILD). Some diseases are strongly associated with current or previous tobacco use, for example, IPF. Pulmonary hemorrhage is far more common in active smokers with Goodpasture disease than in prior or nonsmokers.
- Exposures both at home and in the workplace should be evaluated. These may include exposures to radiation, asbestos, metal dusts, wood dusts, chemicals or fumes, pets, moldy environments, down comforters and/or pillows, and more. Patients should be questioned regarding the degree and duration of their exposures, and the use of respiratory protective equipment.
- Family history should be obtained, specifically as it relates to pulmonary fibrosis, lung disease, or autoimmune disease. Multiple inheritance patterns have been described with ILDs including complex (sarcoidosis), autosomal dominant (tuberous sclerosis), and autosomal recessive (Hermansky–Pudlak syndrome).

Physical Examination
- Extrapulmonary examination in patients with ILD should pay particular attention to findings of systemic diseases that may affect the lungs. These include CTDs, sarcoidosis, tuberous sclerosis, and others.
  - Examples include sclerodactyly, mechanic's hands, Raynaud phenomenon, dry mucous membranes, telangiectasias, skin rashes, facial erythema, papules, eczema, or other skin lesions.
- Cardiac examination should focus on findings suggesting the presence of PH/cor pulmonale including a right ventricular heave, pulmonary artery tap, tricuspid regurgitation holosystolic murmur, right-sided S3, and peripheral edema. These findings are usually indicative of advanced lung disease.
- Clubbing is a very nonspecific finding described in lung diseases, heart diseases, and gastrointestinal (GI) diseases. It can be seen in IPF, sarcoidosis, PLCH, and other ILDs.
- The pulmonary examination in ILDs is nonspecific. Findings may include dry inspiratory crackles, which are best noted posteriorly near the lung bases. Wheezes and inspiratory squeaks may also be noted.

Diagnostic Testing

Diagnostic testing in the evaluation of ILDs typically involves:
- Chest imaging including CXR and high-resolution CT (HRCT) of the chest
- Pulmonary function tests (PFTs)
- Blood testing
- Lung sampling including bronchoscopy and video-assisted thoracic surgery (VATS)

Chest Imaging
- Review of old CXRs is often very helpful in assessing both the rate and extent of change of lung disease over time.
- Up to 10% of CXRs may be normal in patients with ILD; as a result, a normal CXR may not exclude ILD in settings where the clinical suspicion of ILD is very high.
- As a result of the wide variety of ILDs, CXRs may have a highly variable appearance.
- The most common abnormality on CXR in ILD is a reticular pattern of linear opacities that may be localized or form a network involving the lungs diffusely.
- However, nodular opacities, alveolar opacities, mixed alveolar opacities, and reticular opacities and occasionally cystic changes are also seen.
- Extensive fibrosis of the lungs may lead to volume loss in one or both lungs.
- Patients with known or suspected ILDs should undergo CT scanning as the diagnosis of many ILDs relies on HRCT.[60]
- HRCT is a scanning technique that uses thin slice (usually 1-mm thick) images that are obtained and processed using a high-frequency reconstruction algorithm.[60] Scans are obtained with the patient in a supine position during a breath hold at maximal inspiration and then during a breath hold at maximal expiration.
- Prone imaging may be performed in cases where atelectasis obscures the posterior lung bases.
- The pattern on HRCT is important in determining the differential diagnosis of ILD (Table 10-6). Notably, published guidelines exist for the definitive radiologic diagnosis of certain ILDs, specifically IPF.[60]

Pulmonary Function Testing
- PFTs are a noninvasive set of tests that allow for evaluation of lung function, stratification of disease severity, and for monitoring of disease progression over time.
- Complete pulmonary function testing involves spirometry, lung volumes, and diffusing capacity (DLCO), along with resting and exercise pulse oximetry.

TABLE 10-6	Clinical and Radiologic Features of Interstitial Lung Diseases	
	Clinical Features	**HRCT Findings**
UIP	• Insidious onset and progressive dyspnea • Dry cough • Poorly responsive to treatment, poor long-term survival • Variable course punctuated by intermittent exacerbations • Pattern can be associated with connective tissue disease • Older patients >50 y • Male predominance	• UIP on CT or biopsy forms the radiologic basis for diagnosing IPF in the absence of underlying cause • Subpleural, basal predominant reticulation/interstitial thickening • Honeycombing with/without traction bronchiectasis • Heterogeneous (geographic) distribution • Absence of ground glass, consolidation, micronodules, cysts, or air trapping • May have atypical distribution in familial cases
NSIP	• Associated with younger patients • More common in females • Commonly associated with collagen vascular diseases, including scleroderma, rheumatoid arthritis, and antisynthetase syndrome • Response to therapy is variable depending on etiology	• Interstitial thickening, often with peripheral subpleural sparing • Ground-glass infiltrates • Traction bronchiectasis • Homogeneous distribution • In end-stage disease, may develop fibrotic changes and "bronchiolectasis" that resembles UIP
RB-ILD	• Associated with cigarette smoking • Generally responsive to smoking cessation	• Bronchiolocentric ground-glass nodules with an upper lobe predominance
DIP	• Associated with cigarette smoking and occupational exposures • Generally responsive to smoking cessation • May be treated with corticosteroids	• Peripheral ground-glass opacities or consolidation • May have small, well-defined cysts
COP	• Subacute course, often presents as multiple outpatient treatment failures of bronchitis/pneumonia • Often associated with infections or drug exposures • Responsive to prolonged courses of corticosteroids • Often recurs if steroids are withdrawn too rapidly	• Multifocal ground-glass opacities and consolidations • Usually lower lobe predominant • Infiltrates may be migratory on serial imaging • May have "reverse halo" or atoll sign

TABLE 10-6	Clinical and Radiologic Features of Interstitial Lung Diseases (continued)	
	Clinical Features	HRCT Findings
Sarcoidosis	• Dyspnea, cough, and chest pain are common presenting symptoms • Systemic symptoms may be prominent • Approximately 1 in 20 cases are asymptomatic and incidentally detected on CXR • Almost any organ system may be affected	• Perilymphatic nodules • Patchy ground-glass opacities • Reticular infiltrates • Traction bronchiectasis • Progressive massive fibrosis • Hilar or mediastinal lymphadenopathy
Fibrotic HP/ fibrotic HP with honeycombing	• Presents in a similar fashion to UIP/IPF • There may be a history of systemic symptoms (fever, myalgias) • Associated with environmental exposures (birds, molds, hot tubs) but these are identified in <50% of cases	• Reticular abnormality with an upper or mid-lung predominance • Micronodules • Mosaic attenuation/air trapping • Peribronchovascular predominance • Honeycombing may be present in more advanced disease

BAL, bronchoalveolar lavage; COP, cryptogenic organizing pneumonia; DIP, desquamative interstitial pneumonia; HP, hypersensitivity pneumonitis; HRCT, high-resolution CT; ILD, interstitial lung disease; IPF, idiopathic pulmonary fibrosis; NSIP, nonspecific interstitial pneumonia; RB-ILD, respiratory bronchiolitis–associated interstitial lung disease; UIP, usual interstitial pneumonia.

Data from Kadoch MA, Cham MD, Beasley MB, et al. Idiopathic interstitial pneumonias: a radiology-pathology correlation based on the revised 2013 American Thoracic Society-European Respiratory Society classification system. *Curr Probl Diagn Radiol.* 2015;44:15-25; Raghu G, Collard HR, Egan JJ, et al. An official ATS/ERS/JRS/ALAT statement: idiopathic pulmonary fibrosis – evidence-based guidelines for diagnosis and management. *Am J Respir Crit Care Med.* 2011;183:788-824; Webb RW, Higgins CB. *Thoracic Imaging*: Pulmonary and Cardiovascular Radiology. Lippincott Williams & Wilkins; 2005.

• PFTs allow us to determine whether patients have restrictive lung disease, obstructive lung disease, or a mixed pattern of disease. This aids in the differential diagnosis of ILD.
• While most fibrotic ILDs demonstrate a restrictive pattern on PFTs, a number of ILDs may demonstrate obstruction, including smoking-related lung diseases (RB-ILD and PLCH), cystic lung diseases (LAM and BHD), and sarcoidosis.
• DLCO is commonly decreased in patients with ILD but is a nonspecific finding.
• In some cases, the presence of coexisting COPD in patients with ILDs may lead to a mixed pattern of lung disease on PFTs. In other cases, pseudonormalization of PFTs occurs where the combination of restriction and obstruction leads to the finding of "normal" testing. In these cases, a low DLCO may be the only clue that the patient has significant underlying lung disease when the PFTs are reviewed in isolation.

CHAPTER 10

- Resting and exercise pulse oximetry are commonly assessed using a 6MW test.
- Serial PFTs obtained at follow-up visits are a useful way to monitor for disease progression and may have prognostic significance.[61]

Laboratories

- Routine laboratory testing in the evaluation of ILD patients includes CBC, BMP, and LFT testing. These may provide clues to the diagnosis (eosinophilia).
- Many drugs used in the treatment of ILD require regular monitoring of blood counts, renal function, or liver function.
- Serologic testing for CTDs is obtained in all patients with clinical stigmata of CTD.
- Aldolase and creatinine kinase may be tested to evaluate for evidence of myositis in patients with a clinical suspicion for antisynthetase syndrome. In cases where suspicion is high for myositis, panels of muscle-specific antibodies should also be obtained.
- In any patient with a high suspicion for scleroderma or Sjögren disease, an ENA panel should be obtained. ENA panels vary but contain a wide variety of antibodies to screen for CTD.
- In practice, serologic testing is often obtained in a wide range of patients to exclude subclinical CTD. Many centers obtain a minimum of an antinuclear antibody (ANA), rheumatoid factor, and a cyclic citrullinated peptide antibody tests, even patients with suspected IPF, since rheumatoid arthritis ILD often presents with a UIP pattern on HRCT.
- In patients with cystic lung disease on imaging, testing for vascular endothelial growth factor type D (VEGF-D) may be helpful in making the diagnosis of LAM. Levels of VEGF-D > 800 pg/mL in the correct clinical or radiographic setting can be diagnostic of LAM.[62]
- Genetic testing can also be helpful in cystic lung diseases and can screen for tuberous sclerosis–associated LAM (*TSC1* and *TSC2* gene mutations) and BHD (*FLCN*, folliculin gene mutations) where appropriate.

Lung Sampling

- When an extensive evaluation does not result in a confident diagnosis, lung sampling can be considered.
- Bronchoalveolar lavage (BAL) is used to sample the cellular content of the lungs. It has limited utility in the evaluation of ILD.
- BAL is useful in excluding coexisting infection and, in some cases, malignancy. It is also useful in cases where diffuse alveolar hemorrhage or eosinophilic lung disease is suspected.[63]
- Lung biopsy should only be undertaken at centers with expertise in evaluating ILD patients. Generally, biopsy should be reserved for circumstances where the diagnosis is uncertain and clarification would result in a significantly altered approach to management.
- While lung biopsy is desired in many cases, patients with ILD are often considerably physiologically impaired and may not tolerate the procedure.
- Although many patients tolerate lung biopsy well, certain subgroups of patients are predisposed to complications, including decompensation of their ILD following lung biopsy.[64] Patients with IPF may develop disease exacerbations following lung biopsy, resulting in disease progression and even death.
- Two types of lung biopsy are available: transbronchial forceps biopsy (TBBx) and VATS biopsy.
- TBBx is often performed along with BAL during bronchoscopy. It is most useful in cases in which small biopsy samples suffice for diagnosis.

- TBBx has the highest yield in bronchiolocentric ILDs, such as sarcoidosis, berylliosis, and lymphangitic carcinomatosis.[65] It is also useful in cases where eosinophilic pneumonia or pulmonary alveolar proteinosis is suspected.
- TBBx is insufficient for differentiating most idiopathic ILDs, especially between UIP and NSIP, given inadequate sample size.
- However, a recently developed test, the Envisia Genomic Classifier, uses genomic patterns in TBBx samples to distinguish UIP fibrotic lung disease from non-UIP fibrotic lung disease. It is may helpful in well-selected patients with lung fibrosis who would not tolerate VATS biopsy.
- Transbronchial cryobiopsy is a newer option that allows for larger volume tissue sampling without a surgical lung biopsy. Further studies are required to integrate this technique into the ILD diagnostic algorithm.[66]
- In cases with UIP patterns, VATS biopsies are preferred as they yield tissue samples large enough for accurate diagnosis. HRCT should be used to target areas of active disease and avoid lung regions with end-stage fibrosis, which is nondiagnostic.

SPECIFIC ILDs

Idiopathic Pulmonary Fibrosis

- IPF is the most common form of idiopathic interstitial pneumonia.
- The incidence of IPF in the US is estimated to be 7–16 cases per 100,000 population. In older populations (e.g., >65 years), the incidence goes up considerably.[67]
- The pathophysiology is incompletely understood, but alveolar epithelial cell injury and dysregulated tissue repair are thought to play a significant role.
- A history of cigarette smoking is the strongest risk factor associated with IPF. Other risk factors for IPF include age >60 years, male sex, and GERD.[60]
- Increasingly, familial clusters of IPF are being identified and are referred to as familial pulmonary fibrosis (FPF).
- Genetic variant associated with FPF includes those in pulmonary surfactant protein C (*SFTPC*), surfactant protein A2 (*SFTPA2*), and mucin 5B (*MUC5B*).[68]
- Around 15% cases of FPF have short telomere syndrome resulting from mutations in telomere maintenance genes including telomerase RNA component (*TERC*), telomerase reverse transcriptase (*TERT*), and others. Short telomere syndrome can present with bone marrow failure, premature graying, cirrhosis, nail dystrophy, and mucosal leukoplakia.[69]
- Patients with IPF are usually aged 60 years or older.
- They commonly present with slowly progressive dyspnea and nonproductive cough over years to months.
- Extrapulmonary or systemic symptoms are rare.
- Physical examination may reveal dry inspiratory crackles.
  Digital clubbing has been reported in 45%–75% of cases depending on the series.[70]
- A diagnosis of IPF requires:
  ○ exclusion of all other causes of fibrosing lung disease (CTD, HP, sarcoid) and
  ○ a radiographic pattern of definite UIP on HRCT (Table 10-6, Figure 10-3) or
  ○ a UIP pattern on surgical lung biopsy.
- For patients requiring lung biopsy to confirm the diagnosis of IPF, VATS lung biopsy is preferred, as tissue sampling TBBx is diagnostic in less than one-third of cases.[71]
- A multidisciplinary approach employing discussion with pulmonary, radiology, and pathology staff with ILD experience increases diagnostic accuracy.
- Radiographic pattern:
  ○ HRCT is mandatory for imaging ILDs and particularly IPF.

CHAPTER 10

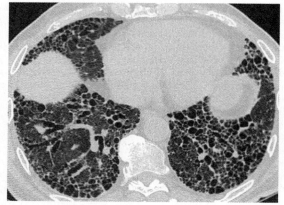

Figure 10-3. Usual interstitial pneumonitis. (Figure courtesy of Dr. Constantine Raptis, Mallinckrodt Institute of Radiology.)

- ○ A pattern of definite UIP on HRCT includes the presence of honeycombing, and subpleural and basilar predominant reticulation. The affected portions of the lung should demonstrate a geographic or heterogeneous involvement. The presence or absence of traction bronchiectasis does not impact the diagnosis.
  - ○ The pattern of a definite UIP on HRCT in the appropriate clinical setting (where other potential causes of ILD have been ruled out) may be sufficient to determine the diagnosis of IPF.
  - ○ In the setting of a FPF, the HRCT pattern may be atypical, often lacking a basal predominance. Even histologically, strictly defined UIP is identified in less than half of FPF cases.[72]
- • Disease-modifying treatment options are limited in IPF (Table 10-7).
  - ○ There is no medical cure for IPF.
  - ○ Most medications studied have not been found to impact disease progression and some have proved dangerous (increased risks of death and hospitalization have been associated with combined use of N-acetylcysteine, azathioprine, and prednisone).[73]
  - ○ Pirfenidone, an oral antifibrotic agent, and nintedanib, an oral tyrosine kinase inhibitor, have both been shown to slow the rate of lung function decline in patients with IPF.[74,75] They may also have a mortality benefit.
  - ○ The most frequent side effects with nintedanib are diarrhea (62% of patients), nausea, and vomiting.
  - ○ The most frequent side effects of pirfenidone are skin rash (30%), photosensitivity, nausea, and diarrhea.
  - ○ Drug-induced liver disease can occur with both agents, and monitoring of liver function tests (LFT) is mandatory with both agents. Elevations in LFTs can be managed with dose adjustments or discontinuation.
- • Pulmonary rehabilitation has been associated with improvements in 6MW distance and quality of life in IPF.[73]
- • Prognosis and clinical course are variable, but those diagnosed with mild, moderate, and severe disease by spirometry have been reported to have median survivals of 55.6, 38.7, and 27.4 months, respectively.[74]

TABLE 10-7	Medical Treatment of Selected Interstitial Lung Diseases
ILD	Potential Therapeutic Interventions[a]
Medication-induced ILD	• Discontinue culprit medication • Corticosteroids
Connective tissue disease–associated ILD (UIP, NSIP, COP)	• Corticosteroids • Immunosuppressive therapy (e.g., cyclophosphamide, azathioprine, mycophenolate, rituximab)
IPF	• Pirfenidone • Nintedanib • Consideration for participation in a clinical trial
DIP, RB-ILD	• Smoking cessation • Corticosteroids (likely of limited benefit)
Sarcoidosis	• Corticosteroids • Immunosuppressive therapy (e.g., methotrexate, azathioprine, infliximab)
HP	• Avoid offending antigens • Corticosteroids (likely of limited benefit) • Antifibrotic therapy • Immunosuppressive therapy

[a]Lung transplantation is a consideration for select patients with end-stage interstitial lung disease.
COP, cryptogenic organizing pneumonia; DIP, desquamative interstitial pneumonia; HP, hypersensitivity pneumonitis; ILD, interstitial lung disease; IPF, idiopathic pulmonary fibrosis; NSIP, nonspecific interstitial pneumonia; RB-ILD, respiratory bronchiolitis–associated interstitial lung disease; UIP, usual interstitial pneumonia.

• Poor prognostic factors for IPF:
  ○ Decline in forced vital capacity of >10% over six months
  ○ Decrease in DLCO of >15% over six months
  ○ Decrease in 6MW distance of >150 m over 12 months[61]
• Exacerbations of IPF are characterized by acute worsening of dyspnea or oxygenation (within 30 days) and new ground-glass opacifications/ consolidations on CT with no evidence of infection, pulmonary embolus, or heart failure.[60]
• Exacerbations are typically treated with high-dose corticosteroids, although their benefit has not been systematically proven. Patients often do not return to their pre-exacerbation baseline after IPF exacerbations and mortality rates are high.[76]
• Lung transplantation remains the ultimate therapy in patients with advanced IPF. Without lung transplantation, outcomes in IPF remain poor. Patients should be referred to a lung transplant program at the time of diagnosis of IPF.

Nonspecific Interstitial Pneumonia

• NSIP can describe both a radiographic pattern on HRCT and pathologic pattern on lung biopsy.
• It is referred to as nonspecific because biopsies, in particular, lack the histologic features characteristic of other idiopathic interstitial pneumonias.
• NSIP is one of the subtypes of idiopathic interstitial pneumonia. However, idiopathic NSIP is rare.

- NSIP is much more commonly secondary to other causes including[77]:
  - CTD: Including scleroderma, Sjögren disease, antisynthetase syndrome, and rheumatoid arthritis. Interstitial pneumonia with autoimmune features is a distinct subcategory of ILD where patients with confirmed NSIP on HRCT or lung biopsy have clinical features of autoimmune disease not conforming to any particular CTD.[78]
  - Drug toxicity: Drugs commonly associated with NSIP including amiodarone, nitrofurantoin, methotrexate, statins, and various chemotherapeutic agents have been associated with development of NSIP.
  - HIV infection: Less common in the age of highly active antiretroviral therapy (HAART).
  - Others: These include fibrotic HP, FPF, graft versus host disease, and IgG4 disease.
- Patients with NSIP tend to be younger than those with IPF and are more commonly female.[79]
- Due to the frequency of secondary causes, NSIP may present with fevers, chills, weight loss, or flu-like symptoms. Symptoms of CTD are also common.
- HRCT demonstrates a combination of ground-glass and reticular opacities often in a peripheral and basal predominant distribution. A peribronchovascular distribution may also be noted. There is often sparing of the immediate subpleural space from involvement, which is relatively specific for NSIP (Table 10-6) (Figure 10-4).
- Other features of NSIP include traction bronchiectasis, centrilobular nodules, air trapping on exhalation imaging and rarely microscopic honeycombing.
- While the diagnosis of idiopathic NSIP may require a surgical lung biopsy, most cases of secondary NSIP do not when the diagnosis is certain from the history, physical examination, and laboratory testing. In cases where lung biopsy is required, VATS biopsy is essential.
- Treatment of CTD-associated NSIP usually involves immunosuppression with steroids, in combination with steroid-sparing agents such as mycophenolate, azathioprine, rituximab, or cyclophosphamide (Table 10-7).

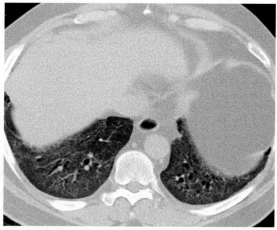

Figure 10-4. Nonspecific interstitial pneumonitis. (Figure courtesy of Dr. Constantine Raptis, Mallinckrodt Institute of Radiology.)

- Management of patients with CTD-related ILD should be undertaken in a multi-disciplinary fashion.
- NSIP from drug toxicity is treated by discontinuation of the offending agent. In some cases, steroid therapy may be required.
- Other secondary causes of NSIP are treated by targeting the primary disease, for example, HIV (HAART) and IgG4 disease (steroids).
- In cases refractory to therapy, lung transplant remains an option in selected instances.
- Patients with NSIP have a significantly better prognosis than those with IPF.[79]

Hypersensitivity Pneumonitis

- HP is a pulmonary syndrome of varying clinical presentation and natural history.
- It is the result of an immune-mediated pulmonary response directed against a plethora of potential inhaled antigens to which an individual is both sensitized and hyperresponsive.
- Hundreds of antigens have been described as causing HP and include bacteria, mycobacteria, fungi, organic proteins, chemicals, and metals.[80]
- Well-described clinical presentations of HP include farmer's lung (exposure to moldy hay) and bird fanciers' disease (exposure to birds).
- Since a minority of people exposed to inhaled antigens manifest with disease, disease expression is thought to be dependent on a complex interaction of antigen dose, intensity and duration of antigen exposure, antigen immunogenicity, and host factors such as genetic susceptibility.
- Currently, the optimal characterization of HP is based on the presence or absence of fibrosis and honeycombing on either HRCT or pathologic samples. The radiologic phenotypes in particular have prognostic significance[81]:
  - HP without fibrosis (median survival >14 years)
  - HP with fibrosis (median survival 7.95 years)
  - HP with fibrosis and honeycombing (median survival 2.8 years)
- Acute forms of HP (corresponding to nonfibrotic disease) may manifest over hours to weeks and are often temporally related to antigen exposure. They present with relatively rapid onset of dyspnea, cough, and chest tightness. In addition, patients may manifest with systemic symptoms including fevers, chills, myalgias, and malaise. Resolution is expected following antigen removal.
- Chronic disease (corresponding to fibrosis and honeycombing) and dyspnea often progress indolently over time and are often associated with dry cough. Unlike IPF, chronic forms of HP can be accompanied by systemic symptoms including anorexia, weight loss, and fatigue.
- A careful and thorough exposure history should be taken and should include inquiry about exposure to birds or bird feathers (including down pillows and comforters), hot tubs (associated with aerosolized mycobacterial exposure), air humidifiers, moldy homes or workplaces, animal furs, epoxies, plant matter, industrial dusts, and chemicals.[82]
- Specific antibody testing for culprit antigens can be sent to specialized labs when indicated, although positive serologies only support exposure to the antigens against which the antibodies are directed and do not necessarily confirm causation.
- The causative exposure/antigen is identified in <50% of cases.
- HRCT findings in nonfibrotic disease include nodular or diffuse ground-glass opacities, mosaic appearance on inspiratory scans, and air trapping on expiratory sequences.[82]
- HRCT findings in fibrotic and honeycomb disease include upper lobe–predominant reticulation in a bronchovascular distribution, mosaic attenuation on inspiratory

scans, air trapping on expiratory sequences, and of course honeycombing (Table 10-6).[82]

- Treatment should involve paying careful attention to identification of the offending antigen because antigen avoidance, when identified, has been associated with significantly improved survival (Table 10-7).[6]
- Corticosteroid therapy has been the classic mainstay of treatment for fibrotic honeycombing disease, although data from randomized clinical trials are lacking.
- In selected cases, a trial of immunosuppression can be attempted with close follow-up.[83]
- Most recently, nintedanib has been proposed as an alternative treatment. This is based on the results of trial looking at the use of nintedanib in progressive fibrosing ILDs.[84]

Sarcoidosis

- Sarcoidosis is a multisystem inflammatory disease most commonly affecting the lungs.
- Other organs are less commonly involved and include the skin, lymph nodes, eyes, heart, and nervous system. However, any organ may be affected by sarcoidosis.[85]
- The cause of sarcoidosis has not been identified, but is likely the interaction of a number of environmental and host genetic factors.[86]
- Sarcoidosis typically occurs in young adults.
- It is more common in African Americans than in Caucasians (3–4 times higher incidence). African Americans also present with earlier onset disease, and with a greater burden of extrapulmonary disease. In addition, African American patients have higher hospitalization rates and higher mortality rates (8–14 times higher).[87]
- In up to 50% of cases, sarcoidosis may be asymptomatic and detected on incidental chest imaging.
- When symptomatic, patients often present with progressive dyspnea, nonproductive cough, or chest pain.
- Extrapulmonary manifestations of sarcoidosis include[88]:
  ○ Ocular disease may include uveitis, retinal disease, conjunctivitis, and lachrymal gland involvement.
  ○ Skin disease may manifest with various rashes including erythema nodosum (raised, red, tender nodules on anterior legs) and lupus pernio (indurated plaques with associated discoloration of the nose, cheeks, lips, and ears).
  ○ Nervous system involvement can manifest as encephalopathy, granulomatous meningitis, mononeuritis multiplex, or a host of other neurologic anomalies.
  ○ Cardiac involvement may result in cardiomyopathy and heart failure, ventricular aneurysms, arrhythmias, and sudden cardiac death.[89] The heart may be the only organ involved in >20% of cases.
  ○ Endocrine involvement can manifest as hypercalcemia and hypercalciuria secondary to dysregulated production of calcitriol.[90]
- Sarcoidosis may also present with two well-described acute clinical syndromes[88]:
  ○ Löfgren syndrome is characterized by arthritis, erythema nodosum, and bilateral hilar lymphadenopathy.[86]
  ○ Heerfordt syndrome presents with a combination of uveitis, parotid gland swelling, fevers, and in some cases facial palsy. It is also known as uveoparotid fever.
- CXR imaging in sarcoidosis may manifest with pulmonary opacities, thoracic lymphadenopathy, or a combination of both. CXR is also used to stage the disease (Table 10-8).

TABLE 10-8	Scadding Staging of Sarcoidosis	
CXR Findings	Frequency at Presentation (%)
Stage 0: Normal	5–15
Stage I: Hilar or mediastinal lymphadenopathy	25–65
Stage II: Hilar or mediastinal lymphadenopathy with pulmonary infiltrates	20–40
Stage III: Pulmonary infiltrates	10–15
Stage IV: End-stage fibrosis	5

Adapted from Maller V, Knipe H. Thoracic sarcoidosis (staging). Accessed March 4, 2021. http://radiopaedia.org/articles/thoracic-sarcoidosis-staging?lang=us

- On HRCT, parenchymal nodules appear in almost 80% of patients. They typically follow a perilymphatic distribution and may coalescence into larger opacities.[86] Other findings may include alveolar opacities, pulmonary fibrosis, and air trapping on expiratory imaging (Table 10-6).
- Laboratory testing should be obtained. Serum calcium, urine calcium, CBC, BMP, and LFTs should all be checked. Abnormalities in these are not diagnostic of sarcoidosis but can help determine extent of disease and organ involvement.
- In the appropriate clinical setting, sarcoidosis is diagnosed by the presence of non-caseating granulomas on biopsy samples of involved organs (commonly the lung, lymph nodes, or skin). The presence of granulomas in more than one organ system is preferable when making the diagnosis.[90]
- Exclusion of other diseases is obligatory when diagnosing sarcoidosis.[90] Excluding infectious disease is of particular importance, especially in patients who reside in areas with endemic fungal or mycobacterial disease, as these can mimic sarcoidosis.
- Treatment of sarcoidosis can be complicated, and referral to pulmonary and other specialists is often necessary.
- For mild disease, symptoms and radiographic changes may remit in the absence of treatment.
- In the setting of more symptomatic or progressive disease, corticosteroids are typically first-line therapy and many patients can be treated with intermittent steroid therapy alone (Table 10-7).
- Patients with more advanced disease or those requiring longer-term steroid therapy may need to be transitioned to steroid-sparing immunosuppression such as methotrexate or azathioprine.
- Tumor necrosis factor alpha antagonists are typically reserved for severe disease that progresses despite the aforementioned therapies.[91]
- Prognosis is highly variable, ranging from indolent self-remitting disease to progressive fibrosis requiring transplantation. As a broad rule, acute onset disease tends toward a better prognosis, while more indolent onset disease may become unremittingly progressive.

Organizing Pneumonia

- OP is a nonspecific pulmonary response to injury characterized by inflammation and proliferation of granulation tissue in the alveoli and terminal bronchioles.
- OP was previously referred to as bronchiolitis obliterans with OP.
- OP may be either:

○ Idiopathic, referred to as COP, and one of the subtypes of idiopathic interstitial pneumonia, or

○ Secondary, and occur in association with CTDs, drug toxicity (e.g., amiodarone, checkpoint inhibitors), infections, inhalational injury (e.g., cocaine, industrial gasses), radiation treatment, and along with other ILDs (e.g., vasculitis).[92]

• Patients often present with dyspnea, cough, fevers, malaise, fatigue, and weight loss lasting weeks to months. These symptoms may mimic pneumonia, and a frequent scenario is a patient presenting with multiple episodes of "pneumonia" unresponsive to antibiotics therapy.

• On HRCT, OP manifests with multifocal patchy consolidation, often in a peripheral or peribronchovascular distribution. The opacities may affect all lung zones and when followed over time may be migratory.[92] The reverse halo or atoll sign is thought to be very specific for OP on HRCT but is not commonly seen (Table 10-6).

• Diagnosis is often suggested through a combination of good history taking and HRCT appearance.

• PFTs are nonspecific and may demonstrate restriction.

• BAL is useful to rule out infection.

• The method of lung biopsy is controversial. While TBBx may make the diagnosis, some feel that they may not be sufficient to detect secondary causes of OP due to the small size of the biopsies. As such, several centers recommend VATS biopsy where OP is suspected.[64]

• Patients normally have good response to treatment with steroids. However, recurrence is common and long-term steroid therapy over 3–6 months is generally recommended. If OP continues without response to treatment or progresses to fibrosis, prognosis is poor.

• In cases associated with other diseases (e.g., vasculitis, CTD), treatment is directed at the underlying cause.

Smoking-Related ILD

Certain ILDs manifest almost exclusively in smokers. These include RB-ILD, DIP, and PLCH.

Respiratory Bronchiolitis Interstitial Lung Disease

• RB-ILD is typically associated with heavy smoking (often 30 pack-years or more).[93]

• It commonly presents in the third to fifth decades of life.

• On HRCT, RB-ILD manifests with centrilobular ground-glass nodules, often with an upper lobe predilection. In some cases, the nodules are more confluent and present as ground-glass opacities (Table 10-6).

• Other changes related to smoking, such as emphysema and bronchial wall thickening, may also be present.[94]

• Symptoms and radiographic findings often improve with smoking cessation (Table 10-7).[94]

Desquamative Interstitial Pneumonia

• DIP may represent a spectrum of disease along with RB-ILD.

• Ninety percent of patients with DIP are heavy smokers.[95]

• The other 10% may have CTD, HIV, or environmental exposures. A congenital form may be seen in children.

• The predominant HRCT finding in DIP is bilateral ground-glass opacity, which may be peripheral, patchy, or diffuse in distribution. It is classically described as

triangular-shaped opacities radiating from the hila to the periphery of the lung; however, this finding is noted in only a minority of patients (Table 10-6).
- Small cystic spaces occasionally develop within the ground-glass opacities.
- Response to smoking cessation is favorable, although some patients may require corticosteroid therapy (Table 10-7).[96]
- The disease occasionally persists despite therapy.

Pulmonary Langerhans Cell Histiocytosis

- Langerhans cell histiocytosis is a rare disorder of unknown etiology.
- It results from abnormal clonal proliferation of Langerhans cells derived from bone marrow precursors.
- Multisystem involvement with extrapulmonary disease involving the skin, central nervous system, skeleton, and other organs is common in children but rare in adults where disease is confined to the lungs.[97]
- PLCH presents in adult smokers between the ages of 20 and 40 years with cough, dyspnea, weight loss, and occasionally spontaneous pneumothorax.[97]
- HRCT demonstrates a combination of nodules and cysts.[63]
- Nodules tend to predominate in early disease. They range from few to innumerable in number and typically have a centrilobular distribution. They may have irregular margins and cavitate to form cysts.
- Cystic lung lesions predominate in later disease. The cysts are characterized by irregular/bizarre margins and have an upper lobe predominance, often sparing the lung bases. They cysts are commonly thin walled but may occasionally be a few millimeters thick.
- Unlike typical ILDs, lung volumes are often preserved.
- The primary therapy for PLCH is smoking cessation. Response to smoking cessation is considered good, with up to 50% of patients demonstrating improvement or resolution.[98]
- Approximately 20% of patients have persistent, progressive disease.
- In these patients, a trail of steroid therapy may be considered, but data for this are lacking.
- In the most resistant forms of disease, chemotherapeutic agents including cladribine and vinblastine have been used with variable success.
- Some patients with PLCH have mutations in the mitogen-activated protein kinase pathway such as *BRAF* V600E. In these patients, targeted therapy with vemurafenib (a BRAF kinase inhibitor) has been used.[98]

Pneumoconioses

- Pneumoconioses are diseases of the lung parenchyma that result from exposure to airborne dusts or fibers including asbestos, silica, beryllium, coal, tin, and others.[99]
- Pneumoconiosis (with the exception of asbestosis) are characterized by upper lobe–predominant nodular patterns on CT that have the potential to conglomerate over time to form large space occupying lesions known as progressive massive fibrosis.

Asbestos-Induced Lung Disease

- Arises from exposure to asbestos, a substance historically used in construction, insulation, and fireproofing materials.
- HRCT findings may range from pleural thickening, pleural plaques (often with calcification), subpleural banding (reticulation running parallel to the pleura), to parenchymal changes resembling UIP. The presence of pleural plaques aids in differentiation from other ILDs, but asbestos-related fibrotic disease can exist in the absence of pleural manifestations.

- Treatment focuses on asbestos avoidance and supportive care.
- Prognosis is good in mild disease, although the risk of lung cancer is significantly increased in the setting of concomitant cigarette use.
- Exposure to asbestos also increases the risk of developing mesothelioma.

Silicosis

- Silicosis results from exposure to crystalline silica, which is found in stone and sand. Foundry workers, construction workers, sandblasters, and glassblowers are at increased risk.[100]
- HRCT typically demonstrates small nodules in the upper and mid zones with hilar adenopathy in a pattern that may resemble those seen in sarcoidosis. This is known as simple silicosis.
- Simple silicosis may progress to complicated silicosis characterized by coalescence of nodules in the perihilar areas of the lung to form conglomerate masses or areas of progressive massive fibrosis.
- Treatment is supportive, although close monitoring for development of TB is warranted given the increased risk of TB in these patients.[101]
- An acute form of silicosis, also known as silicoproteinosis, has been described with episodes of inhalation of high concentrations of silica. It appears as diffuse ground-glass opacities on CXR. Mortality is high.

Berylliosis

- Berylliosis is caused by exposure to beryllium and beryllium compounds.[102]
- Exposure occurs in the aerospace industry, atomic industry, beryllium mining, and fluorescent light bulb manufacturing.
- It is clinically indistinguishable from pulmonary sarcoidosis.

Coal Workers' Pneumoconiosis

- Coals workers' pneumoconiosis (CWP) is caused by inhalation of high carbon coal dust. It is commonly known as "black lung disease."
- HRCT typically demonstrates small nodules in the upper and mid zones. This is known as simple silicosis.[103]
- Simple CWP may progress to complicated CWP characterized by coalescence of nodules in the perihilar areas of the lung to form areas of progressive massive fibrosis.
- Caplan syndrome, also known as rheumatoid pneumoconiosis, is the presence of pulmonary nodules in the lungs of patients diagnosed with rheumatoid arthritis who have also been exposed to coal dust. It has also been described in patients with rheumatoid arthritis exposed to silica.

Cystic Lung Diseases

- Cystic lung diseases are a heterogeneous group of disorders that include LAM, PLCH, BHD, LIP, pulmonary amyloidosis, and light chain deposition disease.
- These diseases are characterized by the presence of cysts on HRCT imaging. Cysts are air-filled lucencies or low attenuation areas with thin (usually ≤2 mm) walls located within normal lung parenchyma.[104]
- The cysts range from few to innumerable in number.
- Cysts should not be confused with emphysema, bullae, pneumatoceles, honeycombing, or cavitary lung lesions.
- The location and thickness of the cyst walls can be helpful for disease differentiation.
  ○ PLCH is generally characterized by upper lobe–predominant cysts with thicker and irregular/bizarre-shaped walls.

- ○ BHD demonstrates larger-sized cysts with a peripheral and basilar distribution, often abutting the pleura.
- ○ LAM, LIP, and amyloidosis most often have a random distribution of cysts.[105]
- Cystic lung diseases are associated with a high incidence of pneumothorax compared to the general population, and pneumothorax is a common presenting complaint.

Lymphangioleiomyomatosis

- LAM is a progressive cystic lung disease seen almost exclusively in women of child-bearing age.
- LAM may develop sporadically or as part of tuberous sclerosis complex (TSC), a neurocutaneous multisystem disorder characterized by multiple benign hamartomas of the skin, brain, kidney, lung, and other organs.[106]
- Men with TSC may also develop LAM.
- Most patients present with progressive dyspnea. Other presentations include pneumothorax, and chylous pleural and abdominal effusions.
- The most common extrapulmonary manifestations of LAM are renal angiomyolipomas (AML)—benign kidney tumors containing blood vessels, smooth muscle, and fatty tissue.[107]
- Lymphangioleiomyomas are another characteristic feature of LAM. They are fluid-filled structures that can be seen in the retroperitoneal space, pelvis, and mediastinum.[106]
- LAM is usually diagnosed based on a combination of clinical presentation and imaging findings including cystic lung disease and renal AMLs.
- VEGF-D levels can be tested, with levels ≥800 pg/mL reliably distinguishing LAM from other cystic lung diseases.[62]
- Genetic testing for tuberous sclerosis (*TSC1* and *TSC2* gene mutations) can be undertaken where clinically indicated.
- In rare cases, lung biopsy may be needed for histopathologic confirmation.[108] This is usually pursued via bronchoscopy and TBBx. Surgical biopsy is no longer commonly performed. Lesions will demonstrate characteristic human melanoma black 45 staining.
- First-line therapy for pulmonary LAM currently is the mammalian target of rapamycin inhibitor, sirolimus, which has been shown to reduce disease progression.[109]
- Everolimus has been shown to be effective in patients who do not tolerate sirolimus.[110]
- Otherwise, supportive care, including oxygen therapy, avoidance of activities that could place patients at higher risk for pneumothorax, and pulmonary rehabilitation are mainstays of therapy.
- In some cases, patients may require evaluation for lung transplantation.

Other Cystic Lung Diseases

- PLCH:
  - ○ PLCH is described in the "Smoking-related ILD" section.
- BHD syndrome is a rare cause of cystic disease associated with skin and renal neoplasms.[111]
  - ○ It is the result of germline mutations in the *FLCN* gene, whose product is folliculin, a putative tumor suppressor protein.
  - ○ Pulmonary cysts in BHD are irregularly shaped and commonly localized to the lung bases, often in a subpleural location.[112]
  - ○ BHD can be diagnosed based on clinical presentation and may be confirmed by skin biopsy showing fibrofolliculomas, a skin hamartoma characteristic of BHD.

- ○ Genetic testing for *FLCN* mutation can also be performed.
- ○ Treatment is supportive, and progression is generally slow.[107]
- Amyloidosis can be associated with cystic lung disease in the setting of underlying systemic amyloidosis or may be organ limited to the lungs (MALT lymphoma). It may also be seen in long-standing CTDs or myeloma.[113]
  - ○ The cysts are variable in size and distribution. They may be associated with tracheal disease or pulmonary nodules, which often calcify.
  - ○ Treatment focuses on the underlying condition.
- LIP is a rare disease, usually associated with CTDs (primarily Sjögren syndrome), lymphoproliferative diseases (e.g., lymphoma), and viral infections (e.g., HIV). Idiopathic cases also occur.[114]
  - ○ Imaging demonstrates irregular cysts, multifocal ground-glass opacities, nodularity, and septal thickening.
  - ○ Treatment and prognosis are variable depending on the underlying condition.

GENERAL MANAGEMENT CONSIDERATIONS

- All ILD patients should be monitored for the development of hypoxemic respiratory failure. Supplemental oxygenation should be provided to maintain oxyhemoglobin saturation by pulse oximetry (SpO_2) ≥ 89% both at rest and with exertion (measured by 6MW testing).
- Smoking cessation/avoidance should be strongly encouraged.
- Patients should avoid occupational/environmental triggers of their ILD, if identified.
- Pulmonary rehabilitation therapy should be prescribed for all patients if they meet eligibility criteria.
- Bone density assessment is recommended for patients receiving chronic systemic corticosteroid therapy, along with periodic reassessment (e.g., every 1–2 years).
- *Pneumocystis jirovecii* pneumonia prophylaxis should be considered in patients receiving chronic steroid therapy,[115] generally at doses of >15 mg prednisone daily.
- Patients on immunosuppressive therapy should have appropriate bloodwork (CBC and/or BMP and/or LFT) monitored periodically.
- Patients should receive vaccinations against pneumococcus and influenza.
- Patients with ILDs should be considered for referral to centers with expertise in the diagnosis and treatment of these conditions, with consideration for participation in ongoing clinical trials.
- ILD increases the risk of PH.[116] Patients with dyspnea out of proportion to their parenchymal lung disease or those with symptoms of right heart failure should be screened with TTE. Although the use of pulmonary vasodilators in this population remains controversial, recent studies have shown improvement in functional status with inhaled treprostinil.[117]
- Several ILDs are associated with an increased incidence of malignancy. (e.g., IPF, asbestosis). Rapid weight loss or radiographic changes (e.g., new solitary nodules or persistent consolidation) should raise suspicion and prompt further workup.
- Goals of care and expectations of therapy should be made clear to all patients.
- Palliative care is an ongoing part of disease management in many ILDs, and hospice care should be discussed with all patients with advanced disease who are not transplant candidates. Open discussions of goals of care are helpful in guiding management of acute exacerbations and progressive disease.[118]

Hemoptysis

GENERAL PRINCIPLES

Hemoptysis is the coughing up of blood or blood-stained mucus. It is a sign of underlying pulmonary pathology. It can be life threatening and requires rapid identification, workup, and treatment.

Definition

- **True hemoptysis** is expectoration of blood from the lower respiratory tract below the glottis.
- **Massive or life-threatening hemoptysis:**
  - Is usually defined by volume per unit time.
  - It is most commonly defined as **>600 mL of blood expectorated per 24 hours.**[119,120]
  - Volumes of >100 mL in 24 hours associated with gas exchange abnormality, airway obstruction, or hemodynamic instability are also considered life threatening.

Classification

Clinically, hemoptysis is usually classified as being **massive/life threatening or not (see above).** It may also be classified by the **anatomic location** of the bleeding.
- Airway
- Parenchyma
- Vascular
- Combination

There are various other classifications in the literature based on appearance, frequency, rate, volume, and potential for clinical consequences of the hemoptysis that may suggest an underlying etiology or predict outcome and thus help guide in diagnosis and management. However, considerable overlap exists in the clinical presentation both within and between etiologies.

Etiology

See Table 10-9.

Epidemiology

The incidence of each cause of hemoptysis varies considerably. Table 10-10 lists some of the most common causes of hemoptysis.[121,122]

Pathophysiology

The source of hemoptysis depends on the etiology and location of the underlying pathologic process.
- **The pulmonary arterial circulation** supplies 99% of all blood flow to the lung parenchyma under low pressure. Disruption can result in minor hemoptysis or more life-threatening hemoptysis due to processes such as vasculitis, diffuse alveolar hemorrhage, pulmonary embolism, acute respiratory distress syndrome, arteriovenous malformation (AVM) rupture, pulmonary artery catheter trauma, severe mitral stenosis, LV failure, or Rasmussen aneurysm (pulmonary artery aneurysm associated with TB).
- **The bronchial arterial circulation** arises from the aorta and intercostal arteries. It supplies high-pressure blood flow to the lungs but accounts for only 1% of pulmonary blood flow. Disruption by a foreign body, tumor invasion, fungal invasion, or

TABLE 10-9	Etiology of Hemoptysis
Location	**Etiology**
Airway	**Bronchitis, bronchiectasis, malignancy**, foreign body, trauma, pulmonary endometriosis, and bronchitiasis
Parenchymal	**Pneumonia, vasculitides, and pulmonary hemorrhage syndromes** (antineutrophil cytoplasmic antibody–positive vasculitis, Goodpasture syndrome, systemic lupus erythematosus, diffuse alveolar hemorrhage, acute respiratory distress syndrome)
Vascular	**Elevated pulmonary venous pressure** (LV failure, mitral stenosis), pulmonary embolism, arteriovenous malformation, pulmonary arterial trauma (i.e., pulmonary arterial catheter balloon overinflation), varices/aneurysms, vasculitides, and pulmonary hemorrhage syndromes
Multiple locations	**Cavitary lung disease** (TB, aspergilloma, lung abscess), thrombocytopenia, disseminated intravascular coagulation, anticoagulants, antiplatelets, cocaine and other inhaled agents, lung biopsy, bronchovascular fistula, bronchopulmonary sequestration, and Dieulafoy disease
Other	Up to 50%. Favorable prognosis, in general. Up to 4% eventually diagnosed with malignancy[3,4]

TABLE 10-10	Epidemiology of Hemoptysis
Etiology	**Incidence (%)**
Bronchitis	2–37
Bronchiectasis	1–37
TB and cavitary lung disease	2–69
Malignancy	2–24
Pneumonia	1–16
Pulmonary embolus	3
Pulmonary edema	4
Idiopathic	2–50

denuded airway mucosa can result in massive, life-threatening hemoptysis. Bleeding from the bronchial circulation may account for up to 88% of all cases of massive hemoptysis.

DIAGNOSIS

Identifying and correcting the underlying pathologic process is the basis of diagnosis and management of hemoptysis (Figure 10-5).

Clinical Presentation

Hemoptysis may present in isolation or accompany other manifestations of an underlying disorder (Table 10-9). The appearance, timing, and volume of hemoptysis can provide important clues to narrowing the differential diagnosis.

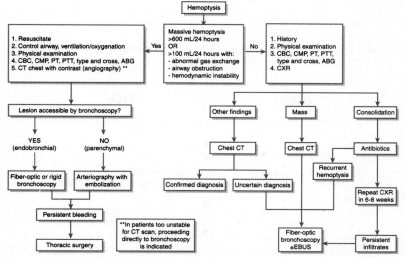

Figure 10-5. Algorithm for evaluation of hemoptysis. ABG, arterial blood gas; CBC, complete blood count; CMP, complete metabolic panel; EBUS, endobronchial ultrasound; PT, prothrombin time; PTT, partial thromboplastin. (Adapted from Earwood JS, Thompson TD. Hemoptysis: evaluation and management. *Am Fam Physician.* 2015;91:243-249.)

- Appearance: Gross blood, blood-tinged sputum, blood-streaking, foamy pink sputum
- Timing: First episode, recurrent episodes, chronic small volumes, acute large volumes
- Volume: Minor, submassive, massive

History
- The most important facts to gather include volume of hemoptysis, patient age, smoking history, prior lung disease, previous malignancy, risk factors for coagulopathy, and prior episodes of hemoptysis.
- Review of systems should focus on symptoms suggesting cardiopulmonary disease, active infection, underlying malignancy, and systemic inflammatory disorders.

Physical Examination
- Obtaining vital signs including oxygen saturation is the first step in patient examination.
- Thereafter, one should pay attention to the patient's general state of health, lung examination noting focal or diffusely abnormal findings such as bronchial breath sounds, crackles, stridor, and/or expiratory wheezes.
- A thorough examination should always be performed, observing any manifestations suggesting underlying cardiopulmonary, infectious, immunologic, or malignant disease.

Differential Diagnosis
One must distinguish between **true hemoptysis** and **pseudohemoptysis**, which comes from the upper airway (above the glottis), or aspirated GI tract bleeding that is later expectorated.

CHAPTER 10

Diagnostic Testing

- A thorough **history and physical examination** is important to provide clues and guidance in additional testing.
- Additional testing is aimed at determining and localizing the bleeding source and identifying the underlying etiology.

Laboratories and Electrocardiography

- Basic lab work including CBC, comprehensive metabolic panel, and coagulation studies are indicated.
- Type and cross-matching of blood are indicated, especially in cases of massive hemoptysis.
- An ABG analysis may be indicated in cases of shortness of breath or respiratory compromise.
- Sputum studies may be helpful in cases of infection and can be analyzed with routine Gram stain and culture, fungal culture, and acid-fast bacilli smear/culture as indicated.
- Serologic studies and urinalysis with microscopy may be clinically indicated based on the suspicion for rheumatologic disease or vasculitis. These may include ANA screen, antineutrophil cytoplasmic antibody (ANCA) screen, including reflex testing to myeloperoxidase and proteinase 3, antiglomerular basement membrane antibodies, complement levels, cryoglobulins, double-stranded DNA antibodies, and others.
- Brain natriuretic peptide or N-terminal pro b-type natriuretic peptide levels may be helpful when cardiac failure is suspected.
- ECG can help assess for underlying cardiac disease.

Imaging

- **Posteroanterior and lateral CXR** are performed in all cases of hemoptysis.
  - **Unfortunately, these may be normal or nonlocalizing in up to 50% of all cases.**[123,124]
  - Furthermore, CXR may be normal in up to 10% of hemoptysis cases caused by bronchogenic carcinoma.[123]
- **Chest CT:** CT should be performed if the diagnosis remains in doubt after initial clinical and CXR evaluation (see Figure 10-5). CT chest can be performed with or without contrast; however, CT angiography is increasingly useful in localizing the source of hemoptysis.
  - Advantages:
    - Can visualize parenchyma, vasculature, and airways to varying extent.
    - **Especially useful for hemoptysis resulting from bronchiectasis, cavitary lung disease, masses, and vascular malformations.**[125]
    - **Can detect up to 96% of CXR-occult malignancies.**[126]
    - CT visualizes tumors with efficacy comparable with bronchoscopy.[127]
    - CT angiography may be better than bronchoscopy in determining the etiology and source of hemoptysis.[128]
    - CT angiography is useful for planning embolization procedures.[129]
  - Disadvantages:
    - CT is less efficacious than bronchoscopy in recognizing subtle bronchial and mucosal lesions.[125]
    - It is nonspecific in cases of parenchymal/alveolar hemorrhage.
    - Delay in treatment places unstable patients at high risk.
- **Echocardiography** may be performed if structural or valvular cardiac disease is suspected.

Diagnostic Procedures

- **Fiber-optic (flexible) bronchoscopy:** Generally **localizes/lateralizes bleeding source** in over two-thirds of cases, depending on the setting.[130]
  - **Indications:**
    - If the source is unclear after initial evaluation and imaging
    - Persistent or recurrent hemoptysis
    - To rule out infection
    - If the clinical presentation suggests an airway abnormality
    - To obtain biopsy specimens, if imaging suggests malignancy or is nonlocalizing in the **presence of at least two risk factors for bronchogenic carcinoma:**
      - Male sex
      - Age >40 years
      - >40 pack-year smoking
      - Duration of hemoptysis >1 week
      - Volume expectorated >30 mL[6,131,132]
    - To identify potential anatomic area for arterial embolization
    - To provide endobronchial treatments
    - To rule out alveolar hemorrhage
  - The timing of bronchoscopy is controversial, although yields increase when performed during or within 48 hours of bleeding.[131]
- **Bronchial and pulmonary arteriography is** performed in the setting of **persistent, recurrent, or massive hemoptysis.**
  - Advantages:
    - Can be both diagnostic and therapeutic via simultaneous **embolization** of the visualized culprit vessel.
    - Useful in hemoptysis of varying degrees in the setting of different etiologies including bronchiectasis, malignancy, aspergilloma, and others.[133]
    - Can be preceded by CT angiography for procedure planning.[129]
  - Disadvantages:
    - **Variable and inexact localization** of the bleeding source depending on clinical setting.[130]
    - Anatomic variability.
    - Bleeding in cases where it is insufficient for contrast extravasation.

TREATMENT

The approach to hemoptysis is primarily aimed at **distinguishing massive/life-threatening hemoptysis from nonmassive hemoptysis**. The three main goals are:
1. to stabilize the patient's airway and hemodynamics,
2. to diagnose the cause and localize the site of hemoptysis, and
3. to decide on need for and type of therapy in each case.

- **Nonmassive hemoptysis** is usually treated conservatively. Treatment may include the following:
  - Reversal of coagulopathy
  - Antitussives
  - Bronchoscopy if recurrent
  - Steroids and/or immunosuppression for rheumatologic conditions
  - Antibiotics for infection (fungal, TB, mycobacteria)
  - Diuretics and/or inotropes for heart disease (LV failure, mitral stenosis)
- **Massive hemoptysis:** management requires urgent action, intensive care monitoring, and an early multidisciplinary approach including an interventional pulmonologist, a thoracic surgeon, and an interventional radiologist (see Figure 10-5).

- ○ **Initial stabilization:**
  - ▪ **Airway management** may require intubation, with a large (>8 mm) endotracheal tube.[134]
    - □ Single-lumen main stem intubation for selective ventilation of unaffected lung.
    - □ Double-lumen endotracheal intubation for selective ventilation of unaffected lung. Should be performed and managed only under appropriately skilled supervision.
  - ▪ **Lateral decubitus positioning** (affected lung down) to minimize aspiration into unaffected lung.
  - ▪ Inhaled tranexamic acid may reduce volume of expectorated blood, reduce hospital length of stay, lead to more frequent resolution of hemoptysis, reduce recurrence rates, and reduce the need for invasive procedures, without increased adverse effects noted. More investigation is needed on this intervention.[135]
  - ○ **Bronchoscopy** with directed airway therapy: **Rigid bronchoscopy** is favored if available because it provides optimal airway access and ventilatory control and easier suctioning and allows for manipulation of instruments.
    - ▪ **Direct tamponade with the distal end of the bronchoscope.**
    - ▪ **Balloon tamponade:** Left in place for 1–2 days. Monitor for ischemic mucosal injury or postobstructive pneumonitis.[136] Fogarty balloons, bronchial blockers, and pulmonary artery catheter balloons have all been described for tamponading bleeding.
    - ▪ **Endobronchial electrocautery.**[137]
    - ▪ **Argon plasma coagulation.**[137,138]
    - ▪ **Endobronchial stent placement.**[139]
    - ▪ **Topical hemostatic agents:** Cold saline, epinephrine, vasopressin, thrombin, and oxidized regenerated cellulose have been used to control bleeding.[140–142]
- • **Arteriography and embolization should be performed early** in massive or recurrent hemoptysis.
  - ○ **Successful embolization in >85% of cases can be achieved** with careful localization.[133,143]
  - ○ Embolization is particularly useful in cystic fibrosis (CF) patients.[144,145]
  - ○ **Treatment failure is usually because of inadequate or incomplete source vessel identification.** Postembolization arteriography may identify additional systemic culprit vessels, most commonly from the intercostal and phrenic arteries.[146]
  - ○ **Rebleeding is common** in embolized patients, occurring in up to 20% of cases over 1 year. Rebleeding appears to be more common in patients with sarcoidosis, malignancy, and aspergilloma.[143,147,148]
  - ○ **Risks** include bronchial or partial pulmonary infarction and, rarely, ischemic myelopathy because of inadvertent embolization of a spinal artery.

Medications

Systemic procoagulants: These are used only in unstable massive hemoptysis as a temporizing measure. Alternatively, they may be required when conventional bronchoscopic, interventional, or surgical therapies are contraindicated and/or unavailable. Examples are administration of factor VII, vasopressin, and aminocaproic acid.

Surgical Management

Emergent surgery has high morbidity and mortality compared with elective surgery following patient stabilization.[119]

- • **Lobectomy or pneumonectomy offers definitive cure.**

○ **Indications: Persistent focal/unilateral massive hemoptysis despite other therapy.** It is particularly useful for stable patients with hemoptysis due to cavitary lung disease, localized bronchogenic carcinoma, AVM, or traumatic injuries.[149]

○ **Contraindications:** Poor pulmonary reserve, advanced malignancy, active TB, diffuse lung disease, or diffuse alveolar hemorrhage.

REFERRAL/CONSULTATION

- Pulmonary (interventional for massive hemoptysis, if available)
- Thoracic surgery
- Interventional radiology

OUTCOME/PROGNOSIS

Mortality depends on etiology and volume of hemoptysis.[119,150,151]
- Mortality may be as high as 80% in cases of massive hemoptysis because of malignancy.
- Mortality tends to be <10% with nonmassive hemoptysis.
- Mortality in patients with bronchiectasis and lung infections is <1%.

Cystic Fibrosis

GENERAL PRINCIPLES

Definition

CF is an **autosomal recessive disorder** caused by mutations of the CF transmembrane conductance regulator gene (*CFTR*), which results in multisystem exocrine organ dysfunction.

Epidemiology

- In the US, >30,000 people are affected by CF, and about 1000 new cases are diagnosed every year.[152,153]
- CF is the most common life-shortening genetic disease in Caucasians; however, the diagnosis should be considered in patients of diverse ethnic backgrounds as well.
- The prognosis of CF has continuously improved, and today >50% of patients with CF in the US are aged ≥18 years.

Etiology

- CF is caused by **mutations in the *CFTR* gene**, a cyclic adenosine monophosphate–regulated chloride channel, which normally maintains hydration of exocrine organ secretions.
- Abnormal CFTR function causes decreased chloride secretion and increased sodium absorption on the surface of epithelial cells, which can result in thickened secretions in the airways, sinuses, pancreatic ducts, biliary tree, intestines, and reproductive tract.
- CFTR mutations are categorized into five classes: (1) **defective synthesis, (2) defective processing and maturation, (3) defective regulation, (4) defective conductance, and (5) reduced function/synthesis.**
- The most common mutation is **F508del**, a class II mutation resulting from the deletion of DNA coding for phenylalanine (F) amino acid at position 508. The

CHAPTER 10

majority of the resultant misfolded protein is destroyed intracellularly and does not reach the cell surface. More than 85% of patients in the US with CF have at least one copy of this mutation.[153]

- To date, >2000 other potentially causative mutations in the CFTR gene have been identified.[153]

Pathophysiology

- The primary pulmonary manifestations of CF are related to the malfunction of chloride transport across the airway epithelium, resulting in diminished airway surface liquid and impaired mucociliary clearance.
- Poor mucociliary clearance, infection, inflammation, and chronic airway obstruction often result in bronchiectasis, chronic infection, respiratory failure, and premature death.
- Similarly, thickened secretions in the pancreatic and biliary ducts lead to maldigestion, malabsorption, and, occasionally, liver disease and diabetes.[154]

DIAGNOSIS

- Today, children with CF are typically diagnosed via newborn screening or during childhood, but there is increasing recognition of milder variants that may not present until later in life.
- In 2018, 62% of new diagnoses were the result of newborn screening.[153] Newborn screening is now routinely performed throughout the US.
- A diagnosis of CF is made when there are:[155]
  ○ Compatible clinical features of CF or
  ○ A positive family history of CF or
  ○ A positive newborn screening test and
  ○ Elevated (>60 mmol/L) sweat chloride or
  ○ Intermediate (30–59 mmol/L) sweat chloride and
    ▪ Presence of two disease-causing mutations in *CFTR* or
    ▪ Abnormal CFTR functional assay
- A diagnosis of **CF-related metabolic syndrome** is made when there is a positive newborn screening test, and an intermediate sweat chloride level without two causative mutations, or a negative (<30 mmol/L) sweat chloride level with two *CFTR* mutations, at least one with unclear phenotypic consequences.
- Although genotyping may assist in the diagnosis, it alone cannot establish or rule out the diagnosis of CF, and the initial test of choice remains the sweat chloride test.

Clinical Presentation

- **Pulmonary manifestations:**
  ○ Cough with purulent sputum production, wheezing, hemoptysis, dyspnea, progressive airflow obstruction, bronchiectasis, and pneumothorax.
- **Extrapulmonary manifestations:**
  ○ Chronic sinusitis, nasal polyposis, pancreatic insufficiency (vitamins A, D, E, and K deficiency), steatorrhea, malnutrition, failure to thrive, meconium ileus, distal intestinal obstruction syndrome, volvulus, intussusception, rectal prolapse, diabetes mellitus, liver cirrhosis, portal hypertension, cholelithiasis, cholecystitis, nephrolithiasis, male infertility (bilateral absence of the vas deferens), epididymitis, growth retardation, hypertrophic pulmonary osteoarthropathy, and osteopenia.

- Older patients with undiagnosed CF often struggle with recurrent sinopulmonary infections, refractory uncontrolled asthma, multiple episodes of pneumonia, unexplained bronchiectasis, recurrent pancreatitis, or male infertility. Diagnosis at an older age is generally associated with milder phenotypes and rarer mutations.

Differential Diagnosis

- **Primary ciliary dyskinesia:** Bronchiectasis, sinusitis, and infertility. Limited GI symptoms and normal sweat chloride levels. Occasionally seen with dextrocardia or situs inversus totalis (Kartagener syndrome).
- **Immunodeficiency (e.g., severe combined immunodeficiency, common variable immunodeficiency):** Recurrent sinus and pulmonary infections but typically no GI symptoms and normal sweat chloride levels.
- **Alpha-1 antitrypsin deficiency:** Early-onset emphysema, airflow obstruction, chronic sputum production, panniculitis, chronic hepatitis, cirrhosis, and hepatocellular carcinoma. Bronchiectasis is a common radiographic feature[156] with normal sweat chloride levels.
- **Shwachman–Diamond syndrome:** Pancreatic insufficiency, cyclic neutropenia, and short stature. May lead to lung disease, but normal sweat chloride levels.[157]
- **Young syndrome:** Bronchiectasis, sinusitis, and azoospermia. Mild respiratory symptoms, lack of GI symptoms, and normal sweat chloride levels.
- **Idiopathic bronchiectasis**

Diagnostic Testing

- **Skin sweat testing** with a standardized quantitative pilocarpine iontophoresis method remains the **gold standard for the diagnosis of CF.**[158]
  - A sweat chloride concentration of ≥60 mmol/L on two separate occasions is consistent with the diagnosis of CF.
  - Intermediate sweat test results (30–59 mmol/L sweat chloride) or nondiagnostic results should lead to repeat sweat testing, genetic testing, or nasal potential difference testing.
  - A normal sweat chloride concentration is generally sufficient to rule out CF, but should be repeated in cases with a high clinical suspicion as normal values can be observed with very uncommon mutations.
  - Sweat testing should be performed at a CF care center to ensure accuracy of results.
  - Abnormal sweat chloride concentrations are rarely detected in non-CF patients.
- **Genetic tests** have detected >2000 putative CF mutations.
  - Two recessive mutations on separate alleles must be present to cause CF.
  - Commercially available CF screens identify >90% of the abnormal genes in a Caucasian Northern European population, although they test for only a minority of the known CF genes. Full gene sequencing is commercially available, but interpretation may be complex. Information about specific mutations and reported clinical phenotype may be found at http://www.cftr2.org/.

Laboratories and Testing

- CXRs often demonstrate hyperinflation with upper lobe–predominant cystic lung disease, bronchiectasis, and mucus plugging.
- High-resolution CT scans may be helpful in evaluating patients with early or mild disease by detecting early airway changes.
- PFTs often demonstrate expiratory airflow obstruction with increased residual volume (air trapping) and total lung capacity (hyperinflation). Impairment of alveolar gas exchange may be present later in the course of disease.

- Sputum cultures typically identify multiple organisms including *Staphylococcus aureus*, nontypeable *Haemophilus influenzae*, *Pseudomonas aeruginosa*, *Stenotrophomonas maltophilia*, and *Burkholderia cepacia* complex. Isolation of mucoid variants of *P. aeruginosa* from the respiratory tract occurs frequently. **Use of special culture media for fastidious organisms is recommended.**
- Nontuberculous mycobacteria (NTM) are also frequently isolated from the airways of persons with CF and may be pathogenic.

TREATMENT

- CF therapy aims to improve quality of life, decrease the number of exacerbations and hospitalizations, reduce the rate of decline in lung function, and decrease mortality.
- **A comprehensive program provided at an accredited CF care center is recommended.**
- Treatment burden can be a significant barrier to proper adherence. The median number of minutes to complete daily therapies is over 90 min/d.

Chronic Therapies
Pulmonary Therapy
- Primarily focused on clearing pulmonary secretions and controlling infection.
- **Inhaled bronchodilators:** β-Adrenergic agonists (such as albuterol, salmeterol, or formoterol). Recommended in all CF patients. Used to treat the reversible component of airflow obstruction and facilitate mucus clearance.
- **Recombinant human DNase** (dornase alpha, Pulmozyme): Digests extracellular DNA, decreasing the viscoelasticity of the sputum. Improves pulmonary function and decreases the incidence of respiratory tract infections that require parenteral antibiotics.[159]
- **Hypertonic saline** (4 mL of inhaled 7% saline): Improves clearance of secretions, results in fewer exacerbations, and improves lung function.[160] Albuterol should be administered prior to reduce bronchospasm.
- **Mechanical airway clearance devices** (oral oscillating device, high-frequency chest oscillation vests): Used in combination with medical therapy to promote airway clearance. Other alternatives include postural drainage with chest percussion and vibration. Exercise is also an excellent form of airway clearance.
- **Immunizations:** Pneumovax and Prevnar 13 are recommended for all patients with CF, as is yearly influenza vaccination.

Antibiotics
- *P. aeruginosa* is the most prevalent organism in CF patients and is associated with significant morbidity and mortality. Over time, the percentage of patients colonized with *P. aeruginosa* (and multidrug-resistant *Pseudomonas*) increases.
- In patients chronically infected with *P. aeruginosa*, the inhaled aerosolized antibiotics tobramycin (300 mg nebulized twice daily) and aztreonam lysinate (75 mg nebulized 3× daily) can be used by alternating 28 days on with 28 days off. These improve pulmonary function, decrease the density of *P. aeruginosa*, and decrease the risk of hospitalization. Continuous alternating inhaled antibiotic therapy has become the standard of care for many patients with chronic *Pseudomonas* infection and pulmonary impairment.

Anti-inflammatory Therapy
- **Azithromycin** (500 mg oral 3×/wk) used chronically shows mild improvement in lung function and reduces days in the hospital for treatment of respiratory

exacerbations. Patients should be screened for NTM before initiation of macrolide antibiotics because chronic monotherapy can lead to macrolide-resistant NTM.

- **Glucocorticoids** used in short courses may be helpful to some patients with asthma-like symptoms, but long-term therapy should be avoided to minimize the side effects.

Restoration of CFTR Function

- Recently, effective modulator therapy has dramatically changed the treatment of CF and changed the disease course for many patients.
- CFTR modulators treat the underlying cause of the disease by correcting protein misfolding, transporting CFTR to the cell surface, and restoring chloride conductance.
- CFTR correctors increase the amount of mature CFTR on the cell surface while potentiators increase the channel-gating activity of CFTR protein.
- The combination of correctors and a potentiator is more effective than either approach alone.
- See Table 10-11 for details regarding the currently Food and Drug Administration–approved CFTR modulators. One should note that the indications for CFTR modulators are constantly changing especially with respect to age cutoffs.

Pulmonary Rehabilitation

- Pulmonary rehabilitation may improve functional status and promote clearance of airway secretions.

Oxygen Therapy and Noninvasive Ventilation

- Oxygen therapy may be indicated based on standard recommendations for the treatment of COPD. Rest and exercise oxygen assessments should be performed as indicated.
- Oxygen may be indicated for patients with a resting $PaO_2 \leq 55$ mm Hg or $SpO_2 \leq 88\%$ at rest or $PaO_2 \leq 59$ mm Hg or $SpO_2 \leq 89\%$ with certain comorbidities (right heart failure, cor pulmonale, or erythrocytosis).
- Nocturnal noninvasive ventilation may be indicated for patients with a daytime resting $PCO_2 > 50$ mm Hg or a nocturnal oxygen saturation <88% for more than 5 minutes on usual daytime oxygen.

Management of Extrapulmonary Manifestations

Pancreatic insufficiency

- Primary management involves **pancreatic enzyme supplementation.** Enzyme dose should be titrated to achieve one to two semisolid stools per day and to maintain adequate growth and nutrition.
- Enzymes are taken immediately before meals and snacks.
- Dosing of pancreatic enzymes should be initiated at 500 units lipase/kg/meal and should not exceed 2500 units lipase/kg/meal.

Vitamin deficiency

- Vitamins A, D, E, and K can all be taken orally with meals and enzymes.
- Iron deficiency anemia requires iron supplementation.

CF-related diabetes mellitus

- Related to pancreatic insufficiency and managed with **insulin**; oral hypoglycemics are not recommended.
- Typical diabetic dietary restrictions are liberalized (high-calorie diet with unrestricted fat) to meet the increased energy requirements of patients with CF and to encourage appropriate growth and weight maintenance.

TABLE 10-11 Currently FDA-Approved CFTR Modulators

CFTR Modulator	FDA-Approved Indications	Mechanism of Action	Clinical Effects	Adverse Effects
Single Therapy				
Ivacaftor (Kalydeco)	>4 mo with responsive partial function CFTR mutations	Potentiator[a]	Improves FEV1 Weight gain Reduces hospitalizations and exacerbation frequency Decreases *Pseudomonas* airway infection Improves sinus disease	Transaminitis[c]
Dual Therapy				
Lumacaftor–ivacaftor (Orkambi)	>2 y with two copies of the F508del mutation	Potentiator plus corrector[b]	[b]Modestly improves FEV1 Reduces hospitalizations and exacerbation frequency	Transaminitis Lumacaftor is a potent inducer of CYP3A Chest discomfort and dyspnea
Tezacaftor–ivacaftor (Symdeko)	>6 y with two copies of the F508del mutation **or** >1 other responsive CFTR mutations	Potentiator plus corrector	Improves FEV1 Reduces hospitalizations and exacerbation frequency	Transaminitis Fewer adverse effects than lumacaftor–ivacaftor
Triple Therapy				
Elexacaftor–tezacaftor–ivacaftor (Trikafta)	>12 y and at least one copy of F508del mutation **or** a responsive CFTR mutation **>90% of patients with CF in the US are eligible for this therapy**	Potentiator plus two correctors	Significantly improves FEV1 (increased by 13.8 points at 4 wk) **63% lower annual rate of exacerbation compared to placebo**	Transaminitis GI upset Elevated bilirubin

General approach to initiation of therapy: If a patient has a genotype that is eligible for more than one therapy, generally recommended to start maximal therapy available for that age group (triple therapy>double therapy> single therapy). Advance therapy when patient meets age criteria for each combination drug. Dose adjustment in Child–Pugh Class B cirrhosis, avoid in Child–Pugh class C disease. Reduce dose when coadministered with CYP3A inhibitors. See package insert. CF, cystic fibrosis; CFTR, CF transmembrane conductance regulator gene; FDA, Food and Drug Administration; FEV1, forced expiratory volume in the first second.
[a]Potentiator: Increases CFTR channel open time at the cell surface.
[b]Corrector: Increases cell surface protein expression by improving the processing and trafficking of CFTR.

- It is recommended that pregnant women with CF undergo screening for gestational diabetes with oral glucose tolerance test at both 12–16 weeks and at 24–48 weeks gestation.

Bowel impaction/distal intestinal obstruction syndrome
- Presents as colicky abdominal pain. Radiographic pattern consistent with a complete or partial obstruction.
- Laxatives such as senna, magnesium citrate, or polyethylene glycol can be tried initially. Refractory cases may require a hypaque enema with visualization of clearance of the obstruction.
- Narcotic use and/or significant dehydration and/or nonadherence with pancreatic enzyme supplementation can precipitate severe bowel obstruction.

CF-related liver disease
- Hepatobiliary manifestations range from mild abnormalities in LFTs to hepatic steatosis or cirrhosis.
- Most cases of cirrhosis are diagnosed during childhood (<18 years).

Osteopenia
- Screening should be routinely performed on patients with CF.
- Managed with calcium, vitamin D supplementation, and bisphosphonate therapy as clinically indicated.

Chronic sinusitis
- Many patients will benefit from chronic **nasal steroid** administration and nasal saline washes.
- Patients whose symptoms cannot be controlled with medical management may benefit from functional endoscopic sinus surgery and nasal polypectomy.

Mental health
- Depression and anxiety are common among patients and caregivers of CF patients and both patients and caregivers should be screened on a regular basis.
- Psychological symptoms are associated with worse adherence, heath-related quality of life, decreased lung function, and lower BMI.

Lifestyle considerations
- When patients with CF have close contact with another individual with CF, there is a risk of aquiring relevant bacterial infections (cross-infection). Nonetheless, robust peer support groups and virtual events exist and are encouraged.
- People with CF should avoid irritating inhaled fumes, dusts, or chemicals, including second-hand smoke.
- A high-calorie diet with vitamin supplementation is typically recommended.
- CF patients should maintain as much activity as possible.
- Although fertility may be decreased in women with CF secondary to thickened cervical mucus, many women with CF have tolerated pregnancy as well. Ideally, pregnancies should be planned to optimize patient status and coordinate care with obstetrics. CF genetic screening should be offered to partners of patients with CF.

Treatment of Acute Exacerbations

- Common CF exacerbation symptoms include increased cough, change in sputum, increased shortness of breath, fevers, weight loss, or reduction in lung function on spirometry.
- When in a healthcare setting, all personnel should implement contact precautions. Of note, patients with previous isolation of *B. cepacia* complex should be cared for in a separate area than those without this species.
- **Antibiotics** are the main treatment for exacerbations.

- Typically, clinicians select antibiotics to which the pathogens are susceptible. However in chronic CF airway infection, it may not be possible to select antibiotics in which all identified pathogens are susceptible.
- *P. aeruginosa* is the most frequent pulmonary pathogen. The standard approach has been to use two antipseudomonal drugs to enhance activity. A combination of an antipseudomonal β-lactam and an aminoglycoside is typically recommended during acute exacerbations.[161] Of note, prior studies have demonstrated that there is no correlation between in vitro susceptibility testing and clinical response to a particular antibiotic.
- The duration of antibiotic therapy is dictated by the clinical response. At least 14 days of antibiotics are typically needed to treat an exacerbation.
- Patients with CF have atypical pharmacokinetics and often require higher drug doses at more frequent intervals during an acute exacerbation.
- Home IV antibiotic therapy is common, but hospitalization may allow better access to comprehensive therapy and diagnostic testing. Oral antibiotics are recommended only for mild exacerbations. The Cystic Fibrosis Foundation (CFF) recommends against the delivery of home antibiotics unless resources and support are equivalent to hospital setting.
- There is insufficient evidence to recommend routine use of steroids in treatment of acute exacerbations.
- Airway clearance should be intensified during an exacerbation.
- Chronic therapies such as bronchodilators, Pulmozyme (dornase), hypertonic saline, pancreatic enzymes, and CFTR modulators should be continued during a hospitalization.
- Other complications that may require hospitalization include:
  - **Hemoptysis:** Basic treatment involves correction of coagulation factors, withholding chest physiotherapy, stopping inhaled antibiotics, and initiation of IV antibiotics. Refractory cases may require bronchial artery embolization.
  - **Pneumothorax:** Unless small pneumothoraces are treated with chest tube placement. Surgical pleurodesis should be considered in cases of recurrent pneumothorax. In general, airway clearance measures that utilize positive pressure should be withheld in cases of a large pneumothorax, as should noninvasive ventilation.

Lung Transplantation

- CF is the third most common indication for lung transplantation worldwide.
- The CF Foundation guidelines recommend lung transplant referral for any patient with CF with:
  - an FEV1 <50% predicted and evidence of rapid decline (20% drop in FEV1 within 12 months)
  - an FEV1 <40% and other evidence of advanced disease (6MW < 400 m, hypoxia, hypercarbia, PH), or
  - any patient with FEV1 <30%.
- All patients undergoing transplant evaluation should be tested for the presence of NTM and *B. cepacia* complex in the sputum. The presence of *Burkholderia cenocepacia* is considered a contraindication to lung transplantation at most transplant centers.

REFERRAL AND FOLLOW-UP

- All persons with CF should be followed at an accredited CF care center.
- Patients with CF generally follow-up as an outpatient every 3 months with PFTs and yearly laboratories including vitamin levels and screening for CF-related diabetes.

- A multidisciplinary team of CF specialists, including physicians, nutritionists, respiratory therapists, and social workers, aid in the routine care of these patients.

OUTCOME/PROGNOSIS

- Predictors of increased mortality include advanced age, female gender, low weight, low FEV1, pancreatic insufficiency, diabetes mellitus, infection with *B. cepacia*, and higher frequency of acute exacerbations.
- With improved therapy, the median survival has been extended to over 47 years.[153]

PATIENT EDUCATION

High-quality information can be found at the CFF website (www.cff.org).

Solitary Pulmonary Nodule

GENERAL PRINCIPLES

- The goal of a careful evaluation of the solitary pulmonary nodule (SPN) is to determine if the lesion is more likely to be **malignant or benign.**
- **A lesion >3 cm has a high likelihood of malignancy and should be treated as such, whereas lesions <3 cm need more careful assessment.**
- Nodules with benign characteristics should be closely followed so that invasive procedures with associated risks can be avoided.
- Identifying early lung cancer is of the utmost importance because there is a >60% survival rate of patients who have a malignant SPN removed.[162]

Definition

An SPN is defined as a rounded lesion <3 cm in diameter. It is completely surrounded by lung parenchyma, unaccompanied by atelectasis, intrathoracic adenopathy, or pleural effusion. Pulmonary nodules <8 mm remain within this definition; however, there is evidence to suggest that these nodules have a lower overall malignancy risk.[162]

Epidemiology

A 2015, California-based, integrated healthcare system's review estimated the incidence of pulmonary nodules to be over 1.5 million. This value is susceptible to errors associated with this form of methodology. However, it does highlight that the incidence of SPN has increased with changes in clinical practice following the National Lung Screening Trial.[163]

Etiology

- Although underlying etiologies for pulmonary nodules are varied, the most important designation clinically is deciphering between a malignant and a nonmalignant process.
- **Malignancy accounts for approximately 40% of SPNs, although this may vary geographically depending on the prevalence of nonmalignant processes such as histoplasmosis.**
- **Granulomas** (both infectious and noninfectious) may account for 50% of undiagnosed SPNs, depending on the prevalence of cancer in the particular population.

CHAPTER 10

- The remaining 10% are composed of **benign neoplasms**, such as **hamartomas** (5%) and a multitude of other causes.

Risk Factors

- **Smoking** is the most important associated risk factor for almost all malignant SPNs.
- For infectious etiologies, an immunocompromised state promotes an increased risk.

Lung Cancer Screening

Screening high-risk patients using low-dose chest CT resulted in a 20% relative reduction in mortality from lung cancer compared to screening with CXR.[164]

DIAGNOSIS

- Diagnosis of the SPN is made radiographically, usually via CXR or CT scan.
- Most frequently, the nodule is noted incidentally on a study performed for other reasons (e.g., chronic cough, chest pain, shortness of breath).

Clinical Presentation

- The majority of SPNs are diagnosed incidentally by radiographic tests done for other reasons, so there may not be overt symptoms.
- There are instances when a nodule may precipitate cough, chest pain, hemoptysis, or sputum production depending on the etiology and location of the SPN.

History

- Ask typical screening questions for malignancy including **weight loss and night sweats.**
- **Hemoptysis** may indicate malignancy but may also prompt investigations for ANCA-associated vasculitis, TB, and hereditary hemorrhagic telangiectasia (HHT).
- Ask about arthritis and arthralgias for possible undiagnosed CTD or sarcoidosis.
- Take an exposure history including recent travel history related to endemic mycoses (histoplasmosis, coccidioidomycosis, etc.) as well as possible TB exposures.
- A history of previous malignancies increases the risk of metastatic disease of the lung.
- Patients who are immunosuppressed from HIV, organ transplant, or chronic steroids have increased risk of infectious causes.
- Smoking is linked to 85% of lung cancers. A patient's risk of lung cancer decreases significantly 5 years after smoking cessation, but never truly returns to baseline.
- An occupational history is important including possible exposure to asbestosis (associated with not only mesothelioma but also non–small-cell lung cancer), silica, beryllium, radon, and ionizing radiation, among others.

Physical Examination

- Although there are no specific physical examination findings related to SPNs, evidence for underlying etiologies might be discovered with a thorough examination.
- Note that signs of weight loss or cachexia are suggestive of malignancy.
- Do a thorough lymph node examination. **A cervical lymph node might provide an easy diagnostic target to determine the etiology of an SPN.**
- Perform a breast examination in women and testicular examination in young men.
- A careful skin examination may reveal telangiectasias, erythema nodosum, rheumatoid nodules, or other findings that might suggest a cause.

Risk Stratification

- The first step in managing an SPN is to stratify the patient in terms of malignancy risk: low-, intermediate-, or high-risk categories (Table 10-12). Risk stratification can be accomplished either qualitatively via clinical judgment or quantitatively using validated risk assessment tools. These approaches appear to be complementary.[165]
- Once the risk of malignancy has been established, further management can proceed, as outlined in Figure 10-6.

Differential Diagnosis

Pulmonary nodules are divided primarily into malignant or benign etiologies, with benign processes further divided into infectious or noninfectious causes (Table 10-13).

Diagnostic Testing

Laboratories
- Routine laboratory testing is seldom helpful unless the history and physical examination strongly suggest an etiology.
- If CTDs or vasculitides are suspected, perform appropriate testing.

TABLE 10-12	Assessment of the Probability of Malignancy		
Assessment Criteria	Low (<5%)	Intermediate (5%–65%)	High (>65%)
Clinical factors alone (determined by clinical judgment and/or use of validated model)	Young, less smoking, no prior cancer, smaller nodule size, regular margins, and/or non–upper lobe location	Mixture of low and high-probability features	Older, heavy smoking, prior cancer, larger size, irregular spiculated margins, and/or upper-lobe location
FDG–PET scan results	Low–moderate clinical probability and low FGD–PET activity	Weak or moderate FDG–PET scan activity	Intensely hypermetabolic nodule
Nonsurgical biopsy results (bronchoscopy or TTNA)	Specific benign diagnosis	Nondiagnostic	Suspicious for malignancy
CT scan surveillance	Resolution or near-complete resolution, progressive or persistent decrease in size, or no growth over ≥2 y (solid nodule) or ≥3–5 y (subsolid nodule)	Nonapplicable	Clear evidence of growth

FDG, 18-fluorodeoxyglucose; PET, positron emission tomography; TTNA, transthoracic needle aspiration.
Reprinted from Gould MK, Donington J, Lynch WR, et al. Evaluation of individuals with pulmonary nodules: when is it lung cancer? Diagnosis and management of lung cancer, 3rd ed—American College of Chest Physicians evidence-based clinical practice guidelines. *Chest*. 2013;143(5):e93s-e120s. Copyright © 2013 The American College of Chest Physicians. With permission.

CHAPTER 10

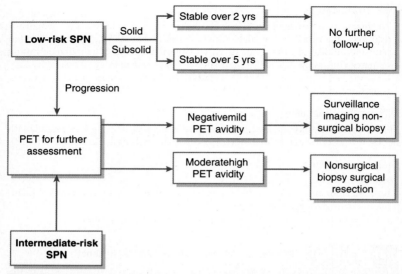

Figure 10-6. Diagnostic and therapeutic management of low- and intermediate-risk pulmonary nodules. PET, positron emission tomography; SPN, solitary pulmonary nodule; yrs, years.

- Hyponatremia may suggest syndrome of inappropriate antidiuretic hormone associated with primary lung cancer, as well as other pulmonary processes.
- Hypercalcemia might suggest lung cancer as well as sarcoidosis.
- Anemia may indicate chronic pulmonary hemorrhage (e.g., HHT) or a chronic inflammatory disease.
- Microbiologic studies, particularly sputum culture, may aid in the diagnosis of an infectious SPN.
- Sputum cytology has limited use because yield is low for peripherally located, small lesions.

Imaging
The mainstay of diagnostic evaluation of an SPN is via radiographic studies, primarily **CXR, chest CT, and positron emission tomography (PET) scan**.
- **CXR:**
  - A previous CXR is an important tool in the initial evaluation of an SPN.
  - If an SPN has been present and unchanged on CXR for >2 years, then further evaluation may not be warranted. **Subsolid** lesions should be followed for longer periods because the volume-doubling time is extended in certain types of non–small-cell lung cancers.
  - If an SPN appears on a new radiograph in <30 days, it is likely not malignant and most likely infectious or inflammatory.
  - There are radiographic findings that make it more likely that a lesion is **benign (calcifications, a laminated appearance)** or more likely **malignant (spiculated, irregular border)** (see Table 10-12).
  - The CXR is easy to obtain and delivers a low dose of radiation; however, it has limitations in the initial characterization, and careful comparisons over time are required for SPN evaluation.

TABLE 10-13	Differential Diagnosis of the Solitary Pulmonary Nodule (SPN)
Malignant	• Primary pulmonary carcinoma (80% of all malignant SPNs) • Primary pulmonary lymphoma • Primary pulmonary carcinoid • Solitary pulmonary metastasis • Melanoma, osteosarcoma, testicular, breast, prostate, colon, and renal cell carcinoma
Benign neoplasms	• Hamartoma (accounts for most benign neoplastic SPNs) • Arteriovenous malformations (consider HHT) • Others, including neural tumors (schwannoma, neurofibroma), fibroma, and sclerosing hemangioma
Granulomas	Infectious • Mycobacterial disease (most commonly TB) and fungal infections (histoplasmosis, coccidioidomycosis, blastomycosis, cryptococcosis, aspergillosis) Noninfectious granulomas associated with vasculitis • Granulomatosis with polyangiitis, eosinophilic granulomatosis with polyangiitis • Noninfectious granulomas not associated with vasculitis • Sarcoid granulomatosis, hypersensitivity pneumonitis, and berylliosis
Other etiologies	Infectious • Bacterial (nocardiosis, actinomycosis, round pneumonia), measles, abscess, septic embolus Noninfectious • Lipoid pneumonia, amyloidosis, subpleural lymph node, rheumatoid nodule, pulmonary scar or infarct, congenital malformations (bronchogenic cyst, sequestration), skin nodule, rib fracture, pleural thickening from mass or fluid

HHT, hereditary hemorrhagic telangiectasia.

- **Chest CT:**
  - Chest CT is now considered the most important radiologic examination for SPN evaluation. With few exceptions, an SPN requires assessment by CT.
  - Accurate volumetric measurement of lesion size allows precise comparison to determine stability or growth.
  - Imaging allows a careful examination of mediastinal lymph nodes.
  - Thin cuts through the lesion are more sensitive than CXR for characterizing calcifications and lamination as well as the margins of the lesion.
- **PET scan:**
  - 18-Fluorodeoxyglucose–PET can help distinguish malignant and benign lesions.
  - PET has a sensitivity of 80%–100% and specificity of 79%–100% for detecting malignancy.
  - **False negatives** can occur in bronchoalveolar carcinoma, carcinoid, and mucinous neoplasms, whereas **false positives** are common in nonmalignant "inflammatory" conditions (infectious and autoimmune processes).

○ A higher incidence of both false-positive and false-negative results occurs in nodules <10 mm, thus discouraging the use of PET scan in this situation.[166]

○ PET scan is most commonly used in the evaluation of low- to moderate-risk indeterminate nodules for further risk stratification (see Figure 10-6).

• **Contrast-enhanced CT:**

○ Techniques are available for using contrast enhancement and measurement of Hounsfield units to risk stratify an SPN for malignancy.

○ A multicenter analysis demonstrated high sensitivity but relatively low specificity for identifying malignant nodules.[167]

○ This method may be an important tool for risk assessment of an indeterminate SPN in centers that have experience with the techniques.

Diagnostic Procedures

• **If a nodule is considered high risk and the patient is an appropriate surgical candidate, then the best approach is to forego biopsy and pursue resection.**

• Any increase in size or density of an SPN on serial imaging warrants additional investigation.

• If a lesion has low-risk characteristics, there is no indication to pursue biopsy and subjecting a patient to an unneeded risk.

• Nonsurgical biopsy via bronchoscopy or transthoracic needle aspiration (TTNA) is typically indicated for patients with a nodule, which has intermediate risk for lung cancer. In addition, for patients in whom surgery represents significant risk secondary to comorbidities, a nonsurgical biopsy may be indicated to demonstrate malignancy prior to surgery or nonsurgical therapy.

• There are primarily two options for biopsy of an SPN: TTNA and flexible bronchoscopy. Choosing either modality is based on nodule and patient factors, as well as institutional experience. These factors include nodule size, location, and finding of emphysema on CT chest.

○ **TTNA:**

▪ This technique is usually performed under the guidance of fluoroscopy, ultrasound, or CT (more common).

▪ This approach is most commonly used for nodules with a peripheral location and without anatomic impediment to a biopsy needle.

▪ Sensitivity of TTNA for the diagnosis of lung cancer is 80%–90% in selected patients.

▪ Specificity for identifying malignancy is high with TTNA; however, there is a significant rate of nondiagnostic biopsies, and sensitivity depends on many factors, including nodule size and distance from the pleura.

▪ A nondiagnostic biopsy does not rule out malignancy.

▪ The complications of TTNA are bleeding (1%), pneumothorax (15%), and 6%–7% incidence of pneumothorax requiring chest tube drainage.[168]

▪ TTNA alone does not provide any additional information regarding the patient's pathological staging.

○ **Bronchoscopy:**

▪ Conventional flexible bronchoscopy is best suited for central airway lesions and has a sensitivity of 88% in malignancy. Advanced bronchoscopic techniques are recommended in the diagnosis of peripheral lesions where their diagnostic yield is superior to that of conventional bronchoscopy.

- Advanced bronchoscopic modalities include radial probe endobronchial ultrasound and electromagnetic navigation, with sensitivities of 73% and 71%, respectively, for the detection of malignancy in peripheral nodules.
- Complete mediastinal and hilar lymph node examination for pathological staging may also be performed during bronchoscopy for peripheral lesion diagnosis, obviating the need for additional procedures.
- The complications of bronchoscopy are bleeding (2%–5%) and pneumothorax (2%–4%).[168]

TREATMENT

- Management of low- and intermediate-risk SPNs is outlined in Figure 10-6.
- Overall treatment strategy is to identify lesions with significant malignancy risk and pursue surgical resection when possible.
- If a specific etiology for the SPN is diagnosed (e.g., a CTD or infection), then treatment is targeted toward the underlying process.

Nonpharmacologic Therapies

- Although **surgical resection is preferable in patients with either a high-risk lesion or biopsy-proven malignancy**, if surgical resection is not an option, other effective therapies exist.
- **Stereotactic radiation** is currently the most widely used therapy in this clinical situation. This mode of external beam therapy aims to decrease collateral radiation–induced damage to adjacent lung tissue.
- There are more experimental approaches, including brachytherapy and radiofrequency ablation, which are currently under development.

Surgical Management

- Surgical resection of an indeterminate SPN is indicated in the following situations:
  - The clinical probability of malignancy is moderate to high (>60%).
  - The nodule is hypermetabolic by PET imaging.
  - The nodule has been proven malignant by biopsy.
  - Patient preference for surgery where the patient is an appropriate surgical candidate.
- A combination of surgical techniques, including VATS, mediastinoscopy, and thoracotomy, can lead to diagnosis (via intraoperative frozen section), staging, and potential cure during a single induction of anesthesia.

MONITORING/FOLLOW-UP

- For a low- or intermediate-risk pulmonary nodule for which resection is not warranted (see Figure 10-6), desired, or possible, routine follow-up with chest CT is standard practice.
- Follow-up of SPN depends on whether it is a solid or subsolid nodule. Solid nodules require 2 years of surveillance, and subsolid nodules require additional years of surveillance to document stability.
- The updated 2017 Fleischner Society recommendations aim toward decreasing the number of chest CT scans for incidentally detected SPN follow-up and to provide greater flexibility to clinicians and patients for shared decision-making.[169]

CHAPTER 10

Pleural Diseases

GENERAL PRINCIPLES

- The pleural lining is a serous membrane covering the lung parenchyma, chest wall, diaphragm, and mediastinum.
- The presence of excess fluid or any amount of gas in the pleural space is abnormal.
- The pleural membrane covering the surface of the lung is known as the visceral pleura; the parietal pleura covers the remaining structures.
- In between the visceral and parietal pleura of each lung is the pleural space, a potential space that contains a thin layer of fluid of approximately 10 mL in volume.
- The parietal pleura secretes approximately 2400 mL of fluid daily, which is reabsorbed by the visceral pleura.[170]

Definition

- A pleural effusion is an accumulation of >10 mL of fluid in the pleural space.
  - A hemothorax refers to a pleural effusion that mainly comprises blood.[171]
  - Chylothorax is a collection of chyle within the pleural space. Chyle is a milky fluid consisting of lymph and fat droplets.[172]
  - A parapneumonic effusion is fluid collection in the pleural space as a result of a pneumonia/consolidation or bronchiectasis. The three types of parapneumonic effusions include uncomplicated effusion, complicated effusion, and empyema.[173,174]
  - An empyema refers to infected fluid within the pleural space.
- A pneumothorax is a collection of air in the pleural space.
  - Primary spontaneous pneumothorax occurs when the lung parenchyma is normal without any obvious underlying lung disease.[175]
  - Secondary spontaneous pneumothorax is a complication of underlying parenchymal lung disease.[175]
  - Sometimes if air is trapped in the pleural space under high pressure, a tension pneumothorax develops, which can be fatal if not recognized and treated.[176,177]

Epidemiology

- More than one million cases of pleural effusion occur annually in the US.
- It is estimated that malignant pleural effusion affects about 150,000 people a year in the US. Congestive heart failure and parapneumonic effusion are the predominant etiologies of pleural effusion in the US.[174]
- Incidence of pneumothorax varies widely by gender, country, and race.

Etiology

- Pleural effusions have a variety of causes and are listed below (Table 10-14).
  - Empyema is generally caused by extension of an infection of the lung or surrounding tissue.
    - Common microbial pathogens are *S. aureus, Streptococcus* species, *H. influenza*, and *oral anaerobes*.
    - Empyemas are frequently polymicrobial in cases where aspiration is suspected, commonly because of oral flora.
  - The three major grouped causes of chylothorax are malignancy (50% of cases),[172,178] trauma (25%), and idiopathic (15%).[179] Other rare causes such as LAM[180] and trauma to thoracic duct account for 10%.

TABLE 10-14	Causes of Pleural Effusion

- Exudates
  - Infections
    - Bacteria
    - TB
    - Fungi
    - Parasites
    - Viruses
    - Mycoplasma
  - Neoplasms
    - Metastatic carcinoma
    - Lymphoma
    - Leukemia
    - Mesothelioma
    - Bronchogenic carcinoma
    - Chest wall tumors
  - Intra-abdominal disease/gastrointestinal
    - Abdominal surgery
    - Pancreatitis
    - Meigs syndrome
    - Intrahepatic abscess
    - Incarcerated diaphragmatic hernia
    - Subdiaphragmatic abscess
    - Esophageal rupture
    - Endoscopic variceal sclerotherapy
    - Hepatitis
  - Collagen vascular diseases/vasculitis
    - Systemic lupus erythematosus
    - Rheumatoid arthritis
    - Drug-induced lupus
    - Sjögren syndrome
    - Granulomatosis with polyangiitis
    - Eosinophilic granulomatosis with polyangiitis
    - Immunoblastic lymphadenopathy
  - Drug-induced pleural disease
    - Nitrofurantoin
    - Dantrolene
    - Methysergide
    - Bromocriptine
    - Procarbazine
    - Amiodarone
  - Pulmonary infarction secondary to thromboembolic disease
  - Miscellaneous
    - Dressler syndrome (postcardiac injury)
    - Sarcoidosis
    - Yellow nail syndrome
    - Trapped lung
    - Radiation therapy
    - Electrical burns

(continued)

TABLE 10-14	Causes of Pleural Effusion (*continued*)

- ■ Iatrogenic injury
- ■ Ovarian hyperstimulation syndrome
- ■ Chronic atelectasis
- ■ Asbestos exposure
- ■ Familial Mediterranean fever
- ■ Urinoma
- ○ Idiopathic
- ○ Lipid laden
  - ■ Chylous
  - ■ Pseudochylous
- ○ Trauma
- • Transudates
  - ○ Increased hydrostatic pressure
    - ■ Congestive heart failure
    - ■ Constrictive pericarditis
    - ■ Superior vena caval obstruction
  - ○ Decreased oncotic pressure
    - ■ Cirrhosis
    - ■ Nephrotic syndrome
    - ■ Hypoalbuminemia
    - ■ Peritoneal dialysis
  - ○ Miscellaneous
    - ■ Acute atelectasis
    - ■ Subclavian catheter misplacement
    - ■ Myxedema
    - ■ Idiopathic

- ■ Seventy-five percent of chylous effusions associated with malignancy are due to lymphoma-related obstruction of pleural lymphatics preventing reabsorption of pleural fluid.[172]
- ■ Trauma as a causative factor of chylothorax includes any cardiothoracic surgical procedure. It may take 1–2 weeks postsurgery for the chylothorax to become apparent.
- ■ In a number of cases, chylothorax results from transdiaphragmatic leakage of chylous ascites.[172] Causes of chylous ascites include nephrotic syndrome, hypothyroidism, and cirrhosis of the liver.[172]
- ○ Hemothorax may result from trauma or an iatrogenic etiology and are rarely spontaneous.[171]
- ○ Other causes of pleural effusion include heart failure, anasarca, and pulmonary embolism.
- • Secondary pneumothorax is often seen in chronic obstructive pulmonary disease, AIDS, CF, TB, *P. jirovecii* pneumonia, sarcoidosis, pulmonary fibrosis, asthma, Marfan disease, LAM, PLCH, trauma, or any cavitary or cystic lung disease.

Pathophysiology

- • Pleural effusions can be categorized as transudates or exudates.
  - ○ Transudates result primarily from passive fluid shifts that occur as a result of changes in the hydrostatic and/or oncotic pressures of the circulation.[181]

- Exudates are indicative of an active pleural process such as inflammation of the pleura or underlying lung tissue.[181]
- There are numerous causes of both transudates and exudates (Table 10-14).[181]
- Primary spontaneous pneumothorax is thought to result from rupture of subpleural apical blebs, with no obvious preceding cause.[182]
- Secondary pneumothorax results from rupture of pathologic lung architecture such as emphysematous bullae, cysts, or cavity formation.[182]

Risk Factors

- Risk factors for pleural effusion reflect those of the underlying causative disease.
- Primary spontaneous pneumothoraces are more common in tall, thin males and recur 50% of the time.
- Marfan disease is associated with a primary spontaneous pneumothorax.[182]

DIAGNOSIS

- Diagnosis of a pleural disease is based on history, physical examination, and radiographic imaging, which includes chest radiography, CT scan, and chest ultrasound.[183]
- Differentiation into a specific pathologic entity is based on history, imaging, and laboratory analysis (chemistry, microbiology, and cytology) of the pleural fluid if present.

Clinical Presentation

- Symptom onset may be chronic, subacute, or acute depending on the rapidity with which the pleural pathology developed (amount of gas or excess pleural fluid).
- If the effusion is very large in nature, it may cause a mass effect progressing to a tension physiology with hemodynamic instability from cardiac tamponade resulting in a life-threatening hypotension.

History

- Dyspnea is the primary symptom of pleural disease, and pain may also be present.
  - Pain is generally pleuritic in nature.
  - Referred pain to the abdomen and ipsilateral shoulder are possible.
- Other symptoms depend on the specific etiology of the pleural disease:
  - Empyema may be associated with fevers, chills, and malaise.
  - Hemothorax may present with signs and symptoms of anemia such as acute or subacute dyspnea.[171]
  - Chylothorax contains large amounts of fat, protein, and lymphocytes, which accounts for nutritional and immunologic deficiencies observed when they are chronic in nature.

Physical Examination

- Decreased expansion on inspiration, dullness to percussion, and decreased or absent breath sounds on auscultation are all consistent with a pleural effusion.
- The examination finding that correlates best with presence of pleural effusion is asymmetric chest wall expansion.
- Asymmetric chest wall appearance, decreased breath sounds, decreased tactile fremitus, and hyperresonance to percussion may be consistent with a large pneumothorax.
- Hypotension may be the presenting sign if there is a mass effect from a large pleural effusion or tension pneumothorax.

Diagnostic Criteria

There are no clinical criteria to definitively diagnose a pleural effusion or pneumothorax and radiographic imaging is generally needed.

Differential Diagnosis

The differential diagnosis for pleural effusion or pneumothorax includes other causes of dyspnea such as pulmonary edema, pneumonia, compressive or resorptive atelectasis, thromboembolic disease, ILD, or central airway obstruction because of benign or malignant disease.

Diagnostic Testing

Radiographic imaging and laboratory testing of pleural fluid are the two most useful diagnostic modalities for diagnosing pleural disease.

Laboratories

* Categorization of pleural fluid as transudative or exudative assists with diagnosis and therapeutic management.[184]
  * Light's criteria compare levels of protein and lactate dehydrogenase in the effusion with those in the patient's serum to determine whether inflammation or fluid shift is responsible for the effusion.[185]
    * If one of the three Light's criteria is met, the effusion is defined as an exudate (Table 10-15).[184,185]
  * Heffner's criteria have similar sensitivity for identifying exudative pleural effusions when compared with Light's criteria and do not require concomitant serum values for comparison (Table 10-15).[186]
* Other useful studies to differentiate the type of pleural effusion include pH, glucose, cell count, Gram stain, culture, and triglycerides. Hematocrit should be sent if hemothorax is suspected.[184]
  * Empyema can be diagnosed by a positive Gram stain or culture.
    * Empyema is also characterized by a low pH and low glucose.
  * Hemothorax is defined by a pleural hematocrit/serum hematocrit of >0.5.
  * Chylothorax is diagnosed by pleural triglycerides >110 mg/dL or by the presence of chylomicrons in the pleural fluid.[172]
    * If chylothorax is suspected and triglycerides are 50–110 mg/dL, a lipoprotein electrophoresis can confirm the presence of chylomicrons.[172]

TABLE 10-15	Criteria for Defining an Effusion

* Light's criteria
  * Pleural fluid protein to serum protein ratio of >0.5
  * Pleural fluid lactate dehydrogenase (LDH) to serum LDH ratio of >0.6
  * Pleural fluid LDH >2/3 serum upper limit of normal
* Heffner criteria
  * Pleural fluid protein >2.9 g/dL
  * Pleural fluid cholesterol >45 mg/dL
  * Pleural fluid LDH > 45% of upper limits of normal serum value

Adapted from Light RW. Clinical manifestations and useful tests. In: Light RW, ed. *Pleural Diseases*. 4th ed. Lippincott Williams and Wilkins; 2001:42-86; Heffner JE, Brown LK, Barbieri CA. Diagnostic value of tests that discriminate between exudative and transudative pleural effusions. *Chest*. 1997;111:970-980.

TABLE 10-16	Helpful Features of Exudative Pleural Effusions

- Malignancy
  - Fluid cytology positive for malignant cells
- TB
  - Pleural fluid is lymphocytic
  - Positive acid-fast bacilli stain is very rare
  - Pleural fluid is sanguineous
- Connective tissue disease
  - Pleural fluid usually lymphocytic and will often have antinuclear antibody positivity
- Pancreatitis
  - Increased amylase
- Infection
  - Gram stain and culture often reveal specific infection
  - Empyema is accompanied by very low glucose and pH and a markedly elevated lactate dehydrogenase
- Drug related
  - Eosinophilic fluid
- Chylothorax
  - Milky fluid, triglyceride level >110 mg/dL
- Hemothorax
  - Sanguineous fluid
  - Hematocrit of pleural fluid is >50% of peripheral blood

- Malignant pleural effusion is diagnosed by a positive fluid cytology, and though highly specific, it is not sensitive. The sensitivity of diagnosis of a malignant pleural effusion increases slightly with subsequent thoracentesis up to three times and with increasing amount of pleural fluid.[187]
- See Table 10-16 for other pleural fluid laboratory values associated with specific pleural effusions.

Imaging
- Chest radiograph is generally the first imaging study obtained when a patient presents with a suspected pleural effusion or pneumothorax.[188]
  - On a posteroanterior chest film, blunting of the costophrenic angle or blurring of the diaphragmatic margin suggests the presence of a pleural effusion.
    - Generally, 200–500 mL of fluid is needed to generate this finding.[189]
  - A lateral decubitus film of the affected side can reveal an effusion of approximately 100 mL and allows for assessment of a free-flowing versus loculated effusion.[188,189]
- CT is more sensitive than routine chest radiography and can detect the presence of even a very small amount of fluid or air in the pleural space as well as the presence of loculations in the pleural fluid.[188]
- Ultrasound is a modality that is increasingly being used to image the pleural space.
  - Ultrasound can detect fluid or air and provides qualitative information regarding pleural fluid and detects small amounts of fluid as well as the presence of septations in the pleural space.
    - Ultrasound findings such as fluid echogenicity and the presence of septations indicate a complex loculated effusion potentially changing management and predicting clinical outcome.
    - Ultrasound guidance is often used to direct treatments such as drainage of fluid or chest tube insertion.

Diagnostic Procedures

- Thoracentesis should be performed for diagnosis in cases of pleural effusion of unknown etiology. Subsequent thoracentesis increase the diagnostic yield depending on the etiology.[187]
- Therapeutic thoracentesis can lead to symptom relief and is indicated for dyspnea.
  - Thoracentesis should generally be performed after ultrasound localization of pleural fluid to decrease risk of complications such as pneumothorax.
  - CXR should be performed after the procedure to rule out a complicating pneumothorax.
  - Hemothorax is a rare complication.

TREATMENT

- Generally, treatment of a pleural effusion depends on the etiology.
  - Transudative pleural effusions are most appropriately managed by treating the underlying cause.
    - Symptomatic treatment may involve drainage of the effusion if the presenting symptom is dyspnea or acute respiratory failure.
  - Exudative pleural effusions should be evaluated for an underlying cause.
    - Treatment may involve drainage of the effusion or even pleurodesis to prevent reaccumulation of fluid.
    - Placement of an indwelling pleural catheter for malignant recurrent pleural effusions or in cases of hepatic hydrothorax refractory to medical therapy may be an option.[190]
- Treatment of pneumothorax generally involves draining the air from the pleural space by insertion of a chest tube.
- Pleurodesis should be considered after the first episode of secondary spontaneous pneumothorax because rates of recurrence are high.[175]

Medications

- Pleural effusions can sometimes be treated with medications depending on the cause.
- Parapneumonic effusions and empyema are treated with antibiotics in conjunction with fluid drainage.[174]
- Transudative pleural effusions can sometimes be treated effectively with diuretics in disease states such as congestive heart failure, anasarca, renal failure, and liver failure.
- There is no medical treatment for pneumothorax.

Nonpharmacologic Therapies

- Pleurodesis involves instillation of a sclerosing agent into the pleural space to cause scarring and restriction of the space itself.
  - This is generally performed for recurrent malignant effusion, recurrent pneumothorax once the lung has reexpanded, occasionally for chylothorax, and after the first episode of secondary spontaneous pneumothorax.[175]
- When other modalities fail, total parenteral nutrition with complete bowel rest can cause chylothoraces to resolve as oral intake results in chyle formation.[172]
  - Medium-chain triglyceride diets have been tried, as chyle is derived from long-chain triglycerides in the diet, though this has yielded mixed results.[172]
- If a pneumothorax is <15% of the hemithorax volume, it is safe to observe and follow-up with radiographic studies.

- High oxygen content (e.g., 100% nonrebreather mask) administration increases the rate of pleural air reabsorption by increasing the nitrogen gradient between the air in the pneumothorax and the pleural capillaries.
- In cases of persistent pneumothorax secondary to a bronchopleural fistula, fiberoptic bronchoscopy with placement of endobronchial valves causing atelectasis of the distal lung may be an option if the bronchopleural fistula has been localized to one location via balloon catheter occlusion.[191]

Surgical Management

- Pleural effusion:
  - Chest tube insertion is often indicated for drainage of large pleural effusions.
  - Other indications for chest tube insertion include empyema, chylothorax, and hemothorax.[171]
  - Thoracentesis can be used as a therapeutic modality.
  - Malignant pleural effusion:
    - Tunneled pleural catheter is used for recurrent malignant pleural effusion and occasionally hepatic hydrothorax refractory to medical management and diuresis.[190]
    - This catheter can be drained at home every other day with attachment to a vacuum-sealed device or gravity collection system.
    - About 30%–50% of patients who have indwelling tunneled pleural catheters in place for malignant pleural effusion may experience auto-pleurodesis, or the cessation of significant additional pleural fluid drainage. In these cases, the indwelling pleural catheters may be removed with a very low likelihood for reaccumulation of pleural fluid on the side where the catheter was placed.[192]
  - Empyema:
    - In cases where chest tube drainage does not effectively drain an empyema and there is continued evidence of infection, VATS with decortication is often indicated.
    - There is a role for intrapleural use of tissue plasminogen activator and recombinant deoxyribonuclease (DNase) in pleural infections. These result in improved fluid drainage and decreased need for surgical intervention.[193]
  - Hemothorax:
    - Requires surgical stabilization in 30% of penetrating injuries and 15% of blunt injuries.[194]
    - Initial output of >1500 mL of blood or continued chest tube output or >200 mL of blood over 2 hours requires surgical intervention.
    - Clotted blood in the pleural space may require VATS to prevent development of empyema or fibrothorax.[195]
  - Chylothorax:
    - For persistent chylothorax, surgical interventions include thoracic duct ligation via VATS in conjunction with pleurectomy or pleurodesis.[195]
    - Pleuroperitoneal shunting is also occasionally performed, though obviously not in cases in which the pleural disease is secondary to chylous ascites.[194]
    - Early surgical intervention for chylothorax should be considered when chest tube output is >1500 mL/d or in a patient with malnourishment or an immunocompromised state.[172]
  - Pneumothorax:
    - Treated with chest tube insertion if they are large, symptomatic, under tension, recurrent, or bilateral.

▫ In extreme circumstances where a large pneumothorax is causing cardiovascular collapse, immediate needle decompression is indicated by inserting a needle in the anterior chest above the nipple line in a parasternal location.

- For recurrent pneumothorax, VATS may be indicated with endoscopic stapling and removal of the bulla or fistula, particularly if there is a bronchopleural fistula.[191]
- Therapeutic success of bronchoscopic management of bronchopleural fistula with endobronchial valves, coils, glue, or sealant has been variable and treatment must be individualized.[191]

SPECIAL CONSIDERATIONS

- The etiology of pleural effusions can often be discerned by their appearance.
  ○ A serous effusion is more likely to be transudative, while an exudative effusion is more likely to have other appearances, frequently with a cloudy or serosanguinous appearance.
  ○ If the fluid appears frankly bloody, a hemothorax should be suspected.
  ○ Pus indicates an empyema.
  ○ Milky white and opalescent pleural fluid is indicative of a chylothorax.
- In cases of massive hemothorax requiring surgical intervention, clamping the chest tube may result in tension hemothorax and cardiovascular collapse.[195]
- Chylothorax is nonirritating and bacteriostatic, thus secondary infection is extremely rare.[194]

COMPLICATIONS

- Disease recurrence.
- Cardiovascular compromise in extreme cases.
- Other complications are disease-specific.

REFERRAL

- Interventional pulmonology may be consulted for the placement of chest tubes, tunneled pleural catheters, or endobronchial valve.
- Surgical consultation may be needed as per the "Surgical Management" section above.

REFERENCES

1. Simonneau G, Montani D, Celermajer DS, et al. Haemodynamic definitions and updated clinical classification of pulmonary hypertension. *Eur Respir J*. 2019;53:1801913.
2. Humbert M, Sitbon O, Chaouat A, et al. Pulmonary arterial hypertension in France: results from a national registry. *Am J Respir Crit Care Med*. 2006;173:1023-1030.
3. Peacock AJ, Murphy NF, McMurray JJ, et al. An epidemiological study of pulmonary arterial hypertension. *Eur Respir J*. 2007;30:104-109.
4. Badesch DB, Raskob GE, Elliott CG, et al. Pulmonary arterial hypertension: baseline characteristics from the REVEAL registry. *Chest*. 2010;137:376-387.
5. Rich S, Dantzker DR, Ayres SM, et al. Primary pulmonary hypertension. A national prospective study. *Ann Intern Med*. 1987;107:216-223.
6. Thenappan T, Shah SJ, Rich S, Gomberg-Maitland M. A USA-based registry for pulmonary arterial hypertension: 1982-2006. *Eur Respir J*. 2007;30:1103-1110.
7. Pengo V, Lensing AW, Prins MH, et al. Incidence of chronic thromboembolic pulmonary hypertension after pulmonary embolism. *N Engl J Med*. 2004;350:2257-2264.

8. Sahay S. Evaluation and classification of pulmonary arterial hypertension. *J Thorac Dis.* 2019;11:S1789-S1799.

9. Morrell NW, Aldred MA, Chung WK, et al. Genetics and genomics of pulmonary arterial hypertension. *Eur Respir J.* 2019;53:1801899

10. McLaughlin VV, Archer SL, Badesch DB, et al. ACCF/AHA 2009 expert consensus document on pulmonary hypertension: a report of the American College of Cardiology Foundation Task Force on expert consensus documents and the American Heart Association—developed in collaboration with the American College of Chest Physicians, American Thoracic Society, Inc., and the Pulmonary Hypertension Association. *Circulation.* 2009;119:2250-2294.

11. Coghlan JG, Denton CP, Grunig E, et al. Evidence-based detection of pulmonary arterial hypertension in systemic sclerosis: the DETECT study. *Ann Rheum Dis.* 2014;73:1340-1349.

12. McGoon M, Gutterman D, Steen V, et al. Screening, early detection, and diagnosis of pulmonary arterial hypertension: ACCP evidence-based clinical practice guidelines. *Chest.* 2004;126:14S-34S.

13. Forfia PR, Fisher MR, Mathai SC, et al. Tricuspid annular displacement predicts survival in pulmonary hypertension. *Am J Respir Crit Care Med.* 2006;174:1034-1041.

14. Lam CS, Roger VL, Rodeheffer RJ, et al. Pulmonary hypertension in heart failure with preserved ejection fraction: a community-based study. *J Am Coll Cardiol.* 2009;53:1119-1126.

15. Hoeper MM, Bogaard HJ, Condliffe R, et al. Definitions and diagnosis of pulmonary hypertension. *J Am Coll Cardiol.* 2013;62:D42-D50.

16. Miyamoto S, Nagaya N, Satoh T, et al. Clinical correlates and prognostic significance of six-minute walk test in patients with primary pulmonary hypertension. Comparison with cardiopulmonary exercise testing. *Am J Respir Crit Care Med.* 2000;161:487-492.

17. Minai OA, Pandya CM, Golish JA, et al. Predictors of nocturnal oxygen desaturation in pulmonary arterial hypertension. *Chest.* 2007;131:109-117.

18. van de Veerdonk MC, Kind T, Marcus JT, et al. Progressive right ventricular dysfunction in patients with pulmonary arterial hypertension responding to therapy. *J Am Coll Cardiol.* 2011;58: 2511-2519.

19. Fisher MR, Forfia PR, Chamera E, et al. Accuracy of Doppler echocardiography in the hemodynamic assessment of pulmonary hypertension. *Am J Respir Crit Care Med.* 2009;179:615-621.

20. Jean-Luc Vachiéry J, Tedford RJ, Rosenkranz S, et al. Pulmonary hypertension due to left heart disease. *Eur Respir J.* 2019;53:1801897.

21. Badesch DB, Abman SH, Ahearn GS, et al. Medical therapy for pulmonary arterial hypertension: ACCP evidence-based clinical practice guidelines. *Chest.* 2004;126:35S-62S.

22. Kim NH, Delcroix M, Jenkins DP, et al. Chronic thromboembolic pulmonary hypertension. *J Am Coll Cardiol.* 2013;62:D92-D99.

23. Ogawa A, Satoh T, Fukuda T, et al. Balloon pulmonary angioplasty for chronic thromboembolic pulmonary hypertension: results of a multicenter registry. *Circ Cardiovasc Qual Outcomes.* 2017;10:e004029.

24. Benza RL, Gomberg-Maitland M, Elliott CG, et al. Predicting survival in patients with pulmonary arterial hypertension: the REVEAL risk score calculator 2.0 and comparison with ESC/ERS-Based risk assessment strategies. *Chest.* 2019;156:323-337.

25. Benza RL, Kanwar MK, Raina A, et al. Development and validation of an abridged version of the REVEAL 2.0 risk score calculator, REVEAL lite 2, for use in patients with pulmonary arterial hypertension. *Chest.* 2021; 159 337-346.

26. Boucly A, Weatherald J, Savale L, et al. Risk assessment, prognosis and guideline implementation in pulmonary arterial hypertension. *Eur Respir J.* 2017;50:1700889.

27. Galiè N, Channick RN, Frantz RP, et al. Risk stratification and medical therapy of pulmonary arterial hypertension. *Eur Respir J.* 2019;53:1801889.

28. Olsson KM, Delcroix M, Ghofrani HA, et al. Anticoagulation and survival in pulmonary arterial hypertension: results from the comparative, prospective registry of newly initiated therapies for pulmonary hypertension (COMPERA). *Circulation.* 2014;129:57-65.

29. Preston IR, Roberts KE, Miller DP, et al. Effect of warfarin treatment on survival of patients with pulmonary arterial hypertension (PAH) in the Registry to Evaluate Early and Long-Term PAH Disease Management (REVEAL). *Circulation.* 2015;132:2403-2411.

30. Bradley EA, Ammash N, Martinez SC, et al. "Treat-to-close": non-repairable ASD-PAH in the adult—results from the North American ASD-PAH (NAAP) multicenter registry. *Int J Cardiol.* 2019;291:127-133.

31. Humbert M, Sitbon O, Chaouat A, et al. Survival in patients with idiopathic, familial, and anorexigen-associated pulmonary arterial hypertension in the modern management era. *Circulation.* 2010;122:156-163.

32. Benza RL, Miller DP, Gomberg-Maitland M, et al. Predicting survival in pulmonary arterial hypertension: insights from the registry to evaluate early and long-term pulmonary arterial hypertension disease management (REVEAL). *Circulation.* 2010;122:164-172.

33. American Academy Sleep Medicine Task Force. Sleep-related breathing disorders in adults: recommendations for syndrome definition and measurement techniques in clinical research. *Sleep.* 1999;22:667-689.

CHAPTER 10

34. Young T, Palta M, Dempsey J, et al. The occurrence of sleep-disordered breathing among middle-aged adults. *N Eng J Med.* 1993;328:1230-1235.

35. Peppard PE, Young T, Barnet JH, et al. Increased prevalence of sleep-disordered breathing in adults. *Am J Epidemiol.* 2013;177:1006-1014.

36. Somers VK, White DP, Amin R, et al. Sleep apnea and cardiovascular disease. *Circulation.* 2008;118:1080-1111.

37. McNicholas WT, Bonsignore MR. Sleep apnoea as an independent risk factor for cardiovascular disease: current evidence, basic mechanisms, and research priorities. *Eur Respir J.* 2007;29:165-178.

38. Young T, Finn L, Peppard PE, et al. Sleep disordered breathing and mortality: eighteen-year follow-up of the Wisconsin sleep cohort. *Sleep.* 2008;31:1071-1078.

39. Marshall NS, Wong KKH, Liu PY, et al. Sleep apnea as an independent risk factor for all-cause mortality: the Busselton health study. *Sleep.* 2008;31:1079-1085.

40. Reichmuth KJ, Austin D, Skatrud JB, Young T. Association of sleep apnea and type II diabetes: a population based study. *Am J Respir Crit Care Med.* 2005;172:1590-1595.

41. Karimi M, Hedner J, Häbel H, et al. Sleep apnea related risks of motor vehicle accidents is reduced by continuous positive airway pressure: Swedish traffic accident registry data. *Sleep.* 2015;38:341-349.

42. Liistro G, Rombaux P, Belge C, et al. High Mallampati score and nasal obstruction are associated risk factors for obstructive sleep apnoea. *Eur Respir J.* 2003;21:248-252.

43. Kapur VK, Auckley DH, Chowdhuri S, et al. Clinical practice guideline for diagnostic testing for adult obstructive sleep apnea: an American Academy of Sleep Medicine clinical practice guideline. *J Clin Sleep Med.* 2017;13:479-504.

44. Kuan YC, Wu D, Huang KW, et al. Effects of modafinil and armodafinil in patients with obstructive sleep apnea: a meta-analysis of randomized controlled trials. *Clin Ther.* 2016;38:874-878.

45. Sigurdson K, Ayas NT. The public health and safety consequences of sleep disorders. *Can J Physiol Pharmacol.* 2007;85:179-183.

46. Buchner NJ, Sanner BM, Borgel J, Rump LC. Continuous positive airway pressure treatment of mild to moderate obstructive sleep apnea reduces cardiovascular risk. *Am J Respir Crit Care Med.* 2007;176:1274-1280.

47. McEvoy RD, Antic NA, Heeley E, et al. CPAP for prevention of cardiovascular events in obstructive sleep apnea. *N Engl J Med.* 2016;375:919-931.

48. Fein AS, Shvilkin A, Shah D, et al. Treatment of obstructive sleep apnea reduces the risk of atrial fibrillation recurrence after catheter ablation. *J Am Coll Cardiol.* 2013;62:300-305.

49. Borel JC, Tamisier R, Dias-Domingos S, et al. Type of mask may impact on continuous positive airway pressure adherence in apneic patients. *PLoS One.* 2013;8:e64382. doi:10.1371/journal.pone.0064382

50. Fietze I, Glos M, Moebus I, et al. Automatic pressure titration with APAP is as effective as manual titration with CPAP in patients with obstructive sleep apnea. *Respiration.* 2007;74:279-286.

51. Nussbaumer Y, Bloch K, Genser T, Thurneer R. Equivalence of autoadjusted and constant continuous positive airway pressure in home treatment of sleep apnea. *Chest.* 2006;129:638-643.

52. Strollo PJ, Soose RJ, Maurer JT, et al. Upper-airway stimulator for obstructive sleep apnea. *N Engl J Med.* 2014;370:139-149.

53. Li KK, Powell NB, Riley RW, et al. Long-term results of maxillomandibular advancement surgery. *Sleep Breath.* 2000;4:137-139.

54. Sher AE, Schechtman KB, Piccirillo JF. Efficacy of modifications of the upper airway in adults with obstructive sleep apnea syndrome. *Sleep.* 1996;19:156-177.

55. Caples SM, Rowley JA, Prinsell JR, et al. Surgical modifications of the upper airway for obstructive sleep apnea in adults: a systematic review and meta-analysis. *Sleep.* 2010;33:1396-1407.

56. Tuomilehto HPI, Seppä JM, Partinen MM, et al. Life style intervention with weight reduction: first-line treatment in mild obstructive sleep apnea. *Am J Respir Crit Care Med.* 2009;179:320-327.

57. Greenberg DL, Lettieri CJ, Eliasson AH. Effects of surgical weight loss on measures of obstructive sleep apnea: a meta-analysis. *Am J Med.* 2009;122: 535-542.

58. Mickelson SA. Preoperative and postoperative management of obstructive sleep apnea patients. *Otolaryngol Clin N Am.* 2007;40:877-889.

59. Travis WD, Costabel U, Hansell DM, et al. An official American Thoracic Society/European Respiratory Society statement: update of the international multidisciplinary classification of the idiopathic interstitial pneumonias. *Am J Respir Crit Care Med.* 2013;188:733-748.

60. Raghu G, Collard HR, Egan JJ, et al. An official ATS/ERS/JRS/ALAT statement—idiopathic pulmonary fibrosis: evidence-based guidelines for diagnosis and management. *Am J Respir Crit Care Med.* 2011;183:788-824.

61. Ley B, Collard HR, King TE Jr. Clinical course and prediction of survival in idiopathic pulmonary fibrosis. *Am J Respir Crit Care Med.* 2011;183:431-440.

62. McCormack FX, Gupta N, Finlay GR, et al. Official American Thoracic Society/Japanese Respiratory Society clinical practice guidelines: lymphangioleiomyomatosis diagnosis and management. *Am J Respir Crit Care Med.* 2016;194:748-761.

63. Meyer KC, Raghu G, Baughman RP. An official American Thoracic Society clinical practice guideline: the clinical utility of bronchoalveolar lavage cellular analysis in interstitial lung disease. *Am J Respir Crit Care Med.* 2012;185:1004-1014.

64. Lettieri CJ, Veerappan GR, Helman DL, et al. Outcomes and safety of surgical lung biopsy for interstitial lung disease. *Chest.* 2005;127:1600-1605.

65. Bradley B, Branley HM, Egan JJ, et al. Interstitial lung disease guideline: the British Thoracic Society in collaboration with the Thoracic Society of Australia and New Zealand and the Irish Thoracic Society. *Thorax.* 2008;63:51-58.

66. Hetzel J, Maldonado F, Ravaglia C, et al. Transbronchial cryobiopsies for the diagnosis of diffuse parenchymal lung diseases: expert statement from the Cryobiopsy Working Group on safety and utility and a call for standardization of the procedure. *Respiration.* 2018;95:188-200.

67. Raghu G, Weycker D, Edelsberg J, et al. Incidence and prevalence of idiopathic pulmonary fibrosis. *Am J Respir Crit Care Med.* 2006;174:810-816.

68. Lawson WE, Loyd JE, Degryse AL. Genetics in pulmonary fibrosis—familial cases provide clues to the pathogenesis of idiopathic pulmonary fibrosis. *Am J Med Sci.* 2011;341:439-443.

69. Snetselaar R, van Moorsel HM, Kazemier KM, et al. Telomere length in interstitial lung diseases. *Chest.* 2015;148:1011-1018.

70. King TE, Jr. Idiopathic pulmonary fibrosis. In: Schwarz MI, King TE, Jr, eds. *Interstitial Lung Disease.* 5th ed. People's Medical Publishing House-USA; 2011:895.

71. Sheth JS, Belperio JA, Fishbein MC, et al. Utility of transbronchial vs surgical lung biopsy in the diagnosis of suspected fibrotic interstitial lung disease. *Chest.* 2017;151:389-399.

72. Leslie KO, Cool CD, Sporn TA, et al. Familial idiopathic interstitial pneumonia: histopathology and survival in 30 patients. *Arch Pathol Lab Med.* 2012;136:1366-1376.

73. Idiopathic Pulmonary Fibrosis Clinical Research Network; Raghu G, Anstrom KJ, King TE Jr, et al. Prednisone, azathioprine, and *N*-acetylcysteine for pulmonary fibrosis. *N Engl J Med.* 2012;366:1968-1977.

74. King TE Jr, Bradford WZ, Castro-Bernardini S, et al. A phase 3 trial of pirfenidone in patients with idiopathic pulmonary fibrosis. *N Engl J Med.* 2014;370:2083-2092.

75. Richeldi L, du Bois RM, Raghu G, et al. Efficacy and safety of nintedanib in idiopathic pulmonary fibrosis. *N Engl J Med.* 2014;370:2071-2082.

76. Hyzy R, Huang S, Myers J, et al. Acute exacerbation of idiopathic pulmonary fibrosis. *Chest.* 2007;132:1652-1658.

77. Nayfeh AS, Chippa V, Moore DR. *Nonspecific interstitial pneumonitis.* In: *StatPearls* [Internet]. StatPearls Publishing; 2021.

78. Fischer A, Antoniou KM, Brown KK, et al. An official European Respiratory Society/American Thoracic Society research statement: interstitial pneumonia with autoimmune features. *Euro Resp J.* 2015;46:976-987.

79. Travis WD, Hunninghake G, King TE Jr, et al. Idiopathic nonspecific interstitial pneumonia: report of an American Thoracic Society project. *Am J Respir Crit Care Med.* 2008;177:1338-1347.

80. Nogueiraa R, Melo N, Novais H, et al. Hypersensitivity pneumonitis: antigen diversity and disease implications. *Pulmonology.* 2019;25:97-108.

81. Salisbury ML, Gu T, Murray S, et al. Hypersensitivity pneumonitis: radiologic phenotypes are associated with distinct survival time and pulmonary function Trajectory. *Chest.* 2019;155:699-711.

82. Raghu G, Remy-Jardin M, Ryerson CJ, et al. Diagnosis of hypersensitivity pneumonitis in adults. An official ATS/JRS/ALAT clinical practice guideline. *Am J Respir Crit Care Med.* 2020;202:e36-e69.

83. Salisbury ML, Myers JL, Belloli EA, et al. Diagnosis and treatment of fibrotic hypersensitivity pneumonia. Where we Stand and where we need to go. *Am J Respir Crit Care Med.* 2017;196:690-699.

84. Flaherty KR, Wells AU, Cottin V, et al. Nintedanib in progressive fibrosing interstitial lung diseases. *N Engl J Med.* 2019;381:1718-1727.

85. Fernández Pérez ER, Swigris JJ, Forssén AV, et al. Identifying an inciting antigen is associated with improved survival in patients with chronic hypersensitivity pneumonitis. *Chest.* 2013;144:1644-1651.

86. Baughman RP, Culver DA, Judson MA. A concise review of pulmonary sarcoidosis. *Am J Respir Crit Care Med.* 2011;183:573-581.

87. Mirsaeidi M, Machado RF, Schraufnagel D, et al. Racial difference in sarcoidosis mortality in the United States. *Chest.* 2015;147:438-449.

88. Crouser ED, Maier LA, Wilson KC, et al. Diagnosis and detection of sarcoidosis. An official American Thoracic Society clinical practice guideline. *Am J Respir Crit Care Med.* 2020;201:e26-e51.

89. Kim JS, Judson MA, Donnino R, et al. Cardiac sarcoidosis. *Am Heart J.* 2009;157:9-21.

90. Joint statement of the American thoracic Society (ATS), the European respiratory Society (ERS) and the world association of sarcoidosis and other granulomatous disorders (WASOG) adopted by the ATS board of Directors and by the ERS Executive Committee, February 1999. Statement on sarcoidosis. *Am J Respir Crit Care Med.* 1999;160:736-755.

CHAPTER 10

91. Schutt AC, Bullington WM, Judson MA. Pharmacotherapy for pulmonary sarcoidosis: a Delphi consensus study. *Respir Med*. 2010;104:717-723.

92. Baque-Juston M, Pellegrin A, Leroy S, et al. Organizing pneumonia: what is it? A conceptual approach and pictorial review. *Diagn Interv Imaging*. 2014;95:771-777.

93. Craig PH, Wells AU, Doffman S, et al. Desquamative interstitial pneumonia, respiratory bronchiolitis and their relationship to smoking. *Histopathology*. 2004;45:275-282.

94. Nakanishi M, Demura Y, Mizuno S, et al. Changes in HRCT findings in patients with respiratory bronchiolitis-associated interstitial lung disease after smoking cessation. *Euro Resp J*. 2007;29:453-461.

95. Carrington CB, Gaensler EA, Coutu RE, et al. Natural history and treated course of usual and desquamative interstitial pneumonia. *N Engl J Med*. 1978;298:801-809.

96. Ryu JH, Colby TV, Hartman TE, Vassallo R. Smoking-related interstitial lung diseases: a concise review. *Eur Respir J*. 2001;17:122-132.

97. Tazi A. Adult pulmonary Langerhans' cell histiocytosis. *Eur Respir J*. 2006;27:1272-1285.

98. Lorillon G, Tazi A. How I manage pulmonary Langerhans cell histiocytosis. *Eur Respir Rev*. 2017;26:170070.

99. Farzaneh MR, Jamshidiha F, Kowsarian S. Inhalational lung disease. *Int J Occup Environ Med*. 2010;1:11-20.

100. American thoracic Society Committee of the Scientific assembly on environmental and occupational health. Adverse effects of crystalline silica exposure. *Am J Respir Crit Care Med*. 1997; 155:761-768.

101. Cullinan P, Reid P. Pneumoconiosis. *Prim Care Respir J*. 2013;22:249-252.

102. Fireman E, Haimsky E, Noiderfer M, et al. Misdiagnosis of sarcoidosis in patients with chronic beryllium disease. *Sarcoidosis Vasc Diffuse Lung Dis*. 2003;20:144-148.

103. Remy-Jardin M, Degreef JM, Beuscart R, et al. Coal worker's pneumoconiosis: CT assessment in exposed workers and correlation with radiographic findings. *Radiology*. 1990;177:363-371.

104. Hansell DM, Bankier AA, MacMahon H, et al. Fleischner Society: glossary of terms for thoracic imaging. *Radiology*. 2008;246:697-722.

105. Park S, Lee EJ. Diagnosis and treatment of cystic lung disease. *Korean J Intern Med*. 2017;32:229-238.

106. O'Mahony AM, Lynn E, Murphy DJ, et al. Lymphangioleiomyomatosis: a clinical review. *Breathe*. 2020;16:200007.

107. Ryu JH, Tian X, Baqir M, Xu K. Diffuse cystic lung diseases. *Front Med*. 2013;7:316-327.

108. Gupta N, Finlay GA, Kotloff RM, et al. Lymphangioleiomyomatosis diagnosis and management: high-resolution chest computed tomography, transbronchial lung biopsy, and pleural disease management. An official American Thoracic Society/Japanese Respiratory Society clinical practice guideline. *Am J Respir Crit Care Med*. 2017;196:1337-1348.

109. McCormack FX, Inoue Y, Moss J, et al. Efficacy and safety of sirolimus in lymphangioleiomyomatosis. *N Engl J Med*. 2011;364:1595-1606.

110. Goldberg HJ, Harari S, Cottin V, et al. Everolimus for the treatment of lymphangioleiomyomatosis: a phase II study. *Euro Resp J*. 2015;46:783-794.

111. Menko FH, van Steensel MA, Giraud S, et al. Birt-Hogg-Dubé syndrome: diagnosis and management. *Lancet Oncol*. 2009;10:1199-1206.

112. Gupta N, Seyama K, McCormack FX. Pulmonary manifestations of Birt-Hogg-Dubé syndrome. *Familial Cancer*. 2013;12:387-396.

113. Zamora AC, White DB, Sykes AG, et al. Amyloid-associated cystic lung disease. *Chest*. 2016;149:1223-1233.

114. Cha SI, Fessler MB, Cool CD, et al. Lymphoid interstitial pneumonia: clinical features, associations and prognosis. *Eur Respir J*. 2006;28:364-369.

115. Yale SH, Limper AH. Pneumocystis carinii pneumonia in patients without acquired immunodeficiency syndrome: associated illness and prior corticosteroid therapy. *Mayo Clin Proc*. 1996;71:5-13.

116. Farkas L, Gauldie J, Voelkel NF, Kolb M. Pulmonary hypertension and idiopathic pulmonary fibrosis: a tale of angiogenesis, apoptosis, and growth factors. *Am J Respir Cell Mol Biol*. 2011;45:1-15.

117. Waxman A, Restrepo-Jaramillo R, Thnappan T, et al. Inhaled Treprostinil in pulmonary hypertension due to interstitial lung disease. *N Engl J Med*. 2021;384:325-334.

118. Bajwah S, Koffman J, Higginson IJ, et al. 'I wish I knew more...' the end-of-life planning and information needs for end-stage fibrotic interstitial lung disease: views of patients, carers and health professionals. *BMJ Support Palliat Care*. 2013;3:84-90.

119. Corey R, Hla KM. Major and massive hemoptysis: reassessment of conservative management. *Am J Med Sci*. 1987;294(5):301-309.

120. Wang K, Mehta A, Turner J, eds. *Flexible Bronchoscopy*. 2nd ed. Wiley-Blackwell; 2004.

121. Abdulmalak C, Cottenet J, Beltramo G, et al. Haemoptysis in adults: a 5-year study using the French nationwide hospital administrative database. *Eur Resp J*. 2015;46:503-511.

122. Hirshberg B, Biran I, Glazer M, Kramer MR. Hemoptysis: etiology, evaluation, and outcome in a tertiary referral hospital. *Chest*. 1997;112:440-444.

123. Poe RH, Israel RH, Marin MG, et al. Utility of fiberoptic bronchoscopy in patients with hemoptysis and a nonlocalizing chest roentgenogram. *Chest.* 1988;93:70-75.

124. Marshall TJ, Flower CDR, Jackson JE. The role of radiology in the investigation and management of patients with haemoptysis. *Clin Radiol.* 1996;51:391-400.

125. McGuinness G, Beacher JR, Harkin TJ, et al. Hemoptysis: prospective high-resolution CT/broncho-scopic correlation. *Chest.* 1994;105:1155-1162.

126. Thirumaran M, Sundar R, Sutcliffe IM, Currie DC. Is investigation of patients with haemoptysis and normal chest radiograph justified? *Thorax.* 2009;64:854-856.

127. Bønløkke S, Guldbrandt LM, Rasmussen TR. Bronchoscopy in patients with haemoptysis and normal computed tomography of the chest is unlikely to result in significant findings. *Danish Med J.* 2015;62:A5123.

128. Chalumeau-Lemoine L, Khalil A, Prigent H, et al. Impact of multidetector CT-angiography on the emergency management of severe hemoptysis. *Eur J Radiol.* 2013;82:e742-e747. doi:10.1016/j.ejrad.2013.07.009

129. Khalil A, Parrot A, Nedelcu C, et al. Severe hemoptysis of pulmonary arterial origin: signs and role of multidetector row CT angiography. *Chest.* 2008;133:212-219.

130. Saumench J, Escarrabill J, Padro L, et al. Value of fiberoptic bronchoscopy and angiography for diagnosis of the bleeding site in hemoptysis. *Ann Thorac Surg.* 1989;48:272-274.

131. Jackson CV, Savage PJ, Quinn DL. Role of fiberoptic bronchoscopy in patients with hemoptysis and a normal chest roentgenogram. *Chest.* 1985;87:142-144.

132. O'Neil KM, Lazarus AA. Hemoptysis. Indications for bronchoscopy. *Arch Intern Med.* 1991;151:171-174.

133. Tom LM, Palevsky HI, Holsclaw DS, et al.Recurrent bleeding, survival, and longitudinal pulmonary function following bronchial artery embolization for hemoptysis in a U.S. adult population. *J Vasc Interv Radiol.* 2015;26:1806-1813.

134. Haponik EF, Fein A, Chin R. Managing life-threatening hemoptysis: has anything really changed. *Chest.* 2000;118:1431-1435.

135. Wand O, Guber E, Guber A, et al. Inhaled tranexamic acid for hemoptysis treatment: a randomized controlled trial. *Chest.* 2018;154:1379-1384.

136. Lordan JL, Gascoigne A, Corris PA. The pulmonary physician in critical care. Illustrative case 7: assessment and management of massive haemoptysis. *Thorax.* 2003;58:814-819.

137. Morice RC, Ece T, Ece F, Keus L. Endobronchial argon plasma coagulation for treatment of hemoptysis and neoplastic airway obstruction. *Chest.* 2001;119:781-787.

138. Tremblay A, Marquette CH. Endobronchial electrocautery and argon plasma coagulation: a practical approach. *Can Respir J.* 2004;11:305-310.

139. Randes JC, Schmidt E, Yung R. Occlusive endobronchial stent placement as a novel management approach to massive hemoptysis from lung cancer. *J Thorac Oncol.* 2008;3:1071-1072.

140. Conlan AA, Hurwitz SS. Management of massive haemoptysis with the rigid bronchoscope and cold saline lavage. *Thorax.* 1980;35:901-904.

141. Tsukamoto T, Sasaki H, Nakamura H. Treatment of hemoptysis patients by thrombin and fibrinogen–thrombin infusion therapy using a fiberoptic bronchoscope. *Chest.* 1989;96:473-476.

142. Valipour A, Kreuzer A, Koller H. Koessler W. Bronchoscopy-guided topical hemostatic tamponade therapy for the management of life-threatening hemoptysis. *Chest.* 2005;127:2113-2118.

143. Swanson KL, Johnson CM, Prakash UB, et al. Bronchial artery embolization: experience with 54 patients. *Chest.* 2002;121:789-795.

144. Brinson GM, Noone PG, Mauro MA, et al. Bronchial artery embolization for the treatment of hemoptysis in patients with cystic fibrosis. *Am J Respir Crit Care Med.* 1998;157:1951-1958.

145. Antonelli M, Midulla F, Tancredi G, et al. Bronchial artery embolization for the management of non-massive hemoptysis in cystic fibrosis. *Chest.* 2002;121:796-801.

146. Chun HJ, Byun JY, Yoo S, et al. Added benefit of thoracic aortography after transarterial embolization in patients with hemoptysis. *Am J Roentgenol.* 2003;180:1577-1581.

147. Syha R, Benz T, Hetzel J, et al. Bronchial artery embolization in hemoptysis: 10-year survival and recurrence-free survival in benign and malignant etiologies—a retrospective study. *RöFo.* 2016;188:1061-1066.

148. Van den Heuvel MM, Els Z, Koegelenberg CF, et al. Risk factors for recurrence of haemoptysis following bronchial artery embolisation for life-threatening haemoptysis. *Int J Tuberc Lung Dis.* 2007;11:909-914.

149. Jean-Baptiste E. Clinical assessment and management of massive hemoptysis. *Crit Care Med.* 2000;28:1642-1647.

150. Bobrowitz ID, Ramakrishna S, Shim YS. Comparison of medical vs. surgical treatment of major hemoptysis. *Arch Intern Med.* 1983;143:1343-1346.

151. Garcia-Olivé I, Sanz-Santos J, Centeno C, et al. Results of bronchial artery embolization for the treatment of hemoptysis caused by neoplasm. *J Vasc Interv Radiol.* 2014;25:221-228.

152. Scotet V, L'Hostis C, Férec C. The changing Epidemiology of cystic fibrosis: incidence, survival and impact of the CFTR gene discovery. *Genes (Basel).* 2020;11:589.

153. Cystic Fibrosis Foundation. *Cystic Fibrosis Foundation Patient Registry 2016 Annual Data Report.* 2017;2018.
154. Rowe SM, Miller S, Sorscher EJ. Cystic fibrosis. *N Engl J Med.* 2005;352:1992-2001.
155. Farrell PM, White TB, Ren CL, et al. Diagnosis of cystic fibrosis: consensus guidelines from the Cystic Fibrosis Foundation. *J Pediatr.* 2017;181S:S4–S15.
156. Parr DG, Guest PG, Reynolds JH, et al. Prevalence and impact of bronchiectasis in alpha1-antitrypsin deficiency. *Am J Respir Crit Care Med.* 2007;176:1215-1221.
157. Burroughs L, Woolfrey A, Shimamura A. Shwachman–Diamond syndrome: a review of the clinical presentation, molecular pathogenesis, diagnosis, and treatment. *Hematol Oncol Clin N Am.* 2009;23:233-248.
158. LeGrys VA, Yankaskas JR, Quittell LM, et al. Diagnostic sweat testing: the cystic fibrosis Foundation guidelines. *J Pediatr.* 2007;151:85-89.
159. Fuchs HJ, Borowitz DS, Christiansen DH, et al. Effect of aerosolized recombinant human DNase on exacerbations of respiratory symptoms and on pulmonary function in patients with cystic fibrosis. The Pulmozyme Study Group. *N Engl J Med.* 1994;331:637-642.
160. Elkins MR, Robinson M, Rose B, et al. A controlled trial of long-term inhaled hypertonic saline in patients with cystic fibrosis. *N Engl J Med.* 2006;354:229-240.
161. Ramsey BW, Davies J, McElvaney NG, et al. A CFTR potentiator in patients with cystic fibrosis and the G551D mutation. *N Engl J Med.* 2011;365:1663-1672.
162. Howington JA, Blum MG, Chang AC, et al. Treatment of stage I and II non-small cell lung cancer: diagnosis and management of lung cancer, 3rd ed—American College of Chest Physicians evidence-based clinical practice guidelines. *Chest.* 2013;143:e278S-e313S. doi:10.1378/chest.12-2359
163. Gould MK, Tang T, Liu IL, et al. Recent trends in the identification of incidental pulmonary nodules. *Am J Respir Crit Care Med.* 2015;192:1208-1214.
164. Aberle DR, Adams AM, Berg CD, et al. Reduced lung-cancer mortality with low-dose computed tomographic screening. *N Engl J Med.* 2011;365:395-409.
165. Balekian AA, Silvestri GA, Simkovich SM, et al. Accuracy of clinicians and models for estimating the probability that a pulmonary nodule is malignant. *Ann Am Thorac Soc.* 2013;10:629-635.
166. Nomori H, Watanabe K, Ohtsuka T, et al. Evaluation of F-18 fluorodeoxyglucose (FDG) PET scanning for pulmonary nodule less than 3 cm in diameter, with special reference to the CT images. *Lung Cancer.* 2004;45:19-27.
167. Swensen SJ, Viggiano RW, Midthun DE, et al. Lung nodule enhancement at CT: multicenter study. *Radiology.* 2000;214:73-80.
168. Gould MK, Donington J, Lynch WR, et al. Evaluation of individuals with pulmonary nodules—when is it lung cancer? Diagnosis and management of lung cancer, 3rd ed: American College of Chest Physicians evidence-based clinical practice guidelines. *Chest.* 2013;143:e93s-e120s. doi:10.1378/chest.12-2351
169. MacMahon H, Naidich DP, Goo JM, et al. Guidelines for management of incidental pulmonary nodules detected on CT images: from the Fleischner Society 2017. *Radiology.* 2017;284:228-243.
170. Staton GW, Ingram RH. Chapter IX. Disorders of the pleura, hila, and mediastinum. In: Dale DC, Federman DD, eds. *Sci Am Medicine 2004.* Accessed May 3, 2005. Available at: http://edmedia.emory.edu/GStaton/Pleura,%20Hila.pdf
171. Jacoby RC, Battistella FD. Hemothorax. *Semin Respir Crit Care Med.* 2001;22:627-630.
172. Doerr CH, Miller DL, Ryu JH. Chylothorax. *Semin Respir Crit Care Med.* 2001;22:617-626.
173. Light RW. A new classification of parapneumonic effusions and empyema. *Chest.* 1995;108:299-301.
174. Light RW, Girard WM, Jenkinson SG, George RB. Parapneumonic effusions. *Am J Med.* 1980;69:507-512.
175. Miller AC, Harvey JE. Guidelines for the management of spontaneous pneumothorax. Standards of care Committee, British Thoracic Society. *BMJ.* 1993;307:114-116.
176. Fraser RS. Pneumothorax. In: Fraser RG, Pare AJ, eds. *Fraser and Pare's Diagnosis of Diseases of the Chest.* 4th ed. WB Saunders; 1999:2781-2794.
177. Jantz MA, Pierson DJ. Pneumothorax and barotraumas. *Clin Chest Med.* 1994;15:75-91.
178. Boylan A, Broaddus VC. Tumors of the pleura. In: Mason RJ, Murray JF, Nadel JA, Broaddus VC, eds. *Murray and Nadel's Textbook of Respiratory Medicine.* 4th ed. Elsevier Health Sciences; 2005:1989-2010.
179. Ferrer JS, Muñoz XG, Orriols RM, et al. Evolution of idiopathic pleural effusion: a prospective, long-term follow-up study. *Chest.* 1996;109:1508-1513.
180. Almoosa KF, Mc Cormack FX, Sahn SA. Pleural disease in lymphangioleiomyomatosis. *Clin Chest Med.* 2006;27:355-368.
181. Heffner JE, Brown LK, Barbieri CA. Diagnostic value of tests that discriminate between exudative and transudative pleural effusions. *Chest.* 1997;111:970-980.
182. Sahn SA, Heffner JE. Spontaneous pneumothorax. *N Engl J Med.* 2000;342:868-874.
183. Sahn SA. State of the art. The pleura. *Am Rev Respir Dis.* 1988;138:184-234.
184. Light RW. Clinical manifestations and useful tests. In: LightRW, ed. *Pleural Diseases.* 4th ed. Lippincott Williams and Wilkins; 2001:42-86.

185. Lee YCG, Light RW. Future directions. In: Light RW, Lee YCG, eds. *Textbook of Pleural Diseases*. Hodder Arnold; 2003:536-541.
186. Light RW, Macgregor MI, Luchsinger PC, Ball WC Jr. Pleural effusions: the diagnostic separation of transudates and exudates. *Ann Intern Med*. 1972;77:507-513.
187. Solooki M. Diagnostic yield of cytology in malignant pleural effusion: impact of volume and repeated thoracentesis. *Eur Resp J*. 2011;38:p3550.
188. Kennedy L, Sahn SA. Noninvasive evaluation of the patient with a pleural effusion. *Chest Surg Clin N Am*. 1994;4:451-465.
189. Woodring JH. Recognition of pleural effusion on supine radiographs: how much fluid is required? *Am J Roentgenol*. 1984;142:59-64.
190. Chen A, Massoni J, Jung D, Crippin J. Indwelling tunneled pleural catheters for the management of hepatic hydrothorax: a pilot study. *Ann Am Thorac Soc*. 2016;13:862-866.
191. Lois M, Noppen M. Bronchopleural fistulas. *Chest*. 2005;128:3955-3965.
192. Heffner JE, Klein JS. Recent advances in the diagnosis and management of malignant pleural effusions. *Mayo Clin Proc*. 2008;83:235-250.
193. Rahman NM, Maskell NA, West A, et al. Intrapleural use of tissue plasminogen activator and DNAase in pleural infection. *N Engl J Med*. 2011;365:518-526.
194. Yeam I, Sassoon C. Hemothorax and chylothorax. *Curr Opin Pulm Med*. 1997;3:310-314.
195. Light RW, Broaddus VC. Pneumothorax, chylothorax, hemothorax, and fibrothorax. In: Murray RF, Nadel JA, eds. *Textbook of Respiratory Medicine*. 3rd ed. Elsevier Science; 2000:2043-2055.

Adverse Drug Reactions

GENERAL PRINCIPLES

Definition

- An **adverse drug reaction** (ADR) is an undesired pharmacological response that occurs when a drug is given for the appropriate purpose.
- The etiology of a drug reaction can be immunologic, toxic, or idiosyncratic in nature.
- Drug allergy is due to an immune response that is mediated by drug-specific antibody or T cells.

Classification

- *Type A* reactions are predictable, often dose dependent, and related to the pharmacokinetics of the drug. They comprise up to 80% of all ADRs (e.g., hepatic failure due to overdose of acetaminophen, sedative side effects of antihistamines, drug–drug interactions, and gastrointestinal bacterial alteration after antibiotics).
- *Type B* reactions are unpredictable and are not related to the dose or the drug's pharmacokinetics. They account for 10%–15% of all ADRs.
  - Immune-mediated adverse reactions can be from a variety of mechanisms. They usually occur on reexposure to the offending drug.
  - **Nonimmunologic reactions** (pseudoallergic or anaphylactoid) are caused by IgE-independent degranulation of mast cells.

Epidemiology

- ADRs are reported to account for 10%–15% of hospitalized patients.[1]
- Mortality from ADRs is significant and ranges from 0.14% to 0.32%.[2]
- Lifetime prevalence of drug-induced anaphylaxis is 0.05%–2%.[1] The most common drugs causing IgE-mediated anaphylaxis are penicillins and anesthetic agents given during the perioperative period. Drug-induced anaphylaxis is seen predominantly in older age group.

Etiology

- **β-Lactam** antibiotics are the most common drug class allergy in United States, which includes penicillins, penicillin derivatives (ampicillin and amoxicillin), cephalosporins, monobactams, and carbapenems. Penicillin allergy is the most prevalent antibiotic allergy of this class. About 8% of patients in healthcare report have a penicillin allergy.[3] About 90% patients with history of penicillin allergy will be able to tolerate penicillins, as most patients outgrow their allergy over time.[4] Given the lower likelihood of having true penicillin allergy, antimicrobial stewardship programs have been developed to decrease use of β-lactam alternatives.
- Hospitalized patients with a history of penicillin allergy have been shown to have a longer hospital stay with increased incidence of vancomycin-resistant *Enterococcus*,

methicillin-resistant *Staphylococcus aureus*, and *Clostridioides difficile* infections compared to patients without a reported penicillin allergy.[5]

- The chemical structure of penicillins results in their high immunogenicity with a reactive β-lactam ring that covalently binds with carrier proteins to form a hapten, which stimulates an immune response.
  - The major determinant of immunogenicity of penicillin is the benzylpenicilloyl form seen in 93% of tissue-bound penicillin.
  - The minor antigenic determinants are all remaining penicillin conjugates. They comprise benzylpenicillin, benzylpenicilloate, and benzylpenilloate.
- The cross-reactivity between β-lactam antibiotics is variable and largely determined by their side-chain structure attached to the β-lactam ring.
  - Risk of a cross-reaction between a penicillin and cephalosporin that do not share the same side chain is <2%. Cross-reactivity between penicillin and monobactams is 0%, between penicillin and carbapenems is <1%, and between cephalosporins and carbapenems is <1%.[6]
  - Patients with **amoxicillin allergy** should avoid cefadroxil, cefprozil, and cefatrizine as all these drugs share same R-group side chain.
  - The monobactam **aztreonam** does share an identical R1-group side chain as ceftazidime and is cross-reactive.
- **Sulfonamide allergy**
  - There is an increase in allergy to sulfonamides in patients with HIV compared to the general population. Trimethoprim–sulfamethoxazole hypersensitivity occurs in 60% of HIV-positive patients compared to 5% of HIV-negative patients.[7]
  - Type I IgE-mediated reactions to sulfonamides are not common. The most frequently seen reaction is a maculopapular rash (T cell–mediated) that develops 7–12 days after initiating the drug. Other reactions include urticaria and, less commonly, anaphylaxis, Stevens–Johnson syndrome (SJS), and toxic epidermal necrolysis (TEN). Cross-reactivity between antibiotic and nonantibiotic sulfa-containing medications is low.[8] Patients with sulfonamide antibiotic allergy were more likely to react to penicillin than a sulfonamide nonantibiotic.[8]
- **NSAIDs** and aspirin can cause IgE-mediated urticaria, angioedema, and anaphylaxis. It can also exacerbate urticaria in patients who have chronic urticaria. Exacerbation of respiratory symptoms in patients with underlying asthma is referred to as aspirin-exacerbated respiratory disease (AERD). AERD is composed of a triad consisting of asthma, NSAID sensitivity, and nasal polyposis. COX2 inhibitors are generally safe to administer in these patients. Aspirin desensitization followed by daily aspirin therapy in AERD patients improves asthma exacerbations, oral steroid use, reduced nasal polyps, and sinus infections. Certain asthma biologics can also be used in patients with AERD.

Pathophysiology

The immunologic mechanisms for drug hypersensitivity are demonstrated in the Gell and Coombs classification of hypersensitivity (Table 11-1).

Risk Factors

Factors that increase a patient's risk of an ADR include size and structure of drug, route of exposure (cutaneous most immunogenic), dose, duration, frequency, gender (women > men), genetic factors (HLA type, history of atopy), prior drug reaction, coexisting medical illnesses, and concurrent medical therapy.

TABLE 11-1	Immunologically Mediated Drug Reactions	
Type of Reaction	Representative Examples	Mechanism
Anaphylactic (type 1)	Anaphylaxis Urticaria Angioedema	IgE-mediated degranulation of mast cells with resultant mediator release
Cytotoxic (type 2)	Autoimmune hemolytic anemia Interstitial nephritis	IgG or IgM antibodies against cell antigens and complement activation
Immune complex (type 3)	Serum sickness Vasculitis	Immune complex deposition and subsequent complement activation
Cell mediated (type 4)	Contact dermatitis Photosensitivity dermatitis	Activated T cells against cell surface–bound antigens

DIAGNOSIS

Clinical Presentation

- A history is essential for making the diagnosis of an allergic drug reaction. Questions should be directed at establishing the following information: sign and symptoms, timing of the reaction, purpose of the drug, other medications the patient is receiving, prior exposure to drug or related drug, and history of other allergic drug reactions.
- Urticaria, angioedema, wheezing, and anaphylaxis are all characteristics of IgE-mediated (type 1) reactions.
  - Symptoms do not typically occur on the first exposure to the medication unless the patient has been exposed to a structurally related medication. On reexposure, however, symptoms tend to manifest acutely (often <1 hour).
  - IgE-mediated reactions tend to worsen with repeated exposure to the offending medication.
  - Non–IgE-mediated reactions (anaphylactoid) can be clinically indistinguishable from IgE-mediated reactions because the final common pathway for their reaction is mast cell degranulation.
- **Maculopapular exanthemas** are the most common cutaneous manifestation of drug allergy.
  - These reactions are mediated by T cells and typically delayed in onset, first occurring between 2 and 14 days of exposure to culprit medications. It can occur sooner with subsequent exposures. Lesions typically begin on the trunk, especially in dependent areas, and spread to the extremities.
  - Rarely, these rashes can progress to a more serious drug reaction involving blistering of the skin and/or end-organ involvement.
- **DRESS (Drug Reaction with Eosinophilia and Systemic Symptoms)** is a serious life-threatening ADR, often presenting as rash and fever with systemic involvement, and can manifest as hepatitis, eosinophilia, pneumonitis, lymphadenopathy, and nephritis.
  - Symptoms tend to present 2–6 weeks after introduction of medication and resolve few weeks to months after stopping the offending agent. Certain viral infections

such as Epstein–Barr virus, human herpesvirus (HHV)-6, HHV-7, and cytomegalovirus are associated with increased risk of complications.

- First described with antiepileptic (carbamazepine) agents but has also been reported to occur with allopurinol, NSAIDs, some antibiotics, and β-blockers.
- **Erythema multiforme (EM), SJS, and TEN** are all serious drug reactions primarily involving the skin.
  - EM is characterized most typically by target lesions. SJS and TEN manifest with varying degrees of sloughing of the skin and mucous membranes (<10% in SJS and >30% in TEN). Risk factors being HIV, hematological malignancy, systemic lupus erythematosus, and bone marrow transplant.
  - **Readmistration or future skin testing with the offending drug is absolutely contraindicated.**

PREVENTION AND TREATMENT

- Acute drug reactions such as anaphylaxis should be treated promptly and **discontinuation** of the suspected drug is the most important initial approach in managing an allergic drug reaction.
- HLA testing may be indicated in susceptible populations for prevention of a severe ADR for some drugs such as abacavir and carbamazepine.
- Future use of the drug in question should **always be avoided** unless there is no therapeutic alternative available.
- If use of the drug must be considered, a careful history of the reaction is helpful in defining the potential risk. Patients may lose their sensitivity to a drug over time, and determining the date of reaction is useful. Symptoms that occur with the start of a drug course are more likely to be IgE-mediated than symptoms that develop several days after the completion of a course.
- The types of symptoms are also important. Toxic reactions (e.g., nausea secondary to macrolide antibiotics or codeine) are not immunologic reactions and do not necessarily predict problems with other members in their respective class.

REFERRAL

- If no alternative drug is available and the patient has a history of an IgE-mediated reaction, the patient should be referred to an allergist for further evaluation.
- The allergist may perform one of several procedures if indicated depending on the medication, type of reaction, and availability of testing reagents.
- **Skin testing** may be performed to assess for the presence of IgE to the medication.
  - Although skin testing may be performed to nearly any medication, sensitivity and specificity of the skin test results have been best established with penicillin.
  - Results of testing to drugs other than penicillin must be interpreted within the clinical context of the case.
- **Graded dose challenge** assesses how the patient tolerates progressively larger doses of medication (e.g., 1/1000, 1/10, and full dose given 20 minutes apart).
- **Drug desensitization** is defined as induction of temporary state of clinical unresponsiveness or tolerance to a suspected drug. It is performed when the patient has an identified IgE-mediated reaction but still requires the medication.
  - The drug must be taken daily at a specified dose to maintain the "desensitized state."

- ○ If a dose of the drug is missed following a desensitization procedure, then the patient will often need to undergo a repeat desensitization as the desensitization state will wane based on half-life of the drug.
- ○ Successful desensitization or graded challenge does not preclude the development of a non–IgE-mediated or delayed reaction (e.g., rash).

Anaphylaxis

GENERAL PRINCIPLES

Definition

Anaphylaxis is a rapidly developing, life-threatening systemic reaction mediated by the release of mast cell and basophil-derived mediators into the circulation. The peak severity is seen usually within 5–30 minutes.

Classification

- **Immunologic anaphylaxis:** IgE mediated (type 1 hypersensitivity) or IgG mediated (rare)
- **Nonimmunologic anaphylaxis.** Previously known as pseudoallergic or anaphylactoid reactions

Epidemiology

Incidence of anaphylaxis is approximately 50–2000 episodes per 100,000 person-years. Fatality is estimated at 0.7%–2% per case of anaphylaxis. In the US, the lifetime prevalence of anaphylaxis is reported to be 1.6%.[9]

Etiology

Immunologic causes
- Foods, especially peanuts, tree nuts, shellfish, finned fish, milk, and eggs
- Insect stings (bees, wasps, and fire ants)
- Medications
- Latex rubber
- Blood products

Nonimmunologic causes
- Radiocontrast media
- Medications (i.e., NSAIDs, opiates, vancomycin, muscle relaxants, rarely ACE inhibitors, and sulfating agents)
- Hemodialysis
- Physical factors (cold temperature or exercise)
- Idiopathic

Pathophysiology

Immunologic
- Anaphylaxis is due to sensitization to an antigen and formation of specific IgE to that antigen. On reexposure, the IgE on mast cells and basophils binds the antigen and cross-links the IgE receptor, which causes activation of the cells with subsequent systemic release of preformed mediators, such as histamine.
- The release of mediators ultimately causes capillary leakage, cellular edema, and smooth muscle contractions resulting in the constellation of physical symptoms.

Nonimmunologic
Non–IgE-mediated anaphylaxis is also mediated by direct degranulation of mast cells and basophils in the absence of immunoglobulins.

Risk Factors

- Persistent asthma: increased risk of fatal anaphylaxis if asthma is uncontrolled.
- Cardiovascular disease: increased risk for death in older age.
- Elevated baseline tryptase indicates possible mast cell disorder. Individuals with **mastocytosis**, a disease characterized by a proliferation of mast cells, are at higher risk for severe anaphylaxis from both IgE- and non–IgE-mediated causes.
- Previous sensitization and formation of antigen-specific IgE with history of anaphylaxis.
- Concomitant use drugs: beta-adrenergic blockers, ACE inhibitors, NSAIDs, alcohol, etc.
- Cofactors such as exercise, fever, acute infection, premenstrual status, and emotional.
- Sensitivity to seafood or iodine does not predispose to radiocontrast media reactions.

Prevention

- **For all types of anaphylaxis, recognition of potential triggers and avoidance are the best prevention.**
- **Self-injectable epinephrine and patient education for all patients with a history of anaphylaxis.**
- Radiocontrast sensitivity reactions: Premedication before procedure include giving prednisone 50 mg PO given 13, 7, and 1 hour before procedure and diphenhydramine 50 mg PO given 1 hour before procedure.
- **Premedication is not 100% effective, and appropriate precautions for handling a reaction should be taken.**
- Red man syndrome from vancomycin: symptoms can usually be prevented by slowing the rate of infusion and premedicating with diphenhydramine (50 mg PO) 30 minutes before start of the infusion as this is a non–IgE-mediated drug reaction.

DIAGNOSIS

Diagnosis is based primarily on history and physical examination and the documentation of the presence of a specific IgE to the suspected allergen (if the trigger is IgE mediated). Confirmation of anaphylaxis can, in some cases, be provided by the laboratory finding of an elevated serum tryptase level. However, the absence of an elevated tryptase level does not exclude anaphylaxis, particularly if food is the suspected cause.

Clinical Presentation

- The clinical manifestations of allergic and nonimmunologic anaphylaxis are the same.
- Manifestations include pruritus, flushing, urticaria, angioedema, respiratory distress (due to laryngeal edema, laryngospasm, or bronchospasm), hypotension, uterine cramping, abdominal cramping, emesis, and diarrhea.
- Most serious reactions occur within minutes after exposure to the antigen, but in some circumstances, the reaction may be delayed for hours. An example is the galactose-α-1,3-galactose allergy that is thought to be triggered by tick bites and is a cause of delayed anaphylaxis (3–6 hours) to red meats including beef, pork, and lamb.
- Some patients experience a biphasic reaction characterized by a recurrence of symptoms after resolution of initial anaphylactic episode. Time range is varied and typically occurs 1–8 hours.

- A few patients have a protracted course that requires several hours to days of continuous supportive treatment.

History

A thorough history is taken to help identify the potential trigger, such as new foods, medications, or other commonly known allergens. Also documenting the time of onset of symptoms—that is, minutes to hours or days after a suspected exposure—can help to classify the type of anaphylaxis.

Physical Examination

- Pay special attention to vital signs: Blood pressure, respiratory rate, and oxygen saturation.
- Airway and pulmonary: Assess for any evidence of laryngeal edema or angioedema. Auscultate lung fields to listen for evidence of wheezing. Continue to assess for need to protect the airway.
- Perform a focused cardiovascular examination.
- Skin: Urticaria or erythema.

Diagnostic Criteria

See Table 11-2 for diagnostic criteria for anaphylaxis.

Differential Diagnosis

- Anaphylaxis due to **preformed IgE and re-exposure:** Medications, insect sting, and foods are the most common causes of anaphylaxis.
- **Exercise-induced anaphylaxis:** anaphylaxis occurs exclusively in association with physical exertion and other cofactors. Triggers include food (wheat, celery, nuts,

TABLE 11-2	Anaphylaxis

Anaphylaxis is likely when one of the following three criteria occurs:

1. Acute skin and/or mucosal symptoms (e.g., hives, pruritus, flushing, lip/tongue/uvula swelling) and one of the following:
   a. Respiratory symptoms (e.g., wheezing, stridor, shortness of breath, hypoxia)
   b. Hypotension or associated end-organ dysfunction (e.g., hypotonia, syncope, incontinence)
2. Exposure to probable allergen for the patient and two or more of the following:
   a. Skin/mucosal tissue involvement
   b. Respiratory symptoms
   c. Hypotension or end-organ dysfunction
   d. Persistent gastrointestinal symptoms (e.g., emesis, abdominal pain)
3. Decreased blood pressure after exposure to known allergen for the patient:
   a. Adults: Systolic blood pressure <90 mm Hg or >30% decrease in systolic blood pressure
   b. Infants and children: Hypotension for age or >30% decrease in systolic blood pressure

Modified from Sampson HA, Munoz-Furlong A, Campbell RL, et al. Second symposium on the definition and management of anaphylaxis: Summary report—Second National Institute of Allergy and Infectious Disease/Food Allergy and Anaphylaxis Network symposium. *J Allergy Clin Immunol.* 2006;117(2):391-397. Copyright © 2006 American Academy of Allergy, Asthma and Immunology. With permission.

seafood) and NSAIDs. Treatment would be to avoid exercise immediately after eating causative foods.

- Causes of **non–IgE-mediated anaphylaxis**
  - **Radiocontrast sensitivity reactions** are thought to be from direct degranulation of mast cells in susceptible patients because of osmotic shifts.
  - **Red man's syndrome** from vancomycin consists of pruritus and flushing of the face and neck.
  - **Mastocytosis.**
  - **Ingestant-related reactions** can mimic anaphylaxis. This is usually due to sulfites or the presence of a histamine-like substance in spoiled fish (scombroidosis).
  - **Flushing syndromes** include flushing due to red man syndrome, carcinoid, vasointestinal peptide (and other vasoactive intestinal peptide–secreting tumors), postmenopausal symptoms, rosacea, use of niacin, and alcohol use.
- Other forms of shock such as hypoglycemic, cardiogenic, septic, and hemorrhagic.
- Vasovagal syncope can be distinguished from anaphylaxis by the presence of bradycardia; however, bradycardia can occur in anaphylaxis because of the Bezold–Jarisch reflex.
- Respiratory diseases such as acute laryngotracheitis and foreign body obstruction in trachea.
- Miscellaneous syndromes such as hereditary angioedema (HAE; C1 esterase inhibitor [C1 INH] deficiency syndrome), pheochromocytoma, neurologic (seizure, stroke), and capillary leak syndrome.
- Neuropsychiatric causes such as panic attacks or vocal cord dysfunction.
- Idiopathic.

Diagnostic Testing

- Epicutaneous skin testing and serum-specific IgE testing when available to identify trigger allergens.
- Serum tryptase peaks at 1 hour after symptoms begin and may be present for up to 4 hours.

TREATMENT

- Early recognition of signs and symptoms of anaphylaxis is a critical first step in treatment.
- **Epinephrine is the medication of choice for treatment of anaphylaxis.**
- **Maintain recumbent position while assessing and starting therapy.**
- **Airway management is a priority.** Supplemental 100% oxygen therapy should be administered. Endotracheal intubation may be necessary. If laryngeal edema is not rapidly responsive to epinephrine, cricothyroidotomy or tracheotomy may be required.
- **Volume expansion with IV fluids may be necessary.**

Medications

Epinephrine should be administered immediately. There are no absolute contraindications for treatment with epinephrine in anaphylaxis.
- Adult: 0.3–0.5 mg (0.3–0.5 mL of a 1:1000 solution) IM in the lateral thigh, repeated at 10- to 15-minute intervals if necessary.
- Child: 1:1000 dilution at 0.01 mg/kg or 0.1–0.3 mL administered IM in the lateral thigh, repeated at 10- to 15-minute intervals if necessary.

- 0.5 mL of 1:1000 solution sublingually in cases of major airway compromise or hypotension.
- 3–5 mL of 1:10,000 solution via central line.
- 3–5 mL of 1:10,000 solution diluted with 10 mL of normal saline via endotracheal tube.
- For protracted symptoms that require multiple doses of epinephrine, an IV epinephrine drip may be useful; the infusion is titrated to maintain adequate BP.

Glucagon could reverse refractory bronchospasm and hypotension in patients who are taking β-adrenergic antagonists. Recommended dosage is 1–5 mg intravenously bolus slowly over 5 minutes followed by an infusion at 5–15 μg/min titrated to clinical response. Monitor for side effects such as nausea and vomiting.

Inhaled β-adrenergic agonists should be used to treat resistant bronchospasm.

Glucocorticoids have no significant immediate effect and may **not** prevent biphasic reactions.

Antihistamines relieve skin symptoms but have no immediate effect on the reaction. They may shorten the duration of the reaction.
- Adult: Diphenhydramine 25–50 mg IM or IV, cetirizine 10 mg oral or IV
- Child: Diphenhydramine 12.5–25.0 mg IM or IV, cetirizine 5–10 mg oral or IV

REFERRAL

Referrals to an allergist for further evaluation should be offered to all patients with a history of anaphylaxis. More importantly, patients with *Hymenoptera* sensitivity should be evaluated to determine eligibility for venom immunotherapy.

Eosinophilia

GENERAL PRINCIPLES

- Eosinophils are granulocytes that developed from bone marrow pluripotent progenitor cells.
- Eosinophil maturation is promoted by interleukins (IL-5, IL-3), and granulocyte-macrophage colony-stimulating factor.
- Eosinophils are normally seen in peripheral tissue such as mucosal tissues in the gastrointestinal and respiratory tracts. They are recruited to sites of inflammation.
- Eosinophils can be involved in a variety of infectious, allergic, neoplastic, and idiopathic diseases.

Definition

- A value >500 eosinophils/μL is defined as having eosinophilia.
- The extent of eosinophilia can be categorized as mild (500–1500 cells/μL), moderate (1500–5000 cells/μL), or severe (>5000 cells/μL).
- The degree of eosinophilia is *not* a reliable predictor of eosinophil-mediated organ damage.

Classification

- Peripheral eosinophilia can be divided into primary, secondary, or idiopathic.
- Primary eosinophilia is seen with hematologic disorders where there may be a clonal expansion of eosinophils (chronic eosinophilic leukemia) or a clonal expansion of cells that stimulate eosinophil production (chronic myeloid or lymphocytic disorders).

- Secondary eosinophilia is also called reactive eosinophilia. It is a polyclonal expansion of eosinophils due to overproduction of IL-5. There are numerous causes such as parasites, allergic diseases, autoimmune disorders, toxins, medications, and endocrine disorders such as Addison disease.
- Idiopathic eosinophilia is considered when primary and secondary causes are excluded.

Hypereosinophilic Syndrome

A proliferative disorder of eosinophils characterized by sustained eosinophilia >1500 cells/μL for ≥1 month documented on two occasions with eosinophil-mediated damage to organs such as the heart, gastrointestinal tract, kidneys, brain, and lung. All other causes of eosinophilia should be excluded to make the diagnosis.[10]

- Hypereosinophilic syndrome (HES) occurs predominantly in men between the ages of 20 and 50 years and presents with insidious onset of fatigue, cough, and dyspnea.
- Approximately 10%–15% HES patients have myeloproliferative disorders. Myeloproliferative variants of HES are characterized by constitutive expression of *FIP1L1/PDGFRA* fusion protein and elevated serum vitamin B_{12} levels.
- Lymphocytic-variant HES (L-HES) accounts for 17%–26% HES patients. Unusual IL-5–producing T cells are found in L-HES.
- Cardiac disease is a major cause of morbidity and mortality in patients with HES. At presentation, patients typically are in the late thrombotic and fibrotic stages of eosinophil-mediated cardiac damage with signs of a restrictive cardiomyopathy and mitral regurgitation. An echocardiogram may detect intracardiac thrombi, endomyocardial fibrosis, or thickening of the posterior mitral valve leaflet. Neurologic manifestations range from peripheral neuropathy to stroke or encephalopathy. Bone marrow examination reveals increased eosinophil precursors.
- **Acute eosinophilic leukemia** is a rare myeloproliferative disorder that is distinguished from HES by several factors: an increased number of immature eosinophils in the blood and/or marrow, >10% blast forms in the marrow, and symptoms and signs compatible with an acute leukemia. Treatment is similar to other leukemias.
- **Lymphoma.** Eosinophilia can present in any T- or B-cell lymphoma. As many as 5% of patients with non-Hodgkin lymphoma and up to 15% of patients with Hodgkin lymphoma have modest peripheral blood eosinophilia. Eosinophilia in Hodgkin lymphoma has been correlated with IL-5 messenger RNA expression by Reed–Sternberg cells.
- **Atheroembolic disease.** Cholesterol embolization can lead to eosinophilia, eosinophiluria, renal dysfunction, livedo reticularis, purple toes, and increased erythrocyte sedimentation rate (ESR).
- **Immunodeficiency.** Hyper-IgE syndrome, autoimmune lymphoproliferative syndrome, and Omenn syndrome can present with recurrent infections, dermatitis, and eosinophilia.

Epidemiology

In industrialized nations, peripheral blood eosinophilia is most often due to atopic disease, whereas helminthic infections are the most common cause of eosinophilia in the rest of the world.

DIAGNOSIS

There are two approaches that are useful for evaluating eosinophilia, either by associated clinical context (Table 11-3) or by degree of eosinophilia (Table 11-4).

TABLE 11-3	Causes of Eosinophilia

Eosinophilia Associated With Atopic Disease

Allergic rhinitis	Atopic dermatitis
Asthma	

Eosinophilia Associated With Pulmonary Infiltrates

Chronic eosinophilic pneumonia	Allergic bronchopulmonary aspergillosis
Acute eosinophilic pneumonia	Coccidioidomycosis
Tropical pulmonary eosinophilia	Löffler syndrome (larvae traveling in lung)

Eosinophilia Associated With Parasitic Infection

Helminths (*Ascaris lumbricoides*, *Strongyloides stercoralis*, hookworm, *Toxocara canis* or *Toxocara cati*, *Trichinella*)

Protozoa (*Dientamoeba fragilis*, *Sarcocystis*, and *Isospora belli*)

Eosinophilia Associated With Primary Cutaneous Disease

Atopic dermatitis	Eosinophilic folliculitis
Eosinophilic fasciitis	Episodic angioedema with anaphylaxis
Eosinophilic cellulitis	

Eosinophilia Associated With Multiorgan Involvement

Drug-induced eosinophilia	Eosinophilic leukemia
Eosinophilic granulomatosis with polyangiitis	Systemic mastocytosis
Hypereosinophilic syndrome	Lymphomas

Miscellaneous Causes

Eosinophilic gastroenteritis	Transplant rejection
Interstitial nephritis	Atheroembolic disease
Eosinophilia myalgia syndrome	Adrenal insufficiency
Retroviral infections (HIV, human T-lymphotropic virus type 1)	

TABLE 11-4	Classification of Eosinophilia Based on the Peripheral Blood Eosinophil Count

Peripheral Blood Eosinophil Count (cells/µL)		
500–2000	2000–5000	>5000
Allergic rhinitis	Intrinsic asthma	Eosinophilia myalgia syndrome
Allergic asthma	Allergic bronchopulmonary aspergillosis	Hypereosinophilic syndrome
Food allergy	Helminthiasis	Episodic angioedema with eosinophilia
Urticaria	Drug reactions	EGPA
Addison disease	Vascular neoplasms	Leukemia
Pulmonary infiltrates with eosinophilia syndromes	Eosinophilic granulomatosis with polyangiitis (EGPA)	
Solid neoplasms	Eosinophilic fasciitis	
Nasal polyposis	HIV	

Clinical Presentation

History

- A history is important in narrowing the differential diagnosis of eosinophilia. It is important to determine if the patient has symptoms of atopic disease (rhinitis, wheezing, rash) or cancer (weight loss, fatigue, fever, night sweats) and to evaluate for other specific organ involvement such as lung, heart, or nerves. Prior eosinophil count can help determine the duration and magnitude of eosinophilia.
- A complete medication list, including over-the-counter supplements, and a full travel, occupational, and dietary history should be obtained.
- Any pet contact should be ascertained for possible exposure to toxocariasis.

Physical Examination

Physical examination should be guided by the history, with a special focus on the skin, upper and lower respiratory tracts, and cardiovascular and neurologic systems.

Laboratories

- Initial laboratory evaluations generally include complete blood count (CBC) with differential and eosinophil count, liver function tests, serum chemistries and creatinine, serum vitamin B_{12} level, troponin, markers of inflammation (e.g., ESR and/or C-reactive protein [CRP]), and urinalysis. Further diagnostic studies are based on clinical presentations and initial findings. Mild **eosinophilia associated with symptoms of rhinitis or asthma** is indicative of underlying atopic disease, which can be confirmed by skin testing.
- Depending on the travel history, **stool examination** for ova and parasites should be done on three separate occasions. Because only small numbers of helminths may pass in the stool and because tissue- or blood-dwelling helminths will not be found in the stool, **serologic tests** for antiparasite antibodies should also be sent. Such tests are available for strongyloidiasis, toxocariasis, and trichinellosis.
- Diagnosis at the time of presentation with Löffler syndrome can be made by detection of *Ascaris* larvae in respiratory secretions or gastric aspirates but not stool.
- Peripheral blood smear and flow cytometry of lymphocyte subpopulations can aid in the diagnosis of hematologic malignancy. Bone marrow biopsy for pathologic, cytogenetic, and molecular testing on bone marrow and/or peripheral blood (e.g., for *FIP1L1/PDGFRA* mutation) may be required. Serum vitamin B_{12} level may be elevated in myeloproliferative neoplasms and autoimmune lymphoproliferative syndrome.
- Evaluation for idiopathic HES should also consist of troponin measurement, echocardiogram, and ECG.
- Immunoglobulin levels are helpful if concerned for an immunodeficiency. Elevated immunoglobulin levels can be found in L-HES.
- A tryptase level is necessary if mastocytosis is considered as a cause of eosinophilia.

Imaging

CXR or CT findings may also help to narrow the differential diagnosis.

- Peripheral infiltrates with central clearing are indicative of chronic eosinophilic pneumonia.
- Diffuse infiltrates in an interstitial, alveolar, or mixed pattern may be seen in acute eosinophilic pneumonia as well as drug-induced eosinophilia with pulmonary involvement.

- Transient infiltrates may be seen in Löffler syndrome, EGPA, or allergic broncho-pulmonary aspergillosis (ABPA).
- Central bronchiectasis is a major criterion in the diagnosis of ABPA.
- A diffuse miliary or nodular pattern, consolidation, or cavitation may be found in cases of tropical pulmonary eosinophilia.
- A CT of the sinuses, nerve conduction studies, and testing for p-ANCA may be helpful in the diagnosis of eosinophilic granulomatosis with polyangiitis (EGPA).

Diagnostic Procedures
- If no other cause of pulmonary infiltrates has been identified, a **bronchoscopy** may be necessary for analysis of bronchoalveolar lavage (BAL) fluid and lung tissue. The presence of eosinophils in BAL fluid or sputum with eosinophilic infiltration of the parenchyma is most typical of acute or chronic eosinophilic pneumonia.
- Skin biopsy will aid in diagnosing the cutaneous eosinophilic diseases and EGPA.

TREATMENT

- Mild eosinophilia with no evidence of end-organ damage may not need treatment.
- Oral steroids are indicated when there is evidence of organ involvement. However, strongyloidiasis must be excluded before administration of steroids to prevent hyperinfection syndrome.
- When a drug reaction is suspected, discontinuation of the drug is both diagnostic and therapeutic. Other treatment options depend on the exact cause of eosinophilia because, with the exception of HES, eosinophilia is a manifestation of an underlying disease.
- **HES:** Patients with marked eosinophilia with no organ involvement may have a benign course. In contrast, those with organ involvement and **FIP1L1/PDGFRA**-associated disease may have an extremely aggressive course without treatment.
  - Monitoring and early initiation of high-dose glucocorticoids should be pursued in all patients except those who have the *FIP1L1/PDGFRA* fusion gene.
  - Patients with the *FIP1L1/PDGFRA* fusion mutation should be started on imatinib mesylate (Gleevec), a tyrosine kinase inhibitor. Treatment should be initiated promptly in these patients to prevent progression of cardiac disease and other end-organ damage. Imatinib has been shown to induce disease remission and halt progression.[11]
  - Hydroxyurea has been the most frequently used effective second-line agent and/or steroid-sparing agent for HES. Interferon-α2b in combination with glucocorticoids has been used to treat L-HES. Hematopoietic cell transplantation may be considered in refractory HES.
  - Mepolizumab, a humanized anti–IL-5 antibody, has shown corticosteroid-sparing effects in FIP1L1/PDGFRA-negative, corticosteroid-responsive subjects with HES.[12]
  - Alemtuzumab, an anti-CD52 antibody (CD52 is expressed on the surface of eosinophils), has been shown to be effective in treatment for patients with refractory idiopathic HES.[13]
- Primary eosinophilia disorders should be followed by a specialist; any cases of unresolved or unexplained eosinophilia warrant evaluation by an allergist/immunologist.

Urticaria and Angioedema

GENERAL PRINCIPLES

Definition

- **Urticaria** (hives) are raised, erythematous, well-demarcated pruritic skin lesions. Central clearing can cause an annular lesion and is often seen after antihistamine use. An individual lesion usually lasts minutes to hours.
- **Angioedema** is swelling of the deep dermis and subcutaneous tissue. It is often painful rather than pruritic and generally lasts less than 48 hours. It can be found anywhere on the body but most often involves the tongue, lips, eyelids, throat, bowels, and/or genitals.

Classification

- **Acute urticaria (with or without angioedema)** is defined as the occurrence of hives and/or angioedema lasting <6 weeks. It can be caused by an allergic reaction to a medication, food, insect sting, or exposure (contact or inhalation) to an allergen. Patients can develop a hypersensitivity to a food, medication, or self-care product that previously had been used without difficulty. In many cases of acute urticaria, no identifiable trigger can be found.
- **Chronic urticaria (with or without angioedema)** is defined as the occurrence of hives and/or angioedema for >6 weeks. There are many possible causes of chronic urticaria and angioedema, including medications, autoimmunity, self-care products, and physical triggers. However, the etiology remains unidentified in >80% of cases.

Epidemiology

- Urticaria is a common condition that affects 15%–24% of the US population at some time in their life. Chronic idiopathic urticaria occurs in approximately 1% of the US population, and there does not appear to be an increased risk in persons with atopy.[14]
- Angioedema occurs in 40%–50% of patients with urticaria.

Etiology

- IgE-mediated: drugs, foods, stinging and biting insects, latex, inhalant, or contact allergens
- Non–IgE-mediated: narcotics, muscle relaxants, radiocontrast, vancomycin, NSAIDs, ACE inhibitors
- Transfusion reactions
- Infections (i.e., viral, bacterial, parasitic)
- Systemic disorders: autoimmune diseases, malignancy, mastocytosis, HES, cryoglobulinemia, and hereditary diseases
- Physical urticaria: dermographism, cold, cholinergic, pressure, vibratory, solar, and aquagenic
- Idiopathic

Pathophysiology

Most forms of urticaria and angioedema are caused by the degranulation of mast cells or basophils and the release of inflammatory mediators. Histamine is the primary mediator and elicits edema (wheal) and erythema (flare). HAE and related syndromes are mediated by the overproduction of bradykinin and are not responsive to antihistamines.

DIAGNOSIS

Diagnosis is based on complete history and physical examination with characteristic skin lesions.

Clinical Presentation

- Patients with an acute urticaria episode present with history of pruritic, raised, erythematous lesions. Individual lesions resolve over a period of 1–24 hours.
- Angioedema usually presents with painful swelling without pruritus. The swelling can take up to 72 hours to resolve.
- Physical urticaria is induced by environmental or physical stimuli. The common triggers are cold, heat, sweating, exercise, pressure, vibration, and sunlight. Dermographism, literally "skin writing," is the most common form of physical urticaria. It affects approximately 4% of the population and can be elicited by briskly stroking or scratching skin.

History

- A detailed history should elicit identifiable triggers and rule out any systemic causes. When the individual skin lesion lasts longer than 48 hours, the diagnosis of urticarial vasculitis must be investigated by a skin biopsy.
- Any changes in environmental exposures, foods, medications, personal care products, etc. should be determined.
- It is important to differentiate from anaphylaxis, which affects organs other than the skin, as this will be treated differently (see "Anaphylaxis" section).

Physical Examination

- Complete examination of the affected and nonaffected skin.
- Urticaria appears as erythematous, raised lesions that blanch with pressure.
- Angioedema appears as swelling; can often involve the face, tongue, extremities, or genitalia; and may be asymmetric.

Differential Diagnosis

- IgE–mediated allergic reaction to drugs, foods, insects, inhalant, or contact allergen.
- Non–IgE–mediated drug and food reactions (i.e., medications including NSAIDs, vancomycin, radioactive iodine, opiates, muscle relaxants, foods including tomatoes and strawberries).
- Pruritic urticarial papules and plaques of pregnancy.
- Mast cell release syndromes (i.e., systemic mastocytosis, cutaneous mastocytosis including urticaria pigmentosa).
- Cutaneous small-vessel vasculitis (i.e., urticarial vasculitis, systemic lupus erythematosus).
- HES.
- Toxic drug eruptions.
- Allergic contact dermatitis (i.e., poison ivy, poison oak).
- Cryopyrin-associated periodic syndromes including familial cold autoinflammatory syndrome and Muckle–Wells syndrome.
- **Angioedema without urticaria** should lead to consideration of specific entities.
  - Use of ACE inhibitors or angiotensin II receptor blockers (ARBs) can be associated with angioedema at any point in the course of therapy and can occur up to 6 weeks after last exposure.
  - **HAE, or C1 INH deficiency,** is inherited in an autosomal dominant pattern; 25% of cases arise from de novo mutations.

○ **Acquired C1 INH deficiency** presents similarly to HAE but is typically associated with an underlying lymphoproliferative disorder, connective tissue disease, or other neoplasias.

Diagnostic Testing

Epicutaneous skin testing and patch testing are only indicated when symptoms are associated with specific triggers.

Laboratories

• Routine laboratory testing in the absence of a clinical history is rarely helpful in determining an etiology in chronic urticaria. Evaluation for systemic disease associated with chronic urticaria includes CBC with differential, CRP or ESR, thyroid-stimulating hormone, renal and hepatic profiles.

• Autologous serum skin testing, assays for basophil histamine release, and autoantibodies to IgE and the high-affinity IgE receptor are available, but the utility of these tests has not been established.

• All patients with **angioedema without urticaria should be screened with a C4 level, which is reduced during and between attacks of HAE.** If the C4 level is reduced, a quantitative and functional C1 INH assay should be performed. Measuring C1 INH levels alone is not sufficient because 15% of patients have normal levels of a dysfunctional C1 INH protein; therefore, it is important to also obtain the functional assay.

• Acquired C1 INH deficiency patients have reduced C1q, C1 INH level and function, and C4 levels due to an autoantibody to C1 INH.

Diagnostic Procedures

• A skin biopsy should be performed if individual lesions persist for >24 hours to rule out urticarial vasculitis.

TREATMENT

• The ideal treatment of acute urticaria with or without angioedema is identification and avoidance of specific causes. **All potential causes should be eliminated.** Most cases of acute urticaria are self-limited and resolve spontaneously.

• Careful consideration should be given to the **elimination or substitution of each prescription or over-the-counter medication** or supplement. If a patient reacts to one medication in a class, the reaction likely will be triggered by all medications in that class. Exacerbating agents (e.g., NSAIDs, opiates, vancomycin, and alcohol) should be avoided because they may induce nonspecific mast cell degranulation and exacerbate urticaria caused by other agents.

Medications

If acute urticaria is associated with additional systemic symptoms such as hypotension, laryngeal edema, or bronchospasm, treatment with epinephrine (0.3–0.5 mL of a 1:1000 solution IM) should be administered immediately. See "Anaphylaxis" section for additional information.

Acute Urticaria and/or Angioedema

• **Second-generation antihistamines** such as cetirizine, fexofenadine, or loratadine should be administered to patients until the hives have cleared. Higher than conventional, US FDA–approved doses may provide more efficacy. A first-generation antihistamine such as hydroxyzine may be added as an evening dose if needed to obtain control in refractory cases. H_2 antihistamines, such as ranitidine, may also be added to the above treatment.

- **Oral corticosteroids** should be reserved for patients with moderate to severe symptoms. Corticosteroids will not have an immediate effect but may prevent relapse.
- If a patient presents with systemic symptoms, self-administered epinephrine should be prescribed for use in the case of anaphylaxis.

Chronic Urticaria
- Use of a second-generation H_1 antihistamine once or twice daily (up to four times daily).
- If no response, then can add H_2 antihistamine, leukotriene receptor antagonist, and/or first-generation H_1 antihistamine or doxepin to be taken at bedtime.
- If continued urticaria, then can choose an alternative such as omalizumab (FDA approved for patient with chronic urticaria that fail H_1 antihistamine therapy), cyclosporine, hydroxychloroquine, dapsone, or other immunosuppressants.
- **Optimal duration of therapy has not been established; tapering medications after 3–6 months of symptom control has been suggested.**

Hereditary and Acquired Angioedema (Disorder of C1 Inhibitor)
- Acute attacks: C1 inhibitor concentrate, icatibant, and ecallantide are first-line agents. If none of the first-line agents are available, fresh frozen plasma can be used. Also pursue symptomatic therapy and rehydration.
- Preventative medications include C1 inhibitor replacement via IV or SC, lanadelumab, berotralstat, attenuated androgens, and antifibrinolytics.

REFERRAL

All patients with chronic urticaria or a history of anaphylaxis should be referred to an allergy specialist for evaluation to identify potential allergic and autoimmune triggers.

Immunodeficiency

GENERAL PRINCIPLES

Definition
- Primary immunodeficiencies (PIDs) are disorders of the immune system that result in an increased susceptibility to infection.
- Secondary immunodeficiencies are also disorders of increased susceptibility to infection but are attributable to an external source.

Classification
PIDs can be organized by the defective immune components with considerable heterogeneity in each disorder.
- **Predominantly antibody deficiencies:** The defect is primarily in the ability to make antibodies.
  - Common variable immune deficiency (CVID)
  - X-linked (Bruton) agammaglobulinemia
  - IgG subclass deficiency
  - Specific antibody deficiency
  - Hyper-IgM syndrome
  - Selective IgA deficiency

- **Combined immunodeficiencies and syndromes:** The defect results in deficiencies in both cellular and humoral immune responses.
  - Severe combined immunodeficiencies
  - DiGeorge syndrome
  - Hyper-IgE (Job) syndrome
- **Defects of innate immunity:** Defects in germline-encoded receptors and downstream signaling pathways.
  - Deficiency of Toll-like receptor signaling
  - Mendelian susceptibility to mycobacterial diseases (MSMD)
  - Natural killer (NK) cell deficiency
  - Phagocytic cell deficiencies
  - Chronic granulomatous disease (CGD)
- **Complement deficiencies**
- **Diseases of immune dysregulation:** Autoimmunity and lymphoproliferation are characteristic manifestations in these disorders.

Epidemiology

- Secondary immunodeficiency syndromes, particularly HIV/AIDS, are the most common immunodeficiency disorders.
- The estimated prevalence of PIDs is approximately 1 in 1200 live births.
- Most PIDs presenting in adulthood are humoral immune defects affecting antibody production.

Etiology

- Predominantly antibody immune deficiencies are thought to be caused by defects in B-cell maturation. Combined immunodeficiencies are caused by defective T-cell–mediated immunity and associated antibody deficiency.
- A variety of genetic mutations have been associated with specific PID syndromes.
- Secondary immunodeficiencies can be caused by medications (chemotherapy, immunomodulatory agents, corticosteroids), infectious agents (e.g., HIV), malignancy, antibody loss (e.g., nephrotic syndrome, protein losing enteropathy, or consumption during a severe underlying infection), autoimmune disease (e.g., systemic lupus erythematosus, rheumatoid arthritis), malnutrition (vitamin D), and other underlying diseases (e.g., diabetes mellitus, cirrhosis, uremia).

DIAGNOSIS

Clinical Presentation

- The hallmark of PID is recurrent infections. Clinical suspicion should be increased by recurrent sinopulmonary infection, deep-seated infections, opportunistic infections, or disseminated infections in an otherwise healthy patient.
- Specific PIDs are often associated with particular types of pathogens (e.g., catalase-positive infections in CGD or MSMD).
- Recurrent urinary tract infections are only rarely associated with PID.
- Patients with PIDs may also present with autoimmunity, immune dysregulation, allergic diseases, and malignancies.
- **Selective IgA deficiency** is the most common immune deficiency, with a prevalence of 1 in 300–500 people.
  - Most patients are asymptomatic. Some may present with recurrent sinus and pulmonary infections. Therapy is directed at early treatment with antibiotics because IgA replacement is not available.

- Associated autoimmune diseases are observed in 20%–30% of cases. Absolute IgA-deficient patients (i.e., <7 mg/dL) are at risk for developing a severe transfusion reaction to blood products including IV immunoglobulin (IVIG), because of the presence of IgE anti-IgA antibodies in some individuals; therefore, these patients should be transfused with washed red blood cells or receive blood products only from IgA-deficient donors.
- **CVID** is the most common symptomatic PID, occurring with a frequency of 1/25,000. It includes a heterogeneous group of disorders in which most patients present in the second to fourth decade of life with recurrent sinus and pulmonary infections and are discovered to have low and dysfunctional IgG, IgA, and/or IgM antibodies with poor response to immunizations.
  - B-cell numbers are often normal, but there is decreased ability to produce immunoglobulin because of the lack of isotype-switched memory B cells. Some patients may also exhibit T-cell dysfunction.
  - CVID is largely idiopathic, although there are molecular defects in the B-cell signaling and development pathways (e.g., TACI, ICOS, BAFF-R, and CD19) with some forms of the disorder.
  - Patients with CVID are particularly susceptible to infection with encapsulated organisms.
  - Patients may have associated gastrointestinal disease or autoimmune abnormalities (most commonly autoimmune hemolytic anemia, idiopathic thrombocytopenic purpura, pernicious anemia, and rheumatoid arthritis).
  - There is an increased incidence of malignancy, especially lymphoid and gastrointestinal malignancy.
  - Therapy consists of IVIG or subcutaneous immunoglobulin (SCIG) replacement therapy as well as prompt treatment of infections with antibiotics.
- **Specific antibody deficiency** is defined as poor or absent antibody responses to polysaccharide antigens (i.e., 23-valent pneumococcal vaccine) in the setting of normal levels of immunoglobulins and IgG subclasses.
  - B-cell numbers and response to protein antigens (i.e., tetanus toxoid and diphtheria toxoid) are usually normal.
  - Patients have increased susceptibility to sinopulmonary infections. Allergic diseases are also common.
  - Therapeutic approaches include adequate antibiotic treatment for infections, pneumococcal conjugate vaccine, and immunoglobulin replacement.
- **X-linked (Bruton) agammaglobulinemia** clinically manifests very similarly to severe CVID and is typically diagnosed in childhood, but can present in adulthood.
  - Patients usually have low levels of all immunoglobulin types and very low levels of B cells.
  - Specific genetic defect is in Bruton tyrosine kinase, which is involved in B-cell maturation.
- **Subclass deficiency.** Deficiencies of each of the IgG subclasses (IgG1, IgG2, IgG3, and IgG4) have been described.
  - These patients present with similar complaints as the CVID patients.
  - Total IgG levels may be normal. A strong association with IgA deficiency exists. There is disagreement as to whether this is a separate entity from CVID. In most cases, there is no need to evaluate IgG subclass levels.
  - Isolated subclass deficiency without recurrent infections is of unknown clinical significance.
- **Hyper-IgM syndrome** is characterized by low IgA and IgG levels with normal or increased IgM and poor antibody function. There are several gene mutations

reported, which cause defective class switching in immunoglobulins. Depending on the mutation, some patients may have poor T-cell function as well, leading to increased opportunistic infections.

- **Hyper-IgE syndrome (Job syndrome)** is characterized by recurrent pyogenic infections of the skin and lower respiratory tract. This syndrome can result in severe abscess and empyema formation. Some forms of the disease are associated with autosomal dominant mutation of *STAT3*.
  - The most common organism involved is *S. aureus*, but other bacteria and fungi have been reported.
  - Patients present with recurrent infections and have associated pruritic dermatitis, coarse (lion-like) facies, growth retardation, scoliosis, retention of primary teeth, and hyperkeratotic nails.
  - Laboratory data reveal the presence of normal levels of IgG, IgA, and IgM but markedly elevated levels of IgE. A marked increase in tissue and blood eosinophils may also be observed.
- **Complement deficiencies** are a broad category of PID characterized by recurrent infections to a range of pathogens.
  - Recurrent disseminated Neisseria infections are associated with a deficiency in the terminal complement system (C5–C9).
  - Systemic lupus–like disorders and recurrent infection with encapsulated organisms have been associated with deficiencies in other components of complement.
  - CH50 and AH50 are useful to screen for deficiencies of the classical pathway and alternative pathway, respectively.
- **CGD** is characterized by defective killing of intracellular pathogens by neutrophils.
  - Patients usually present with frequent infection, often with abscesses, from *S. aureus* and other catalase-positive organisms. *Aspergillus* is a particularly troublesome pathogen for patients with CGD.
  - Diagnosis is made by demonstration of defective respiratory burst with flow cytometry assay using dihydrorhodamine.
- **MSMD** is caused by defects in Th1 immunity and is associated with mutations in genes involved in interferon-γ and IL-12 signaling. Characteristic infections include mycobacterial infections (including typical and atypical *Mycobacterium*) and *Salmonella* infections.

Diagnostic Testing

- Frequent sinopulmonary infections, recurrent and invasive infections requiring IV antimicrobial agents, infections with unusual pathogens, and family history of PID are warning signs for PIDs.
- Initial evaluation should focus on identifying possible secondary causes of recurrent infection such as allergy, medications, and anatomic abnormalities. Workup begins with a CBC with differential, HIV test, quantitative immunoglobulin levels, and complement levels. Often the evaluation will need to include enumeration of lymphocytes by flow cytometry if B-, T-, or NK-cell defects are suspected. Other specialized tests including genetic testing may be needed to make a definitive diagnosis.
- If clinical suspicion is high for an underlying antibody-predominant PID, B-cell function can be assessed by measuring immunoglobulin response to vaccinations. Preimmunization and postimmunization titers for both a protein antigen (i.e., tetanus) and a polysaccharide antigen (i.e., Pneumovax, the unconjugated 23-valent vaccine) are measured because proteins and polysaccharide antigens are handled differently by the immune system.
- Titers of specific antibodies are measured before and at 4–8 weeks after immunization.
- Genetic testing can also be performed.

TREATMENT

• Killed or subcomponent vaccines are safe for most patients with PID, although some patients may not produce full response. Live attenuated vaccines may be contraindicated in some individuals with PID and their families.
• Prophylactic antibiotics may be considered in some PID syndromes to prevent infections.
• IgA deficiency: No specific treatment is available. However, these patients should be promptly treated at the first sign of infection with an antibiotic that covers *Streptococcus pneumoniae* or *Haemophilus influenzae*.
• CVID should be treated with immunoglobulin replacement in forms of IVIG or SCIG. Numerous preparations of immunoglobulin are available, all of which undergo viral inactivation steps. Possible side effects include myalgias, vomiting, chills, and lingering headache (due to immune complex–mediated aseptic meningitis).

REFERRAL

Patients in whom a PID is being seriously considered should undergo evaluation by an allergist/clinical immunologist with expertise in diagnosing and treating PID.

REFERENCES

1. Thong B, Tan TC. Epidemiology and risk factors for drug allergy. *Br J Clin Pharmacol.* 2011;71(5): 684-700.
2. Gomes ER, Demoly P. Epidemiology of hypersensitivity drug reactions. *Curr Opin Allergy Clin Immunol.* 2005;5(4):309-316.
3. Macy E. Penicillin and beta-lactam allergy: epidemiology and diagnosis. *Curr Allergy Asthma Rep.* 2014;14(11):476.
4. Khan DA, Solensky R. Drug allergy. *J Allergy Clin Immunol.* 2010;125(2 suppl 2):126-138.
5. Macy E, Contreras R. Health care use and serious infection prevalence associated with penicillin "allergy" in hospitalized patients: a cohort study. *J Allergy Clin Immunol.* 2014;133(3):790-796.
6. Chiriac AM, Banerji A, Gruchalla RS, et al. Controversies in drug allergy: drug allergy pathways. *J Allergy Clin Immunol Pract.* 2019;7:46-60.
7. Phillips E, Mallal S. Drug hypersensitivity in HIV. *Curr Opin Allergy Clin Immunol.* 2007;7(4):324-330.
8. Strom BL, Schinnar R, Apter AJ, et al. Absence of cross-reactivity between sulfonamide antibiotics and sulfonamide nonantibiotics. *N Engl J Med.* 2003;349(17):1628-1635.
9. Wood RA, Camargo CA Jr, Lieberman P, et al. Anaphylaxis in America: the prevalence and characteristics of anaphylaxis in the United States. *J Allergy Clin Immunol.* 2014;133(2):461.
10. Valent P, Klion AD, Horny HP, et al. Contemporary consensus proposal on criteria and classification of eosinophilic disorders and related syndromes. *J Allergy Clin Immunol.* 2012;130(3):607.e9-612.e9
11. Metzgeroth G, Walz C, Erben P, et al. Safety and efficacy of imatinib in chronic eosinophilic leukaemia and hypereosinophilic syndrome – a phase-II study. *Br J Haematol.* 2008;143(5):707-715.
12. Roufosse FE, Kahn JE, Gleich GJ, et al. Long-term safety of mepolizumab for the treatment of hypereosinophilic syndromes. *J Allergy Clin Immunol.* 2013;131(2):461.e5-467.e5.
13. Strati P, Cortes J, Faderl S, Kantarjian H, Verstovsek S. Long-term follow-up of patients with hypereosinophilic syndrome treated with alemtuzumab, an anti-CD52 antibody. *Clin Lymphoma Myeloma Leuk.* 2013;13(3):287-291.
14. Bernstein JA, Lang DM, Khan DA, et al. The diagnosis and management of acute and chronic urticaria: 2014 update. *J Allergy Clin Immunol.* 2013;133(5):1270.e66-1277.e66

12 Fluid and Electrolyte Management

Maryam Saleem and Steven Cheng

FLUID MANAGEMENT AND PERTURBATIONS IN VOLUME STATUS

- **Total body water (TBW):** Water comprises approximately 60% of lean body weight in men and 50% in women. Two-thirds of TBW is **intracellular fluid** (ICF) and one-third is **extracellular fluid** (ECF). ECF is further subdivided into intravascular and interstitial spaces in a ratio of 1:4.
  - **Example:** For a healthy 70-kg man:

$$TBW = 0.6 \times 70 = 42 \text{ L}$$

  - ICF = 2/3 TBW = 0.66 × 42 = 28 L
  - ECF = 1/3 TBW = 0.33 × 42 = 14 L
  - Intravascular compartment = 0.25 × 14 = 3.5 L
  - Interstitial compartment = 0.75 × 14 = 10.5 L
  - The distribution of water between intravascular and interstitial spaces can be affected by changes to the Starling balance of forces. Low oncotic pressure (i.e., low albumin states) and high hydrostatic pressure (i.e., Na^+-retentive states) increase the movement of fluid from vascular to interstitial compartments, which is an important step in the development of edema.
- **Total body Na^+:** 85%–90% of **total body Na^+** is extracellular and constitutes the predominate solute in the ECF. Changes to the body's total Na^+ content typically results from a loss or gain of this Na^+-rich fluid, leading to contraction or expansion of the ECF space.

The Euvolemic Patient

- In a euvolemic patient, the goal of fluid and electrolyte administration is to maintain homeostasis. The best way to accomplish this is to allow free access to food and oral fluids. Patients who are unable to tolerate oral intake require maintenance fluids to replace renal, gastrointestinal (GI), and insensible fluid losses.
- The decision to provide maintenance IV fluid should be thoughtfully considered and not administered by route. Fluid administration should be reassessed *at least* daily. Patient weight, which may indicate net fluid balance, should be monitored carefully.
- Table 12-1 provides a list of common IV solutions and their contents. By combining the necessary components, one can derive an appropriate maintenance fluid regimen tailored for each patient.

TABLE 12-1	Commonly Used Parenteral Solutions				
IV Solution	Osmolality (mOsm/L)	[Glucose] (g/L)	[Na$^+$] (mEq/L)	[Cl$^-$] (mEq/L)	HCO$_3$ Equivalents (mEq/L)
D5W	278	50	0	0	0
0.45% NaCl[a]	154	_[b]	77	77	0
0.9% NaCl[a]	308	_[b]	154	154	0
3% NaCl	1026	–	513	513	0
Lactated Ringer's[c]	274	_[b]	130	109	28

[a]NaCl 0.45% and 0.9% are half-normal and normal saline, respectively.
[b]Also available with 5% dextrose.
[c]Also contains 4 mEq/L K$^+$, 1.5 mEq/L Ca^{2+}, and 28 mEq/L lactate.
D5W, 5% dextrose in water.

The Hypovolemic Patient

GENERAL PRINCIPLES

Volume depletion generally results from a deficit in **total body Na$^+$** content. Renal causes of Na$^+$ loss include diuresis, salt-wasting nephropathies, and mineralocorticoid deficiency. **Extrarenal** causes include losses from the GI and respiratory tracts, hemorrhage, and severe third spacing of fluid in critically ill patients.

DIAGNOSIS

Clinical Presentation

Mild degrees of volume depletion are often not clinically detectable, whereas larger fluid losses can lead to fatigue, muscle cramps, and postural dizziness. Severe volume depletion can result in mental status changes, oliguria, and hypovolemic shock.

Diagnostic Testing

The following laboratory studies are consistent with volume depletion but are not required for the diagnosis:
• Urine Na$^+$ <15 mEq.
• Fractional excretion of sodium (FeNa) <1%. FeNa can be calculated as ([Urine Na$^+$ × Serum Cr] ÷ [Urine Cr × Serum Na$^+$]) × 100.
• Elevated urine osmolality and serum bicarbonate levels can often be seen.
• Hematocrit and serum albumin may be increased from hemoconcentration.

TREATMENT

• Because it is difficult to estimate **volume deficits**, therapy is largely empiric, requiring frequent reassessments of volume status while resuscitation is under way.
• Mild volume contraction can usually be corrected via the oral route. However, the presence of hemodynamic instability, symptomatic fluid loss, or intolerance to oral administration requires IV therapy.

- The primary therapeutic goal is to protect hemodynamic stability and replenish **intravascular volume** with fluid that will expand the ECF compartment. Na^+-based solutions are ideal for volume resuscitation since the Na is retained in the ECF.
- Intravenous fluid can be administered as boluses for patients with poor cardiac reserve or significant edema. Once the patient is stable, fluids can be administered at a maintenance rate to replace ongoing losses. In patients with hemorrhage or GI bleeding, **blood transfusion** can accomplish both volume expansion and concomitant correction of anemia.

The Hypervolemic Patient

Hypervolemia reflects a surplus of **total body Na^+** resulting in expansion of the ECF compartments. It can be caused by excess retention or reabsorption of Na^+. It is a frequent finding in conditions with impaired circulating volume, such as heart failure and cirrhosis.

DIAGNOSIS

Clinical Presentation

- Expansion of the **interstitial compartment** may result in peripheral edema, ascites, and pleural effusions.
- Expansion of the **intravascular compartment** may result in pulmonary rales, elevated jugular venous pressure, hepatojugular reflux, an S_3 gallop, and elevated blood pressures.
- Because overt signs of hypervolemia may not manifest until 3–4 L of fluid retention, a gradual rise in water weight is often the earliest indication of Na^+ retention.

Diagnostic Testing

- Laboratory studies are generally not needed as hypervolemia is primarily a bedside diagnosis. However, the following findings can be seen in the appropriate clinical contexts:
  - Brain natriuretic peptide may be elevated in patients with heart failure.
  - Urine $[Na^+]$ may be low (<15 mEq/L) in patients with reduced effective circulating volume.
- A CXR may show pulmonary edema or pleural effusions, but clear lung fields do not exclude volume overload.

TREATMENT

Treatment must address not only the ECF volume excess but also the underlying pathologic process. Alleviating the Na^+ excess can be accomplished by the judicious use of diuretics and by limiting Na^+ intake.

Medications

- Diuretics enhance the renal excretion of Na^+ by blocking the various sites of Na^+ reabsorption along the nephron.
  - **Loop diuretics** are commonly used for brisk and immediate diuresis.
  - **Thiazide diuretics** are used for hypertension and states of chronic Na^+ retention.
  - **Potassium-sparing diuretics** have a comparatively small effect but are useful as adjunctive agents.

- Treatment of the underlying disease process is critical to prevent continued Na^+ reabsorption in the kidney. Nephrotic syndrome is discussed in Chapter 13, Renal Diseases. Treatment of heart failure is discussed in Chapter 5, Heart Failure and Cardiomyopathy; and cirrhosis is addressed in Chapter 19, Liver Diseases.

DISORDERS OF SODIUM CONCENTRATION

Hypernatremia and **hyponatremia** are primarily disorders of *water balance* or *water distribution*. A persistent abnormality in $[Na^+]$ requires both an initial challenge to water balance as well as a disturbance of the adaptive response.

Hyponatremia

Hyponatremia is defined as a plasma $[Na^+]$ **<135 mEq/L.**

GENERAL PRINCIPLES

- To maintain a normal $[Na^+]$, the ingestion of water must be matched by the excretion of water. Hyponatremia occurs when this balance is disturbed by the excessive addition of water to the ECF and/or the insufficient removal of water from the ECF.
- Processes which increase the movement of water into the ECF include:
  - **Hyperosmolar hyponatremia.** When an osmotically active solute other than Na^+ accumulates in the ECF, it draws water into the ECF and dilutes the $[Na^+]$. This is most commonly caused by **hyperglycemia**, resulting in a fall in plasma $[Na^+]$ of 1.6–2.4 mEq/L for every 100 mg/dL rise in plasma glucose.[1]
  - **Water intoxication.** Rarely, the ECF water content rises simply because the ingested quantity of water exceeds the capacity for renal water clearance. This is seen in primary polydipsia, beer potomania, and the so-called "tea and toast" diet.
- Processes which impair the clearance of water from the ECF generally involve the antidiuretic hormone (ADH), a hormone which controls water reabsorption in the kidney.
  - **"Appropriate"** ADH secretion occurs with a fall in effective circulating volume. In these conditions, thirst and water retention are stimulated, protecting volume status at the cost of osmolality. This category is classically subdivided into hypovolemic and hypervolemic hyponatremia, based on the associated assessment of ECF status.
  - **"Inappropriate"** secretion of ADH occurs in the absence of osmotic- or volume-related stimuli. Because the renal response to volume expansion remains intact, these patients are typically **euvolemic.** However, because of the rise in TBW, serum concentrations of Na^+ are decreased.
    - Conditions that stimulate ADH secretion independent of volume status or osmolality include nausea, adrenal dysfunction, and hypothyroidism.
    - The **syndrome of inappropriate ADH secretion (SIADH)** occurs in the absence of physiologic stimuli for ADH secretion. It is commonly associated with neuropsychiatric disorders (e.g., meningitis, encephalitis, acute psychosis, cerebrovascular accident, head trauma), pulmonary diseases (e.g., pneumonia, tuberculosis, positive-pressure ventilation, acute respiratory failure), and

malignant tumors (most commonly, small-cell lung cancer). **Pharmacologic agents**, such as selective serotonin reuptake inhibitors, narcotics, antipsychotic agents, chlorpropamide, and NSAIDs, have also been implicated in SIADH.

DIAGNOSIS

Clinical Presentation

The clinical features of hyponatremia are related to the change in water content and the subsequent risk of cerebral edema. The presence and severity of neurologic symptoms depends on both the magnitude and rapidity of decrease in plasma [Na$^+$]. In **acute hyponatremia** (i.e., developing in <2 days), patients may complain of nausea and malaise. As the plasma [Na$^+$] falls further, symptoms may progress to include headache, lethargy, confusion, and obtundation. Stupor, seizures, and coma do not usually occur unless the plasma [Na$^+$] falls acutely below 115 mEq/L. In **chronic hyponatremia** (>3 days in duration), adaptive mechanisms designed to defend cell volume occur and tend to minimize the increase in ICF volume and its symptoms.

Diagnostic Testing

- The underlying cause of hyponatremia can often be ascertained from an accurate history and physical examination, including an assessment of **ECF volume status** and the **effective circulating volume.**
- Three laboratory tests, when used with a clinical assessment of volume status, can narrow the differential diagnosis of hyponatremia: (1) the **plasma osmolality**, (2) the **urine osmolality**, and (3) the **urine [Na$^+$]** (Figure 12-1).
- **Plasma osmolality:** Most patients with hyponatremia have a low plasma osmolality (<275 mOsm/L).
  - Normal serum osmolality suggests **pseudohyponatremia,** a laboratory miscalculation of the plasma sodium content attributed to extremely elevated protein and lipid levels.
  - Elevated serum osmolality suggests **hyperosmolar hyponatremia**, most commonly attributable to hyperglycemia.
- **Urine osmolality:** The appropriate renal response to hypo-osmolality is to excrete a maximally dilute urine.
  - **Low urine osmolality** (urine osmolality <100 mOsm/L and specific gravity <1.003) suggests that renal adaptation is intact but overwhelmed, as seen in primary polydipsia.
  - An elevated urine osmolality indicates that ADH is present, resulting in reabsorption of water.
- **Urine [Na$^+$]** adds laboratory corroboration to the bedside assessment of effective circulating volume and can discriminate between **extrarenal** and **renal losses** of Na$^+$. The appropriate response to decreased effective circulating volume is a urine [Na$^+$] <10 mEq/L. A urine [Na$^+$] of >20 mEq/L suggests a normal effective circulating volume or a Na$^+$-wasting defect.

TREATMENT

- **Rate of correction**
  - In *chronic* hyponatremia, the target rate of correction should not exceed 8 mEq/L over 24 hours.
    - The risk of iatrogenic injury is increased in patients with chronic hyponatremia, since cells adapt to the hypo-osmolar state over time.

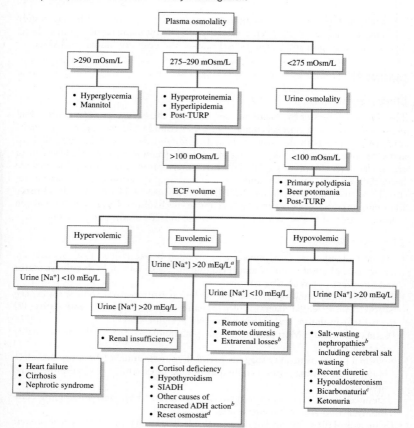

Figure 12-1. Algorithm depicting the diagnostic approach to hyponatremia. ADH, antidiuretic hormone; ECF, extracellular fluid; post-TURP, post–transurethral resection of the prostate syndrome; SIADH, syndrome of inappropriate antidiuretic hormone. [a]Urine [Na+] may be <20 mEq/L with low Na+ intake. [b]See text for details. [c]From vomiting-induced contraction alkalosis or proximal renal tubular acidosis. [d]Urine osmolality may be <100 mOsm/L after a water load.

- The primary risk of overcorrection is the development of central pontine myelinolysis (CPM). CPM results from damage to neurons due to rapid osmotic shifts. In its most overt form, it is characterized by flaccid paralysis, dysarthria, and dysphagia. It can be confirmed by CT scan or MRI of the brain. The risk of precipitating CPM is increased with correction of the [Na+] by 10–12 mEq/L in a 24-hour period.[2] Other risk factors for developing CPM include preexisting hypokalemia, malnutrition, and alcohol use disorder.
  - In *symptomatic* hyponatremia, the serum [Na+] should again be corrected cautiously. A targeted rise in serum [Na+] by 4–6 mEq/L within the first 4–6 hours is generally sufficient to reverse the neurologic sequelae and avoid overcorrection. The total daily correction should still not exceed 8 mEq/d.

- **Type of intervention**
  - In **severe hyponatremia**, hypertonic saline should be used to achieve the correction described above.
    - Hypertonic saline (3% saline) can be given as a continuous infusion in stable severe hyponatremia. A variety of formulas can be used to estimate the infusion rate, but as none of them account for ongoing free water loss, the risk of overcorrection is substantial. A more modest starting rate of 0.25–0.3 ml/kg/h provides a greater margin of safety and can be titrated based on subsequent laboratory data.
    - Alternatively, hypertonic saline can be given in 100 mL boluses (up to three doses as needed). This provides a rapid initial correction, ideal for patients with intracranial lesions or concerns for herniation, while limiting the risk of overcorrection.
    - Since no equation or algorithm can adequately predict dynamic fluctuations in water balance, it is absolutely critical to frequently **recheck laboratory data** to ensure correction at an appropriate rate and adjust fluid administration.
    - Desmopressin acetate (DDAVP) can also be given to prevent overcorrection of hyponatremia, particularly in patients who may have a reversible cause of ADH secretion.
  - In asymptomatic hyponatremia, treatment should be targeted to the cause of the disorder.
    - **Hypovolemic hyponatremia.** In patients with acute hypovolemic hyponatremia, **isotonic** saline can be used to restore the intravascular volume. Because ADH is stimulated by the volume depletion, fluid resuscitation will decrease ADH secretion and facilitate renal elimination of water.
    - **Hypervolemic hyponatremia.** Hyponatremia in congestive heart failure (CHF) and cirrhosis often reflects the severity of the underlying disease. The hyponatremia itself is typically asymptomatic. Definitive treatment requires management of the underlying condition, although restriction of water intake can attenuate the hyponatremia.
    - **SIADH.** In addition to the correction of contributing factors (pneumonia, drugs, etc.), water restriction, solute tablets, and diuretics can also be used.
      - **Water restriction.** This is typically the first-line treatment for SIADH. The amount of fluid restriction depends on the amount of water eliminated by the kidney. A useful guide to the necessary degree of fluid restriction is as follows:
        - If (Urine Na^+ + Urine K^+)/Serum Na^+ <0.5, restrict to 1 L/d.
        - If (Urine Na^+ + Urine K^+)/Serum Na^+ is 0.5–1.0, restrict to 500 mL/d.
        - If (Urine Na^+ + Urine K^+)/Serum Na^+ is >1, the patient has a negative renal free water clearance, and any amount of ingested water may be retained. In such situations, adjunctive therapy is required.
      - **A high dietary solute load** (using salt or urea tablets) can be extremely helpful, particularly since water restriction can be challenging for patients. The obligate water loss that accompanies the excretion of the high dietary solute load helps to alleviate the water retention in SIADH.
      - **Loop diuretics** impair the urinary concentrating mechanism and can enhance free water excretion.
      - **Vasopressin antagonists** promote a water diuresis and may be useful in the therapy of SIADH. Both IV (conivaptan) and oral (tolvaptan) preparations are approved for the treatment of euvolemic hyponatremia. However, given the risks of overcorrection, these agents should be initiated in a closely monitored inpatient setting.

Hypernatremia

GENERAL PRINCIPLES

- Hypernatremia is defined as a plasma $[Na^+]$ >**145 mEq/L** and represents a state of **hyperosmolality** (see "Disorders of Sodium Concentration" section).
- Hypernatremia may be caused by a primary **Na^+ gain** or a **water deficit**, the latter being much more common. Normally, this hyperosmolar state stimulates thirst and the excretion of a maximally concentrated urine. For hypernatremia to persist, one or both of these compensatory mechanisms must be impaired.
- **Impaired thirst response** may occur in situations where access to water is limited, often due to physical restrictions (institutionalized, handicapped, postoperative, or intubated patients) or mental impairment (delirium, dementia).
- **Hypernatremia due to water loss.** The loss of water must occur in excess of electrolyte losses to raise $[Na^+]$.
  - **Nonrenal water loss** may be due to evaporation from the skin and respiratory tract (insensible losses) or loss from the GI tract. Diarrhea is the most common GI cause of hypernatremia. Osmotic diarrhea (induced by lactulose, sorbitol, or malabsorption of carbohydrate) and viral gastroenteritis, in particular, result in disproportional water loss.
  - **Renal water loss** results from either **osmotic diuresis** or **diabetes insipidus (DI).**
    - **Osmotic diuresis** is frequently associated with glycosuria and high osmolar feeds. In addition, increased urea generation from accelerated catabolism, high-protein feeds, and stress-dose steroids can also result in an osmotic diuresis.
    - Hypernatremia secondary to nonosmotic urinary water loss is usually caused by impaired vasopressin secretion **(central diabetes insipidus [CDI])** or resistance to the actions of vasopressin **(nephrogenic diabetes insipidus [NDI]).** Partial defects occur more commonly than complete defects in both types.
    - The most common cause of CDI is destruction of the neurohypophysis from trauma, neurosurgery, granulomatous disease, neoplasms, vascular accidents, or infection. In many cases, CDI is idiopathic.
    - NDI may either be inherited or acquired. Acquired NDI often results from a disruption to the renal concentrating mechanism due to drugs (lithium, demeclocycline, amphotericin), electrolyte disorders (hypercalcemia, hypokalemia), medullary washout (loop diuretics), and intrinsic renal diseases.
- **Hypernatremia due to primary Na^+ gain** occurs infrequently because of the kidney's capacity to excrete the retained Na^+. However, it can rarely occur after repetitive **hypertonic saline** administration or chronic **mineralocorticoid excess.**
- **Transcellular water shift** from ECF to ICF can occur in circumstances of transient intracellular hyperosmolality, as in seizures or rhabdomyolysis.

DIAGNOSIS

Clinical Presentation

- Hypernatremia results in contraction of brain cells as water shifts to attenuate the rising ECF osmolality. Thus, the most severe symptoms of hypernatremia are neurologic, including altered mental status, weakness, neuromuscular irritability, focal neurologic deficits, and, occasionally, coma or seizures. As with hyponatremia, the severity of the clinical manifestations is related to the *acuity* and *magnitude* of the

rise in plasma [Na⁺]. **Chronic hypernatremia** is generally less symptomatic as a result of adaptive mechanisms designed to defend cell volume.
- **CDI and NDI** generally present with complaints of polyuria and thirst. Signs of volume depletion or neurologic dysfunction are generally absent unless the patient has an associated thirst abnormality.

Diagnostic Testing

Urine osmolality and the **response to DDAVP** can help narrow the differential diagnosis for hypernatremia (Figure 12-2).
- The appropriate renal response to hypernatremia is a small volume of concentrated urine (urine osmolality >800 mOsm/L). **Urine osmolality** <800 mOsm/L suggests a defect in renal water conservation.
  - A urine osmolality <300 mOsm/L in the setting of hypernatremia suggests complete forms of CDI and NDI.
  - Urine osmolality between 300 and 800 mOsm/L can occur from partial forms of DI as well as osmotic diuresis. The two can be differentiated by quantifying the daily solute excretion (estimated by the urine osmolality multiplied by urine volume in 24 hours). A daily solute excretion >900 mOsm/L defines an osmotic diuresis.
- **Response to DDAVP.** Complete forms of CDI and NDI can be distinguished by administering the vasopressin analog DDAVP (10 μg intranasally) after careful water restriction. The urine osmolality should increase by at least 50% in complete CDI and does not change in NDI. The diagnosis is sometimes difficult when partial defects are present.

TREATMENT

- **Rate of correction**
  - Aggressive correction of *symptomatic* **hypernatremia** is potentially dangerous, although the risk is not as well defined as overcorrection in hyponatremia. Out of an abundance of caution, the water deficit should be reduced gradually and plasma [Na⁺] levels should be reduced by no more than **10–12 mEq/L/d.**
  - In *chronic* **hypernatremia**, the risk of treatment-related complications may be increased because of the cerebral adaptation to the chronic hyperosmolar state. The plasma [Na⁺] should be lowered at a more moderate rate (between 5 and 8 mEq/L/d).
- **Intervention**
  - The mainstay of management is the administration of water, preferably by mouth or nasogastric tube. Alternatively, 5% dextrose in water (D5W) or quarter NS can be given via IV.
    - The extent of the **free water deficit** can be calculated by the equation:

$$\text{Free water deficit} = \left\{\left([\text{Na}^+] - 140\right)/140\right\} \times (\text{TBW})$$

    - This free water deficit provides a target amount of water that should be replaced to correct the hypernatremia.
    - The rate of water administration can be estimated by dividing this amount by the time frame over which hypernatremia should be normalized to achieve the target rate of correction outlined above.
      - Example: For a 3-L free water deficit that you wish to correct over 24 hours, the D5W can be run at 3 L/24 h = 125 mL/h.

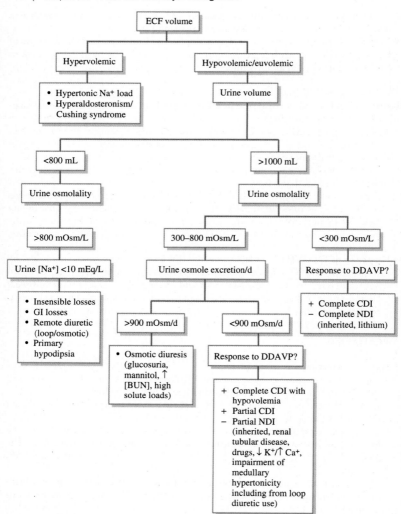

Figure 12-2. Algorithm depicting the diagnostic approach to hypernatremia. BUN, blood urea nitrogen; ↑Ca^+, hypercalcemia; CDI, central diabetes insipidus; DDAVP, desmopressin acetate; ECF, extracellular fluid; GI, gastrointestinal; NDI, nephrogenic diabetes insipidus; ↓K^+, hypokalemia; (+), conditions with increase in urine osmolality in response to desmopressin acetate; (−), conditions with little increase in urine osmolality in response to desmopressin acetate.

  □ It should be noted that this equation does NOT account for ongoing free water losses. Using this equation alone without considering ongoing losses through GI or renal excretion may result in an underestimation of the amount of water required to correct a patient's hypernatremia.

- No single equation adequately captures the dynamic input and output of free water in a patient. Because of this, it is critically important to **recheck laboratory data** to ensure that an appropriate rate of correction is being achieved.
  - Specific therapies for the underlying cause
    - **Hypovolemic hypernatremia.** In patients with mild volume depletion, Na^+-containing solutions such as 0.45% NS can be used to replenish the ECF as well as the water deficit. If patients have severe or symptomatic volume depletion, correction of volume status with **isotonic fluid** should take precedence over correction of the hyperosmolar state. Once the patient is hemodynamically stable, hypotonic fluid can be given to replace the free water deficit.
    - **Hypernatremia from primary Na^+ gain** is unusual. Cessation of iatrogenic Na^+ is typically sufficient.
    - **DI without hypernatremia.** DI is best treated by removing the underlying cause. Despite the renal water loss, DI should not result in hypernatremia if the thirst mechanism remains intact. However, treatment is sometimes required to alleviate symptomatic polyuria.
      - **CDI.** Because the polyuria is the result of impaired secretion of vasopressin, treatment is best accomplished with the administration of DDAVP, a vasopressin analog.
      - **NDI.** A low-Na^+ diet combined with **thiazide** diuretics will decrease polyuria by inducing mild volume depletion. This enhances proximal reabsorption of salt and water, thus decreasing urinary free water loss. Decreasing protein intake will further decrease urine output by minimizing the solute load that must be excreted.

POTASSIUM

- Potassium is the major **intracellular** cation.
- The K^+ intake of individuals on an average Western diet is approximately 1 mEq/kg/d, 90% of which is absorbed by the GI tract. Maintenance of the steady state necessitates matching K^+ excretion with ingestion.
- The elimination of potassium occurs predominately through **renal excretion.** It is highly dependent on the **distal urine flow rate and aldosterone,** both of which enhance Na reabsorption in exchange for K+ secretion in the distal nephron.

Hypokalemia

GENERAL PRINCIPLES

- Hypokalemia is defined as a plasma $[K^+]$ <3.5 mEq/L.
- True hypokalemia may result from one or more of the following: (1) **decreased net intake,** (2) **shift into cells,** or (3) **increased net loss.**
  - **Diminished intake** is seldom the sole cause of K^+ depletion because urinary excretion can be effectively decreased to <15 mEq/d. However, dietary K^+ restriction may exacerbate the hypokalemia from GI or renal loss.
  - **Transcellular shift.** Movement of K^+ into cells may transiently decrease the plasma $[K^+]$ without altering total body K^+ content. These shifts can result from alkalemia, insulin, and catecholamine release. **Hypokalemic periodic paralysis** is a rare

disorder that predisposes patients to transcellular K^+ shifts that result in episodic muscle weakness. The hypokalemic form can be triggered after a carbohydrate-rich meal.

- **Nonrenal K^+ loss.** Hypokalemia may result from the loss of potassium-rich fluids from the lower GI tract. Hypokalemia from the loss of upper GI contents is typically more attributable to renal K^+ secretion from secondary hyperaldosteronism.
- **Renal K^+ loss** accounts for most cases of *chronic* hypokalemia. This may be caused by any of the following factors:
  - **Augmented distal urine flow** occurs commonly with diuretic use and osmotic diuresis (e.g., glycosuria). Bartter and Gitelman syndromes mimic diuretic use and promote renal K^+ loss by the same mechanism.
  - **Hyperaldosteronism** can result in increased renal K^+ loss because aldosterone plays a central role in coupling the reabsorption of sodium with the excretion of potassium.
    - **Primary mineralocorticoid excess** can be the result of an adrenal adenoma or adrenocortical hyperplasia.
    - Cortisol also has an affinity for mineralocorticoid receptors but is typically converted quickly to cortisone, which has markedly less mineralocorticoid activity. Still, if cortisol is present in abundance (Cushing syndrome) or fails to be converted to cortisone (syndrome of mineralocorticoid excess), it may mimic hyperaldosteronism.
    - **Secondary hyperaldosteronism** can be seen in any situation with a decreased effective circulating volume.
    - Constitutive activation of the distal renal epithelial Na^+ channel can mimic hyperaldosteronism. This occurs in a number of monogenic disorders, including **Liddle syndrome**, and leads to hypertension and hypokalemia. Unlike primary or secondary hyperaldosteronism, aldosterone levels are often suppressed in disorders of the epithelial Na^+ channel.

DIAGNOSIS

Clinical Presentation

- The clinical features of K^+ depletion vary greatly and their severity depends in part on the degree of hypokalemia. Symptoms seldom occur unless the plasma [K^+] is <3.0 mEq/L.
- Fatigue, myalgias, and muscular weakness or cramps of the lower extremities are common. Smooth muscle function may also be affected and may manifest with complaints of constipation or frank paralytic ileus. Severe hypokalemia may lead to complete paralysis, hypoventilation, or rhabdomyolysis.

Diagnostic Testing

- When the etiology is not immediately apparent, **renal K^+ excretion** and the **acid–base status** can help identify the cause.
- **Urine K^+.** The appropriate response to hypokalemia is to excrete <25 mEq/d of K^+ in the urine. Urinary K^+ excretion can be measured with a 24-hour urine collection or estimated by multiplying the spot urine [K^+] by the total daily urine output. A spot urine [K^+] may be helpful (urine [K^+] <15 mEq/L suggests appropriate K^+ conservation), but the results can be confounded by a variety of factors.
- **Acid–base status.** Intracellular shifting and renal excretion of K^+ are often closely linked with the acid–base status. Hypokalemia is generally associated with metabolic

alkalosis and can play a critical role in the maintenance of metabolic alkalosis. The finding of metabolic acidosis in a patient with hypokalemia thus narrows the differential significantly, implying lower GI loss, distal renal tubular acidosis (RTA), or the excretion of a nonreabsorbable anion from an organic acid (diabetic ketoacidosis [DKA], hippurate from toluene intoxication).
- **ECG** changes associated with hypokalemia include flattening or inversion of the T wave, a prominent U wave, ST-segment depression, and a prolonged QU interval. Severe K^+ depletion may result in a prolonged PR interval, decreased voltage, and widening of the QRS complex.

TREATMENT

- The **therapeutic goals** are to safely correct the K^+ deficit and to minimize ongoing losses through treatment of the underlying cause. Hypomagnesemia should also be sought in all hypokalemic patients and corrected to allow effective K^+ repletion.
- Correction of the K^+ deficit can be accomplished with either oral or IV therapy.
- **Oral therapy.** It is generally safer to correct the K^+ deficit via the oral route when hypokalemia is mild and the patient can tolerate oral administration. Oral doses of 40 mEq are generally well tolerated and can be given as often as every 4 hours. Traditionally, 10 mEq of potassium salts are given for each 0.10 mEq/L decrement in serum $[K^+]$. However, with increasing severity of hypokalemia, this grossly underestimates the K^+ necessary to normalize *total* K^+ content. Furthermore, as the K^+ shifts back to the intracellular space, it may appear as though K^+ supplementation is doing very little to correct ECF $[K^+]$. In such cases, potassium supplementation should be increased and continued until serum levels rise.
- **IV therapy.** Patients with imminently life-threatening hypokalemia and those who are unable to take anything by mouth require IV replacement therapy with KCl. The maximum concentration of administered K^+ should be no more than 40 mEq/L via a peripheral vein or 100 mEq/L via a central vein. The rate of infusion should not exceed 20 mEq/h unless paralysis or malignant ventricular arrhythmias are present. Rapid IV administration of K^+ should be used judiciously and requires close observation.

Hyperkalemia

GENERAL PRINCIPLES

- Hyperkalemia is defined as a plasma $[K^+]$ >**5.0 mEq/L.**
- **Pseudohyperkalemia** represents an artificially elevated plasma $[K^+]$ due to K^+ movement out of cells immediately before or following venipuncture. Contributing factors include repeated fist clenching, hemolysis, and marked leukocytosis or thrombocytosis.
- True hyperkalemia occurs as a result of one of the following:
  - **Transcellular shift.** Insulin deficiency, hyperosmolality, nonselective β-blockers, digitalis, metabolic acidosis (excluding those from organic acids), and depolarizing muscle relaxants, such as succinylcholine, release K^+ from ICF stores into the ECF compartment. The release of intracellular K+ can also be seen after severe exercise, rhabdomyolysis, and tumor lysis syndrome.
  - **Increased exposure to K^+** is rarely the sole cause of hyperkalemia unless there is an impairment in renal excretion. Foods with a high content of K^+ include salt

substitutes, dried fruits, nuts, tomatoes, potatoes, spinach, bananas, and oranges. Juices derived from these foods may be especially rich sources.

- ○ **Decreased renal K^+ excretion.** In the setting of hyperkalemia, the kidney is capable of generating a significant urinary excretion of K^+. This process can be impaired by a number of processes, including volume depletion, renal injury, adrenal insufficiency, and hyporeninemic hypoaldosteronism (type 4 RTA).
- **Drugs** may also be implicated in the genesis of hyperkalemia through a variety of mechanisms. Common culprits include angiotensin-converting enzyme inhibitors, angiotensin receptor blockers, potassium-sparing diuretics, NSAIDs, and cyclosporine. Heparin and ketoconazole can also contribute to hyperkalemia through the decreased production of aldosterone, although these agents alone are typically insufficient to sustain a clinically significant hyperkalemia.

DIAGNOSIS

Clinical Presentation

- The most serious effect of hyperkalemia is cardiac arrhythmogenesis secondary to potassium's pivotal role in membrane potentials. Patients may present with palpitations, syncope, or even sudden cardiac death.
- Severe hyperkalemia causes partial depolarization of the skeletal muscle cell membrane and may manifest as weakness, potentially progressing to flaccid paralysis and hypoventilation if the respiratory muscles are involved.

Diagnostic Testing

- If the etiology is not readily apparent and the patient is asymptomatic, **pseudohyperkalemia** should be excluded by rechecking laboratory data.
- An assessment of **renal [K^+] excretion** and the **renin–angiotensin–aldosterone axis** can help narrow the differential diagnosis when the etiology is not immediately apparent.
  - ○ Low aldosterone levels suggest either adrenal disease (renin levels elevated) or hyporeninemic hypoaldosteronism (renin levels low; occurs with type 4 RTA).
  - ○ High aldosterone levels, typically accompanied by high renin levels, suggest aldosterone resistance (pseudohypoaldosteronism) but can also be seen in K^+-sparing diuretics.
- **ECG** changes include increased T-wave amplitude or peaked T waves. More severe degrees of hyperkalemia result in a prolonged PR interval and QRS duration, atrioventricular conduction delay, and loss of P waves. Progressive widening of the QRS complex and its merging with the T wave produce a sine wave pattern. The terminal event is usually ventricular fibrillation or asystole.

TREATMENT

Severe hyperkalemia with ECG changes is a medical emergency and requires immediate treatment directed at minimizing membrane depolarization and acutely reducing the ECF [K^+]. **Acute therapy** may consist of some or all of the following (the hypokalemic effect is additive):

- **Calcium gluconate** decreases membrane excitability but does not lower [K^+]. The usual dose is 10 mL of a 10% solution infused over 2–3 minutes. The effect begins within minutes but is short lived (30–60 minutes), and the dose can be repeated if no improvement in the ECG is seen after 5–10 minutes.

- **Insulin** causes K^+ to shift into cells and temporarily lowers the plasma $[K^+]$. A commonly used combination is 10–20 units of regular insulin and 25–50 g of glucose administered IV. Hyperglycemic patients should be given the insulin alone.
- **NaHCO$_3$** is effective for severe hyperkalemia associated with metabolic acidosis. In the acute setting, it can be given as an IV isotonic solution (three ampules of $NaHCO_3$ in 1 L of 5% dextrose).
- **β_2-Adrenergic agonists** promote cellular uptake of K^+. The onset of action is 30 minutes, lowering the plasma $[K^+]$ by 0.5–1.5 mEq/L, and the effect lasts for 2–4 hours. Albuterol can be administered in a dose of 10–20 mg as a continuous nebulized treatment over 30–60 minutes.
- **Longer term** means for $[K^+]$ removal.
  ○ Increasing distal Na^+ delivery in the kidney enhances renal K^+ clearance. This can be achieved with the administration of saline in patients who appear volume depleted. Otherwise, diuretics can be used if renal function is adequate.
  ○ **Cation exchange resins,** such as sodium zirconium cyclosilicate and patiromer, promote the excretion of K^+ in the GI tract and can be used in the management of chronic or resistant hyperkalemia. Both agents appear to be effective, well tolerated, and safe. The usual dose of patiromer is 8.4 g mixed with 100 mL of water, given daily. Sodium zirconium cyclosilicate may have a faster onset of action and is usually initiated at 10 g up to three times/day.
- **Dialysis** should be reserved for patients with renal failure and those with severe life-threatening hyperkalemia who are unresponsive to more conservative measures.
- **Chronic therapy** may involve dietary modifications to avoid high K^+ foods, correction of metabolic acidosis with oral alkali, the promotion of kaliuresis with diuretics, and/or administration of exogenous mineralocorticoid in states of hypoaldosteronism.

CALCIUM

- Approximately 99% of body calcium is in bone; most of the remaining 1% is in the ECF. Nearly 50% of serum calcium is ionized (free), whereas the remainder is complexed to albumin (40%) and anions such as phosphate (10%).
- **Calcium balance** is regulated by **parathyroid hormone** (PTH) and **calcitriol.**
  ○ **PTH** increases serum calcium by stimulating bone resorption, increasing calcium reclamation in the kidney, and promoting renal conversion of vitamin D to calcitriol. Serum calcium regulates PTH secretion by a negative feedback mechanism: Hypocalcemia stimulates and hypercalcemia suppresses PTH release.
  ○ **Calcitriol** [1,25-dihydroxycholecalciferol, 1,25-dihydroxyvitamin D_3, or $1,25(OH)_2D_3$] is the active form of vitamin D. It stimulates intestinal absorption of calcium and is one of many factors that provide feedback to the parathyroid gland.

Hypercalcemia

GENERAL PRINCIPLES

- A serum calcium >**10.3 mg/dL** with a normal serum albumin or an ionized calcium >**5.2 mg/dL** defines hypercalcemia.
- Clinically significant hypercalcemia typically requires both an increase in ECF calcium and a decrease in renal calcium clearance. Underlying disturbances to calcium

metabolism are thus often masked by compensatory mechanisms until the patient develops a concomitant disorder, such as decreased renal clearance from volume depletion. More than 90% of cases are due to **primary hyperparathyroidism** or **malignancy.**

- **Primary hyperparathyroidism** causes most cases of hypercalcemia in *ambulatory* patients.
- **Malignancy** is responsible for most cases of hypercalcemia among *hospitalized* patients. Patients usually have advanced, clinically obvious disease. In these patients, hypercalcemia may develop from stimulation of osteoclast bone resorption from tumor cell products, tumor-derived **PTH-related peptide** (PTHrP), and tumor calcitriol production.
- Less common causes account for about 10% of cases of hypercalcemia and include increased vitamin D activity (exogenous exposure to vitamin D or increased generation of calcitriol in chronic granulomatous diseases), **the milk-alkali syndrome** (acute or chronic development of hypercalcemia, alkalosis, and renal failure from the ingestion of large quantities of calcium-containing antacids), adrenal insufficiency, prolonged immobilization, Paget disease, and acromegaly.

DIAGNOSIS

Clinical Presentation

Clinical manifestations generally are present only if serum calcium exceeds 12 mg/dL and tend to be more severe if hypercalcemia develops rapidly. Most patients with **primary hyperparathyroidism** have asymptomatic hypercalcemia that is found incidentally. Symptoms include renal manifestations (polyuria and nephrolithiasis and risk of renal failure with nephrocalcinosis when calcium level rises above 13 mg/dL), GI symptoms (anorexia, vomiting, constipation), and neurologic symptoms (weakness, fatigue, confusion, stupor, and coma).

Diagnostic Testing

- **Serum calcium** should be interpreted with knowledge of the serum albumin, or an ionized calcium should be measured. **Corrected $[Ca^{2+}]$ = $[Ca^{2+}]$ + {0.8 × (4.0 − [albumin])}.** Many patients with primary hyperparathyroidism will have a calcium level that is chronically within the high-normal range.
- Intact **serum PTH** may be the most important first step in the evaluation of hypercalcemia.
  - ○ Elevations in ECF calcium typically result in suppression of PTH. Thus, the finding of a normal or elevated intact PTH in the setting of hypercalcemia is suggestive of primary hyperparathyroidism.
  - ○ When the intact PTH is appropriately suppressed, **PTHrP** can be measured to investigate possible humoral hypercalcemia of malignancy.
- **$1,25(OH)_2D_3$** levels are elevated in granulomatous disorders, primary hyperparathyroidism, calcitriol overdose, and acromegaly.
- **Serum phosphorus** is often decreased in hyperparathyroidism because of stimulation of phosphaturia, whereas Paget disease and vitamin D intoxication both tend to have increased phosphorus levels.
- **Urine calcium** may be elevated in primary hyperparathyroidism because of a filtered load of calcium that exceeds the capacity for renal reabsorption. If the family history and clinical picture are suggestive, patients with **familial hypocalciuric**

hypercalcemia can be distinguished from patients with primary hyperparathyroidism by documenting a low calcium clearance by 24-hour urine collection (<200 mg calcium per day) or fractional excretion of calcium (<1%).
- **ECG** may reveal a shortened QT interval and, with very severe hypercalcemia, variable degrees of atrioventricular block.

TREATMENT

- **Acute management** of hypercalcemia is warranted if severe symptoms are present or with serum calcium >12 mg/dL. The following regimen is presented in the order that therapy should be given.
  - ○ **Correction of hypovolemia** with 0.9% saline fluid is mandatory in patients who demonstrate volume depletion, because hypovolemia prevents effective calciuresis. Maintenance fluids can be continued after achieving euvolemia to sustain a urine output of 100–150 mL/h. The patient should be monitored closely for signs of volume overload.
  - ○ **IV bisphosphonates** can be used to decrease the liberation of calcium from bone in persistent hypercalcemia. Pamidronate 60 mg is infused over 2–4 hours; for severe hypercalcemia (>13.5 mg/dL), 90 mg can be given over the same duration. A hypocalcemic response is typically seen within 2 days and may persist for 2 weeks or longer. Treatment can be repeated after 7 days if hypercalcemia recurs. Zoledronate is a more potent bisphosphonate that is given as a 4-mg dose infused over at least 15 minutes. Hydration should precede bisphosphonate use. Renal insufficiency is a relative contraindication.
- Other options
  - ○ **Calcitonin** inhibits bone resorption and increases renal calcium excretion. Salmon calcitonin, 4–8 IU/kg IM or SC every 6–12 hours, lowers serum calcium 1–2 mg/dL within several hours in 60%–70% of patients. Although it is less potent than other inhibitors of bone resorption, it has no serious toxicity, is safe in renal failure, and may have an analgesic effect in patients with skeletal metastases.
  - ○ **Glucocorticoids** are effective in hypercalcemia due to hematologic malignancies and granulomatous production of calcitriol. The initial dose is 20–60 mg/d of prednisone or its equivalent. After serum calcium stabilizes, the dose should be gradually reduced to the minimum needed to control symptoms of hypercalcemia.
  - ○ **Denosumab** is a receptor activator of nuclear factor kappa-B ligand inhibitor that can be used in patients with hypercalcemia that is refractory to bisphosphonates or in patients with a contraindication to bisphosphonate therapy, such as patients with chronic kidney disease. It is given at a dose of 120 mg SC weekly for 4 weeks and then monthly.
  - ○ **Dialysis.** Hemodialysis and peritoneal dialysis using low calcium dialysate are effective for patients with very severe hypercalcemia (>16 mg/dL) and CHF or renal insufficiency.
- **Chronic management** of hypercalcemia
  - ○ **Primary hyperparathyroidism.** In many patients, this disorder has a benign course, with minimal fluctuation in serum calcium concentration and no obvious clinical sequelae. Parathyroidectomy is indicated in patients with (1) corrected serum calcium >1.0 mg/dL above the upper limit of normal, (2) creatinine clearance <60 mL/min, (3) age <50 years, and (4) bone density at hip, lumbar spine, or

distal radius >2.5 standard deviations below peak bone mass (T score <−2.5) and/
or previous fragility fracture.[3] Surgical intervention typically has a high success rate
(95%) with low morbidity and mortality.

○ **Medical therapy** may be a reasonable option in asymptomatic patients who are
not surgical candidates. Management consists of liberal oral hydration with a
high-salt diet, daily physical activity to lessen bone resorption, and avoidance of
thiazide diuretics. Oral bisphosphonates and estrogen replacement therapy or raloxifene in postmenopausal women can be considered in the appropriate clinical
context. Cinacalcet, an activator of the calcium-sensing receptor, has also been
shown to reduce PTH secretion and serum calcium levels.

○ **Malignant hypercalcemia.** Bisphosphonate and glucocorticoid therapy with a
calcium-restricted diet (<400 mg/d) can be tried, although these maneuvers rarely
yield long-term success unless the malignancy responds to treatment. **Denosumab**
may be used in patients with persistent hypercalcemia of malignancy in whom
bisphosphonates may be contraindicated because of renal failure.

Hypocalcemia

GENERAL PRINCIPLES

- A serum calcium **<8.4 mg/dL** with a normal serum albumin or an ionized calcium
<4.2 mg/dL defines hypocalcemia.
- **Effective hypoparathyroidism.** Reduced PTH activity can result from decreased
PTH release from autoimmune, infiltrative, or iatrogenic (e.g., post-thyroidectomy)
destruction of parathyroid tissue. Release of PTH is also impaired with both hypomagnesemia (<1 mg/dL) and severe hypermagnesemia (>6 mg/dL).
- **Vitamin D deficiency** lowers total body calcium but does not usually affect serum
calcium levels unless the deficiency is severe because the resultant secondary hyperparathyroidism often corrects serum calcium levels. Significant vitamin D deficiency
can occur in the elderly or those with limited sun exposure, advanced liver disease
(due to decreased synthesis of precursors), and nephrotic syndrome. Reduced activity in vitamin D activation via 1-α-hydroxylase activity can be seen with vitamin
D–dependent rickets and chronic renal insufficiency.
- Serum calcium levels may also be reduced by profound elevations in serum phosphorus or oxalate, which bind with the calcium and deposit in various tissues. Calcium
can also be bound by citrate (during transfusion of citrate-containing blood products or with continual renal replacement using citrate anticoagulation) as well as by
drugs such as foscarnet and fluoroquinolones. Increased binding to albumin can
also be seen in the context of alkalemia, which increases the exposure of negatively
charged binding sites on albumin.

DIAGNOSIS

Clinical Presentation

- Clinical manifestations vary with the degree of hypocalcemia and rate of onset.
- Acute, severe hypocalcemia may cause laryngospasm, confusion, seizures, or vascular collapse with bradycardia and decompensated heart failure.
- Acute, moderate hypocalcemia may cause increased excitability of nerves and muscles, leading to circumoral or distal paresthesias and tetany.

- **Trousseau sign** is the development of carpal spasm when a blood pressure cuff is inflated above systolic pressure for 3 minutes. **Chvostek sign** refers to twitching of the facial muscles when the facial nerve is tapped anterior to the ear. The presence of these signs is known as **latent tetany.**

Diagnostic Testing

- Laboratory data should be used to evaluate the calcium–PTH axis as well as concurrent mineral abnormalities.
- **Albumin** should be measured when there is an abnormality in serum calcium levels to rule out pseudohypocalcemia.
- **Serum PTH** that is low or inappropriately normal in the setting of hypocalcemia is indicative of hypoparathyroidism. A high PTH is often found with vitamin D deficiency, PTH resistance, and hyperphosphatemia.
- **Serum phosphorus** is often helpful in identifying vitamin D deficiency (low calcium, low phosphorus) or intravascular chelation of calcium (low calcium, high phosphorus).
- **Vitamin D** stores are usually assessed by measuring only $25(OH)D_3$ because calcitriol $[1,25(OH)_2D_3]$ levels can be normalized through the compensatory increase of 1-α-hydroxylase activity.
- **Magnesium** deficiency should always be ruled out during management of hypocalcemia.
- **ECG** may show a prolonged QT interval and bradycardia.

TREATMENT

Acute management of symptomatic hypocalcemia requires prompt and aggressive therapy.

- **Phosphorus** must first be checked. In severe hyperphosphatemia (>6.5 mg/dL), administration of calcium will increase the calcium–phosphorus product and may exacerbate the formation of ectopic calcifications. In acute, symptomatic hypocalcemia with severe hyperphosphatemia, dialysis may be needed to acutely manage the mineral abnormalities. If the hypocalcemia is asymptomatic, a reduction of phosphorus should precede aggressive calcium supplementation.
- **Hypomagnesemia,** if present, must be treated first to effectively correct the hypocalcemia.
- **Calcium supplementation.** IV calcium should be reserved for severe or symptomatic hypocalcemia and can be administered as calcium chloride or calcium gluconate. Calcium gluconate is typically favored because of reduced risk of tissue toxicity with extravasation. Calcium gluconate is often prepared as a 10% solution (100 mg of calcium gluconate per mL). One ampule (10 mL) of calcium gluconate thus contains 1000 mg of calcium gluconate and approximately 90 mg of elemental calcium.
- **Chronic management.** Treatment requires calcium supplements and vitamin D or its active metabolite to increase intestinal calcium absorption.
  - **Oral calcium supplements.** Calcium carbonate (40% elemental calcium) or calcium acetate (25% elemental calcium) can be given with the goal administration of 1–2 g of *elemental* calcium PO tid. Calcium supplementation should be given apart from meals to minimize binding with phosphorus and maximize enteric absorption.
  - **Vitamin D.** Simple dietary deficiency can be corrected by the use of ergocalciferol 400–1000 IU/d. A 6- to 8-week regimen of 50,000 IU should be dosed weekly in

those with underlying impairments in vitamin D metabolism (i.e., renal insufficiency) and daily in patients with severe malnutrition or malabsorption.

○ In comparison, **calcitriol** has a much more rapid onset of action. The initial dosage is 0.25 μg daily, and most patients are maintained on 0.5–2.0 μg daily. The dose can be increased at 2- to 4-week intervals. Because calcitriol increases enteric absorption of phosphorus as well as calcium, phosphorus levels should be monitored and oral phosphate binders initiated if phosphorus exceeds the normal range.

PHOSPHORUS

- Approximately 85% of **total body phosphorus** is in bone, and most of the remainder is within cells. Thus, serum phosphorus levels may not reflect total body phosphorus stores.
- **Phosphorus balance** is determined primarily by four factors:
  ○ **PTH** regulates the incorporation and release of minerals from bone stores and decreases proximal tubular reabsorption of phosphate, causing urinary wasting.
  ○ The **phosphate concentration** itself regulates renal proximal reabsorption.
  ○ **Insulin** lowers serum levels by shifting phosphate into cells.
  ○ **Calcitriol** [$1,25(OH)_2D_3$] increases serum phosphate by enhancing intestinal phosphorus absorption.

Hyperphosphatemia

GENERAL PRINCIPLES

- A serum phosphate >**4.5 mg/dL** defines hyperphosphatemia.
- **Hyperphosphatemia** is caused by one of the following:
  ○ **Transcellular shift** occurs in rhabdomyolysis, tumor lysis syndrome, and massive hemolysis as phosphorus is released from cells into the ECF. Metabolic acidosis and hypoinsulinemia reduce phosphorus flux into cells and contribute to the hyperphosphatemia sometimes seen in DKA.
  ○ **Increased intake** leading to hyperphosphatemia usually occurs in the setting of renal insufficiency, either with dietary indiscretion in chronic kidney disease or as an iatrogenic complication. The latter can be seen when Phospho-Soda enemas (e.g., Fleet) or active vitamin D analogs are given to patients with renal insufficiency.
  ○ **Decreased renal excretion** occurs most commonly in the setting of renal failure. Occasionally, hypoparathyroidism and pseudohypoparathyroidism reduce renal phosphorus clearance as well.

DIAGNOSIS

Clinical Presentation

- Signs and symptoms are typically attributable to hypocalcemia and the metastatic calcification of soft tissues. Occasionally, skin deposition can result in severe pruritus. **Calciphylaxis** describes the tissue ischemia that may result from the calcification of smaller blood vessels and their subsequent thrombosis.
- Chronic hyperphosphatemia contributes to the development of renal mineral/bone disorders such as secondary hyperparathyroidism (see Chapter 13, Renal Diseases).

Diagnostic Testing

The elevated serum phosphorus can be accompanied by hypocalcemia as a result of **intravascular chelation** of calcium by phosphorus.

TREATMENT

- **Acute hyperphosphatemia** is treated by increasing renal excretion of phosphorus, and as such, treatment is limited when renal insufficiency is present.
  - **Recovery of renal function** will often correct the hyperphosphatemia in the patient within 12 hours. Saline and/or acetazolamide (15 mg/kg q4h) can be given to further encourage phosphaturia, if needed.
  - **Hemodialysis** may be required, especially if irreversible renal insufficiency or symptomatic hypocalcemia is present.
- **Chronic hyperphosphatemia** is almost always associated with chronic kidney disease. Its management consists of reducing phosphorus intake through dietary modification and the use of phosphate binders. This is discussed more fully in Chapter 13, Renal Diseases.

Hypophosphatemia

GENERAL PRINCIPLES

- A serum phosphate **<2.8 mg/dL** defines hypophosphatemia.
- Hypophosphatemia may be caused by one of the following:
  - **Impaired intestinal absorption** occurs with the malabsorption syndromes, the use of oral phosphate binders, or vitamin D deficiency from any cause. Chronic alcoholism is often associated with poor intake of both phosphate and vitamin D resulting in total body phosphorus depletion.
  - **Increased renal excretion** occurs with high levels of PTH, as seen in hyperparathyroidism. Hypophosphatemia may also occur from osmotic diuresis and disorders of proximal tubular transport such as familial X-linked hypophosphatemic rickets and Fanconi syndrome. In acutely ill patients on continuous renal replacement therapy, the removal of phosphorous by slow continuous dialysis can also result in hypophosphatemia.
  - **Transcellular shift** is stimulated by respiratory alkalosis as well as insulin. The latter is responsible for the paradoxical reduction in phosphorus during treatment of malnutrition with hyperalimentation (**the refeeding syndrome**). The endogenous increase in insulin during treatment shifts phosphorus intracellularly, further reducing serum phosphorus in the malnourished individual. Phosphorus can also be rapidly absorbed into bone following parathyroidectomy for severe hyperparathyroidism (hungry bone syndrome).

DIAGNOSIS

Clinical Presentation

Signs and symptoms typically occur only if total body phosphate depletion is severe. Manifestations include muscle injury (rhabdomyolysis, impaired diaphragmatic function, and heart failure), neurologic abnormalities (paresthesias, dysarthria, confusion, stupor, seizures, and coma), and rarely, hemolysis and platelet dysfunction.

Diagnostic Testing

- The cause is usually apparent from the clinical situation in which the hypophosphatemia occurs. If not, measurement of **urine phosphorus excretion** helps define the mechanism. Renal excretion of >100 mg by 24-hour urine collection or a fractional excretion of phosphate >5% during hypophosphatemia indicates excessive renal loss.
- Low serum **25(OH)D₃** suggests dietary vitamin D deficiency or malabsorption. An elevated **intact PTH** may occur in primary or secondary hyperparathyroidism.

TREATMENT

- **Acute moderate hypophosphatemia** (1.0–2.5 mg/dL) is common in the hospitalized patient and is often due simply to **transcellular shifts**, requiring no treatment if asymptomatic, except correction of the underlying cause.
- **Acute severe hypophosphatemia** (<1.0 mg/dL) may require IV phosphate therapy when associated with serious clinical manifestations. IV preparations include potassium phosphate (1.5 mEq potassium/mmol phosphate) and sodium phosphate (1.3 mEq sodium/mmol phosphate). Extreme care must be taken to avoid hyperphosphatemia, which may lead to hypocalcemia. If hypotension occurs, acute hypocalcemia should be suspected, and the infusion should be stopped or slowed. Further doses should be based on symptoms and on the serum calcium and phosphorus levels, which should be measured every 8 hours.
- **Chronic hypophosphatemia.** Vitamin D deficiency, if present, should be treated first (see "Calcium, Hypocalcemia, Treatment" section) followed by oral supplementation of 0.5–1.0 g elemental phosphorus PO bid to tid. Preparations include Neutra-Phos (250 mg elemental phosphorus and 7 mEq of Na⁺ and K⁺ per capsule) and Neutra-Phos K⁺ (250 mg elemental phosphorus and 14 mEq K⁺ per capsule). Contents of the capsules should be dissolved in water. Fleet Phospho-Soda (815 mg phosphorus and 33 mEq sodium per 5 mL) is an alternative oral agent. Limiting side effects include nausea and diarrhea.

MAGNESIUM

- **Magnesium** plays an important role in neuromuscular function.
- Approximately 60% of body magnesium is stored in bone, and most of the remainder is found in cells. Only 1% is in the ECF. As a result, the serum magnesium is a poor predictor of intracellular and total body stores and may grossly underestimate total magnesium deficits.
- The main determinant of magnesium balance is the **magnesium concentration** itself, which directly influences renal excretion. Hypomagnesemia stimulates tubular reabsorption of magnesium, whereas hypermagnesemia inhibits it.

Hypermagnesemia

GENERAL PRINCIPLES

- A serum magnesium **>2.2 mEq/L** defines hypermagnesemia.
- Most cases of clinically significant hypermagnesemia are **iatrogenic**, occurring with large doses of magnesium-containing antacids or laxatives and during treatment of preeclampsia with IV magnesium. Because renal excretion is the only means of

lowering serum magnesium levels, the presence of significant renal insufficiency can lead to magnesium toxicity even with therapeutic doses of these antacids and laxatives.
- Mild, insignificant elevations in magnesium can occur in end-stage renal disease patients, theophylline intoxication, DKA, and tumor lysis syndrome.

DIAGNOSIS

Clinical Presentation
- Signs and symptoms are usually seen when the serum magnesium level is >4 mEq/L.
- Neuromuscular abnormalities usually include hyporeflexia (usually the first sign of magnesium toxicity), lethargy, and weakness that can progress to paralysis and diaphragmatic involvement, leading to respiratory failure.
- Cardiac findings include hypotension, bradycardia, and cardiac arrest.

Diagnostic Testing
The **ECG** may reveal bradycardia and prolonged PR, QRS, and QT intervals with magnesium levels of 5–10 mEq/L. Complete heart block or asystole may eventually ensue with levels >15 mEq/L.

TREATMENT

- **Prevention.** In the setting of significant renal insufficiency, the inadvertent administration of magnesium-containing medications (e.g., Maalox, magnesium citrate) should be avoided.
- **Asymptomatic hypermagnesemia.** In the setting of normal renal function, normal magnesium levels will quickly be attained with removal of the magnesium load.
- **Symptomatic hypermagnesemia**
  ○ Prompt supportive therapy is critical, including mechanical ventilation for respiratory failure and a temporary pacemaker for significant bradyarrhythmias.
  ○ The effects of hypermagnesemia can be antagonized quickly by the administration of 10% calcium gluconate 10–20 mL IV (1–2 g) over 10 minutes.
  ○ Renal excretion can be encouraged with saline administration. With significant renal insufficiency, hemodialysis is required for definitive therapy.

Hypomagnesemia

GENERAL PRINCIPLES

- A serum magnesium <**1.3 mEq/L** defines hypomagnesemia.
- Hypomagnesemia is most commonly caused by impaired intestinal absorption and increased renal excretion.
  ○ **Decreased intestinal absorption** occurs in malnutrition (chronic alcoholics or any malabsorption syndrome), GI loss (prolonged diarrhea and nasogastric aspiration), and chronic use of proton pump inhibitors, presumably due to impaired intestinal absorption.
  ○ **Increased renal excretion** of magnesium can occur from increased renal tubular flow (as occurs with osmotic diuresis) as well as impaired tubular function (as seen with resolving acute tubular necrosis, loop diuretics, and Bartter and Gitelman syndromes).

- **Drugs.** Several medications similarly induce defects in tubular magnesium transport including aminoglycosides, amphotericin B, cisplatin, pentamidine, and cyclosporine.

DIAGNOSIS

Clinical Presentation
- Neurologic manifestations include lethargy, confusion, tremor, fasciculations, ataxia, nystagmus, tetany, and seizures.
- Atrial and ventricular arrhythmias may occur, especially in patients treated with digoxin.

Diagnostic Testing
- Low serum $[Mg^{2+}]$ in conjunction with an appropriate clinical scenario is sufficient to establish the diagnosis of **magnesium deficiency.** However, because of the slow exchange of magnesium between the bone and intracellular pools, a normal serum level does not exclude total body **magnesium deficiency.**
- The etiology of hypomagnesemia usually is evident from the clinical context, but if there is uncertainty, measurement of **urine magnesium excretion** is helpful. A 24-hour urine magnesium of >2 mEq (or >24 mg) or a fractional excretion of magnesium of >2% during hypomagnesemia suggests **increased renal excretion.** The fractional excretion of magnesium is calculated by:

$$\left(Urine\ Mg^{2+}/Urine\ Cr \right) \div \left[\left(Serum\ Mg^{2+} \times 0.7 \right)/Serum\ Cr \right] \times 100$$

- Hypocalcemia and/or hypokalemia can often be found as a result of hypomagnesemia-induced derangements in mineral homeostasis.
- **ECG** abnormalities may include a prolonged PR and QT interval with a widened QRS. **Torsades de pointes** is the classically associated arrhythmia.

TREATMENT

- In patients with normal renal function, excess magnesium is readily excreted, and there is little risk of causing hypermagnesemia with recommended doses. However, *magnesium must be given with extreme care in the presence of renal insufficiency.*
- The route of magnesium administration depends on whether clinical manifestations from magnesium deficiency are present.
  ○ **Asymptomatic hypomagnesemia** can be treated orally. Numerous preparations exist, including Mag-Ox 400 (240 mg elemental magnesium per 400-mg tablet), UroMag (84 mg per 140-mg tablet), and sustained-release Slow-Mag (64 mg per tablet). Typically, approximately 240 mg of elemental magnesium is administered daily for mild deficiency, whereas more severe hypomagnesemia may require up to 720 mg/d of elemental magnesium. The major side effect is diarrhea.
  ○ **Severe symptomatic hypomagnesemia** should be treated with 1–2 g magnesium sulfate (1 g magnesium sulfate = 96 mg elemental magnesium) IV over 15 minutes. To account for gradual redistribution to severely depleted intracellular stores, replacement therapy may need to be maintained, often for 3–7 days. Serum

magnesium should be measured daily and the infusion rate adjusted to maintain a serum magnesium level of <2.5 mEq/L. Tendon reflexes should be tested frequently because hyporeflexia suggests hypermagnesemia. Reduced doses and more frequent monitoring must be used even in mild renal insufficiency.

ACID–BASE DISTURBANCES

GENERAL PRINCIPLES

- The normal ECF **pH is 7.40 ± 0.03.** Perturbations in pH can occur with changes in the ratio of $\left[HCO_3^-\right]$ to partial pressure of carbon dioxide (pCO_2) as described by the **Henderson–Hasselbalch equation**:

$$pH = 6.1 + \log\left(\left[HCO_3^-\right] \div \left[pCO_2 \times 0.3\right]\right)$$

- Maintenance of pH is essential for normal cellular function. Three general mechanisms exist to keep it within a narrow window:
  - **Chemical buffering** is mediated by $\left[HCO_3^-\right]$ in the ECF and by protein and phosphate buffers in the ICF. The normal $\left[HCO_3^-\right]$ is 24 ± 2 mEq/L.
  - **Alveolar ventilation** minimizes variations in the pH by altering the pCO_2. The normal pCO_2 is 40 ± 5 mm Hg.
  - **Renal H⁺ handling** allows the kidney to adapt to changes in acid–base status via HCO_3^- reabsorption and excretion of titratable acid (e.g., $H_2PO_4^-$) and NH_4^+.
- **Acidemia and alkalemia** refer to processes that lower and raise pH regardless of mechanism. They can be caused by metabolic or respiratory disturbances:
  - **Metabolic acidosis** is characterized by a decrease in the plasma $\left[HCO_3^-\right]$ due to either HCO_3^- loss or the accumulation of acid.
  - **Metabolic alkalosis** is characterized by an elevation in the plasma $\left[HCO_3^-\right]$ due to either H⁺ loss or HCO_3^- gain.
  - **Respiratory acidosis** is characterized by an elevation in pCO_2 resulting from alveolar hypoventilation.
  - **Respiratory alkalosis** is characterized by a decrease in pCO_2 resulting from hyperventilation.

DIAGNOSIS

Analysis should be systematic so that accurate conclusions are drawn and appropriate therapy initiated. Once the acid–base process is correctly identified, further diagnostic studies may be undertaken to determine the precise etiologies at play.
- **Step 1.** Check arterial blood gas. Acidemia is present when pH is <7.37 and alkalemia when pH >7.43.
- **Step 2.** Establish the primary disturbance by determining whether the change in $\left[HCO_3^-\right]$ or pCO_2 can account for the observed deflection in pH.
  - In acidemia, a decreased $\left[HCO_3^-\right]$ suggests metabolic acidosis, and an elevated pCO_2 suggests respiratory acidosis. In alkalemia, an elevated $\left[HCO_3^-\right]$ suggests metabolic alkalosis, whereas a decreased pCO_2 suggests respiratory alkalosis.

CHAPTER 12

○ A **combined disorder** is present when pH is normal, but the pCO_2 and $[HCO_3^-]$ are both abnormal. Changes in both pCO_2 and $[HCO_3^-]$ can cause the change in pH.

• **Step 3.** Determine whether compensation is appropriate.

○ The **compensatory mechanism** is an adaptation to the primary acid–base disturbance intended to stabilize the changing pH. A respiratory process that shifts the pH in one direction will be compensated by a metabolic process that shifts the pH in the other and vice versa.

○ The effect of compensation is to attenuate, *but not completely correct*, the primary change in pH.

○ The expected compensations for the various primary acid–base derangements are given in Table 12-2.

○ An inappropriate compensatory response suggests the presence of a combined disorder.

○ Example: In a patient with metabolic acidosis, respiratory compensation attenuates the metabolic disturbance to pH by lowering pCO_2. However, if the pCO_2 is higher than expected, respiratory compensation is insufficient, revealing a respiratory acidosis with the primary metabolic acidosis. If pCO_2 is lower than expected, compensation is excessive, revealing a concomitant respiratory alkalosis.

• **Step 4.** Determine the **anion gap (AG)**.

○ In normal individuals, the total serum cations are balanced with the total serum anions. Total cations comprise measured cations (MCs) and unmeasured cations, whereas total anions comprise measured anions (MAs) and unmeasured anions (UAs). Certain forms of acidosis are characterized by an increase in the pool of UAs. The **AG** is merely a way of demonstrating the accumulation of this UA.

TABLE 12-2	Expected Compensatory Responses to Primary Acid–Base Disorders	
Disorder	**Primary Change**	**Compensatory Response**
Metabolic acidosis	↓ [HCO32]	↓ pCO_2 1.2 mm Hg for every 1 mEq/L ↓ [HCO32] OR pCO_2 = last two digits of pH
Metabolic alkalosis	↑ [HCO32]	↑ pCO_2 0.7 mm Hg for every 1 mEq/L ↑ [HCO32]
Respiratory acidosis	↑ pCO_2	–
Acute	–	↑ [HCO32] 1.0 mEq/L for every 10 mm Hg ↑ pCO_2
Chronic	–	↑ [HCO32] 3.5 mEq/L for every 10 mm Hg ↑ pCO_2
Respiratory alkalosis	↓ pCO_2	–
Acute	–	↓ [HCO32] 2.0 mEq/L for every 10 mm Hg ↓ pCO_2
Chronic	–	↓ [HCO32] 5.0 mEq/L for every 10 mm Hg ↓ pCO_2

○ > $AG = \left[Na^+\right] - \left[Cl^-\right] + \left[HCO_3^-\right]$. The normal AG is 10 ± 2 mEq/L.

$$UA - UC = MC - MA$$

○ Because total cations = total anions:

$$AG = \text{the excess of unmeasured anions (vs. unmeasured cations)}$$
$$= UA - UC$$

○ Rearranging the equation:

$$MC + UC = MA + UA$$

○ MCs are Na^+; MAs are Cl^- and HCO_3^- .
○ Because albumin is the principal UA, the AG should be corrected if there are gross changes in serum albumin levels.

$$\mathbf{AG_{correct} = AG + \left\{(4 - [albumin]) \times 2.5\right\}}$$

○ An elevated AG suggests the presence of metabolic acidosis with a circulating anion (Table 12-3).

TABLE 12-3	The Four Primary Acid–Base Disorders and Their Common Etiologies		
	Acidosis		**Alkalosis**
Metabolic	Gap • Ketoacids (starvation, alcoholic, diabetic) • Exposures (methanol, ethylene glycol, salicylates) • Lactic acid (shock, drug related) • Profound uremia		Generation • Loss of H^+-rich fluids (GI loss) • Contraction alkalosis • Alkali administration
	Nongap • Nonrenal HCO_3^- loss (diarrhea) • Renal $HCO_3 2$ loss (type 2 RTA) • ↓ H secretion (type 1 RTA) • Hypoaldosteronism (type 4 RTA)		Maintenance • Volume contraction • Chloride depletion • Hypokalemia
		Type 1 RTA / **Type 2 RTA** / **Type 4 RTA**	
	Serum [K]	↓ or nl / ↓ or nl / ↑	
	Serum [HCO₃]	<10 / 15–20 / >15	
	Urine pH	>5.3 / Varies / <5.3	
Respiratory	Depression of respiratory center Neuromuscular failure Lung disease		CNS stimulation Hypoxemia Anxiety

CNS, central nervous system; GI, gastrointestinal; nl, normal; RTA, renal tubular acidosis.

- **Step 5.** Assess the delta gap.
  - To maintain a stable total anion content, every increase in an UA should be met with a decrease in HCO_3^-. Comparing the change in the AG (ΔAG) with the change in the $\left[HCO_3^-\right]$ $\left(\Delta\left[HCO_3^-\right]\right)$ is a simple way of making sure that each change in the AG is accounted for.
  - If the $\Delta AG = \Delta\left[HCO_3^-\right]$, this is a simple AG metabolic acidosis.
  - If the $\Delta AG > \Delta\left[HCO_3^-\right]$, the $\left[HCO_3^-\right]$ did not decrease as much as expected. This is a metabolic alkalosis **and** AG metabolic acidosis. **Example:** A patient with DKA has been vomiting before admission. He has an AG of 20 and an $\left[HCO_3^-\right]$ of 20. His ΔAG = 10 and $\Delta\left[HCO_3^-\right]$ = 4, revealing an AG metabolic acidosis (DKA) with a metabolic alkalosis (vomiting).
  - If the $\Delta AG < \Delta\left[HCO_3^-\right]$, the $\left[HCO_3^-\right]$ decreased more than expected. This is a nongap metabolic acidosis **and** AG metabolic acidosis. **Example:** A patient is admitted with fevers and hypotension after a prolonged course of diarrhea. She has an AG of 15 and an $\left[HCO_3^-\right]$ of 12. Her ΔAG is 5 and her $\Delta\left[HCO_3^-\right]$ is 12, revealing a nongap metabolic acidosis (diarrhea) and an AG metabolic acidosis (lactic acidosis).

Metabolic Acidosis

GENERAL PRINCIPLES

- The causes of a metabolic acidosis can be divided into those that cause an **elevated AG** and those with a **normal AG.** Many of the causes seen in clinical practice can be found in Table 12-3.
- AG acidosis results from exposure to acids, which contribute an UA to the ECF. Common causes are DKA, lactic acidosis, and toxic alcohol ingestions.
- Non-AG acidosis can result from the loss of $\left[HCO_3^-\right]$ from the GI tract. Renal causes due to renal excretion of $\left[HCO_3^-\right]$ or disorders of renal acid handling are referred to collectively as **RTAs.**
- Enteric $\left[HCO_3^-\right]$ loss occurs most commonly in the setting of severe diarrhea.
- The three forms of RTA correlate with the three mechanisms that facilitate renal acid handling: proximal bicarbonate reabsorption, distal H^+ secretion, and generation of NH_3, the principle urinary buffer. Urinary buffers reduce the concentration of free H^+ in the filtrate, thus attenuating the back leak of H^+, which occurs at low urinary pH.
  - **Proximal (type 2) RTA** is caused by impaired proximal tubular HCO_3^- reabsorption. Causes include inherited mutations (cystinosis), heavy metals, drugs (tenofovir, ifosfamide, carbonic anhydrase inhibitors), and multiple myeloma and other monoclonal gammopathies.
  - **Distal (type 1) RTA** results from impaired distal H^+ secretion. This may occur because of impairment in H^+ secretion, as seen with a variety of autoimmune (Sjögren syndrome, lupus, rheumatoid arthritis) or renal disorders. Hypercalciuria is another main cause of distal RTA in adults. It can also be caused by a back leak of H^+ due to increased membrane permeability, as seen with amphotericin B.
  - **Distal hyperkalemic (type 4) RTA** may result from either low aldosterone levels or from aldosterone resistance. The resulting hyperkalemia reduces the availability

of NH_3 to buffer urinary H^+. Hyporeninemic hypoaldosteronism is seen with some frequency in patients with diabetes. Certain drugs, including NSAIDs, β-blockers, and cyclosporine, have also been implicated.

DIAGNOSIS

The first step in narrowing the differential diagnosis for a metabolic acidosis is to calculate the **AG**.
- The specific cause of an **elevated AG** can usually be determined by clinical history. However, specific laboratory studies are available to identify certain anions such as lactate, acetoacetate, acetone, and β-hydroxybutyrate. (It should be noted that the use of nitroprusside to detect ketones may fail to identify ketoacidosis due to β-hydroxybutyrate.) The presence of an alcohol (methanol, ethanol, ethylene glycol) can also be determined with laboratory assays. Clinical suspicion for toxic alcohol ingestion is corroborated by an increased **osmolal gap.** This gap is the difference between measured and calculated serum osmolality:

$$[Osm]_{meas} - \{([Na^+] \times 2) + ([glucose] \div 18) + ([BUN] \div 2.8)\}$$

- If a **normal AG** is present, the GI HCO_3^- losses can be differentiated from RTAs via the **urine anion gap** (UAG). The **UAG** is the difference between the major measured anions and cations in urine: $[Na^+]_u + [K^+]_u - [Cl^-]_u$. Because NH_4^+ is the major unmeasured urinary cation, a negative UAG reflects high NH_4^+ excretion, an appropriate response to a metabolic acidosis. Conversely, a positive UAG signifies low NH_4^+ excretion, which in the face of a metabolic acidosis suggests a defect in distal renal acidification.
- Serum $[K^+]$ and urine pH can be helpful in distinguishing between the RTAs.
  - Types 1 and 2 are typically associated with hypokalemia, whereas type 4 is characterized by hyperkalemia.
  - Urine pH is low (usually <5.3) in type 4 RTA because the defect is in the generation of the NH_3 buffer, and the mechanism for H^+ secretion is intact. In contrast, urine pH is inappropriately high in type 1 RTA (urine pH >5.3). In type 2 RTA, the urine pH is variable. It is elevated during the initial bicarbonaturia, when filtered bicarbonate exceeds the threshold for reabsorption, and low when the filtered load is below this threshold.

TREATMENT

- **Ketoacidosis** attributable to ethanol abuse and starvation can be corrected with the resumption of caloric intake through oral intake or dextrose-containing fluids and by correction of any volume depletion that may be present. The treatment of DKA is described in Chapter 23, Diabetes Mellitus and Related Disorders.
- **Lactic acidosis** will resolve once the underlying cause is treated and tissue perfusion is restored. Often, this involves aggressive therapeutic maneuvers for the treatment of shock as described in Chapter 8, Critical Care. The administration of alkali does not appear to have clear benefit in lactic acidosis and may lead to rebound metabolic alkalosis once the underlying cause is managed. Its use in dire circumstances or severe acidosis remains controversial.
- Management of toxic ingestions is described in Chapter 28, Toxicology.

- **Normal AG metabolic acidosis.** Treatment with NaHCO$_3$ is appropriate for patients with a normal AG metabolic acidosis. The HCO$_3^-$ deficit can be calculated in mEq:

$$HCO_3^- \text{ deficit} = \left\{ 0.5 \times \text{lean weight} \times \left[24^- \left(HCO_3^- \right) \right] \right\}$$

  However, this assumes a volume of distribution equal to 50% of total body weight. In reality, the distribution of HCO$_3^-$ increases with the severity of the acidosis and may exceed 100% of total body weight in very severe acidosis. It should be noted that the standard 650-mg tablet of oral NaHCO$_3$ provides only 7 mEq of HCO$_3^-$, whereas one ampule of IV NaHCO$_3$ contains 50 mEq. Still, parenteral NaHCO$_3$ should always be prescribed with caution because of the potential adverse effects, including pulmonary edema, hypokalemia, and hypocalcemia.
- **Treatment of the RTAs.** Correction of the chronic acidemia with alkali administration is warranted to prevent its catabolic effect on bone and muscle.
  - In *distal (type 1) RTA*, correction of the metabolic acidosis requires oral HCO$_3^-$ replacement on the order of 1–2 mEq/kg/d with NaHCO$_3$ or sodium citrate. Potassium citrate replacement may be necessary for patients with hypokalemia, nephrolithiasis, or nephrocalcinosis. Underlying conditions should be sought and treated.
  - In *proximal (type 2) RTA*, much larger amounts of alkali (10–15 mEq/kg/d) are required to reverse the acidosis. Administration of potassium salts minimizes the degree of hypokalemia associated with alkali therapy.
  - Management of *type 4 RTA* requires correction of the underlying hyperkalemia. This consists of dietary K$^+$ restriction (40–60 mEq/d) and possibly a loop diuretic with or without oral NaHCO$_3$ (0.5–1 mEq/kg/d). Mineralocorticoid administration (fludrocortisone, 50–200 µg PO daily) should be used in patients with primary adrenal insufficiency and may be considered in other causes of hypoaldosteronism.

Metabolic Alkalosis

GENERAL PRINCIPLES

- Development of a persistent metabolic alkalosis requires both generation (an inciting cause) and maintenance (a persistent impairment of the corrective renal response).
- Generation often occurs with a primary increase in the plasma $\left[HCO_3^- \right]$ and may be due to either **HCO$_3^-$ gain** from alkali administration or, more commonly, **excessive H$^+$ loss.** The latter may result from the loss of H$^+$-rich fluids, including upper GI secretions. **Contraction alkalosis** refers to the contraction of volume around a fixed content of bicarbonate.
- Maintenance requires a concomitant impairment in renal HCO$_3^-$ excretion because the kidney normally has a large capacity to excrete HCO$_3^-$. This occurs as a result of a **decreased glomerular filtration rate** or enhanced tubular HCO$_3^-$ reabsorption from **chloride depletion, volume contraction,** and **hypokalemia.** A decrease in filtered chloride is sensed by the macula densa and, as a result of tubuloglomerular feedback, reduces filtered HCO$_3^-$ and stimulates aldosterone release. It also limits adaptive distal HCO$_3^-$ secretion. Metabolic alkalosis is often described as being **chloride responsive** or **chloride unresponsive.**

DIAGNOSIS

Clinical Presentation

Because key causes of metabolic alkalosis are related to volume contraction, patients may present with signs of volume depletion. Occasionally, patients demonstrate hypertension or mild ECF expansion as a result of mineralocorticoid excess.

Diagnostic Testing

- The etiology of metabolic alkalosis is often obvious from the history. Common causes include loss of upper GI secretions through vomiting or excessive urinary H⁺ loss from diuretics.
- Urine electrolytes are generally useful in identifying the etiology of a metabolic alkalosis when the history and physical examination are unrevealing.
  - A **urine [Cl⁻]** <20 mEq/L is consistent with **chloride-responsive** metabolic alkalosis and usually indicates volume depletion. A urine [Cl⁻] >20 mEq/L indicates a chloride-unresponsive cause (see Table 12-3).
  - Urine [Na⁺] is not reliable in predicting the effective circulating volume in these conditions because *bicarbonaturia obligates renal Na⁺ loss* even in volume depletion.
- **Serum potassium** levels are often low in metabolic alkalosis because of transcellular shifts. Furthermore, hypokalemia contributes to alkalosis by increasing tubular H⁺ secretion and Cl⁻ wasting.

TREATMENT

- **Chloride-responsive** metabolic alkaloses are most effectively treated with saline resuscitation until euvolemia is achieved. The increase in filtered chloride leads to improved renal handling of the bicarbonate load.
- **Chloride-unresponsive** metabolic alkaloses do not respond to saline administration and are often associated with a normal or expanded ECF volume.
  - Mineralocorticoid excess can be managed with a K⁺-sparing diuretic (amiloride or spironolactone) and repletion of the K⁺ deficit.
  - The alkalosis from excessive alkali administration will quickly resolve once the HCO_3^- load is withdrawn, assuming normal renal function.
  - Given that the presence of hypokalemia will continue to perpetuate some degree of alkalosis regardless of other interventions, potassium must be repleted in all cases of metabolic alkalosis.
  - Acetazolamide can be used if the alkalosis persists despite the above interventions or if saline administration is limited by a patient's volume overload. This therapy promotes bicarbonaturia, although renal K⁺ loss is enhanced as well. Acetazolamide can be dosed at 250 mg q6h × 4 or as a single dose of 500 mg.
  - Severe alkalemia (pH >7.70) with ECF volume excess and/or renal failure can be treated with isotonic (150 mEq/L) HCl administered via a central vein. The amount of HCl required can be calculated as follows: (0.5 × lean weight in kg) × ($\left[HCO_3^- \right]$ −24). Correction should occur over 8–24 hours.

Respiratory Acidosis

GENERAL PRINCIPLES

The causes of respiratory acidosis can be divided into hypoventilation from (1) **respiratory center depression**, (2) **neuromuscular failure**, (3) **decreased respiratory system compliance**, (4) **increased airway resistance**, and (5) **increased dead space** (see Table 12-3).

Diagnosis

• Symptoms of respiratory acidosis result from changes in the cerebrospinal fluid (CSF) pH. A very severe hypercapnia may be well tolerated if it is accompanied by renal compensation and a relatively normal pH. Conversely, a modest rise in pCO_2 can be very symptomatic if acute.
• Initial symptoms and signs may include headache and restlessness, which may progress to generalized hyperreflexia/asterixis and coma.

TREATMENT

• Treatment is directed at correcting the underlying disorder and improving ventilation (see Chapter 10, Pulmonary Diseases).
• Administration of $NaHCO_3$ to improve the acidemia may *paradoxically worsen the pH* in situations of limited ventilation. The administered HCO_3^- will combine with H^+ in the tissues and form pCO_2 and water. If ventilation is fixed, this extra CO_2 generated cannot be blown off and worsening of hypercapnia will result. Therefore, HCO_3^- should, in general, be avoided in *pure* respiratory acidoses.

Respiratory Alkalosis

GENERAL PRINCIPLES

The common causes of hyperventilation resulting in respiratory alkalosis are given in Table 12-3.

DIAGNOSIS

Clinical Presentation

• The rise in CSF pH that occurs with **acute respiratory alkalosis** is associated with a significant reduction in cerebral blood flow that may lead to light-headedness and impaired consciousness. Generalized membrane excitability can result in seizures and arrhythmias. Symptoms and signs of acute hypocalcemia (see "Calcium, Hypocalcemia, Clinical Presentation" section) may be evident from the abrupt fall in ionized calcium that can occur.
• **Chronic respiratory alkalosis** is usually asymptomatic because a normal pH is well defended by compensation.

Diagnostic Testing

The rise in pH from **acute respiratory alkalosis** can cause a reduced ionized calcium, a profound hypophosphatemia, and hypokalemia.

TREATMENT

- Treatment of respiratory alkalosis should focus on identifying and treating the underlying disease.
- In intensive care unit patients, this may involve changing the ventilator settings to decrease ventilation (see Chapter 8, Critical Care).

REFERENCES

1. Hillier TA, Abbott RD, Barrett EJ. Hyponatremia: evaluating the correction factor for hyperglycemia. *Am J Med*. 1999;106:399-403.
2. Sterns RH, Cappuccio JD, Silver SM, et al. Neurologic sequelae after treatment of severe hyponatremia: a multicenter perspective. *J Am Soc Nephrol*. 1994;4:1522-1530.
3. Bilezikian JP, Khan AA, Potts JT Jr, et al. Guidelines for the management of asymptomatic primary hyperparathyroidism: summary statement from the third international workshop. *J Clin Endocrinol Metab*. 2009;94:335-339.

CHAPTER 12

13 Renal Diseases

Blessing Osondu and Seth Goldberg

Evaluation of the Patient With Renal Disease

DIAGNOSIS

Clinical Presentation
- Most patients with renal disease are asymptomatic. Renal disease is often initially discovered because of abnormal routine laboratory data, specifically an elevated serum creatinine (Cr) level. An abnormal urinalysis or sediment, with proteinuria, hematuria, or pyuria, may also indicate renal disease, requiring further evaluation.
- The presentation of acute kidney injury (AKI) can be quite variable, ranging from constitutional symptoms of generalized malaise to more concerning symptoms such as worsening hypertension, dependent or generalized edema, decreasing urine output, foamy urine, weight changes, or poor appetite. With advanced chronic kidney disease (CKD), patients may start to experience nausea, vomiting, a metallic taste in the mouth, and lethargy. A wide range of electrolyte abnormalities including hyperkalemia, hypocalcemia, hyperphosphatemia, and metabolic acidosis may also develop.

Diagnostic Testing
During the initial evaluation of a patient with renal disease, it is important to determine if there is a need for emergent dialysis by obtaining pertinent laboratory and imaging studies. Additional testing is then performed to identify the underlying etiology.

Basic diagnostic testing
- A basic evaluation includes electrolytes (with calcium and phosphorus), Cr, blood urea nitrogen (BUN), and albumin. When Cr is stable over days to weeks, it can be used to calculate an estimated glomerular filtration rate (eGFR). eGFR can be calculated using the Chronic Kidney Disease Epidemiology Collaboration (CKD-EPI) equation or the Modification of Diet in Renal Disease (MDRD) formula. Historically, these equations have incorporated a modifier for race. However, with the growing acknowledgment that race is a social construct, and not a biologic one, the American Society of Nephrology and the National Kidney Foundation have advocated for removing this variable.
- With both equations, CKD is not diagnosed when the eGFR is >60 mL/min/1.73 m^2 unless other evidence of renal damage (e.g., proteinuria) is present for at least 3 months.
- Use of cystatin C to estimate the GFR can more accurately classify patients in the eGFR range of 45–60 mL/min/1.73 m^2, although this has not been shown to improve outcomes or to provide better predictions of risk.[1]
- Unlike the complex formulae described above, the Cockcroft–Gault equation can be calculated manually, and yields an estimated creatinine clearance, which is equal to ([140 − age]/[serum creatinine in mg/dL]) × (weight in kg/72). The equation should be multiplied by 0.85 for women.

- These equations are not helpful in estimating renal function when the creatinine is not in steady state.

Urine studies

- Routine urine studies include a urine dipstick (for protein, blood, glucose, leukocyte esterase, nitrites, pH, and specific gravity) as well as a freshly voided specimen for microscopic examination of urine sediment (cells, casts, and crystals). The urine sample is centrifuged at 2100 rpm for 5 minutes, and then most of the supernatant is poured off. The pellet is resuspended by gently tapping the side of the tube.
- **Proteinuria and albuminuria** can be estimated from a spot urine protein-to-creatinine ratio or albumin-to-creatinine ratio in patients whose serum creatinine level is in the steady state. The ratio is expressed in milligrams of protein or albumin per gram of creatinine. The 2012 KDIGO guidelines have revised the definition for albuminuria based on the urinary albumin-to-creatinine ratio as being normal to mildly increased (A1, <30 mg/g), moderately increased (A2, 30–300 mg/g), and severely increased (A3, >300 mg/g).[2] These values can serve as a useful prognostic tool for adverse events. The term microalbuminuria is no longer used. A normal ratio for proteinuria is <250 mg/g. A 24-hour urine collection for protein can be obtained when the serum Cr is not at a stable baseline.
- **Hematuria**, which is defined as more than three red blood cells (RBCs) per high-power field on an unspun specimen, can represent an infectious, inflammatory, or malignant process anywhere along the urinary tract. Dysmorphic RBCs (with rounded protuberances) are suggestive of a glomerular source of injury. These may be accompanied by RBC casts formed within the tubules. The absence of RBCs in a patient with a positive dipstick for blood suggests hemolysis or rhabdomyolysis, forms of pigment nephropathy.
- **White blood cells** (WBCs) in the urine represent an infectious or inflammatory process. This may be seen with urinary tract infection (UTI), kidney parenchymal infections such as pyelonephritis or abscess, or acute interstitial nephritis (AIN). WBC casts can accompany WBCs in the urine and are suggestive of AIN and pyelonephritis but can also be seen as part of an active sediment in inflammatory glomerular diseases.
- Additional biochemistry tests can be ordered to evaluate for specific etiologies and will be discussed in the individual sections below.

Imaging

- **Renal ultrasonography** can be helpful in acute and chronic kidney diseases. It can document the presence of two kidneys, assess organ size and distribution of renal cysts, and identify hydronephrosis in the setting of obstruction. Small kidneys (<9 cm) generally reflect chronic disease. Diseases including diabetes, HIV, deposition disorders, and polycystic kidney disease are associated with large kidneys (generally >13 cm). A discrepancy in kidney size of >2 cm suggests chronic disease in a unilateral kidney, such as that seen in renal artery stenosis with atrophy of the affected kidney. Retroperitoneal fibrosis can encase the ureters and prevent dilation despite the presence of an obstruction.
- **CT with contrast** has less utility in the evaluation of kidney disease because the iodinated contrast dye can be nephrotoxic. However, noncontrast helical CT scanning has become the test of choice in evaluating nephrolithiasis.
- **MRI and magnetic resonance angiography (MRA)** can be helpful in evaluating renal masses, detecting renal artery stenosis, and diagnosing renal vein thrombosis. Unlike standard arteriography, MRA does not require the administration of nephrotoxic contrast agents but does employ gadolinium-based contrast agents, which are associated with the development of nephrogenic systemic fibrosis (NSF) in patients

with advanced kidney disease or dialysis dependence.[3] Guidelines that limit the use of gadolinium in at-risk patients have decreased the incidence of NSF.

* **Radionuclide scanning** uses technetium isotopes to assess the contribution of each kidney to the overall renal function, providing important information if unilateral nephrectomy is being considered for malignancy or for living donation. Renal scanning is also useful in transplantation, where renal uptake and excretion of the tracer can be followed.

Diagnostic procedures

* **Kidney biopsy** should be considered in adults with unexplained proteinuria, hematuria, or renal dysfunction. It can determine diagnosis, classify disease, guide therapy, and provide prognostic relevance in many settings, particularly in the evaluation of glomerular or deposition diseases. Biopsy of a renal transplant allograft may be necessary to distinguish allograft rejection from medication toxicity and other causes of renal dysfunction. Biopsy is unlikely to provide useful diagnostic information when the kidneys are very small, suggestive of advanced chronicity and fibrotic kidneys. This scenario also carries an increased risk of postprocedural bleeding, and biopsy should generally be avoided in these cases.
* Preparative measures for native kidney biopsy include avoiding aspirin, NSAIDs, and antiplatelet agents for 5–7 days. Blood pressure must be controlled, and anticoagulation must be reversed before the procedure. Ultrasonography (to document the presence of two kidneys and assess size and location) and urinalysis or urine culture to exclude infection should also be performed prior to the procedure. If uremic platelet dysfunction is suspected by abnormal platelet function assays, IV desmopressin acetate (DDAVP at 0.3 µg/kg) can be infused 30 minutes before biopsy. Patients on dialysis should not receive heparin immediately after the biopsy. If body habitus precludes a percutaneous approach, a transjugular renal biopsy can be performed.
* A hemoglobin drop of approximately 10% is common after the procedure. Difficulty voiding after the procedure may represent urethral clot obstructing the flow of urine.

Acute Kidney Injury

GENERAL PRINCIPLES

Definition

According to the KDIGO 2012 guidelines, AKI is defined and categorized by varying Cr elevations or decreases in urine output.[4]

* Stage 1 AKI is defined as a Cr 1.5–1.9 times baseline (known or presumed to have occurred within the prior 7 days), an increase in Cr ≥ 0.3 mg/dL within 48 hours, or a urine output <0.5 mL/kg/h for 6–12 hours.
* Stage 2 AKI is defined as a Cr 2–2.9 times baseline or a urine output <0.5 mL/kg/h for at least 12 hours.
* Stage 3 AKI is defined as a Cr ≥ 3 times baseline, a Cr increase of ≥4 mg/dL, initiation of renal replacement therapy, urine output <0.3 mL/kg/h for at least 24 hours, or anuria for at least 12 hours.

Classification

Renal failure can be classified as oliguric or nonoliguric based on the amount of urine output. Cutoffs of approximately 500 mL/d or 25 mL/h for 6–12 hours are frequently used in clinical practice.

Etiology

The etiology of AKI should be determined when possible. It can be classified based on the anatomic location of the physiologic defect. **Prerenal** disease involves a disturbance of renal perfusion, whereas **postrenal** disease involves obstruction along the urinary collecting system. **Intrinsic** renal disease involves the tubules, glomeruli, microvasculature, or interstitium of the kidneys. Table 13-1 lists some of the common causes of AKI.

Prerenal

- The term **prerenal azotemia** implies that the inherent function of the kidneys is preserved, in the setting of renal hypoperfusion and reduced GFR. States of decreased effective circulating blood volume, resulting from intravascular volume depletion, low cardiac output, or disordered vasodilation (hepatic cirrhosis), may also result in prerenal azotemia.
- When the cause is true volume depletion, presentation involves a history of excessive volume loss or reduced intake. The physical examination may reveal dry mucous membranes, poor skin turgor, and orthostatic vital signs (drop in blood pressure by at least 20/10 mm Hg or an increase in heart rate by 10 bpm after standing from a seated or lying position). The central venous pressure is typically <8 cm H_2O.
- Low cardiac output causes prerenal azotemia via a drop in the effective circulating volume despite being in a state of total body volume overload. Sympathetic and neurohormonal activation stimulates the renin–angiotensin–aldosterone system (RAAS) for sodium reclamation, as well as driving antidiuretic hormone (ADH), promoting further water retention. This can lead to an increased reabsorption of urea nitrogen in relation to creatinine, and patients present with a prerenal pattern on laboratory investigations (BUN:Cr ratio >20, urine sodium <20 mEq/L, fractional excretion of sodium <1%). In heart failure, diuresis may paradoxically improve the prerenal azotemia by unloading the ventricles and improving cardiac function and renal perfusion (see Chapter 5, Heart Failure and Cardiomyopathy). The use of ultrafiltration (UF) was evaluated and found to be inferior to pharmacologic therapies, resulting in more adverse events in the treatment of acute decompensated heart failure.[5]

TABLE 13-1	Causes of Acute Renal Failure	
Prerenal	**Intrinsic**	**Postrenal**
Hypovolemia	Tubular: Ischemic ATN, toxic ATN (contrast, pigment, uric acid)	Urethral obstruction
Hypotension (including sepsis)		Ureteral obstruction (bilateral, or unilateral if solitary kidney)
Loss of autoregulation (NSAIDs, RAAS blockers)	Vascular: Glomerulonephritis, dysproteinemia, thrombotic microangiopathy (HUS, TTP), atheroembolic disease	
Abdominal compartment syndrome	Interstitial: Acute interstitial nephritis, pyelonephritis	
Renal artery stenosis		
Heart failure		
Hepatic cirrhosis		

ATN, acute tubular necrosis; HUS, hemolytic uremic syndrome; RAAS, renin–angiotensin–aldosterone system; TTP, thrombotic thrombocytopenic purpura.

- Hepatic failure with splanchnic vasodilation, venous pooling, and ascites formation diminishes the effective circulating volume. RAAS activation along with ADH secretion will produce a prerenal pattern on laboratory investigations, despite being in a state of total body volume overload. This can progress to **hepatorenal syndrome** (HRS), which is characterized by a rise in serum creatinine of >1.5 mg/dL that is not reduced with administration of albumin (1 g/kg of body weight) and after a minimum of 2 days off diuretics. The diagnosis of HRS should be made in the absence of shock, nephrotoxic agents, or findings of renal parenchymal disease (e.g., active urinary sediment on urine microscopy).[6] Spontaneous bacterial peritonitis, aggressive diuresis, gastrointestinal bleeding, or large-volume paracentesis can precipitate HRS in patients with liver cirrhosis. Management of the renal disease is supportive, and if definitive treatment of the liver disorder (either through recovery or via transplantation) can occur, renal recovery is common. Temporizing measures include treatment of the underlying precipitating factor (e.g., peritonitis, gastrointestinal bleeding, hypotension) and withholding diuretics or other offending agents. Dialytic support can be used as a bridge to transplantation in appropriate candidates, with anticipation of renal recovery if the period of dialysis dependence is shorter than 6 weeks.
- Simultaneous liver kidney (SLK) transplant should be considered if the candidate meets specific criteria published in 2016 by the US Organ Procurement and Transplant Network (OPTN) and the United Network for Organ Sharing (UNOS). These include CKD with a GFR ≤35 mL/min/1.73 m², sustained AKI with a GFR ≤25 mL/min/1.73 m², or dialysis dependence for at least 6 weeks. Patients with the diagnosis of a metabolic disease that would place a renal allograft at risk of failing, such as primary hyperoxaluria, atypical hemolytic uremic syndrome (HUS) from mutations in factor H or factor I, familial non-neuropathic systemic amyloidosis, or methylmalonic aciduria, would also be candidates for SLK.[7] Additional treatment options are discussed further in Chapter 19, Liver Diseases.
- In the volume-depleted patient, certain medications can affect the ability of the kidney to autoregulate blood flow and maintain GFR. NSAIDs inhibit the counterbalancing vasodilatory effects of prostaglandins at the afferent arteriole and can induce AKI in volume-depleted patients. Angiotensin-converting enzyme (ACE) inhibitors and angiotensin receptor blockers (ARBs) can cause efferent arteriolar vasodilation and a drop in the GFR.
- Abdominal compartment syndrome from intestinal ischemia, obstruction, or massive ascites can compromise flow through the renal vasculature via increased intra-abdominal pressure (IAP). An IAP >20 mm Hg, measured via a pressure transducer attached to the bladder catheter in a patient who is sedated, supports the diagnosis.

Postrenal
- Postrenal injury occurs when the flow of urine is obstructed within the collecting system. Common causes include **prostatic enlargement, bilateral kidney stones, or malignancy** (e.g., extrinsic compression by a mass, retroperitoneal fibrosis). The increased intratubular hydrostatic pressure leads to the diminished GFR. Bilateral involvement (or unilateral obstruction to a solitary functioning kidney) is generally required to produce a significant change in the Cr level. When this diagnosis is suspected, a renal ultrasound should be obtained early to evaluate for hydronephrosis. Note that hydronephrosis may be less pronounced when there is concomitant volume depletion or if retroperitoneal fibrosis has encased the ureters, preventing their dilation. Therefore, if this diagnosis is still suspected, renal ultrasound should be repeated after the patient has received adequate volume repletion.

- Treatment depends on the level of obstruction. When urethral flow is impeded (often by prostatic enlargement in men), placement of a bladder catheter can be both diagnostic and therapeutic; a **postvoid residual urine volume >300 mL** suggests the diagnosis. When the upper urinary tract is involved, urologic or radiologic decompression may be necessary, with stenting or placement of percutaneous nephrostomy tubes.
- Relief of bilateral obstruction is frequently followed by a **postobstructive diuresis.** Serum electrolytes need to be closely monitored if polyuria ensues, and replacement of approximately half of the urinary volume with 0.45% saline is recommended.
- Crystals may cause micro-obstructive uropathy within the tubules. IV acyclovir and the protease inhibitor indinavir can induce AKI by this mechanism. The urine may show evidence of crystals, although sometimes not until urine flow is re-established. Treatment is typically supportive after the offending agent is discontinued. As with resolution of other forms of obstructive uropathy, a polyuric phase may occur.

Intrinsic Renal

Causes of intrinsic renal failure can be divided anatomically into tubular, glomerular/vascular, and interstitial categories. Disease can be primarily renal in nature or part of a systemic process.

- **Tubular**
  - **Ischemic acute tubular necrosis (ATN)** is the most common cause of renal failure in the hospital setting, especially in the intensive care unit, and is the end result of any process that leads to significant hypoperfusion of the kidneys, including sepsis, hemorrhage, or any prolonged prerenal insult.
    - The injury results in the sloughing of renal tubular cells, with this cellular debris congealing in a matrix of Tamm–Horsfall protein to form granular casts. The casts have a "muddy brown" appearance and are strongly suggestive of ATN in the appropriate clinical context. The fractional excretion of sodium (FE_{Na}) (>1%) and fractional excretion of urea (FE_{Urea}) (>35%) are typically elevated as the tubules lose their ability to concentrate the urine. However, these calculations are not specific to ATN.
    - Management of ATN is supportive, with avoidance of further nephrotoxic insults. Fluid management is aimed at maintaining euvolemia. Volume deficits, if present, should be corrected. If there are signs of volume overload and oliguria, a furosemide stress test may predict the severity of AKI. A single furosemide dose of 1.0 or 1.5 mg/kg (depending on prior furosemide exposure) is administered, and the urine output in the first 2 hours is measured. A 2-hour urine output of less than 200 mL offers the best combination of sensitivity and specificity and has a good predictive capacity to identify those patients who will progress to advanced stages of AKI. Patients must be euvolemic or hypervolemic to qualify for this test and should not be on pressor support.[8] Continuing diuretic therapy if a response is seen has not been shown to hasten recovery but can simplify overall management.
    - Recovery from ATN may take days to weeks to occur but can be expected in >85% of patients with previously normal renal function. Dialysis may be necessary to bridge the time to recovery.
  - Toxic ATN can result from endogenous chemicals (e.g., hemoglobin, myoglobin pigments) or medications (e.g., iodinated contrast, aminoglycosides, combination of vancomycin and piperacillin/tazobactam). These forms share many of the diagnostic features of ischemic ATN.
    - **Iodinated contrast** is a potent renal vasoconstrictor and is toxic to renal tubules. When renal injury occurs, the Cr typically rises 24–48 hours after exposure and

CHAPTER 13

peaks in 3–5 days. Risk factors for contrast nephropathy include underlying CKD, age >75 years, diabetes, volume depletion, heart failure, higher contrast volumes, and use of hyperosmolar contrast. Preventative measures include periprocedural IV volume expansion and discontinuation of diuretics within 24 hours of the procedure. Normal saline at 150 mEq/L can be given at 3 mL/kg/h for 1 hour before exposure, then at 1 mL/kg/h for 6 hours after the procedure. In a large randomized controlled trial, sodium bicarbonate was not found to be superior to normal saline, whereas acetylcysteine was equivocal to placebo and therefore is not recommended.[9]

- **Aminoglycoside nephrotoxicity** is typically nonoliguric, occurs from direct toxicity to the proximal tubules, and results in the renal wasting of potassium and magnesium. Replacement of these electrolytes may become necessary. A similar pattern of potassium and magnesium loss is seen in cisplatin toxicity. A prolonged exposure to the aminoglycoside of at least 5 days is required. Peak and trough levels correlate poorly with the risk of developing renal injury. Risk may be minimized by avoiding volume depletion and by using the extended-interval dosing method (see Chapter 15, Antimicrobials).

- **Pigment nephropathy** results from direct tubular toxicity by hemoglobin and myoglobin. Vasoconstriction may also play a role. The diagnosis may be suspected by a positive urine dipstick test for blood but an absence of RBCs on microscopic examination. In **rhabdomyolysis**, the creatine kinase level is elevated to at least 10 times the upper limit of normal with a disproportionate rise in the serum Cr. Potassium and phosphorus may also be elevated in the setting of muscle breakdown. Aggressive IV fluid administration with normal saline should be initiated immediately, and large volumes are required to replace the fluid lost into necrotic muscle tissue. Urinary alkalinization with intravenous sodium bicarbonate is not generally recommended as it may worsen the hypocalcemia.

- In **tumor lysis syndrome**, there is rapid death of cancer cells either spontaneously or in response to treatment. In addition to the elevated Cr, there is typically hyperuricemia, hyperphosphatemia, and hypocalcemia. A ratio of urine uric acid to urine Cr that is >1 is consistent with acute uric acid nephropathy, as is the finding of uric acid crystals in the urine sediment. Prophylaxis with allopurinol 600 mg can decrease uric acid production. Rasburicase (15 mg/kg IV) is highly effective at depleting uric acid levels and can be given as prophylaxis or as treatment. Alkalinization of the urine should be avoided if hyperphosphatemia is present because this could increase the risk of calcium phosphate precipitation in the urine.

- **Glomerular/vascular**
  - The finding of **dysmorphic urinary RBCs, RBC casts, or proteinuria in the nephrotic range (>3.5 g/d)** would strongly suggest the presence of a glomerular disease. Glomerular diseases are described individually in further detail in later sections of this chapter.
  - A subset of glomerular diseases can present with rapidly deteriorating renal function, termed **rapidly progressive glomerulonephritis.** This describes a type of presentation rather than a specific disease. A nephritic picture is common, with RBC casts, edema, and hypertension. Crescent formation is seen in >50% of glomeruli, suggesting inflammation and cellular proliferation. For those deemed to have salvageable renal function, management typically consists of high-dose corticosteroids and cyclophosphamide or other potent immunosuppressive agents.
  - **Thrombotic microangiopathy** (TMA) is a general term encompassing a broad spectrum of disease resulting in hemolytic anemia, platelet consumption, and

intracapillary thrombi, with associated endothelial cell injury. Differentiating among the various causes of this entity can allow for better targeted therapy. **Hemolytic uremic syndrome** (HUS) results from diarrheal bacterial toxins (e.g., Shiga and Shiga-like toxin) that cause direct injury to the endothelial cells. **Thrombotic thrombocytopenic purpura** (TTP) can result from a reduced activity of ADAMTS13 (due to deficiency or inhibitory antibodies) leading to von Willebrand factor–rich microthrombi secondarily affecting arterioles and capillaries of a variety of organs. **Atypical HUS** has been described in patients with mutations or inhibitors in proteins that regulate the complement cascade, such as factor H and factor I, responsive to treatment with eculizumab, a C5 inhibitor.[10] Malignant hypertension and a variety of medications (e.g., mitomycin C, clopidogrel, gemcitabine, tacrolimus) have also been associated with TMA. Classification, diagnosis, and therapy are discussed in Chapter 20, Disorders of Hemostasis and Thrombosis.

- ○ **Atheroembolic disease** can be seen in patients with diffuse atherosclerosis after undergoing an invasive aortic or other large artery manipulation, including cardiac catheterization, coronary arterial bypass grafting, aortic aneurysm repair, and placement of an intra-aortic balloon pump. Physical findings may include retinal arteriolar plaques, lower extremity livedo reticularis, and areas of digital necrosis. Peripheral eosinophilia and hypocomplementemia may be present, and WBC casts may be found in the urine sediment. However, in many cases, the only laboratory abnormality is a rising Cr that follows a stepwise progression. Renal biopsy shows cholesterol clefts in the small arteries. Anticoagulation may worsen embolic disease and should be avoided if possible. No specific treatment is available. Many patients progress to CKD and even to end-stage renal disease (ESRD).

- **Interstitial**
  - ○ **Acute interstitial nephritis** (AIN) involves an acute inflammation of the renal parenchyma. The causes of AIN are broad and include medications (in >70% of cases), infectious agents, and systemic diseases. β-Lactam antibiotics are the most frequently cited causative agents, but nearly all antibiotics can be implicated. Other medications, such as proton pump inhibitors, 5-aminosalicylates, and allopurinol, have been associated with AIN. NSAIDs can produce a chronic interstitial nephritis with nephrotic range proteinuria. Streptococcal infections, leptospirosis, and sarcoidosis have also been implicated in AIN. The classic triad of **fever, rash, and eosinophilia** is seen in less than one-third of patients, and its absence does not exclude the diagnosis. Pyuria and WBC casts on urine microscopy are also suggestive of AIN. The time course typically requires exposure for at least 5–10 days before renal impairment occurs.
  - ○ **Treatment is principally withdrawal of the offending agent. Renal recovery typically ensues, although the time course is variable, and temporary dialytic support may be necessary** in severe cases. A short course of prednisone at 1 mg/kg/d may hasten recovery.[11]
  - ○ Parenchymal infections with **pyelonephritis** or **renal abscesses** are uncommon causes of AKI. Bilateral involvement is usually necessary to induce a rise in Cr. Urine findings include pyuria and WBC casts, and antibiotic therapy is guided by culture results.

DIAGNOSIS

- Uncovering the cause of AKI requires careful attention to the events preceding the rise in Cr. In the hospitalized patient, blood pressure patterns, irregular cardiac rhythms, hydration status, medications, and iodinated contrast use must be

CHAPTER 13

investigated. Antibiotic dose and duration as well as PRN medications should not be overlooked.

- Evidence of ongoing hypovolemia or hypoperfusion is suggestive of prerenal disease but may have progressed to an acute tubular injury pattern. Most causes of postrenal disease are identified on ultrasound by dilation of the collecting system or by massive urine output upon placement of a bladder catheter. However, obstruction cannot be completely ruled out even if not identified on imaging, especially in the setting of early obstruction or volume depletion. Patients may need volume resuscitation and an ultrasound repeated in several days if renal function does not improve.

- **Urinary casts** point toward an intrinsic cause of AKI. Granular casts ("muddy brown") suggest ATN, WBC casts suggest an inflammatory or infectious interstitial process, and RBC casts strongly suggest glomerular disease. Identification of crystals in the urine sediment may be supportive of kidney disease related to intoxication of ethylene glycol, uric acid excretion, tumor lysis syndrome, or medications such as acyclovir and indinavir. This underscores the importance of examining urinary sediment in the evaluation of AKI.

- Various laboratory parameters can be used to differentiate prerenal states from ATN in oliguric patients and are summarized in Table 13-2. The basis for these tests is to evaluate tubular integrity, which is preserved in prerenal disease but lost in ATN. In states of hypoperfusion, the kidneys should avidly reabsorb sodium, resulting in a low FE_{Na}: $FE_{Na} = ([U_{Na} \times P_{Cr}]/[P_{Na} \times U_{Cr}]) \times 100$, where U is urine and P is plasma.

- **A value <1% suggests renal hypoperfusion with intact tubular function.** Loop diuretics and metabolic alkalosis can induce natriuresis, increase the FE_{Na}, and mask the presence of renal hypoperfusion. The FE_{Urea} can instead be calculated in these settings, where a value of <35% suggests a prerenal process.

- Contrast and pigment nephropathy can result in a low FE_{Na} because of early vasoconstriction ("prerenal" drop in glomerular perfusion), as can glomerular diseases because of intact tubular function. The FE_{Na} also has limited utility when AKI is superimposed on CKD because the underlying tubular dysfunction makes the test difficult to interpret.

- With hypoperfusion, the urine is typically concentrated, containing an osmolality >500 mOsm/kg and a high specific gravity (>1.020). In ATN, concentrating ability is lost and the urine is usually isosmolar to the serum (isosthenuria). In the blood, the ratio of BUN to Cr is normally <20:1, and an elevation is consistent with hypovolemia.

- •The FE_{Na} should not be used alone to determine the cause of AKI, but instead interpreted in the context of the patient and clinical scenario.

TABLE 13-2	Laboratory Findings in Oliguric Acute Kidney Injury					
Diagnosis	BUN:Cr	FE_{Na} (%)	Urine Osmolality (mOsm/kg)	Urine Na	Urine SG	Sediment
Prerenal azotemia	>20:1	<1	>500	<20	>1.020	Bland
Oliguric ATN	<20:1	>1	<350	>40	Variable	Granular casts

ATN, acute tubular necrosis; BUN, blood urea nitrogen; Cr, creatinine; FE_{Na}, fractional excretion of sodium; SG, specific gravity.

TREATMENT

- Disease-specific therapies are covered in their respective sections. In general, treatment of AKI is primarily supportive in nature. **Volume status** should be evaluated to correct for hypovolemia or hypervolemia. Volume deficits, if present, should be corrected, after which the goal of fluid management should be to keep input equal to output. In the oliguric volume-overloaded setting, a trial of diuretics (usually high-dose loop diuretics in a bolus or as a continuous drip) may simplify management, although it has not been shown to hasten recovery.
- Electrolyte imbalances should be corrected in the setting of AKI. **Hyperkalemia**, when mild (<6 mEq/L), may be treated with dietary potassium restriction and potassium-binding resins (e.g., sodium polystyrene sulfonate, sodium zirconium cyclosilicate). When further elevated or accompanied by ECG abnormalities, immediate medical therapy is indicated with calcium gluconate, insulin and glucose, inhaled β-agonists, and possibly bicarbonate (see Chapter 12, Fluid and Electrolyte Management). Severe hyperkalemia that is refractory to medical management is an indication for urgent dialysis.
- Mild **metabolic acidosis** can be treated with oral sodium bicarbonate, 650–1300 mg three times daily. Severe acidosis (pH <7.2) can be temporized with IV sodium bicarbonate but requires monitoring for volume overload, rebound alkalosis, and hypocalcemia. Acidosis that is refractory to medical management is an indication for urgent dialysis.

SPECIAL CONSIDERATIONS

- Patients with AKI require daily assessment to determine the need for renal replacement therapy. Severe acidosis, hyperkalemia, or volume overload refractory to medical management mandates the initiation of dialysis. Certain drug and alcohol intoxications (methanol, ethylene glycol, or salicylates) should be treated with hemodialysis. Uremic pericarditis (with a friction rub) or encephalopathy should also be treated promptly with renal replacement therapy. Patients suffering from acute oliguric renal failure who are not expected to recover promptly may benefit from earlier initiation of dialysis.
- In the absence of one of these acute indications, the timing of initiating dialytic therapy is less certain. Two studies analyzed this subject in ICU patients in a randomized controlled fashion with somewhat contradictory results. Starting dialytic support in patients with a threefold elevation in Cr or a Cr of 4 mg/dL or greater did not show improved outcomes as compared to delaying dialysis until a traditional indication developed.[12] A smaller study, however, did show a survival advantage for patients beginning dialysis with a two- to threefold increase in Cr, as compared to patients with more severe elevations.[13]

Glomerulopathies

GENERAL PRINCIPLES

- Glomerular diseases traditionally have been classified based on the clinical presentation as existing on a spectrum with the nephrotic syndrome on one end (characterized by proteinuria >3.5 g/d and accompanied by hypoalbuminemia, hyperlipidemia, and edema), and the nephritic syndrome on the other end (characterized by hematuria, hypertension, edema, and renal insufficiency). Although most have overlapping features, specific diseases do have a tendency to feature one syndrome over the other, related to the predominant histologic site of glomerular injury. In most cases, a kidney biopsy will be necessary to determine the most specific diagnosis, a step that is crucial for treatment.

- Minimal change disease (MCD), focal segmental glomerulosclerosis (FSGS), and membranous nephropathy (MN) typically present with nephrotic features. IgA nephropathy, postinfectious glomerulonephritis, anti-GBM antibody disease, and antineutrophil cytoplasmic antibody (ANCA)-associated vasculitis typically present with nephritic features. Membranoproliferative glomerulonephropathy (MPGN) can present with overlapping features of both nephrotic and nephritic disease.

- Nephrotic diseases typically show injury along the filtration barrier, with thickening of the glomerular basement membrane (GBM) or fusion of the podocyte foot processes. By comparison, nephritic diseases generally show varying degrees of mesangial cell proliferation and mesangial deposition. With more aggressive disease, cellular or fibrous crescents may be seen within Bowman capsule.

- When a nephrotic process is suspected, it may be useful to check antinuclear antibodies (ANA), complement levels (C3, C4), cryoglobulins, and viral serologies (HIV, hepatitis B and C, parvovirus, cytomegalovirus [CMV], Epstein–Barr virus [EBV]). It is important to review the medication profile and rule out malignancy or other systemic infectious or inflammatory conditions. A serum protein electrophoresis (SPEP) and urine immunofixation can be performed in proteinuric patients to evaluate for a monoclonal gammopathy and should be suspected when a large protein–albumin gap is present.

- When a nephritic process is suspected, testing for anti-GBM antibodies, ANCA, and anti-streptolysin-O (ASO) titers may be helpful in narrowing the differential diagnosis. As with nephrotic processes, testing for ANA, C3, C4, cryoglobulins, and viral serologies can also provide useful information.

- Complement levels may be decreased in certain nephritic disorders, such as postinfectious glomerulonephritis, lupus nephritis, MPGN, C3 glomerulopathy, and subacute bacterial endocarditis. Others, such as IgA nephropathy, ANCA vasculitis, and anti-GBM antibody disease, typically have normal complement levels.

TREATMENT

- Many disorders share similar features, and general therapeutic maneuvers can be addressed as a group. Specific therapies for individual glomerular diseases are discussed later in the chapter.

- Glomerular disease presenting with proteinuria should be treated with **ACE inhibitors or ARBs** to reduce intraglomerular pressure if there are no concerns for hyperkalemia and if the serum creatinine is stable. Efficacy can be monitored by serial urine protein to Cr ratios. Electrolytes and Cr should be checked within 1 week of treatment initiation or an increase in dose to document stability of renal function and potassium. A Cr increase within the range of 0.1–0.3 mg/dL (or up to 30% of baseline) is acceptable and if greater, then renal artery stenosis should be ruled out. Modest dietary protein restriction to 0.8 g/kg/d may slow progression, but this remains controversial.

- Edema and volume overload can usually be effectively managed with **diuretics** combined with **sodium restriction.** Aggressive treatment of hypertension can also slow the progression of renal disease.

- Hyperlipidemia associated with nephrotic syndrome responds to dietary modification and **statins (3-hydroxy-3-methylglutaryl–coenzyme A [HMG-CoA] reductase inhibitors).**
- Nephrotic syndrome is associated with a hypercoagulable state and can predispose patients to thromboembolic complications. Deep venous thrombi and renal vein thrombosis may occur and should be treated with heparin followed by long-term oral anticoagulation.
- Anticoagulation is absolutely indicated in the setting of deep venous thrombosis or pulmonary embolism. Prophylactic anticoagulation should be considered in severely nephrotic patients with a serum albumin <2.0–2.5 g/dL and additional risk factors that could predispose them to clotting (e.g., family history of clots, immobilization).[14] Exact mechanisms of thrombosis remain controversial but likely include urinary loss of antithrombotic proteins and increased synthesis of clotting factors.
- When **immunosuppression** is considered, the risk of therapy should always be weighed against the potential benefit. Renal salvageability should be addressed, and patients with advanced kidney disease on presentation who are unlikely to benefit from such treatment may be better served by avoiding the risks of high-dose immunosuppression. Cytotoxic agents (e.g., cyclophosphamide) require close monitoring of WBC counts, checked at least weekly at the initiation of therapy. Dose adjustments may be needed to maintain the WBC count >3500 cells/μL. Rituximab, a monoclonal antibody directed against CD20, has shown promise in a variety of immune-mediated disorders, including severe lupus nephritis, MN, and ANCA-associated vasculitis.[15] Other immunosuppressive agents include calcineurin inhibitors (e.g., tacrolimus, cyclosporine) and mycophenolate mofetil. Therapeutic plasma exchange has a role in only specific circumstances as described in more detail below.

Minimal Change Disease

GENERAL PRINCIPLES

Epidemiology

MCD is the most common cause of nephrotic syndrome in children but has a second peak in adults aged 50–60 years. Typically, there is sudden onset of proteinuria with hypertension and edema, although renal insufficiency is unusual.

Associated Conditions

Secondary forms of MCD may accompany certain malignancies (Hodgkin disease and solid tumors being the most common) and therefore, patients in the appropriate age group should undergo further cancer screening. A form of interstitial nephritis associated with NSAID use may also be associated with MCD.

DIAGNOSIS

The kidney biopsy reveals normal glomeruli on light microscopy and negative immunofluorescence. Electron microscopy shows complete foot process effacement. This may have a similar appearance to early onset FSGS and thus be difficult to differentiate.

TREATMENT

- In adults, treatment with high-dose oral prednisone at 1 mg/kg daily (not exceeding 80 mg/d) or 2 mg/kg on alternate days (not exceeding 120 mg, every other day) may induce

CHAPTER 13

remission (i.e., decrease in proteinuria) after a minimum of 4 weeks, but can require up to 16 weeks of therapy. Prednisone can then be tapered off over a 6-month period.

- Relapse may occur in up to 75% of adults. Reinstitution of prednisone is often effective. If the patient is steroid dependent or steroid resistant, cytotoxic agents may be needed, with cyclophosphamide 2 mg/kg/d or chlorambucil 0.2 mg/kg/d. Cyclosporine 3–5 mg/kg/d or mycophenolate mofetil 1000 mg twice a day for 2 years can be considered as alternative therapies.[16] Rituximab may be beneficial in frequently relapsing or glucocorticoid-dependent MCD.[17]

Focal Segmental Glomerulosclerosis

GENERAL PRINCIPLES

- FSGS is not a single disease but rather a pattern of glomerular injury with various mechanisms. It typically presents with nephrotic syndrome, hypertension, and sometimes renal insufficiency.
- FSGS can be classified into primary (idiopathic) and secondary forms.[18] Secondary forms of FSGS are associated with obesity, vesicoureteral reflux, sickle cell disease, medications (pamidronate, α-interferon, tyrosine kinase inhibitors), and infections (HIV, parvovirus, CMV, EBV).

DIAGNOSIS

The kidney biopsy reveals segmental sclerosis of some glomeruli under light microscopy. The degree of interstitial fibrosis and tubular atrophy (rather than glomerular scarring) correlates with prognosis. Immunofluorescence shows deposition of IgM and C3 in areas of sclerosis, representing areas of trapped immune deposits. Electron microscopy shows effacement of the podocyte foot processes similar to that seen in MCD. Lesions can be classified into distinct histomorphologic variants, though their clinical significance is uncertain. The tip variant tends to have the most favorable prognosis while the collapsing variant is associated with the poorest outcomes.

TREATMENT

Management is similar to MCD. For patients with nephrotic range proteinuria, a trial of high-dose oral prednisone at 1 mg/kg daily (not exceeding 80 mg daily) or 2 mg/kg on alternate days (not exceeding 120 mg, every other day) may induce remission and then be tapered off over a 6-month period. Patients who relapse after a period of apparent responsiveness may benefit from a repeat course of steroids. Nonresponders and relapsers may respond to treatment with cyclosporine 5 mg/kg/d. Cyclophosphamide and mycophenolate mofetil can also be used. Induction of a complete remission (<0.3 g/d of proteinuria) or a partial remission (50% reduction in proteinuria and <3.5 g/d) is associated with significantly slower loss of renal function.

Membranous Nephropathy

GENERAL PRINCIPLES

- MN usually presents with heavy proteinuria and nephrotic syndrome. Disease progression is variable, with one-third remitting spontaneously, one-third progressing to ESRD, and one-third with an intermediate course.

- Secondary etiologies of MN include autoimmune or collagen vascular diseases (systemic lupus erythematosus [SLE] class V, Sjögren syndrome, rheumatoid arthritis), infection (viral hepatitis, syphilis), and medications (penicillamine, NSAIDs, mercury, gold). Malignancy may also play a role; patients with MN should undergo age-appropriate cancer screening.

DIAGNOSIS

Kidney biopsy shows thickening of the GBM without significant hypercellularity on light microscopy. Also seen are "spikes" along the GBM on silver stain, representing areas of normal basement membrane interposed between subepithelial deposits. On immunofluorescence, there is granular staining along the GBM with IgG and C3. On electron microscopy, subepithelial deposits are seen. Antibodies to the podocyte antigen phospholipase A_2 receptor have been implicated in 70% of adult idiopathic MN. Antibodies against thrombospondin type-1 domain-containing 7A (THSD7A) are seen in 10% of patients with MN and have been linked to malignancy.[19] Additional podocyte antigens are currently being investigated.

TREATMENT

- Up to 30% of patients with MN will go into spontaneous remission.[20] KDIGO guidelines recommend conservative therapy as an initial approach with ACE inhibitors or ARBs for proteinuria and blood pressure control, diuretics for volume management, with or without anticoagulation. Because of the generally favorable prognosis, specific therapy should be reserved for patients at higher risk for progression (e.g., heavy proteinuria, reduced GFR, male gender, age >50 years, hypertension).
- When immunosuppression is considered, a variety of regimens have been studied. One option is to use alternating months of a corticosteroid and a cytotoxic agent for 6 months (prednisone 0.5 mg/kg/d for months 1, 3, and 5, and cyclophosphamide 2.5 mg/kg/d for months 2, 4, and 6).[21]
- Rituximab has been shown to provide a more durable remission when compared to cyclosporine at 24 months of treatment.[22]

Diabetic Nephropathy

GENERAL PRINCIPLES

Diabetic nephropathy (DN) is the most common cause of ESRD in the United States. Risk factors include smoking, family history of ESRD, hypertension, and poor glycemic control. The degree of albuminuria also correlates with the risk of progression to ESRD. Early disease is characterized by glomerular hyperfiltration with an elevated GFR, followed by a linear decline that may progress to ESRD.

DIAGNOSIS

Diagnostic Testing

Kidney biopsy is not usually performed in patients who present with classic DN unless the rate of renal decline is more rapid than would be anticipated, or to rule out other causes of nephrotic syndrome. Histology for DN shows glomerular sclerosis with nodular mesangial expansion (Kimmelstiel–Wilson nodules) on light microscopy. Immunofluorescence does not reveal immune deposition. Electron microscopy may show GBM thickening.

TREATMENT

Tight glycemic control was associated with better outcomes in patients with type 1 diabetes mellitus; the benefit was not as profound in patients with type 2 diabetes mellitus.[23] Specific hyperglycemic therapy is discussed further in Chapter 23, Diabetes Mellitus and Related Disorders. An ACE inhibitor or ARB is considered the first-line agent in the treatment of hypertension in diabetic patients and can improve proteinuria. Studies combining ACE inhibitors with an ARB or the direct renin inhibitor aliskiren have shown worse renal and cardiovascular outcomes.[24] Metformin should not be started in patients with a GFR <45 mL/min/1.73 m^2 due to a risk of lactic acidosis. Sodium–glucose cotransporter-2 (SGLT2) inhibitors (empaglifozin, canaglifozin, dapaglifozin) have been studied extensively among patients with diabetes mellitus and CKD with estimated GFR of ≥30 mL/min/1.73 m^2 and are shown to decrease the risk of a sustained decline in renal function, progression to ESRD, or death from renal or cardiovascular causes.[25] SGLT2 inhibitors should be avoided in patients with active foot ulcers, lower extremity ischemia, or advanced liver disease.

Deposition Disorders/Dysproteinemias

GENERAL PRINCIPLES

Dysproteinemias, including those observed in multiple myeloma, encompass **amyloidosis, light chain deposition disease (LCDD), heavy chain deposition disease (HCDD)**, and **monoclonal immunoglobulin deposition disease**. These disorders can affect the kidney in a variety of ways, including glomerular or tubular deposition, formation of insoluble protein casts in the tubules (micro-obstructive cast nephropathy), or through hypercalcemia and volume depletion. Glomerular deposition is typically associated with heavy proteinuria due to overflow as well as disruption of the filtration barrier integrity.

DIAGNOSIS

Diagnostic Testing

Diagnosis is suggested by an abnormal monoclonal protein found on SPEP or urine immunofixation, or an imbalance in the κ/λ serum free light chain ratio. Routine urine dipstick tests for negatively charged albumin, and therefore may miss the positively charged Ig chains, unless glomerular involvement has led to a generalized protein leakage. In some cases, all of these tests are negative and only tissue biopsy can make the diagnosis.

- Biopsy of the kidney can show characteristic deposits. For amyloidosis, these appear as Congo Red–positive β-pleated fibrils of 10 nm in diameter under electron microscopy. Immunofluorescence can identify the specific Ig chains for amyloidosis (more likely to be lambda light chains), LCDD (more likely to be kappa light chains), and HCDD. **Fibrillary glomerulopathy** and **immunotactoid glomerulopathy** are distinct deposition diseases that are characterized by Congo Red–negative deposits. The fibrils of fibrillary glomerulopathy (12–20 nm) are typically thicker than those for amyloid, whereas the microtubules of immunotactoid glomerulopathy are even thicker (20–60 nm) with a visible lumen in cross section. Immunotactoid glomerulonephropathy has a strong association with myelodysplastic disorders.

- When cast nephropathy develops in a dysproteinemic disorder, the biopsy shows enlarged tubules filled with proteinaceous material. Immunofluorescence can identify the specific components of these casts.

TREATMENT

Chemotherapy aimed at the underlying disease can be effective in reversing renal disease; this may be particularly important in myeloma when cast nephropathy is present on biopsy. Small studies have previously suggested renal benefit with plasmapheresis to accomplish an aggressive reduction in light chain burden. However, with improvements in chemotherapeutic options, there is no significant benefit of plasmapheresis or high-cutoff hemodialysis for short-term outcomes when compared to conventional supportive measures.[26] There is no specific treatment for fibrillary or immunotactoid glomerulopathy, although treatment of underlying malignancy, if identified, may slow renal disease progression.

Membranoproliferative Glomerulonephritis

GENERAL PRINCIPLES

MPGN can present with nephrotic syndrome, nephritic syndrome, or a combination of both. Traditional MPGN is distinguished by having an immunoglobulin-mediated basis, while nonimmunoglobulin forms are now categorized under a distinct **C3 glomerulopathy** classification.[27] Primary idiopathic MPGN is uncommon. Hepatitis C accounts for most cases of secondary MPGN and can be seen in association with cryoglobulinemia. Other secondary causes include HIV, SLE, chronic infections, and various malignancies.

DIAGNOSIS

Clinical Presentation

- MPGN results from immune complex–mediated activation of the classical complement pathway, with the finding of both immunoglobulin and complement on immunofluorescence staining of the biopsy specimen. IgM and C3 are most commonly seen, particularly in hepatitis C–associated cases.
- The separately classified entity, C3 glomerulopathy, encompasses **C3 glomerulonephritis (C3GN)**, and **dense deposit disease (DDD)**, defined by the dominant staining for C3 on immunofluorescence, in the absence of immunoglobulin. The antibody C3 nephritic factor may be present in C3GN, stabilizing the C3-convertase and promoting complement consumption. This leads to a disorganized regulation of the alternate pathway. Deficiencies of complement regulators (factor H, factor I, complement factor H–related proteins), antibodies against the complement regulators, or a gain of function mutation in factor B may also activate the complement cascade. DDD also shows complement deposition in the absence of immunoglobulin but is characterized by electron dense deposits in the GBM.

Diagnostic Testing

In MPGN, the kidney biopsy shows diffuse mesangial proliferation and hypercellularity on light microscopy, with "lobulization" of the glomerular tuft, giving it a "cauliflower" appearance. Accumulation of debris along the filtration barrier may lead to a damage–repair cycle that results in duplication of the GBM, giving a double-contour or "tram track" appearance on silver stain. Immunofluorescence can show granular mesangial and capillary wall deposits of Ig in the immune complex–mediated forms, whereas only the C3 staining is positive in C3GN or DDD. Electron microscopy can show subendothelial or intramembranous deposits.

TREATMENT

- In adult idiopathic MPGN, treatment with immunosuppression has not shown a consistent benefit, although this may have been a result of lumping together diseases with dissimilar pathophysiology under an older classification scheme.
- Treatment of the secondary forms is targeted at the underlying disease. However, in aggressive forms where there is rapid deterioration of renal function in the presence of cryoglobulins, plasmapheresis may help slow down disease progression and stabilize renal function. Case series have demonstrated a potential role of the anti-C5 monoclonal antibody eculizumab in the treatment of C3 glomerulopathy.[28,29]

IgA Nephropathy/Henoch–Schönlein Purpura

GENERAL PRINCIPLES

- IgA nephropathy is a result of abnormal glycosylation of the hinge region of immunoglobulin A. This results in autoantibodies which interact with abnormally glycosylated protein and cause glomerular disease. Although serum IgA levels do not correlate with disease activity, events that potentially lead to overproduction (concurrent upper respiratory infection) or decreased clearance (hepatic cirrhosis) may predispose to development of this disease.
- This disease process is typically idiopathic, characterized by a nephritic picture with microscopic (and less commonly, macroscopic) hematuria and nonnephrotic range proteinuria.
- Presentation is usually in the second or third decade of life, often following a slowly progressive course. Multiple forms of pathology exist, from mild lesions and mesangial proliferation to global sclerosis resulting in progression to ESRD.
- Henoch–Schönlein purpura is a related disorder that may represent a systemic form of the disease, with vasculitis of the skin (palpable purpura of the lower trunk and extremities), gastrointestinal tract, and joints.

DIAGNOSIS

Diagnostic Testing

Kidney biopsy shows increased mesangial cellularity on light microscopy, with predominant IgA and C3 deposition on immunofluorescence. On electron microscopy, there are electron dense deposits in the mesangium.

TREATMENT

- Aggressiveness of therapy depends on the severity of disease. For patients with a benign course, conservative management with ACE inhibitors or ARBs is recommended. The benefit of omega-3 fatty acid fish oil remains controversial.
- For patients with persistent proteinuria of >1 g/d despite maximally tolerated RAAS blockade, corticosteroids have been shown to provide benefit with reduction of proteinuria and slowed decline in GFR.[30] Long-term sustained benefit with immunosuppression is less well-established.[31] The incidence of adverse events was higher in subjects receiving immunosuppression rather than conservative therapy alone, thus treatment decisions need to be individualized.

Postinfectious Glomerulonephropathy

GENERAL PRINCIPLES

- Postinfectious glomerulonephropathy classically presents as nephritic syndrome, with hematuria, hypertension, edema, and renal insufficiency. Proteinuria may be present and is usually in the subnephrotic range.
- This entity is classically associated with streptococcal infection, which typically affects children under the age of 10, after a latent period of 2–4 weeks from onset of pharyngitis or skin infection. However, bacterial endocarditis, visceral abscesses, and ventriculoperitoneal shunt infections can also lead to this immune complex–mediated disease.
- Low complement levels are usually seen. ASO titers may be elevated serially, as may anti-DNase B antibodies in streptococcal-associated disease.

DIAGNOSIS

Kidney biopsy reveals hump-shaped subepithelial deposits on electron microscopy corresponding to the deposits on immunofluorescence (C3 dominant, or C3 and IgG co-dominant staining). There is widespread mesangial proliferation and infiltration of polymorphonuclear neutrophils.

TREATMENT

Treatment is primarily supportive. Resolution of the underlying infection typically leads to renal recovery in 2–4 weeks, even in cases requiring dialysis. A brisk diuresis should be anticipated in the recovery period and electrolytes should be carefully monitored.

Lupus Nephritis

GENERAL PRINCIPLES

Lupus nephritis (LN) can manifest as proteinuria of varying degrees with dysmorphic RBCs and RBC casts and renal insufficiency. Positive lupus serology (e.g., ANA, anti–double-stranded DNA antibodies, anti-histone antibodies, anti-Smith antibodies) and hypocomplementemia (especially low C3) are often present during acute flares. The anti-Smith antibody is specific for SLE.

DIAGNOSIS

- Renal biopsy can provide diagnostic and prognostic information. The International Society of Nephrology/Renal Pathology Society classification has six major categories based on histologic appearance.[32]
  - Class I (minimal mesangial LN) does not show mesangial hypercellularity, though mesangial deposits may be seen in immunofluorescence and electron microscopy.
  - Class II (mesangial proliferative LN) is characterized by mesangial hypercellularity (four or more nuclei in nonhilar region) or matrix expansion, primarily with mesangial deposits on immunofluorescence and electron microscopy.
  - Class III (focal LN) shows glomerular lesions (including endocapillary or extracapillary hypercellularity, necrosis, crescents) with mesangial and subendothelial deposits, involving <50% of glomeruli.
  - Class IV (diffuse LN) shows glomerular lesions (including endocapillary or extracapillary hypercellularity, necrosis, crescents) with mesangial and subendothelial deposits involving ≥50% of glomeruli.
  - Class V (membranous LN) has features resembling MN with >50% of glomeruli showing subepithelial deposits with or without mesangial hypercellularity. This may occur in conjunction with class III or class IV disease.
  - Class VI (advanced sclerosis LN) with ≥90% globally sclerosed glomeruli.
- Immunofluorescence is usually positive for IgG, IgA, IgM, C1q, and C3, for the "full-house" fluorescence pattern. It is also important to note that these classes could switch, and biopsy is necessary to classify LN patients prior to treatment.

TREATMENT

Aggressiveness of therapy takes into consideration the renal and extrarenal manifestations of the disease.

- Class I LN rarely requires specific treatment, and therapy is directed at the extrarenal manifestations. There are usually no long-term adverse effects on kidney function.
- For class II LN, therapy depends on the amount of proteinuria and the degree of extrarenal manifestations. When proteinuria is <1 g/d, routine management and monitoring is typically sufficient. However, if there is significant proteinuria >3 g/d, treatment with corticosteroids or calcineurin inhibitors may be required.
- For class III, IV, or V LN, treatment can be divided into initial induction therapy and maintenance therapy.
- Initial induction therapy for aggressive disease is with corticosteroids (IV methylprednisolone 5–10 mg/kg for 3 days followed by oral prednisone 0.5–1.0 mg/kg/d tapered over 6–12 months according to patient's clinical response) PLUS either cyclophosphamide or mycophenolate mofetil.
- Cyclophosphamide can be given IV or PO, though more recent studies utilize the IV route due to a lower cumulative dose. A standard regimen is 0.5–1.0 g/m^2 monthly for 6 months, although a more recent study in European patients found comparable efficacy with a lower cumulative dose, given as 500 mg IV every 2 weeks for 3 months[33]
- Mycophenolate mofetil (2–3 g daily in divided doses) was compared to cyclophosphamide for induction therapy, with no significant difference in the response rate at 6 months[34]

- For maintenance therapy, mycophenolate mofetil (1–2 g/d in divided doses) with low-dose corticosteroids (less than 10 mg/day of prednisone) was shown to be superior to azathioprine (1.5–2.5 mg/kg/d) combined with corticosteroids.[35]
- Rituximab therapy has also been shown to have treatment efficacy in lupus nephritis refractory to standard therapy. When combined with corticosteroids and mycophenolate mofetil, however, it did not show improved clinical outcomes after 1 year.[36]
- Treatment course should be closely followed to ensure remission by monitoring renal function, proteinuria, hematuria, complement levels, and auto-antibody levels.

Pulmonary–Renal Syndromes

GENERAL PRINCIPLES

Several distinct clinical entities make up the pulmonary–renal syndromes with vasculitic involvement of the alveolar and glomerular capillaries. Typically, this results in rapidly progressive renal failure with concurrent pulmonary involvement in the form of alveolar hemorrhage. A nephritic picture predominates, with dysmorphic RBCs and RBC casts in the urine. Arthralgias, abdominal pain, and fever may represent other systemic manifestations.

DIAGNOSIS

- In **anti-GBM antibody disease**, circulating antibody to the α-3 subunit of the noncollagenous (NCI) domain of type IV collagen is deposited in the basement membrane of glomeruli, resulting in linear staining on immunofluorescence. **Goodpasture syndrome** includes pulmonary involvement with damage to the alveolar basement membrane and can present with life-threatening alveolar hemorrhage. The presence of anti-GBM antibody in the serum supports the diagnosis, and 10%–30% of patients will also have a positive ANCA serology. This disease is more common in Caucasian patients, with peak age of 20–30 years and another peak at 60–70 years.
- In **granulomatosis with polyangiitis** (GPA), vasculitic lesions involve the small vessels of the kidneys and may also involve the lungs, skin, and gastrointestinal tract. As in anti-GBM antibody disease, pulmonary hemorrhage may be life-threatening. Biopsy findings include small-vessel vasculitis with noncaseating granuloma formation in the kidneys, lungs, or sinuses.
  - GPA is part of a group of diseases known as **ANCA-associated vasculitis**, or pauci-immune glomerulonephritis (referring to the absence of immunostaining deposits), which includes eosinophilic granulomatosis with polyangiitis (EGPA) and microscopic polyangiitis (MPA).
  - In GPA, there is a positive cytoplasmic ANCA (c-ANCA) directed against serine proteinase-3 (PR3) in 80%–90% of cases, whereas in MPA and EGPA, there is a positive perinuclear ANCA (p-ANCA) directed against myeloperoxidase (MPO) in 60% of cases.

TREATMENT

- In anti-GBM antibody disease, the goal of therapy is to clear and suppress production of the pathogenic antibodies. Treatment is with daily total volume (4 L) plasmapheresis for approximately 14 days PLUS oral cyclophosphamide 2 mg/kg/d for 3 months PLUS glucocorticoids (IV methylprednisolone 500 to 1000 mg/d IV for 3 days followed by oral prednisone, 1 mg/kg/d based on ideal body weight not exceeding a total of 80 mg/day with a slow taper off by 6 months). Serial measurement of the anti-GBM antibody level is useful to monitor therapy; the treatment goal is to achieve an undetectable level.

- Poor response to therapy is predicted by the presence of oliguria, Cr >5.7 mg/dL, or dialysis dependence on presentation. Even if the likelihood of renal recovery is low, evidence of pulmonary involvement warrants aggressive therapy.

- Management of ANCA-associated vasculitis includes corticosteroids (IV methylprednisolone 1 g/d for 3 days followed by prednisone 1 mg/kg/d not exceeding a total of 80 mg/d, tapered over 3–6 months), and either cyclophosphamide (15 mg/kg IV every 2 weeks for three doses then every 3 weeks for 3–6 months, or as 1.5–2 mg/kg/d PO for 3–6 months) or rituximab (either as 375 mg/m^2 weekly for 4 weeks, or as 1 g with two doses 14 days apart) to induce remission. Azathioprine can be substituted once remission is achieved (2 mg/kg/d). Methotrexate (15–25 mg/wk) was not found to be safer than azathioprine.[37] Mycophenolate mofetil (1.5–3 g/d in divided doses) was less efficacious in maintaining remission than azathioprine.[38] Maintenance therapy is continued for a duration dictated by the individual patient's clinical course, though a typical course may extend 12–24 months after a stable remission has been achieved.

- In a recent study, there was no benefit with the addition of plasma exchange.[39] This study also reported noninferiority of a reduced dose of prednisone (0.5 mg/kg/d not exceeding a total of 40 mg/d) as compared to the standard regimen.

- Double-strength sulfamethoxazole–trimethoprim given twice daily has been shown to reduce extrarenal relapses and to prevent *Pneumocystis (carinii) jirovecii* infection in patients on high-dose immunosuppression.

Polycystic Kidney Disease

GENERAL PRINCIPLES

- Autosomal dominant polycystic kidney disease (ADPKD) is a hereditary disorder resulting in cystic enlargement of the kidneys. The incidence is estimated to be 1 in 500 to 1000 live births. Approximately 20% of patients with ADPKD do not have a positive family history. ADPKD currently accounts for up to 10% of patients with ESRD.

- There are two well-described mutations in the polycystin genes, PKD1 and PKD2 which encode for polycystin (PC) 1 and 2, respectively. PKD1 is more common, accounting for approximately 85% of ADPKD. PKD2 is associated with later progression of disease.

- The mechanism by which cysts form is unclear; a proposed "two-hit" hypothesis implicates a second somatic mutation that inactivates the wild-type allele in individual cells. The polycystin gene products localize to the primary cilium of the apical membrane of tubular cells. Disordered cell division and aberrant planar cell polarity may lead to overgrowth of the tubular segment, eventually pinching off from the rest of the collecting system and forming discrete cysts. In abnormal cells, cyclic AMP imparts a proliferative phenotype as well as inducing chloride extrusion into the cyst lumen.

DIAGNOSIS

Clinical Presentation

- Hypertension is an early feature of ADPKD and occurs even prior to a reduction in the GFR in approximately 60% of patients. As the affected tubules enlarge, they impinge on the blood flow to neighboring glomeruli, rendering them ischemic. This in turn leads to RAAS activation and systemic hypertension. Onset of kidney failure is highly variable, with half of patients reaching ESRD by the age of 60.

- Kidney stones develop in approximately 25% of patients with ADPKD, with a higher proportion of uric acid composition as compared to the general population.
- Cerebral aneurysms, hepatic cysts, mitral valve prolapse, and colonic diverticula are found in association with ADPKD. As cysts enlarge, they may result in a palpable flank mass. Gross hematuria and pain may indicate cyst hemorrhage into the collecting system. Flank pain may also be caused by cyst infection or stretching of the renal capsule.

Diagnostic Testing

- Differentiation from other renal cystic diseases (acquired cystic kidney diseases, medullary sponge kidney, medullary cystic kidney disease, glomerulocystic kidney disease) can be made by the presence of enlarged cystic kidneys rather than shrunken or normal-sized cystic kidneys.
- Ultrasonography reveals multiple cysts. In the setting of a positive family history, a diagnosis of ADPKD can be made from ultrasound findings, with criteria differing according to age. Three or more cysts (unilateral or bilateral) are required for diagnosis in patients between the ages of 15 and 39. From ages 40 to 59, two or more cysts in each kidney are required. From age 60 and older, more than four cysts in each kidney are required to make the diagnosis.
- Patients with a family history of cerebral aneurysms or with symptoms attributable to a cerebral aneurysm should undergo evaluation with brain MRI/MRA; imaging can be performed without the use of gadolinium contrast.
- Genetic testing may be considered if patients have equivocal imaging results or a definitive diagnosis is required.

TREATMENT

- Treatment of hypertension consists of reduction in sodium intake and pharmacologic therapy when indicated. A large randomized controlled trial of patients with ADPKD suggested improved preservation of renal function at blood pressure targets of 95–110/60–75, but tolerability was limited by symptomatic hypotension.[40] Thus, guidelines for blood pressure control in patients with ADPKD are similar to those in other patients with CKD, targeting a systolic pressure of <120 mm Hg using standardized office measurements.
- In 2018, tolvaptan was approved in the United States for treatment of ADPKD. Blockade of the vasopressin-2 receptor inhibits cyclic AMP production. Large randomized controlled trials of tolvaptan have revealed a reduction of the cyst growth rate and a decreased rate of GFR decline as compared to placebo.[41,42] Treatment can be offered to patients with a GFR above 25 mL/min/1.73 m^2 and evidence of disease progression (e.g., GFR decline, enlarged kidney volume, increased kidney length). Of note, subjects between the ages of 56 and 65 who were enrolled in the clinical trial did not show a benefit beyond that of placebo. Polyuria and polydipsia are frequently experienced by patients on this medication, and it may limit dose escalation to the goal of 90 mg in the morning and 30 mg in the afternoon. Close monitoring of hepatic enzymes is mandatory, with measurements at baseline, at 2 weeks, 4 weeks, monthly through the first 18 months, then every 3 months afterward.
- Gross hematuria from cyst hemorrhage can usually be managed with bed rest, hydration, and analgesia. Resolution may take 5–7 days.

CHAPTER 13

- Cyst infections are generally treated with antibiotics that achieve good penetration into the cysts. Sulfamethoxazole–trimethoprim and ciprofloxacin are the antibiotics of choice. The absence of bacterial growth in the urine does not rule out infection as the cystic fluid does not necessarily communicate with the rest of the collecting system.
- Pain that persists without an obvious hemorrhagic or infectious cause may respond to targeted cyst drainage or cyst reduction surgery. Drained cysts do tend to recur, limiting the long-term efficacy of this procedure.

Nephrolithiasis

GENERAL PRINCIPLES

Nephrolithiasis is more common in men than women by a 2:1 ratio, with a peak age at the third to fourth decade. There are certain medical conditions that predispose patients to kidney stones, including diabetes mellitus, hypertension, metabolic syndrome, distal renal tubular acidosis, gout, and ADPKD.

- **Calcium-based stones** are the most common type of kidney stones (80%). Among these, the most common type is mixed calcium oxalate and calcium phosphate followed by calcium oxalate alone, and then calcium phosphate alone. These stones are radiopaque. Calcium oxalate stones can be found in acidic or alkaline urine and can be dumbbell shaped or appear as paired pyramids (giving them an envelope appearance when viewed on end). Calcium phosphate stones can appear as elongated, blunt crystals and form in alkaline urine.
- **Uric acid stones** (10%) develop in conditions that promote an acidic urine, such as what is observed in patients with the metabolic syndrome. Hyperuricosuric states such as gout and myeloproliferative disorders are also associated with uric acid stones, though the predominant risk factor for their precipitation is an acidic environment. These stones are radiolucent, and the crystals can exhibit a variety of shapes, with needles and rhomboid forms being the most common.
- **Struvite stones** (10%) are also known as "triple phosphate" stones, with phosphate being present in its trivalent form and combining with three cations, ammonium, magnesium, and calcium. They are radiopaque and can extend to fill the renal pelvis, taking on a staghorn configuration. On microscopy, struvite crystals have a characteristic coffin-lid shape. They develop in alkaline urine associated with urea-splitting organisms (e.g., *Proteus, Klebsiella, Serratia, Haemophilus, Pseudomonas*) and are more commonly seen in patients with anatomic abnormalities (e.g., vesicoureteral reflux, obstruction of the pelviureteric junction, ureteral stricture).
- **Cystine stones** (<1%) are uncommon and form as a result of an autosomal recessive disorder, in which the renal epithelium has a decreased ability to reabsorb the dibasic amino acids cystine, ornithine, lysine, and arginine. Among these, only cystine is highly insoluble and precipitates to form stones in acidic urine. These stones have an intermediate radiolucency and appear as hexagonal crystals in the urine.

DIAGNOSIS

Clinical Presentation

The clinical presentation of kidney stones varies based on the location and the size of the stone. Some stones are completely asymptomatic, and others may present with flank pain at the costovertebral angle radiating to the groin, genitals, or suprapubic area. Patients may also present with hematuria, dysuria, and urinary urgency. Nondysmorphic RBCs may be noted under urine microscopy. Oliguria and AKI are uncommon but can result if there is bilateral obstruction or if a solitary functioning kidney is affected.

Diagnostic Testing

- Basic laboratory investigations include urine (culture, pH, microscopy) and serum (calcium, phosphate, parathyroid hormone [PTH], magnesium, uric acid) studies. Urine should be strained and passed stones analyzed for composition.
- A kidney ultrasound is safe, relatively inexpensive, and readily available but may miss stones that are <3 mm. Plain abdominal films may reveal radiopaque stones composed of calcium salts, struvite, or cystine, but may miss small stones, those that are obscured by other structures, or radiolucent uric acid stones. Noncontrast CT scanning has replaced other imaging modalities as the study of choice for suspected nephrolithiasis in an acute presentation.
- Certain patients may require a more extensive evaluation, including a detailed dietary history and a 24-hour urine collection for volume, calcium, sodium, phosphate, uric acid, citrate, oxalate, and cystine, and pH measurement. A history of recurrent stone or bilateral stone diseases, family history of stones, and presence of inflammatory bowel diseases or other malabsorptive processes should prompt a more detailed evaluation. This collection should not be done during an acute episode in a hospitalized patient but rather reserved for when the patient is on their usual outpatient diet.

TREATMENT

- General treatment of an acute event consists of **volume expansion** to increase urine output as well as analgesia. If the stone is obstructing outflow or accompanied by infection, removal is indicated with urgent urologic or radiologic intervention.
- After passage of a stone, treatment is directed at **prevention of recurrent stone formation.** Regardless of stone type, the foundation of therapy is maintenance of high urine output (2–3 L/d) and a low-sodium diet (2–2.3 g/d or 80–100 mmol/d).
- For calcium oxalate stones, an age-appropriate dietary calcium intake with no added calcium supplements is recommended. If hypercalciuria is present, adherence to a low-sodium diet should be ensured, with the addition of a thiazide diuretic as the next step. If hypocitraturia is present, potassium citrate (10–60 mEq/d in divided doses) can be started; lemon juice (4 ounces mixed with a liter of water) is an alternate strategy that has been studied, though consistent long-term benefit has not been proven. Oxalate-rich foods (e.g., spinach, rhubarb) should be avoided if hyperoxaluria is present.
- Uric acid stones can be prevented or reduced in size by urinary alkalinization, preferentially with potassium citrate 10–60 mEq/d in divided doses to target a urine pH of 6–6.5. A low-protein diet is advised. In patients who do not respond to urine alkalinization with potassium citrate, reduction in uricosuria can be targeted with xanthine oxidase inhibitors (allopurinol or febuxostat).
- Struvite stones frequently require surgical intervention for their removal. Monthly urine cultures should be obtained, and if positive, aggressive antibiotic treatment is indicated. Any anatomical abnormality identified as a causative factor for struvite stones should be corrected when possible.

CHAPTER 13

- Cystine stones require extensive urinary alkalinization to a pH of 7.0–7.5 to induce solubility, aggressive sodium restriction (<2 g/d), and high fluid intake of 3.5–5 L/d. Tiopronin can further increase solubility through breakage and exchange of disulfide bonds. Side effects include loss of taste, fever, rash, arthritis, proteinuria, myelosuppression, and hepatotoxicity.

Management of Chronic Kidney Disease

GENERAL PRINCIPLES

- CKD is classified based on the GFR and albuminuria. Based on the GFR (Figure 13-1), it can be divided into five stages: G1 (GFR ≥90 mL/min/1.73 m^2), G2 (GFR 60–89), G3 (subdivided into G3a with a GFR 45 to 59 and G3b with a GFR 30–44), G4 (GFR 15–29), and G5 (GFR <15 not on renal replacement therapy). For G1 and G2, additional evidence of renal disease, such as proteinuria, needs to be present for at least 3 months. Definitions for albuminuria are based on the urinary albumin-to-creatinine ratio as described earlier in the chapter. GFR, degree of albuminuria, etiology of CKD, and other risk factors should be considered together as these predict clinical outcomes and help in planning for renal replacement therapy.
- Patients are usually asymptomatic until significant renal function is lost (late stage G4 and stage G5). However, complications including hypertension, anemia, and mineral bone disorders (renal osteodystrophy and secondary hyperparathyroidism) often develop during stage G3 and thus should be investigated and addressed before patients become symptomatic.

Prognosis of CKD by GFR and Albuminuria Categories: KDIGO 2012				Persistent albuminuria categories Description and range		
				A1	A2	A3
				Normal to mildly increased	Moderately increased	Severely increased
				<30 mg/g <3 mg/mmol	30-300 mg/g 3-30 mg/mmol	>300 mg/g >30 mg/mmol
GFR categories (mL/min/1.73 m^2) Description and range	G1	Normal or high	≥90			
	G2	Mildly decreased	60-89			
	G3a	Mildly to moderately decreased	45-59			
	G3b	Moderately to severely decreased	30-44			
	G4	Severely decreased	15-29			
	G5	Kidney failure	<15			

Figure 13-1. Stages of chronic kidney disease. CKD, chronic kidney disease; GFR, glomerular filtration rate. (Reprinted from Summary of recommendation statements. *Kidney Int Suppl (2011).* 2013;3(suppl):5–14. Copyright © 2013 International Society of Nephrology. With permission.)

- In the setting of CKD, initiation of dialysis based solely on a target GFR has not shown a mortality benefit.[43] Dialysis should be started before the worsening of the patient's metabolic or nutritional status.

Risk Factors

- **Decreased renal perfusion** can lead to a decline in GFR. This can occur with true volume depletion or diminished effective circulating volume (e.g., congestive heart failure, liver cirrhosis with ascites). **NSAIDs** can be particularly deleterious in this setting because they block renal autoregulatory mechanisms which preserve GFR. ACE inhibitors or ARBs also produce a reversible decrement in GFR through alterations in hemodynamics.
- **Uncontrolled hypertension** leads to hyperfiltration, which may lead to worsening proteinuria and further damage to the glomeruli.
- **Albuminuria** has also been identified as a risk factor for progression of renal disease. A prognostic scale has been developed incorporating both the GFR and degree of albuminuria to predict the likelihood to renal failure (see Figure 13-1).
- **Nephrotoxic agents**, such as iodinated contrast agents and aminoglycosides, should be avoided when possible. Careful attention to drug dosing is mandatory, frequently guided by the estimated GFR or CKD stage. Drug levels should be monitored where appropriate.
- Patients undergoing coronary angiography are at particular risk for worsening CKD. **Contrast nephropathy** and **atheroembolic disease** are potential complications of coronary angiography, and the risks and benefits of the procedure must be weighed with the patient before proceeding.
- **UTI** or **obstruction** should be considered in all patients with an unexplained drop in renal function.
- Worsening **renal artery stenosis** may also lead to a more rapid decline in GFR as well as sudden worsening of previously controlled hypertension.
- **Renal vein thrombosis** may occur as a complication of nephrotic syndrome and can exacerbate CKD. Hematuria and flank pain may be present.
- The **APOL1 gene** has been linked to a major health disparity in patients with African ancestry, with a cumulative lifetime risk of reaching ESRD approximately 7.5% compared to 2% in patients with European ancestry. The high-risk genotypes include homozygous G1/G1, homozygous G2/G2, and compound heterozygous G1/G2. African American patients with or without diabetes mellitus with two APOL1 risk alleles have a faster rate of CKD progression and increased likelihood of developing ESRD.[44]
- Other risk factors include high BMI, history of cardiovascular disease, and smoking.

TREATMENT

Treatment of CKD is focused on addressing the risk factors mentioned above: dietary modification, blood pressure control, adequate treatment of associated conditions, and ultimately, preparation for renal replacement therapy.

- **Dietary recommendations**
  - **Sodium restriction** to <2 g/d is recommended for patients with CKD and hypertension. Restriction to <2 g/d should also be used if heart failure or refractory hypertension is present.
  - **Fluid restriction** is generally not required in CKD patients and, if excessive, may lead to volume depletion and hypernatremia. Restriction is appropriate in patients with dilutional hyponatremia.

- There is currently no benefit to show that strict **dietary protein** restriction is indicated as a treatment to slow progression of CKD.
- **Potassium should be restricted** to 60 mEq/d in individuals with hyperkalemia. Tomato-based products, bananas, potatoes, and citrus drinks are high in potassium and should be avoided in these patients.
- **Dietary phosphate restriction** should be to 800–1000 mg/d. Dairy products, dark colas, nuts, and processed meat should be avoided in hyperphosphatemia. Oral binders (calcium carbonate or acetate, lanthanum carbonate, sevelamer carbonate) can be taken with meals if dietary restrictions are unable to control phosphate levels.
- **Smoking** accelerates CKD progression and patients should be counseled about the importance of tobacco cessation.
- **Hypertension**
  - Uncontrolled hypertension accelerates the rate of decline of renal function. The 2021 KDIGO guidelines recommend targeting a systolic blood pressure of <120 mm Hg using standardized office measurements for patients with CKD.[45]
  - **ACE inhibitors** or **ARBs** should be used preferentially in the CKD population. They lower intraglomerular pressure and possess renal protective properties beyond their antihypertensive effect, particularly in proteinuric states. Because of their effects on intrarenal hemodynamics, a 30% rise in serum Cr should be anticipated and tolerated; a further rise should prompt a search for possible renal artery stenosis. The Cr and serum potassium should be checked approximately 1 week after a dose adjustment. Combined therapy with ACE inhibitors and ARBs is not recommended because of an increased risk of hyperkalemia and AKI without statistical benefit in mortality or long-term renal protection.[46]
  - **Diuretics** are also beneficial in achieving euvolemia in hypertensive CKD patients. Thiazide diuretics become less effective as the GFR falls below 30 mL/min, whereas loop diuretics retain their efficacy, although higher doses may be required for the desired effect.
- **Albuminuria and proteinuria**
  Blood pressure control, and RAAS inhibition specifically, has been shown to decrease albuminuria and CKD progression.
- **Metabolic acidosis**
  - As renal function deteriorates, the kidneys are unable to appropriately excrete sufficient acid, resulting in metabolic acidosis (mixed high and normal anion gap). To compensate, alkaline buffer is released from bone but can ultimately worsen bone mineral disease.
  - Oral bicarbonate tablets (650 or 1300 mg twice or three times daily) to keep serum bicarbonate level of ≥22 mEq/L have been shown to slow CKD progression.[47]
- **Hyperlipidemia**
  - Therapy with statins combined with ezetimibe has shown improved cardiovascular outcomes with fewer major atherosclerotic events in patients with moderate to severe CKD and in the dialysis population, although the benefit in patients on dialysis was less.[48] Use of lipid-lowering therapy is appropriate in patients with atherosclerotic disease at all stages of CKD.
  - In 2014, KDIGO clinical practice guidelines recommended a statin with ezetimibe in adults aged 50 and older with a GFR <60 mL/min/1.73 m^2, but not for patients receiving dialysis or transplant recipients. An escalating statin dose in those not meeting LDL cholesterol targets was not recommended.[49]
- **Diabetes mellitus**
  - KDOQI guideline recommends a target HbA1C of 7% to prevent progression of CKD as well as micro- and macrovascular complications.

- ○ SGLT2 inhibitors have been extensively studied and now reported to have reno-protective outcomes as well as cardiovascular benefits in patients with or without albuminuria with a GFR of ≥30 mL/min/1.73 m^2.[25]
- **Anemia**
  - ○ A normocytic anemia is common in CKD and should be evaluated once the GFR falls below 60 mL/min/1.73.
  - ○ Alternate causes for an anemia should be sought in the appropriate setting and iron stores assessed. If the transferrin saturation is ≤30% and there is no evidence of iron overload (ferritin <500 ng/mL), consideration should be given to iron repletion with an intravenous preparation of iron. Options include iron dextran (1000 mg once with test dose of 25 mg), ferric gluconate (125 mg, eight doses), or iron sucrose (200 mg, five doses). IV iron use should be avoided in patients with active infections.
  - ○ Erythropoiesis-stimulating agents (ESAs), such as epoetin and darbepoetin, can effectively reduce but do not prevent the need for RBC transfusions. ESA therapy increases the risk of stroke, thrombotic and cardiovascular events, and can worsen outcomes in patients with malignancy. These agents should not be started in CKD unless the hemoglobin is <10 g/dL, other causes of anemia such as iron deficiency are addressed, and reduction in transfusions is a goal. The minimum dose that maintains the hemoglobin above the need for transfusion and below 11 g/dL should be used. Targeting higher levels of hemoglobin has been associated with increased cardiovascular mortality, and this risk may be related to the higher doses of ESA.[50] When stable doses of ESAs are used, hemoglobin should be monitored every 3 months.
- **Mineral bone disorders**
  - ○ CKD bone mineral disorders increase in prevalence as the GFR declines through stage G3 and more advanced disease. They include disorders of bone turnover and secondary hyperparathyroidism.
  - ○ **Osteitis fibrosa cystica** is associated with secondary hyperparathyroidism and increased bone turnover, resulting in bone pain and increased fracture risk. Adynamic bone disease is a low-turnover state with suppressed PTH levels. Osteomalacia can involve deposition of aluminum into bone and is less commonly seen today with the decreased use of aluminum-based phosphate binders.
  - ○ In CKD, starting in stage G3, vitamin D deficiency, low calcium, and elevated phosphate can all contribute to **secondary hyperparathyroidism.** The general goal of therapy is to suppress PTH toward normal while maintaining normal serum calcium and phosphate. This can be addressed in three steps: repletion of vitamin D stores (25-OH vitamin D), control of dietary phosphate with binders, and administration of active vitamin D (1,25-dihydroxyvitamin D or an analogue).
    - Deficient stores (25-OH vitamin D <30 ng/mL) should be corrected with oral ergocalciferol 50,000-IU capsules weekly or every other week or cholecalciferol 2000–4000 IU daily. The duration of treatment depends on severity of the deficiency, with levels <5 ng/dL warranting at least 12 weeks of treatment. Once at goal, maintenance therapy can rely on either monthly ergocalciferol 50,000 IU or daily cholecalciferol 1000–2000 IU.
    - Phosphate control can be difficult as GFR declines, even with appropriate dietary restriction. Phosphate binders inhibit gastrointestinal absorption. Calcium-based binders are effective when given with meals as calcium carbonate (200 mg of elemental calcium per 500-mg tablet) or calcium acetate (169 mg of elemental calcium per 667-mg tablet). In general, the total daily elemental calcium

CHAPTER 13

administered should be <1500 mg. Lanthanum carbonate and sevelamer carbonate are non-calcium-based alternatives. Ferric citrate and sucroferric oxyhydroxide are approved for use as phosphorus binders for patients on dialysis.

- Active vitamin D (1,25-dihydroxyvitamin D) and its synthetic analogues are potent suppressors of PTH and can be administered if serum PTH remains elevated. Options include daily calcitriol (0.25–1 μg), paricalcitol (1–5 μg), or doxercalciferol (1–5 μg). Calcium levels need to be monitored regularly and doses adjusted to avoid hypercalcemia.
- Cinacalcet is a calcimimetic that acts on the parathyroid gland to suppress PTH release. It should be used only in dialysis patients and usually in conjunction with active vitamin D because it may induce significant hypocalcemia and is relatively ineffective as monotherapy.

- **Preparation for renal replacement therapy**
  - Patients should be counseled at an early stage to determine preferences for renal replacement therapies, including hemodialysis, peritoneal dialysis (PD), and eligibility for renal transplantation.
  - In CKD stage G4, preparation for the creation of a permanent vascular access for hemodialysis should be initiated by protecting the nondominant forearm from IV catheters, blood pressure measurements, and blood draws. Timely referral for vein mapping and to a vascular access surgeon can facilitate arteriovenous (AV) access.
  - Certain immunizations are recommended for patients with CKD including the hepatitis B vaccine for all adults with a GFR < 30 mL/min/1.73 m^2 and the polyvalent pneumococcal vaccine for all adults with CKD irrespective of the stage. Other vaccines can be given per routine.

RENAL REPLACEMENT THERAPIES

Approach to Dialysis

TREATMENT

- **Modalities**
  - Renal replacement therapy is indicated when conservative medical management is unable to control the metabolic derangements of kidney disease. This applies to the acute and chronic settings. Common acute indications include **hyperkalemia**, **metabolic acidosis**, and **volume overload** that are refractory to medical management. Uremic **encephalopathy** or **pericarditis**, as well as certain **intoxications** (methanol, ethylene glycol, or salicylates), can all be indications for urgent dialysis. In the chronic setting, renal replacement therapy is typically begun before deterioration of the metabolic or nutritional status of the patient.
  - Dialysis works by solute diffusion and water transport across a selectively permeable membrane. In hemodialysis, blood is pumped counter-currently to a dialysis solution within an extracorporeal membrane. This can be performed intermittently (3–4 hours during the day) or in a continuous 24-hour fashion depending on hemodynamic stability or goals of therapy.
  - PD uses the patient's peritoneal membrane as the selective filter, and dialysis fluid is instilled into the peritoneal cavity.
  - Transplantation offers the best long-term survival and replaces the filtration and endocrine functions of the native kidney. However, long-term immunosuppression comes with its own risks.

- **Diffusion**

  The selectively permeable membrane contains pores that allow electrolytes and other small molecules to pass by diffusion while preventing movement of larger molecules and cellular components of the blood. Movement relies on the molecular size and the concentration gradient. Potassium, urea, Cr, and other waste products of metabolism pass into the dialysis solution while alkaline buffers (bicarbonate or lactate) enter the blood from the dialysis solution.

- **Ultrafiltration/convection**

  ○ Removal of volume is termed ultrafiltration. It can be achieved in hemodialysis via a transmembrane hydrostatic pressure that removes excess fluid from the blood compartment. In PD, water follows its osmotic gradient into the relatively hyperosmolar dialysis solution (usually with dextrose providing the osmotic driving force).

  ○ As water is removed from the vascular compartment, it drags along solute in proportion to its concentration in the blood. This usually accounts for only a small fraction of the total clearance but can be significantly increased if a physiologic "replacement fluid" is infused into the patient concurrently to prevent hypovolemia, a process termed convective clearance. This strategy is frequently employed by continuous hemodialysis modalities.

Hemodialysis

GENERAL PRINCIPLES

- Hemodialysis is by far the most common form of renal replacement therapy in the United States. Intermittent hemodialysis (IHD) typically runs for 3–4 hours per session and is performed three times weekly. Outpatient, in-center hemodialysis for ESRD generally uses this modality, although variations are available for patients undergoing home treatments.

- Continuous renal replacement therapy (CRRT) can be used in specialized circumstances, particularly when the patient's hemodynamic status would not tolerate the rapid fluid shifts of IHD. Although less efficient (with slower blood flow) and with slower UF rates, CRRT can achieve equivalent clearances of both solute and fluid compared to IHD due to its continuous, 24-hour nature. The slower blood flows may necessitate anticoagulation (with either systemic heparin or regional citrate) to prevent the filter from clotting. Continuous modalities require specialized nursing and an intensive care setting.

  ○ There are various modalities of CRRT, including continuous venovenous hemodiafiltration (CVVHDF) and continuous venovenous hemodialysis (CVVHD). None of these modalities have been shown to be superior to the others.

  ○ In CVVHDF, blood is slowly pumped counter-currently to a dialysis solution (allowing for diffusive clearance), and a replacement fluid (an isotonic physiologic solution devoid of uremic toxins and other waste products) is infused into the circuit to balance most of the ultrafiltrate (convective clearance). CVVHD does not utilize a replacement fluid and thus convective clearance is not performed.

- Sustained low-efficiency dialysis uses intermediate treatment lengths (8–12 hours), allowing for adequate clearances, while patients can spend a significant portion of the day off the machine to allow for non-bedside testing, procedures, and physical therapy.

- **Prescription and adequacy**
  - IHD typically runs for 3–4 hours and can ultrafilter 3–4 L safely in hemodynamically stable patients. In the chronic setting, IHD is generally performed three times weekly, although the longer interdialytic interval on the weekend has been associated with a heightened mortality risk.[51] In the acute setting, the appropriate interval is not clearly defined, although a three times weekly schedule is likely adequate and remains common practice.
  - Adequacy is assessed by calculating BUN clearance, which serves as a surrogate marker of the "uremic factors." The urea reduction ratio can be calculated by the following:

$$\text{URR} = \left[\left(\text{predialysis BUN} - \text{postdialysis BUN} \right) / \left(\text{predialysis BUN} \right) \right] \times 100$$

  - A reduction rate of ≥65% is considered adequate in the chronic setting.[52] An adequacy target is less well defined for AKI. Intensive daily hemodialysis was not shown to be superior to standard three times weekly treatments.[53]
  - Clearance is measured differently in CRRT in which dialytic therapy spans over 24 hours, effectively providing an extracorporeal "GFR." Drug dosing needs to be adjusted accordingly; an estimate of this clearance can be calculated by the sum of the dialysis fluid, replacement fluid, and net UF rates converted into milliliters per minute. For most circumstances, this approximates a clearance of 20–50 mL/min.
  - With CRRT, the net UF rate can be adjusted as needed, according to the patient's hemodynamic status. Electrolyte levels (particularly calcium and phosphorus) should be monitored very carefully to ensure they remain within the desired ranges. Ionized calcium levels are especially important to follow when regional citrate anticoagulation is being used.
  - Phosphate, which is predominantly intracellular, is generally poorly removed by IHD; however, in CRRT, there is continuous efflux of this anion, and significant hypophosphatemia can occur.

COMPLICATIONS

- Nontunneled catheters are typically placed in the internal jugular or femoral vein and carry the same risks as other central venous catheters (infection, bleeding, pneumothorax). They are almost exclusively used in the inpatient setting and are typically used for up to 1–2 weeks. Tunneled catheters have lower rates of infection and can be used for 6 months while a more definitive access is maturing (AV fistula or graft).
  - Fevers and rigors, particularly during dialysis, should prompt a search for an infectious cause, and empiric antibiotic coverage for staphylococci and gram-negative bacteria should be administered.
  - The catheter should then be replaced after a period of defervescence and sterilization of the blood (at least 48 hours). Documented bacteremia should be treated with antibiotics for at least several weeks.
- Thrombosis of an AV fistula or graft can frequently be recanalized by thrombolysis or thrombectomy. Stenotic regions can be evaluated by a fistulogram, and treatment may encompass angioplasty or stent deployment.
- Intradialytic hypotension is most commonly due to intravascular volume depletion from rapid UF. Antihypertensive medications may also contribute. Infectious causes should be considered in the appropriate setting. Acute treatment of hypotension includes infusion of normal saline (as 200-mL boluses) and reduction of the UF rate.

- Dialysis disequilibrium is an uncommon syndrome that may occur in severely uremic patients undergoing their first several treatments. Rapid toxin clearance is thought to result in cerebral edema by osmolar shifts and can present as nausea, emesis, headache, confusion, or seizures. Occurrence can be prevented or ameliorated by initiating patients on dialysis with slower blood flow rates, slower dialysate flow rates, and shorter treatments.

Peritoneal Dialysis

GENERAL PRINCIPLES

- There are two modalities in use: manual exchanges and automated cycler exchanges.
  - The manual modality, also called continuous ambulatory peritoneal dialysis (CAPD), has the patient instill dialysis fluid into the peritoneum for a specified length of time, after which the dialysate is drained and replaced by another dwell.
  - The automated modality, also called continuous cycling peritoneal dialysis (CCPD), typically operates overnight where a machine runs a preprogrammed set of exchanges while the patient sleeps. A final fill usually remains in the peritoneum and is carried during the daytime for continued solute exchange.
- Both PD modalities require strict adherence to sterile technique, and careful patient selection is necessary.
- **Prescription and adequacy**
  - The choice between CAPD and CCPD usually depends on patient preference and on the transport characteristics of the peritoneal membrane. Manual exchanges (i.e., CAPD) can be used as a backup modality, particularly in the hospital where nurse staffing or machine availability may be limited.
  - In writing PD orders, the following variables must be specified: dwell volume, dwell time, number of exchanges, and dextrose concentration of the dialysis solution. The dwell volume is typically between 2 and 3 L, and can vary based on patient characteristics. The dextrose concentration can be 1.5%, 2.5%, or 4.25%, providing the osmotic gradient for fluid removal. Higher dextrose concentrations allow for greater UF but also lead to more inward glucose diffusion and worsening hyperglycemia. Icodextrin is a glucose polymer preparation that can be used in longer dwell because it is minimally absorbed and thus maintains an effective osmotic gradient up to 18 hours. Commercially available PD solutions may have color-coded tabs with which patients may be more familiar rather than the actual concentrations (yellow for 1.5%, green for 2.5%, red for 4.25%).
  - PD is less efficient than conventional hemodialysis. However, given its continuous nature, solute clearance and UF can approximate that of other modalities. Larger volumes and more frequent exchanges can assist with solute exchange. Increasing the concentration of dextrose can promote greater UF in volume-overloaded patients.
  - Residual renal function is very important in the PD population, and avoidance of nephrotoxins should be practiced.[54]

COMPLICATIONS

- **Peritonitis** is a common complication of PD and can be serious with up to 6% of peritonitis episodes resulting in death. It is diagnosed when at least two of the following are present: diffuse abdominal pain and/or cloudy dialysate effluent, a

dialysate effluent WBC count of >100 cells/μL (after a dwell time of at least 2 hours) with >50% neutrophils, and a positive dialysate effluent culture.
- Empiric intraperitoneal antibiotics should cover for both gram-positive and gram-negative organisms, with vancomycin or a first-generation cephalosporin PLUS a third-generation cephalosporin or an aminoglycoside.[55]
- The intraperitoneal route is the preferred method of administration, unless the patient is overtly septic, in which case IV antibiotics should be used. Antibiotics can be tailored once culture results are known and should be continued for 2–3 weeks. Multiple organisms, particularly if gram negative, should prompt a search for intestinal perforation.
- Tunnel or exit site infections may present with local erythema, tenderness, or purulent drainage, although crusting at the exit site alone does not necessarily indicate infection. Treatment can be with oral cephalosporins (gram positive) or fluoroquinolones (gram negative). However, infections can be difficult to eradicate, and catheter removal may be required with a temporary transition to hemodialysis.
- Failure of PD fluid to drain is termed outflow failure. This may result from kinking of the catheter, constipation, or plugging of the catheter with fibrin strands. Conservative treatment should aim at resolving constipation if present, instilling heparin (500 units/L) into the PD fluid, or infusing alteplase (1 mg/mL) into the catheter.
- Small hernias are at particularly high risk for incarceration and should be corrected surgically while the patient is temporarily treated with hemodialysis. Fluid leaks can lead to abdominal wall and genital edema and typically result from anatomic defects. Hydrothorax usually occurs on the right side and can be diagnosed by a markedly elevated glucose concentration in the pleural fluid. Pleurodesis can eliminate the potential space and permit continuation of PD.
- **Sclerosing encapsulating peritonitis** is a complication of long-term PD. The peritoneal membrane becomes thickened and entraps loops of bowel, leading to symptoms of bowel obstruction. A bloody drainage may be present. Treatment is supportive with the focus on bowel rest and surgical lysis of adhesions. A trial of immunosuppression with prednisone 10–40 mg/d may have limited benefit.
- Hyperglycemia results from the systemic absorption of glucose from the dialysis fluid. Because peritoneal uptake of insulin is unpredictable, treatment with subcutaneous insulin is preferred.
- Unlike hemodialysis, patients on PD tend to experience hypokalemia, likely due to a continuous potassium exodus in the dialysate as well as from an intracellular shift from the increased endogenous insulin production. Oral replacement with low dose supplementation (10–20 mEq/d of potassium chloride) is usually sufficient. Potassium dietary restrictions may also be liberalized.
- Protein loss can be high, and the dietary protein intake should be 1.2–1.3 g/kg/d. Episodes of peritonitis can make the membrane even more susceptible to protein losses.

Transplantation

GENERAL PRINCIPLES

- Renal transplantation offers patients an improved quality of life and survival as compared to other renal replacement modalities.
- Pretransplant evaluation focuses on cardiopulmonary status, vascular sufficiency, and human lymphocyte antigen typing. Structural abnormalities of the urinary tract

need to be addressed. Contraindications include many malignancies, active infection, or significant cardiopulmonary disease.

- In adult recipients, the renal allograft is placed in the extraperitoneal space, in the anterior lower abdomen. Vascular anastomosis is typically to the iliac vessels, whereas the ureter is attached to the bladder through a muscular tunnel to approximate sphincter function.

- Immunosuppression protocols vary among institutions. A typical regimen would include prednisone along with a combination of a calcineurin inhibitor (cyclosporine or tacrolimus) and an antimetabolite (mycophenolate derivative, azathioprine, or rapamycin).

- Evaluation of allograft dysfunction frequently requires kidney biopsy. Current laboratory and radiologic tests cannot reliably distinguish acute rejection from drug toxicity, the two most common causes of a rising Cr in the transplant population. Posttransplant lymphoproliferative disease, interstitial nephritis, and infections such as CMV, *Polyomavirus* (BK virus), and pyelonephritis may present similarly to acute allograft dysfunction and should be excluded.

- Complications and long-term management of transplant recipients are discussed further in Chapter 17, Solid Organ Transplant Medicine.

REFERENCES

1. Shardlow A, McIntyre NJ, Fraser SDS, et al. The clinical utility and cost impact of cystatin C measurement in the diagnosis and management of chronic kidney disease: a primary care cohort study. *PLoS Med.* 2017;14:e1002400. doi:10.1371/journal.pmed.1002400.
2. Levey AS, Eckardt KU, Tsukamoto Y, et al. Definition and classification of CKD. *Kidney Int.* 2013;3(1):19-62.
3. Daftari Besheli L, Aran S, Shagdan K, et al. Current status of nephrogenic system fibrosis. *Clin Radiol.* 2014;69:661-668.
4. Khwaja A. KDIGO clinical practice guidelines for acute kidney injury. *Nephron Clin Pract.* 2012;120(4):c179-c184.
5. Bart BA, Goldsmith SR, Lee KL, et al. Ultrafiltration in decompensated heart failure with cardiorenal syndrome. *N Engl J Med.* 2012;367:2296-2304.
6. Gines P, Schrier RW. Renal failure in cirrhosis. *N Engl J Med.* 2009;361:1279-1290.
7. Formica RN, Aeder M, Boyle G, et al. Simultaneous liver-kidney allocation policy: a proposal to optimize appropriate utilization of scarce resources. *Am J Transplant.* 2016;16(3):758-766.
8. Chawla LS, Davison DL, Brasha-Mitchell E, et al. Development and standardization of a furosemide stress test to predict the severity of acute kidney injury. *Crit Care.* 2013;17(5):R207.
9. Weisbord SD, Gallagher M, Jneid H, et al. Outcomes after angiography with sodium bicarbonate and acetylcysteine. *N Engl J Med.* 2018;378:603-614.
10. Noone D, Waters A, Pluthero FG, et al. Successful treatment of DEAP-HUS with eculizumab. *Pediatr Nephrol.* 2014;29:841-851.
11. González E, Gutiérrez E, Galeano C, et al. Early steroid treatment improves the recovery of renal function in patients with drug-induced acute interstitial nephritis. *Kidney Int.* 2008;73(8):940-946.
12. Gaudry S, Hajage D, Schortgen F, et al. Initiation strategies for renal-replacement therapy in the intensive care unit. *N Engl J Med.* 2016;375:122-133.
13. Zarbock A, Kellum JA, Schmidt C, et al. Effect of early vs delayed initiation of renal replacement therapy on mortality in critically ill patients with acute kidney injury: the ELAIN randomized clinical trial. *JAMA.* 2016;315:2190-2199.
14. Lin R, McDonald G, Jolly T, et al. A systematic review of prophylactic anticoagulation in nephrotic syndrome. *Kidney Int Rep.* 2020;5(4):435-447.
15. Stone JH, Merkel PA, Spiera R, et al. Rituximab versus cyclophosphamide for ANCA-associated vasculitis. *N Engl J Med.* 2010;363:221-232.
16. Day CJ, Cockwell P, Lipkin GW, et al. Mycophenolate mofetil in the treatment of resistant idiopathic nephrotic syndrome. *Nephrol Dial Transplant.* 2002;17(11):2011-2013.
17. Munyentwali H, Bouachi K, Audard V, et al. Rituximab is an efficient and safe treatment in adults with steroid-dependent minimal change disease. *Kidney Int.* 2013;83:511-516.
18. De Vriese AS, Sethi S, Nath KA, et al. Differentiating primary, genetic, and secondary FSGS in adults: a clinicopathologic approach. *J Am Soc Nephrol.* 2018; 29(3):759-774.

CHAPTER 13

19. Hoxha E, Beck LH Jr, Weich T, et al. An indirect immunofluorescence method facilitates detection of thrombospondin type I domain-containing 7A-specific antibodies in membranous nephropathy. *J Am Soc Nephrol* 2017;28(2):520-531.

20. Schieppati A, Mosconi L, Perna A, et al. Prognosis of untreated patients with idiopathic membranous nephropathy. *N Engl J Med.* 1993;329(20):85-89.

21. Ponticelli C, Altieri P, Scolari F, et al. A randomized study comparing methylprednisolone plus chlorambucil versus methylprednisolone plus cyclophosphamide in idiopathic membranous nephropathy. *J Am Soc Nephrol.* 1998;9(3):444-450.

22. Fervenza FC, Appel GB, Barbour SJ, et al. Rituximab or cyclosporine in the treatment of membranous nephropathy. *N Engl J Med.* 2019;381(1):36-46.

23. Action to Control Cardiovascular Risk in Diabetes Study Group; Gerstein HC, Miller ME, et al. Effects of intensive glucose lowering in type 2 diabetes. *N Engl J Med.* 2008;358(24):2545-2559.

24. Yusuf S, Teo KK, Pogue J, et al. Telmisartan, ramipril, or both in patients at high risk for vascular events. *N Engl J Med.* 2008;358:1547-1559.

25. Tuttle KR, Brosius FC, Cavender MA, et al. SGLT2 inhibition for CKD and cardiovascular disease in type 2 diabetes: report of a scientific workshop sponsored by the National Kidney Foundation. *Am J Kidney Dis.* 2021;70(1):1-16.

26. Bridoux F, Carron PL, Pegourie B, et al. Effect of high-cutoff hemodialysis vs conventional hemodialysis on hemodialysis independence among patients with myeloma cast nephropathy: a randomized clinical trial. *JAMA.* 2017;318:2099-2110.

27. Sethi S, Fervenza FC. Membranoproliferative glomerulonephritis – a new look at an old entity. *N Engl J Med.* 2012;366:1119-1131.

28. Daina E, Noris M, Remuzzi G. Eculizumab in a patient with dense-deposit disease. *N Engl J Med.* 2012;366:1161-1163.

29. Welte T, Arnold F, Kappes J, et al. Treating C3 glomerulopathy with eculizumab. *BMC Nephrol.* 2018;19(1):7.

30. Lv J, Zhang H, Wong MG, et al. Effect of oral methylprednisolone on clinical outcomes in patients with IgA nephropathy: the TESTING randomized clinical trial. *JAMA.* 2017;318(5): 432-442.

31. Rauen T, Eitner F, Fitzner C, et al. Intensive supportive care plus immunosuppression in IgA nephropathy. *N Engl J Med.* 2015;373(23):2225-2236.

32. Bajema IM, Wilhelmus S, Alpers CE, et al. Revision of the International Society of Nephrology/Renal Pathology Society classification for lupus nephritis: clarification of definitions, and modified National Institutes of Health activity and chronicity indices. *Kidney Int.* 2018;93(4):789-796.

33. Houssiau FA, Vasconcelos C, D'Cruz D, et al. Immunosuppressive therapy in lupus nephritis: the Euro-Lupus Nephritis Trial, a randomized trial of low-dose versus high-dose intravenous cyclophosphamide. *Arthritis Rheum.* 2002;46(8):2121-2131.

34. Appel GB, Contreras G, Dooley MA, et al. Mycophenolate mofetil versus cyclophosphamide for induction treatment of lupus nephritis. *J Am Soc Nephrol.* 2009;20(5):1103-1112.

35. Dooley MA, Jayne D, Ginzler EM, et al. Mycophenolate versus azathioprine as maintenance therapy for lupus nephritis. *N Engl J Med.* 2011;365:1886-1895.

36. Rovin BH, Furie R, Latinis K, et al. Efficacy and safety of rituximab in patients with active proliferative lupus nephritis: the Lupus Nephritis Assessment with Rituximab study. *Arthritis Rheum.* 2012;64(4):1215-1226.

37. Pagnoux C, Mahr A, Hamidou MA, et al. Azathioprine or methotrexate maintenance for ANCA-associated vasculitis. *N Engl J Med.* 2008;359(26):2790-2803.

38. Hiemstra TF, Walsh M, Mahr A, et al. Mycophenolate mofetil vs azathioprine for remission maintenance in antineutrophil cytoplasmic antibody-associated vasculitis: a randomized controlled trial. *JAMA.* 2010;304(21)2381-2388.

39. Walsh M, Merkel PA, Peh CA, et al. Plasma exchange and glucocorticoids in severe ANCA-associated vasculitis. *N Engl J Med.* 2020;382(7):622-631.

40. Schrier RW, Abebe KZ, Perrone RD, et al. Blood pressure in early autosomal dominant polycystic kidney disease. *N Engl J Med.* 2014;371:2255-2266.

41. Torres VE, Chapman AB, Devuyst O, et al. Tolvaptan in patients with autosomal dominant polycystic kidney disease. *N Engl J Med.* 2012;367:2407-2418.

42. Torres VE, Chapman AB, Devuyst O, et al. Tolvaptan in later-stage autosomal dominant polycystic kidney disease. *N Engl J Med.* 2017;377:1930-1942.

43. Cooper BA, Branley P, Bulfone L, et al. A randomized, controlled trial of early versus late initiation of dialysis. *N Engl J Med.* 2010;363:609-619.

44. Parsa A, Kao WHL, Xie D, et al. APOL1 risk variants, race, and progression of chronic kidney disease. *N Engl J Med.* 2013;369(23):2183-2196.

45. Kidney Disease: Improving Global Outcomes (KDIGO) Blood Pressure Work Group. KDIGO 2021 clinical practice guideline for the management of blood pressure in chronic kidney disease. *Kidney Int.* 2021;99(3S):S1-S87.

46. Fried LF, Emanuele N, Zhang JH, et al. Combined angiotensin inhibition for the treatment of diabetic nephropathy. *N Engl J Med.* 2013;369:1892-1903.
47. Hultin S, Hood C, Campbell KL, et al. A systematic review and meta-analysis on effects of bicarbonate therapy on kidney outcomes. *Kidney Int Rep.* 2020;6(3):695-705.
48. Baigent C, Landray MJ, Reith C, et al. The effects of lowering LDL cholesterol with simvastatin plus ezetimibe in patients with chronic kidney disease (Study of Heart and Renal Protection): a randomised placebo-controlled trial. *Lancet.* 2011;377:2181-2192.
49. Wanner C, Tonelli M. KDIGO clinical practice guidelines for lipid management in CKD: summary of recommendation statements and clinical approach to the patient. *Kidney Int.* 2014;85(6):1303-1309.
50. Solomon SD, Uno H, Lewis EF, et al. Erythropoietic response and outcomes in kidney disease and type 2 diabetes. *N Engl J Med.* 2010;363:1146-1155.
51. Foley RN, Gilbertson DT, Murray T, Collins AJ. Long interdialytic interval and mortality among patients receiving hemodialysis. *N Engl J Med.* 2011;365:1099-1107.
52. Eknoyan G, Beck GJ, Cheung AK, et al. Effect of dialysis dose and membrane flux in maintenance hemodialysis. *N Engl J Med.* 2002;347:2010-2019.
53. Palevsky PM, Zhang JH, O'Connor TZ, et al. Intensity of renal support in critically ill patients with acute kidney injury. *N Engl J Med.* 2008;359:7-20.
54. Paniagua R, Amato D, Vonesh E, et al. Effects of increased peritoneal clearances on mortality rates in peritoneal dialysis: ADEMEX, a prospective, randomized, controlled trial. *J Am Soc Nephrol.* 2002;13:1307-1320.
55. Li PK, Szeto CC, Piraino B, et al. ISPD peritonitis recommendations: 2016 update on prevention and treatment. *Perit Dial Int.* 2016;36(5):481-508.

CHAPTER 13

14 Treatment of Infectious Diseases

Miguel A. Chavez, Nigar Kirmani, and
Stephen Y. Liang

Principles of Therapy

GENERAL PRINCIPLES

- Infections are caused by bacteria, viruses, fungi, or parasites and can involve any organ system.
- Rising antimicrobial resistance is an urgent problem. Antimicrobials should be used carefully and only when indicated. Antimicrobial stewardship combats drug resistance, avoids adverse effects, and curbs excess cost.
- Infectious disease consultation reduces mortality and can aid with diagnosis and management of complicated infectious diseases and monitoring of antimicrobial therapy.[1]

DIAGNOSIS

- **History and physical examination** are critical, particularly for diagnostic dilemmas such as fever of unknown origin (FUO). Eliciting exposures, sexual history, travel history, and recreational activities informs and helps broaden the differential diagnosis.
- **Aerobic, anaerobic, fungal, or acid-fast bacilli (AFB) microbiologic cultures** should be performed on patient specimens as indicated. The microbiology laboratory should be consulted if fastidious organisms with special growth requirements are suspected to ensure appropriate transport and processing of cultures.
- **Gram stain, fungal stain, or AFB stain** from potentially infected patient specimens can facilitate rapid presumptive diagnosis and guide empiric antibiotic selection.
- **Rapid diagnostic testing** (e.g., polymerase chain reaction [PCR]) can provide early identification of an infectious etiologic agent and/or presence of antibiotic resistance genes (e.g., mecA gene).
- **Antimicrobial susceptibility testing** of cultures facilitates selection of antimicrobial agents.

TREATMENT

- **Choice of initial antimicrobial therapy**
  - Overuse of antimicrobials has led to the emergence of antimicrobial-resistant organisms, some with few treatment options. Therefore, the first question to ask is, "Does an infection exist that needs to be treated?"
  - Empiric antimicrobial therapy should be directed against the most likely infecting organism(s).

- Knowing antimicrobial susceptibility patterns is essential in selecting empiric therapy. Antibiograms provide important insight into trends in local antimicrobial resistance.
- Drug allergies, previous microbiologic cultures, and prior antimicrobial exposure help guide antimicrobial selection.
- De-escalate to an antimicrobial regimen with the narrowest spectrum of activity once the infectious etiologic agent is identified and susceptibility data are available.
- **Timing for the initiation of antimicrobial therapy**
  - In acute clinical scenarios, empiric therapy should begin immediately, ideally after appropriate microbiologic cultures have been obtained. Emergent therapy is indicated in patients with sepsis, meningitis, or rapidly progressive necrotizing infections, and in those with febrile neutropenia or asplenia.
  - In clinically stable patients, empiric antimicrobials can be withheld pending further evaluation, allowing for more targeted therapy.
- **Antimicrobial route and dosing administration**
  - Patients with serious infections should receive IV antimicrobial agents. Oral therapy is acceptable in less urgent circumstances if adequate drug concentrations can be achieved at the site of infection.
  - Renal and hepatic function should guide antimicrobial dosing regimens. Some antimicrobials require serum drug monitoring and dosing weight.
  - Always assess for drug–drug interactions before starting treatment to avoid adverse events and ensure effectiveness of therapy.
- **Assessment of outcomes on antimicrobial therapy**
  - If there is concern for potential treatment failure, ask the following questions:
    - Is the isolated organism the etiologic agent? Is there a superinfection?
    - Has an appropriate antimicrobial regimen been selected? Is there treatment adherence?
    - Are adequate concentrations of the antimicrobial achieved at the site of infection?
    - Has adequate source control been accomplished?
- **Duration of therapy**
  - Use the shortest duration of therapy for the infection identified.
  - Treatment of acute uncomplicated infections should be continued until the patient is afebrile and clinically well, usually for a minimum of 72 hours.
  - Some infections (e.g., endocarditis, septic arthritis, osteomyelitis) require prolonged therapy.

SPECIAL CONSIDERATIONS

- **Immunosuppression**
  - In patients living with HIV/AIDS, solid organ or hematopoietic stem cell transplant (HSCT) recipients, patients undergoing chemotherapy, and patients receiving glucocorticoids or other immune-modulating agents, consider opportunistic infections. Neutropenic patients require broader empiric antimicrobial therapy.
- **Pregnancy or postpartum**
  - There are no Class A antimicrobials. Penicillins and cephalosporins (Class B) are frequently used. **Tetracyclines and fluoroquinolones are contraindicated.** Sulfonamides and aminoglycosides should not be used if alternative agents are available.
  - Many antimicrobials are excreted in breast milk and should be used with caution in breast-feeding women.

TOXIN-MEDIATED INFECTIONS

Clostridioides difficile Infection

GENERAL PRINCIPLES

The most frequently implicated antimicrobials associated with *Clostridioides difficile* infection (CDI) include clindamycin, fluoroquinolones, broad-spectrum penicillins, and cephalosporins.

DIAGNOSIS

Clinical Presentation

- Symptoms range from mild or moderate watery diarrhea to severe and potentially fatal pseudomembranous colitis. Abdominal pain, cramping, low-grade fever, and leukocytosis are often present.
- Fulminant disease can manifest as colonic ileus or toxic megacolon leading to bowel perforation.

Differential Diagnosis

Antibiotic-associated osmotic diarrhea without CDI should be considered and will resolve after withdrawal of the antibiotic.

Diagnostic Testing

Testing for CDI is recommended in patients with unexplained and new-onset diarrhea (≥3 unformed stools in 24 hours). Diagnosis is made by detection of toxigenic *C. difficile* in diarrheal stool through nucleic acid amplification test (NAAT) or enzyme immunoassay.

TREATMENT

- For an initial episode of CDI (severe or nonsevere), treatment should consist of vancomycin 125 mg PO q6h for 10 days or fidaxomicin 200 mg PO q12h for 10 days and discontinuation of the offending antibiotic if possible.[2]
- For fulminant infections complicated by ileus, toxic megacolon, hypotension, or shock, surgery consultation should be obtained along with treatment consisting of vancomycin 500 mg PO or by nasogastric tube q6h in combination with metronidazole 500 mg IV q8h. If ileus is present, consider adding rectal instillation of vancomycin. In some cases, colectomy may be necessary.[2]
- Endpoint of therapy is cessation of diarrhea; **do not retest stool for toxin clearance.**
- Avoid antimotility agents in severe disease.
- Recurrence is common and is treated with pulsed-tapered oral vancomycin or fidaxomicin if not previously used.
- Fecal microbiota transplantation may be considered for patients with multiple recurrences despite appropriate antibiotic treatment.[2]

Tetanus

GENERAL PRINCIPLES

- Caused by *Clostridium tetani* toxin from wound contamination with spores.
- Tetanus is best prevented by immunization. For high-risk wounds, additional prophylaxis with human tetanus immunoglobulin 250 units IM is recommended.[3]

DIAGNOSIS

Diagnosis is clinical. Classically presents with intensely painful muscle spasms and rigidity, followed by autonomic dysfunction. Symptoms often begin in the face (trismus, risus sardonicus) and neck muscles. Delirium and high fever are usually absent.

TREATMENT

- Passive immunization with human tetanus immunoglobulin 3000–6000 units IM (in divided doses with part infiltrated around the wound) to neutralize unbound toxin is warranted. Active immunization with tetanus toxoid should be given at a separate site.
- Surgical debridement of the wound is critical.
- Antibiotic therapy, usually consisting of metronidazole 500 mg IV q6–8h or penicillin G 2–4 million units IV q4–6h, for 7–10 days is recommended.
- Benzodiazepines or neuromuscular blocking agents may be used to control spasms.

TOXIC SHOCK SYNDROME

Toxic shock syndrome (TSS) is a life-threatening systemic disease caused by exotoxin superantigens produced by *Staphylococcus aureus* or group A β-hemolytic *Streptococcus* (GABHS) (Table 14-1).

Staphylococcal TSS

GENERAL PRINCIPLES

Most often associated with colonization of surgical wounds, burns, vaginitis, or tampon use in young women. Cases are also seen after nasal packing for epistaxis. Mortality is low (<3%) in menstrual cases.

DIAGNOSIS

- Diagnosis is made based on clinical and laboratory data.
- Typical findings include fever, hypotension, and a macular desquamating erythroderma of the palms and soles. Vomiting, diarrhea, myalgias, weakness, shortness of breath, and altered mental status may be early signs of multiorgan failure.
- Blood cultures are usually negative but help rule out alternative pathogens. Alternative diagnosis such as Rocky Mountain spotted fever (RMSF) and leptospirosis should also be considered and ruled out with appropriate testing.

CHAPTER 14

TABLE 14-1	Treatment of Toxic Shock Syndromes		
Etiology	Antibiotic Therapy	Adjunctive Therapy	Notes
Group A β-hemolytic *Streptococcus* (GABHS)	Penicillin G 4 million units IV q4h + clindamycin 900 mg IV q8h for 10–14 d	IVIG 1 g/kg on day 1, then 0.5 g/kg on days 2 and 3	Surgical debridement is almost always indicated for necrotizing infections. Clindamycin is added to decrease toxin production.
Staphylococcus aureus	Oxacillin 2 g IV q4h or vancomycin 1 g IV q12h + clindamycin 900 mg IV q8h for 10–14 d	IVIG as per GABHS may be useful in severe cases, but higher doses may be needed	Surgical debridement may be necessary for wounds. Tampons and other foreign bodies should be removed and avoided in future, especially if TSST-1 antibody titers are negative.

IVIG, intravenous immunoglobulin; TSST-1, toxic shock syndrome toxin 1.

TREATMENT

See Table 14-1.

Streptococcal TSS

GENERAL PRINCIPLES

Associated with invasive GABHS infections, particularly necrotizing fasciitis or myositis (80% of cases). Mortality is much higher (30%–70%) compared to staphylococcal TSS.

DIAGNOSIS

• Initial presentation is typically abrupt onset of severe diffuse or localized pain. Systemic manifestations are otherwise similar to staphylococcal TSS, but the desquamating erythroderma is much less common.
• Blood cultures are usually positive, and antistreptolysin O titers are elevated.

TREATMENT

See Table 14-1.

SKIN, SOFT-TISSUE, AND BONE INFECTIONS

Purulent Skin and Soft-Tissue Infections (Furuncles, Carbuncles, Abscesses)

GENERAL PRINCIPLES

Methicillin-resistant *S. aureus* (MRSA) and methicillin-sensitive *S. aureus* (MSSA) account for 25%–50% of cases.

TREATMENT

- Incision and drainage (I&D) alone is usually adequate, especially for abscesses measuring <5 cm.
- Antibiotic therapy is needed for extensive disease; systemic illness; rapid progression with associated cellulitis; comorbid diseases (diabetes mellitus); immunosuppression, location on face, hand, or genitalia; or lack of response to I&D.
- Empiric antibiotic therapy should cover community-acquired MRSA. Oral antibiotics include clindamycin 300–450 mg q8h, trimethoprim–sulfamethoxazole (TMP–SMX) 1–2 double-strength tablets q12h, doxycycline 100 mg q12h, and linezolid 600 mg q12h.
- Duration of antibiotic therapy is usually 5–7 days.[4]

Nonpurulent Skin and Soft-Tissue Infections (Erysipelas and Cellulitis)

ERYSIPELAS

General Principles

Erysipelas appears as a painful, superficial, erythematous, sharply demarcated lesion that usually affects the lower extremities. In normal hosts, GABHS is responsible for this infection.

Treatment

Penicillin V 250–1000 mg PO q6h or penicillin G 1.0–2.0 million units IV q6h, depending on the severity of illness. In patients who are penicillin allergic, macrolides and clindamycin are alternatives.

CELLULITIS

General Principles

- Common organisms include β-hemolytic streptococci and *S. aureus* (MSSA and MRSA).
- Severe cellulitis is sometimes seen after exposure to fresh (*Aeromonas hydrophila*) or salt (*Vibrio vulnificus*) water.

CHAPTER 14

Treatment

- If streptococci or MSSA are suspected, a β-lactam antibiotic (cephalexin or dicloxacillin 500 mg PO q6h) or clindamycin can be used.
- If there is a strong concern for community-acquired MRSA, empiric antibiotic coverage may consist of clindamycin, doxycycline, or linezolid. TMP–SMX can also be used in combination with a β-lactam antibiotic (e.g., cephalexin) to provide streptococcal coverage.
- Coverage for waterborne pathogens should initially consist of ceftazidime 2 g IV q8h, cefepime 2 g IV q8h, or ciprofloxacin 750 mg PO q12h in combination with doxycycline 100 mg IV/PO q12h.

Complicated Skin and Soft-Tissue Infections

GENERAL PRINCIPLES

Deep soft-tissue infections, surgical and traumatic wound infections, large abscesses, complicated cellulitis, and infected ulcers and burns fall under this classification.

DIAGNOSIS

Cultures of abscesses and surgical debridement specimens should be obtained to guide antibiotic therapy.

TREATMENT

Patients should be hospitalized to receive IV antibiotics (including MRSA coverage) and undergo surgical intervention as necessary. Vancomycin 15–20 mg/kg IV q12h, linezolid 600 mg PO/IV q12h, daptomycin 4 mg/kg IV qday, clindamycin 900 mg IV q8h, and ceftaroline 600 mg IV q12h are all acceptable antibiotic options.[4]

Infected Decubitus Ulcers and Limb-Threatening Diabetic Foot Ulcers

GENERAL PRINCIPLES

- Infections are usually polymicrobial. **Superficial swab cultures are unreliable.** Instead, deep tissue cultures obtained after wound debridement are preferred.
- Osteomyelitis is a frequent complication and should be excluded.

TREATMENT

- Wound care and debridement are important first-line therapies.
- **Mild diabetic foot infections** are usually due to *S. aureus* and streptococci and can be treated with cephalexin or amoxicillin–clavulanate (875 mg/125 mg PO q12h).[5] If MRSA is suspected, either TMP–SMX or doxycycline is recommended.
- **Moderate to severe infections** require systemic antibiotics covering *S. aureus* (including MRSA), anaerobes, and enteric gram-negative organisms. Options include vancomycin plus a β-lactam/β-lactamase inhibitor combination, a carbapenem, or vancomycin with metronidazole combined with either ciprofloxacin or a third-generation cephalosporin.

Necrotizing Fasciitis

GENERAL PRINCIPLES

- This is an infectious disease emergency with high mortality manifested by extensive soft-tissue infection and thrombosis of the microcirculation with resulting necrosis. Infection spreads quickly along fascial planes and may be associated with sepsis or TSS. Fournier gangrene is necrotizing fasciitis of the perineum.
- Bacterial etiology is either mixed (aerobic and anaerobic organisms) or monomicrobial (GABHS or *S. aureus*, including community-acquired MRSA).

DIAGNOSIS

Clinical Presentation

May present initially like simple cellulitis rapidly progressing to necrosis with dusky, hypoesthetic skin and bulla formation in association with severe pain. Pain out of proportion to examination should raise concern for necrotizing fasciitis.

Diagnostic Testing

- Diagnosis is clinical. High suspicion should prompt **immediate surgical exploration** where lack of resistance to probing is diagnostic.
- Cultures of operative specimens and blood should be obtained. Creatinine kinase may be elevated.
- CT and plain films may demonstrate gas and fascial edema early in the disease process.

TREATMENT

- Aggressive surgical debridement is critical, along with IV antibiotics and volume support.
- Initial broad-spectrum empiric antibiotic therapy should consist of a β-lactam/β-lactamase inhibitor, high-dose penicillin, carbapenem, or fluoroquinolone in combination with clindamycin. Vancomycin should also be added until MRSA can be excluded.

Anaerobic Myonecrosis (Gas Gangrene)

GENERAL PRINCIPLES

Usually due to *Clostridium perfringens*, *Clostridium septicum*, *S. aureus*, GABHS, or other anaerobes.

TREATMENT

Treatment requires prompt surgical debridement and combination antimicrobial therapy with IV penicillin plus clindamycin. A third-generation cephalosporin, ciprofloxacin, or an aminoglycoside should be added until a gram-negative infection can be excluded.

CHAPTER 14

Osteomyelitis

GENERAL PRINCIPLES

Osteomyelitis is an inflammatory process caused by an infecting organism that can lead to bone destruction. It should be considered when skin or soft-tissue infections overlie the bone and when localized bone pain accompanies fever or sepsis.

DIAGNOSIS

- Diagnosis is made by detection of exposed bone through a skin ulcer or by imaging with plain films, bone scintigraphy, or MRI.
- Biopsy and cultures of the affected bone should be performed (before initiation of antimicrobials when possible) for pathogen-directed therapy.
- Erythrocyte sedimentation rate and C-reactive protein are usually markedly elevated and can be used to monitor response to therapy.

TREATMENT

- See Table 14-2.
- Parenteral β-lactam antibiotics (oxacillin, cefazolin) are effective against MSSA. Vancomycin, daptomycin, and linezolid are used to treat MRSA osteomyelitis. Oral agents capable of achieving reasonable bone levels include TMP–SMX, clindamycin, and doxycycline.
- Gram-negative osteomyelitis can be treated with parenteral or oral fluoroquinolones, which have excellent bone penetration and bioavailability, or with a third-generation cephalosporin.
- The optimal duration of antibiotic therapy is uncertain. Cure typically requires at least 4–6 weeks of high-dose antimicrobial therapy. Parenteral therapy should be given initially; oral regimens may be considered after 2–3 weeks if the pathogen is susceptible and adequate bactericidal levels can be achieved.

CENTRAL NERVOUS SYSTEM INFECTIONS

Meningitis

GENERAL PRINCIPLES

- Meningitis (inflammation of the meninges) is caused by bacterial, viral, or fungal infections or by noninfectious causes including medications.
- Bacterial meningitis is a medical emergency and requires immediate therapy without delay for diagnostic procedures. Rapid initiation of antimicrobial treatment decreases mortality.
- *Streptococcus pneumoniae* is the most common bacterial etiology in adults, followed by *Neisseria meningitidis*, group B *Streptococcus*, and *Haemophilus influenzae*. *Listeria monocytogenes* is more frequent in the elderly and in immunocompromised hosts.
- Health care–associated meningitis (after neurosurgical procedures or head trauma) and intraventricular shunt infections are caused by staphylococci (*S. aureus* and coagulase-negative staphylococci) and gram-negative bacilli (especially *Pseudomonas aeruginosa*).

TABLE 14-2	Treatment of Osteomyelitis	
Etiology of Osteomyelitis	Organism	Treatment Considerations
Acute hematogenous	• *Staphylococcus aureus*	• Antibiotic therapy alone may be sufficient if no foreign body present.
Vertebral	• *S. aureus* • Gram-negative bacilli • *Mycobacterium tuberculosis*	• Biopsy off antibiotics (preferred) to guide therapy. • Antibiotic therapy alone may be sufficient.
Associated with a contiguous focus of infection	• *S. aureus* • Gram-negative bacilli • Coagulase-negative staphylococci (surgical site infections) • Anaerobes/polymicrobial (infected sacral decubitus ulcers, diabetics)	• Diabetics and patients with peripheral vascular disease seldom are cured with antibiotics alone. Revascularization, debridement, or amputation is often required. • Long-term, suppressive antimicrobial therapy can be used if surgery is not feasible. • Hyperbaric oxygen may be a useful adjunct.
Presence of an orthopedic device	• *S. aureus* • Coagulase-negative *Staphylococcus* species	• Rarely eradicated by antimicrobials alone, and typically requires removal of the device. • If removal is impossible, the addition of rifampin 300 mg PO q8-12h is recommended and long-term, suppressive antimicrobial therapy may be needed.
Associated with hemoglobinopathies	• *S. aureus* • *Salmonella* species	
Chronic osteomyelitis	• Gram-negative pathogens (necrotic sequestrum) • *S. aureus*	• Surgical removal of sequestrum is recommended in addition to antibiotics.
Culture-negative osteomyelitis	• Review above pathogens	• Empiric therapy should cover *S. aureus* and all other likely pathogens.

CHAPTER 14

DIAGNOSIS

Clinical Presentation

• Meningitis should be considered in any patient with fever and stiff neck or neurologic symptoms, especially altered mental status.
• **Aseptic meningitis** (meningitis with negative bacterial cultures) is usually milder and may be preceded by upper respiratory symptoms or pharyngitis. Enteroviruses,

and occasionally arboviruses, are the most common cause; drugs such as NSAIDs and TMP–SMX are less common causes.
• Bacterial, viral, and noninfectious etiologies cannot be distinguished clinically.

Diagnostic Testing

Diagnosis requires a **lumbar puncture (LP)** with measurement of opening pressure; cerebrospinal fluid (CSF) protein, glucose, and cell count with differential; and Gram stain with culture (Table 14-3). Blood cultures should also be obtained. Head CT scan before LP is **not** necessary for immunocompetent patients unless there are focal neurologic abnormalities, seizures, or diminished level of consciousness.[6]
• In bacterial meningitis, CSF shows a neutrophilic pleocytosis, elevated protein, and low glucose. In **aseptic meningitis**, a lymphocytic CSF pleocytosis is common (although neutrophils may predominate early), along with a normal glucose. CSF PCR can detect enteroviruses, herpes simplex virus (HSV), and HIV. CSF lymphocytosis with profoundly decreased glucose level should prompt a workup for tuberculous or fungal meningitis.
• Depending on the clinical scenario, other useful CSF studies include Venereal Disease Research Laboratory to diagnose neurosyphilis, acid-fast stain and culture, cryptococcal antigen (CrAg) and fungal culture, and arbovirus antibodies.

TREATMENT

• High-dose parenteral antimicrobial therapy should be started **immediately after LP.** An empiric regimen should be based on patient risk factors and Gram stain of the CSF.
• In patients aged 2–50 years, ceftriaxone 2 g IV q12h or cefotaxime 2 g IV q4–6h and vancomycin 15–20 mg/kg IV q8–12h are recommended.

TABLE 14-3	Typical Cerebrospinal Fluid Findings in Meningitis[6]				
	Opening Pressure (mm H_2O)	White Cells (/μL)	Glucose (mg/dL)	Protein (mg/dL)	Laboratory Diagnosis
Normal	<180	0–5	50–75	15–40	None
Bacterial meningitis	↑	100–5000 neutrophils	<40	100–500	Gram stain, culture
Tuberculous meningitis	↑	50–300 lymphocytes	<45	50–300	Acid-fast bacilli smear, culture, polymerase chain reaction (PCR) for *Mycobacterium tuberculosis*
Cryptococcal meningitis	↑↑	20–500 lymphocytes	<40	>45	Cryptococcal antigen, India ink stain, fungal culture
Viral meningitis	↑	10–1000 lymphocytes	Normal	50–100	Virus-specific PCR

- Ampicillin 2 g IV q4h should be added for **patients older than 50 years** to cover *L. monocytogenes.*
- Immunocompromised patients should receive vancomycin plus ampicillin plus cefepime 2 g IV q8h or meropenem 2 g IV q8h.
- In the postneurosurgical setting, after head **trauma** or for intraventricular shunt infection, vancomycin and ceftazidime 2 g IV q8h or cefepime is indicated.
- Empiric regimens should be **narrowed** once cultures are known.
- **Dexamethasone** 0.15 mg/kg IV q6h started just before or with initial antibiotics and continued for 4 days reduces the risk of a poor neurologic outcome in meningitis caused by *S. pneumoniae.* Glucocorticoids should not be used for other pathogens.
- **Therapy for specific infections**
  - For *S. pneumoniae*, initial therapy consists of ceftriaxone plus vancomycin. Vancomycin is discontinued if the isolate is susceptible to ceftriaxone (minimum inhibitory concentration [MIC] <0.5 µg/mL). For penicillin-sensitive isolates (MIC <0.06 µg/mL), penicillin G 4 million units IV q4h can be used. Start dexamethasone early.
  - For *N. meningitidis*, high-dose ceftriaxone or cefotaxime is used. If the isolate is susceptible (MIC <0.1 µg/mL), penicillin can be used. Alternatives are meropenem and chloramphenicol. Patients should be placed in **droplet isolation** for 24 hours after starting treatment. Close contacts (household contacts; healthcare personnel performing procedures placing them in close contact with secretions [e.g., endotracheal intubation] without the use of appropriate personal protective equipment) should receive prophylaxis with either ciprofloxacin 500 mg PO once; rifampin 600 mg PO q12h for 2 days; or ceftriaxone 250 mg IM once. Terminal component complement deficiency (C5–C9) should be ruled out in patients with recurrent meningococcal infections.
  - *L. monocytogenes* meningitis occurs in immunosuppressed adults, pregnant women, and the elderly. Treatment is with ampicillin 2 g IV q4h for at least 3 weeks. Use TMP–SMX (TMP 5 mg/kg IV q6h) or meropenem (2 g IV q8h) in penicillin-allergic patients.
  - **Gram-negative bacillary meningitis** is usually a complication of head trauma or neurosurgical procedures. High-dose ceftazidime or cefepime 2 g IV q8h is used for *P. aeruginosa.* Ceftriaxone or cefotaxime may be used for susceptible pathogens. Alternatives include meropenem and ciprofloxacin.
  - ***S. aureus* meningitis** can result from high-grade bacteremia, extension from a parameningeal focus, or recent neurosurgical procedure. Vancomycin should be used in penicillin-allergic patients and for methicillin-resistant isolates. Oxacillin or nafcillin 2 g IV q4h is the drug of choice for MSSA; ceftriaxone is an alternative. First- and second-generation cephalosporins do not penetrate the CSF and are **not** used.
  - For **enteroviral** meningitis, the treatment is supportive care. Acyclovir 10 mg/kg IV q8h is used to treat **HSV meningitis**.

Encephalitis

GENERAL PRINCIPLES

- Encephalitis is inflammation of the brain parenchyma, usually due to a viral infection.
- **HSV-1** is the most common and important cause of sporadic infectious encephalitis. Others include arboviruses such as West Nile virus (WNV), enteroviruses, other herpesviruses, and rabies.

CHAPTER 14

- Nonviral causes include *Mycobacterium tuberculosis*, syphilis, fungi, *Mycoplasma pneumoniae*, and *Bartonella henselae*. In the summer months, tick-borne illness (e.g., *Ehrlichia*, RMSF, and Lyme disease) should be considered.
- Noninfectious causes include vasculitis, collagen vascular disease, paraneoplastic syndromes, and acute disseminated encephalomyelitis, seen after infection or immunization.

DIAGNOSIS

Clinical Presentation

Presenting complaints include fever, **altered mental status**, and neurologic abnormalities, such as personality change or seizures, usually without meningeal signs.

Diagnostic Testing

- CSF analysis should include PCR testing for HSV and enteroviruses and measurement of CSF and serum arbovirus IgM antibodies for WNV. A positive PCR for HSV-1 confirms the diagnosis, but a negative PCR does not rule it out. Other PCR tests (*Ehrlichia, Bartonella, Mycoplasma*, varicella–zoster virus, cytomegalovirus) are sent if there is clinical suspicion.
- MRI may show temporal lobe enhancement in HSV encephalitis.

TREATMENT

- Acyclovir 10 mg/kg IV q8h should be started on **all** patients with suspected encephalitis and continued for 14–21 days, until HSV is definitively ruled out. Delayed therapy increases the risk of poor neurologic outcomes.
- Treatment of other viral causes is mainly supportive.
- Antibiotic therapy for presumed bacterial meningitis (see above) should be initiated if clinically indicated and discontinued once CSF cultures are negative. Doxycycline 100 mg q12h should be added if there is suspicion for tick-borne illness.[7]

Brain Abscess

GENERAL PRINCIPLES

- Brain abscess in the immunocompetent host is usually bacterial in origin and the result of spread from a contiguous focus (mastoiditis, sinusitis, dental infection), septic emboli from endocarditis, bacteremia, trauma, or surgery.
- Infection is often polymicrobial, with viridans streptococci, *S. aureus*, and anaerobes being the most common pathogens; staphylococci and gram-negative bacilli predominate after surgery. *Streptococcus anginosus* is especially associated with abscess formation. In immunocompromised hosts, etiologies include invasive fungal infection, *Nocardia*, and TB; in HIV-infected patients, toxoplasmosis is a leading consideration.[8]

DIAGNOSIS

- Diagnosis is radiographic, with ring-enhancing lesions seen on MRI or CT scan.
- A microbiologic etiology should be determined by aspiration, biopsy, or surgery.

TREATMENT

- Empiric therapy should cover the most likely pathogens based on the primary infection site. A third-generation cephalosporin (ceftriaxone) combined with metronidazole and vancomycin is started in immunocompetent hosts and narrowed when culture data are available. Use cefepime or ceftazidime instead of ceftriaxone after neurosurgical procedures or head trauma.
- Neurosurgical consultation is imperative for drainage; cultures **must** be sent to enable pathogen-directed therapy, as a prolonged course of antibiotic therapy is often needed.
- Follow-up imaging to assess improvement determines length of therapy.

Neurocysticercosis

- Neurocysticercosis should be suspected in patients from Mexico and Central and South America who present with seizures.
- Ingested eggs of *Taenia solium* differentiate into larvae, which disseminate to brain and other tissues and form cysts.
- Brain imaging reveals characteristic multiple unilocular cysts that eventually calcify.
- Treatment consists of anticonvulsants, albendazole or praziquantel, with concomitant glucocorticoids to decrease the inflammatory response, and/or surgery.[9]

BLOODSTREAM INFECTIONS AND CATHETER-RELATED BLOODSTREAM INFECTIONS

Bloodstream Infections

GENERAL PRINCIPLES

- Bloodstream infections (BSIs) are a major cause of morbidity and mortality despite available antimicrobials and supportive care.
- Community-acquired BSI is defined by positive blood cultures obtained in the outpatient setting or <48 hours into the patient's hospital stay.
- Transient bacteremia can occur with brushing teeth, dental work, or other mucosal disrupting procedures, but it is typically asymptomatic and self-limiting.
- Positive blood cultures resulting from contamination by skin or environmental flora do not represent true infection and should be assessed based on clinical presentation.
- *S. aureus*, *S. epidermidis* (coagulase-negative staphylococci), aerobic gram-negative species, and *Candida* spp. are the most common organisms associated with BSI and catheter-related bloodstream infections (CRBSI).

DIAGNOSIS

- Diagnosis of BSI is made based on clinical criteria and blood culture results. Blood cultures should be obtained in patients with sepsis, including those with shaking chills and fever, and in infections associated with a high likelihood of bacteremia (e.g., endovascular infections, vertebral osteomyelitis and discitis, epidural abscess, meningitis, septic arthritis). Patients with low likelihood of bacteremia (e.g., uncomplicated cases of cystitis, cellulitis, or community-acquired pneumonia [CAP]) should not have blood cultures drawn.

- Prior to initiation of antimicrobials, at least two sets of blood cultures (each set consisting of aerobic and anaerobic bottles) should be taken from separate venipuncture sites.
- Careful identification of the source of bacteremia and potential metastatic sites of infection based on history and physical examination is warranted.

TREATMENT

- Recommendations for empiric and definitive treatment for BSI are outlined in Table 14-4.
- Duration of therapy will depend on the pathogen and whether the infection is complicated or uncomplicated and should start from the date of the first negative blood culture.
- Source control to eradicate the source of bacteremia is essential.

Catheter-Related Bloodstream Infections

GENERAL PRINCIPLES

- Vascular catheters should be removed when no longer needed for care.
- Subclavian central venous catheters (CVCs) are associated with lower CRBSI rates than internal jugular CVCs, whereas femoral CVCs have the highest rates and should be avoided or removed within 72 hours of placement.
- SC tunneling and use of antiseptic-impregnated CVCs may further reduce the incidence of CRBSI. Routine exchange of a CVC over a guide wire is not recommended.

DIAGNOSIS

Clinical Presentation

CRBSI should be suspected in any febrile patient with a vascular catheter. Clinical findings include local inflammation or phlebitis at the catheter insertion site, sepsis, endophthalmitis, lack of another source of bacteremia, and resolution of fever after catheter removal.

Diagnostic Testing

Diagnosis is similar to that of BSI. At least two sets of peripheral blood cultures should be obtained prior to initiation of antibiotics. One of the sets may be drawn from the catheter if obtaining two sets peripherally is not feasible.

TREATMENT

- Recommendations for empiric and definitive treatment for CRBSI are outlined in Table 14-4.
- Duration of therapy depends on the pathogen, whether the infection is complicated or uncomplicated, and should start from the date of the first negative blood culture or removal of the infected CVC, whichever occurred later.
- **Catheter removal** is always preferable.[10] At a minimum, it is recommended that the catheter be removed in the following situations:
  - Hemodynamic instability or persistent BSI despite >72 hours of appropriate antimicrobial therapy.

TABLE 14-4	Treatment of Common Pathogens Associated With Bloodstream Infections and Catheter-Related Bloodstream Infections	
Organism	Treatment	Other Considerations
Empiric therapy	• Vancomycin 15–20 mg/kg IV q12h. The dose should be adjusted to achieve a vancomycin trough between 15 and 20 µg/mL. • Gram-negative bacilli should be covered based on the clinical syndrome and likelihood of presence. β-Lactam/β-lactamase inhibitor[a] or ceftriaxone 2 g IV qday are alternatives. Coverage against *Pseudomonas* should be considered based on local microbiological data and the severity of disease. Fourth-generation cephalosporins,[b] piperacillin/tazobactam, or carbapenems[c] are options. • Patient with risk factors for candidemia or yeasts identified on blood cultures should be treated with an echinocandin (e.g., micafungin 100 mg IV qday).	• Antimicrobials should be tailored once species identification and susceptibilities are known. • Gram stain or molecular diagnosis can guide initial empiric therapy.
Staphylococcus aureus	• **MSSA:** Oxacillin 2 g IV q4h or cefazolin 1–2 g IV q8h. • **MRSA:** First line is vancomycin 15–20 mg/kg IV q12h with a target vancomycin trough between 15 and 20 µg/mL. Linezolid 600 mg PO/IV q12h or daptomycin 6 mg/kg IV qday are alternatives. • Routine use of gentamicin for synergy in *S. aureus* bacteremia is not recommended. • The recommended duration of therapy is generally 4–6 weeks. A 2-week course is acceptable for uncomplicated MRSA bacteremia, as defined by a negative TEE, negative blood cultures, and defervescence within 72 hours of starting effective therapy, absence of prosthetic material (e.g., pacemaker, valve), and no evidence of metastatic infection.	• Infectious Diseases consultation. • Source control if possible: Drainage of abscess, removal of hardware or IV catheter. • TTE in all patients. TEE should be considered in those with suspicion of endocarditis. • Repeat blood cultures to demonstrate clearance of bacteremia.

TABLE 14-4	Treatment of Common Pathogens Associated With Bloodstream Infections and Catheter-Related Bloodstream Infections (*continued*)	
Organism	Treatment	Other Considerations
Coagulase-negative staphylococci	• CoNS can be considered blood culture contaminants if isolated on single blood culture set. Correlate clinically. • First line is vancomycin 15–20 mg/kg IV q12h with a target vancomycin trough between 15 and 20 µg/mL. • Definitive treatment is based on susceptibilities similar to *S. aureus* depending on the organism if it is methicillin-susceptible or resistant. • Duration of therapy is 7–14 days depending on the source of infection.	• TTE only in those with suspicion of endocarditis or persistent positive blood cultures. • Repeat blood cultures to demonstrate clearance of bacteremia.
Streptococcus spp.	• Definitive treatment should be guided by antibiotic susceptibility testing. • Penicillin-susceptible: Penicillin G 12–18 million units IV qday or ceftriaxone 2 g IV qday. • Penicillin-resistant: Vancomycin 15 mg/kg IV q12h.	• TTE only in those with suspicion of endocarditis or persistent positive blood cultures. • Repeat blood cultures to demonstrate clearance of bacteremia. • Colonoscopy is recommended in those with *Streptococcus gallolyticus* bacteremia without clear source.
Enterococcus spp.	• Ampicillin-susceptible: Ampicillin 2 g IV q4h. • Ampicillin-resistant: Vancomycin 15 mg/kg IV q12h. • Ampicillin-resistant AND vancomycin-resistant: Infectious Diseases consultation recommended. Empiric treatments include linezolid 600 mg IV/PO q12h or daptomycin 6 mg/kg IV qday. • Duration of treatment should be 7–14 days.	• TTE only in those with suspicion of endocarditis or persistent positive blood cultures. • Repeat blood cultures to demonstrate clearance of bacteremia.

TABLE 14-4	Treatment of Common Pathogens Associated With Bloodstream Infections and Catheter-Related Bloodstream Infections (continued)	
Organism	Treatment	Other Considerations
Gram-negative bacilli	• Definitive treatment should be guided by antibiotic susceptibility testing. • Duration may range from 7 to 14 days. • Resistant gram-negative bloodstream infection may require consultation with an Infectious Diseases specialist.	• Repeat blood cultures to demonstrate clearance of bacteremia is not necessary if patient is clinically improving but should be considered if IV catheter or hardware is present.
Candida spp.	• Micafungin 100 mg IV qday in cases of moderate to severe illness pending species identification. • Fluconazole 400 mg IV/PO qday may be appropriate for stable patients who have not had any recent azole exposure. • Duration of antifungal treatment should be for 14 days after the first negative blood culture.	• Infectious Diseases consultation is recommended. • TTE in all patients. • Ophthalmology consultation is advised to look for Candida endophthalmitis.

MRSA, methicillin-resistant Staphylococcus aureus; MSSA, methicillin-sensitive Staphylococcus aureus; TEE, transesophageal echocardiography; TTE, transthoracic echocardiography.
[a]β-Lactam/β-lactamase inhibitors: Ampicillin/sulbactam 1.5–3 g IV q6h, piperacillin/tazobactam 3.75–4.5 g IV q6h.
[b]Fourth-generation cephalosporin: Cefepime 1 g IV q8h.
[c]Carbapenems: Meropenem 1 g IV q8h.

    ○ Any CRBSI involving S. aureus, most gram-negative bacilli, fungi, or mycobacteria.
    ○ Insertion site or tunnel site infection (pus or significant inflammation at the site).
    ○ Evidence of endocarditis or metastatic infection.
• Antibiotic lock therapy in combination with an extended course of antibiotics may be an option in certain situations where catheter salvage is absolutely necessary.

CARDIOVASCULAR INFECTIONS

Infective Endocarditis

GENERAL PRINCIPLES

Etiology
• Infective endocarditis (IE) is presumed to result from injury to the valvular endothelium or endocardium, exposing subendothelial collagen to which platelets, fibrin, and eventually bacteria adhere.

- Native valve infective endocarditis (NVIE) is usually caused by gram-positive cocci. *S. aureus* is the most common pathogen followed by viridans group streptococci, enterococci, and coagulase-negative staphylococci. Increasing rates of *S. aureus* bacteremia have contributed to a rising incidence of **acute bacterial endocarditis (ABE)** and health care–associated endocarditis (related to IV catheters and invasive procedures).
- *Enterococcus* species cause 5%–10% of cases of **subacute bacterial endocarditis (SBE).**
- Bacteremia from distant foci of infection or dental procedures are frequent seeding events.
- *Streptococcus gallolyticus* (former *S. bovis*) bacteremia and endocarditis are associated with lower gastrointestinal tract disease, including neoplasms. Groups B and G streptococcal endocarditis may also be associated with large intestinal pathology.
- Gram-negative and fungal IEs occur infrequently and are usually associated with injection drug use or prosthetic heart valves.
- Early prosthetic valve endocarditis (PVE) (within the first year of surgery) commonly occurs in the first 2 months and is typically caused by *S. aureus*, coagulase-negative staphylococci, gram-negative bacilli, and *Candida* spp. Late-onset PVE is caused by the same organisms seen in NVIE.
- Coagulase-negative staphylococci (e.g., *Staphylococcus epidermidis*) primarily occur in patients with prosthetic heart valves, although NVIE is increasing, particularly in healthcare settings. *Staphylococcus lugdunensis* is associated with a high rate of perivalvular extension and metastatic spread, resembling *S. aureus* clinically.
- **HACEK** is an acronym for a group of fastidious, slow-growing, gram-negative bacteria (*Haemophilus, Aggregatibacter, Cardiobacterium, Eikenella,* and *Kingella* species) that account for 5%–10% of community-acquired cases of IE.

Risk Factors

Acquired structural heart disease (e.g., degenerative valve disease, rheumatic heart disease), congenital disease (e.g., bicuspid aortic valve, ventricular septal defect), injection drug use, prosthetic heart valves, intravascular devices, chronic hemodialysis, and a prior history of endocarditis are predisposing factors for endocarditis.

DIAGNOSIS

The modified Duke criteria (Tables 14-5 and 14-6) incorporate microbiologic, pathologic, echocardiographic, and clinical findings and are widely used but should not replace clinical judgment.

Clinical Presentation

- Clinical presentation is variable, ranging from acute sepsis, commonly seen in ABE, to an indolent low-grade febrile illness, malaise, and anorexia in SBE.
- Fever and heart murmur are the two signature features.
- Local complications include valvular destruction, perivalvular extension, and heart failure.
- Embolic phenomena to microvascular sites (splinter hemorrhage, petechiae, Janeway lesions) or large vessels can occur. Metastatic infection can cause infarcts to organs such as the brain (stroke), kidneys, spleen, and lungs.
- Immune complex-mediated manifestations (nephritis, arthralgias, Osler nodes; or false positive serology of rheumatoid factor, syphilis) are more commonly seen in SBE.

TABLE 14-5	Modified Duke Criteria for the Diagnosis of Infective Endocarditis[11]

Major Criteria

Positive Blood Cultures

1. Two separate blood cultures with viridans group streptococci, *Streptococcus gallolyticus* (formerly *bovis*), *Staphylococcus aureus*, HACEK group, or community-acquired enterococci, in the absence of a primary focus of infection.
2. Persistently positive blood cultures: At least two blood cultures drawn more than 12 h apart **OR** all of three or a majority of four separate blood cultures, drawn 1 h apart.
3. Single positive blood culture for *Coxiella burnetii* or antiphase 1 IgG antibody titer ≥1:800.

Evidence of Endocardial Involvement

Positive echocardiogram for IE, such as:

1. Oscillating intracardiac mass on a valve or supporting structure, in the path of regurgitant jets, or on implanted material in the absence of another anatomic explanation
2. Abscess
3. New partial dehiscence of a prosthetic valve
4. New valvular regurgitation (change in preexisting murmur not sufficient)

Minor Criteria

1. Predisposing heart condition or IV drug use
2. Fever ≥38°C (100.4°F)
3. Vascular phenomena: Arterial emboli, septic pulmonary infarcts, mycotic aneurysm, intracranial or conjunctival hemorrhage, Janeway lesions
4. Immunologic phenomena: Glomerulonephritis, Osler nodes, Roth spots, rheumatoid factor
5. Microbiologic evidence: Positive blood culture but not meeting major criteria **OR** serologic evidence of infection with an organism consistent with IE

HACEK, *Haemophilus*, *Aggregatibacter*, *Cardiobacterium*, *Eikenella*, *Kingella*; IE, infective endocarditis.
Modified from Li JS, Sexton DJ, Mick N, et al. Proposed modifications to the Duke criteria for the diagnosis of infective endocarditis. *Clin Infect Dis.* 2000;30(4):633-638, by permission of Oxford University Press.

CHAPTER 14

• **PVE** must be considered in any patient with persistent bacteremia after heart valve surgery or new valve dehiscence with secondary hemolysis.

Diagnostic Testing

• The most reliable diagnostic criterion for IE and a major Duke criterion is persistent bacteremia in a compatible clinical setting. Three blood cultures should be taken from separate sites drawn 30 minutes apart before empiric antimicrobial therapy is initiated to maximize pathogen recovery. Blood cultures are negative in 10%–15% of patients, most commonly because of prior receipt of antibiotics.
• Echocardiography plays an important role in establishing the diagnosis of IE and determining the need for surgical intervention.

TABLE 14-6	Definition of Infective Endocarditis (IE) by Modified Duke Criteria[11]
Definite IE	
Pathologic criteria:	
Microorganism demonstrated by culture or histology of a vegetation or intracardiac abscess **OR**	
Confirmed histology showing active endocarditis	
Clinical criteria:	
Two major criteria **OR**	
One major and three minor criteria **OR**	
Five minor criteria	
Possible IE	
One major and one minor criteria **OR**	
Three minor criteria	
Rejected IE	
Firm alternative diagnosis **OR**	
Resolution of manifestations with therapy for ≤4 d **OR**	
No pathological evidence at surgery or autopsy after antibiotic therapy ≤4 d	

Modified from Li JS, Sexton DJ, Mick N, et al. Proposed modifications to the Duke criteria for the diagnosis of infective endocarditis. *Clin Infect Dis.* 2000;30(4):633-638, by permission of Oxford University Press.

- Patients with IE and vegetations seen by transthoracic echocardiography (TTE) are at higher risk of embolism, heart failure, and valvular disruption. However, a negative TTE cannot rule out IE, having a sensitivity of 50%–60%.
- Transesophageal echocardiography has higher sensitivity (90%) and should be the first test in patients with prosthetic valves or complicated IE (i.e., perivalvular abscess). In every other situation, TTE should be performed first.[12]
- True **culture-negative IE** is rare and usually caused by fastidious pathogens that do not grow in standard blood culture media. These include *Coxiella burnetii* (Q fever), *Bartonella, Brucella, Tropheryma whipplei* (Whipple disease), *Legionella*, and fungi. Empiric therapy can be initiated despite negative cultures. Serological or molecular testing should be performed if blood cultures are negative and there are epidemiological clues for the pathogens above.
- ^{18}F-fluorodeoxyglucose cardiac positron emission tomography plus CT may be useful in cases of suspected PVE. Its role in native valve IE remains to be determined.

TREATMENT

- **IE** often requires empiric antimicrobial treatment before culture results become available. Initial treatment for *S. aureus* should consist of vancomycin 15 mg/kg IV q12h. Infectious diseases consultation is advised to help define an antimicrobial regimen. Therapy should then be modified based on culture and susceptibility data. For methicillin-sensitive isolates, oxacillin 2 g IV q4h is superior to vancomycin.
- In selected cases of **SBE** where the patient is clinically stable, therapy can usually be delayed until culture data and susceptibilities are available.
- **Antibiotic therapy for specific organisms** is described in Table 14-7.

TABLE 14-7	Treatment of Endocarditis Caused by Specific Organisms[12]		
Organism	Antibiotic Regimen	Duration	Notes
Viridans Group Streptococci and *Streptococcus gallolyticus*			
MIC <0.12 µg/mL	• Penicillin G (12–18 million units IV qday) or ceftriaxone (2 g IV qday) ± gentamicin (3 mg/kg IV qday) for the first 2 wk • Vancomycin (15 mg/kg IV q12h)	4 wk If used, gentamicin is given only during the first 2 wk	• PVE, major embolic, or extended symptoms require a 6-wk course of treatment + gentamicin. • Gentamicin may be ototoxic and nephrotoxic.
MIC 0.12–0.5 µg/mL	• Penicillin G (4 million units IV q4h) or ceftriaxone + gentamicin • Vancomycin if PCN allergic + gentamicin	4 wk total with 2 wk of gentamicin	• Vancomycin is reserved for patients with true β-lactam allergy and unable to be desensitized.
MIC >0.5 µg/mL	• Treat as enterococcal endocarditis	6 wk	
Enterococcus Species			
Penicillin-susceptible	• Ampicillin (2 g IV q4h) + gentamicin (3 mg/kg ideal body weight in 2–3 equally divided doses) • Ampicillin + ceftriaxone (2 g IV q12h)	4–6 wk	• If high-level gentamicin resistance, substitute streptomycin (15 mg/kg IV qday IV in two divided doses based on ideal body weight) or ceftriaxone (4 g IV qday in two divided doses).
Penicillin-resistant	• Vancomycin (15 mg/kg IV q12h) + gentamicin (3 mg/kg in 3 equally divided doses)	6 wk	
Vancomycin (VRE) and ampicillin resistant	• Linezolid (600 mg IV/PO q12h) • Daptomycin (≥10–12 mg/kg qday)	≥6 wk	• This should be managed in conjunction with an Infectious Diseases consultant.
Staphylococcus aureus			
NVE MSSA	• Oxacillin or nafcillin (2 g IV q4h) • Cefazolin (2 g IV q8h) if penicillin allergy without anaphylaxis	6 wk	• Initial 3–5 d gentamicin for synergy may not be beneficial. • Penicillins are superior to vancomycin, and desensitization is preferred when possible.

(continued)

TABLE 14-7	Treatment of Endocarditis Caused by Specific Organisms[12] *(continued)*		
Organism	**Antibiotic Regimen**	**Duration**	**Notes**
Right-sided only NVE MSSA (IV drug user)	• Oxacillin or nafcillin (2 g IV q4h) • Cefazolin (2 g IV q8h) if penicillin allergy without anaphylaxis	≥2 wk	• 2 wk is only recommended in patients without cardiac complications, or embolic events other than pulmonary emboli. • CK must be monitored in patients on daptomycin.
NVE, MRSA	• Vancomycin (15 mg/kg IV q12h) or daptomycin (≥8 mg/kg IV qday)	6 wk	
Staphylococcus Species (Prosthetic Valve)			
MSSA/MSSE	• Oxacillin + rifampin (300 mg PO q8h) + gentamicin (3 mg/kg per 24 h IV in 2 or 3 equally divided doses)	≥6 wk total	Gentamicin given only during the first 2 wk.
MRSA/MRSE	• Vancomycin + rifampin + gentamicin	≥6 wk total	Gentamicin given only during the first 2 wk.
HACEK organisms	• Ceftriaxone (2 g IV qday) Alternatives: • Ampicillin (2 g IV q4h) • Ciprofloxacin (400 mg IV q12h)	4 wk for NVE 6 wk for PVE	HACEK stands for _Haemophilus, Aggregatibacter, Cardiobacterium, Eikenella,_ and _Kingella._
Culture-negative IE	Consultation with an infectious diseases specialist to define the most appropriate choice of therapy is recommended		

Baseline and weekly audiometry recommended for patients receiving aminoglycosides for >7 days. Monitor aminoglycoside and vancomycin levels. Goal vancomycin trough levels are 15–20 µg/mL.

CK, creatinine kinase; IE, infective endocarditis; MIC, minimum inhibitory concentration; MRSA, methicillin-resistant _Staphylococcus aureus_; MRSE, methicillin-resistant _Staphylococcus epidermidis_; MSSA, methicillin-sensitive _Staphylococcus aureus_; MSSE, methicillin-sensitive _Staphylococcus epidermidis_; NVE, native valve endocarditis; PCN, penicillin; PVE, prosthetic valve endocarditis; VRE, vancomycin-resistant _Enterococcus_.

- **Standard care consists of targeted IV antimicrobials for 4–6 weeks, starting from the day that source control and blood culture clearance are achieved.**[12]
- **PVE** requires aggressive combination of antimicrobials for at least 6 weeks or longer and surgery because of the increased risk for treatment failure and relapse. Initial empiric therapy pending culture data include the addition of rifampin and gentamicin to improve biofilm penetration.

• Transition to oral therapy can be considered in selected patients after an initial IV course but additional trials are needed to validate this approach in other clinical settings.
• **Response to antimicrobial therapy**
  ○ Clinical improvement is frequently seen within 3–10 days of initiating therapy.
  ○ Blood cultures should be obtained daily until clearance of bacteremia has been documented.
  ○ Persistent or recurrent fever usually represents extensive cardiac infection but also may be due to septic emboli, drug hypersensitivity, or subsequent nosocomial infection.

Surgical Management

• Indications for surgery in patients with **NVIE** include persistent vegetation after systemic embolization; mobile vegetations ≥10 mm; ≥1 embolic event in the first 2 weeks of treatment or increase in the size of the vegetation despite antimicrobial therapy; refractory heart failure and aortic or mitral regurgitation with ventricular failure; heart block, annular or aortic abscess, fistula, or perforation; infection with fungi or other highly resistant organisms; and persistent bacteremia or fever lasting >5–7 days, provided that other sites of infection and fever have been excluded.
• For **PVE**, besides the indications listed above, valve dehiscence, intracardiac fistula, severe prosthetic valve dysfunction resulting in heart failure, and relapsing PVE also warrant surgery.[12]

SPECIAL CONSIDERATIONS

American Heart Association recommendations for prophylaxis for IE are outlined in Table 14-8.

Myocarditis

GENERAL PRINCIPLES

• Myocarditis is an inflammatory disease of the myocardium often but not always caused by an infectious agent.
• Causes of infectious myocarditis include viruses, bacteria, rickettsia, fungi, and parasites.
• Viruses are the most frequent etiologic organism and include enteroviruses (coxsackie B and echovirus), adenovirus, human herpesvirus 6, parvovirus B19, and many others.

CLINICAL PRESENTATION

Chest pain, elevated cardiac enzymes (e.g., troponin), fever, and diffuse ST-segment abnormalities on EKG are the classical manifestations of infectious myocarditis.

DIAGNOSIS

• The diagnostic "gold standard" is endomyocardial biopsy for histological, immunological, and immunohistochemical criteria, including specific viral PCR.
• Cardiac MRI can be useful for diagnosis and monitoring of disease progression.
• Viral culture and serologic testing are rarely helpful.

CHAPTER 14

TABLE 14-8	Endocarditis Prophylaxis[13]

I. Endocarditis prophylaxis is recommended for the following cardiac conditions: prosthetic valves; previous endocarditis; unrepaired cyanotic congenital heart disease or repaired congenital heart disease with prosthetic material during the first 6 mo after procedure, or with residual defects at or adjacent to the site of the prosthetic device; and cardiac valvulopathy in transplant recipients.

II. Regimens for dental, oral, or respiratory tract procedures (including dental extractions, periodontal or endodontic procedures, professional teeth cleaning, bronchoscopy with biopsy, rigid bronchoscopy, surgery on respiratory mucosa, and tonsillectomy):

Standard prophylaxis	Amoxicillin 2 g PO 1 h before procedure
Unable to take PO	Ampicillin 2 g IM or IV, or cefazolin or ceftriaxone 1 g IM or IV within 30 min before procedure
Penicillin-allergic patient	Clindamycin 600 mg PO, or cephalexin 2 g PO, or clarithromycin or azithromycin 500 mg PO 1 h before procedure
Penicillin allergic and unable to take PO	Clindamycin 600 mg IV, or cefazolin or ceftriaxone 1 g IV within 30 min before procedure

III. Gastrointestinal and genitourinary procedures do not require routine use of prophylaxis. High-risk patients infected or colonized with enterococci should receive amoxicillin, ampicillin, or vancomycin to eradicate the organism before urinary tract manipulation.

IV. Prophylaxis is recommended for procedures on infected skin, skin structures, or musculoskeletal tissue ONLY for patients with cardiac conditions outlined above. An antistaphylococcal penicillin or cephalosporin should be used.

TREATMENT

Supportive care is the mainstay of treatment. NSAIDs should be avoided. The role of IV immunoglobulin and antiviral agents in viral-mediated myocarditis remains anecdotal.[14]

Pericarditis

GENERAL PRINCIPLES

- A diagnosis of acute pericarditis (inflammation of the pericardium) can be made with at least two of the following four criteria: pleuritic chest pain, pericardial rub, new widespread ST-segment elevation or PR depression, and new or worsening pericardial effusion.
- Viruses are the most common infectious etiology. Staphylococci, *S. pneumonia*, *M. tuberculosis*, and histoplasmosis are occasional causes.

TREATMENT

- If an infectious etiology is identified, specific treatment should be initiated. The role of antiviral therapies in viral pericarditis remains unclear.

- Aspirin (750–1000 mg q8h for 1–2 weeks) or NSAIDs (ibuprofen 600 mg q8h for 1–2 weeks) are recommended as first-line therapy for acute pericarditis.
- Adjuvant colchicine (0.5 mg PO qday [<70 kg] or q12h [≥70 kg] for 3 months) is also recommended as first-line therapy.[15]

UPPER RESPIRATORY TRACT INFECTIONS

Pharyngitis

GENERAL PRINCIPLES

- Viruses are the most common cause of pharyngitis. GABHS pharyngitis is responsible for merely 5%–15% of cases in adults, with other bacteria responsible to a lesser extent. Unfortunately, 60% of adults with pharyngitis receive antibiotics.
- **Acute HIV infection** should be considered in the setting of pharyngitis with atypical lymphocytosis and negative *Streptococcus* and Epstein–Barr virus testing. Suppurative complications including **peritonsillar or retropharyngeal abscess** should be considered in the patient with severe unilateral pain, muffled voice, trismus, and dysphagia.

DIAGNOSIS

Clinical Presentation

Fever, cervical lymphadenopathy, tonsillar exudates, and throat pain are the most common clinical manifestations. Distinguishing bacterial from viral pharyngitis on clinical grounds alone is difficult.

Diagnostic Testing

- Diagnostic testing is usually reserved for symptomatic patients with exposure to a case of streptococcal pharyngitis, those with signs of significant infection (fever, tonsillar exudates, and cervical adenopathy) or whose symptoms persist despite symptomatic therapy, and patients with a history of rheumatic fever. Testing for SARS-CoV-2 should be considered.
- Rapid antigen detection testing (RADT) is useful for diagnosing **GABHS** (>90% sensitivity and specificity), which requires antimicrobial therapy to prevent suppurative complications and rheumatic fever. A negative test does not reliably exclude GAS, making throat culture necessary if clinical suspicion is high.
- Serology for **Epstein–Barr virus** (e.g., heterophile agglutinin or monospot) and examination of a peripheral blood smear for atypical lymphocytes should be performed when infectious mononucleosis is suspected.
- A NAAT pharyngeal swab for gonococcal pharyngitis is recommended in those with risk factors for sexual transmitted diseases, particularly receptive oral intercourse.

TREATMENT

- Most cases of pharyngitis are self-limited and do not require antimicrobial therapy.
- Treatment for **GABHS** is indicated with a positive culture or RADT, if the patient is at high risk for development of rheumatic fever, or if the diagnosis is strongly suspected, pending culture results. Treatment options include penicillin V 500 mg PO q12h for 10 days, clindamycin 300 mg PO q8h for 10 days, azithromycin

CHAPTER 14

500 mg PO on day 1 followed by 250 mg qday on days 2–5, or benzathine penicillin G 1.2 million units IM as a one-time dose.[16] In some communities, up to 15% of the **GABHS** isolates are resistant to macrolides.

- Gonococcal pharyngitis is treated with ceftriaxone 500 mg IM as a single dose, plus doxycycline for 7 days or a single dose of azithromycin (if the patient is pregnant) if coinfection with chlamydia is identified.

Epiglottitis

GENERAL PRINCIPLES

- Epiglottitis is a respiratory emergency, as inflammation of the epiglottis can lead to airway obstruction.
- *H. influenzae* type B, *S. pneumoniae*, *S. aureus*, and GABHS are common bacterial causes of epiglottitis, although viral and fungal pathogens may also be implicated.

DIAGNOSIS

Clinical Presentation

Fever, sore throat, odynophagia, drooling, muffled voice, and dysphagia in a patient with a normal oropharyngeal examination should prompt a clinical diagnosis of epiglottitis. Inspiratory stridor is a sign of impending respiratory compromise.

Diagnostic Testing

- Throat and blood cultures are useful in determining the etiology.
- Soft-tissue lateral radiographs of the neck may demonstrate the "thumb print" sign.
- Bedside ultrasound can aid in the diagnosis and show the "alphabet P sign."
- Definitive diagnosis is made by visualization of the epiglottis with direct laryngoscopy.

TREATMENT

- Airway stabilization is the priority; otolaryngology consultation is recommended in all suspected cases.
- Antimicrobial therapy should include an agent that is active against *H. influenzae*, such as ceftriaxone 2 g IV qday or cefotaxime 2 g IV q6-8h. Vancomycin or clindamycin should be added if there is concern for MRSA. Glucocorticoids are often also given.

Rhinosinusitis

GENERAL PRINCIPLES

- **Acute rhinosinusitis** is most frequently caused by upper respiratory viruses. Bacterial pathogens, such as *S. pneumoniae*, *H. influenzae*, *Moraxella catarrhalis*, and anaerobes, are involved in <2% of cases and should be considered only if symptoms persist for >10 days. In immunosuppressed patients, fungal causes (i.e., *Mucor*, *Rhizopus*, and *Aspergillus* species) should be considered.
- **Chronic rhinosinusitis** may be caused by any of the etiologic agents responsible for acute sinusitis, as well as *S. aureus*, *Corynebacterium diphtheriae*, and many anaerobes (e.g., *Prevotella* spp., *Veillonella* spp.). Possible contributing factors include asthma, nasal polyps, allergies, or immunodeficiency.

DIAGNOSIS

Clinical Presentation

- **Acute rhinosinusitis** presents with purulent nasal discharge, nasal obstruction, facial or dental pain, and sinus tenderness with or without fever, lasting <4 weeks.
- **Chronic rhinosinusitis** is defined by symptoms lasting >12 weeks including mucopurulent drainage, nasal obstruction, facial pain or pressure, and decreased sense of smell with documented signs of inflammation.

Diagnostic Testing

- Diagnosis requires objective evidence of mucosal disease, usually with rhinoscopy and nasal endoscopy. If radiological imaging is done, limited sinus CT should be used. Plain films are not recommended.
- When performed, sinus cultures should be obtained by nasal endoscopy or sinus puncture. Nasal swabs are not helpful.

TREATMENT

- The goals of medical therapy for acute and chronic rhinosinusitis are to control infection, reduce tissue edema, facilitate drainage, maintain patency of the sinus ostia, and break the pathologic cycle that leads to chronic sinusitis.
- **Acute rhinosinusitis**
  - **Symptomatic treatment** is the mainstay of therapy, including oral decongestants and analgesics with or without a short course of topical decongestant or intranasal glucocorticoid.[17]
  - **Empiric antibiotic therapy** is indicated only for severe persistent symptoms (≥10 days) or failure of symptomatic therapy. First-line therapy should consist of a 5- to 7-day course of amoxicillin–clavulanate 875 mg/125 mg PO q12h. Doxycycline or a respiratory fluoroquinolone (e.g., moxifloxacin, levofloxacin) may be used as alternative therapy in case of β-lactam allergy or primary treatment failure. TMP–SMX and macrolides are not recommended for empiric therapy due to high rates of resistance.
- **Chronic rhinosinusitis.** Treatment usually includes topical and/or systemic glucocorticoids; the role of antimicrobial agents is unclear. If antibiotics are prescribed, amoxicillin–clavulanate is considered first line; clindamycin can be used in the setting of penicillin allergy. Some chronic cases may require endoscopic surgery.

LOWER RESPIRATORY TRACT INFECTIONS

Acute Bronchitis

GENERAL PRINCIPLES

Acute bronchitis involves inflammation of the bronchi, most often caused by viruses such as coronavirus, rhinovirus, influenza, or parainfluenza. Uncommon causes include *M. pneumoniae*, *Chlamydophila pneumoniae*, and *Bordetella pertussis*. Unfortunately, 60%–90% of patients with acute bronchitis are given antibiotics.

DIAGNOSIS

Clinical Presentation

Symptoms include cough with or without sputum production lasting >5 days sometimes with associated wheezing or rhonchi on physical examination. Up to half of the patients have purulent sputum production; however, fever is uncommon.

Diagnostic Testing

- Diagnosis is made clinically. Sputum cultures are not recommended.
- COVID-19 should be ruled out.
- In febrile, systemically ill, or older patients with abnormal vital signs, pneumonia should be evaluated for radiographically, and diagnostic tests for influenza should be performed depending on the season and local disease trends.
- Cough lasting >2 weeks in an adult should be evaluated for pertussis with a nasopharyngeal swab for culture or PCR.

TREATMENT

- Treatment is symptomatic and should be directed toward controlling cough (dextromethorphan 15 mg PO q6h).
- Multiple studies have shown no benefit in antimicrobial therapy for generally healthy patients with acute, non–pertussis-related bronchitis.
- Pertussis treatment consists of azithromycin 500 mg PO single dose followed by 250 mg PO qday for 4 more days, or clarithromycin 500 mg PO q12h for 14 days. Cases should be reported to the local health department for contact tracing and administration of postexposure prophylaxis of contacts with azithromycin when indicated.

Influenza Virus Infection

GENERAL PRINCIPLES

Influenza is an acute febrile respiratory illness, readily transmissible and associated with outbreaks of varying severity during the winter months.

DIAGNOSIS

Clinical Presentation

In immunocompetent patients, influenza virus infection causes an acute, self-limited febrile illness associated with headache, myalgias, cough, coryza, and malaise. These symptoms may last up to 2 weeks.

Diagnostic Testing

Diagnosis is usually made clinically during influenza season, with confirmation by nasopharyngeal swab for rapid antigen testing, PCR (higher sensitivity), or direct fluorescent antibody test and culture.

TREATMENT

- Treatment is usually symptomatic.
- Antiviral medications may shorten the duration of illness but must be initiated within 24–48 hours of the onset of symptoms to be effective in immunocompetent

patients.[18] Antiviral therapy should not be withheld from patients presenting >48 hours after symptom onset requiring hospitalization or at high risk for complications (see "Complications").

- ○ The **neuraminidase inhibitors** (oseltamivir 75 mg PO q12h or zanamivir 10 mg inhaled q12h, each for 5 days, or peramivir, 600 mg single dose IV) are approved by the US Food and Drug Administration for the treatment of influenza A and B.
- ○ **M2 inhibitors** (amantadine and rimantadine, each 100 mg PO q12h) are **not** recommended due to high rates of resistance.
- ○ Circulating strains change annually with varying resistance patterns to both classes of antivirals. **Treatment decisions must be based on annual resistance data**, available from the Centers for Disease Control and Prevention (CDC) (http://www.cdc.gov).
- **Vaccination** is the most reliable prevention strategy. Annual vaccination is recommended for all individuals 6 months of age and older. Efficacy of vaccination varies annually from 50% to 90% depending on prevailing outbreak and circulating influenza strains.

COMPLICATIONS

- Adults older than 65 years, residents of nursing homes and other long-term care facilities, pregnant women (and those up to 2 weeks postpartum), and patients with chronic medical conditions (e.g., pulmonary disease, cardiovascular disease, active malignancy, diabetes mellitus, chronic renal insufficiency, chronic liver disease, immunosuppression including HIV and transplantation, morbid obesity) are at greater risk of complications.
- Influenza pneumonia and secondary bacterial pneumonia, typically due to *S. aureus*, are the most common complications of influenza infection.
- Viral antigenic drift and shift can cause emergence of strains with enhanced virulence or the potential for pandemic spread, requiring modified therapy or heightened infection control measures.

Coronavirus Disease 2019 (COVID-19)

GENERAL PRINCIPLES

- COVID-19 is caused by a novel coronavirus, Severe Acute Respiratory Syndrome coronavirus 2 (SARS-CoV-2) that has spread globally. Infection can be asymptomatic or manifest with a wide range of symptoms, ranging from mild respiratory disease to acute hypoxic respiratory failure requiring mechanical ventilation support.
- SARS-CoV-2 is a single-stranded RNA virus transmitted through respiratory droplets during talking, coughing, or sneezing. There is an increased risk of infection with prolonged exposure to an infected person (being within 6 ft for at least 15 minutes) or shorter exposures to individuals who are symptomatic.[19]

DIAGNOSIS

Clinical Presentation

- The mean incubation period for COVID-19 is 5 days (interquartile range of 2–7 days).
- Mild to moderate COVID-19 symptoms include cough, shortness of breath, fever, anosmia, ageusia, myalgias, and gastrointestinal symptoms.

CHAPTER 14

- Severe disease will most commonly present with acute hypoxic respiratory failure. In addition, patients can develop acute kidney injury, liver dysfunction, bleeding and coagulation dysfunction, and septic shock.

Diagnostic Testing

Diagnosis is made using RT-PCR testing via nasal swab. Given possible false negative results, a presumptive diagnosis can be made with compatible clinical, laboratory, and imaging findings.

TREATMENT

- Strategies to treat COVID-19 are rapidly evolving. For updated recommendations, consult World Health Organization (www.who.int), CDC (www.cdc.gov), and National Institutes of Health (https://www.covid19treatmentguidelines.nih.gov/) treatment guidelines available online.
- **Dexamethasone** 6 mg PO qday for 10 days or until discharge is recommended for severely ill patients with COVID-19 requiring oxygen and/or ventilatory support. If dexamethasone is not available, it is reasonable to use other glucocorticoids at equivalent doses although data are limited.
- **Remdesivir** is a novel nucleotide analog with in vitro activity against SARS-CoV-2. It has been shown to reduce time to recovery and possibly mortality in those requiring supplemental oxygen.
- Convalescent plasma from individuals who have recovered from COVID-19 may provide passive immunity. The available evidence is unclear about its role in the treatment of COVID-19.
- Monoclonal antibodies developed to neutralize SARS-CoV-2 are still being studied in clinical trials.
- Supportive management of acute hypoxic respiratory failure and ARDS should be followed in severe disease.
- **Vaccination** is the most reliable prevention strategy to decrease symptomatic cases, hospitalization, and deaths.

COMPLICATIONS

- Adults older than 65 years, residents of nursing homes and other long-term care facilities, and patients with chronic medical conditions (e.g., pulmonary disease, cardiovascular disease, active malignancy, diabetes mellitus, chronic renal insufficiency, chronic liver disease, morbid obesity) are at greater risk of complications and death.
- Secondary bacterial pneumonia is uncommon. Use of steroids can cause reactivation of underlying infections in those with epidemiological risk factors such as strongyloidiasis, histoplasmosis, etc. Secondary fungal infections with *Aspergillus* spp. or COVID-19–associated pulmonary aspergillosis (CAPA) have been reported.

Community-Acquired Pneumonia

GENERAL PRINCIPLES

- The predominant organism involved is *S. pneumoniae*; other bacterial etiologies are *H. influenzae* and *M. catarrhalis*. Pneumonia caused by atypical agents, such as *Legionella pneumophila*, *C. pneumoniae*, or *M. pneumoniae*, cannot be reliably distinguished clinically. Influenza, SARS-CoV-2, and other respiratory viruses may also cause pneumonia in adults.

- Community-acquired MRSA is an important cause of severe, necrotizing pneumonia.
- Patients aged 65 years or older, and those with certain medical conditions, should receive the pneumococcal vaccination with both the 23-valent and the 13-valent vaccine, as recommended per CDC guidelines.[20]

DIAGNOSIS

Clinical Presentation

- The presentation of CAP is extremely variable. Fever and respiratory symptoms, including cough with sputum production, dyspnea, and pleuritic chest pain, are common in immunocompetent patients. Signs include tachypnea, rales, or evidence of consolidation on auscultation.
- CAP presents acutely, over a matter of hours to days. If a patient has symptoms for more than 2–3 weeks, particularly if accompanied by weight loss or night sweats, this should raise the question of an alternate diagnosis, such as mycobacterial or fungal infection.

Diagnostic Testing

- Prior to antibiotic therapy, sputum Gram stain and culture of an adequate sputum sample and blood cultures before antibiotic therapy should be obtained in all patients who are going to be hospitalized, and, if disease is severe, urinary antigen tests for *S. pneumoniae* and *L. pneumophila*.
- Nasopharyngeal swab for influenza, SARS-CoV-2, or other virus detection by PCR, and respiratory samples for atypical pathogens should be sent in selected cases.
- If TB is suspected, sputum for acid-fast stain and culture should be obtained, and the patient should be placed on airborne isolation.
- Chest radiography should be performed and may reveal lobar consolidation, interstitial infiltrates, or cavitary lesions, confirming the diagnosis.
- Fiberoptic bronchoscopy may be used for detection of less common organisms, especially in immunocompromised patients, or if the patient is not responding to adequate therapy.

TREATMENT

- All patients should be assessed for hospitalization and evaluated for comorbid factors, oxygenation, and severity of illness using validated severity scales such as the Pneumonia Severity Index or CURB-65.
- Antibiotics should be given as soon as CAP is diagnosed, ideally within 4 hours of arrival to the hospital, as delays lead to higher mortality. Antibiotic therapy should be narrowed once a specific microbiologic etiology has been identified.
- **Empiric antibiotic therapy** with an emphasis on targeting likely pathogens based on comorbidities and other risk factors is described in Table 14-9.[21]
- **Thoracentesis** of pleural effusions should be performed, with analysis of pH, cell count, Gram stain and bacterial culture, protein, and lactate dehydrogenase (LDH) (see Chapter 10, Pulmonary Diseases). Empyemas should be drained.

CHAPTER 14

TABLE 14-9	Empiric Treatment for Community-Acquired Pneumonia

Outpatient Regimens

No comorbidities[a] or risk factors for MRSA or *Pseudomonas aeruginosa*[b]

- Monotherapy with amoxicillin 1000 mg PO q8 hours OR doxycycline 100 mg PO q12 hours for at least 5 d
- Monotherapy with azithromycin 500 mg PO on first day, then 250 mg qday on day 2–5

With comorbidities[a]

- Combination therapy with amoxicillin/clavulanate 875 mg/125 mg PO q12 hours, cefpodoxime 200 mg PO q12 hours, OR cefuroxime 500 mg PO q12 hours for at least 5 d PLUS doxycycline or azithromycin
- Monotherapy with a respiratory fluoroquinolone (e.g., levofloxacin 750 mg PO qday, moxifloxacin 400 mg PO qday)

Inpatient Regimens

Nonsevere

- β-Lactam (ampicillin–sulbactam 1.5–3 g IV q6 hours, ceftriaxone 1–2 g IV qday, cefotaxime 1–2 g IV q8 hours, or ceftaroline 600 mg IV q12 hours) PLUS macrolide (e.g., azithromycin)
- Monotherapy with respiratory fluoroquinolone (e.g., levofloxacin, moxifloxacin)

Severe disease

- β-Lactam PLUS macrolide
- β-Lactam PLUS fluoroquinolone

Prior respiratory isolation of MRSA or *P. aeruginosa*

- MRSA: Expand empiric coverage with vancomycin 15 mg/kg IV q12 hours (adjusted based on levels and renal clearance) or linezolid 600 mg IV/PO q12 hours regardless of disease severity.
- *P. aeruginosa*: Expand empiric coverage with piperacillin–tazobactam 4.5 g IV q6 hours, cefepime 2 g IV q8 hours, ceftazidime 2 g IV q8 hours, imipenem 500 mg IV q6 hours, meropenem 1 g IV q8 hours, or aztreonam 2 g IV q8 hours regardless of disease severity.
- Obtain cultures (and/or nasal PCR for MRSA, if available) to help tailor antibiotic therapy.

Recent hospitalization and receipt of parenteral antibiotics in the preceding 90 d and locally validated risk factors for MRSA or *P. aeruginosa*

- Nonsevere disease: Obtain cultures (and/or nasal PCR for MRSA, if available) but do not expand coverage unless MRSA and/or *P. aeruginosa* is identified.
- Severe disease: Expand empiric coverage for MRSA and/or *P. aeruginosa* and obtain cultures (and nasal PCR for MRSA, if available) to help tailor antibiotic therapy.

MRSA, methicillin-resistant *Staphylococcus aureus*; PCR, polymerase chain reaction.
Adapted from Metlay JP, Waterer GW, Long AC, et al. Diagnosis and treatment of adults with community-acquired pneumonia. An official clinical practice guideline of the American Thoracic Society and Infectious Diseases Society of America. *Am J Respir Crit Care Med.* 2019;200(7):e45-e67.
[a]Chronic heart, lung, liver, or renal disease; diabetes mellitus; alcoholism; malignancy; or asplenia.
[b]Prior respiratory isolation of MRSA or *P. aeruginosa* or recent hospitalization AND receipt of parenteral antibiotics in the preceding 90 days.

Lung Abscess

GENERAL PRINCIPLES

- Lung abscess typically results from aspiration of oral flora.
- Polymicrobial infections are common and involve oral anaerobes (*Prevotella* spp., *Peptostreptococcus, Fusobacterium, Bacteroides* spp., and *Actinomyces* spp.). Microaerophilic streptococci (*S. anginosus group*), enteric gram-negative bacilli (*Klebsiella pneumoniae*), and *S. aureus*, including community-acquired MRSA, are less frequent causes.
- Risk factors include periodontal disease and conditions that predispose patients to aspiration of oropharyngeal contents (alcohol intoxication, sedative use, seizures, stroke, and neuromuscular disease).

DIAGNOSIS

Clinical Presentation

Infections are indolent and may be reminiscent of pulmonary TB, with fever, chills, night sweats, weight loss, dyspnea, and cough productive of putrid or blood-streaked sputum for several weeks.

Diagnostic Testing

- Chest radiography is sensitive and typically reveals infiltrates with cavitation and air–fluid levels in dependent areas of the lung, such as the lower lobes or the posterior segments of the upper lobes. Chest CT can provide additional anatomic detail.
- Respiratory isolation and sputum testing for TB should be performed on all patients with cavitary lung lesions.

TREATMENT

- Antibiotic therapy should consist of clindamycin or a β-lactam/β-lactamase inhibitor (ampicillin–sulbactam, piperacillin–tazobactam, amoxicillin–clavulanate) or a carbapenem (ertapenem). For MRSA cavitary lung lesions, linezolid or vancomycin should be used. Metronidazole monotherapy is ineffective due to the presence of microaerophilic nonculturable organisms in the oral microbiota; thus, it should be combined with penicillin.
- Percutaneous drainage or surgical resection is rarely necessary and should be reserved for antibiotic-refractory disease, usually involving large abscesses (>6 cm) or infections with resistant organisms.

Tuberculosis

GENERAL PRINCIPLES

- Approximately 1.7 billion people are infected with TB; although <15% progress to active disease.[22] Most US cases occur in foreign-born individuals and result from reactivation of prior infection.
- Multidrug-resistant TB (resistance to both rifampin and isoniazid) has increased among immigrants from Southeast Asia, sub-Saharan Africa, the Indian subcontinent, and Eastern Europe. Extensively drug-resistant tuberculosis (MDR-TB plus resistance to fluoroquinolones and at least one of the three injectable second-line drugs) is becoming increasingly prevalent in sub-Saharan Africa.

CHAPTER 14

- High risk of TB exposure occurs among household contacts, prisoners, the homeless, injection drug users, and immigrants from high-prevalence countries.
- Latent tuberculosis infection (LTBI) refers to someone who has infection but not disease (clinical and radiological evidence of active disease). The **lifetime** risk of progression to active disease is 10% (5% within 2 years of infection and an additional 5% thereafter). In poorly controlled HIV and other immunosuppressed patients, the **annual** progression rate from latent to active TB is 10%. Adequate treatment of LTBI can reduce the risk of disease up to 90%.[23]

DIAGNOSIS

Clinical Presentation

- The most frequent clinical presentation is pulmonary disease. Symptoms are often indolent and may include cough for >14 days, hemoptysis, dyspnea, fever, night sweats, weight loss, or fatigue. Misdiagnosis and treatment with a fluoroquinolone for presumed CAP can lead to treatment delay and fluoroquinolone resistance.
- Extrapulmonary disease can present as cervical lymphadenopathy, genitourinary disease, osteomyelitis, miliary dissemination, meningitis, peritonitis, or pericarditis.

Diagnostic Testing

- Chest radiography may reveal focal infiltrates, nodules, cavitary lesions, miliary disease, pleural effusions, or hilar/mediastinal lymphadenopathy. Reactivation disease classically involves the upper lobes.
- Three sputum specimens should be sent for AFB smears and cultures. A diagnosis of active TB is made with a positive AFB smear, a positive NAAT for *M. tuberculosis* complex, or positive culture. Nontuberculous mycobacteria (NTM) may be positive on smear but negative on NAAT. AFB smear sensitivity can be up to 90%, if three sputum samples are tested.
- All patients with confirmed or suspected TB should undergo HIV testing.
- *M. tuberculosis* can take several weeks to grow in culture, so if the clinical suspicion is high, presumptive therapy even with negative smears may be indicated until cultures are negative.
- Antimicrobial susceptibility testing should be performed on all initial isolates and on isolates obtained from patients who do not respond to standard therapy. Rapid detection of rifampin resistance, possible with molecular techniques (Cepheid Gene Xpert MTB/RIF), correlates with MDR-TB. Genetic testing on direct specimens is also available for select cases through the CDC (molecular detection of drug resistance).
- LTBI may be diagnosed by a positive tuberculin skin test (TST) or interferon-γ release assay (IGRA). Current guidelines recommend IGRA testing in all individuals 5 years or older, rather than TST.[24] Available IGRAs include QuantiFERON-TB assay and T-SPOT.TB assay, both approved by the FDA. IGRAs are not affected by prior Bacillus Calmette–Guérin vaccination and have specificity of >95% and sensitivity of 80%–90% for diagnosis of LTBI.

TREATMENT

Active TB

- Hospitalized patients with active TB should be placed in airborne isolation in a **negative-pressure room.** Healthcare personnel should use an N95 or powered air purifying respiratory during patient care.

- The local health department should be notified of all TB cases so that contacts can be identified and directly observed therapy (DOT) administered when the patient is discharged. DOT is essential to ensure adherence and prevent emergence of drug resistance.
- **Multidrug anti-TB treatment regimens** are required because drug resistance develops when a single drug is administered. Extended therapy is necessary because of the prolonged generation time of mycobacteria.
- The **intensive phase** of therapy (first 8 weeks) for uncomplicated pulmonary TB should consist of four drugs (RIPE): **rifampin** (**RIF**, 10 mg/kg; maximum, 600 mg PO qday), **isoniazid** (**INH** 5 mg/kg; maximum, 300 mg PO qday), **pyrazinamide** (**PZA**, 15–25 mg/kg; maximum, 2 g PO qday), and **ethambutol** (**EMB**, 15–25 mg/kg PO qday). Pyridoxine (vitamin B_6) 25–50 mg PO qday should be used with INH to prevent sensory neuropathy. If the isolate proves to be **fully susceptible** to INH and RIF, then EMB can be dropped and INH, RIF, and PZA continued to complete this initial phase.
- The **continuation phase** consists of 16 weeks of INH and RIF to reach a standard total of 6 months of therapy for pulmonary TB. Patients at high risk for relapse (cavitary pulmonary disease or positive AFB cultures after 2 months of therapy) should be treated for an additional 28 weeks beyond the 8-week initial phase, for a total of 9 months.
- Daily therapy is the most efficacious regimen and it is recommended in patients with HIV. Thrice weekly therapy can be considered in the continuation phase.
- Therapy for **pregnant women** or **multidrug-resistant TB** often requires individualized drug regimens, and consultation with an expert in the treatment of TB is strongly recommended.
- **Extrapulmonary disease** in adults can be treated in the same manner as pulmonary disease, with 6-month regimens, except for bone and joint infection (9–12 months) and central nervous system (CNS) TB (12 months).[25]
- **Glucocorticoids** in combination with antituberculous drugs are only recommended in tuberculous meningitis but not routinely for tuberculous pericarditis. Prednisone 1 mg/kg (maximum, 60 mg) PO qday or dexamethasone 12 mg IV qday is tapered over several weeks.

Latent TB

- Chemoprophylaxis for LTBI should be administered only after active disease has been ruled out by clinical assessment and chest radiography.
- Risk factors for progression include a positive conversion within 2 years of a previously negative TST or IGRA; a history of untreated TB or radiographic evidence of previous fibrotic disease (calcified granulomas in the absence of fibrosis do not confer increased risk); patients with HIV infection, diabetes mellitus, end-stage renal disease, hematologic or lymphoreticular malignancy, chronic malnutrition, or silicosis or who are receiving immunosuppressive therapy; and close contacts (household members) of patients with active disease who have been diagnosed with LTBI.
- Persons with advanced **HIV** infection or other severely immunocompromised states (e.g., transplant) who have had known contact with a patient with active TB should be treated for LTBI.
- INH 300 mg PO qday for 6–9 months is the most studied regimen for LTBI who have risk factors for progression to active disease, regardless of age. However, <60% of patients complete the 9-month treatment course.
- Other recommended options include RIF 600 mg qday for 4 months, or INH 900 mg PO plus rifapentine 900 mg PO (with dose adjustment for patients <50 kg) once weekly for 3 months. RIF monotherapy has lower risk of hepatotoxicity compared to INH monotherapy.[26]

CHAPTER 14

Monitoring

- **Response to therapy.** Patients with initial positive sputum AFB smears should submit sputum for AFB smear and culture every 1–2 weeks until AFB smears become negative. Sputum should then be obtained monthly until two consecutive negative cultures are documented. Conversion of cultures from positive to negative is the most reliable indicator of response to treatment. Continued symptoms or persistently positive cultures after 3 months of treatment should raise the suspicion of drug resistance or lack of adherence and prompt referral to an expert in the treatment of TB. Referral to the public health department is recommended to ensure adherence by DOT and to monitor for medication-related complications.
- **Adverse reactions** (see Chapter 15 section on antimycobacterial agents). Regular clinical and laboratory evaluation is recommended to identify early signs of adverse reactions.

GASTROINTESTINAL AND ABDOMINAL INFECTIONS

Infectious Gastroenteritis

Infectious gastroenteritis is also addressed in Chapter 18, Gastrointestinal Diseases.

TREATMENT

- Fluid and electrolyte replacement is the mainstay of therapy.
- Antimotility agents should be avoided in dysenteric diarrhea.
- Antibiotics can be used in dysenteric diarrhea for severe disease, bloody stools, and in high-risk patients.[27]
- Azithromycin 1 g single dose or 500 mg PO qday for 3 days, ciprofloxacin 750 mg PO single dose or 500 mg q12h for 3 days, and levofloxacin 500 mg PO single dose or qday for 3 days are often used.
- Antibiotics are contraindicated in enterohemorrhagic *Escherichia coli*, as they increase the risk of hemolytic uremic syndrome.
- Traveler's diarrhea can be treated with ciprofloxacin or TMP–SMX without stool testing.
- Treat empirically if there is suspicion for CDI.

Chronic Diarrhea

Chronic diarrhea is also addressed in Chapter 18, Gastrointestinal Diseases.

TREATMENT

- Giardiasis is diagnosed by stool antigen testing or microscopic examination. Treatment is tinidazole 2 g PO single dose or nitazoxanide 500 mg PO q12h for 3 days or metronidazole 500 mg PO q12h for 7 days.
- Amebiasis is diagnosed by stool microscopy, antigen testing, and serology. Treatment is metronidazole 500 mg q8h for 7–10 days or tinidazole 2 g qday for 3 days, followed by iodoquinol or paromomycin to eradicate cysts.

Intra-Abdominal Infection

- Intra-abdominal infections occur because of inflammation or disruption of the gastrointestinal tract and can be low risk (uncomplicated) or high risk (complicated).
- Infections are typically polymicrobial with enteric gram-negative bacilli (e.g., *E. coli*, *Klebsiella* spp.), *Enterococcus* spp., and especially anaerobes such as *Bacteroides fragilis*.
- Low-risk community-acquired infection includes acute diverticulitis, colitis, or appendiceal abscess.
- High-risk community infections occur in patients at risk for adverse outcomes or resistant pathogens (e.g., age >70 years, comorbidities, immunocompromised, delayed source control).
- Health care–associated infections (HAIs) may be caused by multidrug-resistant organisms (MDROs) and require additional antibiotics if ESBL-producing organisms or MRSA are a consideration.

TREATMENT

- Start empiric antibiotics promptly. See Table 14-10.
- Source control with abscess drainage or surgical resection is critical.[28]
- Avoid clindamycin, cefoxitin, and moxifloxacin due to increased resistance among *B. fragilis*.

TABLE 14-10	Empiric Therapy Examples for Intra-Abdominal Infections[28]

Oral Regimens
- Amoxicillin–clavulanate 875 mg/125 mg PO q12h
- Ciprofloxacin 500–750 mg PO q12h + metronidazole 500 mg PO q8h
- Moxifloxacin 400 mg PO qday

Parenteral Regimens

Low risk—no concern for *Pseudomonas aeruginosa*
- Ertapenem 1 g IV q24h
- Ceftriaxone 1–2 g IV qday + metronidazole 500 mg IV q8h
- Piperacillin/tazobactam 4.5 g IV q6h

High risk—concern for *P. aeruginosa*
- Piperacillin/tazobactam 4.5 g IV q6h
- Cefepime 1–2 g IV q8h + metronidazole 500 mg IV q8h
- Ciprofloxacin 400 mg IV q8–12h + metronidazole 500 mg IV q8h
- Meropenem 1 g IV q8h or imipenem–cilastatin 500 mg IV q6h

Concern for vancomycin-resistant *Enterococcus* spp.[a]
- Add linezolid 600 mg PO/IV q12h or daptomycin 6–8 mg/kg IV qday to above regimens

Concern for yeast[a]
- Add echinocandin (e.g., micafungin 100 mg IV qday) or fluconazole 400 mg PO/IV qday to above regimens

[a]If isolated from a sterile site.

CHAPTER 14

Peritonitis

GENERAL PRINCIPLES

- **Primary** or **spontaneous bacterial peritonitis (SBP)** is a common complication of cirrhosis and ascites. *E. coli*, *K. pneumonia*, and *S. pneumoniae* are common pathogens. *M. tuberculosis* and *Neisseria gonorrhoeae* (Fitz-Hugh–Curtis syndrome) also can occasionally cause primary peritonitis (see Chapter 16, Sexually Transmitted Infections, Human Immunodeficiency Virus, and Acquired Immunodeficiency Syndrome).
- **Secondary peritonitis** may be caused by a perforated viscus or contiguous spread from a visceral infection, usually resulting in an *acute* surgical abdomen.
- Peritonitis related to **peritoneal dialysis** is addressed in Chapter 13, Renal Diseases.

DIAGNOSIS

Clinical Presentation
SBP may present with abdominal pain without fever. SBP should be ruled out with a diagnostic paracentesis in patients with cirrhosis and ascites presenting with gastrointestinal bleeding, encephalopathy, acute kidney injury, or other decompensation of liver disease. Patients with secondary peritonitis present with abdominal tenderness and peritoneal signs.

Diagnostic Testing
- Send blood cultures and ascites fluid for culture (directly inoculate culture bottles at bedside), cell count, and differential. **SBP** is diagnosed when ascites fluid has >250 neutrophils/mm^3.
- Diagnosis of **secondary peritonitis** is made clinically and with imaging to evaluate for free air (perforation) and the source of infection. Blood cultures should be obtained.

TREATMENT

- First-line treatment for SBP includes either a third-generation cephalosporin (e.g., ceftriaxone 2 g IV qday) or a fluoroquinolone (e.g., ciprofloxacin 400 mg IV q12h). Administration of IV albumin on days 1 and 3 of treatment may improve survival.[29]
- Treatment should be continued for 5 days. Extended courses may be needed for *P. aeruginosa* or resistant organisms.
- **SBP prophylaxis** with a fluoroquinolone or TMP–SMX should be initiated after the first episode of SBP or after variceal bleeding.
- **Secondary peritonitis** may require surgical intervention if there is perforation or intra-abdominal abscess. Anaerobic coverage with metronidazole 500 mg IV q8h should be added to above antibiotics. Antibiotics are continued until imaging demonstrates resolution of the abscess.

Hepatobiliary Infections

GENERAL PRINCIPLES

- **Acute cholecystitis** is associated with cholelithiasis and is caused by intestinal flora including *E. coli*, *Klebsiella*, *Enterobacter*, etc. Acalculous cholecystitis occurs in 5%–10% of cases.
- **Ascending cholangitis** is a fulminant infectious complication of an obstructed common bile duct, often following pancreatitis or cholecystitis.

DIAGNOSIS

Clinical Presentation

Tenderness and guarding of the right upper quadrant (RUQ) on deep inspiration (Murphy sign) is a common sign of a hepatobiliary infection. Ascending cholangitis presents as the **Charcot triad** of fever, RUQ pain, and jaundice. **Reynolds pentad** adds symptoms of confusion and hypotension and warrants rapid intervention. Bacteremia and shock are common.

Diagnostic Testing

- Elevated liver enzymes in a cholestatic pattern suggests acute cholangitis.
- Diagnosis of biliary tract infections is usually made by imaging with ultrasonography. Cholescintigraphy using technetium-99m hydroxy iminodiacetic acid scanning (also referred to as HIDA scan) and CT scanning may also be useful.
- Endoscopic retrograde cholangiopancreatography serves as diagnostic and therapeutic intervention for common bile duct obstruction and allows for stone extraction and/or biliary stent insertion.

TREATMENT

- Management of **acute cholecystitis** includes parenteral fluids, restricted PO intake, analgesia, and surgery. Advanced age, severe disease, or complications such as gallbladder ischemia or perforation, peritonitis, or bacteremia mandate broad-spectrum antibiotics such as ampicillin/sulbactam 3 g IV q6h, piperacillin/tazobactam 3.375 g IV q6h, ertapenem 1 g IV qday, or meropenem 500 mg IV q8h. Immediate surgery is indicated for severe or complicated disease but may be delayed up to 6 weeks if there is an initial response to medical therapy. After cholecystectomy, perioperative antibiotics may be discontinued.[30]
- **Ascending cholangitis** requires aggressive supportive care, including broad-spectrum antibiotics as above. Surgical or endoscopic decompression and drainage is necessary. Development of an abscess requires surgical drainage.

Other Infections

- **Viral hepatitis** (see Chapter 19, Liver Diseases)
- ***Helicobacter pylori*–associated disease** (see Chapter 18, Gastrointestinal Diseases)

CHAPTER 14

GENITOURINARY INFECTIONS

- Urinary tract infections (UTIs) can be uncomplicated or complicated, depending on host factors and underlying conditions. Diagnostic and therapeutic approaches to adult genitourinary infections are determined by gender-specific anatomic differences, prior antimicrobial exposures, and the presence of catheters, stents, etc. Infections are primarily caused by Enterobacterales (*E. coli*, *Proteus mirabilis*, and *K. pneumoniae*) and *Staphylococcus saprophyticus*.
- Workup includes urinalysis and microscopic examination of a fresh, unspun, clean-voided, or catheterized urine specimen. Pyuria (positive leukocyte esterase or ≥ 8 leukocytes per high-power field) or bacteriuria (positive nitrites or ≥ 1 organism per oil immersion field) suggests active infection if compatible symptoms are present. A high number of epithelial cells indicate an inadequate sample. A urine Gram stain can be helpful in guiding initial antimicrobial choices. Quantitative culture often yields $>10^5$ bacteria colony-forming units (CFU)/mL, but colony counts as low as 10^2–10^4 bacteria/mL may indicate infection in women with acute dysuria.

Asymptomatic Bacteriuria

- Asymptomatic bacteriuria is defined as the isolation of $>10^5$ CFU/mL of a single bacterial species in a specimen (men, catheters) or two consecutive specimens (women) in appropriately collected urine obtained from a person **without** symptoms of urinary infection.
- **Asymptomatic bacteriuria** is of limited clinical significance and **should not be treated except in pregnant women or patients undergoing urologic surgery**. Pregnant women should have screening urine culture near the end of the first trimester and be treated if positive. Treatment is **not** recommended for asymptomatic bacteriuria in the elderly, diabetics, institutionalized patients, spinal cord injury patients, or catheterized patients.

Cystitis

- Uncomplicated cystitis is defined as infection of the bladder or lower urinary tract in otherwise healthy, nonpregnant women.
- Complicated cystitis is defined as infection in patients with anatomic abnormalities, obstruction, immunosuppression, pregnancy, indwelling catheters, or unusual pathogens.
- Recurrent cystitis can occur in women, either due to reinfection or recurrence.[31]

DIAGNOSIS

Clinical Presentation

- Lower UTI is diagnosed based on history of dysuria, urgency, frequency, or suprapubic pain associated with pyuria and bacteriuria on urinalysis and urine culture. Fever is more likely if there is pyelonephritis.
- Dysuria without pyuria in sexually active patients warrants consideration of sexually transmitted infection (see Chapter 16, Sexually Transmitted Infections, Human Immunodeficiency Virus, and Acquired Immunodeficiency Syndrome).

Diagnostic Testing

- **Acute uncomplicated cystitis in women**. Many women are treated empirically without a urine culture. A pretreatment urine culture is recommended for patients at risk for antimicrobial resistance, or for patients at risk for more serious infection such as those with underlying urological abnormalities or immunosuppression.
- **Sterile pyuria**. Prior antimicrobials may result in negative urine cultures. Differential diagnosis includes chronic interstitial nephritis, interstitial cystitis, or infection with atypical organisms including *Chlamydia trachomatis*, *Ureaplasma urealyticum*, *N. gonorrhoeae*, or rarely, *M. tuberculosis*. Specific cultures of the endocervix for sexually transmitted infections should be performed.

TREATMENT

- See Tables 14-11 and 14-12.
- Posttreatment urine culture is unnecessary unless symptoms do not improve within 48 hours. Foreign bodies including stents and catheters should ideally be removed if feasible.
- **Recurrent cystitis in women** is usually due to reinfection (with a different organism). Risk factors include frequency of intercourse and spermicide use in young women and urologic abnormalities such as incontinence and cystocele in older women. Relapses (with the original infecting organism) that occur within 2 weeks of cessation of therapy should be treated similar to the original episode of cystitis.
- Prophylaxis may be considered for patients with frequent reinfection using continuous or postcoital antibiotics. Estrogen therapy in postmenopausal women may also have a role in prevention; cranberry products have not been shown to help.

Genitourinary Infections in Men

CYSTITIS

Cystitis is uncommon in young men and recurrence should prompt evaluation for prostatitis; *E. coli* is the most frequent pathogen. Risk factors include urologic abnormality, anal intercourse, and lack of circumcision. Pyuria may also be an indication of sexually transmitted infections. A pretreatment urinalysis and culture should be sent. Other urologic studies are appropriate when treatment fails, in recurrent infections, or when pyelonephritis occurs.

PROSTATITIS

- **Acute prostatitis** usually presents with fever, chills, dysuria, pelvic pain, obstructive symptoms, and a boggy, tender prostate on examination. It is caused by *E. coli* and other gram-negative organisms. Diagnosis is made by physical examination, urinalysis, and culture. Prostatic massage is contraindicated as it can lead to bacteremia.
- **Chronic prostatitis** is defined as the presence of urinary symptoms for >3 months. It is often noninfectious. Chronic bacterial prostatitis is caused by enteric gram-negative organisms. Symptoms include frequency, dysuria, urgency, perineal discomfort, and recurrent UTIs. Urine cultures should be obtained when the patient is symptomatic. Referral to a urologist for quantitative cultures before and after prostatic massage may be necessary. Transrectal ultrasound can be used if prostatic abscess is suspected.

CHAPTER 14

TABLE 14-11	Empiric Therapy for Urinary Tract Infections[31]	
Disease	Empiric Therapy	Notes
Simple Cystitis		
Women	*First line:* • TMP–SMX × 3 d • Nitrofurantoin × 5 d • Fosfomycin × 1 dose *Alternative:* • FQ (not first line) × 3 d *Pregnancy:* • Nitrofurantoin × 7 d • Cephalexin × 7 d • Cefuroxime axetil × 7 d	• Choose antibiotics based on local susceptibility patterns. • Extend therapy to 7 d for diabetics and older patients. • Oral β-lactams have lower efficacy; avoid if early pyelonephritis is suspected. • Treat asymptomatic bacteriuria in pregnancy.
Men	*First line:* • TMP–SMX • FQ	• Treat 7–14 d. • Avoid nitrofurantoin and β-lactam in men due to low tissue concentrations.
Pyelonephritis, complicated UTI	*Outpatient, mild–moderate illness:* • FQ × 7 d • Third-generation cephalosporin IV or IM once followed by FQ or TMP–SMX *Inpatient, severe illness:* • Third- or fourth-generation cephalosporin[a] • β-Lactam/β-lactamase inhibitor[b] • FQ • Carbapenems[c]	• Consider IV until afebrile followed by outpatient oral therapy in stable patients to complete 10–14 d. • Can consider shortening if complicating factor is resolved (i.e., removal of stone). • Do not use FQ in pregnancy.
Recurrent cystitis	*Postcoital prophylaxis:* TMP–SMX SS × 1 or nitrofurantoin 100 mg × 1 or cephalexin 250 mg × 1 *Continuous prophylaxis:* TMP–SMX 0.5 SS qday or every other day × 6 mo or nitrofurantoin 50–100 mg qhs × 6 mo	• Topical vaginal estrogen in postmenopausal women. • Methenamine hippurate may have a role in preventing recurrent UTI. Addition of vitamin C to maintain an acidified urine can be offered.

DS, double strength; FQ, fluoroquinolone; GU, genitourinary; SS, single strength; TMP, trimethoprim; TMP–SMX, trimethoprim–sulfamethoxazole; UTI, urinary tract infection.
[a]Third- or fourth-generation cephalosporins include ceftriaxone 1–2 g IV qday (third-generation) or cefepime 1 g IV q8h (fourth-generation).
[b]β-Lactam/β-lactamase inhibitors: Piperacillin/tazobactam 3.75–4.5 g IV q6h.
[c]Carbapenems: Meropenem 1 g IV q8h.

TABLE 14-12	Dosing Examples for Urinary Tract Infections	
Class	Oral (Less Severe)	Parenteral (More Severe)
Folate inhibitors	• TMP–SMX DS 160 mg/800 mg PO q12h • Trimethoprim 100 mg PO q12h	N/A
Fluoroquinolone	• Ciprofloxacin 250–500 mg PO q12h • Levofloxacin 250–750 mg PO qday	• Ciprofloxacin 400 mg IV q12h • Levofloxacin 250–750 mg IV qday
β-Lactam/β-lactamase inhibitor	• Amoxicillin–clavulanate 500 mg/125 mg PO q12h or q8h	• Ampicillin–sulbactam 1.5–3 g IV q6h • Piperacillin–tazobactam 3.375–4.5 g IV q6h
Cephalosporins	• Cephalexin 200–500 mg PO q6h • Cefpodoxime proxetil 100 mg PO q12h	• Cefazolin 1 g IV q8h • Ceftriaxone 1 g IV qday • Cefepime 1 g IV q8h
Carbapenems	N/A	• Ertapenem 1 g IV q8h • Imipenem 500 mg IV q6h • Meropenem 1 g IV q8h
Aminoglycoside	N/A	• Gentamicin 5 mg/kg qday
Fosfomycin[a]	• Fosfomycin 3 g PO once	N/A
Nitrofurantoin[a]	• Nitrofurantoin 100 mg PO q12h	N/A

DS, double strength; N/A, not applicable; TMP–SMX, trimethoprim–sulfamethoxazole.
[a]Uncomplicated cystitis.

Treatment

- **Acute bacterial prostatitis** should be treated with a 4- to 6-week course of either ciprofloxacin 500 mg PO q12h or TMP–SMX 160 mg/800 mg (double strength) PO q12h.
- Chronic prostatitis is difficult to treat. Culture-positive **chronic bacterial prostatitis** should receive prolonged therapy (for at least 6 weeks with a fluoroquinolone or TMP–SMX).

EPIDIDYMITIS

Epididymitis presents as a unilateral scrotal ache with swollen and tender epididymis on examination. Causative organisms are usually *N. gonorrhoeae* or *C. trachomatis* in sexually active young men and gram-negative enteric organisms in older men. Diagnosis and therapy should be directed according to this epidemiology, with NAAT testing and ceftriaxone and doxycycline in young men, and levofloxacin in older men.[32]

PYELONEPHRITIS

Pyelonephritis is infection of the kidney, usually due to ascending infection from the lower urinary tract. The causative agents are typically Enterobacterales such as *E. coli*,

Klebsiella spp., or *Proteus* spp. The incidence of MDRO is rising, especially in patients with recent use of broad-spectrum antibiotics, exposure to healthcare facilities, or travel to areas with high rates of MDROs.

Diagnosis

Clinical Presentation

Patients present with fever, chills, flank pain, nausea/vomiting, and costovertebral angle tenderness, often along with cystitis symptoms. Patients may present with sepsis or multiorgan dysfunction, especially if they have urinary obstruction and recent instrumentation or are elderly or diabetic.

Diagnostic Testing

- Urinalysis reveals significant bacteriuria, pyuria, red blood cells, and occasional leukocyte casts. A urine culture should always be sent. Blood cultures should be obtained in hospitalized patients as bacteremia may be present in 15%–20% of cases, especially in severely ill, elderly, and immunocompromised patients.
- Imaging may be considered if symptoms persist despite 48–72 hours of appropriate antibiotics or for suspected urinary tract obstruction. Ultrasonography or CT scan may demonstrate the presence of obstruction, a renal abscess, or renal calculi, which may require more invasive management.

Treatment

- Start empiric antibiotics promptly. See Tables 14-11 and 14-12.
- Patients with **severe illness** and pregnant patients should be treated initially with IV therapy. Patients with **mild to moderate illness** who can tolerate oral medications can be managed as outpatients.

FUNGAL AND ATYPICAL ORGANISMS

- Clinical presentations are varied and not pathogen specific. Consider systemic mycoses in normal hosts with unexplained chronic pulmonary pathology, chronic meningitis, lytic bone lesions, chronic skin lesions, FUO, or cytopenias. In immunocompromised patients, besides the above presentations, the development of new pulmonary, cutaneous, funduscopic, or head and neck signs and symptoms should prompt consideration of fungal and other atypical pathogens.
- Mycoses can often be identified by considering epidemiologic clues (many are geographically restricted), site of infection, inflammatory response, and microscopic fungal appearance. These infections can be complex and difficult to treat, and infectious disease consultation is recommended in all cases.
- Antifungal agents have variable doses, depending on severity of infection and the patient's renal and hepatic function. Lipid formulations of amphotericin B are preferred over the deoxycholate formulation due to its more favorable toxicity profile. Significant drug–drug interactions exist between azole antifungals and many other medications, including immunosuppressant drugs. Loading doses of azole antifungals may be recommended in certain circumstances. Because treatment may be prolonged (weeks to months), it is recommended to check therapeutic levels of several antifungals to minimize toxicity. Levels may be checked for flucytosine, itraconazole, posaconazole, and voriconazole but not for isavuconazole or fluconazole.
- For details on treatment of fungal pathogens, *Nocardia*, and *Actinomyces*, see Table 14-13.

TABLE 14-13	Treatment of Fungal Infections, *Nocardia*, and *Actinomyces*
Pathogen and Therapy	**Additional Comments**
***Candida* spp.** *Mucosal* • Thrush: Clotrimazole troche, nystatin suspension, or Fluc 100–200 mg qday × 7–14 d • Esophageal: Fluc 200 mg qday × 14–21 d • Vaginal: Topical azole × 3–7 d or Fluc 150 mg PO once • Frequent recurrence: Fluc 150 mg/wk × 6 mo *Invasive candidiasis* • Empirical treatment: Echinocandin • Targeted: Based on species and susceptibilities • Average duration: 14 d	• *Prophylaxis*: May be beneficial in select patients with solid organ transplant, chemotherapy-induced neutropenia, or stem cell transplants. • *Complicated infection*: Duration may be extended if metastatic foci present or continued neutropenia.
Cryptococcus neoformans *Nonmeningeal, local, or mild–moderate disease* • Fluc 400 mg PO/IV qday × 6–12 mo *Meningeal, disseminated, or moderately severe–severe disease* • Induction phase: Amb + 5-FC × 2 wk • Consolidation phase: Fluc 400 mg PO qday × 8 wk • Continuation phase: Fluc 200 mg qday × 6–12 mo	• Perform LP to rule out meningitis. • HIV: Initiate ART 2–10 wk after starting Tx. Continue Fluc 200 mg PO qday for at least 12 mo and until CD4 count ≥100 for 6 mo. • Check baseline CSF opening pressure. If ≥25 cm of CSF, reduce by 50% (up to 30 mL). Perform daily serial LPs if pressure elevated (≥25 cm H_2O).
Histoplasma capsulatum *Pulmonary* • Acute, mild–moderate: Observation. May undergo Tx if symptoms >1 mo • Acute, moderately severe to severe: Amb for 1–2 wk or until clinically improved, then Itra for 12 wk • Chronic cavitary: Itra for 12–24 mo *Progressive disseminated histoplasmosis (PDH)* • Mild–moderate: Itra for 12 mo • Moderately severe to severe: Amb for 1–2 wk or until clinically improved, then Itra for 12 mo *Mediastinal fibrosis* • Antifungal treatment is not recommended	• HIV: Itra 200 mg PO qday ppx in areas of high endemicity if CD4 count <150. • PDH: Check urine antigen levels during/after Tx to monitor for relapse. • TDM for itraconazole is recommended.

CHAPTER 14

(continued)

TABLE 14-13	Treatment of Fungal Infections, *Nocardia*, and *Actinomyces* (*continued*)
Pathogen and Therapy	**Additional Comments**
Blastomyces dermatitidis *Pulmonary or disseminated extrapulmonary* • Mild to moderate: Itra for 6–12 mo • Moderately severe to severe: Amb for 1–2 wk or until clinically improved, then Itra for 6–12 mo • Immunosuppressed: Treat as severe disease for 12 mo *CNS:* Amb for 4–6 wk then Fluc 800 mg PO qday for 12 mo *Suppression:* Itra lifelong if continued immunosuppression	• For CNS disease, Itra or Vori can be used instead of Fluc.
Coccidioides immitis *Pulmonary* • Uncomplicated pneumonia, asymptomatic pulmonary nodule: May not need Tx. If Tx, Fluc 400 mg PO qday for 3–6 mo • Diffuse pneumonia: Amb for 1–2 wk or until clinically improved, then Fluc 400 mg PO qday for 12 mo *Disseminated/extrapulmonary* • Nonmeningeal: Fluc 800–1200 mg IV/PO qday • Meningeal: Fluc 800–1200 mg IV/PO qday—if not improving, consider intrathecal Amb; followed by Fluc lifelong	• Can follow serum CF titers during/after treatment. Rising titers suggest recurrence. • Consider surgery if pulmonary cavitary disease >2 yr or rupture. • HIV: Continue Tx until CD4 count ≥250. • After meningeal disease improves, lifelong Fluc. • Hydrocephalus may require shunt for decompression.
Sporothrix *Lymphocutaneous/cutaneous:* Itra × 3–6 mo *Severe systemic* • Pulmonary/disseminated/osteoarticular: Amb for 1–2 wk or until clinically improved, then Itra for 12 mo • Meningeal: Amb for 4–6 wk then Itra for 12 mo	• If no initial response, can use higher doses of Itra or add topical saturated solution of potassium iodide.

TABLE 14-13	Treatment of Fungal Infections, *Nocardia*, and *Actinomyces* (*continued*)
Pathogen and Therapy	**Additional Comments**

Aspergillus

Pulmonary aspergilloma: Surgical resection or arterial embolization in cases of severe hemoptysis

Invasive pulmonary aspergillosis: Vori for at least 6–12 wk until lesions and immunosuppression resolve

Invasive sinonasal aspergillosis: Amb or Vori. Surgical debridement is adjunctive and often required for cure

Allergic bronchopulmonary aspergillosis: Itra or intermittent steroids may decrease exacerbations

Prophylaxis: Posa in high-risk patients may be considered

- Amb to cover mucormycosis as initial therapy for sinus disease pending confirmation of diagnosis.
- If immunosuppression recurs, may need to restart ppx or Tx.

Mucormycosis

Cutaneous, rhinocerebral: Aggressive surgical resection and debridement with clean margins followed + Amb at upper dose range until improvement

Pulmonary: Amb

- Mortality is very high in immunosuppressed patients with disseminated disease.
- Posa and Isa are alternative Tx, after initial induction therapy with Amb.

Nocardia

Cutaneous: TMP–SMX

Severe infection (including CNS): Induction regimen typically includes two or three drugs including TMP–SMX, imipenem or linezolid for 4–6 wk with stepdown to oral therapy for 6–12 mo

Suppression/prophylaxis: TMP–SMX

- TMP–SMX is drug of choice but typically combined with other agents in disseminated disease.
- Use susceptibility results to guide treatment.

Actinomyces

Penicillin G 18–24 million units IV per day × 4–6 wk then penicillin VK 1 g PO tid × 6–12 mo

- Surgery or drainage may be helpful in some cases.
- Clindamycin or doxycycline can be used if penicillin allergy.

5-FC, flucytosine; Amb, amphotericin B; ART, antiretroviral therapy; CF, complement fixation; CNS, central nervous system; CSF, cerebrospinal fluid; Fluc, fluconazole; Isa, isavuconazole; Itra, itraconazole; LP, lumbar puncture; Posa, posaconazole; ppx, prophylaxis; TDM, therapeutic drug monitoring; TMP–SMX, trimethoprim–sulfamethoxazole; Tx, treatment; Vori, voriconazole.

CHAPTER 14

Candidiasis

GENERAL PRINCIPLES

- *Candida* species are the most common cause of invasive fungal infections in humans.
- *Candida* species are considered part of the normal microbiota of the gastrointestinal and genitourinary tract; however, infections ranging from uncomplicated **mucocutaneous candidiasis** to life-threatening **invasive candidiasis** affecting any organ can occur.
- Mucocutaneous disease may resolve after elimination of the causative condition (e.g., antibiotic therapy) or may persist and progress in the setting of deficiencies with cell-mediated immunity that occur in conditions such as AIDS.
- Invasive disease is often associated with concurrent antibiotic use, contraceptive use, neutropenia, cytotoxic therapy, and indwelling foreign bodies. In the US, *Candida* is the fourth most common cause of BSI overall, and the leading cause of nosocomial BSI. Serious complications of candidemia include skin lesions, ocular disease, endocarditis, and osteomyelitis.[33]

DIAGNOSIS

- Any *Candida* species can be responsible for the syndromes above, but *Candida albicans* is the most common species. Diagnosis of **mucocutaneous candidiasis** is usually based on clinical findings but can be confirmed by a potassium hydroxide preparation of exudates.
- Identification of the *Candida* species is important because some species are more resistant to the azole antifungal agents than others. Cultures can be obtained in refractory cases or to diagnose **invasive candidiasis** by performing blood or tissue cultures.

TREATMENT

See Table 14-13.

Cryptococcosis

GENERAL PRINCIPLES

- *Cryptococcus neoformans* is a ubiquitous yeast associated with soil and pigeon excrement.
- Disease is principally meningeal (headache and mental status changes) and pulmonary (ranging from asymptomatic nodular disease to fulminant respiratory failure). Disseminated disease can involve any organ with predilection for the CNS, lungs, skin (umbilicated lesions mimicking molluscum), bone, and prostate.
- Infection typically affects patients with impaired cellular immunity and carries high morbidity and mortality. Although rare, infection in patients with end-stage liver disease has been associated with higher mortality compared to HIV-positive patients and should be considered when symptoms of cryptococcosis are present.

DIAGNOSIS

- Diagnosis via culture and histology tissue evaluation with the use of specific fungal stains are considered the gold standard.

- CrAg testing by latex agglutination or lateral flow assay is highly sensitive and specific in both serum and CSF.
- Distinguishing between disseminated disease and localized pulmonary and asymptomatic disease is fundamental to guide therapy. Any patient with CNS disease, positive blood cultures, or elevated serum CrAg and those with severe pulmonary disease should be considered to have disseminated disease. Disseminated disease warrants an LP to exclude coexistent CNS involvement. Always measure opening pressure, as elevated opening pressure (≥25 cm H_2O) has poor prognostic implications and must be managed with decompression, usually with serial LP or a lumbar drain.[34]

TREATMENT

Treatment is dependent on the patient's immune function and site of infection (see Table 14-13). **Management of elevated intracranial pressure is critical.** Infectious disease consultation is recommended and has been associated with decreased 90-day mortality.

Histoplasmosis

GENERAL PRINCIPLES

- *Histoplasma capsulatum* var. *capsulatum* is a dimorphic fungus (yeast in tissues; mold in the environment) that grows in soil contaminated by bat or bird droppings.[35]
- *Histoplasmosis* is the most common endemic mycosis diagnosed in the US. The highest areas of endemicity are along the Ohio and Mississippi River Valleys. Histoplasmosis is also common throughout Latin America.

DIAGNOSIS

- Clinical manifestations are extremely varied, including acute flu-like symptoms, chronic granulomatous pulmonary disease, or fulminant multiorgan failure in immunocompromised patients.
- Diagnosis is based on culture or histopathology, antigen assay (urine, blood, or CSF), or antibody detection assays using a complement fixation (CF) test, with titers of 1:8 seen in most patients and titers ≥1:32 highly suggestive of active infection. The urine antigen assay is the most sensitive test for detecting acute and disseminated disease and is helpful in following response to therapy. Antibody assays are useful in subacute and chronic disease; antigen assays are less sensitive.

TREATMENT

See Table 14-13.

Blastomycosis

GENERAL PRINCIPLES

- *Blastomyces dermatitidis* is dimorphic fungus that is endemic to the Ohio and Mississippi River valleys, as well as the Upper Midwestern, South Central, and Southeastern US.

CHAPTER 14

- The organism commonly disseminates, affecting the lungs, skin, bone, brain, and genitourinary tract. Aggressive pulmonary and CNS disease can occur in both immunocompromised and immunocompetent patients.

DIAGNOSIS

Definitive diagnosis is based on culture. Presumptive diagnosis can be made by histopathology and visualization of characteristic yeast forms, or antigen assay in serum or urine. Of note, antigen assay can cross-react with *Histoplasma* species. Serologic studies can also cross-react with *Histoplasma* and *Cryptococcus* species and are unreliable for diagnosis.

TREATMENT

See Table 14-13.

Coccidioidomycosis

GENERAL PRINCIPLES

- *Coccidioides immitis* is a dimorphic fungus that is endemic to the Southwestern US and Central America.
- Disease is usually a self-limited pulmonary syndrome, responsible for up to 25% of all CAP in endemic regions. Less common manifestations are chronic pulmonary illness and disseminated disease, which can affect the meninges, bones, joints, and skin. Risk factors for development of severe or disseminated disease include immunocompromising conditions, African or Filipino ancestry, diabetes, and pregnancy.

DIAGNOSIS

- Diagnosis requires culture, histopathology, or positive CF serology.
- Serum CF titer of 1:16 or greater suggests extrathoracic dissemination.
- **LP** should be performed for culture and CF serology, to rule out CNS involvement in persons with worsening, or persistent headache, altered mental status, unexplained nausea or vomiting, or new focal neurologic deficit.[36]
- **Skin testing** should only be used for epidemiologic purposes to evaluate exposure.

TREATMENT

See Table 14-13.

Aspergillosis

GENERAL PRINCIPLES

- *Aspergillus* species are ubiquitous environmental fungi that cause a broad spectrum of disease, usually affecting the respiratory system and sinuses.
- **Pulmonary aspergillomas** arise in the setting of preexisting bullous lung disease and are easily recognized by characteristic radiographic presentation and *Aspergillus* serology.

- **Invasive aspergillosis (IA)** is a serious condition associated with vascular invasion, thrombosis, and ischemic infarction of involved tissues and progressive disease after hematogenous dissemination. IA is usually seen in severely immunocompromised patients, especially allogeneic HSCT recipients.
- **Allergic bronchopulmonary aspergillosis** is a chronic relapsing and remitting respiratory syndrome associated with *Aspergillus* colonization.

DIAGNOSIS

- Diagnosis can be very difficult given the varied manifestations of IA, and a high index of suspicion should be applied to patients with prolonged severe immunosuppression.
- Radiographic findings can be highly suggestive of pulmonary IA, particularly the halocrescent sign on CT.
- Histopathology/cytology and culture examination of tissue and fluid specimens is recommended.
- Serum and bronchoalveolar lavage (BAL) galactomannan assay are accurate markers for the diagnosis of IA and can be followed prospectively in at-risk patients (e.g., hematologic malignancy, HSCT).[37]

TREATMENT

See Table 14-13.

Sporotrichosis

GENERAL PRINCIPLES

Sporothrix schenckii is a globally endemic fungus that causes disease following traumatic inoculation with soil or plant material; most cases are occupational. Infection can also be associated with spread from infected cats or other digging animals.

DIAGNOSIS

Clinical Presentation

- Lymphocutaneous disease is the usual manifestation with localization to skin and soft tissues following the lymphatic vessels proximal to the primary lesion (sporotrichoid pattern or nodular lymphangitis). Differential diagnoses include infection due to *S. aureus*, nontuberculous mycobacteria, tularemia, and *Nocardia* spp.
- Pulmonary and disseminated forms of the infection are rarely seen from inhalation of the fungus.

Diagnostic Testing

Diagnosis requires culture or histopathologic demonstration of yeast in tissue or body fluids.[38]

TREATMENT

See Table 14-13.

Mucormycosis

GENERAL PRINCIPLES

- Zygomycetes are a class of ubiquitous environmental fungi found in decaying organic substrates. They have been reclassified into two orders, Mucorales and Entomophthorales.
- Mucorales contains the genera most commonly involved in human disease. These include *Mucor* spp., *Rhizopus* spp., and *Cunninghamella* spp. Disease manifestations vary depending on the affected organ, but the main clinical presentations include sinus (rhino-orbital or rhinocerebral), pulmonary, cutaneous, gastrointestinal, and disseminated infections. Angioinvasion and multiorgan infarction are rapidly progressive. Risk factors include immunosuppression, iron overload, high-dose glucocorticoid therapy, penetrating trauma, and poorly controlled diabetes, especially in the setting of ketoacidosis.

DIAGNOSIS

- Clinical manifestations vary depending on which organ is affected. Invasive mucormycosis is devastating with rapid development of tissue necrosis from vascular invasion and thrombosis.
- Diagnosis requires tissue culture and silver stain with care to avoid disrupting fungal architecture.
- Head CT or MRI is helpful in head and neck disease to identify involved structures.
- Sinus endoscopy should be performed if there is concern for invasive fungal sinusitis.

TREATMENT

See Table 14-13.

Nocardiosis

GENERAL PRINCIPLES

- *Nocardia* is a ubiquitous group of aerobic gram-positive branching filamentous bacteria that causes severe local and disseminated disease in the setting of impaired cell-mediated immunity. *Nocardia* can be differentiated from *Actinomyces* by AFB stain, as mycolic acid is present in the cell wall and it can grow under aerobic conditions.
- Typical infection tends to be pulmonary infiltrate, abscess, or empyema, but dissemination is common and tends to favor CNS infection, causing abscess.

DIAGNOSIS

- Clinical presentation can be acute, subacute, or chronic pneumonia.
- Chest imaging can reveal a variety of findings such as infiltrates, nodules, pleural effusions, or cavities.[39]
- Diagnosis requires sputum or tissue Gram stain and culture (including AFB), often needing multiple samples because yields are low.

- Brain MRI is recommended to evaluate for concurrent CNS infection in patients with pulmonary disease.

TREATMENT

See Table 14-13.

Actinomycosis

GENERAL PRINCIPLES

Actinomyces is a microaerophilic gram-positive bacillus that usually causes soft-tissue swelling of the oropharynx, face, or neck, typically over or underneath the mandible (orocervicofacial actinomycosis). Pulmonary and gastrointestinal disease can also be seen. Classic infections are chronic, indurated soft-tissue lesions associated with draining fistulae that pass through tissue planes. Unlike *Nocardia*, infection due to *Actinomyces* is not limited to immunocompromised hosts.

DIAGNOSIS

Clinical presentation varies depending on what site is affected. Orocervicofacial infection is the most common form. Rare sites include the CNS and bones. Diagnosis is made by histopathology (gram-positive branching bacilli) or observation of "sulfur granules" in drainage.[40]

TREATMENT

See Table 14-13.

Nontuberculous Mycobacteria

- NTM are ubiquitous environmental organisms that cause a spectrum of disease primarily involving the lungs (80%), skin and soft tissues, lymph nodes, and disseminated disease. Susceptibility testing and an infectious disease consultation are recommended to guide treatment. Different species are commonly associated with specific clinical presentations:
  - **Pulmonary infection:** *Mycobacterium avium* complex (isolated in 85% of the cases), *Mycobacterium kansasii*, and *Mycobacterium abscessus* are the most common pathogens involved.
  - **Skin, soft-tissues, and bone infection:** *Mycobacterium fortuitum*, *Mycobacterium chelonae*, *Mycobacterium scrofulaceum*, *Mycobacterium marinum* ("fish tank granuloma"), and *Mycobacterium ulcerans* (Buruli ulcer).
  - **Lymphadenitis:** *M. avium* complex and *M. scrofulaceum*.
  - **Disseminated:** *M. avium*, *M. kansasii*, *M. abscessus*, *M. chelonae*, and *Mycobacterium haemophilum* (see Chapter 16, Sexually Transmitted Infections, Human Immunodeficiency Virus, and Acquired Immunodeficiency Syndrome).[41]
- *Mycobacterium leprae* is classified separately from other NTM because of its potential for human-to-human transmission. When rarely encountered in the US, it is associated with exposure to armadillos. Clinically, typical findings include hypopigmented anesthetic skin lesions.

CHAPTER 14

TICK-BORNE INFECTIONS

- Tick-borne infections are common during the summer months in many areas of the US; prevalence of specific diseases depends on the local population of vector ticks and animal reservoirs.
- Coinfection with multiple tick-borne infections can occur and should be considered when patients present with overlapping syndromes (e.g., Lyme disease with cytopenias).
- Risk should be assessed by outdoor activity in endemic regions rather than the report of a tick bite, which often goes unnoticed.

Lyme Disease

GENERAL PRINCIPLES

- Lyme borreliosis is a systemic illness of variable severity caused by the spirochete *Borrelia burgdorferi* and is the most common vector-borne disease in the US. It is seen in endemic regions, including the northeastern US coast, the upper Midwest, and northern California.
- Prophylactic doxycycline 200 mg PO (single dose) is recommended within 72 hours of removal of a high-risk tick bite meeting the following criteria: (1) an *Ixodes* spp. tick was identified, (2) the bite occurred in a highly endemic region, and (3) the tick was attached for ≥36 hours.[42]

DIAGNOSIS

Clinical Presentation

Lyme disease has three distinct clinical stages, following an incubation period of 7–10 days:
- Stage 1 (early local disease) is characterized by mild constitutional symptoms and erythema *migrans*, a slowly expanding macular rash >5 cm in diameter, classically with central clearing (often not seen). This may be difficult to differentiate from Southern tick–associated rash illness, caused by the bite of the lone star tick (*Amblyomma americanum*), which presents with an erythema *migrans*–like lesion in the Midwest and Southern US.
- Stage 2 (early disseminated disease) occurs within several weeks to months and includes multiple erythema *migrans* lesions, neurologic symptoms (e.g., seventh cranial nerve palsy, meningoencephalitis), cardiac symptoms (atrioventricular block, myopericarditis), and asymmetric oligoarticular arthritis, most commonly affecting the knee.
- Stage 3 (late disease) occurs after months to years and includes chronic dermatitis, neurologic disease, and asymmetric monoarticular or oligoarticular arthritis. Chronic fatigue is not seen more frequently in patients with Lyme borreliosis than in control subjects.

Diagnostic Testing

Diagnosis rests on clinical suspicion in the appropriate setting but can be supported by two-tiered testing (e.g., enzyme immunoassay or indirect fluorescent antibody test followed by IgM and IgG immunoblots) with acute and convalescent serologies. In the acute phase of the illness, sensitivity of the serological testing is below 50%.

TREATMENT

- Treatment depends on stage and severity of disease. Oral therapy (doxycycline 100 mg PO q12h, amoxicillin 500 mg PO q8h, or cefuroxime axetil 500 mg PO q12h for 10–21 days) is used for early localized or disseminated disease without neurologic or cardiac involvement. The same agents, given for 28 days, are recommended for late Lyme disease. Doxycycline has the added benefit of covering potential coinfection with ehrlichiosis. In the setting of true β-lactam allergy and if doxycycline cannot be given, macrolides are an alternative with a lower cure rate (~80%).
- Parenteral therapy (e.g., ceftriaxone 2 g IV qday, cefotaxime 2 g IV q8h, penicillin G 3–4 million units IV q4h) for 14–21 days is preferred over oral therapy for severe neurologic or cardiac disease, regardless of the stage.[42]

Rocky Mountain Spotted Fever

GENERAL PRINCIPLES

RMSF is an acute febrile illness caused by *Rickettsia rickettsii* and transmitted by a variety of ticks, most commonly *Dermacentor variabilis* (dog tick). The regions with highest endemicity include the South Atlantic (North and South Carolina and Virginia) and South Central US (Oklahoma, Arkansas, and Tennessee).

CLINICAL PRESENTATION

The classic triad of fever, headache, and rash is often not present in the early phases of the disease. The typical petechial rash with centripetal distribution (starting on the distal extremities and extending to the trunk) will be present in <50% of patients in the first 3 days of illness, but develops in >90% between the third and fifth days of illness. Presumptive diagnosis can be based on the clinical syndrome and warrants immediate treatment.

DIAGNOSIS

Acute and convalescent serologies support the diagnosis; however, early treatment may abolish the appearance of antibodies in the convalescent phase. PCR or immunostaining of tissue samples, such as skin biopsies, are highly specific.

TREATMENT

Antibiotic treatment of choice is doxycycline 100 mg IV/PO q12h for 7 days or continued for 3 days after the patient defervesce. Chloramphenicol is an alternative.

OUTCOME/PROGNOSIS

If treatment is delayed, RMSF is the most likely tick-borne illness to result in death or serious sequelae.[43]

Ehrlichiosis and Anaplasmosis

GENERAL PRINCIPLES

Ehrlichiosis and anaplasmosis are systemic tick-borne infections caused by obligate intracellular bacteria of the *Anaplasmataceae* family. Two similar syndromes are recognized:
- **Human monocytic ehrlichiosis** (HME), caused by *Ehrlichia chaffeensis* and transmitted by the lone star tick, is endemic to the Southern and South Central US.
- **Human granulocytic anaplasmosis** (HGA), caused by *Anaplasma phagocytophilum*, is found in the same regions as Lyme disease and shares the same tick vector (*Ixodes* spp.).

DIAGNOSIS

Clinical Presentation

Clinical onset of illness usually occurs 1 week after tick exposure with fever, headache, myalgias, and arthralgias. Rash is uncommon in adults. Leukopenia, thrombocytopenia, and elevated liver transaminases are important clues to the diagnosis. Severe disease can result in respiratory failure, renal insufficiency, and meningoencephalitis. CNS involvement is uncommon in HGA.

Diagnostic Testing

- Identification of morulae in circulating monocytes (HME) or granulocytes (HGA) on a blood smear is uncommonly seen but diagnostic.
- Acute and convalescent serologies obtained 3–6 weeks apart remain the diagnostic gold standard, but cross-reactivity among *Ehrlichia* spp. and reduced antibody response due to early treatment are common.
- PCR of the blood has high specificity (60%–85%) and sensitivity (60%–90%).

TREATMENT

Treatment should be started promptly based on clinical suspicion. Doxycycline 100 mg PO/IV q12h for 7–10 days is the drug of choice. Rifampin 300 mg PO q12h for 7–10 days is an option for patients with contraindications to doxycycline therapy. Lack of defervescence after 72 hours of treatment suggests an alternative diagnosis.[43]

Tularemia

GENERAL PRINCIPLES

- Tularemia is caused by the gram-negative bacteria *Francisella tularensis* and is endemic to the South Central US. It is associated with exposure to infected animals (particularly rabbits) and transmitted via tick bite or aerosolized droplets.
- *F. tularensis* is one of the most infectious pathogens known, with as few as 10 organisms necessary to cause disease. Due to its extreme infectivity, ease of dissemination, and capacity to cause illness with subsequent death, tularemia is considered a potential bioterrorism agent.

DIAGNOSIS

Clinical Presentation

Fever and malaise occur 2–5 days after exposure. Three clinical presentations are recognized, depending on the route of transmission: ulceroglandular (painful regional lymphadenitis with a skin ulcer), typhoidal (systemic disease with high fever and hepatosplenomegaly), and pneumonia. Systemic and pneumonic diseases have high mortality if not treated promptly.

Diagnostic Testing

- Culture isolation in blood, sputum, or pleural fluid lacks sensitivity. Before sending specimens, the microbiology laboratory must be notified given the high infectivity of *F. tularensis* (biosafety level 3 facilities are required).
- Acute and convalescent serologic studies provide a retrospective diagnosis.

TREATMENT

Aminoglycosides are the treatment of choice. Streptomycin 1 g IM q12h or gentamicin 5 mg/kg IV divided q8h for 10 days are preferred. Doxycycline 100 mg IV/PO q12h for 14 days is an alternative but is more likely to result in relapse. Ciprofloxacin 500–750 mg PO q12h for 14–21 days is also an alternative.[44]

Babesiosis

GENERAL PRINCIPLES

- Babesiosis is a malaria-like illness that is caused by the intraerythrocytic parasite *Babesia microti*, a tick-borne protozoan.
- Coinfection with Lyme disease can occur because both are transmitted by the same tick vector (*Ixodes* spp.).

DIAGNOSIS

- Clinical disease ranges from subclinical to severe, with fever, chills, myalgias, and headache. Complications of severe disease include renal failure, respiratory distress, and multiorgan dysfunction.
- Hemolytic anemia, elevated LDH, transaminitis, and thrombocytopenia are typical laboratory findings.
- Diagnosis is made by visualization of the parasite in erythrocytes on thin blood smears.
- Blood PCR is the most sensitive test.

TREATMENT

- For mild disease, atovaquone 750 mg PO q12h plus azithromycin 500 mg PO on day 1, then 250 mg qday for 7–10 days, is the treatment of choice.
- Severe disease (organ dysfunction, parasitemia >5% or immunosuppressed) should be treated with clindamycin 600 mg IV q8h plus quinine 650 mg PO q8h for 7–10 days. Exchange transfusion may also be needed.

CHAPTER 14

• Longer durations of therapy may be necessary in patients with persistent symptoms or until parasitemia has cleared.[45]

Heartland and Bourbon Virus

GENERAL PRINCIPLES

Bourbon and Heartland viruses are rare systemic emerging tick-borne infections recently identified in the Midwest and Southern US.

CLINICAL PRESENTATION

• *Heartland virus disease*: Fever, malaise, headache, **diarrhea, leukopenia, and thrombocytopenia.**[46]
• *Bourbon fever*: Fever, malaise, headache, **nausea, vomiting, and maculopapular rash.** Bone marrow suppression and acute respiratory distress syndrome reflect severe disease.[47]

DIAGNOSIS

Protocols exist facilitating testing through state health departments and the CDC.

TREATMENT

No specific treatments for Bourbon or Heartland virus infection exist. Treatment is supportive.

MOSQUITO-BORNE INFECTIONS

Arboviruses

GENERAL PRINCIPLES

• Arboviruses are arthropod-borne viruses; their major vectors are mosquitoes and ticks. Vector control is important for disease control.
• The leading cause of arboviral disease in the US is WNV; other viruses (La Crosse, Powassan, St. Louis encephalitis, Eastern equine encephalitis) cause sporadic outbreaks.
• Infections usually occur in the summer months, and most are subclinical. Encephalitis is the most common clinical syndrome.
• Worldwide, Zika virus, chikungunya, and dengue are major causes of morbidity and mortality.

West Nile Virus

WNV causes over 95% of neuroinvasive arboviral infections in the US. It is transmitted by *Culex* mosquitoes. Infections peak in late summer and early fall.

DIAGNOSIS

Clinical Presentation

- Most infections are asymptomatic. Symptomatic cases range from a mild febrile illness to aseptic meningitis, fulminant encephalitis, or a poliomyelitis-like presentation with flaccid paralysis. Extrapyramidal symptoms can occur. Long-term neurologic sequelae are common with severe disease.
- Risk factors for neuroinvasive disease include age older than 60 years, malignancy, diabetes, organ transplantation, and genetic factors.

Diagnostic Testing

Diagnosis is usually clinical or by CSF and serum WNV-specific IgM. Serum WNV IgG antibodies persist for years and suggest previous infection. Cross-reactivity with the less common St. Louis encephalitis virus occurs.

TREATMENT

Treatment for arboviral meningoencephalitides is mostly supportive.[48]

Chikungunya

GENERAL PRINCIPLES

Chikungunya virus is transmitted to humans by the bite of an infected *Aedes* mosquito. It is endemic to Africa, Asia, Europe, and the Caribbean.

DIAGNOSIS

Infection should be considered in travelers from endemic areas who present with fever and polyarthralgia.

Clinical Presentation

Fever and malaise are the earliest symptoms progressing to polyarthralgia 2–5 days after onset of fever. Multiple distal joints are involved, with pain that can be disabling. Maculopapular rash may appear. Relapsing joint pain for several months can occur in some patients.

Diagnostic Testing

PCR in the first week of disease can confirm acute infection. Acute and convalescent serology can also be helpful for diagnosis.

TREATMENT

Supportive care with rest and anti-inflammatory agents.[49]

Dengue

- Dengue virus is transmitted by *Aedes* mosquitoes. It is endemic in Asia, the Pacific, Africa, South and Central America, and the Caribbean.

CHAPTER 14

- Most cases in the US involve travelers, but local outbreaks have occurred in Texas and Florida (Key West). There are five different dengue virus serotypes (DENV 1–5); infection with one does not protect against others. Higher immune response can happen on subsequent exposures to DENV serotypes.

DIAGNOSIS

Clinical Presentation

Incubation period is 4–10 days. Fever, headache, myalgia, bone pain, rash, leukopenia, and thrombocytopenia are the predominant symptoms. Increased vascular permeability and plasma leakage lead to dengue hemorrhagic fever characterized by bleeding manifestations. Hypotension and circulatory collapse occur in dengue shock syndrome.

Diagnostic Testing

Virus can be detected by PCR during the first 5 days, and by acute and convalescent serology later in the course of illness.

TREATMENT

Maintenance of adequate intravascular volume is critical. There is no antiviral treatment; avoid aspirin and NSAIDs.[50]

Zika Virus

- In addition to the bite of the *Aedes* mosquito, Zika can also be transmitted sexually, via blood transfusion, or from a pregnant mother to her fetus.
- Since 2007, large outbreaks of Zika infection have occurred in the Pacific Islands, Central/South America, Mexico, Africa, and Asia. Most cases in the US have involved travelers; however, mosquito-borne transmission has occurred in Texas and Florida.

DIAGNOSIS

Clinical Presentation

Most infections are asymptomatic. Fever, maculopapular rash, conjunctivitis, arthralgias, and headache are common. Complications include neurologic disease (including Guillain–Barré syndrome) and microcephaly and fetal loss in pregnant women (congenital Zika infection).

Diagnostic Testing

PCR testing for acute infection, and acute and convalescent serology for recent infection.

TREATMENT

Treatment is symptomatic.[51] Pregnant women should avoid travel to Zika-infected areas. Consult the CDC website for updated information at https://wwwnc.cdc.gov/travel/page/zika-information.

Malaria

GENERAL PRINCIPLES

- Malaria is endemic to most of the tropical and subtropical world, with 229 million infections and 409,000 deaths in 2019. It is transmitted by the female *Anopheles* mosquito. Five species cause human disease: *Plasmodium falciparum, Plasmodium vivax, Plasmodium ovale, Plasmodium malariae,* and *Plasmodium knowlesi.*
- Travel advice and chemoprophylaxis regimens can be found at http://www.cdc.gov/travel/.

DIAGNOSIS

Clinical Presentation
- Patients present with nonspecific symptoms, including fever, headache, and myalgias.
- *P. falciparum* malaria, the most severe form, is associated with high mortality. Complicated, or severe, falciparum malaria is diagnosed if there is hyperparasitemia (>5%), cerebral malaria, hypoglycemia, lactic acidosis, renal failure, acute respiratory distress syndrome, or coagulopathy.
- Paroxysmal fever every other day can be seen in *P. vivax* and *P. ovale,* and every 3 days with *P. malariae.*

Diagnostic Testing
- Malaria should be excluded in all persons with fever who have traveled to an endemic area.
- Diagnosis is made by visualization of parasites on Giemsa-stained thick and thin blood smears, preferably obtained during febrile episodes.
- Rapid diagnostic tests targeting antigens common to all *Plasmodium* species as well those specific to *P. falciparum* are available but should be confirmed with microscopy.

TREATMENT

- Treatment should be started as soon as possible and is dependent on the type of malaria, severity, and risk of chloroquine resistance. Updated information from the CDC can be found at http://www.cdc.gov/travel/ and http://www.cdc.gov/malaria.
- **Uncomplicated malaria (*P. falciparum, P. ovale, P. vivax, P. malariae,* and *P. knowlesi*) from chloroquine-sensitive areas:**
  - Chloroquine 600 mg base PO single dose followed by 300 mg base PO at 6, 24, and 48 hours.
- **Uncomplicated *P. falciparum* from chloroquine-resistant areas and *P. vivax* from Indonesia or Papua New Guinea:**
  - Artemether–lumefantrine (20 mg artemether, 120 mg lumefantrine) 4 tablets PO at 0 and 8 hours, followed by 4 tablets q12h × 2 days.
  - Quinine sulfate 542 mg base PO q8h plus doxycycline 100 mg PO q12h or clindamycin 20 mg base/kg/d divided into three daily doses for 7 days.
  - Atovaquone–proguanil (250 mg atovaquone/100 mg proguanil) four tablets PO qday for 3 days.
- **P. ovale or P. vivax:** Add primaquine phosphate 30 mg base PO qday for 14 days to prevent relapse, after ruling out glucose-6-phosphate dehydrogenase deficiency.

• **Complicated severe malaria (most commonly *P. falciparum*):** Artesunate 3 mg/kg IV (first dose) followed by 3 mg/kg IV at 12 and 24 hours, followed by 3 mg/kg IV qday for 3 days. If IV artesunate is not available commercially, an emergency request can be made to the CDC Malaria Branch (weekdays: 770-488-7788; after-hours: 770-488-7100). While waiting for IV artesunate, start oral medication (artemether–lumefantrine, atovaquone–proguanil, or quinine plus doxycycline or clindamycin).[52]

ZOONOSES

For **avian and swine influenza, anthrax, and plague,** see the "Bioterrorism and Emerging Infections" section below.

Cat Scratch Disease (Bartonellosis)

GENERAL PRINCIPLES

B. henselae is facultative intracellular, coccobacillus that can be transmitted from animals to humans through a bite or scratch. Other *Bartonella* spp. are transmitted by vectors (e.g., fleas, lice) and include *B. bacilliformis* (Carrión disease) and *B. quintana* (trench fever).

CLINICAL PRESENTATION

• Cat scratch disease is usually a self-limiting disease with few papulopustular lesions appearing 3–30 days after a cat bite or scratch, followed by regional lymphadenitis (usually cervical or axillary) and mild constitutional symptoms. Atypical presentations include oculoglandular disease (Parinaud syndrome), encephalopathy, retinitis (stellate exudates), arthritis, FUO, and culture-negative endocarditis.
• In immunocompromised hosts, especially HIV-infected patients with a CD4 count <200 cells/mL, it can cause bacillary angiomatosis (angioproliferative nodules involving the skin and multiple organs) and peliosis hepatis (hepatosplenic cystic lesions).

DIAGNOSIS

Diagnosis is made by exclusion of other causes of lymphadenitis, detection of high antibody titers to *B. henselae*, PCR of infected tissue, or histopathological visualization of the bacilli using Warthin–Starry stain.

TREATMENT

• Localized cat scratch disease spontaneously resolves in 2–4 months without treatment. If antimicrobial therapy is prescribed, azithromycin 500 mg PO single dose followed by 250 mg PO qday for 4 more days is recommended.
• Needle aspiration of suppurative lymph nodes may provide symptomatic relief.[53]
• Culture-negative endocarditis due to *B. henselae* is discussed in the "Cardiovascular Infections" section.

- Ventilator-associated pneumonia (VAP) is defined as HAP developing >48–72 hours after endotracheal intubation and mechanical ventilation.
- In addition to new or progressive pulmonary infiltrate, patients may present with fever, purulent respiratory secretions, tachypnea, and hypoxia.

Diagnostic Testing

- Diagnosis is made by clinical criteria as well as microbiologic testing.
- Noninvasive respiratory sampling (e.g., spontaneous expectoration, sputum induction, nasotracheal suctioning) is recommended to establish a microbiologic diagnosis of HAP prior to initiating empiric treatment. Likewise, noninvasive sampling comprised of endotracheal aspiration with semiquantitative culture can serve as first step over bronchoscopy aspirates (e.g., BAL, blind bronchial sampling) to aid in diagnosis of VAP.[57]

TREATMENT

- Initial empiric antimicrobial therapy should cover *S. aureus* (including MRSA) and *P. aeruginosa.* Targeted therapy should be based on culture results and in vitro sensitivity testing.[58]
- Empyemas require drainage.

Catheter-Associated Urinary Tract Infection

GENERAL PRINCIPLES

- Catheter-associated urinary tract infection (CAUTI) is the most common HAI.
- *E. coli,* other gram-negative Enterobacterales, *P. aeruginosa*, gram-positives (staphylococci, enterococci), and yeast are commonly isolated from catheterized urine.
- Aseptic technique during insertion of a catheter is of utmost importance for prevention of CAUTI as well as **prompt removal of the catheter** when no longer needed.

DIAGNOSIS

Clinical Presentation

Fever is the most common symptom. Suprapubic and/or flank pain are helpful localizing symptom, although nonspecific presentations (e.g., altered mental status) are also possible.

Diagnostic Testing

- Urinalysis and urine culture should be performed before starting antibiotics. Diagnosis requires identification of $\geq 10^3$ CFU/mL of a single uropathogen or ≥ 1 species of bacteria in urine cultures obtained from patients with indwelling catheters or from a midstream collection if a catheter has been removed within the past 48 hours.
- Pyuria and bacteriuria occur in **all** in patients with chronic indwelling catheters and **should not be treated** in absence of symptoms (unless there are complicating factors, as mentioned previously).

TREATMENT

- Symptomatic CAUTI should be managed with removal or exchange of the catheter and treatment with 7–10 days of antibiotic therapy.
- Candiduria should be treated with catheter removal and should **not** be treated unless the patient is immunocompromised and at high risk for candidemia.[59]

BIOTERRORISM AND EMERGING INFECTIONS

- Changing patterns in human behavior and demographics, natural phenomena, and microbial evolution lead to new infections within a population or increased incidence or geographic range of known pathogens (emerging infections) (Table 14-14). Included in this category are several highly fatal and easily produced microorganisms, which have the potential to be used as agents of bioterrorism and produce substantial illness in large populations via an aerosol route of exposure. Most of these diseases are rare, so a high index of suspicion is necessary to identify the first few cases.
- A bioterrorism-related outbreak should be considered if an unusually large number of patients present simultaneously with a respiratory, gastrointestinal, or febrile rash syndrome; if several otherwise healthy patients present with unusually severe disease; or if an unusual pathogen for the region is isolated.

Anthrax

GENERAL PRINCIPLES

Spores from the gram-positive *Bacillus anthracis* germinate at the site of entry into the body.

DIAGNOSIS

Clinical Presentation

- **Cutaneous anthrax** (<2% case fatality rate), also known as "woolsorters disease," usually results from skin contact with spores from infected animals or animal products (e.g., wool, hides). Infection is characterized by a painless black eschar with surrounding tissue edema.
- **Systemic anthrax can assume the following forms:**
  - **Inhalational anthrax** (45% case fatality rate) stems from inadvertent aerosolization of spores from contaminated animal products or an intentional release such as a bioterrorism event. Infection presents initially with an influenza-like illness, gastrointestinal symptoms, or both, followed by fulminant respiratory distress and multiorgan failure.
  - **Gastrointestinal anthrax** (≥40% case fatality rate) commonly results from consumption of undercooked infected animal meat. Symptoms include nausea, vomiting, abdominal pain, ascites, and gastrointestinal hemorrhage related to necrotic mucosal ulcers.

TABLE 14-14	Emerging Infectious Diseases		
Pathogen	Epidemiology	Clinical Presentation and Diagnosis	Management
ESKAPE pathogens *Enterococcus faecium* *Staphylococcus aureus* *Klebsiella pneumoniae* *Acinetobacter baumannii* *Pseudomonas aeruginosa* *Enterobacter* species	Group of antibiotic-resistant bacteria that are the leading cause of nosocomial infections worldwide. They are selected by inappropriate antimicrobial use. Most are MDROs via acquired plasmid-mediated resistance (e.g., colistin resistance by the *mcr-1* gene).	Multiple clinical presentations, but most commonly cause nosocomial BSI, VAP, IAI, and hardware-associated infections. Diagnosis is based on cultures with susceptibility testing and/or detection of β-lactamase, carbapenemase, PBP2A, or other mechanism or resistance via molecular or biochemical tests.	Treatment is organism-specific and should be based on antimicrobial susceptibility testing results. An ID consultation should always be obtained as this has shown to decrease mortality in these infections.[1]
Candida auris	Multidrug-resistant *Candida* i.e., hard to identify in the laboratory. Commonly misidentified as *Candida haemulonii*.	Health care–associated BSI, wound, and ear infections. Fungal cultures with susceptibilities allow the diagnosis.	Pending susceptibilities and echinocandin should be used. Consultation with an ID specialist is highly recommended.
Zoonotic influenza viruses	Emergence of influenza A strains previously confined to avian/swine host via antigenic shifts, with the potential to cause a pandemic. Acquired via exposure to infected live or dead poultry/pigs (e.g., live animal markets).	Ranges from a mild upper respiratory infection (fever and cough) to a rapid progression to severe pneumonia, ARDS, shock, and even death. Nasopharyngeal swab for PCR is the most sensitive diagnostic test. If PCR is not available, a rapid antigen detection immunoassay should be done.	A neuraminidase inhibitor (oseltamivir) for a minimum of 5 d is the treatment of choice. Infection control measures and close communication with public health authorities are critical.

(continued)

CHAPTER 14

TABLE 14-14	Emerging Infectious Diseases *(continued)*		
Pathogen	Epidemiology	Clinical Presentation and Diagnosis	Management
Vaccine-preventable diseases	The antivaxxer movement has contributed to the rise of preventable infections in countries with established vaccination programs.	See "Lower Respiratory Tract Infections" section in this chapter for details about pertussis. Measles presents with high fever, coryza, cough, conjunctivitis, and small white spots inside the cheeks (Koplik spots). After several days, a descending rash affecting palms and soles appears. Specific serological and/or PCR testing establish the diagnosis.	Prevention through vaccination per recommended ACIP guidelines is key. Patients with measles should be placed on respiratory isolation. Close contacts of patients with *Bordetella pertussis* should receive antimicrobial prophylaxis with a macrolide.
Viral hemorrhagic fever **Filoviruses** (Ebola and Marburg) **Flaviviruses** (dengue, yellow fever) **Bunyaviruses** (hantaviruses, Congo–Crimean hemorrhagic fever, Rift Valley fever) **Arenaviruses** (South American hemorrhagic fever, Lassa fever)	Caused by many different RNA viruses in endemic areas. Most are transmitted by aerosol or contact with infected body fluids. Ebola has been shown to also have sexual transmission via semen.	Fever, headache, joint and muscle aches, diarrhea/vomiting, and unexplained bleeding or bruising are common to all of these infections. Specific serological and/or molecular testing will establish the diagnosis.	There is currently no antiviral drug licensed by the FDA for any of these infections. CYD–TDV (Dengvaxia) vaccine has been approved for use in dengue-endemic territories, only in children of middle-school age, and with previous laboratory evidence of DENV infection. The vaccine is not approved for travelers. WHO endorses the use of the recombinant vesicular stomatitis virus vaccine for the Zaire Ebola virus, if an Ebola outbreak occurs.

ARDS, acute respiratory distress syndrome; BSI, bloodstream infection; FDA, Food and Drug Administration; IAI, intra-abdominal infections; ID, Infectious Diseases; MDRO, multidrug-resistant organism; PBP2A, penicillin-binding protein 2A; PCR, polymerase chain reaction; VAP, ventilator-associated pneumonia; WHO, World Health Organization.

○ **Anthrax meningitis** (nearly always fatal) can arise from cutaneous, inhalational, or gastrointestinal anthrax, manifesting with parenchymal brain hemorrhage, seizures, delirium, or coma.

Diagnostic Testing

Diagnosis of inhalational disease is suggested by a widened mediastinum without infiltrates on chest radiograph and confirmed by blood culture and PCR. Notify local infection control and public health department immediately for confirmed cases.

TREATMENT

- Empiric therapy for systemic anthrax with possible or confirmed meningitis is ciprofloxacin 400 mg IV q8h and meropenem 2 g IV q8h and linezolid 600 mg IV q12h for 2–3 weeks until clinically stable. Transition to oral therapy with ciprofloxacin 500 mg PO q12h *or* doxycycline 100 mg PO q12h *and* one other active agent can occur thereafter and continued to complete a total 60-day course of antimicrobial therapy to reduce the risk of delayed spore germination.
- Systemic anthrax with meningitis excluded should be treated with ciprofloxacin 400 mg IV q8h *and* clindamycin 900 mg IV q8h or linezolid 600 mg IV q12h for 2 weeks until clinically stable, followed by transition to oral therapy to complete a total 60-day course of antimicrobial therapy as above. Antitoxin, including monoclonal antibodies (raxibacumab, obiltoxaximab) and anthrax immunoglobulin, may be requested from the CDC in select circumstances to treat inhalational anthrax in combination with antimicrobial therapy.
- Uncomplicated cutaneous anthrax can be treated with oral ciprofloxacin 500 mg q12h *or* doxycycline 100 mg q12h for 7–10 days for naturally acquired cases and 60 days for bioterrorism-related cases.
- Postexposure prophylaxis for individuals at risk for inhalational anthrax consists of oral ciprofloxacin 500 mg q12h or doxycycline 100 mg q12h for 60 days after exposure.[60]

Plague

GENERAL PRINCIPLES

- Plague is caused by the gram-negative bacillus *Yersinia pestis.*
- Naturally acquired plague occurs rarely in the Southwestern US after exposure to infected animals (e.g., through scratches, bites, direct handling, inhalation of aerosolized respiratory secretions) and via rodent flea bites.

DIAGNOSIS

Clinical Presentation

There are three forms of plague.
- **Bubonic:** Local painful lymphadenitis (bubo) and fever (14% case fatality rate).
- **Septicemic:** Can cause peripheral necrosis and disseminated intravascular coagulation (DIC) ("black death"). Usually from progression of bubonic disease (30%–50% case fatality rate).

- **Pneumonic:** Severe pneumonia with hemoptysis preceded by initial influenza-like illness (57% case fatality rate, nearing 100% when treatment is delayed). Pneumonic disease can be transmitted from person to person and would be expected after inhalation of aerosolized *Y. pestis*.

Diagnostic Testing

Diagnosis is confirmed by isolation of *Y. pestis* from blood, sputum, or CSF. Treat all diagnostic samples as highly infectious. Notify local infection control and public health departments immediately.

TREATMENT

- Treatment should start at first suspicion of plague because rapid initiation of antibiotics improves survival. Agents of choice are streptomycin 1 g IM q12h; gentamicin 5 mg/kg IV/IM qday *or* a 2 mg/kg loading dose and then 1.7 mg/kg IV/IM q8h, with appropriate monitoring of drug levels; or doxycycline 100 mg PO/IV q12h. Alternatives include ciprofloxacin and chloramphenicol. Oral therapy can be started after clinical improvement, for a total course of 10–14 days.
- Postexposure prophylaxis is indicated after unprotected face-to-face contact with patients with known or suspected pneumonic plague and consists of doxycycline 100 mg PO q12h or ciprofloxacin 500 mg PO q12h for 7 days.

Botulism

GENERAL PRINCIPLES

- Botulism results from intoxication with botulinum toxin, produced by the anaerobic gram-positive bacillus *Clostridium botulinum.*
- Modes of acquisition include ingestion of the neurotoxin from improperly canned food and contamination of wounds with *C. botulinum* from the soil. Inhalational botulism could result from an intentional release of aerosolized toxin.
- Mortality is low when botulism is recognized early but may be very high in the setting of mass exposure and limited access to mechanical ventilation equipment.

DIAGNOSIS

- The classic triad consists of an absence of fever, clear sensorium, and symmetric descending flaccid paralysis with cranial nerve involvement, beginning with ptosis, diplopia, and dysarthria, and progressing to loss of gag reflex and diaphragmatic function with respiratory failure, followed by diffuse skeletal muscle paralysis. Sensation remains intact. Paralysis can last from weeks to months.
- Diagnosis is confirmed by detection of toxin in serum. Notify local infection control and public health departments.

TREATMENT

- Treatment is primarily supportive and may require mechanical ventilation in the setting of respiratory failure. Wound botulism requires extensive surgical debridement.

- Further progression of paralysis can be halted by early administration of botulinum antitoxin, available through the state public health department or the CDC. Antitoxin is reserved only for cases where there is a high suspicion for botulism based on clinical presentation and exposure history. Routine postexposure prophylaxis with antitoxin is not recommended because of the high incidence (10%) of hypersensitivity reactions and limited supply.

Viral Hemorrhagic Fevers

GENERAL PRINCIPLES

- This syndrome is caused by many different RNA viruses, including filoviruses (Ebola and Marburg), flaviviruses (dengue, yellow fever), bunyaviruses (Hantaviruses, Congo–Crimean hemorrhagic fever [CCHF], Rift Valley fever [RVF]), and arenaviruses (South American hemorrhagic fevers, Lassa fever) (Table 14-14).
- The 2014-16 West African Ebola virus disease (EVD) epidemic and subsequent outbreaks in Central Africa demonstrate that sustained human-to-human transmission of EVD is possible in vulnerable populations.
- Case fatality rates are variable but can be as high as 90% for EVD in resource-limited settings.

DIAGNOSIS

Clinical Presentation

- Early symptoms include fevers, myalgias, and malaise, with varying severity and symptomatology depending on the virus, but all can severely disrupt vascular permeability and cause DIC. Thrombocytopenia, leukopenia, and hepatitis are common.
- Vomiting and severe diarrhea leading to significant dehydration and mortality, as evidenced by the West African EVD epidemic, can also be a prominent feature.[61]

Diagnostic Testing

- Diagnosis requires consideration of epidemiology and patient risk factors, especially travel to endemic areas.
- Serology performed by reference laboratories can confirm diagnosis. Notify local infection control and public health departments immediately.

TREATMENT

- Treatment is primarily supportive with attention to infection control.
- A recombinant vesicular stomatitis virus–Zaire Ebola virus vaccine offered protection against EVD after exposure during the West African EVD epidemic. Preexposure vaccination is recommended for adults who are at high risk for occupational exposure.[62]
- Monoclonal antibodies have been approved for the treatment of EVD.
- Exposed contacts should monitor temperature twice daily for 3 weeks. Postexposure prophylaxis with oral ribavirin can be administered to febrile CCHF, Lassa, and RVF contacts.

CHAPTER 14

REFERENCES

1. Burnham JP, Olsen MA, Stwalley D, Kwon JH, Babcock HM, Kollef MH. Infectious diseases consultation reduces 30-day and 1-year all-cause mortality for multidrug-resistant organism infections. *Open Forum Infect Dis.* 2018;5(3):ofy026.
2. McDonald LC, Gerding DN, Johnson S, et al. Clinical practice guidelines for Clostridium difficile infection in adults and children: 2017 update by the Infectious Diseases Society of America (IDSA) and Society for Healthcare Epidemiology of America (SHEA). *Clin Infect Dis.* 2018;66(7):e1-e48.
3. Liang JL, Tiwari T, Moro P, et al. Prevention of pertussis, tetanus, and diphtheria with vaccines in the United States: recommendations of the Advisory Committee on Immunization Practices (ACIP). *MMWR Recomm Rep.* 2018;67(2):1-44.
4. Stevens DL, Bisno AL, Chambers HF, et al. Practice guidelines for the diagnosis and management of skin and soft tissue infections: 2014 update by the Infectious Diseases Society of America. *Clin Infect Dis.* 2014;59(2):147-159.
5. Lipsky BA, Berendt AR, Cornia PB, et al. 2012 Infectious Diseases Society of America clinical practice guideline for the diagnosis and treatment of diabetic foot infections. *Clin Infect Dis.* 2012;54(12):e132-e173.
6. Tunkel AR, Hartman BJ, Kaplan SL, et al. Practice guidelines for the management of bacterial meningitis. *Clin Infect Dis.* 2004;39(9):1267-1284.
7. Tunkel AR, Glaser CA, Bloch KC, et al. The management of encephalitis: clinical practice guidelines by the Infectious Diseases Society of America. *Clin Infect Dis.* 2008;47(3):303-327.
8. Brouwer MC, Coutinho JM, van de Beek D. Clinical characteristics and outcome of brain abscess: systematic review and meta-analysis. *Neurology.* 2014;82(9):806-813.
9. White AC, Coyle CM, Rajshekhar V, et al. Diagnosis and treatment of neurocysticercosis: 2017 clinical practice guidelines by the Infectious Diseases Society of America (IDSA) and the American Society of Tropical Medicine and Hygiene (ASTMH). *Am J Trop Med Hyg.* 2018;98(4):945-966.
10. Mermel LA, Allon M, Bouza E, et al. Clinical practice guidelines for the diagnosis and management of intravascular catheter-related infection: 2009 update by the Infectious Diseases Society of America. *Clin Infect Dis.* 2009;49(1):1-45.
11. Li JS, Sexton DJ. Proposed modifications to the Duke criteria for the diagnosis of infective endocarditis. *Clin Infect Dis.* 2000;30(4):633-638.
12. Baddour LM, Wilson WR, Bayer AS, et al. Infective endocarditis in adults: diagnosis, antimicrobial therapy, and management of complications – a scientific statement for healthcare professionals from the American Heart Association. *Circulation.* 2015;132(15):1435-1486.
13. Wilson W, Taubert KA, Gewitz M, et al. Prevention of endocarditis. Guidelines from the American heart association fever, endocarditis, and Kawasaki disease committee, Council on cardiovascular disease in the young, and the Council on clinical Cardiology, Council on cardiovascular surgery and anesthesia, and the quality of care and outcomes research interdisciplinary working group. *Circulation.* 2007;116(15):1736-1754.
14. Caforio AL, Pankuweit S, Arbustini E, et al. Current state of knowledge on aetiology, diagnosis, management, and therapy of myocarditis: a position statement of the European Society of Cardiology Working Group on Myocardial and Pericardial Diseases. *Eur Heart J.* 2013;34(33):2636-2648, 2648a-2648d.
15. Adler Y, Charron P, Imazio M, et al. 2015 ESC guidelines for the diagnosis and management of pericardial diseases – the task force for the diagnosis and management of pericardial diseases of the European Society of Cardiology (ESC) endorsed by: the European Association for Cardio-Thoracic Surgery (EACTS). *Eur Heart J.* 2015;36(42):2921-2964.
16. Shulman ST, Bisno AL, Clegg HW, et al. Clinical practice guideline for the diagnosis and management of group A streptococcal pharyngitis: 2012 update by the Infectious Diseases Society of America. *Clin Infect Dis.* 2012;55(10):1279-1282.
17. Rosenfeld RM, Piccirillo JF, Chandrasekhar SS, et al. Clinical practice guideline (update): adult sinusitis executive summary. *Otolaryngol Head Neck Surg.* 2015;152(4):598-609.
18. Fiore AE, Fry A, Shay D, et al. Antiviral agents for the treatment and chemoprophylaxis of influenza – recommendations of the Advisory Committee on Immunization Practices (ACIP). *MMWR Recomm Rep.* 2011;60(1):1-24.
19. Wiersinga WJ, Rhodes A, Cheng AC, et al. Pathophysiology, transmission, diagnosis, and treatment of coronavirus disease 2019 (COVID-19): a review. *JAMA.* 2020;324(8):782-793.
20. Kim DK, Riley LE, Hunter P. Advisory committee on immunization practices recommended immunization schedule for adults aged 19 years or older – United States, 2018. *MMWR Morb Mortal Wkly Rep.* 2018;67(5):158-160.
21. Metlay JP, Waterer GW, Long AC, et al. Diagnosis and treatment of adults with community-acquired pneumonia. An official clinical practice guideline of the American Thoracic Society and Infectious Diseases Society of America. *Am J Respir Crit Care Med.* 2019;200(7):e45-e67.
22. World Health Organization. *Global Tuberculosis Report 2020.* World Health Organization; 2021.

23. Zenner D, Beer N, Harris RJ, Lipman MC, Stagg HR, van der Werf MJ. Treatment of latent tuberculosis infection: an updated network meta-analysis. *Ann Intern Med.* 2017;167(4):248-255.

24. Lewinsohn DM, Leonard MK, LoBue PA, et al. Official American thoracic society/infectious diseases society of America/Centers for disease control and prevention clinical practice guidelines: diagnosis of tuberculosis in adults and children. *Clin Infect Dis.* 2017;64(2):111-115.

25. Blumberg HM, Burman WJ, Chaisson RE, et al. American thoracic society/Centers for disease control and prevention/infectious diseases society of America: treatment of tuberculosis. *Am J Respir Crit Care Med.* 2003;167(4):603-662.

26. Nahid P, Dorman SE, Alipanah N, et al. Official American thoracic society/Centers for disease control and prevention/infectious diseases society of America clinical practice guidelines: treatment of drug-susceptible tuberculosis. *Clin Infect Dis.* 2016;63(7):e147-e195.

27. Riddle MS, DuPont HL, Connor BA. ACG clinical guideline: diagnosis, treatment, and prevention of acute diarrheal infections in adults. *Am J Gastroenterol.* 2016;111(5):602-622.

28. Mazuski JE, Tessier JM, May AK, et al. The surgical infection society revised guidelines on the management of intra-abdominal infection. *Surg Infect.* 2017;18(1):1-76.

29. Runyon BA; AASLD. Introduction to the revised American Association for the Study of Liver Diseases Practice Guideline management of adult patients with ascites due to cirrhosis 2012. *Hepatology.* 2013;57(4):1651-1653.

30. Gomi H, Solomkin JS, Schlossberg D, et al. Tokyo Guidelines 2018: antimicrobial therapy for acute cholangitis and cholecystitis. *J Hepatobiliary Pancreat Sci.* 2018;25(1):3-16.

31. Gupta K, Hooton TM, Naber KG, et al. International clinical practice guidelines for the treatment of acute uncomplicated cystitis and pyelonephritis in women: a 2010 update by the Infectious Diseases Society of America and the European Society for Microbiology and Infectious Diseases. *Clin Infect Dis.* 2011;52(5):e103-e120.

32. Naber KG, Bergman B, Bishop MC, et al. EAU guidelines for the management of urinary and male genital tract infections. Urinary Tract Infection (UTI) working group of the Health Care Office (HCO) of the European Association of Urology (EAU). *Eur Urol.* 2001;40(5):576-588.

33. Pappas PG, Kauffman CA, Andes DR, et al. Clinical practice guideline for the management of candidiasis: 2016 update by the Infectious Diseases Society of America. *Clin Infect Dis.* 2016;62(4):e1-e50.

34. Perfect JR, Dismukes WE, Dromer F, et al. Clinical practice guidelines for the management of cryptococcal disease: 2010 update by the Infectious Diseases Society of America. *Clin Infect Dis.* 2010;50(3):291-322.

35. Wheat LJ, Azar MM, Bahr NC, Spec A, Relich RF, Hage C. Histoplasmosis. *Infect Dis Clin North Am.* 2016;30(1):207-227.

36. Galgiani JN, Ampel NM, Blair JE, et al. 2016 Infectious Diseases Society of America (IDSA) clinical practice guideline for the treatment of coccidioidomycosis. *Clin Infect Dis.* 2016;63(6):e112-e146.

37. Patterson TF, Thompson GRIII, Denning DW, et al. Practice guidelines for the diagnosis and management of aspergillosis: 2016 update by the Infectious Diseases Society of America. *Clin Infect Dis.* 2016;63(4):e1-e60.

38. Kauffman CA, Bustamante B, Chapman SW, Pappas PG; Infectious Diseases Society of America. Clinical practice guidelines for the management of sporotrichosis: 2007 update by the Infectious Diseases Society of America. *Clin Infect Dis.* 2007;45(10):1255-1265.

39. Ambrosioni J, Lew D, Garbino J. Nocardiosis: updated clinical review and experience at a tertiary center. *Infection.* 2010;38(2):89-97.

40. Kononen E, Wade WG. Actinomyces and related organisms in human infections. *Clin Microbiol Rev.* 2015;28(2):419-442.

41. Koh WJ. Nontuberculous mycobacteria-overview. *Microbiol Spectr.* 2017;5(1). doi:10.1128/microbiolspec.TNMI7-0024-2016.

42. Lantos PM, Rumbaugh J, Bockenstedt LK, et al. Clinical practice guidelines by the Infectious Diseases Society of America (IDSA), American Academy of Neurology (AAN), and American College of Rheumatology (ACR): 2020 guidelines for the prevention, diagnosis and treatment of Lyme disease. *Clin Infect Dis.* 2021;72(1):1-8.

43. Biggs HM, Behravesh CB, Bradley KK, et al. Diagnosis and management of tickborne rickettsial diseases: Rocky mountain spotted fever and other spotted fever group Rickettsioses, ehrlichioses, and anaplasmosis - United States. *MMWR Recomm Rep.* 2016;65(2):1-44.

44. Nigrovic LE, Wingerter SL. Tularemia. *Infect Dis Clin North Am.* 2008;22(3):489-504, ix.

45. Vannier E, Krause PJ. Human babesiosis. *N Engl J Med.* 2012;366(25):2397-2407.

46. Pastula DM, Turabelidze G, Yates KF, et al. Notes from the field: Heartland virus disease – United States, 2012-2013. *MMWR Morb Mortal Wkly Rep.* 2014;63(12):270-271.

47. Kosoy OI, Lambert AJ, Hawkinson DJ, et al. Novel thogotovirus associated with febrile illness and death, United States, 2014. *Emerg Infect Dis.* 2015;21(5):760-764.

48. Petersen LR, Brault AC, Nasci RS. West Nile virus: review of the literature. *JAMA.* 2013;310(3):308-315.

49. Weaver SC, Lecuit M. Chikungunya virus and the global spread of a mosquito-borne disease. *N Engl J Med.* 2015;372(13):1231-1239.

CHAPTER 14

50. World Health Organization. *Dengue: Guidelines for Diagnosis, Treatment, Prevention and Control.* New Edition. World Health Organization; 2009.
51. Petersen LR, Jamieson DJ, Powers AM, Honein MA. Zika virus. *N Engl J Med.* 2016;374(16):1552-1563.
52. Centers for Disease Control and Prevention. *Treatment of Malaria: Guidelines for Clinicians (United States).* Accessed May 8, 2021. https://www.cdc.gov/malaria/resources/pdf/Malaria_Treatment_Guidelines.pdf
53. Rolain JM, Brouqui P, Koehler JE, Maguina C, Dolan MJ, Raoult D. Recommendations for treatment of human infections caused by Bartonella species. *Antimicrob Agents Chemother.* 2004;48(6):1921-1933.
54. McBride AJ, Athanazio DA, Reis MG, Ko AI. Leptospirosis. *Curr Opin Infect Dis.* 2005;18(5):376-386.
55. Pappas G, Akritidis N, Bosilkovski M, Tsianos E. Brucellosis. *N Engl J Med.* 2005;352(22):2325-2336.
56. Eldin C, Melenotte C, Mediannikov O, et al. From Q fever to Coxiella burnetii infection: a paradigm change. *Clin Microbiol Rev.* 2017;30(1):115-190.
57. Kalil AC, Metersky ML, Klompas M, et al. Management of adults with hospital-acquired and ventilator-associated pneumonia: 2016 clinical practice guidelines by the Infectious Diseases Society of America and the American Thoracic Society. *Clin Infect Dis.* 2016;63(5):e61-e111.
58. Liu C, Bayer A, Cosgrove SE, et al. Clinical practice guidelines by the Infectious Diseases Society of America for the treatment of methicillin-resistant *Staphylococcus aureus* infections in adults and children. *Clin Infect Dis.* 2011;52(3):e18-e55.
59. Hooton TM, Bradley SF, Cardenas DD, et al. Diagnosis, prevention, and treatment of catheter-associated urinary tract infection in adults: 2009 international clinical practice guidelines from the Infectious Diseases Society of America. *Clin Infect Dis.* 2010;50(5):625-663.
60. Swartz MN. Recognition and management of anthrax – an update. *N Engl J Med.* 2001;345(22):1621-1626.
61. Bah EI, Lamah MC, Fletcher T, et al. Clinical presentation of patients with Ebola virus disease in Conakry, Guinea. *N Engl J Med.* 2015;372(1):40-47.
62. Choi MJ, Cossaboom CM, Whitesell AN, et al. Use of Ebola vaccine: recommendations of the advisory committee on immunization practices, United States, 2020. *MMWR Recomm Rep.* 2021;70(1):1-12.

15 Antimicrobials

David J. Ritchie, Nigar Kirmani, and Daniel T. Ilges

Introduction

As microbial resistance is increasing among many pathogens, a review of institutional as well as local, regional, national, and global susceptibility trends can assist in the development of empiric therapy regimens. Antimicrobials should be modified based on results of culture and sensitivity testing to definitive therapy agent(s) that have the narrowest spectrum possible. In many cases, shorter durations of therapy have been shown to be as effective as traditionally longer courses. As many oral agents have excellent bioavailability, switching from parenteral to oral therapy whenever possible is recommended. Several antibiotics have major drug interactions or require alternate dosing in renal or hepatic insufficiency, or both. For antiretroviral, antiparasitic, and antihepatitis agents, see Chapter 16, Sexually Transmitted Infections, Human Immunodeficiency Virus, and Acquired Immunodeficiency Syndrome; Chapter 14, Treatment of Infectious Diseases; and Chapter 19, Liver Diseases, respectively.

ANTIMICROBIAL AGENTS

Penicillins

GENERAL PRINCIPLES

- Penicillins (PCNs) irreversibly bind PCN-binding proteins (PBPs) in the bacterial cell wall, ultimately causing osmotic rupture and death. Acquired resistance in many bacterial species through alterations in PBPs or expression of hydrolytic enzymes has limited their use.
- PCNs remain among the drugs of choice for syphilis and infections caused by PCN-sensitive streptococci and enterococci, methicillin-sensitive *Staphylococcus aureus* (MSSA), *Listeria monocytogenes, Pasteurella multocida*, and *Actinomyces.*

TREATMENT

- **Aqueous PCN G** (2–5 million units IV q4h or 12–30 million units daily by continuous infusion) is an IV preparation of PCN G and the drug of choice for most PCN-susceptible streptococcal infections and neurosyphilis.
- **Procaine PCN G** is an IM repository form of PCN G that can be used as an alternative treatment for neurosyphilis at a dose of 2.4 million units IM daily in combination with probenecid 500 mg PO qid for 10–14 days.
- **Benzathine PCN** is a long-acting IM repository form of PCN G that is used for treating early latent syphilis (<1 y duration [one dose, 2.4 million units IM]) and

late latent syphilis (unknown duration or >1 y [2.4 million units IM weekly for three doses]). It is occasionally given for group A streptococcal pharyngitis and prophylaxis after acute rheumatic fever.

- **PCN V** (250–500 mg PO q6h) is an oral formulation of PCN that is typically used to treat group A streptococcal pharyngitis.
- **Ampicillin** (1–3 g IV q4–6h) is the drug of choice for treatment of infections caused by susceptible *Enterococcus* species or *L. monocytogenes.* Oral ampicillin (250–500 mg PO q6h) may be used for uncomplicated sinusitis, pharyngitis, otitis media, and urinary tract infections (UTIs), but oral amoxicillin is generally preferred.
- **Ampicillin–sulbactam** (1.5–3.0 g IV q6h) combines ampicillin with the β-lactamase inhibitor sulbactam in a 2:1 ratio, thereby extending the spectrum to include MSSA, anaerobes, and many Enterobacterales. The sulbactam component also has unique activity against some strains of *Acinetobacter.* The agent is appropriate for treatment of head and neck infections; upper and lower respiratory tract infections; genitourinary tract infections; and abdominal, pelvic, and polymicrobial soft tissue infections, including those due to human or animal bites.
- **Amoxicillin** (250–1000 mg PO q8h, 875 mg PO q12h, or 775 mg extended-release q24h) is an oral antibiotic similar to ampicillin that is used for uncomplicated sinusitis, pharyngitis, otitis media, community-acquired pneumonia (CAP), and UTIs.
- **Amoxicillin–clavulanic acid** (875 mg PO q12h, 500 mg PO q8h, 90 mg/kg/d divided q12h [Augmentin ES-600 suspension], or 2000 mg PO q12h [Augmentin XR]) is an oral antibiotic similar to ampicillin/sulbactam that combines amoxicillin with the β-lactamase inhibitor clavulanate. It is useful for treating complicated sinusitis and otitis media and for prophylaxis of human or animal bites after appropriate local treatment.
- **Nafcillin, oxacillin** (1–2 g IV q4–6h), and **dicloxacillin** (250–500 mg PO q6h) are penicillinase-resistant synthetic PCNs that are drugs of choice for treating MSSA infections. Dose reduction of nafcillin should be considered in concomitant hepatic and renal impairment.
- **Piperacillin–tazobactam** (3.375 g IV q6h or 4.5 g IV q6h for *Pseudomonas*) combines piperacillin with the β-lactamase inhibitor tazobactam. This combination is active against most Enterobacterales, *Pseudomonas*, MSSA, ampicillin-sensitive enterococci, and anaerobes, making it useful for intra-abdominal and complicated polymicrobial soft tissue infections. Combination with vancomycin IV can increase risk of nephrotoxicity.

SPECIAL CONSIDERATIONS

Adverse events: All PCN derivatives have been associated with anaphylaxis, interstitial nephritis, elevated liver function tests (LFTs), anemia, leukopenia, thrombocytopenia, and phlebitis. Prolonged high-dose therapy (>2 wk) is typically monitored with weekly serum creatinine and complete blood count (CBC). Monitoring LFTs is especially important with oxacillin/nafcillin, as these agents can cause hepatitis. All patients should be asked about PCN, cephalosporin, or carbapenem allergies. These agents should not be used in patients with a reported serious PCN allergy without prior skin testing, desensitization, or both.

Cephalosporins

GENERAL PRINCIPLES

- Cephalosporins exert their bactericidal effect by interfering with cell wall synthesis by the same mechanism as PCNs.
- These agents are clinically useful because of their broad spectrum of activity and low toxicity profile. All cephalosporins are devoid of clinically significant activity against enterococci when used alone. Within this class, only ceftaroline is active against methicillin-resistant *S. aureus* (MRSA).

TREATMENT

- **First-generation cephalosporins** have activity against MSSA, streptococci, *Escherichia coli*, and many *Klebsiella* and *Proteus* species. These agents have limited activity against other enteric gram-negative bacilli and anaerobes. **Cefazolin** (1–2 g IV/IM q8h) is the most commonly used parenteral preparation, and **cephalexin** (250–500 mg PO q6h) and **cefadroxil** (500 mg–1 g PO q12h) are oral preparations. These agents are commonly used for treating skin/soft tissue infections, UTIs, MSSA infections, and for surgical prophylaxis (cefazolin IV).
- **Second-generation cephalosporins** have expanded coverage against enteric gram-negative rods and can be divided into above-the-diaphragm and below-the-diaphragm agents.
  - **Cefuroxime** (1.5 g IV/IM q8h) is useful for treatment of infections above the diaphragm. This agent has reasonable MSSA and streptococcal activity in addition to an extended spectrum against gram-negative aerobes and can be used for skin/soft tissue infections, complicated UTIs (cUTIs), and some community-acquired respiratory tract infections. It does not cover *Bacteroides fragilis*.
  - **Cefuroxime axetil** (250–500 mg PO q12h), **cefprozil** (250–500 mg PO q12h), and **cefaclor** (250–500 mg PO q12h) are oral second-generation cephalosporins typically used for bronchitis, sinusitis, otitis media, UTIs, local soft tissue infections, and oral step-down therapy for pneumonia or cellulitis responsive to parenteral cephalosporins.
  - **Cefoxitin** (1–2 g IV q4–8h) and **cefotetan** (1–2 g IV q12h) are useful for treatment of infections below the diaphragm. These agents, also known as cephamycins, have activity against gram negatives and anaerobes, including *B. fragilis*, and are commonly used for intra-abdominal or gynecologic surgical prophylaxis and infections, including diverticulitis and pelvic inflammatory disease.
- **Third-generation cephalosporins** cover aerobic gram-negative bacilli and retain significant activity against streptococci and MSSA (except ceftazidime). Ceftazidime is the only third-generation cephalosporin that is useful for treating serious *Pseudomonas aeruginosa* infections. Some of these agents (ceftriaxone, ceftazidime) have substantial central nervous system (CNS) penetration and are useful in treating meningitis when given at high doses (see Chapter 14, Treatment of Infectious Diseases). Third-generation cephalosporins are not reliable for the treatment of serious infections caused by organisms producing AmpC β-lactamases regardless of the

results of susceptibility testing. These resistant pathogens should generally be treated empirically with carbapenems or cefepime.

- ◦ **Ceftriaxone** (1–2 g IV/IM q12–24h) can be used as empiric therapy for pyelonephritis, urosepsis, pneumonia, intra-abdominal infections (combined with metronidazole), gonorrhea, and meningitis. It can also be used for osteomyelitis, septic arthritis, endocarditis, and skin/soft tissue infections caused by susceptible organisms. **Ceftriaxone** 2 g IV q12h in combination with ampicillin IV is appropriate for treatment of ampicillin-susceptible *Enterococcus faecalis* endocarditis, especially when aminoglycosides need to be avoided.
- ◦ **Cefpodoxime proxetil** (100–400 mg PO q12h), **cefdinir** (300 mg PO q12h), **ceftibuten** (400 mg PO q24h), and **cefditoren pivoxil** (200–400 mg PO q12h) are oral third-generation cephalosporins useful for the treatment of bronchitis and complicated sinusitis, otitis media, and UTIs. These agents can also be used as step-down therapy for CAP. **Cefixime** (400 mg PO once) is no longer recommended as a first-line therapy for gonorrhea but may be used as alternative therapy for gonorrhea with a close 7-day test-of-cure follow-up.
- ◦ **Ceftazidime** (1–2 g IV/IM q8h) may be used for treatment of infections caused by susceptible strains of *P. aeruginosa* and other susceptible gram-negative bacilli, but lacks clinically significant activity against MSSA.
- **The fourth-generation cephalosporin cefepime** (500 mg–2 g IV/IM q8–12h) has excellent aerobic gram-negative coverage, including *P. aeruginosa* and other bacteria producing AmpC β-lactamases. Its gram-positive activity is similar to that of ceftriaxone. **Cefepime** is routinely used for empiric therapy in febrile neutropenic patients. It also has a prominent role in treating infections caused by antibiotic-resistant gram-negative bacteria and some infections involving both gram-negative and gram-positive aerobes in most sites. Anaerobic coverage should be added where anaerobes are suspected.
- **Ceftaroline** (600 mg IV q12–8h) is a cephalosporin with anti-MRSA activity. **Ceftaroline's** unique MRSA activity stems from its affinity for PBP2a, the same cell wall component that renders MRSA resistant to all other β-lactams. **Ceftaroline** has similar activity to ceftriaxone against gram-negative pathogens, with virtually no activity against *Pseudomonas*, *Acinetobacter*, and other organisms producing AmpC β-lactamase, extended-spectrum β-lactamase (ESBL), or *Klebsiella pneumoniae* carbapenemase (KPC).
- **Novel cephalosporins and combination agents** include **ceftolozane–tazobactam** and **ceftazidime–avibactam**, as well as the novel siderophore cephalosporin **cefiderocol**. A summary of activity of new gram-negative beta-lactams is provided in Table 15-1.
  - ◦ **Ceftolozane–tazobactam** (1.5–3 g tazobactam IV q8h) combines ceftolozane, a novel cephalosporin, and the β-lactamase inhibitor tazobactam in a 2:1 ratio. This agent is approved by the U.S. Food and Drug Administration (FDA) for treatment of complicated intra-abdominal infections (in combination with metronidazole), cUTIs, including pyelonephritis, and hospital-acquired/ventilator-associated bacterial pneumonia (HABP/VABP). Ceftolozane–tazobactam has excellent activity against gram-negative bacteria, including many *P. aeruginosa* that are resistant to other antipseudomonal β-lactam antibiotics. Ceftolozane–tazobactam is also active against some ESBL-producing organisms, but is not reliably active against MSSA, enterococci, and anaerobes.
  - ◦ **Ceftazidime–avibactam** (2.5 g IV q8h) contains ceftazidime in combination with the novel β-lactamase inhibitor avibactam. This agent is FDA-approved for

TABLE 15-1	Activity of Novel Gram-Negative Antibiotics versus Resistant Organisms					
Antibiotic	ESBL	KPC	OXA-48	MBL	CRPA	CRAB
Imipenem/relebactam	X	X			X	
Ceftolozane/tazobactam	X				X	
Ceftazidime/avibactam	X	X	X		X	
Meropenem/vaborbactam	X	X				
Cefiderocol	X	X	X	X	X	X

CRAB, carbapenem-resistant *Acinetobacter baumannii*; CRPA, carbapenem-resistant *Pseudomonas aeruginosa*; ESBL, extended-spectrum β-lactamase; KPC, *Klebsiella pneumoniae* carbapenemase; MBL, metallo-β-lactamases; OXA-48, oxacillinase-48.

treatment of cUTIs, complicated intra-abdominal infections (in combination with metronidazole), and HABP/VABP. Ceftazidime–avibactam is broadly active against gram-negative bacteria, including some *P. aeruginosa* that are resistant to other antipseudomonal β-lactams. This agent is also active against ESBL- and AmpC-producing strains and possesses unique activity against KPC- and OXA-48-producing carbapenem-resistant Enterobacterales (CRE). Ceftazidime–avibactam is not active against metallo-β-lactamase (MBL)-producing CRE as monotherapy, but may be useful in combination with aztreonam for the treatment of these infections. Ceftazidime–avibactam is not reliably active against MSSA, enterococci, and anaerobes.

○ **Cefiderocol** (2g IV q8h) is a novel siderophore cephalosporin with broad coverage of gram-negative bacilli, including CRE, *Stenotrophomonas*, *Acinetobacter*, and *Pseudomonas* species resistant to other β-lactam antibiotics. This agent chelates free iron to enter cells via iron active transport channels, resulting in high concentrations in the periplasmic space, where cefiderocol binds to PBPs to disrupt cell wall synthesis. Cefiderocol is FDA-approved for the treatment of cUTI, including pyelonephritis, and HABP/VABP. Cefiderocol is stable to hydrolysis by most β-lactamases, including AmpC, ESBL, KPC, OXA-48, and MBLs; however, cefiderocol does **not** possess reliable activity against gram-positive pathogens and anaerobes.

SPECIAL CONSIDERATIONS

Adverse events: All cephalosporins have been rarely associated with anaphylaxis, interstitial nephritis, elevated LFTs, anemia, thrombocytopenia, and leukopenia. **PCN-allergic patients may have a cross-hypersensitivity reaction to cephalosporins.** These agents should not be used in a patient with a reported severe PCN allergy (i.e., anaphylaxis, hives) without prior skin testing or desensitization, or both. Prolonged therapy (>2 wk) is typically monitored with a weekly serum creatinine and CBC. Because of its biliary elimination, ceftriaxone may cause biliary sludging. Cefepime has been associated with CNS side effects, including delirium and seizures, especially when given at high doses in individuals with renal impairment.

Monobactams

GENERAL PRINCIPLES

Aztreonam (1–2 g IV/IM q6–12h) is a monobactam that is **only active against aerobic gram-negative bacteria**, including *P. aeruginosa*. It is useful in patients with known serious β-lactam allergy because there is no apparent cross-reactivity. Aztreonam is also available in an inhalational dosage form (75 mg inhaled q8h for 28 d) to improve respiratory symptoms in cystic fibrosis patients infected with *P. aeruginosa*.

Carbapenems

GENERAL PRINCIPLES

Imipenem–cilastatin (500 mg–1 g IV/IM q6–8h), **meropenem** (1–2 g IV q8h or 500 mg IV q6h), and **ertapenem** (1 g IV q24h) are the currently available carbapenems in the United States. Carbapenems exert their bactericidal effect by interfering with cell wall synthesis, similar to PCNs and cephalosporins, and are active against many gram-positive and most gram-negative bacteria, including anaerobes. They are among the antibiotics of choice for infections caused by organisms producing AmpC or ESBLs. Imipenem–cilastatin is the most active carbapenem against ampicillin-susceptible *E. faecalis* and can also be used for treating *Nocardia* and some atypical mycobacterial infections.

TREATMENT

- Carbapenems are important agents for treatment of many antibiotic-resistant bacterial infections at most body sites. These agents are commonly used for severe polymicrobial infections, including Fournier gangrene, intra-abdominal catastrophes, and sepsis in immunocompromised hosts.
- Notable bacteria that are **resistant** to carbapenems include ampicillin-resistant enterococci, MRSA, *Stenotrophomonas*, and KPC- and MBL-producing gram-negative organisms. In addition, ertapenem does not provide reliable coverage against *P. aeruginosa*, *Acinetobacter*, or enterococci; therefore, imipenem or meropenem would be preferred for empiric treatment of nosocomial infections when these pathogens are suspected. **Meropenem** is the preferred carbapenem for treatment of CNS infections.
- **Meropenem–vaborbactam** (4 g IV q8h) contains meropenem plus the novel boron-based β-lactamase inhibitor vaborbactam. This agent is FDA-approved for treatment of cUTIs. Meropenem–vaborbactam has unique activity against KPC-producing Enterobacterales, but not against MBL-producing strains. Notably, vaborbactam does not appreciably enhance the activity of meropenem against *Pseudomonas* or *Acinetobacter* species. Because of the meropenem component, this agent is reliably active against MSSA and anaerobes. Of note, the standard recommended dose of meropenem–vaborbactam contains 2 g of meropenem, a dose previously reserved for CNS infections.
- **Imipenem–cilastatin–relebactam** (1.25 g IV q6h) combines the activity of imipenem–cilastatin with relebactam, a novel β-lactamase inhibitor similar to avibactam. Notably, each 1.25 g contains 500 mg of imipenem, 500 mg of cilastatin, and 250 mg of relebactam. This agent is FDA-approved for cUTIs, including pyelonephritis,

complicated intra-abdominal infections, and HABP/VABP. Compared to imipenem–cilastatin alone, imipenem–cilastatin–relebactam does offer additional activity against *Pseudomonas* and KPC-producing CRE.

SPECIAL CONSIDERATIONS

- **Adverse events:** Carbapenems can precipitate seizure activity, especially in older patients, individuals with renal insufficiency, and patients with preexisting seizure disorders or other CNS pathology, and should be avoided in these patients unless there is no alternative therapy. Like cephalosporins, carbapenems have been rarely associated with anaphylaxis, interstitial nephritis, elevated LFTs, anemia, and leukopenia.
- **Patients who are allergic to PCNs/cephalosporins may have a cross-hypersensitivity reaction to carbapenems,** and these agents should be avoided in patients with severe PCN allergy without prior skin testing, desensitization, or both. Prolonged therapy (>2 wk) is typically monitored with a weekly serum creatinine, LFTs, and CBC.
- Carbapenems also possess a unique drug interaction with valproic acid and derivatives, resulting in reduced concentrations of these anti-epileptic medications. This, together with the aforementioned CNS toxicity, can precipitate seizures in individuals with epilepsy on valproic acid derivatives. Concomitant use should be considered a contraindication.

Aminoglycosides

GENERAL PRINCIPLES

Aminoglycosides exert their bactericidal effect by binding to the bacterial ribosome, causing misreading during translation of bacterial messenger RNA into proteins. These drugs are often used in combination with cell wall–active agents (i.e., β-lactams and vancomycin) for treatment of some severe infections caused by gram-positive and gram-negative aerobes. Use in combination with cell wall–active antibiotics can lead to synergistic killing. Aminoglycosides do not have activity against anaerobes, and their activity is impaired in the low pH/low oxygen environment of abscesses. Cross-resistance among aminoglycosides is common, but not absolute, and susceptibility testing with each aminoglycoside is recommended. Use of these antibiotics is limited by **significant nephrotoxicity and ototoxicity**.

TREATMENT

- Traditional dosing of aminoglycosides involves daily divided dosing with the upper end of the dosing range reserved for life-threatening infections. Peak and trough concentrations should be obtained with the third or fourth dose and then every 3–4 days, along with regular serum creatinine monitoring. **Increasing serum creatinine or peak/troughs out of the acceptable range requires immediate attention.**
- **Extended-interval dosing of aminoglycosides** is an alternative method of administration in patients without significant renal impairment and is more convenient for most indications. Extended-interval doses are provided in the following specific drug sections. A drug concentration is obtained 6–14 hours after the first dose, and a nomogram (Figure 15-1) is utilized to determine the subsequent dosing interval.

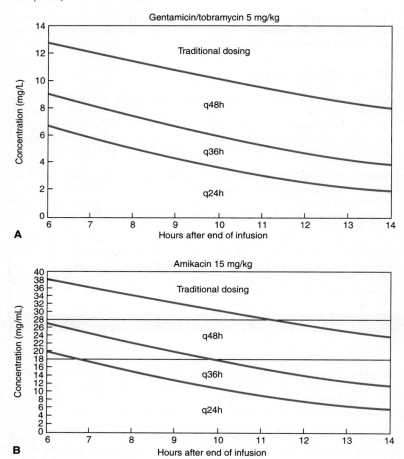

Figure 15-1. Nomograms for extended-interval aminoglycoside dosing. A, Gentamicin/tobramycin. B, amikacin.

Drug concentrations 6–14 hours after the prior dose should be monitored at least every week; serum creatinine should be checked at least thrice weekly. In patients who are not responding to therapy, a 12-hour concentration should be checked, and if that concentration is undetectable, extended-interval dosing should be abandoned in favor of traditional dosing.

- For **obese patients** (actual weight >20% above ideal body weight [IBW]), an obese dosing weight (IBW + 0.4 × [actual body weight − IBW]) should be used for determining doses for both traditional and extended-interval methods. Traditional dosing, rather than extended-interval dosing, should be used for patients with endocarditis, burns that cover more than 20% of the body, anasarca, and creatinine clearance (CrCl) of <30 mL/min.

- **Gentamicin and tobramycin** traditional dosing is administered with an initial loading dose of 2 mg/kg IV (2–3 mg/kg in the critically ill), followed by 1.0–1.7 mg/kg IV q8-12h (peak, 3–10 µg/mL; trough, <1 µg/mL). Extended-interval dosing is administered with an initial loading dose of 5 mg/kg, with the subsequent dosing interval determined by a nomogram (see Figure 15-1). Tobramycin is also available as an inhaled agent for adjunctive therapy for patients with cystic fibrosis or bronchiectasis complicated by *P. aeruginosa* infection (300 mg inhalation q12h).
- **Amikacin** has an additional unique role for mycobacterial and *Nocardia* infections. Traditional dosing is an initial loading dose of 5.0–7.5 mg/kg IV (7.5–9.0 mg/kg in the critically ill), followed by 5 mg/kg IV q8h or 7.5 mg/kg IV q12h (peak, 20–35 µg/mL; trough, <10 µg/mL). Extended-interval dosing is 15 mg/kg, with the subsequent dosing interval determined by a nomogram (see Figure 15-1).
- **Plazomicin**, the newest aminoglycoside, is FDA-approved for treatment of cUTI. Plazomicin's spectrum of activity is similar to other aminoglycosides, with increased activity against CRE. Plazomicin is dosed at 15 mg/kg IV q24h, and dose adjustments for obese patients are recommended as above. Goal serum trough levels are <3 µg/mL. Doses may also be adjusted by area-under-the-curve (AUC) pharmacokinetic calculations. An extended-interval dosing nomogram is not available, and doses should **not** be adjusted utilizing existing nomograms for other aminoglycosides.

SPECIAL CONSIDERATIONS

- **Nephrotoxicity** is the major adverse effect of aminoglycosides. Nephrotoxicity is potentially reversible when detected early but can be permanent. Aminoglycosides should be used cautiously or avoided, if possible, in patients with decompensated kidney disease. Concomitant administration of aminoglycosides with other known nephrotoxic agents (i.e., amphotericin B, foscarnet, NSAIDs, pentamidine, polymyxins, cidofovir, and cisplatin) should be avoided if possible.
- **Ototoxicity** (vestibular or cochlear) is another possible adverse event that necessitates baseline and weekly hearing tests with extended therapy (>14 d).

Vancomycin

TREATMENT

- **Vancomycin** (usual starting dose is 15 mg/kg IV q12h) is a glycopeptide antibiotic that interferes with cell wall synthesis by binding to D-alanyl-D-alanine precursors that are critical for peptidoglycan cross-linking in most gram-positive bacterial cell walls. Vancomycin is bactericidal for staphylococci but bacteriostatic for enterococci.
- Vancomycin-resistant *Enterococcus faecium* (VRE) and vancomycin intermediate-resistant *S. aureus* (VISA) present increasing treatment challenges. Vancomycin-resistant *S. aureus* has been reported but remains rare. Indications for use are listed in Table 15-2.
- The **goal trough** concentration is 15–20 µg/mL for treatment of serious infections. Lower troughs of 10–20 µg/mL may be appropriate for less severe infections.
- Dose adjusting to a **target AUC: Minimum inhibitory concentration (MIC) range** of 400–600 mg*h/L, assuming an MIC of 1 mg/L, is recommended for the treatment of serious MRSA infections where pharmacokinetic monitoring and adjustments can be provided quickly and reliably.

TABLE 15-2	Indications for Vancomycin Use
Treatment of serious infections caused by documented or suspected MRSA
Treatment of serious infections caused by ampicillin-resistant, vancomycin-sensitive enterococci
Treatment of serious infections caused by gram-positive bacteria in patients who are allergic to other appropriate therapies
Surgical prophylaxis for placement of prosthetic devices at institutions with known high rates of MRSA or in patients who are known to be colonized with MRSA
Empiric use in suspected gram-positive meningitis until an organism has been identified and sensitivities confirmed
Oral treatment of *Clostridioides difficile* colitis

MRSA, methicillin-resistant *Staphylococcus aureus*.

SPECIAL CONSIDERATIONS

- Vancomycin is typically administered by IV infusion at ≥1 hour per gram per dose. Rapid infusion rates can cause vancomycin infusion reaction, a histamine-mediated reaction characterized by flushing and redness of the upper body. Vancomycin infusion reaction can be adequately managed by premedicating with antihistamines, such as diphenhydramine.
- **Adverse events:** Nephrotoxicity, neutropenia, thrombocytopenia, and rash may also occur.

Fluoroquinolones

GENERAL PRINCIPLES

- Fluoroquinolones exert their bactericidal effect by inhibiting bacterial enzymes DNA gyrase and topoisomerase IV, which are critical for DNA replication. These antibiotics are well absorbed orally, with serum concentrations that approach those of parenteral administration, making them ideal candidates for switching from IV to PO formulations.
- Concomitant administration with aluminum- or magnesium-containing antacids, sucralfate, bismuth, oral iron, oral calcium, oral zinc, and metallic cation–containing enteral nutrition preparations can markedly impair absorption of oral fluoroquinolones.

TREATMENT

- **Ciprofloxacin** (250–750 mg PO q12h, 500 mg PO q24h [Cipro XR], or 200–400 mg IV q8–12h) and **ofloxacin** (200–400 mg IV or PO q12h) are active against gram-negative aerobes including many AmpC-producing pathogens. These agents are commonly used for UTIs, pyelonephritis, infectious diarrhea, prostatitis, and intra-abdominal infections (with metronidazole). Ciprofloxacin has the most reliable activity against *P. aeruginosa* of all quinolones. However, ciprofloxacin has relatively poor activity against gram-positive pathogens and anaerobes and should not be used as empiric monotherapy for CAP, skin/soft tissue infections, or intra-abdominal infections.

- **Levofloxacin** (250–750 mg PO/IV q24h), **moxifloxacin** (400 mg PO/IV q24h daily), and **gemifloxacin** (320 mg PO q24h daily) have improved coverage of streptococci but generally less gram-negative activity than ciprofloxacin (except levofloxacin, which does cover *P. aeruginosa*). Moxifloxacin has been used as monotherapy of intra-abdominal infections because of its antianaerobic activity, although resistance among *B. fragilis* is increasing. Each of these agents is useful for treatment of sinusitis, bronchitis, CAP, and UTIs (except moxifloxacin, which is only minimally eliminated in the urine). Some of these agents have activity against mycobacteria and have a potential role in treating drug-resistant tuberculosis (TB) and atypical mycobacterial infections. Levofloxacin may be used as an alternative for treatment of chlamydial urethritis.
- **Delafloxacin** (300 mg IV q12h or 450 mg PO q12h) is FDA-approved for acute bacterial skin and skin structure infections and CAP. This agent is active against some MRSA, streptococci, some enterococci, gram-negative bacteria (including *Pseudomonas*), and anaerobes. Unlike other fluoroquinolones, delafloxacin does not appear to prolong the QTc interval on the electrocardiogram and may be less prone to causing phototoxicity and CNS adverse effects than other fluoroquinolones.

SPECIAL CONSIDERATIONS

- **Adverse events** include nausea, CNS disturbances (headache, restlessness, and dizziness, especially in the elderly), rash, and phototoxicity. These agents can cause prolongation of the QTc interval (excluding delafloxacin) and should not be used in patients who are receiving class I or class III antiarrhythmics, in patients with known electrolyte or conduction abnormalities, or with other medications that prolong the QTc interval or induce bradycardia. These agents should also be used with caution in the elderly, in whom asymptomatic conduction disturbances are more common. Fluoroquinolones should not be routinely used in patients younger than 18 years or in pregnant or lactating women because of the risk of arthropathy in pediatric patients. They may also cause tendinitis or tendon rupture, especially of the Achilles tendon, particularly in elderly. Peripheral neuropathy, myasthenia gravis exacerbations, and abdominal aortic aneurysms may also rarely occur. An increase in the international normalized ratio may occur when used concurrently with warfarin.
- **This class of antimicrobials has major drug interactions.** Before initiating use of these agents, it is necessary to review concomitant medications.

Macrolides and Lincosamides

GENERAL PRINCIPLES

- Macrolide and lincosamide antibiotics are bacteriostatic agents that block protein synthesis in bacteria by binding to the 50S subunit of the bacterial ribosome.
- This class of antibiotics has activity against gram-positive cocci, including streptococci and staphylococci, and some upper respiratory gram-negative bacteria, but minimal activity against enteric gram-negative bacilli.

TREATMENT

- Macrolides are commonly used to treat pharyngitis, otitis media, sinusitis, and bronchitis, especially in PCN-allergic patients, and are among the drugs of choice for treating *Legionella*, *Chlamydia*, and *Mycoplasma* infections. Azithromycin and clarithromycin can be used as monotherapy for outpatient CAP and have a unique role in the treatment and prophylaxis against *Mycobacterium avium* complex (MAC) infections. Many PCN-resistant strains of pneumococci are also resistant to macrolides.
- **Clarithromycin** (250–500 mg PO q12h or 1000 mg XL PO q24h) has enhanced activity against some respiratory pathogens (especially *Haemophilus*). It is commonly used to treat bronchitis, sinusitis, otitis media, pharyngitis, skin/soft tissue infections, and CAP. It has a prominent role in treating MAC infection and is an important component of regimens used to eradicate *Helicobacter pylori* (see Chapter 18, Gastrointestinal Diseases).
- **Azithromycin** (500 mg PO for 1 day, then 250–500 mg PO q24h for 4 days; 500 mg IV q24h) has a similar spectrum of activity as clarithromycin and is commonly used to treat bronchitis, sinusitis, otitis media, pharyngitis, skin/soft tissue infections, and CAP. It has a prominent role in MAC prophylaxis (1200 mg PO every week) and treatment (500–600 mg PO q24h) in HIV patients. It is also commonly used to treat *Chlamydia trachomatis* infections (1 g PO single dose). A major advantage of azithromycin is that it has much fewer drug interactions than erythromycin and clarithromycin.
- **Clindamycin** (150–450 mg PO q6–8h or 600–900 mg IV q8h) is a lincosamide (related to macrolides), with activity against staphylococci and streptococci, as well as anaerobes, including *B. fragilis*. It has excellent oral bioavailability (90%) and penetrates well into the bone and abscess cavities. It is also used for treatment of aspiration pneumonia and lung abscesses. Clindamycin has activity against some MRSA and can be used for skin and soft tissue infections caused by susceptible strains of this organism. Clindamycin may be used in combination therapy for invasive streptococcal and clostridial infections to decrease toxin production. It may also be used for treatment of suspected anaerobic infections of the head and neck (peritonsillar or retropharyngeal abscesses, necrotizing fasciitis), although metronidazole is used more commonly for intra-abdominal infections (clindamycin has less reliable activity against *B. fragilis*). Clindamycin has additional uses, including treatment of babesiosis (in combination with quinine), toxoplasmosis (in combination with pyrimethamine), and *Pneumocystis jirovecii* pneumonia (in combination with primaquine).

SPECIAL CONSIDERATIONS

Adverse events: Macrolides and clindamycin are associated with nausea, abdominal cramping, and LFT abnormalities. Liver function profiles should be checked intermittently during extended therapy. Hypersensitivity reactions with prominent skin rash are more common with clindamycin, as is pseudomembranous colitis secondary to *Clostridioides difficile*. Clarithromycin and azithromycin may cause QTc interval prolongation and myasthenia gravis exacerbations. **Clarithromycin has major drug interactions** caused by inhibition of the cytochrome P450 (CYP) system.

Sulfonamides and Trimethoprim

GENERAL PRINCIPLES

Sulfadiazine, sulfamethoxazole, and trimethoprim slowly kill bacteria by inhibiting folic acid metabolism. This class of antibiotics is most commonly used for uncomplicated UTIs, sinusitis, and otitis media. Some sulfonamide-containing agents also have unique roles in the treatment of *P. jirovecii, Nocardia, Toxoplasma*, and *Stenotrophomonas* infections.

TREATMENT

- **Trimethoprim** (100 mg PO q12h) is occasionally used as monotherapy for treatment of UTIs. Trimethoprim is more often used in the combination preparations outlined below. Trimethoprim in combination with dapsone is an alternate therapy for mild *P. jirovecii* pneumonia.
- **Trimethoprim–sulfamethoxazole** is a combination antibiotic (IV or PO) with a 1:5 ratio of trimethoprim to sulfamethoxazole. The IV preparation is dosed at 5 mg/kg IV q8h (based on the trimethoprim component) for serious infections. The oral preparations (160 mg trimethoprim/800 mg sulfamethoxazole per double-strength [DS] tablet) are extensively bioavailable, with similar drug concentrations obtained with IV and PO formulations. The combination has a broad spectrum of activity but does not cover *P. aeruginosa*, anaerobes, or *Streptococcus pyogenes*. It is the treatment of choice for *P. jirovecii* pneumonia, *Stenotrophomonas maltophilia*, *Tropheryma whipplei*, and *Nocardia* infections. It is commonly used for treating sinusitis, otitis media, bronchitis, prostatitis, and UTIs (one DS tab PO q12h). Trimethoprim–sulfamethoxazole is active against MRSA and is widely used for uncomplicated cases of skin/soft tissue infections caused by this organism (often two DS tabs PO q12h). It is used as *P. jirovecii* pneumonia prophylaxis in HIV-infected patients, solid organ transplant patients, bone marrow transplant patients, and in patients receiving fludarabine. IV therapy is routinely converted to the PO equivalent for patients who require prolonged therapy.
  For serious infections, such as *Nocardia* brain abscesses, drug levels should be monitored. Sulfamethoxazole peaks (goal 100–150 µg/mL) and troughs (goal 50–100 µg/mL) should be monitored and doses adjusted accordingly. In patients with renal insufficiency, doses can be adjusted according to trimethoprim peaks (goal 5–10 µg/mL). Prolonged therapy can cause bone marrow suppression, which can be managed with leucovorin (5–10 mg PO q24h) until cell counts normalize.
- **Sulfadiazine** (1.0–1.5 g PO q6h) in combination with pyrimethamine (200 mg PO followed by 50–75 mg PO q24h) and leucovorin (10–20 mg PO q24h) is the regimen of choice for toxoplasmosis. Sulfadiazine is also occasionally used to treat *Nocardia* infections.

SPECIAL CONSIDERATIONS

Adverse events: These drugs are associated with cholestatic jaundice, bone marrow suppression, hyperkalemia (with trimethoprim/sulfamethoxazole), hyponatremia, obstructive uropathy, interstitial nephritis, "false" elevations in serum creatinine, and severe hypersensitivity reactions (including Stevens-Johnson syndrome). Nausea is common with higher doses. **All patients should be asked whether they are allergic**

to **"sulfa drugs,"** and specific commercial names should be mentioned (e.g., Bactrim or Septra). Hemolysis in the setting of glucose-6-phosphate dehydrogenase deficiency may also occur.

Tetracyclines

GENERAL PRINCIPLES

- Tetracyclines are bacteriostatic antibiotics that bind to the 30S ribosomal subunit and block protein synthesis.
- These agents have unique roles in the treatment of *Rickettsia*, *Ehrlichia*, *Chlamydia*, and *Mycoplasma* infections. They are used as therapy for most tick-borne infections, including Lyme disease–related arthritis, alternate therapy for syphilis, and therapy for *P. multocida* infections in PCN-allergic patients. The tetracycline derivatives also have activity against some multidrug-resistant (MDR) gram-negative pathogens and may be used in this setting based on results of susceptibility testing.

TREATMENT

- **Tetracycline** (250–500 mg PO q6h) is commonly used for severe acne and in some *H. pylori* eradication regimens. It has largely been replaced by doxycycline for other infections (see below).
- **Doxycycline** (100 mg PO/IV q12h) is the most commonly used tetracycline and is standard therapy for *C. trachomatis*, Rocky Mountain spotted fever, ehrlichiosis, and psittacosis. This agent also has a role in the treatment of CAP and uncomplicated skin and skin structure infections (including infections caused by MRSA, but not *S. pyogenes*), as well as malaria prophylaxis.
- **Minocycline** (200 mg IV/PO × 1 dose, then 100 mg IV/PO q12h) is similar to doxycycline in its spectrum of activity and clinical indications. Among the tetracyclines, minocycline is most likely to provide coverage against *Acinetobacter*. Minocycline can also be used for treating pulmonary nocardiosis, cervicofacial actinomycosis, and *S. maltophilia* infections.
- **Tigecycline** (100–200 mg IV × 1 dose, then 50–100 mg IV q12h) is a tetracycline derivative further classified as a glycylcycline. Tigecycline has broad spectrum of activity against most gram-positive, gram-negative, and anaerobic bacteria, except *P. aeruginosa* and some *Proteus* spp. It may be used for treatment of infections due to susceptible strains of VRE and some MDR gram-negative bacteria, including CRE. Owing to a high volume of distribution and low achievable blood concentrations, tigecycline should not be used to treat primary bacteremia. Tigecycline should generally be avoided when alternative options are available due to a noted increase in all-cause mortality based on a meta-analysis of phase 3 and 4 clinical trial data. Dose adjustment in severe hepatic impairment is indicated.
- **Omadacycline** (200 mg IV × 1 dose, then 100 mg IV q24h or 450 mg PO daily × 2 doses, then 300 mg PO q24h) is a tetracycline derivative FDA-approved for CAP and skin and skin structure infections. This agent can overcome some tetracycline resistance mechanisms, resulting in broad-spectrum activity against gram-positive (including MRSA and VRE), gram-negative, and atypical organisms, as well as anaerobes.
- **Eravacycline** (1 mg/kg IV q12h) is another tetracycline derivative FDA-approved for complicated intra-abdominal infections. This agent has a broad spectrum of activity

similar to omadacycline, including activity against MDR and other tetracycline-resistant pathogens; however, eravacycline has better activity against *Acinetobacter* compared to omadacycline. Eravacycline should **not** be used for the treatment of UTI owing to poor urinary concentrations and subsequent failure to demonstrate noninferiority in clinical trials. This agent is a minor substrate of CYP3A4, resulting in the potential for drug interactions. Dose adjustment is indicated in severe hepatic impairment.

SPECIAL CONSIDERATIONS

- **Adverse events:** Nausea, vomiting, and photosensitivity are common side effects, so patients should be warned about direct sun exposure. Rarely, these medications are associated with pseudotumor cerebri and pancreatitis. **They should not routinely be given to children or to pregnant or lactating women** because they can cause tooth enamel discoloration in the developing fetus and young children. Minocycline is also associated with vestibular disturbances. Oral formulations of tetracyclines may cause esophageal ulceration if not properly swallowed.
- Aluminum- and magnesium-containing antacids and preparations that contain oral calcium, oral iron, or other metallic cations can significantly impair oral absorption of tetracycline and other oral tetracycline derivatives and should be avoided within 2 hours of each dose.

Oxazolidinones

GENERAL PRINCIPLES

Oxazolidinones block assembly of bacterial ribosomes and inhibit protein synthesis. These agents demonstrate high oral bioavailability, allowing for PO therapy when available, and do not require dose adjustments for hepatic or renal dysfunction.

TREATMENT

- **Linezolid** (600 mg IV/PO q12h) has potent activity against gram-positive bacteria, including drug-resistant enterococci, staphylococci, and streptococci, but not against gram-negative bacteria. Linezolid is useful for treating serious infections caused by VRE, as an alternative to vancomycin for treatment of some MRSA infections, and as oral treatment of MRSA infections when IV access is unavailable. Linezolid should generally be avoided for catheter-related bloodstream or catheter site infections.
- **Tedizolid** (200 mg PO/IV q24h) is the newest oxazolidinone antibiotic available. It is FDA-approved for treating skin/soft tissue infections. Tedizolid's spectrum of activity is similar to linezolid, although tedizolid covers some linezolid-resistant *Enterococcus* spp.

SPECIAL CONSIDERATIONS

- **Adverse events** associated with linezolid include diarrhea, nausea, and headache. Myelosuppression, most commonly thrombocytopenia, occurs frequently in patients who receive ≥2 weeks of therapy. Thus, weekly CBC monitoring is indicated. Prolonged therapy has also been associated with peripheral and optic neuropathy. Lactic acidosis may also rarely occur. Adverse events associated with tedizolid are similar to linezolid, although its propensity to cause neuropathies and hematologic toxicities with prolonged use is unknown.

- Linezolid has **several important drug interactions.** It is a mild monoamine oxidase inhibitor and can cause serotonin syndrome when used in combination with other serotonergic agents. Patients should be advised to avoid selective serotonin reuptake inhibitors, other antidepressants, fentanyl, cyclobenzaprine, and meperidine while on linezolid. Ideally, patients should be off antidepressants for at least a week before initiating linezolid. Coadministration of pseudoephedrine with linezolid can elevate blood pressure and should also be avoided. Tedizolid appears less likely to inhibit monoamine oxidase as compared with linezolid; however, patients on serotonergic agents were excluded from tedizolid phase III clinical trials.

Lipoglycopeptides

TREATMENT

Telavancin (7.5–10 mg/kg q24–48h, based on CrCl) is a lipoglycopeptide antibiotic that is FDA-approved for treatment of HABP and VABP caused by *S. aureus* and for complicated skin/soft tissue infections. Telavancin is broadly active against gram-positive bacteria, including MRSA, VISA, heteroresistant VISA, daptomycin- and linezolid-resistant *S. aureus*, streptococci, vancomycin-sensitive enterococci, and some gram-positive anaerobes. The agent is not active against gram-negative bacteria, vancomycin-resistant *S. aureus*, and VRE.

SPECIAL CONSIDERATIONS

Adverse events include nausea, vomiting, metallic or soapy taste, foamy urine, and nephrotoxicity (which necessitates serial monitoring of serum creatinine). Prehydration with normal saline may mitigate the nephrotoxicity observed with the use of this drug. Telavancin can also cause a minor prolongation of the QTc interval. Women of childbearing potential require a negative serum pregnancy test prior to receiving telavancin because of teratogenic effects noted in animals.

Long-Acting Lipoglycopeptides

GENERAL PRINCIPLES

Long-acting lipoglycopeptides are bactericidal antibiotics that inhibit bacterial cell wall biosynthesis, similar to vancomycin. Their spectrum of activity includes gram-positive aerobic pathogens only. These agents are characterized by extremely long terminal half-lives and are currently FDA-approved for skin/soft tissue infections.

TREATMENT

- **Dalbavancin** (1500 mg single dose or 1000 mg IV on day 1 followed by 500 mg IV on day 8 to complete the course of therapy) has a terminal half-life of 346 hours. Dalbavancin is active against staphylococci (including MRSA), streptococci, and enterococci. Susceptibility to dalbavancin can be reliably inferred from vancomycin.

- **Oritavancin** (1200 mg IV administered once to complete therapy) has a terminal half-life of 245 hours. Oritavancin is active against staphylococci (including MRSA), streptococci, and enterococci (including VRE).

SPECIAL CONSIDERATIONS

Adverse events include nausea, diarrhea, vomiting, headache, dizziness, pruritus, and infusion-related reactions. In clinical trials, more dalbavancin-treated patients had alanine LFT elevation greater than three times the upper limit of normal than patients treated with a comparative agent. Dalbavancin may also cause acute kidney injury.

Colistin and Polymyxin B

TREATMENT

Colistimethate sodium (colistin; 300 mg IV × 1, then 180 mg IV q12h) and **polymyxin B** (15,000–25,000 units/kg/d IV divided q12h) are bactericidal polypeptide antibiotics that kill gram-negative bacteria by disrupting the cell membrane. These drugs are typically active against CRE and *P. aeruginosa*, but have recently been replaced by newer, safer β-lactam antibiotics (outlined above). Notably, these agents are inactive against *Proteus, Providencia, Burkholderia,* and *Serratia.*

SPECIAL CONSIDERATIONS

- **These medications should only be given under the guidance of an experienced clinician and as last-line agents** due to significant nephrotoxicity (~30%) and CNS toxicity (~10%). Inhaled colistin (75–150 mg q12h via nebulizer) is better tolerated than the IV formulation, generally causing only mild upper airway irritation, and has some effectiveness as adjunctive therapy for MDR *P. aeruginosa* or *Acinetobacter* pulmonary infections.
- **Adverse events** with parenteral therapy include paresthesias, slurred speech, peripheral numbness, tingling, and significant dose-dependent nephrotoxicity. The dosage should be carefully reduced in patients with renal insufficiency because overdosage can result in neuromuscular blockade and apnea. Serum creatinine should be monitored daily early in therapy and then at a regular interval for the duration of therapy. Concomitant use with aminoglycosides, other known nephrotoxins, or neuromuscular blockers should be avoided.

Cyclic Lipopeptide

TREATMENT

Daptomycin (4 mg/kg IV q24h for skin and skin structure infections; 6–12 mg/kg IV q24h for bloodstream infections) is the only FDA-approved cyclic lipopeptide. The drug exhibits rapid bactericidal activity against a wide variety of gram-positive bacteria, including enterococci, staphylococci, and streptococci. Daptomycin is FDA-approved for treatment of skin/soft tissue infections as well as *S. aureus* bacteremia and right-sided endocarditis. The drug should **not** be used to treat lung infections as activity is decreased in the presence of pulmonary surfactant. Nonsusceptibility to daptomycin can develop during treatment, making it imperative that susceptibility of isolates be verified.

SPECIAL CONSIDERATIONS

Adverse events include gastrointestinal disturbances, injection site reactions, elevated LFTs, and eosinophilic pneumonitis. Serum creatine phosphokinase (CK) should be monitored at baseline and weekly because daptomycin has been associated with skeletal muscle effects, including rhabdomyolysis. Patients should also be monitored for signs of muscle weakness and pain, and the drug should be discontinued if these symptoms develop in conjunction with marked CK elevations (5–10 times the upper limit of normal with symptoms or 10 times the upper limit of normal without symptoms). Concomitant use of statins should be avoided, if possible, because of the potential increased risk of myopathy.

Nitroimidazole

TREATMENT

- **Metronidazole** (250–750 mg PO/IV q6–12h) is only active against anaerobic bacteria and some protozoa. The drug exerts its bactericidal effect through accumulation of toxic metabolites that interfere with multiple biologic processes. It has excellent tissue penetration, including abscess cavities, bone, and the CNS.
- It has greater activity against gram-negative than gram-positive anaerobes but is active against *Clostridium perfringens* and *Clostridioides difficile*; however, it is no longer a preferred treatment for *C. difficile* colitis. Metronidazole is a treatment of choice for bacterial vaginosis and can be used in combination with other antibiotics to treat intra-abdominal infections and brain abscesses. Protozoal infections that are routinely treated with metronidazole include *Giardia*, *Entamoeba histolytica*, and *Trichomonas vaginalis*. Dose reduction may be warranted for patients with decompensated liver disease.

SPECIAL CONSIDERATIONS

Adverse events include nausea, dysgeusia, disulfiram-like reactions to alcohol, and mild CNS disturbances (headache, restlessness). Rarely, metronidazole causes peripheral neuropathy, encephalopathy, and seizures.

Uncomplicated UTI Agents

GENERAL PRINCIPLES

Nitrofurantoin and oral **fosfomycin** are unique in their pharmacokinetic profiles, which result in high urinary, but minimal blood concentrations. These agents should only be used in the treatment of **uncomplicated** UTIs and should **not** be used for pyelonephritis or other systemic infections.

TREATMENT

- **Nitrofurantoin** (50–100 mg PO macrocrystals q6h or 100 mg PO dual-release formulation q12h for 5 d) is metabolized by bacteria into toxic intermediates that inhibit multiple bacterial processes, resulting in bactericidal activity. The agent is indicated for the treatment of uncomplicated UTIs except those caused by *Proteus*, *P. aeruginosa*, *Morganella*, or *Serratia*. Notably, nitrofurantoin can also be effective for uncomplicated VRE UTIs. Nitrofurantoin should be avoided in patients with renal dysfunction due to increased adverse events (outlined below).

- **Fosfomycin** (3 g sachet dissolved in cold water PO once) is a bactericidal oral antibiotic that kills bacteria by inhibiting an early step in cell wall synthesis. It has a spectrum of activity that includes most urinary tract pathogens, including *P. aeruginosa*, enterococci (including VRE), and some MDR Enterobacterales. Oral fosfomycin is most useful for treating uncomplicated UTIs caused by susceptible strains of *E. coli* or *E. faecalis*.

SPECIAL CONSIDERATIONS

- **Adverse events for nitrofurantoin** consist primarily of nausea, which can be mitigated by taking with food. Rarely, neurotoxicity, hepatotoxicity, and pulmonary fibrosis, especially with prolonged use in the setting of renal dysfunction. Thus, it should not be used in patients with CrCl <30 mL/min. Patients should be warned that their urine may become brown secondary to the medication. Probenecid decreases the concentration of nitrofurantoin in the urine and should be avoided.
- **Adverse events for fosfomycin** include diarrhea. It should not be taken with metoclopramide, which interferes with fosfomycin absorption.

Streptogramin

TREATMENT

Quinupristin/dalfopristin (7.5 mg/kg IV q8h) is the only FDA-approved drug in the streptogramin class. This agent exerts its bacteriostatic effect by binding to the 50S bacterial ribosomal subunit, thereby inhibiting bacterial protein synthesis. Quinupristin/dalfopristin has activity against antibiotic-resistant gram-positive organisms, including VRE, MRSA, and MDR strains of *Streptococcus pneumoniae*; however, quinupristin/dalfopristin is inactive against *E. faecalis*.

SPECIAL CONSIDERATIONS

Adverse events include the possibility of severe arthralgias and myalgias, which occur frequently and can necessitate discontinuation of therapy. Injection site pain and thrombophlebitis are common. It has also been associated with elevated LFTs and requires dose adjustment in patients with hepatic impairment. Quinupristin/dalfopristin is similar to clarithromycin with regard to drug interactions.

Pleuromutilin

TREATMENT

Lefamulin (150 mg IV q12h or 600 mg PO q12h) is the first systemic pleuromutilin antibiotic FDA-approved as an alternative agent for treatment of CAP in patients without structural lung disease. Lefamulin exerts its antibacterial effect through interactions with the 50S subunit of the bacterial ribosome, resulting in inhibition of bacterial protein synthesis and cell death. The agent is active against *S. aureus* (including MRSA), *S. pneumoniae, Haemophilus influenzae, Legionella pneumophila, Mycoplasma pneumoniae,* and *Chlamydophila pneumoniae*. Lefamulin is not active against Enterobacterales, *Pseudomonas*, and most anaerobes. Dose adjustment is indicated in severe hepatic impairment. Lefamulin is extensively metabolized via CYP3A4, resulting in the potential for **drug interactions** with agents that significantly inhibit or induce this enzyme.

SPECIAL CONSIDERATIONS

Adverse events include diarrhea (especially with the oral formulation), nausea, vomiting and headache. Infusion-site pain and phlebitis may occur with IV administration. Lefamulin can also prolong the QT interval and should be avoided in patients at risk of QTc prolongation or in combination with other QT-prolonging agents.

ANTIMYCOBACTERIAL AGENTS

Effective therapy of TB requires combination chemotherapy to prevent the emergence of resistant organisms and maximize efficacy. Increased resistance to antituberculous agents has led to the use of more complex regimens and has made susceptibility testing an integral part of TB management (see Chapter 14, Treatment of Infectious Diseases).

Isoniazid

TREATMENT

Isoniazid (INH; 300 mg PO q24h) exerts bactericidal effects by interfering with the synthesis of lipid components of the mycobacterial cell wall. INH is a component of most TB treatment regimens and can be given twice a week in directly observed therapy (15 mg/kg/dose; 900 mg maximum). INH remains the drug of choice for treatment of latent TB infection (300 mg PO q24h for 9 mo or combined with rifapentine in a 12-wk regimen).

SPECIAL CONSIDERATIONS

Adverse events primarily consist of elevations in LFTs (~20%). This effect can be idiosyncratic but is usually seen with advanced age, underlying liver disease, or concomitant consumption of alcohol and may be potentiated by rifampin. Transaminase elevations to greater than threefold the upper limit of the normal range necessitate holding therapy. Patients with known liver dysfunction should have weekly LFTs monitored during the initial stage of therapy. INH also antagonizes vitamin B_6 metabolism and can potentially cause peripheral neuropathy. INH should always be coadministered with pyridoxine 25–50 mg PO daily to minimize the risk of neuropathies, especially in the elderly and pregnant women, as well as in patients with diabetes, renal failure, alcoholism, and seizure disorders.

Rifamycins

GENERAL PRINCIPLES

Rifamycins exert bactericidal activity on susceptible mycobacteria by inhibiting DNA-dependent RNA polymerase, thereby halting transcription.

TREATMENT

- **Rifampin** (rifampicin; 600 mg PO q24h or twice a week) is an integral component of most TB treatment regimens. It is also active against many gram-positive and gram-negative bacteria. Rifampin is used as adjunctive therapy in staphylococcal prosthetic valve endocarditis (300 mg PO q8h) and prosthetic bone and joint infections (450 mg PO q12h) and for prophylaxis of close contacts of patients with *Neisseria meningitidis* infection (5 mg/kg PO q12h × 4 doses). The drug is well absorbed orally and is widely distributed throughout the body including the cerebrospinal fluid (CSF).
- **Rifabutin** (300 mg PO q24h) is primarily used to treat TB and MAC infections in HIV-positive patients on antiretroviral therapy because it has fewer drug–drug interactions and less deleterious effects on protease inhibitor metabolism than rifampin (see Chapter 16, Sexually Transmitted Infections, Human Immunodeficiency Virus, and Acquired Immunodeficiency Syndrome).
- **Rifapentine** (600–900 mg PO one to two times weekly) is primarily used in combination with isoniazid for 12-week once-weekly treatment of latent TB infection, but can also be used for the treatment of active TB. Doses are adjusted based on body weight and active versus latent infection.

SPECIAL CONSIDERATIONS

Adverse events include rash, GI disturbances, hematologic disturbances, hepatitis, and interstitial nephritis. Patients should also be warned about reddish-orange discoloration of body fluids, including contact lenses. Uveitis has also been associated with rifabutin. **This class of antibiotics has major drug interactions** based on CYP enzyme inhibition. Concomitant medications should be screened for drug interactions prior to starting therapy with a rifamycin.

Pyrazinamide

TREATMENT

Pyrazinamide (15–30 mg/kg PO q24h [maximum, 2 g] or 50–75 mg/kg PO twice a week [maximum, 4 g/dose]) kills mycobacteria by an unknown disruption of membrane transport. It is well absorbed orally and widely distributed throughout the body, including the CSF. Pyrazinamide is typically used for the first 2 months of therapy during treatment of active TB.

SPECIAL CONSIDERATIONS

Adverse events include hyperuricemia and hepatitis.

Ethambutol

TREATMENT

Ethambutol (15–25 mg/kg PO q24h or 50–75 mg/kg PO twice a week; maximum, 2.4 g/dose) is bacteriostatic and inhibits arabinosyltransferase (involved in cell wall synthesis). It is commonly utilized in treatment regimens of active TB as well as MAC infections in patients with and without HIV. Doses should be reduced in the presence of renal dysfunction.

SPECIAL CONSIDERATIONS

Adverse events may include **optic neuritis**, which manifests as decreased red-green color perception, decreased visual acuity, or visual field deficits. Baseline and monthly visual examinations should be performed during therapy. Renal function should also be carefully monitored because drug accumulation in the setting of renal insufficiency can increase risk of ocular effects.

Streptomycin

GENERAL PRINCIPLES

Streptomycin is an aminoglycoside that can be used as a substitute for ethambutol and for drug-resistant TB. It does not adequately penetrate the CNS and should not be used for TB meningitis.

ANTIVIRAL AGENTS

Current antiviral agents only suppress viral replication. Viral containment or elimination requires an intact host immune response. Anti-HIV agents will be discussed in Chapter 16, Sexually Transmitted Infections, Human Immunodeficiency Virus, and Acquired Immunodeficiency Syndrome.

Anti-Influenza Agents

GENERAL PRINCIPLES

Zanamivir, oseltamivir, and peramivir are neuraminidase inhibitors that block influenza A and B neuraminidases. Neuraminidase activity is necessary for successful viral egress and release from infected cells. **Baloxavir** is an endonuclease inhibitor that inhibits influenza gene transcription.

TREATMENT

• **Zanamivir** (10 mg [two inhalations] q12h for 5 d, started within 48 h of the onset of symptoms) is an inhaled neuraminidase inhibitor that is active against influenza A and B. It is indicated for treatment of uncomplicated acute influenza infection in adults and children 7 years of age or older who have been symptomatic for <48 hours. It is also indicated for influenza prophylaxis in patients aged 5 years and older. **Adverse events** such as headache, GI disturbances, dizziness, and upper respiratory symptoms are sometimes reported. Bronchospasm, a decline in lung function, or both, may occur in patients with underlying respiratory disorders and may require a rapid-acting bronchodilator for control.

• **Oseltamivir** (75 mg PO q12h × 5 d) is an orally administered neuraminidase inhibitor that is active against influenza A and B. It is indicated for treatment of uncomplicated acute influenza in adults and children 1 year of age or older who have been symptomatic for up to 2 days. This agent is also indicated for prophylaxis of influenza A and B in adults and children 1 year of age or older. Dose adjustment for renal function is indicated.
Adverse events include nausea, vomiting, and diarrhea. Dizziness, headache, and other neuropsychiatric events (e.g., confusion, delirium, hallucination, and/or self-injury) may also occur.

• **Peramivir** (600 mg IV × 1 dose) is an IV neuraminidase inhibitor that is active against influenza A and B. It is FDA-approved for single-dose treatment of acute, uncomplicated influenza in adults who have been symptomatic for up to 2 days. The agent has not been proven to be effective for serious influenza requiring hospitalization but is often given daily for up to 10 days in hospitalized patients unable to tolerate or absorb oral oseltamivir.
Adverse events include diarrhea and rarely skin reactions, behavioral disturbances, neutrophils <1000/μL, hyperglycemia, CK elevation, and LFT elevation.

• **Baloxavir marboxil** (<80 kg: 40 mg × 1 dose; ≥80 kg: 80 mg × 1 dose started within 48 h of the onset of symptoms) is a first-in-class oral prodrug that inhibits influenza virus gene transcription, thereby preventing viral replication. It is FDA-approved for both treatment and postexposure prophylaxis of seasonal influenza caused by influenza A or B and should be given as a single dose within 48 hours of symptoms or exposure.
Adverse events are rare but include diarrhea and rash.

SPECIAL CONSIDERATIONS

These drugs have shown modest activity in clinical trials, with a 1- to 2-day improvement in symptoms in patients who are treated within 48 hours of the onset of influenza symptoms. At the onset of each influenza season, a consultation with local health department officials is recommended to determine the most effective antiviral agent. Although oseltamivir, zanamivir, and baloxavir are effective for prophylaxis of influenza, annual influenza vaccination remains the most effective method for prophylaxis in all high-risk patients and health care workers (see Appendix A, Immunizations and Postexposure Therapies).

Antiherpetic Agents

GENERAL PRINCIPLES

Antiherpetic agents are nucleotide analogs that inhibit viral DNA synthesis. All antiherpetic agents require dose adjustment for renal dysfunction. For ease of classification, antiherpetic agents include those that cover herpes simplex virus (HSV) 1 and 2, and varicella-zoster virus (VZV). Antiviral agents with activity against cytomegalovirus (CMV) will be covered below.

TREATMENT

- **Acyclovir** (400 mg PO q8h for HSV, 800 mg PO five times a day for localized VZV infections, 5–10 mg/kg IV q8h for severe HSV infections, and 10 mg/kg IV q8h for severe VZV infections and HSV encephalitis) is active against HSV and VZV. It is indicated for treatment of primary and recurrent genital herpes, severe herpetic stomatitis, and HSV encephalitis. Acyclovir can be used as prophylaxis in patients who have frequent HSV recurrences (400 mg PO q12h). It is also used for HSV ophthalmicus, disseminated primary VZV in adults (significant morbidity compared to the childhood illness), and severe disseminated primary VZV in children. IV acyclovir should be dosed using IBW in patients with obesity.

  Adverse events. Reversible crystalline nephropathy may occur; preexisting renal failure, dehydration, and IV bolus dosing increase the risk of this effect. Rare cases of CNS disturbances, including delirium, tremors, and seizures, may also occur, particularly with high doses in patients with renal failure and in the elderly.

- **Valacyclovir** (1000 mg PO q8h for VZV, 1000 mg PO q12h for initial episode of genital HSV, and 500 mg PO q12h or 1000 mg PO q24h for suppression of recurrent episodes of genital HSV) is an orally administered prodrug of acyclovir used for the treatment and prevention of HSV infections and for treatment of VZV. Valacyclovir's bioavailability is roughly three to five times higher than oral acyclovir, resulting in less frequent dosing. A 1000 mg oral dose of valacyclovir is equivalent to 5 mg/kg of IV acyclovir.

  Adverse events include GI upset, headache, rash, and rarely CNS disturbances. High doses (8 g/d) have been associated with development of hemolytic-uremic syndrome/thrombotic thrombocytopenic purpura in immunocompromised patients.

- **Famciclovir** (500 mg PO q8h for VZV, 250 mg PO q8h for the initial episode of genital HSV infection, and 250 mg PO q12h for suppression of recurrent episodes of genital HSV) is an orally administered antiviral agent used for the treatment of acute VZV reactivation and for treatment or suppression of genital HSV infections. **Adverse events** include headache, nausea, and diarrhea.

Anticytomegalovirus Agents

TREATMENT

- **Ganciclovir** (5 mg/kg IV q12h for 14–21 d for induction therapy, followed by 5 mg/kg IV q24h) is a nucleoside analogue that inhibits DNA synthesis in the same manner as acyclovir. It has activity against HSV and VZV but is reserved for the treatment of CMV infections given its toxicity profile. Ganciclovir is widely distributed in the body, including the CSF. It is indicated for treatment of CMV retinitis and other serious CMV infections in immunocompromised patients (e.g., transplant and AIDS patients).

  Adverse events: Neutropenia is the main therapy-limiting adverse effect and may require treatment with granulocyte colony-stimulating factor for management (300 μg SC daily to weekly). Thrombocytopenia, rash, confusion, headache, nephrotoxicity, and GI disturbances may also occur. A CBC and basic metabolic profile should be monitored weekly while the patient is receiving therapy. Concomitant use of other agents with nephrotoxic or bone marrow suppressive effects should be avoided, if possible.

- **Valganciclovir** (900 mg PO q12–24h) is the oral prodrug of ganciclovir. This agent has substantial bioavailability and can be used for treatment of CMV retinitis and other systemic CMV infections. A 900 mg oral dose of valganciclovir is equivalent to 5 mg/kg of IV ganciclovir. Adverse events are the same as those for ganciclovir.
- **Foscarnet** (60 mg/kg IV q8h or 90 mg/kg IV q12h for 14–21 d as induction therapy, followed by 90–120 mg/kg IV q24h as maintenance therapy for CMV; 40 mg/kg IV q8h for acyclovir-resistant HSV and VZV) is used to treat acyclovir-resistant HSV/VZV infections and ganciclovir-resistant CMV infections. It can be used in patients who are not tolerating or not responding to ganciclovir.
  Adverse events: Nephrotoxicity is the major dose-limiting toxicity. CrCl, electrolytes (PO_4, Ca^{2+}, Mg^{2+}, and K^+), and serum creatinine should be checked at baseline and at least twice weekly while on therapy. Normal saline (500–1000 mL) should be given before and during infusions to minimize nephrotoxicity. Foscarnet should be avoided in patients with a serum creatinine of >2.8 mg/dL or baseline CrCl of <50 mL/min. Concomitant use of other nephrotoxins should be avoided. Foscarnet chelates divalent cations and can cause tetany even with normal serum calcium levels. Use of foscarnet with pentamidine can cause severe hypocalcemia. Other side effects include seizures, phlebitis, rash, and genital ulcers. **Prolonged therapy with foscarnet should be monitored by physicians who are experienced with administration of home IV therapy and can systematically monitor patients' laboratory results.**
- **Cidofovir** (5 mg/kg IV q wk for 2 wk as induction therapy, followed by 5 mg/kg IV q14d chronically as maintenance therapy) is used primarily to treat systemic CMV infections in patients who are not responding to ganciclovir or foscarnet.
  - **Adverse events:** The most common adverse event is nephrotoxicity. Cidofovir should be avoided in patients with a CrCl of <55 mL/min, a serum creatinine >1.5 mg/dL, significant proteinuria, or a recent history of receipt of other nephrotoxic medications.
  - **Each cidofovir dose should be administered with probenecid** (2 g PO 3 h before the infusion and then 1 g at 2 and 8 h after the infusion) along with 1 L normal saline IV 1–2 h before the infusion to minimize nephrotoxicity. Patients should have a serum creatinine and urine protein checked before each dose of cidofovir is given. This drug requires systematic monitoring of laboratory studies and close physician follow-up.
- **Letermovir** (480 mg IV or PO q24h) is a CMV DNA terminase inhibitor that is FDA-approved for CMV prophylaxis in allogeneic hematopoietic stem cell transplant through 100 days posttransplant. It has been anecdotally utilized for treatment of CMV infection, although this is not an established indication. Significant drug interactions exist and should be determined prior to starting therapy. Letermovir is contraindicated with pimozide and ergot alkaloids. Concomitant use of cyclosporine mandates dose reduction of letermovir to 240 mg q24h.
  Adverse events are rare but include GI upset, headache, and peripheral edema.

Anti-COVID-19 Agents

TREATMENT

Remdesivir (200 mg IV × 1, then 100 mg IV q24h × 5–10 days) is a SARS-CoV-2 nucleotide analog RNA polymerase inhibitor that is FDA-approved for treatment of COVID-19 disease necessitating hospitalization. Remdesivir should not be routinely administered to patients with an estimated GFR <30 mL/min due to risk of the drug's delivery vehicle accumulating. The main **adverse events** of importance include the potential for hypersensitivity reactions during and after drug administration and hepatic transaminase elevations.

ANTIFUNGAL AGENTS

Amphotericin B Formulations

GENERAL PRINCIPLES

Amphotericin B is fungicidal by interacting with ergosterol and disrupting the fungal cell membrane. Reformulation of this agent in various lipid vehicles has decreased some of its adverse side effects. Amphotericin B formulations are not effective for *Pseudallescheria boydii, Candida lusitaniae*, or *Aspergillus terreus* infections.

TREATMENT

- **Amphotericin B deoxycholate** (0.3–1.5 mg/kg q24h as a single infusion over 2–6 h) was once widely used but has now been supplanted by lipid-based formulations of the drug as a result of their improved tolerability.
- **Lipid complexed preparations** of amphotericin B, including liposomal amphotericin B (LAmB; 3–6 mg/kg IV q24h) and amphotericin B lipid complex (5 mg/kg IV q24h), have decreased nephrotoxicity and are generally associated with fewer infusion-related reactions than amphotericin B deoxycholate. LAmB has the most FDA-approved uses and appears to be the best tolerated lipid amphotericin B formulation overall.

SPECIAL CONSIDERATIONS

- The major **adverse event** of all amphotericin B formulations, including the lipid formulations, is **nephrotoxicity.** Patients should receive 500 mL of normal saline before and after each infusion to minimize nephrotoxicity. Concomitant administration of other nephrotoxins should be avoided if possible.
- Common **infusion-related effects** include fever/chills, nausea, headache, and myalgias. Premedication with 500–1000 mg of acetaminophen and 50 mg of diphenhydramine may control many of these symptoms. More severe reactions may be prevented by premedication with hydrocortisone 25–50 mg IV. Intolerable infusion-related chills can be managed with meperidine 25–50 mg IV.
- Amphotericin B therapy is associated with **potassium and magnesium wasting** that generally requires supplementation. Serum creatinine and electrolytes (including Mg^{2+} and K^+) should be monitored at least two to three times a week.

Azoles

GENERAL PRINCIPLES

Azoles are fungistatic agents that inhibit ergosterol synthesis, a key component of fungal cell membranes.

TREATMENT

- **Fluconazole** (100–800 mg PO/IV q24h) is the drug of choice for many *Candida* infections, such as UTIs, thrush, vaginal candidiasis (150-mg single dose), esophagitis, peritonitis, hepatosplenic infection, and severe disseminated candidal infections (e.g., candidemia). It is the treatment of choice for consolidation therapy of cryptococcal meningitis following an initial 14-day course of a lipid amphotericin B formulation in combination with flucytosine or as a second-line agent for primary treatment of cryptococcal meningitis (400–800 mg PO q24h for 8 wk, followed by 200 mg PO q24h thereafter for chronic maintenance treatment). Fluconazole does not have activity against *Candida krusei*, *Aspergillus*, or other invasive mold infections. *Candida glabrata* has intrinsically low susceptibility to fluconazole and determination of the MIC is required.
- **Itraconazole** (200 mg q8h × 3 d, then 200–400 mg PO q24h or super-bioavailable [SUBA] 130 mg po q8h × 3 d, then 130 mg PO q24h) is a triazole with broad-spectrum antifungal activity. It is primarily used to treat dimorphic mold infections, including the endemic mycoses (coccidioidomycosis, histoplasmosis, and blastomycosis) and sporotrichosis. It is an alternative therapy for *Aspergillus* and can also be used to treat infections caused by dermatophytes, including onychomycosis of the toenails and fingernails.
  - The traditional capsules require adequate gastric acidity for absorption and, therefore, should be taken with food or carbonated beverage. The liquid formulation is preferred as it is not significantly affected by gastric acidity and is better absorbed on an empty stomach. SUBA-itraconazole is a new highly bioavailable capsule that can be administered without regard to meals.
  - All formulations of itraconazole exhibit negative ionotropic effects and can cause or exacerbate congestive heart failure. Use should be avoid in individuals with preexisting heart failure.
  - Therapeutic drug monitoring is indicated with itraconazole. Doses should be titrated to achieve a steady-state trough >1 μg/mL (sum of itraconazole and its hydroxy metabolite).
- **Posaconazole** (delayed-release [DR] tablet and IV doses are 300 mg PO/IV q12h on day 1, followed by 300 mg PO/IV q24h; oral suspension dose is 200 mg PO q8h for prophylaxis and 100–400 mg PO q12–24h for oropharyngeal candidiasis treatment) is an oral azole agent that is used for prophylaxis of invasive aspergillosis and candidiasis in hematopoietic stem cell transplant patients with graft-versus-host disease or in patients with hematologic malignancies experiencing prolonged neutropenia from chemotherapy as well as treatment of oropharyngeal candidiasis. It has also been used for treatment of mucormycosis, although it is not FDA-approved for this use.
  - Each suspension dose should be administered with a full meal, liquid supplement, or acidic carbonated beverage (e.g., ginger ale). Acid-suppressive therapy may reduce absorption of the oral suspension, but not the DR tablets.
  - Rifabutin, phenytoin, and cimetidine reduce posaconazole concentrations and should not be used concomitantly.
  - Posaconazole increases bioavailability of cyclosporine, tacrolimus, and midazolam, necessitating dosage reductions of these agents. Dosage reduction of vinca alkaloids, statins, and calcium channel blockers should also be considered.
  - Terfenadine, astemizole, pimozide, cisapride, quinidine, and ergot alkaloids are contraindicated with posaconazole.

○ Therapeutic drug monitoring is recommended when using posaconazole at treatment doses. Doses should be adjusted to obtain a target trough of >1.25 µg/mL when used for active treatment.

• **Voriconazole** (loading dose of 6 mg/kg IV [two doses 12 h apart], followed by a maintenance dose of 4 mg/kg IV q12h or 200 mg PO q12h [100 mg PO q12h if <40 kg]) is a triazole antifungal with a wide range of activity against pathogenic fungi. It is active against all clinically important species of *Aspergillus*, as well as *Candida* (including most non-*albicans*), *Scedosporium apiospermum*, and *Fusarium* spp.

○ It is the treatment of choice for most forms of invasive aspergillosis, for which it demonstrates response rates of 40%–50% and superiority over conventional amphotericin B.

○ Voriconazole is extensively metabolized via the **CYP enzyme system**, including enzymes 2C19, 2C9, and 3A4, resulting in several **clinically significant drug interactions** that must be considered. In particular, rifampin, rifabutin, and carbamazepine (reduced drug levels), and sirolimus (increased drug levels) are contraindicated with voriconazole. Concomitantly administered cyclosporine, tacrolimus, and warfarin can be coadministered but require more careful monitoring.

○ Owing to extensive drug interactions and genetic variations in CYP2C19 metabolism, therapeutic drug monitoring is required to ensure safe and efficacious use of voriconazole. Doses should be titrated to achieve a steady-state trough of 1–5.5 µg/mL.

• **Isavuconazonium sulfate**, the prodrug of **isavuconazole** (372 mg isavuconazonium sulfate [equivalent to 200 mg isavuconazole] PO/IV q8h for 48 h, then 372 mg isavuconazonium sulfate [equivalent to 200 mg isavuconazole] PO/IV q24h), is an azole with broad-spectrum antifungal activity that is FDA-approved for treatment of invasive aspergillosis and invasive mucormycosis.

○ The oral formulation has a 98% oral bioavailability that is unaffected by food.

○ Unlike all other azoles, isavuconazole is not associated with QTc prolongation, but rather QTc shortening.

○ Rifampin, carbamazepine, long-acting barbiturates, and St. John's wort significantly reduce isavuconazole concentrations and are contraindicated.

○ High-dose ritonavir and ketoconazole can significantly increase isavuconazole concentrations and are contraindicated.

SPECIAL CONSIDERATIONS

Adverse effects of all azoles include nausea, diarrhea, and rash. Hepatitis is a rare but serious complication. LFTs should be monitored regularly with chronic use and especially with compromised liver function. Azoles can prolong the QTc interval (excluding isavuconazole) and should be avoided with concomitant QTc prolonging agents. The IV formulations of voriconazole and posaconazole should be used with caution in patients with a CrCl <50 mL/min due to theoretical risk cyclodextrin vehicle accumulation. Voriconazole can commonly cause transient visual disturbances and hallucinations with high trough concentration, as well as phototoxicity. **This class of antibiotics has major drug interactions.**

Echinocandins

GENERAL PRINCIPLES

This class of antifungals inhibits the enzyme (1,3)-β-D-glucan synthase that is essential in fungal cell wall synthesis.

TREATMENT

- **Caspofungin acetate** (70 mg IV loading dose, followed by 50 mg IV q24h) has fungicidal activity against most *Aspergillus* and *Candida* spp., including azole-resistant *Candida* strains. Caspofungin does not have activity against *Cryptococcus, Histoplasma, Blastomyces, Coccidioides*, or Mucorales. It is FDA-approved for treatment of candidemia and refractory invasive aspergillosis and as empiric therapy in febrile neutropenia.

  Metabolism is primarily hepatic, although the CYP enzyme system is not significantly involved. An increased maintenance dosage is necessary with the use of drugs that induce hepatic metabolism (e.g., efavirenz, nelfinavir, phenytoin, rifampin, carbamazepine, dexamethasone). The maintenance dose should be reduced to 35 mg for patients with moderate hepatic impairment; however, no dose adjustment is necessary for renal failure.

- **Micafungin sodium** (50–150 mg IV q24h) is used for candidemia, esophageal candidiasis, and as fungal prophylaxis for patients undergoing hematopoietic stem cell transplantation. The spectrum of activity is similar to that of anidulafungin and caspofungin. There may be clinically insignificant increases in serum concentrations of sirolimus and nifedipine. Micafungin may increase cyclosporine concentrations in about 20% of patients. No change in dosing is necessary in renal or hepatic dysfunction.

- **Anidulafungin** (100–200 mg IV loading dose, followed by 50–100 mg IV q24h) is useful for treatment of candidemia and other systemic *Candida* infections (intra-abdominal abscess and peritonitis) as well as esophageal candidiasis. The spectrum of activity is similar to that of caspofungin and micafungin. Anidulafungin is not a substrate inhibitor or inducer of CYP isoenzymes and does not have clinically relevant drug interactions. No dosage change is necessary in renal or hepatic insufficiency.

SPECIAL CONSIDERATIONS

Adverse events: Fever, rash, nausea, elevated LFTs, histamine-related reactions, phlebitis at the injection site, and delirium are possible but infrequent adverse reactions.

Miscellaneous

- **Flucytosine** (25 mg/kg PO q6h) exerts its fungicidal effects on susceptible *Candida* and *Cryptococcus* species by interfering with DNA synthesis. Main clinical uses are in the treatment of cryptococcal meningitis and severe *Candida* infections in combination with amphotericin B, which results in synergy. This agent should not be used as monotherapy, apart from treatment of fluconazole-resistant *Candida* cystitis, because of risk for rapid emergence of resistance.
  - **Adverse events** include dose-related bone marrow suppression and bloody diarrhea due to intestinal flora conversion of flucytosine to 5-fluorouracil.
  - Peak drug concentrations, drawn 1 hour after oral administration, should be kept between 50 and 100 μg/mL. Close monitoring of serum concentrations and dose adjustments are critical in the setting of renal insufficiency. LFTs should be obtained at least once weekly.

- **Terbinafine** (250 mg PO q24h for 6–12 wk) is an allylamine antifungal agent that kills fungi by inhibiting ergosterol synthesis. It is FDA-approved for the treatment of onychomycosis of the fingernails (6 wk of treatment) or toenails (12 wk of treatment). It is not generally used for systemic infections.

  Adverse events include headache, GI disturbances, rash, LFT abnormalities, and taste disturbances. This drug should not be used in patients with hepatic cirrhosis or a CrCl of <50 mL/min. It does not significantly inhibit the metabolism of cyclosporine (15% decrease) or warfarin.

16 Sexually Transmitted Infections, Human Immunodeficiency Virus, and Acquired Immunodeficiency Syndrome

Joseph N. Cherabie, Rachel M. Presti, and Hilary E. L. Reno

SEXUAL HISTORY AND GENDER-AFFIRMING CARE

Taking a Sexual History

- A sexual history should be taken during initial and subsequent primary care visits, preventive exams, or when signs or symptoms of a sexually transmitted infection (STI) are present as part of the routine medical examination.
- Providers should discuss: partners (number and gender identity), types of sexual practices, use of protection from STIs, history of previous STIs, and pregnancy preferences.
- Providers should use inclusive language without making assumptions. An example opening line is, "What are the genders of your sexual partners?"

Transgender Medicine

GENERAL PRINCIPLES

Transgender is an umbrella term used to describe people with a gender identity that differs from the sex that they were assigned at birth. Transgender medicine is aimed at addressing and minimizing disparities in care for transgender and nonbinary people. In the field of HIV and STIs, providing gender-affirming care is especially important for the health of transgender and nonbinary persons.

Definition

- Gender, gender identity: one's self identification as male or female with influence of societal structures, cultural expectations, and personal interactions.
- Sex: assigned at birth based on appearance of external genitalia.
- Gender expression: the manner in which an individual expresses their gender.

- Sexual orientation: enduring sexual attraction to male partners, female partners, transgender partners, gender diverse partners, or some/all.
- Gender diverse/nonbinary: individuals who do not identify with the gender binary (e.g., male or female).
- Pronouns: words used to refer to individuals based on their identity; one example of gender-neutral pronouns is the singular they/them/their pronouns instead of he/him/his.

Epidemiology

- It is estimated that transgender people represent 0.6% of the US population.
- In national surveys, as many as one-third of transgender people postpone medical care because of concerns of disrespect, discrimination, or lack of access to knowledgeable providers.
- Transgender people have a much higher prevalence of HIV than the general population, with transgender individuals having a 13× greater risk of HIV than the adult population globally. According to current estimates in the United States, 42% of transgender women are living with HIV, and 62% of Black/African American transgender women are living with HIV.[1]

MANAGEMENT

- A safe and welcoming environment should be provided through staff training, knowledge of terminology, gender-neutral bathrooms, and changes to medical forms to include gender assessment questions as recommended by the Williams Institute in their Best Practices Guide.[2]
- Assumptions about gender, sexual orientation, sexual practices, or pronouns should not be made and each patient should be individually assessed for vulnerability to HIV and STIs.
- For more resources about transgender health care, look at the WPATH guidelines, the UCSF's Center of Excellence for Transgender Health, and Fenway Health's National LGBT Health Education Center.
  - WPATH: https://www.wpath.org/publications/soc
  - UCSF Center of Excellence for Transgender Health: http://transhealth.ucsf.edu/protocols
  - National LGBT Health Education Center: https://www.lgbthealtheducation.org

SEXUALLY TRANSMITTED INFECTIONS: ULCERATIVE DISEASES

Current STI treatment guidelines are found at www.cdc.gov/std. Treatment options for each infection can be found in Table 16-1.

Genital Herpes

GENERAL PRINCIPLES

Genital herpes is caused by **herpes simplex virus (HSV)**, types 1 and 2, usually type 2. The proportion of herpes caused by HSV-1 continues to increase among women and men who have sex with men (MSM). HSV-2 is more likely to recur and may require suppressive therapy.

TABLE 16-1	Treatment of Sexually Transmitted Infections	
Infection	**Recommended Regimen(s)**	**Alternative Regimens and Notes**
Genital ulcer disease		
Herpes simplex		
First episode	• Acyclovir 400 mg PO three times a day × 7–10 d • Valacyclovir 1 g PO two times a day × 7–10 d • Famciclovir 250 mg PO three times a day × 7–10 d	
Recurrent episodes	• Acyclovir 800 mg two times a day × 5 d or 800 mg PO three times a day × 2 d • Valacyclovir 1 g PO once a day × 5 d or 500 mg PO two times a day × 3 d • Famciclovir 1 g PO two times a day × 1 d or 125 mg PO two times a day × 5 d or 500 mg once, then 250 mg two times a day × 2 d	In patients with HIV: • Acyclovir 400 mg PO three times a day × 5–10 d • Valacyclovir 1 g PO twice a day × 5–10 d • Famciclovir 500 mg PO twice a day × 5–10 d
Suppressive therapy	• Acyclovir 400 mg PO twice a day • Valacyclovir 500 mg or 1 g PO once daily • Famciclovir 250 mg PO twice daily	In patients with HIV: • Acyclovir 400–800 mg PO twice to three times a day • Valacyclovir 500 mg PO twice a day • Famciclovir 500 mg PO twice a day
Syphilis		
Primary, secondary, or nonprimary, nonsecondary syphilis <1 y	• Benzathine penicillin G 2.4 million units IM single dose	Penicillin-allergic: • Doxycycline 100 mg PO twice daily × 14 d
Syphilis of unknown duration or late >1 y, tertiary	• Benzathine penicillin G 2.4 million units IM once weekly × 3 doses	• Doxycycline 100 mg PO twice daily × 28 d
Neurosyphilis	• Aqueous crystalline penicillin G 18–24 million U/d (as 3–4 million units every 4 h or continuous infusion) × 10–14 d	• Procaine penicillin 2.4 million units IM once daily + probenecid 500 mg PO four times daily × 10–14 d
Pregnancy	• Penicillin is the recommended treatment—desensitize if necessary	

(continued)

TABLE 16-1	Treatment of Sexually Transmitted Infections (*continued*)	
Infection	Recommended Regimen(s)	Alternative Regimens and Notes
Chancroid	• Azithromycin 1 g PO single dose • Ceftriaxone 250 mg IM single dose	• Ciprofloxacin 500 mg PO twice daily × 3 d • Erythromycin base 500 mg PO twice daily × 7 d • Some resistance has been reported for these regimens
Lymphogranuloma venereum	• Doxycycline 100 mg PO twice daily × 21 d	• Erythromycin base 500 mg PO four times a day × 21 d • Azithromycin 1 g PO weekly × 3 weeks and test of cure 4 weeks after treatment
Vaginitis/vaginosis		
Trichomonas	• Metronidazole 500 mg PO twice a day × 7 days	• Tinidazole 2 g PO single dose
For people with a penis with trichomonas	• Metronidazole 2 g PO × 1	
Bacterial vaginosis	• Metronidazole 500 mg PO twice daily × 7 d • Clindamycin cream 2% intra-vaginal at bedtime × 7 d • Metronidazole gel 0.75% intravaginal once a day for 5 d	• Tinidazole 2 g PO once daily × 2 d or 1 g PO once daily × 5 d • Clindamycin 300 mg PO twice daily × 7 d • Clindamycin ovules 100 mg intravaginal × 3 d • Secnidazole 2 g oral granules × 1 dose
Candidiasis	• Intravaginal azoles in variety of strengths for 1–7 d • Fluconazole 150 mg PO × 1	
Severe candidiasis	• Fluconazole 150 mg PO every 72 h × 2–3 doses	• Intravaginal azoles for 7–14 d • Culture and sensitivi-ties may be helpful
Recurrent candidi-asis (four or more episodes in a year)	• Fluconazole 100, 150, or 200 mg PO every 72 h × 7–14 d followed by once weekly × 6 mo	

TABLE 16-1	Treatment of Sexually Transmitted Infections *(continued)*	
Infection	**Recommended Regimen(s)**	**Alternative Regimens and Notes**
Urethritis/cervicitis		
Gonorrhea	• Ceftriaxone 500 mg IM once + doxycycline 100 mg PO twice daily × 7 d if *Chlamydia trachomatis* not ruled out. If testing for *C. trachomatis* is negative no need for concurrent treatment • Azithromycin 1 g PO once is alternative treatment for concurrent *C. trachomatis* infection	• Gentamicin 240 mg IM + azithromycin 2 g PO once • Cefixime 800 mg PO × 1 + doxycycline 100 mg PO twice daily × 7 d if chlamydia not excluded • Oral cephalosporin treatment is not recommended as long as ceftriaxone is available
Disseminated gonococcal infection	• Ceftriaxone 1 g IM or IV daily • Can switch to PO after 24–48 h if substantial improvement, treat for at least 7 d	• Cefotaxime 1 g IV every 8 h • Ceftizoxime 1 g IV every 8 h + azithromycin 1 g PO × 1
Chlamydia	• Doxycycline 100 mg PO twice daily × 7 d	• Azithromycin 1 g PO once (less efficacious in rectal infections) • Levofloxacin 500 mg PO daily × 7 d or ofloxacin 300 mg PO twice daily × 7 d • Retesting is recommended in 3 mo
Mycoplasma genitalium	• If macrolide resistance testing not available, doxycycline 100 mg PO twice daily × 7 d, followed by moxifloxacin 400 mg PO daily × 7 d • If macrolide resistance testing available, doxycycline 100 mg PO twice daily × 7 d then azithromycin 1 g PO × 1 followed by 500 mg PO × 3 d (macrolide sensitive) or moxifloxacin 400 mg PO × 7 d (macrolide resistant)	

(continued)

CHAPTER 16

TABLE 16-1	Treatment of Sexually Transmitted Infections (*continued*)	
Infection	**Recommended Regimen(s)**	**Alternative Regimens and Notes**
Pelvic inflammatory disease		
Outpatient	• Ceftriaxone 500 mg IM once + doxycycline 100 mg PO twice daily × 14 d + metronidazole 500 mg orally twice daily × 14 d	• Cefoxitin 2 g IM + probenecid 1 g PO once can be substituted for ceftriaxone
Inpatient	• Ceftriaxone 1 g IV, cefoxitin 2 g IV every 6 h, or cefotetan 2 g IV every 12 h + doxycycline 100 mg PO twice daily × 14 d + metronidazole 500 mg PO or IV twice daily × 14 d	• Clindamycin 900 mg IV every 8 h + gentamicin 2 mg/kg loading dose, then 1.5 mg/kg every 8 h • Ampicillin–sulbactam 3 g IV every 6 h + doxycycline 100 mg IV then PO twice daily × 14 d

See *cdc.gov/std/* for the current sexually transmitted infection treatment guidelines.

DIAGNOSIS

- Infection is characterized by painful grouped vesicles in the genital and perianal regions that rapidly ulcerate and form shallow tender lesions.
- The initial episode may be associated with inguinal adenopathy, fever, headache, myalgias, and aseptic meningitis; recurrences are usually less severe. Highest rates of transmission are with active lesions; however, asymptomatic shedding of virus is frequent and can lead to transmission.
- Confirmation of HSV infection requires culture or polymerase chain reaction (PCR). Clinical presentation is often adequate for diagnosis.

Syphilis

GENERAL PRINCIPLES

- Syphilis is caused by the spirochete *Treponema pallidum*.
- There is a high rate of HIV coinfection in patients with syphilis, from 40% to 70%, and HIV infection should be excluded with appropriate testing.[2]
- Syphilis can have an atypical course in HIV-infected patients; treatment failures and progression to neurosyphilis are more frequent in this population.
- Syphilis rates in the United States are increasing since the year 2000, especially among MSM.

DIAGNOSIS

Clinical Presentation

- **Primary syphilis** develops within several weeks of exposure and manifests as one or more painless, indurated, superficial ulcerations (chancre).
- **Secondary syphilis** develops 2–10 weeks after the chancre resolves and may produce a rash (usually involves palms and soles), mucocutaneous lesions, adenopathy, and constitutional symptoms.
- **Tertiary syphilis** follows between 1 and 20 years after infection and includes cardiovascular and gummatous disease.
- **Neurologic syphilis** (general paresis, tabes dorsalis, meningovascular, ocular, or otologic syphilis) is usually a late manifestation, but can occur earlier. Ocular syphilis can occur with any stage of syphilis, is increasingly common, and can lead to blindness. Eye manifestations of syphilis include uveitis and retinitis. All patients with syphilis should be evaluated for eye complaints as well as neurological complaints. Otosyphilis is also increasing in prevalence.[3]
- **Congenital syphilis** occurs by vertical transmission from infected mothers and results in stillbirth in up to 40% of pregnancies and has increased by 279% from 2015 to 2019.[4] Infected neonates may develop fetal hydrops, rash, hepatomegaly, myocarditis, neurologic disease, and other varied presentations.

Diagnostic Testing

- In **primary syphilis**, dark-field microscopy of lesion exudates, when available, may reveal spirochetes. A nontreponemal serologic test (e.g., rapid plasma reagin [RPR] or Venereal Disease Research Laboratory [VDRL]) should be confirmed with a treponemal-specific test (e.g., fluorescent treponemal antibody absorption or *T. pallidum* particle agglutination).
- Reverse sequence testing (measuring an enzyme-linked immunosorbent assay or multiplex flow immunoassay before a quantitative RPR) is used by some jurisdictions and may detect early primary syphilis that may otherwise be missed with traditional screening.
- Diagnosis of **secondary syphilis** is made on the basis of positive serologic studies and the presence of a compatible clinical illness.
- **Syphilis, early nonprimary, nonsecondary** is a serologic diagnosis in the absence of symptoms when the patient has been serologically positive for <1 year.
- **Syphilis of unknown duration or latent syphilis** is a serologic diagnosis in the absence of symptoms when the patient has been serologically positive for >1 year or for unknown duration.
- To exclude **neurosyphilis**, a lumbar puncture (LP) should be performed in all patients with neurologic symptoms. For patients with ophthalmic or otosyphilis, LP is indicated if they also have other neurological signs or symptoms. Additionally, some experts recommend LP in patients living with HIV (PLWH) with evidence of tertiary disease, treatment failure, or late syphilis; however, treatment based on abnormal LP findings in the absence of signs or symptoms of neurosyphilis in PLWH and clinical outcomes are not improved.[5] VDRL should be performed on cerebrospinal fluid (CSF), although sensitivity is low and a negative VDRL does not rule out neurosyphilis.
- Response to treatment should be monitored with nontreponemal serologic tests at 3, 6, and 12 months after treatment. In patients with HIV, tests should be checked every 3 months after treatment for 1 year. Inadequate treatment response after

treatment is defined as a lack of fourfold decline in RPR titer at 12 months after primary, secondary or early latent syphilis, or at 24 months after late latent or syphilis of unknown duration.

- For neurosyphilis, no need for repeat CSF exam at 6 months if adequate RPR response and no neurological signs or symptoms are present.

Chancroid

GENERAL PRINCIPLES

Chancroid is caused by *Haemophilus ducreyi*.

DIAGNOSIS

- Chancroid produces a painful genital ulcer and tender suppurative inguinal lymphadenopathy.
- Identification of the organism is difficult and requires special culture media.

Lymphogranuloma Venereum

GENERAL PRINCIPLES

Lymphogranuloma venereum is caused by *Chlamydia trachomatis* (serovars L_1, L_2, or L_3).

DIAGNOSIS

- It manifests as a painless genital ulcer, followed by heaped up, matted inguinal lymphadenopathy. Proctocolitis with pain and discharge can occur with anal infection and has been increasingly seen in the United States.[6,7]
- The diagnosis is based on clinical suspicion and *C. trachomatis* nucleic acid antibody testing (NAAT), if available.

SEXUALLY TRANSMITTED INFECTIONS: VAGINITIS AND VAGINOSIS

Trichomoniasis

DIAGNOSIS

Clinical Presentation

- Clinical symptoms of infection by *Trichomonas vaginalis* include malodorous purulent vaginal discharge, dysuria, and genital inflammation.
- Examination reveals profuse frothy discharge and cervical petechiae.
- *T. vaginalis* is often asymptomatic, especially in males.

Diagnostic Testing

- NAATs and antigen detection tests are available to detect *T. vaginalis* and offer improved sensitivity over the traditional visualization of motile trichomonads on a saline wet mount of vaginal discharge.
- Elevated vaginal pH (≥4.5) is usually seen.

Bacterial Vaginosis

GENERAL PRINCIPLES

The replacement of normal lactobacilli with anaerobic bacteria in the vagina leads to bacterial vaginosis (BV). Although not sexually transmitted, BV increases risk of STI and HIV infections.

DIAGNOSIS

Three of the following criteria are needed to make the diagnosis (Amsel criteria):
- Homogenous, thin, white discharge
- Presence of clue cells on microscopic examination
- Elevated vaginal pH (≥4.5)
- Fishy odor associated with vaginal discharge before or after addition of 10% potassium hydroxide (KOH) (whiff test)

Vulvovaginal Candidiasis

GENERAL PRINCIPLES

Vulvovaginal candidiasis is not generally considered an STI but commonly develops in the setting of antibiotic therapy. Recurrent infections may be a presenting manifestation of unrecognized HIV infection.

DIAGNOSIS

- Thick, cottage cheese–like vaginal discharge in conjunction with intense vulvar inflammation, pruritus, and dysuria is often present.
- Vaginal pH is normal.
- Definitive diagnosis requires visualization of fungal elements on a KOH preparation of the vaginal discharge.

TREATMENT

- Therapy is often initiated on the basis of the clinical presentation.
- Fluconazole failure may indicate the presence of a **non–*Candida albicans* species.**

Cervicitis/Urethritis

GENERAL PRINCIPLES

Cervicitis and urethritis are frequent presentations of infection with ***Neisseria gonorrhoeae* or *C. trachomatis***, and occasionally *Mycoplasma genitalium*, *Neisseria meningitidis*, and *T. vaginalis*. These infections often coexist, and clinical presentations can be identical.

DIAGNOSIS

Clinical Presentation

- People with a vagina presenting with urethritis, cervicitis, or both complain of mucopurulent vaginal discharge, dyspareunia, and dysuria.
- People with a penis presenting with urethritis may have dysuria and purulent penile discharge.
- Most infections are asymptomatic.
- Disseminated gonococcal infection (DGI) can present with fever, tenosynovitis, vesicopustular skin lesions, and polyarthralgias. DGI may also manifest solely as septic arthritis of the knee, wrist, or ankle (see Chapter 25, Arthritis and Rheumatologic Diseases).
- If urethritis or cervicitis is persistent, consider *M. genitalium*.

Diagnostic Testing

- A NAAT performed on endocervical, vaginal, urethral (men), urine, or extragenital samples is recommended to make the diagnosis of *C. trachomatis* or *N. gonorrhoeae* infection. In the case of *N. gonorrhoeae*, a Gram stain of endocervical or urethral discharge with gram-negative intracellular diplococci can rapidly establish the diagnosis. Of note, *N. meningitidis* may appear similar on gram stain but will have negative NAAT for *N. gonorrhoeae*. Culture can be performed on urethral or endocervical swab specimens.
- Recommendations for testing include NAAT testing at extragenital sites of sexual contact (pharynx, rectum), especially in MSM and transgender persons. Not testing all exposed sites misses the majority of infections in certain populations.
- In addition to NAAT studies, patients with suspected DGI should have blood cultures drawn. In the setting of septic arthritis, synovial fluid analysis and culture is indicated.
- NAATs for *M. genitalium are* available and should be considered for persistent urethritis/cervicitis following proper testing and treatment for *C. trachomatis*.

TREATMENT

Because of increasing resistance concerns, treatment options for *N. gonorrhoeae* infection are reduced (see Table 16-1).

Pelvic Inflammatory Disease

GENERAL PRINCIPLES

Pelvic inflammatory disease (PID) is an upper genital tract infection in women, usually preceded by cervicitis. Long-term consequences of untreated PID include chronic pain, increased risk of ectopic pregnancy, and infertility.

DIAGNOSIS

Clinical Presentation

Symptoms can range from mild pelvic discomfort and dyspareunia to severe abdominal pain with fever, which may signal complicating perihepatitis (Fitz-Hugh–Curtis syndrome) or tubo-ovarian abscess.

Diagnostic Testing

- Cervical motion tenderness or uterine or adnexal tenderness, vaginal discharge or friability, and the presence of many white blood cells per low-power field on a saline preparation of vaginal or endocervical fluid are consistent with a diagnosis of PID.
- NAATs or culture of endocervical specimens should be obtained to identify *C. trachomatis* or *N. gonorrhoeae* infection.
- All women diagnosed with PID should be screened for HIV infection.

TREATMENT

Severely ill, pregnant, and HIV-infected women with PID should be hospitalized. Patients unable to tolerate oral antibiotics also warrant admission. See Table 16-1.

HUMAN IMMUNODEFICIENCY VIRUS AND ACQUIRED IMMUNODEFICIENCY SYNDROME

HIV Type 1

GENERAL PRINCIPLES

Definition

HIV type 1 is a retrovirus that predominantly infects lymphocytes that bear the CD4 surface protein, as well as coreceptors belonging to the chemokine receptor family (CCR5 or CXCR4), which, if left untreated, can cause AIDS.

Classification

Diagnosis of AIDS by the Centers for Disease Control and Prevention (CDC) classification is made on the basis of CD4 cell count <200 cells/μL, CD4 percentage <14%, or development of one of the 25 AIDS-defining conditions.[8]

Epidemiology

- HIV type 1 is common throughout the world. By the most recent estimates, over 38 million people worldwide are living with HIV or AIDS, with a significant burden of disease in sub-Saharan Africa.[9]
- In the United States, 1.2 million people are estimated to be infected with HIV with 14% of these people unaware of their infection. The CDC estimates there are nearly 40,000 new infections in the United States every year.
- Despite comprising only 14% of the population in the United States, African Americans account for nearly 42% of all new cases of HIV in this country. Hispanics are also disproportionately affected by HIV representing 27% of new HIV diagnoses. Women comprise approximately 19% of new HIV infections.[10]

- MSM remains the population most heavily affected by HIV in the United States. Of all new HIV infections in 2009, 69% were MSM.[11]
- **HIV type 2** is endemic to regions in West Africa. It is characterized by much slower progression to AIDS and intrinsic resistance to non-nucleoside reverse transcriptase inhibitors (NNRTIs).

Pathophysiology

- After entering the host cell, viral RNA is reverse transcribed into DNA using the HIV **reverse transcriptase.** This viral DNA is inserted into the host genome through the activity of the viral **integrase.** The host cell machinery is then used to produce the relevant viral proteins, which are appropriately truncated by a viral **protease.** Infectious viral particles bud away to infect other CD4 lymphocytes.
- Most infected cells are killed by the host CD8 T-cell response.
- Long-lived latently infected cells persist, especially memory T cells.
- Infection usually leads to CD4 T-cell depletion and **impaired cell-mediated immunity** over a period of 8–10 years.
- Without treatment, >90% of infected patients will progress to AIDS, which is characterized by the development of opportunistic infections (OIs), wasting, and viral-associated malignancies.

Risk Factors

- The virus is primarily transmitted sexually but also via parenteral and perinatal exposure.
- The risk of transmission is low through blood transfusions (1 in 1.4 million). Sharing needles or needlestick injuries result in transmission in 50 per 10,000 exposures.
- Among sexual practices, unprotected anal receptive intercourse carries the highest risk of transmission (138 per 10,000 exposures), followed by insertive anal intercourse, vaginal receptive intercourse, and vaginal insertive intercourse. Oral intercourse carries a low risk of transmission.

Prevention

- HIV transmission can be prevented by multiple prevention methods including regular condom use (internal or external) for vaginal, oral, and anal intercourse, HIV pre- and postexposure prophylaxis, and needle and syringe programs.
- Postexposure prophylaxis (PEP), or the provision of antiretroviral therapy (ART) after needlestick injury or high-risk sexual exposure, can prevent infection. Regimens normally consist of two to three ART drugs taken over 28-day course.
- Preexposure prophylaxis (PrEP), or continuous ART in HIV-negative patients, has proven to decrease the rate of HIV transmission. The current guidelines recommend the use of PrEP for the following high-risk groups:[12]
  ○ MSM
  ○ Heterosexual HIV-discordant couples
  ○ Those with multiple sexual partners with inconsistent condom use
  ○ Commercial sex workers
  ○ IV drug users
  ○ A combination of emtricitabine–tenofovir disoproxil fumarate (TDF/FTC) was the first approved regimen for PrEP. Emtricitabine–tenofovir alafenamide (TAF/FTC) has been recently approved by the U.S. Food and Drug Administration (FDA) and has better renal and bone side effect profile. Before starting PrEP, it is essential to document a negative HIV test, no signs or symptoms of acute HIV infection, hepatitis B status (if positive, stopping PrEP can cause fulminant

hepatitis and death), and normal renal function. These patients should be followed every 3 months for repeat HIV testing as well as STI screening, risk reduction counseling, and every 6 months monitoring of renal function.

DIAGNOSIS

Clinical Presentation

- Acute retroviral syndrome is experienced by up to 75% of patients and is similar to other acute viral illnesses such as infectious mononucleosis due to Epstein–Barr virus (EBV) or cytomegalovirus (CMV) infection. Common presenting symptoms of acute retroviral syndrome are fever, sore throat, nonspecific rash, myalgias, headache, and fatigue.
- As the acute illness resolves spontaneously, many people present to care only after OIs (see later section for clinical presentations) occur late in infection once significant immune compromise has occurred (CD4 count <200 cells/µL). Late presentation can be avoided by routine screening.

History

Initial evaluation of persons with a confirmed HIV infection should include the following measures:
- Complete history with emphasis on previous OIs, viral coinfections, and other complications.
- Psychological and psychiatric history. Depression and substance use are common and should be identified and treated as necessary.
- Family and social support assessment.
- Assessment of knowledge and perceptions regarding HIV is also crucial to initiate ongoing education regarding the nature and ramifications of HIV infection.

Physical Examination

A complete physical examination is important to evaluate for manifestations of immune compromise. Initial findings may include the following:
- Oral findings: thrush (oral candidiasis), hairy leukoplakia, aphthous ulcers
- Lymphatic system: generalized lymphadenopathy
- Skin: psoriasis, seborrheic dermatitis, eosinophilic folliculitis, Kaposi sarcoma, molluscum contagiosum, *Cryptococcus*
- Abdominal examination: evidence of hepatosplenomegaly
- Genital examination: presence of ulcers, genital warts, vaginal discharge, and rectal discharge
- Neurologic examination: presence of sensory deficits and cognitive testing

Diagnostic Criteria

- The updated CDC guidelines for laboratory screening published in 2017 recommend the use of the fourth-generation assay, an antigen/antibody test that involves the detection of the p24 antigen as well as antibodies to HIV-1 and HIV-2. The p24 antigen is a viral capsid protein that can be detected as early as 4–10 days from acute infection, up to 2 weeks earlier than the antibody tests alone. An eclipse phase of infection, during which no testing is positive, still exists for up to 7 days after exposure.
- If the fourth-generation assay is positive, then a differentiation test for HIV-1 and HIV-2 antibodies is performed as a reflex test.

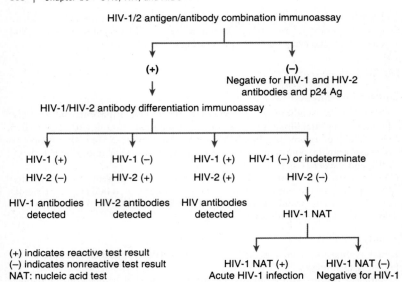

Figure 16-1. Recommended laboratory HIV testing algorithm for serum or plasma specimens. (From Centers for Disease Control and Prevention. *Laboratory Testing for the Diagnosis of HIV Infection: Updated Recommendations.* https://stacks.cdc.gov/view/cdc/50872.)

- If the HIV-1 and HIV-2 antibody differentiation test is negative for both HIV-1 and HIV-2, then nucleic acid amplification testing (NAAT) of HIV-1 RNA via PCR should be performed (Figure 16-1). If the NAAT is positive, this indicates acute infection. Viral loads during acute infection are typically in the range of several million copies per milliliter, so a viral load <1000 copies/mL should be repeated to confirm infection.

Diagnostic Testing

The CDC recommends that **all persons age 13–64 years be offered HIV testing in all health-care settings using an opt-out format.**[13]

- **Persons at high risk should be screened for HIV infection at least annually. High-risk groups include** IV drug users, MSM, sexual partners of a known HIV patient, persons involved in sex trading and their sexual partners, persons with STIs, persons who have multiple sexual partners or who engage in unprotected intercourse, persons who consider themselves at risk, and persons with findings that are suggestive of HIV infection. More frequent screening (every 3–6 months) is sometimes indicated.
- Other groups for whom HIV testing is indicated are:
  - Pregnant women (opt-out screening)
  - Patients with active tuberculosis (TB)
  - Donors of blood, semen, and organs
  - Persons with occupational exposures (e.g., needlesticks) and source patients of the exposures

Laboratories

- **Complete blood count** and **comprehensive metabolic panel** with assessment of liver and kidney parameters, as well as **urinalysis** to evaluate for proteinuria and glycosuria.
- **CD4 cell count** (normal range, 600–1500 cells/µL) and CD4 percentage. Significant immune deficiency requiring prophylactic antibiotics occurs with CD4 <200 cells/µL.
- **Virologic markers:** Plasma HIV RNA predicts the rate of disease progression.
- **Fasting lipid panel:** HIV is associated with an increased risk of metabolic syndrome and cardiovascular disease. Lipids can be affected by several antiretrovirals.
- **Hemoglobin A1c** as HIV as well as ART can have effects on blood glucose metabolism and lead to higher rates of diabetes.
- **TB testing by interferon-γ release assay.**
- **Syphilis screening by the traditional or reverse algorithms.**
- **Hepatitis A, B (HBsAg, HBsAb, HBcAb), and C serologies.**
- **Chlamydia/gonococcal urine/cervical NAAT** for all patients. If patients report receptive anal sex, **rectal NAATs for gonorrhea and *Chlamydia*** are recommended. For those reporting receptive oral sex, **pharyngeal NAAT for gonorrhea** should be obtained.
- **Cervical Papanicolaou smear** (most commonly using the thin prep method).
- **HIV drug resistance testing** for reverse transcriptase and protease genes at baseline and with treatment failure. Integrase gene resistance testing should be performed for those failing integrase inhibitor–based regimens.
- **HLA B5701** for patients in whom one is considering the use of abacavir.
- **CCR5** tropism testing for patients in whom one is considering the use of maraviroc.
- **Glucose-6-phosphate dehydrogenase (G6PD) level** on initiation of care or before starting therapy with an oxidant drug in those with a predisposing ethnic background.

TREATMENT

Immunizations

- From "Primary Care Guidelines for the Management of Persons Infected with Human Immunodeficiency Virus: 2020 Update by the HIV Medicine Association of the Infectious Diseases Society of America."[14]
- Antibody response to vaccines is improved with undetectable HIV viral load and higher CD4 count.
- For a list of recommended vaccinations and indications, please refer to the *Washington Manual of Outpatient Internal Medicine*.

Medications
ART

- **Current recommendations from the International AIDS Society-USA** for the initiation of ART are to treat everyone infected with HIV, regardless of CD4 count.[15]
- In the case of patients with TB or cryptococcal meningitis, ART initiation may be slightly delayed to reduce the risk of immune reconstitution inflammatory syndrome (IRIS).
- Treatment decisions should be individualized by patient readiness, drug interactions, adherence issues, drug toxicities, comorbidities, and the level of risk indicated by CD4 T-cell counts.

- People who could become pregnant, especially if pregnant, should receive optimal ART to reduce the risk of vertical transmission.
- Maximal and durable suppression of HIV replication is the goal of therapy once it is initiated. **ART** should be individualized and closely monitored by measuring plasma HIV viral load. Reductions in plasma viremia correlate with increased CD4 cell counts and prolonged AIDS-free survival. Isolated viral "blips" (<200 copies/mL) are not indicative of virologic failure, but confirmed virologic rebound should trigger an evaluation of adherence, drug interactions, and viral resistance.
- Once viral suppression is obtained, risk for transmission to serodiscordant partner is nearly zero, leading to the new phrase "undetectable = untransmittable".
- Any change in ART increases future therapeutic constraints and potential drug resistance.
- **Antiretroviral drugs:** Approved antiretroviral drugs are grouped into five categories. Experts currently recommend using three active drugs from at least two different classes to maximally and durably suppress HIV viremia.
  - **Nucleotide and nucleoside reverse transcriptase inhibitors (NRTIs)** constrain HIV replication by incorporating into the elongating strand of DNA, causing chain termination. All nucleoside analogs have been associated with **lactic acidosis**, presumably related to mitochondrial toxicity, although current recommended NRTIs have low incidence.
  - **Non-nucleoside reverse transcriptase inhibitors (NNRTIs)** inhibit HIV by binding noncompetitively to the reverse transcriptase. Side effects of NNRTIs include rash, hepatotoxicity, and Stevens–Johnson syndrome (more likely with nevirapine). Central nervous system (CNS) side effects are commonly experienced with the use of efavirenz.
  - **Integrase strand transfer inhibitors (INSTIs)** target DNA strand transfer and integration into a human genome. They tend to have better safety and tolerability profiles than other classes and are associated with a rapid decrease in viral load after initiation. However, in mid-2018, the FDA and the World Health Organization announced that cases of neural tube defects have been reported in babies of women with HIV who were on treatment with dolutegravir at the time of conception. The information comes from an interim analysis of an observational study of ART in Botswana. At the time of this writing, the CDC recommends that alternative regimens be considered in women of childbearing age and women be appropriately counseled. Raltegravir is the only other INSTI for which there are data on pregnant women, and higher rates of birth defects were not seen. Elvitegravir requires coadministration of the pharmacologic booster, cobicistat, which leads to increased incidence of gastrointestinal (GI) intolerance. Integrase inhibitors have also been associated with increased weight gain in recent studies, most evident with dolutegravir and bictegravir, especially among women and people of African descent. Because of its interaction with the cytochrome P450 system, **cobicistat has important drug interactions** that should be evaluated. Cabotegravir is available as a long-acting injectable ART. Few drug interactions exist with the other INSTIs: raltegravir, dolutegravir, and bictegravir.
  - **Protease inhibitors (PIs)** block the action of the viral protease required for protein processing late in the viral cycle. GI intolerance is one of the most commonly encountered adverse effects. These agents have also been associated with metabolic abnormalities such as glucose intolerance, increased cholesterol and triglycerides, and body fat redistribution. Boosting with ritonavir or cobicistat is a common practice to achieve better therapeutic concentrations. Owing to its metabolism via

cytochrome P450, **boosted PIs have important drug interactions,** and concomitant medications should be reviewed carefully.

- ○ **HIV entry inhibitors** target different stages of the HIV entry process. Two drugs are available in this class. **Enfuvirtide (T-20)** is a fusion inhibitor that prevents the fusion of the virus into the host cell. T-20 is only available for use as an SC injection, 90 mg bid. The most frequent side effect for T-20 is a significant local site reaction after the injection. **Maraviroc** is a CCR5 receptor blocker. Initiation of CCR5 inhibitor requires baseline determination of HIV coreceptor tropism (CCR5 or CXCR4).

- **Initial therapy:** ART should be started in an outpatient setting by a physician with expertise in the management of HIV infection. Adherence is the key factor for success. Treatment should be individualized and adapted to the patient's lifestyle and comorbidities. Any treatment decision influences future therapeutic options because of the possibility of drug cross-resistance. **Potent initial ART generally consists of a combination of two NRTIs, plus usually an NNRTI, an INSTI, or a boosted PI. INSTI-based regimens are optimal for initial therapy and are preferred. It should be noted that many of the first-line regimens are coformulated as single-tablet daily regimens. TAF is a new formulation of TDF that is less likely to cause renal toxicity or bone mineral density issues but may be linked to increased weight gain and blood glucose issues, especially when taken with INSTIs.**

- **Treatment monitoring:** After starting or changing ART, the viral load should be checked at 4–6 weeks with an expected 10-fold reduction ($1.0 \log_{10}$) and suppression to <50 copies/mL by 24 weeks of therapy. The regimen should then be reassessed if response to treatment is inadequate. When the HIV RNA becomes undetectable and the patient is on a stable regimen, monitoring can be done every 3–6 months.

- **Treatment failure** is defined as less than a log (10-fold) reduction of the viral load 4–6 weeks after starting a new antiretroviral regimen, failure to reach an undetectable viral load after 6 months of treatment, detection of the virus after initial complete suppression of viral load (which suggests development of resistance), or persistent decline of CD4 cell count or clinical deterioration. Confirmed treatment failure should prompt changes in ART based on results of genotype testing. In this situation, at least two of the drugs should be substituted with other drugs that have no expected cross-resistance. **HIV resistance testing** at this stage may help determine a salvage regimen in patients with prior ART. The importance of adherence should be stressed. Referral to an HIV specialist is highly recommended in this situation.

- **Drug interactions:** Antiretroviral medications, especially PIs, have multiple drug interactions. **PIs and cobicistat both inhibit and induce the P450 system,** and thus interactions are frequent with other inhibitors of the P450 system, including macrolides (erythromycin, clarithromycin) and antifungals (ketoconazole, itraconazole), as well as other inducers such as rifamycins (rifampin, rifabutin) and anticonvulsants (phenobarbital, phenytoin, carbamazepine). Cobisistat can increase concentrations of intranasal corticosteroids with beclomethasone preferred as safer alternative. **Drugs with narrow therapeutic indices that should be avoided or used with extreme caution** include antihistamines (although loratadine is safe), antiarrhythmics (flecainide, encainide, quinidine), long-acting opiates (fentanyl, meperidine), long-acting benzodiazepines (midazolam, triazolam), warfarin, 3-hydroxy-3-methylglutaryl–coenzyme A reductase inhibitors (pitavastatin is the safest), and oral contraceptives. Sildenafil concentrations are increased, whereas methadone and theophylline concentrations are decreased with concomitant administration of certain PIs and NNRTIs.

Complications

Complications of ART: The long-term use of antiretrovirals has been associated with toxicity, the pathogenesis of which is only partially understood at this time.

- **Hyperlipidemia,** especially hypertriglyceridemia, is associated mainly with PIs (especially ritonavir). Improvement has been seen after treatment with atorvastatin, pravastatin, pitavastatin, and/or gemfibrozil.
- **Peripheral insulin resistance, impaired glucose tolerance, and hyperglycemia** have been associated with the use of PI-based regimens, mainly indinavir and ritonavir. Hyperglycemia has also been noted with INSTI regimens, especially when coformulated with TAF compared to TDF. Lifestyle changes or changing ART can be considered in these cases.
- **Osteopenia and osteoporosis** are well described in HIV-infected individuals. The pathogenic mechanism of this problem is likely related to the inflammatory milieu of HIV itself, although the use of TDF may contribute. TAF is recommended over TDF in at-risk patients.
- **Osteonecrosis,** particularly of the hip, has been increasingly associated with HIV disease.
- **Lipodystrophy syndrome** is an alteration in body fat distribution and can be stigmatizing to individuals. Changes consist of the accumulation of visceral fat in the abdomen, neck (buffalo hump), and pelvic areas, and/or the depletion of SC fat, causing facial or peripheral wasting. Lipodystrophy has been associated in particular with older PIs and NRTIs and is uncommon with currently recommended regimens.
- **Lactic acidosis** with liver steatosis is a rare but sometimes fatal complication associated with NRTIs. The mechanism appears to be part of mitochondrial toxicity. Higher rates of lactic acidosis have been reported with the use of the older drugs stavudine and didanosine.
- **Weight gain** has been seen with INSTI-based regimens, especially among women and Black individuals. Weight grain is higher when coformulated with TAF compared to TDF.

SPECIAL POPULATIONS

Pregnancy

- Maximally suppressive ART during pregnancy is critical in preventing vertical transmission.
- Current guidelines recommend that all HIV-infected partners in a couple planning pregnancy should attain virologic suppression before attempting conception.[16]
- Periconception PrEP for the HIV-uninfected partner may provide additional protection to reduce the risk of sexual transmission and should be discussed with the couple.
- If a pregnant person is already suppressed on ART and is tolerating that regimen, they should be maintained on current ART regardless of the agents (including efavirenz). However, consideration should be given to avoiding dolutegravir in pregnancy until more data are available. Boosted darunavir should also be avoided because of low drug levels in pregnancy.
- ART-naïve pregnant people should be started on a combination regimen of TDF/FTC with boosted atazanavir daily, boosted darunavir twice daily, or raltegravir twice daily (especially if early in pregnancy). An alternative is Complera (combined

rilpivirine, TDF, FTC) if started early in pregnancy, CD4 > 200, and viral load <100,000 copies/mL.

- Intrapartum IV zidovudine should be given to patients during labor, although it is not required for those with consistent undetectable viral loads in late pregnancy.
- Cesarean delivery should be scheduled for women with HIV viral loads >1000 in late pregnancy.
- ART should be continued after delivery, consistent with current guidelines to treat everyone to prevent disease progression and HIV transmission.
- Neonatal zidovudine prophylaxis should be given for 4 weeks if the patient has maintained virologic suppression. Neonatal prophylaxis using zidovudine and nevirapine with or without lamivudine should be offered if the mother did not receive antepartum suppressive ART.

Acute HIV Infection

ART given immediately after diagnosing acute infection may provide additional benefits.

- The initiation of early ART in acute infection will suppress the extraordinarily high viral loads seen at this time and reduce further transmission of HIV.
- Early ART may reduce the reservoir of latent virus.
- Early ART maintains immune function and may allow for immunologic control of HIV off ART in resource-limited settings.

Hepatitis

- High rates of coinfection with HBV and hepatitis C virus (HCV) occur in HIV-infected patients.
- Several HIV ART medications (tenofovir, emtricitabine, and lamivudine) also have activity against HBV. Any plan to treat HBV in coinfected patients should ensure that the regimen is fully active against both HIV and HBV. Discontinuation of ART that has been suppressing unrecognized HBV disease can result in reactivation of HBV with resultant acute, and sometimes fatal, HBV infection.
- HCV therapy is rapidly evolving, and a complete delineation of treatment is available in Chapter 19, Liver Diseases.
- Newer directly acting HCV agents appear to be as effective in HIV-infected patients as in monoinfected HCV patients; however, there are significant drug–drug interactions that should be considered, particularly with PI-based therapy, efavirenz, and therapy using the boosting agent cobicistat.

Aging

- With the success of ART, HIV-related mortality is decreasing and HIV-infected persons are experiencing prolonged survival approaching the national survival average.
- In 2018, the CDC estimated that 51% of HIV-infected persons were over the age of 50.
- HIV infection is associated with premature end-organ disease, and thus many of the comorbidities associated with aging may be exacerbated in this growing population, including cardiovascular disease, insulin resistance and diabetes, osteoporosis, neurocognitive impairment, and physical frailty.
- Certain non–AIDS-defining cancers are more common in HIV-infected patients, including anal cancer, lung cancer, and hepatocellular carcinoma. The extent to which this is due to HIV infection versus other risk factors such as smoking, HPV, and HBV/HCV coinfection is unclear.

- The role of long-term HIV infection and ART use in these comorbidities is poorly understood, although the use of NNRTI and PI drug classes is associated with lipid profiles that may exacerbate cardiovascular disease.[17] Higher rates of smoking and alcohol use also exacerbate these comorbidities.

REFERRAL

- All HIV-positive patients should be referred to a HIV specialist, if possible.
- Counseling regarding contraception, safer sex practices, medication adherence, and proper health maintenance is essential.
- Social work referral is important to ensure adequate social support system including housing, mental health assistance, and substance abuse treatment.

Opportunistic Infections

GENERAL PRINCIPLES

- Potent ART has decreased the incidence, changed the manifestations, and improved the outcome of OIs. However, OIs are still a common presentation of unrecognized HIV infection.
- A clinical syndrome associated with the immune enhancement induced by potent ART, **IRIS**, generally presents as local inflammatory reactions. Unmasking IRIS is when a patient develops symptoms of an OI while on ART treatment with no previous symptoms or indications of the patient having that OI previous to immune reconstitution. Paradoxical IRIS is when a patient is known to have a particular OI and worsens while on ART with immune reconstitution. Examples include recurrent symptoms of cryptococcal meningitis, paradoxical reactions with TB reactivation, localized *Mycobacterium avium* complex (MAC) adenitis, aggravation of hepatitis viral infection, and CMV vitreitis soon after the initiation of potent ART.
- In the case of IRIS, ART is usually continued, and the addition of low-dose steroids might decrease the degree of inflammation. TB and cryptococcal meningitis are the only OIs for which delay of starting ART is recommended to prevent IRIS.
- Additional details with updates may be found in the Guidelines for the Prevention and Treatment of Opportunistic Infections in HIV-Infected Adults and Adolescents.[18]

TREATMENT

- **Prophylaxis for OIs** can be divided into primary and secondary prophylaxis.
- **Primary prophylaxis** is established before an episode of OI occurs. Institution of primary prophylaxis depends on the level of immunosuppression as judged by the patient's CD4 cell count and percentage (Table 16-2).
- **Secondary prophylaxis** is instituted after an episode of infection has been adequately treated. Most OIs will require extended therapy.
- **Withdrawal of prophylaxis:** Recommendations suggest withdrawing primary and secondary prophylaxis for most OIs if sustained immunologic recovery has occurred (CD4 cell counts consistently >150–200 cells/μL).[18]

TABLE 16-2	Opportunistic Infection Prophylaxis	
Opportunistic Infection	Indications for Prophylaxis	Medications
PJP	CD4 <200 cells/μL	TMP-SMX DS or SS PO daily (preferred) or three times per week
		Alternatives: dapsone,[a] atovaquone, aerosolized pentamidine
Toxoplasmosis[b]	CD4 <100 cells/μL	TMP-SMX DS PO daily (preferred) or three times per week
		Alternatives: combination of dapsone + pyrimethamine and leucovorin; atovaquone
Mycobacterium avium complex[c]	CD4 <50 cells/μL	Azithromycin 1200 mg PO weekly
		Alternatives: clarithromycin or rifabutin

DS, double strength; PJP, Pneumocystis jirovecii pneumonia; TMP-SMX, trimethoprim-sulfamethoxazole.
[a]Glucose-6-phosphate dehydrogenase (G6PD) testing should be done for dapsone.
[b]If toxoplasmosis IgG is positive.
[c]Not recommended if patient is on effective ART.

PULMONARY SYNDROMES

Pneumocystis Jirovecii Pneumonia

GENERAL PRINCIPLES

Pneumocystis jirovecii pneumonia is the most common OI in patients with AIDS characterized by subacute progressive dyspnea.

DIAGNOSIS

Positive direct immunofluorescent stain from induced sputum samples or bronchoalveolar lavage fluid. Alternatively, histopathologic demonstration of organisms in tissue is also adequate for diagnosis. Chest radiography typically shows diffuse, bilateral ground-glass interstitial infiltrates, but it can also have a variety of atypical appearances.

TREATMENT

• **Trimethoprim-sulfamethoxazole (TMP-SMX)** is the treatment of choice. The dosage is 15–20 mg/kg of the TMP component IV daily, divided q6–8h for severe cases, with a switch to oral therapy when the patient's condition improves. Total

duration of therapy is 21 days. Prednisone should be added with severe disease as defined below. For patients who cannot receive TMP-SMX, the following alternatives are available:
- For mild to moderately severe disease (arterial oxygen tension [PaO_2] >70 mm Hg or alveolar arterial oxygen gradient [$P(A–a)O_2$] <35 mm Hg):
  - TMP, 15 mg/kg PO q8h, and dapsone, 100 mg PO daily. G6PD deficiency should be ruled out before dapsone is used.
  - Clindamycin, 600 mg IV or PO q8h, plus primaquine, 30 mg PO daily. G6PD deficiency should be ruled out before primaquine is used.
  - Atovaquone, 750 mg PO q12h. This drug should be administered with meals to increase absorption.
- For severe disease (PaO_2 <70 mm Hg or $P[A–a]O_2$ ≥35 mm Hg):
  - Prednisone taper should be added. The most frequently prescribed prednisone regimen is 40 mg PO bid on days 1–5 and 40 mg daily on days 6–10, followed by 20 mg on days 11–21.
  - IV pentamidine is used in cases when all other options are exhausted and requires close monitoring for side effects.
- Primary prophylaxis is indicated (see Table 16-2). Secondary PCP prophylaxis can be discontinued if the CD4 count is >200 cells/μL for more than 3 months in patients responding to ART.

Mycobacterium Tuberculosis

GENERAL PRINCIPLES

Mycobacterium tuberculosis is more frequent among HIV-infected patients. Primary or reactivated disease is common.

DIAGNOSIS

- Clinical manifestations depend on the level of immunosuppression. Patients with higher CD4 cell counts tend to exhibit classic presentations with **apical cavitary disease.**
- Profoundly immunosuppressed patients may demonstrate atypical presentations that can resemble disseminated primary infection, with diffuse or localized pulmonary infiltrates and hilar lymphadenopathy.
- Extrapulmonary dissemination is more common in patients with HIV.

TREATMENT

- For treatment recommendations, see Chapter 14, Treatment of Infectious Diseases.
- Current recommendations suggest the **substitution of rifabutin for rifampin** in patients who are receiving concomitant ART, especially PIs. The dosage for rifabutin needs readjustment due to many significant interactions. In subjects who are ART naïve, ART can be delayed for a few weeks after TB-specific therapy is started.

FEBRILE SYNDROMES

Mycobacterium Avium Complex Infection

GENERAL PRINCIPLES

MAC infection is the most commonly occurring mycobacterial infection in AIDS patients and is responsible for significant morbidity in patients with advanced disease (CD4 cell count <50 cells/μL).

DIAGNOSIS

Clinical Presentation
- Disseminated infection with fever, weight loss, night sweats, and GI complaints is the most frequent presentation.
- MAC infection can result in bacteremia in AIDS patients.

Diagnostic Testing
- Anemia and an elevated alkaline phosphatase level are the usual laboratory abnormalities.
- Mycobacterial blood cultures should be sent in suspected cases.

TREATMENT

- Initial therapy should include a **macrolide** (i.e., clarithromycin, 500 mg PO bid) and **ethambutol**, 15 mg/kg PO daily.
- Rifabutin, 300 mg PO daily, an aminoglycoside 10–15 mg/kg IV daily, or a fluoroquinolone can be added in severe cases or patients not on effective ART, and based on susceptibilities.
- Utility of disseminated MAC prophylaxis was recently under debate given prophylaxis toxicity and effectiveness of modern ART; however currently both the US Department of Health and Human Services and the International Antiviral Society of USA recommend against primary prophylaxis if effective ART is initiated immediately and viral suppression achieved (AIIa recommendation). Primary prophylaxis is only currently recommended if patients are not receiving ART and CD4 counts <50 cells/mm^3.
- Secondary prophylaxis for disseminated MAC can be discontinued if the CD4 count has a sustained increase of >100 cells/μL for 6 months or longer in response to ART, and if 12 months of therapy for MAC is completed and there are no symptoms or signs attributable to MAC.

Histoplasma Capsulatum Infections

GENERAL PRINCIPLES

- The severity of infection depends on the degree of the patient's immunosuppression.
- Histoplasmosis often occurs in AIDS patients who live in endemic areas such as the Mississippi and Ohio River Valleys.
- Such infections are usually disseminated at the time of diagnosis.

DIAGNOSIS

- Suspect histoplasmosis in patients with fever, hepatosplenomegaly, and weight loss.
- Pancytopenia develops because of bone marrow involvement.
- Diagnosis is made by a positive culture or biopsy demonstrating 2–4 μm budding yeast, but the urine and serum *Histoplasma* antigens can also be used for diagnosis and to monitor treatment.

TREATMENT

- Disseminated disease is treated with **liposomal amphotericin B**, 3 mg/kg IV daily for 2 weeks or until the patient clinically improves, followed by **itraconazole**, 200 mg PO bid indefinitely.
- CNS disease is initially treated with **liposomal amphotericin B**, 5 mg/kg IV daily for 4–6 weeks, before starting itraconazole.
- Itraconazole absorption should be documented by a serum drug level. Liquid itraconazole is preferred because of improved absorption; however, it can be expensive and difficult to obtain.
- Discontinuation of itraconazole is possible if sustained increase in CD4 count is observed >100–200 cells/μL for more than 6 months.

Coccidioides Immitis Infection

GENERAL PRINCIPLES

- Coccidioidomycosis often occurs in AIDS patients who live in endemic areas such as the southwestern United States, Central America, and South America.
- Infection may be limited to pneumonia or disseminated with possible involvement of CNS, skin, bones, and joints.

DIAGNOSIS

- Suspect coccidioidomycosis in patients with fever, cough, night sweats, joint pains, and travel to an endemic area.
- Diagnosis is made by a positive culture or biopsy demonstrating 20–70 μm spherules; serum serological tests can also aid in the diagnosis.

TREATMENT

- Disseminated disease is treated with **liposomal amphotericin B**, 4–6 mg/kg IV daily for 2 weeks or until the patient clinically improves, followed by fluconazole or itraconazole for at least 12 months.
- CNS disease is initially treated with **fluconazole** 800–1200 mg daily; liposomal amphotericin may be added to the initial regimen. Treatment with fluconazole is continued lifelong.

Other Endemic Fungi

Although not listed as AIDS-defining illnesses, patients with advanced HIV are at risk for other endemic fungi depending on which the region they live. This includes Blastomycosis in the upper Midwest United States, Paracoccidioidomycosis in Central and South America, and *Talaromyces* (formerly *Penicillium*) in Southeast Asia, as well as other endemic fungi.

CENTRAL NERVOUS SYSTEM AND RETINAL DISEASE

Cryptococcus Neoformans

GENERAL PRINCIPLES

- The severity of infection depends on the degree of the patient's immunosuppression.
- **Cryptococcal meningitis** is the most frequent CNS fungal infection in AIDS patients.

DIAGNOSIS

- Patients with CNS infection usually present with headaches, fever, and possibly mental status changes, but presentation can be more subtle.
- Cryptococcal infection can also present as pulmonary or cutaneous disease.
- Diagnosis is based on **LP** results and on the determination of latex cryptococcal antigen, which is usually positive in the serum and the CSF.
- **CSF opening pressure** should always be measured to assess the possibility of elevated intracranial pressure.

TREATMENT

- Initial treatment is with liposomal **amphotericin** dosed at 3–4 mg/kg/d IV, and **flucytosine**, 25 mg/kg PO q6h for at least 2 weeks, followed by **fluconazole**, 400 mg PO daily for at least 8 weeks and then 200 mg PO daily, either lifelong or until immune reconstitution occurs. Fluconazole can be discontinued in those who are asymptomatic with regard to signs and symptoms of cryptococcosis and have a sustained increase (>6 months) in their CD4+ counts to ≥200 cells/μL.
- Repeat LPs (removing up to 30 mL CSF until the pressure is <20–25 cm H_2O) may be required to relieve elevated intracranial pressure.
- The 5-flucytosine level should be monitored during therapy to avoid toxicity.
- Alternative initial therapy is with amphotericin B deoxycholate, 0.7 mg/kg/d IV, and flucytosine, 25 mg/kg PO q6h.
- In persons who have persistent elevation of intracranial pressure, a temporary lumbar drain is indicated.

Toxoplasma Gondii

DIAGNOSIS

Toxoplasmosis typically causes multiple CNS **mass lesions** and presents with encephalopathy and focal neurologic findings.

Diagnostic Testing

Laboratories

Disease represents reactivation of a previous infection, and the serologic workup is usually positive.

Imaging

- MRI of the brain is the best radiographic technique for diagnosis.
- Often the diagnosis relies on response to empiric treatment, as seen by a reduction in the size of the mass lesions.

TREATMENT

- **Sulfadiazine,** 25 mg/kg PO q6h, plus **pyrimethamine**, 200 mg PO on day 1, followed by 50–75 mg PO daily (based on body weight), is the therapy of choice.
- **Leucovorin,** 10–25 mg PO daily, should be added to prevent hematologic toxicity.
- For patients who are allergic to sulfonamides, clindamycin, 600 mg IV or PO q8h, can be used instead of sulfadiazine.
- Doses are reduced after 6 weeks of therapy.
- Secondary prophylaxis can be discontinued among patients with a sustained increase in CD4 count >200 cells/µL for more than 6 months as a result of response to ART and if the initial therapy is complete and there are no symptoms or signs attributable to toxoplasmosis.

Varicella-Zoster Virus

DIAGNOSIS

- Varicella-zoster virus may cause typical dermatomal lesions or disseminated infection including retinal necrosis.
- It may cause encephalitis, which is more common with ophthalmic distribution of facial nerve.

TREATMENT

Acyclovir, 10–15 mg/kg IV q8h for 7–14 days, is the recommended therapy. For milder cases, administration of acyclovir (800 mg PO five times a day), famciclovir (500 mg PO tid), or valacyclovir (1 g PO tid) for 1 week is usually effective.

JC Virus

DIAGNOSIS

- It is associated with **progressive multifocal leukoencephalopathy** (PML). The symptoms include mental status changes, weakness, and disorders of gait.
- Characteristic periventricular and subcortical white matter lesions are seen on MRI.

TREATMENT

Potent ART has improved the survival of patients with PML.

CMV Retinitis

GENERAL PRINCIPLES

CMV retinitis accounts for 85% of CMV disease in patients with AIDS. It commonly develops in a setting of profound CD4 depletions (CD4 cell count <50 cells/μL).

DIAGNOSIS

- CMV viremia can be detected by PCR and is usually present in end-organ disease but can also be seen in the absence of end-organ disease.
- The diagnosis of CMV retinitis is made based on characteristic findings during ophthalmoscopic examination. Patients may report floaters, scotomata, or peripheral visual field defects.

TREATMENT

- Treatment of CMV retinitis can be local or systemic and is administered in two phases, induction and maintenance.
- **Ganciclovir** is given at an induction dosage of 5 mg/kg IV bid for 14–21 days and a maintenance dosage of 5 mg/kg IV daily indefinitely (unless immune reconstitution occurs). The most common side effect of ganciclovir is **myelotoxicity**, resulting in neutropenia. The neutropenia may respond to granulocyte colony-stimulating factor therapy. An intraocular ganciclovir implant is effective but does not provide systemic CMV therapy.
- **Valganciclovir,** a ganciclovir prodrug, has drug levels equivalent to those of IV ganciclovir. For induction, 900 mg PO bid for 14–21 days is given, followed by 900 mg once a day. **Treatment is indefinite unless immunologic recovery occurs.** Adverse effects are similar to those of ganciclovir.
- Alternatives include **IV foscarnet and IV cidofovir.** These drugs carry a significant risk of **nephrotoxicity**; therefore, adequate hydration and electrolyte monitoring (including calcium) are required.
- For other **invasive CMV diseases**, the optimal therapy is with IV ganciclovir, PO valganciclovir, IV foscarnet, or a combination of two drugs (in persons with prior anti-CMV therapy), for at least 3–6 weeks. Foscarnet has the best CSF penetration and is the drug of choice for CMV encephalitis and myelopathy. Long-term maintenance therapy is indicated.

ESOPHAGITIS

Candida

GENERAL PRINCIPLES

- The severity of infection depends on the degree of the patient's immunosuppression.
- Candidiasis is common in the HIV-infected host.
- Other causes of esophagitis include HSV, CMV, and *Histoplasma*.

DIAGNOSIS

Location of infection can be oral, esophageal, or vaginal.

TREATMENT

- Oral and vaginal candidiasis usually responds to local therapy with troches or creams (**nystatin** or **clotrimazole**).
- For patients who do not respond or who have esophageal candidiasis, **fluconazole**, 100–200 mg PO daily for 14–21 days, is the treatment of choice.

SPECIAL CONSIDERATIONS

Fluconazole-resistant candidiasis is increasing, especially in patients with advanced disease who have been receiving antifungal agents for prolonged periods. Endoscopic sampling with culture and resistances may be beneficial in refractory cases.
- **Caspofungin or micafungin,** echinocandins, can be considered for refractory cases.
- **Itraconazole** oral suspension (200 mg bid) is occasionally effective, as is **posaconazole** oral solution, and posaconazole is generally better tolerated than itraconazole. **Voriconazole** may also be useful.

DIARRHEA

Cryptosporidium

DIAGNOSIS

- *Cryptosporidium* causes chronic watery diarrhea with malabsorption in HIV-infected patients.
- Diagnosis is based on the visualization of the parasite in an acid-fast stain or direct immunofluorescence of stool.

TREATMENT

- No effective specific therapy has been developed as ART is essential.
- **Nitazoxanide,** 500 mg PO bid, may be effective.

Cyclospora, Cystoisospora, Microsporidia, and Campylobacter Jejuni

DIAGNOSIS

These organisms cause chronic diarrhea. Microsporidia can also cause biliary tree disease in patients with advanced infection.

TREATMENT

- *Cyclospora* is treated with **TMP-SMX**, one double-strength (DS) tablet PO bid for 7–10 days. *Cystoisospora* (formerly *Isospora)* is treated with **TMP-SMX**, one DS tablet PO qid for 10 days, followed by chronic suppression with TMP-SMX, one DS tablet PO daily.

- Microsporidia caused by *Enterocytozoon bieneusi* is treated with optimized ART. For other species, **albendazole**, 400 mg PO bid can be given. Relapses are common when therapy is stopped.
- *Campylobacter jejuni* is treated with either azithromycin, 500 mg PO daily, or ciprofloxacin, 500–750 mg PO bid for 5 days.

ASSOCIATED NEOPLASMS

Kaposi Sarcoma

GENERAL PRINCIPLES

Kaposi sarcoma is caused by coinfection with human herpesvirus-8, also called Kaposi sarcoma–associated herpesvirus.

DIAGNOSIS

In AIDS patients, it commonly presents as cutaneous lesions, but can be disseminated. The GI tract and lungs are the usual visceral organs involved.

TREATMENT

Mild disease is treated with optimization of ART. Severe disease is treated with chemotherapy plus ART. Liposomal doxorubicin is first-line chemotherapy. Cryotherapy or radiation may be useful as well.

Lymphoma

GENERAL PRINCIPLES

- Lymphomas commonly associated with AIDS are non-Hodgkin lymphoma, CNS and systemic lymphoma, and lymphomas of B-cell origin.
- **EBV** appears to be the associated pathogen.

DIAGNOSIS

- Primary CNS lymphomas are common and can be multicentric.
- Diagnosis is based on clinical symptoms, the presence of enhancing brain lesions, brain biopsy, and a positive EBV-PCR of the CSF.
- Other OIs need to be ruled out.
- Other potential extranodal sites of involvement including bone marrow, GI tract, and liver require tissue biopsy to confirm the diagnosis.

TREATMENT

Treatment involves **chemotherapy** and **radiation**. May respond to corticosteroids alone.

Cervical and Perianal Neoplasias

GENERAL PRINCIPLES

- Both HIV-infected men and women are at high risk for HPV-related disease.
- Certain HPV subtypes such as 16 and 18 are oncogenic.
- Cancer can also arise from perianal condyloma acuminata.
- Unvaccinated males and females ages 9–26 should be given the HPV vaccination series. Current guidelines recommend offering HPV vaccine up to 45 years of age in those who have not been previously vaccinated.

DIAGNOSIS

- Screening for vaginal dysplasia with a Papanicolaou smear is indicated every 6 months during the first year and, if results are normal, annually thereafter.
- Screening for anal intraepithelial neoplasms is currently under evaluation and is recommended by some experts in populations such as MSM, any patient with a history of anogenital condylomas, and women with abnormal vulvar or cervical histology.[19]

TREATMENT

Refer to Chapter 22, Cancer, for specific treatments of these neoplasms.

SEXUALLY TRANSMITTED INFECTIONS IN PATIENTS WITH HIV

For treatment, see Table 16-1.

Genital Herpes

HIV-infected individuals are more likely to have prolonged and severe disease as well as treatment failures due to the development of resistance. Treatment guidelines are slightly different for HIV-infected patients. See Table 16-1.

Genital Warts

GENERAL PRINCIPLES

Genital warts are caused by HPV. Different serotypes have been associated with the lesions, notably types 6 and 11. Other common HPV types (16, 18, 31, and 33) are associated with malignant transformation in different anatomic sites. Genital warts in HIV-infected persons are typically more resistant to treatment and have a higher chance of recurrence.[19]

DIAGNOSIS

Diagnosis is made on the basis of physical examination and history. In some situations, biopsy of the lesions may be necessary.

TREATMENT

Local therapy is aimed at the removal of the warts. HPV vaccination is recommended in women and men ages 9–45 (see previous section on immunizations).

Syphilis

See the section on STIs for more complete information.

Additional Resources

- www.aidsinfo.nih.gov
- www.hivmedicationguide.com
- www.thebody.com
- www.cdc.gov/hiv
- www.hivinsite.ucsf.edu
- www.std.uw.edu
- www.hiv.uw.edu

REFERENCES

1. Centers for Disease Control and Prevention. *HIV Infection, Risk, Prevention, and Testing Behaviors Among Transgender Women—National HIV Behavioral Surveillance, 7 U.S. Cities, 2019-2020*. HIV Surveillance Special Report 27http://www.cdc.gov/hiv/library/reports/hiv-surveillance.html. 2021. Accessed September 20 2021.
2. The GenIUSS Group. *Best Practices for Asking Questions to Identify Transgender and Other Gender Minority Respondents on Population-Based Surveys*. CAThe Williams Institute; 2014. https://williamsinstitute.law.ucla.edu/wp-content/uploads/geniuss-report-sep-2014.pdf
3. Ghanem KG, Ram S, Rice PA. The modern epidemic of syphilis. *N Engl J Med*. 2020;382(9):845-854. PMID: 32101666. doi: 10.1056/NEJMra1901593
4. *Centers for Disease Control and Prevention - Sexually Transmitted Diseases Surveillance Report 2019*. Published April 2021. https://www.cdc.gov/std/statistics/2019/default.htm
5. Workowski KA, Bachmann LH, Chan PA, et al. Sexually transmitted infections treatment guidelines, 2021. *MMWR Recomm Rep*. 2021;70(No. RR-4):1-187. doi:10.15585/mmwr.rr7004a1
6. Ward H, Martin I, Macdonald N, et al. Lymphogranuloma venereum in the United Kingdom. *Clin Infect Dis*. 2007;44(1):26-32.
7. De voux A, Kent JB, Macomber K, et al. Notes from the field: cluster of lymphogranuloma venereum cases among men who have sex with men—Michigan, August 2015-April 2016. *MMWR Morb Mortal Wkly Rep*. 2016;65(34):920-921.
8. 1993 revised classification system for HIV infection and expanded surveillance case definition for AIDS among adolescents and adults. *MMWR Recomm Rep*. 1992;41(RR-17):1-19.
9. World Health Organization. *HIV/AIDS: Data and Statistics*. Updated July 2021. https://www.who.int/data/gho/data/themes/hiv-aids
10. Centers for Disease Control and Prevention. Accessed April 2022. http://www.cdc.gov/hiv/group/gender/women/diagnoses.html
11. Centers for Disease Control and Prevention. Accessed April 2022. https://www.cdc.gov/hiv/group/msm/index.html
12. Centers for Disease Control and Prevention: *US Public Health Service: Preexposure Prophylaxis for the Prevention of HIV Infection in the United States—2017 Update – A Clinical Practice Guideline*. 2018. https://www.cdc.gov/hiv/pdf/risk/prep/cdc-hiv-prep-guidelines-2017.pdf
13. DiNenno EA, Prejean J, Irwin K, et al. Recommendations for HIV screening of gay, bisexual, and other men who have sex with men — United States, 2017. *MMWR Morb Mortal Wkly Rep*. 2017;66:830-832. doi:10.15585/mmwr.mm6631a3
14. Thompson MA, Horberg MA, Agwu AL, et al. Primary care guidance for persons with human immunodeficiency virus: 2020 update by the HIV medicine association of the infectious diseases society of America. *Clin Infect Dis*. 2020;73(11):e3572-e3605. doi:10.1093/cid/ciaa1391
15. International Antiviral Society-USA. *Guidelines*. 2020. http://www.iasusa.org/guidelines/

16. U.S. Department of Health and Human Services. *Recommendations for the Use of Antiretroviral Drugs in Pregnant Women with HIV Infection and Interventions to Reduce Perinatal HIV Transmission in the United States*. 2020. http://aidsinfo.nih.gov/guidelines/html/3/perinatal-guidelines/0

17. Friis-møller N, Weber R, Reiss P, et al. Cardiovascular disease risk factors in HIV patients–association with antiretroviral therapy. Results from the DAD study. *AIDS*. 2003;17(8):1179-1193.

18. Panel on Opportunistic Infections in Adults and Adolescents with HIV. *Guidelines for the Prevention and Treatment of Opportunistic Infections in Adults and Adolescents with HIV: Recommendations from the Centers for Disease Control and Prevention, the National Institutes of Health, and the HIV Medicine Association of the Infectious Diseases Society of America*. Accessed February 1, 2021. http://aidsinfo.nih.gov/contentfiles/lvguidelines/adult_oi.pdf

19. Centers for Disease Control and Prevention. *Human Papillomavirus (HPV)*. 2017. http://www.cdc.gov/std/hpv/treatment.htm

17 Solid Organ Transplant Medicine

Rowena Delos Santos and Wut Yi Hninn

Solid Organ Transplant Basics

GENERAL PRINCIPLES

- Solid organ transplantation is a **treatment, not a cure**, for end-stage organ failure of the kidney, liver, pancreas, heart, and lung. Small intestine and vascularized composite allografts are performed in smaller numbers at specialized centers throughout the country. The benefits of organ replacement coexist with the risks of the immediate procedure followed by the risks of chronic immunosuppression. Thus, not all patients with organ failure are transplant candidates.
- Organs from **deceased donors** remain in short supply, with increasing waiting times for potential recipients. **Living donor transplants** are common in kidney transplantation and are being evaluated in liver and lung transplantations as a partial solution to this shortage. Xenotransplantation (transplantation of animal tissue into humans) is not currently a viable option.
- **Immunologic considerations** between donor and recipient prior to the transplant must be fully evaluated including ABO compatibility, HLA typing, cross-matching, and some degree of immune response testing for the proposed donor. Newer protocols using desensitization techniques have had some success in overcoming these immunologic barriers, such as a desensitization protocol for ABO incompatibility in living donor kidney transplantations.

DIAGNOSIS

- For indications and contraindications of heart, lung, kidney, and liver transplantations, see chapters devoted to these organs.
- **Transplant recipient patient evaluation:** Evaluation of a transplant recipient with medical or surgical problems should encompass details of the patient's organ transplant and treatment. Thus, the following should always be reviewed when taking a history from an organ transplant recipient:
  - Cause of organ failure
  - Treatment for organ failure prior to transplantation
  - Type and date of transplant
  - Cytomegalovirus (CMV) and Epstein–Barr virus (EBV) serology of donor and recipient
  - Induction immunosuppression, particularly use of antibody-based induction therapy
  - Initial allograft function (e.g., nadir creatinine, forced expiratory volume in 1 second [FEV_1], ejection fraction, synthetic function, and transaminases)
  - Current allograft function
  - Complications of transplantation (e.g., surgical problems, acute rejection, delayed graft function, infections, chronic organ dysfunction)
  - Current immunosuppression regimen and recent drug levels

TREATMENT

- **Immunosuppression:** Immunosuppressive medications are used to promote acceptance of a graft (induction therapy), to prevent rejection (maintenance therapy), and to reverse episodes of acute rejection (rejection therapy). These agents are associated with immunosuppressive effects, immunodeficiency toxicities (e.g., infection and malignancy), and nonimmune toxicities (e.g., nephrotoxicity, diabetes mellitus, bone disease, gout, hyperlipidemia, cardiovascular disease, or neurotoxicity).[1,2] Many variables factor into the choice and dose of drug and the guidelines for each specific organ are different.
- **Glucocorticoids:** Glucocorticoids are immunosuppressive and anti-inflammatory. Their mechanisms of action include inhibition of cytokine transcription, induction of lymphocyte apoptosis, downregulation of adhesion molecules and major histocompatibility complex expression, and modification of leukocyte trafficking.
  - Side effects of chronic glucocorticoid therapy are well-known.
  - Steroids are tapered rapidly in the immediate posttransplant period to achieve maintenance doses of 0.1 mg/kg or less.
  - Steroid-free immunosuppression, rapid steroid tapering, and steroid withdrawal are developed to minimize side effects.
  - For most long-term transplant recipients, increases in glucocorticoid therapy (i.e., stress dosing) are not indicated for routine surgery or illness.[3]
- **Calcineurin inhibitors (CNIs):** CNIs inhibit T-lymphocyte activation and proliferation. **They remain the most commonly used immunosuppressant, despite their side effect of nephrotoxicity** (Table 17-1). IV CNIs should be avoided because of their extreme toxicity.
- **Antimetabolites: Inhibition of DNA synthesis**

TABLE 17-1	Calcineurin Inhibitors	
	Tacrolimus (Macrolide Antibiotic)	Cyclosporine (Cyclic 11-Amino Acid Peptide Derived From a Fungus)
Mechanism of action	Reduce IL-2, IL-3, IL-4, CD40L, GMCSF transcription	Reduce IL-2, IL-3, IL-4, CD40L, GMCSF transcription
Drug start dose and trough level goal		
Starting dose	0.1–0.15 mg/kg PO bid	3–8 mg/kg divided bid
Higher initial goal trough	7–10 ng/mL	250–300 ng/mL
Maintenance longer term goal trough	7–10 ng/mL	75–150 ng/mL
Side effects	More neurotoxic and diabetogenic than CsA, alopecia, hyperkalemia, glucose intolerance, tremors, gout, and rarely, thrombotic microangiopathy	Gingival hyperplasia, hirsutism, hypertension, glucose intolerance, hyperlipidemia, hyperkalemia, gout, tremors and, rarely, thrombotic microangiopathy

- ○ **Azathioprine (AZA)** is a purine analog that is metabolized by the liver to 6-mercaptopurine (active drug), which in turn is catabolized by xanthine oxidase. Azathioprine inhibits DNA synthesis and thereby suppresses lymphocyte proliferation. The major dose-limiting toxicity of this agent is myelosuppression, which is typically reversible after dose reduction or discontinuation of the drug. The usual maintenance dose is 1.5–2.5 mg/kg/d in a single dose. Drug levels are generally not obtained. Azathioprine is generally considered safe in pregnancy. It has major drug interactions with allopurinol and febuxostat; the azathioprine dose needs to be reduced 50%–75% to prevent severe myelosuppression.
- ○ **Mycophenolic acid (MPA)** inhibits inosine monophosphate dehydrogenase selectively in monocytes. This enzyme is the rate-limiting enzyme of guanine nucleotide synthesis, which is critical for de novo purine synthesis in both T and B lymphocytes. Two forms are available: mycophenolate mofetil (which is converted to the active metabolite, MPA) and enteric-coated mycophenolate sodium. Adverse effects of MPA commonly include gastrointestinal disturbances (nausea, diarrhea, and abdominal pain) and hematopoietic side effects (leukopenia and thrombocytopenia).
- ○ Antacids that contain magnesium and aluminum interfere with the absorption of MPA.
- ○ Proton pump inhibitors can also interfere with the bioavailability of mycophenolate mofetil, but not enteric-coated MPA, which is absorbed in the small intestine.
- ○ MPA is not used in pregnancy because of its teratogenicity.
- ○ The usual dose is 1–2 g daily in divided doses, although lesser doses may be used with concomitant tacrolimus compared with cyclosporine (CsA), because of enterohepatic circulation affecting MPA levels. Additionally, the dosage of MPA should be reduced in chronic renal impairment. Drug levels can be measured, but the clinical utility of monitoring MPA levels has not been determined.
- • Antiproliferative agents: mTOR inhibitors
  - ○ **Sirolimus and everolimus** inhibit the activation of a regulatory kinase, the mammalian target of rapamycin (mTOR), thus prohibiting T-cell progression from the G_1 to the S phase of the cell cycle. mTOR signaling also affects monocytes/macrophages, dendritic cells, natural killer (NK) cells, and endothelial cells. Thus, mTOR inhibition may lead to clinical effects related to its antiproliferative, antiviral, anti-inflammatory, and antitumor effects.
  - ○ Unlike the CNIs, mTOR inhibitors do not affect cytokine transcription but inhibit cytokine- and growth factor–induced cell proliferation.
  - ○ The major adverse effects include hyperlipidemia (hypertriglyceridemia), anemia, proteinuria, impaired wound healing, cytopenias, peripheral edema, oral ulcers, and gastrointestinal symptoms.
  - ○ Although not directly nephrotoxic, mTOR inhibitors may enhance the vasoconstriction of CNIs and potentiate their nephrotoxicity.
  - ○ Sirolimus interacts with CsA metabolism, making monitoring of both drugs difficult.
  - ○ The typical dose of sirolimus is 2–5 mg daily in a single dose. Everolimus is administered at 0.75–1.50 mg twice daily. Therapeutic drug monitoring is being perfected, with current trough levels between 5 and 15 ng/mL for sirolimus and 3 and 8 ng/mL for everolimus most commonly being used.
  - ○ Sirolimus should be avoided if SCr is more than 2 mg/dL and urine protein is more than 500 mg. It should also be avoided immediately postoperatively because it is associated with poor wound healing, delayed graft function (kidney transplant), anastomotic bronchial dehiscence (lung transplant), and hepatic artery

thrombosis (liver transplant). Limited data are available regarding use of everolimus in the immediate postoperative period.

○ Sirolimus is not used in pregnant women because of teratogenicity in animal models.

○ mTOR inhibitors have been effective in reducing intimal proliferation and obliterative vasculopathy in heart transplantation and have been approved as chemotherapy in advanced renal cell, breast, and other malignancies.

• **Biologic agents**
  ○ Polyclonal antibodies
    ▪ Antithymocyte globulin is produced by injecting human thymocytes into animals and collecting sera. This process generates antibodies against a wide variety of human immune system antigens. When subsequently infused into human patients, T lymphocytes are depleted by complement-mediated lysis and clearance of antibody-coated cells by the reticuloendothelial system. Lymphocyte function is also disrupted by blocking and modulating the expression of cell surface molecules by the antibodies.
    ▪ Important **adverse effects** include fever, chills, arthralgias, myelosuppression, serum sickness, and, rarely, anaphylaxis. Two preparations are available: horse antithymocyte globulin (ATGAM) and rabbit antithymocyte globulin (Thymoglobulin). Current literature suggests that rabbit antithymocyte globulin is more efficacious. These drugs can be used at the time of transplantation to promote engraftment ("induction") or as a subsequent treatment for acute rejection. The long-term risk of increased malignancy, particularly lymphoma, remains a concern.
    ▪ IV immunoglobulin (IVIG) is pooled from several thousand plasma donors to create a product that is IgG rich. Immunomodulatory and anti-inflammatory effects are associated with high dose (1–2 g/kg), but common mechanisms including direct binding to natural antibodies, immunomodulatory proteins, pathogens, inhibition of complement fixation on target tissue, and stimulation of anti-inflammatory pathways are also involved. Because of these effects, IVIG is used in the treatment of antibody-mediated rejection and desensitization of preformed HLA or ABO antibodies. Side effects include flushing, myalgias, chills, headache, and, rarely, anaphylaxis.
  ○ Monoclonal antibodies
    ▪ **Alemtuzumab (Campath 1H)** is a humanized monoclonal antibody against CD52, which is present on B and T cells, macrophages, and NK cells. It can cause significant lymphopenia for up to 6–12 months after dosing, which has led to its use in B-CLL and multiple sclerosis. In kidney transplants, it was used off label as an induction agent.
    ▪ **Basiliximab (Simulect)** is a humanized anti–interleukin-2 receptor (IL-2 receptor or CD25) monoclonal antibody that competitively inhibits the IL-2 receptor and thereby inhibits proliferation of activated T cells. This drug is administered as induction therapy at the time of transplantation and is associated with few side effects.
    ▪ **Belatacept** is a fusion protein (human IgG bound to CTLA4), which competitively binds to CD80/86 on antigen-presenting cells (APCs). This agent blocks T-cell costimulation between CD80/86 on APCs and CD28 on T cells and downregulates the T cell response. This agent is FDA indicated for use as a substitute for CNIs for long-term use as rejection prophylaxis posttransplant. It is contraindicated for use in liver transplantation and in recipients seronegative for EBV because of increased posttransplant lymphoproliferative disease (PTLD) in EBV-seronegative recipients.
    ▪ **Rituximab**, a chimeric monoclonal antibody against the B-cell protein CD20, leads to B cell depletion through complement-dependent cytotoxicity, growth

arrest, and apoptosis. This medication can suppress B cell counts for up to 6–9 months. Side effects such as fever, bronchospasm, and hypotension are attributed to cytokine release. Rituximab also carries the risk of hepatitis B reactivation in patients positive for hepatitis B surface antigen or hepatitis B core antibody. Therefore, prior to starting treatment, patients should be screened for hepatitis B by checking hepatitis B surface antigen and core antibody.

○ Infection prophylaxis

- **Immunization:** Pneumococcal and hepatitis B vaccination should be given to the recipient at the time of pretransplant evaluation. Influenza A vaccination should be administered yearly. Live vaccines should be avoided after transplantation and also in a live donor if organ donation is imminent. Varicella vaccination in seronegative patients if no contraindication for live vaccine and hepatitis A vaccination (particularly in liver transplant candidates) should be considered before transplant. A new inactivated varicella vaccine can be given prior to and after transplantation. Vaccination against SARS-CoV-2 should be encouraged to all pre- and posttransplant patients.

- **Trimethoprim-sulfamethoxazole** prevents urinary tract infections, *Pneumocystis jirovecii* pneumonia, and *Nocardia* infections. Prophylaxis is recommended for 6–12 months posttransplant. In sulfa-allergic patients, dapsone, aerosolized pentamidine, and atovaquone are suitable alternatives.

- **Acyclovir** prevents reactivation of herpes simplex virus (HSV) and varicella-zoster virus but is less effective in CMV prophylaxis. HSV can be a serious infection in immunosuppressed individuals, and some form of prophylaxis should be used during the first year. Patients with recurrent HSV infections (oral or genital) should be considered candidates for long-term prophylaxis. Lifetime acyclovir should be considered in EBV-seronegative patients who receive an EBV-positive organ.

- **Ganciclovir** or **valganciclovir** prevents reactivation of CMV infection when administered to patients who were previously CMV seropositive, received a CMV-positive organ, or both. Typically, these antivirals are administered for 3–12 months following transplantation. CMV hyperimmune globulin or IV ganciclovir can also be used for this purpose. Alternatively, patients can be monitored for the presence of CMV replication in the bloodstream by polymerase chain reaction before symptoms develop and can be treated preemptively.

- **Fluconazole** can be given to patients with a high risk of systemic fungal infections or recurrent localized fungal infections. Fluconazole increases CsA and tacrolimus levels (see "Treatment" under the "Solid Organ Transplant Basics" section).

- **Nystatin suspension**, **clotrimazole** troches, or weekly **fluconazole** are used to prevent oropharyngeal candidiasis (thrush).

GRAFT REJECTION

Acute Rejection, Kidney

GENERAL PRINCIPLES

Most episodes of acute rejection occur within the first year after transplantation. The low incidence of acute rejection today necessitates a careful search for inadequate drug levels, nonadherence, or less common forms of rejection (such as antibody-mediated rejection or plasma cell rejection). Late acute rejection (>1 year after transplantation) is often a result of inadequate immunosuppression or patient nonadherence.

Definition

An immunologically mediated acute deterioration in renal function associated with specific pathologic changes on renal biopsy including lymphocytic interstitial infiltrates, tubulitis, and arteritis (cellular rejection) and/or glomerulitis, capillaritis, and positive staining of the peritubular capillaries for the complement component C4d (antibody-mediated rejection).

Epidemiology

Kidney allograft rejection currently occurs in ~10% of patients. Patients who do not receive induction therapy have a 20%–30% incidence of acute rejection.

DIAGNOSIS

Diagnosis of acute renal allograft rejection is made by percutaneous renal biopsy after excluding prerenal azotemia, CNI nephrotoxicity (trough and/or peak levels and associated signs), infection (urinalysis and culture), obstruction (renal ultrasound), and surgical complications such as urine leak (renal scan). Newer techniques evaluating early markers of acute rejection in the blood and urine are under investigation.

Clinical Presentation

Manifestations include an elevated serum creatinine, decreased urine output, increased edema, or worsening hypertension. Initial symptoms are often absent, only laboratory evaluation will show a rise in creatinine. Constitutional symptoms (fever, malaise, arthralgia, painful or swollen allograft) are uncommon in current practice.

Differential Diagnosis

Differential diagnosis varies with duration after transplantation (Table 17-2).

TABLE 17-2	Differential Diagnosis of Renal Allograft Dysfunction	
>1 wk After Transplant	**<3 mo After Transplant**	**>3 mo After Transplant**
Acute tubular necrosis	Acute rejection	Prerenal azotemia
Hyperacute rejection	Calcineurin inhibitor toxicity	Calcineurin inhibitor toxicity
Accelerated rejection	Prerenal azotemia	Acute rejection (nonadherence, low levels)
Obstruction	Obstruction	Obstruction
Urine leak (ureteral necrosis)	Infection	Recurrent renal disease
Arterial or venous thrombosis	Interstitial nephritis	De novo renal disease
Atheroemboli	Recurrent renal disease	Renal artery stenosis (anastomotic or atherosclerotic)
	BK virus nephropathy	BK virus nephropathy

Acute Rejection, Lung

GENERAL PRINCIPLES

- Of the solid organ transplants, the lung is one of the most immunogenic organs.
- The majority of patients have at least one episode of acute rejection. Multiple episodes of acute rejection predispose to the development of chronic rejection (bronchiolitis obliterans syndrome).
- **Lung transplant rejection** occurs most commonly in the first few months after transplantation.

DIAGNOSIS

Diagnosis is generally made by fiberoptic bronchoscopy with bronchoalveolar lavage and transbronchial biopsies.

Clinical Presentation

Manifestations are nonspecific and include fever, dyspnea, and a nonproductive cough. The chest radiograph is typically unchanged and is generally nondiagnostic even when abnormal (perihilar infiltrates, interstitial edema, pleural effusions). Change in pulmonary function testing is not specific for rejection, but a 10% or greater decline in FVC and/or FEV_1 is clinically significant.

Differential Diagnosis

It is important to distinguish rejection from infection because although the symptoms are similar, the treatments are markedly different.

Acute Rejection, Heart

GENERAL PRINCIPLES

Heart transplant recipients typically have 2–3 episodes of acute rejection in the first year after transplantation with a 50%–80% chance of having at least one rejection episode, most commonly in the first 6 months.

DIAGNOSIS

- Diagnosis is established by endomyocardial biopsy performed during routine surveillance or as prompted by symptoms. Noninvasive techniques have not demonstrated sufficient sensitivity and specificity to replace the endomyocardial biopsy. Repeated endomyocardial biopsies predispose to severe tricuspid regurgitation.
- Manifestations may include symptoms and signs of left ventricular dysfunction, such as dyspnea, paroxysmal nocturnal dyspnea, orthopnea, syncope, palpitations, new gallops, and elevated jugular venous pressure. Many patients are asymptomatic. Acute rejection can also be associated with a variety of tachyarrhythmias (atrial more often than ventricular).

CHAPTER 17

Acute Rejection, Liver

GENERAL PRINCIPLES

- Many liver transplant recipients are maintained on minimal immunosuppression. Acute rejection typically occurs within the first 3 months after transplant and often in the first 2 weeks after the operation. Acute rejection in the liver is generally reversible and does not portend as serious adverse outcomes as in other organs. Recurrent viral hepatitis is a much more frequent and morbid problem.
- **Liver transplant recipients** commonly experience acute allograft rejection, with at least 60% having one episode.

DIAGNOSIS

Diagnosis is made by liver biopsy after technical complications are excluded.

Clinical Presentation

Manifestations can range from a slight elevation in transaminases to signs and symptoms of liver failure including fever, malaise, altered mental status, anorexia, abdominal pain, ascites, elevated bilirubin, and elevated transaminases.

Differential Diagnosis

Differential diagnosis of early liver allograft dysfunction includes primary graft nonfunction, preservation injury, vascular thrombosis, and biliary anastomotic leak or stenosis. These disorders should be excluded clinically or by Doppler ultrasonography. Causes of late allograft dysfunction include rejection, recurrent hepatitis B or C, CMV infection, EBV infection, cholestasis, or drug toxicity.

Acute Rejection, Pancreas

GENERAL PRINCIPLES

- The majority of rejection episodes occur within the first 6 months after transplant. Unlike other organs, clinical findings and biochemical markers correlate poorly with rejection. In particular, if hyperglycemia occurs because of rejection, it is often late, severe, and irreversible. Because 80% of pancreas transplants are performed with a simultaneous kidney transplant of the same immunologic status, renal allograft function and histopathology can be valuable surrogates for diagnosis of pancreas allograft rejection.
- Most pancreas transplants are done with quadruple immunosuppression, consisting of an induction agent and triple maintenance immunosuppression, including corticosteroids. One-year posttransplant acute rejection rates range between 20% and 30%; this contributes significantly to early and late graft loss.

DIAGNOSIS

At time of surgery, the exocrine (digestive enzymes) secretions of the pancreas can be drained into the recipient's intestine (enteric drainage) or into the bladder (bladder drainage). Serum amylase and lipase are used in both the enteric- and bladder-drained recipient to monitor for rejection, but lack specificity. For the bladder-drained allograft, a fall in urinary amylase correlates with rejection. However, allograft biopsy remains the gold standard, demonstrating septal, ductal, and acinar inflammation and endotheliitis. If a recipient received a simultaneous kidney transplant from the same donor, the creatinine and renal biopsy may also be used to diagnose rejection, although isolated pancreas or kidney rejection may rarely occur.

Clinical Presentation
Manifestations may be absent with only a slight elevation in serum amylase and lipase or fall in urinary amylase (bladder drained). Hyperglycemia is a late manifestation of rejection.

Differential Diagnosis
Differential diagnosis of hyperglycemia includes thrombosis (affecting 7% of recipients), islet cell drug toxicity, steroid effect, infection, development of insulin resistance, or recurrent autoimmune disease. Differential diagnosis of elevated serum lipase includes graft pancreatitis, peripancreatic fluid/infection, obstruction, dehydration, and PTLD.

Chronic Allograft Dysfunction

GENERAL PRINCIPLES

- Chronic allograft dysfunction accounts for the vast majority of late graft losses and is the major obstacle to long-term graft survival.
- Chronic allograft dysfunction (formerly chronic rejection) is a slowly progressive, insidious decline in function of the allograft characterized by gradual vascular and ductal obliteration, parenchymal atrophy, and interstitial fibrosis.

DIAGNOSIS

- Diagnosis is challenging and generally requires a biopsy. The rejection process is mediated by immune and nonimmune factors.
- The manifestations of chronic rejection are unique to each organ system.

TREATMENT

To date, no effective therapy is available for established immune-mediated chronic allograft dysfunction. Some patients, particularly those with renal transplants, will require a second solid organ transplant. Current investigational strategies are aimed at prevention.

BIOMARKERS

- The incidence of acute rejection varies between allograft types. Current recommended routine markers/imaging (i.e., serum creatinine in kidney transplant and echocardiogram in heart transplant) are not sensitive enough to detect graft damage in the early stages of rejection. There are limitations of invasive biopsy for routine surveillance. Noninvasive biomarkers could serve as predictive factors for rejection for early identification of allograft injury and prompt early intervention.

- Unbiased high-throughput gene expression profiling technologies and donor-derived cell-free DNA testing are other tools that can help provide further information into the health of an allograft. These technologies are available in kidney and heart transplant, but not currently available for other organ transplants.[4]

Complications

GENERAL PRINCIPLES

- Infections
  - Posttransplant infections are a significant cause of morbidity and, in some cases, mortality for transplant recipients. Types of infections vary depending on the time since transplantation (Table 17-3).[5]
  - **CMV infection** from reactivation of CMV in a seropositive recipient or new infection from a CMV-positive organ can lead to a wide range of presentations from a mild viral syndrome to allograft dysfunction, invasive disease in multiple organ systems, and even death. CMV-seronegative patients who receive a CMV-seropositive organ are at substantial risk, particularly in the first year.
    - Because of the potential progression and severity of untreated disease, treatment is indicated in viremic transplant patients without tissue diagnosis of invasive disease. Seroconversion with a positive IgM titer or a fourfold increase in IgM or IgG titer suggests acute infection; however, many centers now use polymerase chain reaction–based diagnostic techniques from blood samples, and treatment is usually administered in the patient with evidence of viremia. Common treatment options include oral valganciclovir, 450–900 mg PO bid, or IV ganciclovir, 2.5–5.0 mg/kg bid for 3–4 weeks or until clearance of the virus. Both drugs are adjusted for renal function. Hyperimmune globulin is also used with ganciclovir for patients with organ involvement.
    - Foscarnet and cidofovir are more toxic alternatives and should be reserved for ganciclovir-resistant cases.
  - **Hepatitis B and C:** Chronic hepatitis B or hepatitis C or cirrhosis were once considered contraindications to nonhepatic transplant because immunosuppression increases viral replication in organ transplant recipients. However, advances in medical treatment have created opportunities for a substantial number of patients to be effectively treated prior to transplantation.[6]
    - **Hepatitis B** reactivation can cause fulminant hepatic failure even in patients with no evidence of viral DNA replication prior to transplantation. In liver transplantation, the risk of recurrent hepatitis B virus infection can be reduced by the administration of hepatitis B immunoglobulin during and after transplantation. Lamivudine therapy initiated before transplantation to lower viral load leads to decreased likelihood of recurrent hepatitis B virus.
    - **Hepatitis C** progresses slowly in nonhepatic transplants, and the effect of immunosuppression on mortality because of liver disease remains to be determined. Hepatitis C nearly always recurs in untreated liver transplant recipients whose original disease was due to hepatitis C. Therapy for hepatitis C virus with directed antiviral therapy can achieve a sustained virologic response and clearance of the virus.
  - **EBV** plays a role in the development of PTLD. This life-threatening lymphoma is treated by withdrawal or reduction in immunosuppression and aggressive chemotherapy.

TABLE 17-3	Timing and Etiology of Posttransplant Infections	
Time Period	Infectious Complication	Etiology
<1 mo after transplant	Nosocomial pneumonia, wound infection, urinary tract infection, catheter-related sepsis, biliary, chest, or other drainage catheter infection	Bacterial or fungal infections
1–6 mo after transplant	Opportunistic infections	Cytomegalovirus
		Pneumocystis jirovecii
		Aspergillus spp.
		Toxoplasma gondii
		Listeria monocytogenes
		Strongyloides stercoralis
		West Nile virus
		Varicella-zoster virus (VZV)
	Reactivation of preexisting infections	*Mycobacteria* spp.
		Endemic mycoses
		Viral hepatitis
>6 mo after transplant	Community-acquired infections	Bacterial
		Tick-borne disease
		Influenza
		Metapneumovirus
		Norovirus
	Chronic progressive infection	Reactivated VZV (zoster)
		Hepatitis B
		Hepatitis C
		HIV
		Cytomegalovirus
		Epstein–Barr virus
		Papillomavirus
		Polyomavirus (BK)
	Opportunistic infections	*P. jirovecii*
		L. monocytogenes
		Nocardia asteroides
		Cryptococcus neoformans
		Aspergillus spp.
		West Nile virus

- **Other viruses:** The role other viruses, such as human herpesvirus (HHV)-6, HHV-7, HHV-8, and polyomavirus (BK and JC), play in causing posttransplant infections is an area of active investigation. Notably, BK virus is known to cause interstitial nephritis, resulting in renal allograft loss and occasionally ureteral stricture, resulting in obstruction. Because BK virus nephropathy results primarily from reactivation of latent BK in the transplanted organ, this is rarely seen in nonrenal transplant recipients.

- ○ **Fungal and parasitic infections**, such as *Cryptococcus, Mucor*, aspergillosis, and *Candida* spp., result in increased mortality after transplantation. A high degree of suspicion is imperative to diagnose and treat these infections. The role of prophylaxis with oral fluconazole has not been established.
- **Renal disease:** Chronic allograft dysfunction is the leading cause of allograft loss in renal transplant recipients. Chronic CNI (CsA or tacrolimus) nephrotoxicity may also lead to chronic kidney disease and end-stage renal disease (ESRD), requiring dialysis or transplantation in recipients of other solid organ transplants. The incidence of ESRD secondary to CNI toxicity in recipients of solid organ transplants is at least 10%, and the incidence of significant chronic kidney disease approaches 50%.
- **Malignancy** occurs in transplant patients with an overall incidence 3–4 times higher than the general population (age-matched). Cancers with an increased risk of fivefold or greater compared with the general population are Kaposi sarcoma, non-Hodgkin lymphoma, and skin, lip, vulvar, anal, and liver cancer, illustrating the oncogenic potential of associated viral infections and the role of normal immune function in surveillance and clearance of malignant cells.
  - ○ **Skin and lip cancers** are the most common de novo malignancies (40%–50%) seen in transplant recipients, with an incidence 10–250 times that of the general population. Risk factors include immunosuppression, UV radiation, and human papillomavirus infection. These cancers develop at a younger age, and they are more aggressive in transplant patients. Protective clothing, sunscreens, and avoiding sun exposure are recommended. Examination of the skin is the principal screening test and early diagnosis offers the best prognosis.
  - ○ **PTLD** accounts for one-fifth of all malignancies after transplantation, with an incidence of approximately 1%. This is 30- to 50-fold higher than in the general population, and the risk increases with the use of antilymphocyte therapy for induction or rejection. The majority of these neoplasms are large-cell non-Hodgkin lymphomas of the B-cell type. PTLD results from EBV-induced B-cell proliferation in the setting of chronic immunosuppression. The EBV-seronegative recipient of a seropositive organ is at greatest risk. The presentation is often atypical and should always be considered in the patient with new symptoms. Diagnosis requires a high index of suspicion followed by a tissue biopsy. Treatment includes reduction or withdrawal of immunosuppression and chemotherapy.

SPECIAL CONSIDERATIONS

- **Important drug interactions** are always a concern. Before prescribing a new medication, always investigate drug interactions.
- The combination of **allopurinol/febuxostat and azathioprine** should be avoided because of the risk of profound myelosuppression.
- CsA and tacrolimus are metabolized by cytochrome P450 (3A4). Therefore, CsA and tacrolimus levels are decreased by drugs that induce cytochrome P450 activity, such as rifampin, isoniazid, barbiturates, phenytoin, and carbamazepine. Conversely, CsA and tacrolimus levels are increased by drugs that compete for cytochrome P450, such as verapamil, diltiazem, nicardipine, azole antifungals, erythromycin, and clarithromycin. Similar effects are seen with sirolimus and everolimus.

- **Tacrolimus and CsA** should not be taken together due to increased risk of severe nephrotoxicity.
- Lower doses of MPA should be used with tacrolimus or sirolimus.
- Concomitant administration of CsA and sirolimus may result in up to a twofold increase in sirolimus levels; CsA and sirolimus should be dosed 4 hours apart.

REFERENCES

1. Wiseman AC. Immunosuppressive medications. *Clin J Am Soc Nephrol*. 2016;11(2):332-343.
2. Halloran PF. Immunosuppressive drugs for kidney transplantation. *N Engl J Med*. 2004;351:2715-2729.
3. Marik PE, Varon J. Requirement of perioperative stress doses of corticosteroids: a systematic review of the literature. *Arch Surg*. 2008;143(12):1222-1226.
4. Yang JYC, Sarwal MM. Transplant genetic and genomics. *Nat Rev Genet*. 2017;18(5):309-326.
5. Fishman JA, Rubin RH. Infection in organ- transplant recipients. *N Engl J Med*. 1998;338(24):1741-1751 (Table 17-2).
6. Huskey J, Wiseman AC. Chronic viral hepatitis in kidney transplantation. *Nat Rev Nephrol*. 2011;7:156-165.

CHAPTER 17

Gastrointestinal Bleeding

GENERAL PRINCIPLES

Acute gastrointestinal (GI) bleeding is a common clinical problem that results in substantial morbidity, healthcare resource utilization, and costs, especially when it develops in hospitalized patients.[1]
- **Overt GI bleeding** is the passage of fresh or altered blood in emesis or stool.
- **Occult GI bleeding** refers to a positive fecal occult blood test (stool guaiac or fecal immunochemical test) or iron deficiency anemia without visible blood in the stool.
- **Obscure GI bleeding** consists of GI blood loss of unknown origin that persists or recurs after negative initial esophagogastroduodenoscopy (EGD) and ileocolonoscopy.[2]

DIAGNOSIS

Clinical Presentation

History
- Hematemesis, coffee-ground emesis, and/or aspiration of blood or coffee-ground material from a nasogastric (NG) tube indicate an upper GI source of blood loss.
- **Melena**, black sticky stool with a characteristic odor, usually suggests an upper GI source, although small bowel and right-sided colonic bleeds can also result in melena.
- Various shades of **bloody stool (hematochezia)** are seen with distal small bowel or colonic bleeding, depending on the rate of blood loss and colonic transit. Rapid upper GI bleeding can present with hematochezia, typically associated with hemodynamic compromise.
- **Anorectal bleeding** usually results in bright red blood coating the exterior of formed stool or with wiping, and can be associated with distal colonic symptoms (e.g., rectal urgency, straining, or pain with defecation).
- **Anemia** from blood loss can cause fatigue, weakness, abdominal pain, pallor, or dyspnea.
- Estimation of the amount of blood loss is often inaccurate. If the baseline hematocrit is known, the drop in hematocrit provides a rough estimate of blood loss.
- **Coagulation abnormalities** can propagate bleeding from a preexisting lesion in the GI tract. Disorders of coagulation (e.g., liver disease, von Willebrand disease, vitamin K deficiency, and disseminated intravascular coagulation) can influence the course of GI bleeding (see Chapter 20, Disorders of Hemostasis and Thrombosis).
- **Medications** known to affect the coagulation process or platelet function include warfarin, heparin, low-molecular-weight heparin, aspirin, nonsteroidal anti-inflammatory drugs (NSAIDs), P2Y12 receptor blockers (e.g., clopidogrel [Plavix],

prasugrel [Effient], ticagrelor [Brilinta], ticlopidine [Ticlid]), thrombolytic agents, glycoprotein IIb/IIIa receptor antagonists (abciximab [ReoPro], eptifibatide [Integrilin], tirofiban [Aggrastat]), direct thrombin inhibitors (e.g., argatroban, bivalirudin, dabigatran etexilate), and direct factor Xa inhibitors (e.g., rivaroxaban [Xarelto], apixaban).

- **NSAIDs and aspirin** can result in mucosal damage anywhere in the GI tract. Therefore, dual antiplatelet therapy (e.g., clopidogrel plus aspirin) or concomitant aspirin and anticoagulation with warfarin can escalate the risk for GI bleeding by both initiating and propagating bleeding.

Physical Examination

- **Color of stool:** Direct examination of spontaneously passed stool or on **digital rectal examination (DRE)** may help localize the level of bleeding. DRE may also identify anorectal abnormalities including anal fissures, which induce extreme discomfort during the DRE.
- Fresh blood on an **NG aspirate** may indicate ongoing upper GI bleeding requiring urgent endoscopic attention, but hemodynamic status is equally important.[3] The aspirate should be considered positive only if blood or dark particulate matter ("coffee grounds") is seen; **hemoccult testing of NG aspirate has no clinical utility. NG tube** placement is not required in the evaluation of a patient with alternate conclusive evidence of acute GI bleeding. A negative NG aspirate does not rule out bleeding from a duodenal source. An NG tube may help clear the stomach of blood and clots to facilitate visualization during endoscopy, but it does not obviate the need for airway protection with massive bleeding.
- **Orthostatic hemodynamic changes** (drop in systolic BP of >20 mm Hg, rise in pulse rate of >10 bpm) are seen with loss of 10%–20% of the circulatory volume; supine hypotension suggests a >20% loss. Hypotension with a systolic BP of <100 mm Hg or baseline tachycardia >100 bpm suggests significant hemodynamic compromise that requires urgent volume resuscitation.[4]

Diagnostic Testing

Laboratories

- Complete blood cell (CBC) count
- Coagulation parameters (international normalized ratio [INR], partial thromboplastin time)
- Blood group, cross-matching of two to four units of blood
- Comprehensive metabolic profile (creatinine, blood urea nitrogen, liver function tests)

Diagnostic Procedures

- **Endoscopy**
  - **Esophagogastroduodenoscopy (EGD),** with high diagnostic accuracy and therapeutic capability, is the preferred investigative test in upper GI bleeding. Volume resuscitation or blood transfusion should precede endoscopy in hemodynamically unstable patients. Patients with ongoing bleeding or at risk for an adverse outcome benefit most from urgent EGD, whereas stable patients can undergo endoscopy electively during the hospitalization. Hemodynamically stable patients should undergo endoscopy within 24 hours. A clinical trial demonstrated endoscopy within 6 hours did not improve mortality, but patients with ongoing hemodynamic instability after resuscitation were excluded.[5] Promotility agents given 30 minutes prior to EGD (IV erythromycin 125–250 mg or IV metoclopramide

CHAPTER 18

10 mg) may empty the stomach of blood and clots to improve visibility for EGD, but endoscopy should not be delayed.[6] Routine second-look EGD after hemostasis has no proven benefit in reducing surgical intervention or overall mortality.[7]

- ○ **Colonoscopy** can be performed after a rapid bowel purge in clinically stable patients; the purge solution can be infused through an NG tube when not tolerated orally. While diagnostic yield is highest with colonoscopy performed within 24 hours of presentation, patient outcome does not necessarily improve. Therapeutic colonoscopy, however, may reduce transfusion requirements, need for surgery, and length of hospital stay.[8] All patients with acute lower GI bleeding from an unknown source should eventually undergo colonoscopy during the initial hospitalization, regardless of the initial mode of investigation.
- ○ **Anoscopy** may be useful in the detection of internal hemorrhoids and anal fissures but does not replace the need for colonoscopy.
- ○ **Push enteroscopy** allows evaluation of the proximal small bowel beyond reach of a standard EGD, especially if no source is found on careful colonoscopy.[9]
- ○ **Capsule endoscopy** is most useful after the upper gut and the colon have been thoroughly examined and the bleeding source is suspected in the small bowel.[9]
- ○ **Single- and double-balloon enteroscopy** allow visualization of most of the small bowel through either an antegrade or retrograde approach, typically performed when capsule endoscopy localizes bleeding to the small bowel.[9] Balloons at the endoscope tip and overtube can be consecutively inflated and deflated to facilitate deep insertion into the small bowel.
- ○ **Intraoperative enteroscopy** may assist endoscopic therapy or surgical resection of an actively bleeding source in the small bowel but carries a high risk of complications.
- **Tagged red blood cell (RBC) scanning** involves labeling RBCs with technetium-99m that may extravasate into the bowel lumen with active bleeding, detected as pooling of the radioactive tracer on gamma camera scanning, to identify the potential bleeding site. Bleeding rates of 0.2 mL/min can be detected.
- **CT angiography (CTA)** can localize bleeding exceeding 0.3 mL/min before catheter angiography and has an advantage over CT enterography.[9] Tagged RBC and CTA are particularly useful in unstable active bleeding precluding urgent colonoscopy.
- **Angiography** demonstrates extravasation of the dye into the intestine when bleeding rates exceed 0.5 mL/min. Angiography is often performed after bleeding is initially localized by other means. Selective cannulation and infusion of vasopressin vasoconstrict the bleeding vessel; alternatively, the bleeding vessel can be embolized.

TREATMENT

- **Restoration of intravascular volume:** Two large-bore (16- to 18-gauge) IV lines or a central venous line should be urgently placed to provide IV fluid resuscitation. The rate at which fluid can be delivered is proportional to the diameter of the catheter and inversely proportional to its length (i.e., a 22-gauge peripheral catheter delivers fluid at a rate of 35 mL/min compared to 154.7 mL/min with a 16-gauge catheter).[10] Importantly, despite their utility in delivering vasopressors and other essential medications for critical care, a typical triple lumen central venous catheter cannot deliver fluids as quickly as an 18-gauge peripheral IV (69.4 mL/min vs. 98.1 mL/min).[10] A wide bore, short central line is ideal for resuscitating patients in hemorrhagic shock.

- **Packed RBC transfusion** should be utilized when hemoglobin is less than 7 g/dL since a higher transfusion target is associated with increased mortality.[11] A higher threshold for initiating transfusion should be considered in patients with cardiovascular disease. In patients presenting with hemorrhagic shock, however, O-negative blood or simultaneous multiple-unit transfusions should be used if available and continued until hemodynamic stability is achieved.
- **Oxygen administration:** Supplemental oxygen enhances the oxygen-carrying capacity of blood and should be considered in acute GI bleeding.
- **Correction of coagulopathy:** Coagulopathy (INR > 1.5) or thrombocytopenia should ideally be corrected in patients with GI bleeding, but endoscopy should not be delayed.[12] An elevated INR can be treated with vitamin K, fresh frozen plasma (FFP), or intravenous prothrombin complex concentrate (PCC). Reversal agents are available for many antithrombotic agents (vitamin K, FFP, PCC for warfarin; idarucizumab [Praxbind] for the direct thrombin inhibitor dabigatran; andexanet alfa [AndexXa] for factor Xa inhibitors [e.g., apixaban, edoxaban, rivaroxaban]). The decision to reverse coagulopathy should be individualized, considering the severity of bleeding and the risk of thrombosis with reversal. In patients with cirrhosis, INR does not adequately reflect coagulation status; thus, attempts to correct INR can increase portal pressure and worsen bleeding.[13] Rotational thromboelastometry may be helpful to guide resuscitation, if available.
- **Endotracheal intubation** protects the airway and prevents aspiration in obtunded patients with massive hematemesis and in active variceal bleeding.
- **Risk stratification:** Validated risk stratification tools, such as the Rockall and Glasgow-Blatchford scores, may be helpful to identify patients that can be safely discharged.[14]

Medications

- **Nonvariceal upper GI bleeding:** High-dose proton pump inhibitors (PPI) (80 mg IV bolus followed by 8 mg/h continuous infusion) reduce rebleeding and mortality in patients with peptic ulcers with high-risk stigmata (active bleeding or nonbleeding visible vessel, see Table 18-1).[15,16] Twice-daily IV bolus dosing (40 mg IV twice

TABLE 18-1	Forrest Classification of Peptic Ulcers		
Class	Lesion	Risk of Rebleeding	Comments
IA	Spurting	55%	Requires endoscopic therapy, treat with IV PPI for 72 h
IB	Oozing		Requires endoscopic therapy, treat with IV PPI for 72 h
IIA	Nonbleeding visible vessel	43%	Requires endoscopic therapy, treat with IV PPI for 72 h
IIB	Adherent clot	22%	May be treated endoscopically, treat with IV PPI for 72 h
IIC	Flat pigmented spot	10%	Low risk, does not require endoscopic therapy
III	Clean base	5%	Low risk, does not require endoscopic therapy

PPI, proton pump inhibitor.

daily) may provide sufficient acid suppression compared to an infusion.[17] High-dose PPI should be initiated at presentation with suspected upper GI bleeding, which decreases the need for endoscopic hemostasis, though it does not prevent rebleeding.[18] Patients with high-risk stigmata should continue high-dose PPI for 72 hours, then transitioned to twice-daily oral PPI for 14 days, followed by once daily. Patients without high-risk stigmata may start oral PPI after endoscopy. All patients found to have peptic ulcers should be tested for **Helicobacter pylori** and treated with eradication therapy if positive (see Peptic Ulcer Disease section).

- **Variceal bleeding:** Infusion of **octreotide** (an octapeptide that mimics endogenous somatostatin) acutely reduces portal pressures and controls variceal bleeding, improving the diagnostic yield and therapeutic success of subsequent endoscopy. Octreotide should be initiated immediately (50- to 100-μg bolus, followed by infusion at 25–50 μg/h) and continued for 3–5 days if variceal hemorrhage is confirmed on EGD.[19] Prophylactic antibiotics (third-generation cephalosporins or fluoroquinolones) should be administered to patients with cirrhosis and variceal bleeding because antibiotics reduce bacterial infections, rebleeding, and mortality.[20]

- **Thalidomide** may be an effective approach for refractory chronic bleeding from GI vascular malformations.[21] Some patients with chronic GI bleeding from arteriovenous malformations are managed with iron supplementation (PO or IV) and as-needed transfusions, reserving endoscopy for acute bleeding with hemodynamic instability.

Nonpharmacologic Therapies

- **Endoscopic therapy**
  - **Therapeutic endoscopy** offers the advantage of endoscopic hemostasis and should be performed early in acute upper GI bleeding (within 12–24 hours).
  - **Variceal ligation** or **banding** is the endoscopic therapy of choice for esophageal varices, with endotracheal intubation for airway protection if bleeding is massive or the patient is obtunded.[19] Variceal banding can provide both primary and secondary prophylaxis of variceal bleeding, with benefits similar to those from β-blocker therapy alone.[22] Complications include superficial ulceration, dysphagia, and transient chest discomfort.
  - **Sclerotherapy** is also effective but is used mostly when variceal banding is not technically feasible.

- **Transjugular intrahepatic portosystemic shunt (TIPS):** An expandable metal stent is deployed between the hepatic veins and the portal vein to reduce portal venous pressure in refractory esophageal and/or gastric variceal bleeding from portal hypertension. Early TIPS reduces treatment failure and mortality in acute variceal bleeding.[23] Encephalopathy may occur in up to 25% of patients and is treated medically (see Chapter 19, Liver Diseases). If variceal bleeding recurs or if gastric varices redevelop, duplex Doppler ultrasound can assess for TIPS stenosis.

- **Balloon-occluded retrograde transvenous obliteration (BRTO):** Gastric varices are obliterated by interventional radiographic access through a patent gastrorenal shunt.[24]

- **Angiography** (see above) can be used for bleeding peptic ulcers not amenable to endoscopic therapy or when endoscopic therapy fails.

Surgical Management

- **Emergent total colectomy** may rarely be required for massive, unlocalized, colonic bleeding; this should be preceded by EGD to rule out a rapidly bleeding upper source whenever possible. Certain lesions (e.g., neoplasia, Meckel diverticulum) require surgical resection for a cure.

- Angiography is typically attempted prior to surgery for peptic ulcer bleeding not amenable to endoscopic therapy. Perforation necessitates surgical consultation.
- **Total or partial colectomy** may be required for ongoing or recurrent diverticular bleeding.
- **Splenectomy** is curative in bleeding gastric varices from splenic vein thrombosis.
- **Shunt surgery** (portacaval or distal splenorenal shunt) is now rarely performed with the wide availability of TIPS, but it remains a consideration in patients with good hepatic reserve.

SPECIAL CONSIDERATIONS

Cardiac Patients and Gastrointestinal Bleeding

- Timing of restarting antiplatelet or antithrombotic therapy following a GI bleed should be individualized based on the risk of rebleeding from the bleed source and the risk of thrombotic events. In general, these agents should be restarted as soon as possible given that a thrombotic event can be more devastating than recurrent bleeding. A randomized clinical trial showed that restarting aspirin immediately after endoscopic hemostasis was associated with reduced mortality, despite a not significant increase in recurrent bleeding.[25] PPI should be continued while patients are on antiplatelet or antithrombotic medication.
- **PPI prophylaxis** decreases the risk of GI bleeding, without significant increase in major cardiovascular events in patients on dual antiplatelet therapy.[26] Despite concerns that PPIs competitively inhibit the cytochrome P450 enzyme that activates clopidogrel, randomized controlled trials have not substantiated higher vascular events with concurrent use of clopidogrel and PPI.[26]
- **Left ventricular assist devices (LVADs)** are associated with GI bleeding from angiodysplastic lesions, making EGD or push enteroscopy the initial investigation of choice.[27]

Dysphagia and Odynophagia

GENERAL PRINCIPLES

- **Oropharyngeal dysphagia** consists of difficulty in transferring food from the mouth to the esophagus, often associated with nasopharyngeal regurgitation and aspiration. Neuromuscular and, less commonly, structural disorders involving the pharynx and proximal esophagus are typical causes.[28]
- **Esophageal dysphagia** is the sensation of impairment in passage of food down the tubular esophagus. Etiologies include obstructive processes (e.g., webs, rings, esophagitis, neoplasia) or esophageal motor disorders.[29]
- **Odynophagia** is pain on swallowing food and fluids and may indicate the presence of esophagitis, particularly infectious esophagitis or pill esophagitis.

DIAGNOSIS

Oropharyngeal Dysphagia

- A detailed neurologic examination is the first diagnostic step. **Barium videofluoroscopy (modified barium swallow)** evaluates the oropharyngeal swallow mechanism and may identify laryngeal penetration.

CHAPTER 18

- Ear, nose, and throat examination; flexible nasal endoscopy; and imaging studies may identify structural etiologies.
- Laboratory tests for polymyositis, myasthenia gravis, and other neuromuscular disorders are performed when neurologic or structural etiologies are not evident.

Esophageal Dysphagia

- **EGD** is the initial test of choice as it identifies mucosal and structural abnormalities, allows tissue sampling (to evaluate for esophageal eosinophilia or for conclusive diagnosis of suspected neoplasia), and offers the option of dilation, which should be performed for most esophageal strictures.[30,31]
- **Esophageal manometry,** preferably **high-resolution manometry (HRM)**, should be performed when other studies are normal or suggest an esophageal motility disorder. The image-based paradigm of Clouse plots on HRM has simplified testing procedures, allowing for easier analysis, and improved diagnostic utility over conventional manometry.[32] Provocative maneuvers during HRM can prevent under- and overdiagnosis of motility disorders.
- **Endoluminal functional lumen imaging probe (FLIP)** evaluates compliance and distensibility of the esophagus and esophagogastric junction, with the potential for higher sensitivity in the detection of esophageal outflow obstruction compared with manometry. FLIP utilizes impedance planimetry during volume-controlled distention of a compliant balloon to measure cross-sectional area, from which a distensibility index is calculated.[33]
- **Barium swallow** defines anatomy and identifies subtle rings and strictures, which may only be seen with a barium pill or a solid barium bolus.[34]
- Acute esophageal obstruction is best investigated with endoscopy. Barium studies should not be performed when esophageal obstruction is suspected because barium can obscure visualization during endoscopy and may take several days to clear. If a contrast study is needed, water-soluble contrast should be used.

TREATMENT

- Modification of diet and swallowing maneuvers directed by a speech pathologist improve especially oropharyngeal dysphagia. Patients with dysphagia are advised to chew their food well and eat foods of soft consistencies.
- Enteral feeding through a gastrostomy tube is indicated when frank tracheal aspiration is identified on attempted swallowing.
- Endoscopic retrieval of an obstructing food bolus relieves acute dysphagia. This is typically followed by further evaluation, including esophageal biopsies, and subsequent endoscopy for dilation.
- Nutrition needs to be addressed in patients with prolonged dysphagia causing weight loss.

Medications

- Mucosal inflammation from reflux disease can be treated with acid suppression.
- Odynophagia generally responds to specific therapy when the cause is identified (e.g., PPIs for reflux disease, antimicrobial agents for infectious esophagitis). Viscous lidocaine swish-and-swallow solutions may afford symptomatic relief.
- Anticholinergic medication (e.g., transdermal scopolamine) helps drooling of saliva.
- **Glucagon** (2–4 mg IV bolus) or sublingual **nitroglycerin** can be attempted in acute food impaction, but meat tenderizer should not be administered.

Nonpharmacologic Therapies

- Esophageal dilation is performed for strictures, rings, and webs.[31] Empiric bougie dilation may provide symptomatic benefit even when a defined narrowing is not identified in some settings, especially when dysphagia is localized to the high neck, and eosinophilic esophagitis has been excluded.
- Pneumatic dilation of the lower esophageal sphincter (LES) and peroral endoscopic myotomy (POEM) are options for achalasia management (see Esophageal Motor Disorders section). Botulinum toxin injection into the LES provides temporary symptom relief in achalasia and esophageal outflow obstruction from motor etiologies.[31]
- Esophageal stent placement can alleviate dysphagia from inoperable neoplasia.

Nausea and Vomiting

GENERAL PRINCIPLES

- Nausea and vomiting may result from side effects of medications, systemic illnesses, central nervous system (CNS) disorders, and primary GI disorders.
- Vomiting that occurs during or immediately after a meal can result from acute pyloric stenosis (e.g., pyloric channel ulcer) or from functional disorders, while vomiting within 30–60 minutes after a meal may suggest gastric or duodenal pathology. Delayed vomiting of undigested food from a previous meal can suggest gastric outlet obstruction or gastroparesis.
- Symptoms of gastroparesis may be indistinguishable from functional dyspepsia and chronic functional nausea and vomiting with normal gastric emptying.[35]

DIAGNOSIS

- **Bowel obstruction and pregnancy should be ruled out.**
- **Medication lists** should be carefully scrutinized for potential offenders, and systemic illnesses (acute and chronic) should be evaluated as etiologies or contributing factors.
- Endoscopy and/or imaging should be considered in the setting of nonresolving or "red flag" symptoms, such as hematemesis or weight loss.

TREATMENT

- Correction of fluid and electrolyte imbalances is an important supportive measure.
- Oral intake should be limited to clear liquids, if tolerated. Many patients with self-limited illnesses require no further therapy.
- NG decompression may be required for patients with bowel obstruction or protracted nausea and vomiting of any etiology.
- Enteral feeding through jejunal tubes or, rarely, total parenteral nutrition (TPN) may be necessary to supplement nutrient intake.

Medications

Empiric pharmacotherapy (Table 18-2) is often initiated while investigation is in progress or when the etiology is thought to be self-limited.

- **Phenothiazines and related agents:** Prochlorperazine and promethazine are often used as first-line agents in nausea. Drowsiness is a common side effect, and acute dystonic reactions or other extrapyramidal effects may occur.

CHAPTER 18

TABLE 18-2	Commonly Used Antiemetics		
Medication	Dosage	Receptor Target	Comments
Diphenhydramine	25–50 mg PO q6h 10–50 mg IV q6h	Histamine (H_1)	May cause sedation
Dimenhydrinate	50–100 mg PO q4h	Histamine (H_1)	May cause sedation
Meclizine	25–50 mg PO q4h	Histamine (H_1)	Often used for motion-sickness; may cause sedation
Promethazine	12.5–25 mg PO, IM or PR q4-6h	Histamine (H_1)	Drowsiness, dystonic reactions; risk of extra-pyramidal symptoms
Scopolamine	1.5 mg q72h transdermal	Muscarinic (M1)	May cause dry mouth, drowsiness
Prochlorperazine	5–10 mg PO qid 2.5–10 mg IV q4h. Max dose 40 mg/d	Dopamine (D2)	Prolongs QT
Haloperidol[a]	0.5–2 mg PO or IV q6-8h	Dopamine (D2)	Prolongs QT; risk of extrapyramidal symptoms including acute dystonia
Metoclopramide	10 mg PO or IV q6h	Dopamine (D2) Serotonin ($5\text{-}HT_3$)	Risk of extrapyramidal symptoms; not recommended for long-term use
Ondansetron	4–8 mg PO or IV q8h	Serotonin ($5\text{-}HT_3$)	Prolongs QT
Olanzapine[a]	5–10 mg daily	Dopamine (D2) Serotonin ($5\text{-}HT_2$)	Used for chemotherapy-induced nausea; prolongs QT, may cause sedation
Aprepitant	125 mg PO prior to chemotherapy, 80 mg PO on days 2 and 3	Neurokinin-1 (NK1)	Used for chemotherapy-induced nausea; many drug–drug interactions
Lorazepam[a]	0.5–2 mg PO q6h	GABA-A	Does not prolong QT
Dexamethasone[a]	4–8 mg IV once	Mechanism unclear	Used for chemotherapy-induced nausea; may cause insomnia, mood changes

[a]Considered off-label use.

- **Dopamine antagonists:** Metoclopramide is a prokinetic agent with central antiemetic effects. Drowsiness and extrapyramidal reactions may occur, and a warning has been issued by the US Food and Drug Administration (FDA) regarding the risk of permanent **tardive dyskinesia** with high-dose and/or long-term use.[36] Tachyphylaxis may limit long-term efficacy. Domperidone is an alternate agent that does not cross the blood–brain barrier and therefore has no CNS side effects; however, it is not uniformly available.
- **Antihistaminic agents**: Diphenhydramine, dimenhydrinate, and meclizine are most useful for nausea and vomiting related to motion sickness but may also be useful for other causes.
- **Serotonin 5-hydroxytryptamine-3 (5-HT₃) receptor antagonists: Ondansetron** is effective in chemotherapy-associated emesis. It can also be used in emesis that is refractory to other medications, especially the sublingual formulation.
- **Neurokinin-1 (NK-1) receptor antagonist: Aprepitant** is an alternative agent intended for chemotherapy-induced nausea and vomiting.
- **Lorazepam, haloperidol,** and **olanzapine** are other medications with antiemetic effect.

Diarrhea

GENERAL PRINCIPLES

- **Acute diarrhea** consists of abrupt onset of ≥3 unformed bowel movements in conjunction with associated symptoms such as tenesmus, fecal urgency, increased flatulence, nausea, or vomiting.[37] Infectious agents, toxins, and drugs are the major causes of acute diarrhea. In hospitalized patients, pseudomembranous colitis, antibiotic- or drug-associated diarrhea, and fecal impaction should be considered.[38]
- **Chronic diarrhea** consists of passage of loose stools with or without increased stool frequency and urgency for more than 4 weeks.[39]

DIAGNOSIS

- Most acute infectious diarrheal illnesses last less than 24 hours and are likely caused by viruses; therefore, stool studies are unnecessary in short-lived episodes without fever, dehydration, or presence of blood or pus in the stool.[38]
- Stool cultures, *Clostridioides difficile* toxin assay, ova and parasite examinations, and sigmoidoscopy or colonoscopy may be warranted in patients with severe, prolonged, atypical symptoms, or in immunocompromised patients.
- The **fecal osmotic gap** [290−2(stool Na⁺ + stool K⁺)] can be calculated in patients with chronic diarrhea and voluminous watery stools. The osmotic gap is **<50 mOsm/kg in secretory diarrhea** but **>125 mOsm/kg in osmotic diarrhea.**
- A positive fecal occult blood test or fecal leukocyte test suggests inflammatory diarrhea.
- **Steatorrhea** is traditionally diagnosed by demonstration of fat excretion in stool of >7 g/d in a 72-hour stool collection while the patient is on a 100-g/d fat diet. Sudan staining of a stool specimen is an alternate test; >100 fat globules per high-power field (HPF) is abnormal.
- Laxative screening should be considered when chronic diarrhea remains undiagnosed.

Clinical Presentation

- **Acute diarrhea**
  - **Viral enteritis** and **bacterial infections** with *Escherichia coli* and *Shigella*, *Salmonella*, *Campylobacter*, and *Yersinia* spp. constitute the most common causes.
  - **Pseudomembranous colitis** is usually seen in the setting of antimicrobial therapy and is caused by toxins produced by *C. difficile*.[40]
  - **Giardiasis** is confirmed by identification of *Giardia lamblia* trophozoites in the stool, in duodenal aspirate, or in small bowel biopsy specimens. A stool immuno-fluorescence assay is also available for rapid diagnosis.
  - **Amebiasis** may cause acute diarrhea, especially in travelers to areas with poor sanitation and in men who have sex with men. Stool examination for trophozoites or cysts of *Entamoeba histolytica* or a serum antibody test confirms the diagnosis.
  - **Medications** that can cause acute diarrhea include laxatives, antacids, cardiac medications (e.g., digitalis, quinidine), colchicine, and antimicrobial agents; symptoms typically respond to discontinuation.
  - **Graft-versus-host disease** should be considered when diarrhea develops after organ transplantation, especially bone marrow transplantation; **sigmoidoscopy with biopsies** should be pursued to confirm this diagnosis.[41]
- **Chronic diarrhea:** After a careful history, a thorough physical examination, and routine laboratory tests, chronic diarrhea can typically be classified into one of the following categories: watery diarrhea (secretory or osmotic), inflammatory diarrhea, or fatty diarrhea (steatorrhea).[39]

TREATMENT

- Adequate hydration, including IV hydration in severe cases, is the most important treatment in managing diarrheal diseases. Oral rehydration salt (ORS) solutions are World Health Organization (WHO) recommended for optimized water absorption. High-sugar beverages should be avoided because they can exacerbate fluid losses in the absence of sufficient salt. Commercially prepared solutions are available in developed countries (e.g., Pedialyte).
- Antibiotic-associated diarrhea and *C. difficile* infections can be prevented by restricting high-risk antibiotic use and prescribing antibiotics based on sensitivity analysis.
- Symptomatic therapy is offered in simple self-limiting GI infections where diarrhea is frequent or troublesome, while diagnostic workup is in progress, when specific management fails to improve symptoms, and/or when a specific etiology is not identified.
  - **Loperamide, opiates** (tincture of opium, belladonna, and opium capsules), and **anticholinergic agents** (diphenoxylate and atropine [Lomotil]) are the most effective nonspecific antidiarrheal agents.
  - **Pectin** and **kaolin** preparations (bind toxins) and **bismuth subsalicylate** (antibacterial properties) are also useful in symptomatic therapy of acute diarrhea.
  - **Bile acid–binding resins** (e.g., cholestyramine) are beneficial in bile acid–induced diarrhea.
  - **Octreotide** is useful in hormone-mediated secretory diarrhea but can also be of benefit in refractory diarrhea.

Medications

- **Empiric antibiotic therapy** is only recommended in patients with moderate to severe disease and associated systemic symptoms while awaiting stool cultures. Antibiotics can increase the possibility of hemolytic-uremic syndrome associated with Shiga toxin–producing *E. coli* infections (*E. coli* O157:H7), especially in children and the elderly.[42]

- Oral **vancomycin** or **fidaxomicin** are the antibiotics of choice for pseudomembranous colitis. **Metronidazole** can be used intravenously together with **vancomycin** in fulminant disease with hypotension, shock, or ileus. **Fecal microbiota transplant** is a novel treatment option.[43]
- Symptomatic amebiasis is treated with **metronidazole**, followed by **paromomycin** or **iodoquinol** to eliminate cysts.
- Therapy for giardiasis consists of metronidazole or tinidazole, with quinacrine representing an alternative agent.

SPECIAL CONSIDERATIONS

- **Opportunistic agents**, including cryptosporidium, microsporidium, cytomegalovirus (CMV), *Mycobacterium avium* complex, and *Mycobacterium tuberculosis*, may cause **diarrhea in patients with advanced HIV** (CD4 counts <50 cells/μL). However, *C. difficile* may be the most commonly identified bacterial pathogen.[44]
- Other causes of diarrhea in this population include sexually transmitted infections (e.g., syphilis, gonorrhea, chlamydia, herpes simplex virus [HSV]) and non–sexually transmitted infections (e.g., amebiasis, giardiasis, salmonellosis, shigellosis). Intestinal lymphoma and Kaposi sarcoma can also cause diarrhea.
- Stool studies (ova and parasites, culture), endoscopic biopsies, and serologic testing may assist in diagnosis. Management consists of specific therapy if pathogens are identified; symptomatic measures may be of benefit in idiopathic cases.
- Severe *C. difficile* infection can precipitate **toxic megacolon**, which necessitates surgical consultation.

Constipation

GENERAL PRINCIPLES

Definition
Constipation consists of infrequent and incomplete bowel movements, which can be associated with straining and passage of pellet-like stools.

Etiology
- Recent changes in bowel habits may suggest an organic cause, whereas long-standing constipation is more likely to be functional.
- **Medications** (e.g., calcium channel blockers, opiates, anticholinergics, iron supplements, barium sulfate) and systemic diseases (e.g., diabetes mellitus, hypothyroidism, systemic sclerosis, myotonic dystrophy) may contribute.
- Female gender, older age, lack of exercise, low caloric intake, low-fiber diet, and disorders that cause pain on defecation (e.g., anal fissures, thrombosed external hemorrhoids, pelvic floor dyssynergia) are other risk factors.[45]

DIAGNOSIS

- Colonoscopy and barium studies help rule out structural disease and are particularly important in individuals >45–50 years without prior colorectal cancer screening or with alarm features such as anemia, blood in the stool, or new-onset symptoms.[45]
- Colonic transit studies, anorectal manometry, and defecography are reserved for resistant cases without a structural explanation after initial workup.

CHAPTER 18

TREATMENT

- Regular exercise and adequate fluid intake are nonspecific measures.
- Increased **dietary fiber** intake (20–30 g/d) is useful. Fecal impaction should be resolved before fiber supplementation is initiated.
- **Laxatives**
  - **Emollient laxatives** such as docusate sodium, 50–200 mg PO daily, and docusate calcium, 240 mg PO daily, allow water and fat to penetrate the fecal mass. Mineral oil (15–45 mL PO q6–8h) can be given orally or by enema.
  - **Stimulant laxatives** such as castor oil, 15 mL PO, stimulate intestinal secretion and increase intestinal motility. Anthraquinones (cascara, 5 mL PO daily; senna, one tablet PO daily to qid) stimulate the colon by increasing fluid and water accumulation in the proximal colon. Bisacodyl (10–15 mg PO at bedtime, 10-mg rectal suppositories) stimulates colonic peristalsis and is an effective and well-tolerated option for chronic constipation.[45]
  - **Osmotic laxatives** include nonabsorbable salts or carbohydrates that cause water retention in the lumen of the colon. Magnesium salts include milk of magnesia (15–30 mL q8–12h) and magnesium citrate (200 mL PO) and need to be avoided in renal failure. Lactulose (15–30 mL PO bid–qid) can cause bloating as a side effect.
  - **Lubiprostone** (8–24 µg PO bid), a selective intestinal chloride channel activator, moves fluid into the bowel lumen and stimulates peristalsis.[45,46]
  - **Linaclotide** (145–290 µg PO qday) and **plecanatide** (3 mg PO qday) are guanylate cyclase C receptor agonists and also move fluid into the intestinal lumen as their mechanism of action.[47,48]
  - **Prucalopride** is a selective serotonin receptor agonist and a prokinetic agent that is approved for chronic constipation.[46]
- **Enemas:** Sodium biphosphate (Fleet) enemas can be used for mild to moderate constipation and for bowel cleansing before sigmoidoscopy; these should be avoided in renal failure. Tap water enemas (1 L) are also useful. Oil-based enemas (mineral oil, cottonseed colace) as well as Hypaque enemas can be used in refractory constipation.
- **Polyethylene glycol** in powder form (Miralax 17 g PO daily to bid) can be used regularly or intermittently for the treatment of constipation.
- **Subcutaneous or oral methylnaltrexone, oral alvimopan, oral naloxegol, and oral naldemedine** are peripherally acting µ-opioid receptor antagonists (PAMORAs) that provide rapid relief of opioid-induced constipation.[49]
- **Bowel-cleansing agents:** Patients should be placed on a clear liquid diet the previous day and kept nothing by mouth (NPO) for 6 hours or overnight prior to colonoscopy. Patients may experience mild abdominal discomfort, nausea, and vomiting with the bowel preparation.
  - An iso-osmotic **polyethylene glycol solution** (PEG, GoLYTELY, or NuLYTELY 1 gallon, administered at a rate of 8 oz every 10 minutes) is commonly used as a bowel-cleansing agent before colonoscopy. Lower volume preparations, such as PEG (2 L or 0.5 gallon) with ascorbic acid or other laxatives, are alternatives.[50]
  - **Sodium phosphate** (Fleet phosphosoda, 20–45 mL with 10–24 oz liquid, taken the day before and morning of the procedure), a hyperosmotic solution, draws fluid into the gut lumen and produces bowel movements in 0.5–6.0 hours. It is also available in pill form (Visicol or OsmoPrep, 32–40 tablets, taken at the rate of 3–4 tablets every 15 min with 8 oz fluid). Adverse reactions include severe dehydration, hyperphosphatemia, hypocalcemia, hypokalemia, hypernatremia,

and acidosis. A dreaded rare complication is **acute phosphate nephropathy**, where calcium phosphate deposits cause irreversible dysfunction of renal tubules resulting in renal failure. Consequently, sodium phosphate is only used in limited instances.

- ○ **Split preparations:** Proximity of bowel preparation to procedure time improves effectiveness of cleansing and visualization during the procedure. Splitting bowel preparation into two doses, with one dose administered the evening prior and the second dose administered the morning of the procedure, can improve bowel cleansing.[51]
- ○ **Two-day bowel preparation** is sometimes indicated in elderly or debilitated individuals when conventional bowel preparation is contraindicated, not tolerated, or ineffective. This consists of magnesium citrate (120–300 mL PO) administered on two consecutive days while the patient remains on a clear liquid diet; bisacodyl (30 mg PO or 10-mg suppository) is administered on both days.
- ○ **Tap water enemas** (1-L volume) can cleanse the distal colon when colonoscopy is indicated in patients with proximal bowel obstruction.
- Other options: **Biofeedback therapy** and **sacral nerve stimulation** can be effective for idiopathic constipation resistant to medical treatment.[52]

LUMINAL GASTROINTESTINAL DISORDERS

Gastroesophageal Reflux Disease

GENERAL PRINCIPLES

Gastroesophageal reflux disease (GERD) is defined as symptoms and/or complications resulting from reflux of gastric contents into the esophagus and more proximal structures.

DIAGNOSIS

Clinical Presentation

- Typical esophageal symptoms of GERD include **heartburn** and **regurgitation.** GERD can also present as **chest pain**, so it is important to exclude a cardiac source before initiating GI evaluation.[53]
- **Extraesophageal manifestations** of GERD can include cough, laryngitis, asthma, and dental erosions.
- Symptom response to a therapeutic trial of PPIs can be diagnostic, but a negative response does not exclude GERD.[54]

Differential Diagnosis

Other disorders that can result in esophagitis include the following:

- **Eosinophilic esophagitis (EoE)**, characterized by eosinophilic infiltration of esophageal mucosa, is increasingly recognized as an etiology for foregut symptoms.
  - ○ Atopy (i.e., allergic rhinitis, eczema, asthma) is common, and food allergens may trigger the process.
  - ○ **Dysphagia** is prominent, but symptoms can also mimic GERD.
  - ○ Common EGD findings include furrows, luminal narrowing, corrugations, and whitish plaques in the esophageal mucosa. The following establish a diagnosis of EoE: (1) symptoms related to esophageal dysfunction (such as dysphagia or food

impaction), (2) ≥15 eosinophils per HPF on esophageal biopsies, and (3) exclusion of secondary causes of esophageal eosinophilia (such as GERD).[55]

○ First-line therapy for EoE consists of either **PPIs**, which also treats concomitant GERD, or **topical steroids** (swallowed fluticasone, 880–1760 μg/d in two to four divided doses; or swallowed budesonide, 2 mg/d in two to four divided doses).[56] Yield of food allergen testing is typically low. Elimination of trigger foods can include a 6-food elimination diet (eggs, milk, soy, gluten, tree nuts, seafood), although 2-food elimination (milk, gluten) may provide adequate benefit. Dysphagia that persists despite mucosal healing can be due to strictures that can benefit from careful endoscopic dilation. Patients who do not respond to topical steroids may benefit from longer courses or higher doses of topical steroids, systemic steroids, elimination diet trials, or esophageal dilation.[56] Biologic agents are being investigated as management options.

• **Infectious esophagitis** typically presents with dysphagia or odynophagia and is seen most often in immunocompromised states (e.g., AIDS, organ transplant recipients), esophageal stasis (abnormal motility [e.g., achalasia, scleroderma], mechanical obstruction [e.g., strictures]), malignancy, diabetes mellitus, and antibiotic use; however, it can rarely occur in the normal healthy host. The presence of typical oral lesions (thrush, herpetic vesicles) may suggest an etiologic agent.

○ *Candida* **esophagitis** is the most common esophageal infection, typically seen in esophageal stasis, impaired cell-mediated immunity from immunosuppressive therapy (e.g., with steroids or cytotoxic agents), malignancies, or AIDS. Endoscopic visualization of typical whitish plaques has near 100% sensitivity for diagnosis. Empiric antifungal agents are appropriate when concurrent oropharyngeal thrush is present, reserving endoscopy for nonresponse to therapy. **Fluconazole** 100–200 mg/d or **itraconazole** 200 mg/d for 14–21 days is recommended as initial therapy for *Candida* esophagitis; nystatin (100,000 units/mL, 5 mL tid for 3 weeks) and clotrimazole troches (10 mg four to five times a day for 2 weeks) are alternatives for oropharyngeal candidiasis. For infections refractory to azoles, a short course of parenteral **amphotericin B** (0.3–0.5 mg/kg/d) can be considered.[57]

○ **HSV esophagitis** is characterized by small vesicles and well-circumscribed ulcers on endoscopy and typical giant cells on histopathology. Viral antigen or DNA can be identified by immunofluorescent antibodies. Treatment consists of **acyclovir** (400–800 mg PO five times a day for 14–21 days or 5 mg/kg IV q8h for 7–14 days). **Famciclovir** and **valacyclovir** are alternate agents. The condition is usually self-limited in immunocompetent hosts.[57]

○ **CMV esophagitis**, which occurs almost exclusively in immunocompromised hosts, can cause erosions or frank ulcerations. **Ganciclovir** (5 mg/kg IV q12h) or **foscarnet** (90 mg/kg IV q12h for 3–6 weeks) can be used as initial therapy. Oral **valganciclovir** may also be effective.

○ Symptomatic relief can be achieved with 2% viscous **lidocaine** swish and swallow (15 mL PO q3–4h PRN) or **sucralfate** slurry (1 g PO qid).

• **Chemical esophagitis**

○ Ingestion of caustic agents (e.g., alkalis, acids) or medications such as oral potassium, doxycycline, quinidine, iron, NSAIDs, aspirin, and bisphosphonates can result in mucosal irritation and damage. The offending medication should be discontinued if possible. Mucosal coating agents (e.g., sucralfate) and acid-suppressive agents may help.

○ With caustic ingestions, cautious early EGD can evaluate the extent and degree of mucosal damage, and CT can rule out transmural esophageal necrosis or perforation in the setting of mucosal necrosis.[58] A second caustic agent to neutralize the first is contraindicated.

Diagnostic Testing

- **Endoscopy** with biopsies is primarily indicated for avoiding misdiagnosis of alternate causes of esophageal symptoms (e.g., EoE), identification of complications, and evaluation of treatment failures. **Alarm symptoms** of dysphagia, odynophagia, early satiety, weight loss, or bleeding should prompt endoscopy.[30]
- **Ambulatory pH or pH impedance monitoring** can be used to quantify esophageal acid exposure and reflux events and/or to assess reflux-symptom correlation in patients with ongoing symptoms despite acid suppression (especially if endoscopy is negative) or those with atypical symptoms. pH impedance testing detects all reflux events regardless of pH and is best performed off PPI therapy to increase yield; abnormal studies can predict symptomatic response to medical and surgical antireflux therapy. In patients with known GERD and ongoing symptoms despite PPI, pH impedance monitoring can be performed on maximal PPI therapy.[59]
- **Esophageal manometry**, particularly HRM, may identify motor processes contributing to refractory symptoms.

TREATMENT

Medications

- Intermittent or prophylactic over-the-counter **antacids, H_2 receptor antagonists (H_2RAs)**, and **PPIs** are effective with mild or intermittent symptoms.
- **PPIs** are more effective than standard-dose H_2RAs and placebo in symptom relief and endoscopic healing of GERD. Modest gain is achieved by doubling the PPI dose in severe esophagitis or persistent symptoms. Continuous long-term PPI therapy is effective in maintaining remission of GERD symptoms, but the dose should be decreased after 8–12 weeks to the lowest dose that achieves symptom relief.[54] Abdominal pain, headache, and diarrhea are common side effects. Bone demineralization, enteric infections, community-acquired pneumonia, and reduced circulating levels of vitamin B_{12} are reported in observational studies, but conclusive cause-and-effect data are lacking, and benefits of PPI therapy continue to outweigh risks in patients with proven GERD.[60]
- Standard doses of **H_2RAs** can result in symptomatic benefit and endoscopic healing in up to half of patients. Dosage adjustments are required in renal insufficiency.
- Reflux inhibitors consist of γ-aminobutyric acid (GABA) type B receptor agonists that block transient LES relaxations. **Baclofen**, the prototype agent, reduces reflux events, but central side effects can be limiting.[61]

Surgical Management

- Indications for surgical **fundoplication** include the need for continuous PPIs, nonadherence, or intolerance to medical therapy in patients who are good surgical candidates, ongoing nonacid reflux despite adequate medical therapy, and patient preference for surgery.[54] When symptoms are controlled on PPI therapy, medical therapy and fundoplication are equally effective. Although fundoplication could provide better symptom control and quality of life in the short term, new postoperative symptoms and surgical failure can also occur.[54,62]
- Typical GERD symptoms, PPI response, elevated esophageal acid exposure, and correlation of symptoms to reflux events on ambulatory reflux monitoring predict a higher likelihood of a successful surgical outcome.

CHAPTER 18

- Patients with medical treatment failures need careful evaluation to determine whether symptoms are indeed related to acid reflux before surgical options are considered; these patients often have other diagnoses including EoE, esophageal motor disorders, visceral hypersensitivity, and functional heartburn.[54,61]
- Potential complications of surgery include dysphagia, inability to belch, gas-bloat syndrome, and bowel symptoms including flatulence, diarrhea, and abdominal pain.
- In patients with obesity, GERD symptoms improve from a **roux-en-Y gastric bypass**; however, a sleeve gastrectomy can worsen GERD symptoms and should not be offered to obese individuals with GERD.

Lifestyle/Risk Modification

- Patients with nocturnal GERD symptoms may benefit from elevating the head of the bed and avoiding meals within 2–3 hours before bedtime.
- Weight loss may benefit certain overweight patients with GERD.
- Lifestyle modifications alone are unlikely to resolve symptoms in the majority of GERD patients and should be recommended in conjunction with medications.

COMPLICATIONS

- **Esophageal erosion and ulceration** (esophagitis) can rarely lead to overt bleeding and iron deficiency anemia.
- **Strictures** can form when esophagitis heals, leading to dysphagia. Endoscopic dilation and maintenance PPI therapy typically resolve dysphagia from strictures.
- **Barrett esophagus (BE)** is a reflux-induced change from normal squamous esophageal epithelium to specialized intestinal metaplasia and carries a 0.5% per year risk of progression to esophageal adenocarcinoma. Endoscopic screening for BE should be considered for patients with GERD who are at high risk (long duration of GERD symptoms, ≥50 years of age, male gender, Caucasian); patients with BE should undergo periodic surveillance every 3–5 years in the absence of dysplasia. If dysplasia is found in the setting of BE, endoscopic therapy (usually radiofrequency ablation) is preferred to surveillance or surgery.[63]

Esophageal Motor Disorders

GENERAL PRINCIPLES

Definition

- **Achalasia** is the most significant motor disorder of the esophagus, characterized by incomplete LES relaxation with swallowing and lack of adequate peristaltic contractions of the esophageal body.[32,64]
- **Esophagogastric junction outflow obstruction** is a heterogeneous condition that includes incomplete achalasia-like disorders and structural processes (e.g., strictures, tight fundoplication, obstructing hiatus hernia).[32]
- **Esophageal hypermotility disorders** consist of **diffuse esophageal spasm**, characterized by premature, nonperistaltic contractions in the esophageal body, and **hypercontractile disorder** with exaggerated esophageal body contractions.[32]
- **Esophageal hypomotility disorders** are characterized by ineffective, or absent esophageal peristalsis, and can be associated with reflux symptoms and/or increased reflux burden.

DIAGNOSIS

Clinical Presentation

- Dysphagia, regurgitation, chest pain, and weight loss are typical achalasia symptoms. Aspiration pneumonia can also occur.
- Diffuse esophageal spasm and other spastic disorders may have obstructive symptoms (dysphagia, regurgitation) but also perceptive symptoms (chest pain) from heightened esophageal sensitivity.
- LES hypomotility diminishes barrier function, and esophageal body hypomotility affects esophageal clearance of refluxed material, which can lead to prolonged reflux exposure and reflux complications.

Diagnostic Testing

- **Esophageal HRM** represents the gold standard for the diagnosis of esophageal motor disorders.[34] HRM features categorize achalasia into three subtypes that have symptomatic and therapeutic implications.[32]
- **Barium radiographs** (timed upright barium swallow) may demonstrate a typical appearance of a dilated intrathoracic esophagus with impaired emptying, an air–fluid level, absence of gastric air bubble, and tapering of the distal esophagus with a bird's beak appearance in achalasia. A beaded or corkscrew appearance may be seen with diffuse esophageal spasm. A dilated esophagus with an open LES and free gastroesophageal reflux may be seen with severe esophageal hypomotility.
- **Endoscopy** may help exclude a stricture or neoplasia of the distal esophagus in presumed achalasia and spastic disorders. Hypomotility disorders may also manifest a dilated esophagus but with a gaping gastroesophageal junction and evidence of reflux disease.

TREATMENT

Medications

- **Smooth muscle relaxants** such as nitrates or calcium channel blockers administered immediately before meals may provide short-lived symptom relief in spastic disorders and achalasia, but symptom response is suboptimal and side effects can be limiting. Phosphodiesterase inhibitors may provide benefit in hypercontractile disorders but are contraindicated in coronary disease.
- **Botulinum toxin** injection at endoscopy can improve dysphagia for several weeks to months in achalasia and spastic disorders with incomplete LES relaxation.[64] This approach may be useful in elderly and frail patients who are poor surgical risks or as a bridge to more definitive therapy.
- **Neuromodulators** (e.g., low-dose tricyclic antidepressants [TCAs]) may improve perceptive symptoms (such as chest pain) associated with spastic motor disorders and achalasia.
- **Antisecretory therapy** with a PPI is recommended for reflux associated with esophageal hypomotility disorders. No specific promotility therapy exists. Antireflux surgery should be approached with caution in advanced hypomotility disorders.

Surgical Management

Disruption of the circular muscle of the LES using **pneumatic dilation** or surgical incision **(Heller myotomy)** can result in durable symptom relief in achalasia, with comparable symptom outcomes.[64] Gastroesophageal reflux can result, which can be treated with lifelong acid suppression or concurrent partial fundoplication during

CHAPTER 18

myotomy. Esophageal perforation occurs in 3%–5% of patients with pneumatic dilation. **POEM** is minimally invasive with similar short-term symptom improvement but incidence of reflux is higher compared with surgical myotomy.[64]

COMPLICATIONS

- Complications of achalasia include aspiration pneumonia and weight loss.
- Achalasia is associated with a 0.15% risk of squamous cell cancer of the distal esophagus, a 33-fold higher risk relative to the non-achalasia population.

Peptic Ulcer Disease

GENERAL PRINCIPLES

Definition

Peptic ulcer disease (PUD) consists of mucosal breaks in the stomach and duodenum when corrosive effects of acid and pepsin overwhelm mucosal defense mechanisms. Other locations include the esophagus, small bowel adjacent to gastroenteric anastomoses, and within a Meckel diverticulum.

Etiology

- *Helicobacter pylori*, a spiral, Gram-negative, urease-producing bacillus, is responsible for at least half of all PUD and the majority of ulcers that are not due to NSAIDs.
- PUD can develop in 15%–25% of **chronic NSAID and aspirin** users. Past history of PUD, age >60 years, concomitant corticosteroid or anticoagulant therapy, high-dose or multiple NSAID therapy, and presence of serious comorbid medical illnesses increase risk for PUD.[65]
- A gastrin-secreting tumor or **gastrinoma** accounts for <1% of all peptic ulcers.
- Gastric cancer or lymphoma may manifest as a gastric ulcer.
- When none of these etiologies are evident, PUD is designated idiopathic. Most idiopathic PUD could be due to undiagnosed *H. pylori* or undetected NSAID use.
- Cigarette smoking doubles the risk for PUD; it delays healing and promotes recurrence.

DIAGNOSIS

Clinical Presentation

- Epigastric pain or dyspepsia may be presenting symptoms; however, symptoms are not always predictive of the presence of ulcers. Epigastric tenderness may be elicited on abdominal palpation. Ten percent may present with a complication (see Complications).
- The presence of **alarm symptoms** (weight loss, early satiety, bleeding, anemia, persistent vomiting, epigastric mass, and lack of response to PPI) should prompt an EGD to assess for PUD or other diagnoses including gastric cancer.

Diagnostic Testing

- **Endoscopy** is the gold standard for diagnosis of peptic ulcers because it allows direct visualization and tissue sampling for *H. pylori* or cancer.
- **Stool *H. pylori* antigen testing** has good sensitivity and specificity for the diagnosis of *H. pylori* infection and can confirm eradication of *H. pylori* after treatment.

- **Serum *H. pylori* antibody testing** may identify previous or current infection, but both false negative and false positive results are possible. Since the antibody remains detectable as long as 18 months after successful eradication it cannot be used to document successful treatment.
- **Rapid urease assay** (e.g., *Campylobacter*-like organism [CLO] test) and histopathologic examination of endoscopic biopsy specimens diagnose *H. pylori* in patients undergoing endoscopy but may be falsely negative in patients on PPI therapy.
- **Carbon-labeled urea breath testing** is the most accurate noninvasive test for diagnosis, with sensitivity and specificity of 95%; it is often used to document successful eradication after therapy of *H. pylori* infection.[66]

TREATMENT

Medications

- Regardless of etiology, **acid suppression** forms the mainstay of therapy of PUD. Gastric ulcers are typically treated for 12 weeks and duodenal ulcers for 8 weeks.
- Oral PPI or H_2RA therapy will suffice in most instances. Dosage adjustment of H_2RAs is necessary in renal insufficiency. Cimetidine can impair metabolism of many drugs, including warfarin anticoagulants, theophylline, and phenytoin.
- *H. pylori* is a carcinogen and thus should be eradicated in any patient that tests positive. *H. pylori* is treated with a combination of acid suppression and antibiotics. Several regimens are available (Table 18-3).[67,68] Quadruple therapy with a PPI, bismuth, metronidazole, and tetracycline has replaced clarithromycin-based triple therapy as first-line. Patients that have had previous exposure to macrolides should not be treated with clarithromycin-based regimens, and those with fluoroquinolone exposure should not be treated with levofloxacin-based regimens. Eradication should be documented with an *H. pylori* stool antigen test. Failure of two antibiotic regimens should prompt sensitivity testing.
- NSAIDs and aspirin should be avoided when possible; if continued, maintenance PPI therapy and/or a mucosal protective agent (misoprostol, 400–800 μg/d) is recommended.[69]
- **Sucralfate** coats the eroded mucosal surface without blocking acid secretion and can be used as an adjunct to PPI when foregut mucosa is severely ulcerated. Side effects include constipation and reduction of bioavailability of certain drugs (e.g., cimetidine, digoxin, fluoroquinolones, phenytoin, and tetracycline) when administered concomitantly.
- **Antacids** can be useful as supplemental therapy for pain relief in PUD.
- **Nonpharmacologic measures:** Cessation of cigarette smoking should be encouraged. Alcohol in high concentrations can damage the gastric mucosal barrier, but no evidence exists to link alcohol with ulcer recurrence.

Surgical Management

Surgery is still occasionally required for intractable symptoms, GI bleeding refractory to endoscopic therapy, Zollinger–Ellison syndrome, and complicated PUD (i.e., perforation, gastric outlet obstruction). Surgical options vary depending on the location of the ulcer and the presence of complications.

SPECIAL CONSIDERATIONS

- **Zollinger–Ellison syndrome** is caused by a gastrin-secreting non–β islet cell tumor of the pancreas or duodenum. Multiple endocrine neoplasia type I can be associated with this syndrome in one-quarter to one-third of patients.[70] The resultant

TABLE 18-3	Regimens Used for Eradication of *Helicobacter pylori*
Medications and Doses	**Comments**
Tetracycline (500 mg qid), metronidazole (250 mg qid), bismuth (525 mg qid), and PPI[a] for 14 d	Bismuth-containing quadruple therapy; first line
Clarithromycin (500 mg bid), amoxicillin (1 g bid), and PPI[a] for 14 d	Second-line therapy, acceptable first line if low *H. pylori* clarithromycin resistance
Metronidazole (500 mg bid), amoxicillin (1 g bid), and PPI[a]	Second-line therapy in setting of prior macrolide exposure
Clarithromycin (500 mg bid), metronidazole (500 mg bid), and PPI[a]	Therapy for penicillin-allergic patients
Clarithromycin (500 mg bid), amoxicillin (1 g bid), metronidazole (500 mg bid), and PPI[a]	Concomitant therapy; first line
Amoxicillin (1 g bid) and PPI[a] for 5–7 d, followed by clarithromycin (500 mg bid), metronidazole (500 mg bid), and PPI[a] for another 5–7 d	Sequential therapy; first line
Amoxicillin (1 g bid) and PPI[a] for 7 d, followed by amoxicillin (1 g bid), clarithromycin (500 mg bid), metronidazole (500 mg bid), and PPI[a] for another 7 d	Hybrid therapy; first line
Levofloxacin (250 mg bid), amoxicillin (1 g bid), and PPI[a]	Levofloxacin triple therapy; first line
Amoxicillin (1 g bid) and PPI[a] for 5–7 d, followed by levofloxacin (250 mg bid), metronidazole (500 mg bid), and PPI[a]	Fluoroquinolone sequential therapy; first line
Amoxicillin (1 g bid), rifabutin (150 or 300 mg daily) and PPI[a] for 10 d	Salvage therapy
Bismuth (525 mg qid), levofloxacin (250 mg bid), and amoxicillin (1 g bid) and PPI[a]	Salvage therapy
Bismuth (525 mg qid), levofloxacin (250 mg bid), tetracycline (500 mg qid), and PPI[a]	Salvage therapy
Bismuth (525 mg qid), levofloxacin (250 mg bid), metronidazole (250 mg qid), and PPI[a]	Salvage therapy
Bismuth (525 mg qid), clarithromycin (500 mg bid), tetracycline (500 mg qid), and PPI[a]	Salvage therapy
Two antibiotics selected by sensitivity testing on culture, bismuth (525 mg qid), and PPI[a]	Culture-guided therapy (if failed two regimens)

Duration of therapy: 10–14 days unless otherwise stated. When using salvage regimens after initial treatment failure, choose drugs that have not been used before. PPI, proton pump inhibitor.
[a]Standard doses for PPI: omeprazole 20 mg, lansoprazole 30 mg, pantoprazole 40 mg, rabeprazole 20 mg, all twice a day. Esomeprazole is used as a single 40-mg dose once a day.

hypersecretion of gastric acid can cause multiple PUD in unusual locations, ulcers that fail to respond to standard medical therapy, or recurrent PUD after surgical therapy. Diarrhea and GERD symptoms are common.

• Gastric acid output is typically >15 mEq/L, and gastric pH is <1.0. A fasting serum gastrin level while off acid suppression for at least 5 days serves as a screening test in patients who make gastric acid; a value >1000 pg/mL is seen in 90% of patients with Zollinger–Ellison syndrome. When serum gastrin is elevated but <1000 pg/mL, a secretin stimulation test may demonstrate a paradoxical 200-pg increment in serum gastrin level after IV secretin in patients with gastrinomas.[70] High-dose PPIs are used for medical management. Specialized nuclear medicine scans (octreotide and dotatate) can be useful in localizing the neoplastic lesion for curative resection. Long-term survival is often related to underlying comorbidity rather than metastatic gastrinoma.

COMPLICATIONS

• **GI bleeding** (see Cardiac Patients and Gastrointestinal Bleeding section).
• **Gastric outlet obstruction** can occur with ulcers close to the pyloric channel and can manifest as nausea and vomiting, sometimes several hours after meals. Plain abdominal radiographs can show a dilated stomach with an air–fluid level. NG suction can decompress the stomach while fluids and electrolytes are repleted intravenously. Recurrence is common, and endoscopic balloon dilation or surgery is often necessary for definitive correction.
• **Perforation** occurs infrequently and usually necessitates emergent surgery. Perforation may occur in the absence of previous symptoms of PUD. A plain upright radiograph of the abdomen may demonstrate free air under the diaphragm. CT scan is usually diagnostic.
• **Pancreatitis** can result from ulcers in the posterior wall of the stomach or duodenal bulb penetrating the pancreas. The pain becomes severe and continuous, radiates to the back, and is no longer relieved by antisecretory therapy. Serum amylase may be elevated. CT scanning is usually diagnostic. Surgery is often required.

MONITORING/FOLLOW-UP

• Repeat EGD or upper GI series should be performed 8–12 weeks after initial diagnosis of all gastric ulcers to document healing; nonhealing ulcers should be biopsied to evaluate for a malignant ulcer.
• Duodenal ulcers are almost never malignant; therefore, documentation of healing is unnecessary in the absence of symptoms.

Inflammatory Bowel Disease

GENERAL PRINCIPLES

• **Ulcerative colitis (UC)** is an idiopathic chronic inflammatory disease of the colon and rectum, characterized by continuous mucosal inflammation from the rectum to varying extents proximally.
• **Crohn disease (CD)** is characterized by transmural inflammation of the gut wall and can affect any part of the tubular GI tract.

DIAGNOSIS

Clinical Presentation

- Both disorders can present with diarrhea, weight loss, and abdominal pain. UC typically presents with bloody diarrhea. CD can also present with fistula formation, strictures, abscesses, or bowel obstruction.
- **Extracolonic manifestations** of inflammatory bowel disease (IBD) include arthritis, primary sclerosing cholangitis, and ocular and skin lesions.

Diagnostic Testing

- **Endoscopy** remains the preferred method for diagnosis. UC is characterized by continuous inflammation from the rectum and extending varying distances into the colon. Endoscopy may demonstrate colonic involvement in CD (erosions or ulcers with a patchy distribution and skip lesions); ileoscopy during colonoscopy may demonstrate terminal ileal involvement. Video capsule endoscopy may help identify small bowel CD. **Histopathology** demonstrates chronic mucosal inflammation with crypt abscesses and cryptitis in UC. Noncaseating granulomas are classic for CD but are not always seen.
- Cross-sectional **imaging studies** (CT and MRI scans) as well as contrast radiography (small bowel follow-through series, barium enema) are useful to evaluate for complications of CD such as strictures, fistulas, and abscesses.
- **Serologic markers** play a limited role as adjuncts for diagnosis. Anti-*Saccharomyces cerevisiae* antibodies are typically seen in CD, and perinuclear antineutrophil cytoplasmic antibodies (p-ANCA) are seen in UC. C-reactive protein (CRP) and erythrocyte sedimentation rate (ESR) may be elevated but do not always correlate with disease activity.
- *C. difficile* **colitis** is more frequent in IBD patients compared with non-IBD populations; therefore, **stool studies** are warranted to look for this organism with disease flares. **CMV superinfection** can occur in patients on immunosuppressive agents and can be diagnosed by histopathology during endoscopy.

TREATMENT

Medications

Treatment is based on the severity of disease, location, and associated complications. Management aims are to resolve the acute presentation and reduce future recurrences. Both UC and CD can be categorized into three categories of severity for management purposes.

- **Mild to moderate disease:** Patients have little to no weight loss and good functional capacity and are able to maintain adequate oral intake. UC patients have less than four bowel movements daily with no rectal bleeding or anemia, whereas CD patients have little or no abdominal pain. Aminosalicylates (5-ASA) should be used to induce remission in patients with mild to moderate UC (see Table 18-4).[71] Patients with left-sided colitis may respond to topical therapies. Patients who achieve remission with 5-ASAs should continue to take them but may be able to use a lower dose. This class of medications has not been consistently shown to be effective in CD.[72] Ileal-release budesonide may be required to induce remission in patients with mild-moderate CD.
- **Moderate to severe disease** refers to CD patients who fail to respond to treatment for mild to moderate disease or those with significant weight loss, anemia, fever,

TABLE 18-4	Medications for Inflammatory Bowel Disease		
Medication	Dosing	Mechanism of Action	Comments
5-ASA			Not consistently effective for CD
Sulfasalazine	0.5 g bid-1.5 g qid	Metabolized to 5-ASA and a sulfa-pyridine moiety	Significant side effects from sulfapyridine moiety; especially effective for IBD arthropathy
Mesalamine	Varies by brand	Active component of sulfasalazine	Also available in suppository or enema for distal UC
			Rarely can cause paradoxical worsening of colitis
Asacol[a]	800–1600 mg PO tid	Released at a pH of 7 in the distal ileum	
Pentasa[a]	0.5–1.0 g PO qid	Time- and pH-dependent release mechanism distributes in the small bowel and colon	
Apriso[a]	1.5 g PO qday	pH-dependent release distributes throughout the colon	
Lialda[a] (multimatrix delivery system)	1.2–2.4 g PO qday–bid	Sustained release throughout the colon despite decreased frequency of administration	
Balsalazide (Colazal)	1.5 g bid–2.25 tid	Bacterial cleavage to mesalamine by colonic bacteria	
Olsalazine (Dipentum)	500 mg bid	5-ASA dimer cleaved by colonic bacteria	
Antibiotics			Used to treat fistulizing CD and abscesses
Metronidazole	250–500 mg PO tid		Risk of neuropathy
Ciprofloxacin	500 mg PO bid		Risk of tendon rupture

(continued)

CHAPTER 18

TABLE 18-4	Medications for Inflammatory Bowel Disease *(continued)*		
Medication	Dosing	Mechanism of Action	Comments
Corticosteroids		Multiple immuno-suppressing effects	Should NOT be used as maintenance therapy. Topical therapy can be used for distal disease
Methylprednisolone	60 mg IV qday		
Prednisone	40–60 mg qday		
Budesonide	9 mg qday	pH-controlled release delivers drug to ileum and ascending colon (Entocort[b]) Multimatrix system preferentially acts on colon (Uceris[b]) Topical formulations can be used for distal disease	May reduce side effects due to first-pass metabolism
Immunomodulators			
6-Mercaptopurine	1.0–1.5 mg/kg/d PO	Purine analog, causes preferential suppression of T-cell activation and antigen recognition	Checking thiopurine methyltransferase (TPMT) enzyme activity prior to starting therapy identifies patients at risk for dangerous cytopenias 6-Thioguanine (6-TG) metabolite levels assess adequacy of dosing; high 6-methyl mercaptopurine (6-MMP) levels predict hepatotoxicity

TABLE 18-4	Medications for Inflammatory Bowel Disease (*continued*)		
Medication	Dosing	Mechanism of Action	Comments
Azathioprine	1.5–2.5 mg/kg/d PO	S-imidazole precursor of 6-MP	Risk of hepatosplenic T-cell lymphoma with thiopurines, especially in young men
Methotrexate	15–25 mg IM or PO weekly	Inhibits DNA synthesis	May cause nausea/vomiting, hepatotoxicity
Biologics			
Infliximab (Remicade)	5 mg/kg IV infusions at weeks 0, 2, and 6, followed by maintenance infusions every 4–8 weeks	Monoclonal antibody against tumor necrosis factor-alpha (anti–TNF-α)	Risk of opportunistic infections, reactivation of TB and HBV with all anti–TNF-α agents
Adalimumab (Humira)	160 mg SC at week 0, then 80 mg SC at week 2, followed by 40 mg SC every 1–2 weeks	Anti–TNF-α	
Certolizumab pegol (Cimzia)	400 mg SC at weeks 0, 2, and 4, followed by maintenance doses every 4 weeks	Anti–TNF-α	
Golimumab (Simponi)	200 mg SC at week 0, then 100 mg SC at week 2 and every 4 weeks thereafter	Anti–TNF-α	Only approved for UC
Vedolizumab (Entyvio)	300-mg infusions at weeks 0 and 2, followed by infusions every 4–8 weeks	Monoclonal antibody against $\alpha4\beta7$ integrin, prevents T cell migration to inflammation. $\alpha4\beta7$ is specific to GI tract	Good safety profile because of gut specificity

CHAPTER 18

(*continued*)

TABLE 18-4	Medications for Inflammatory Bowel Disease	*(continued)*	
Medication	Dosing	Mechanism of Action	Comments
Natalizumab (Tysabri)	300-mg infusions at weeks 0, 4, and 8, followed by monthly infusions thereafter	Monoclonal antibody to α-4 integrin. In contrast to α4β7, α-4 is found in and outside the GI tract	Risk of JC polyomavirus reactivation causing progressive multifocal leukoencephalopathy has limited its use
Ustekinumab (Stelara)	Weight-dependent dosing of 260–520-mg infusion at week 1, followed by 90-mg subcutaneous maintenance injections every 8 weeks	Monoclonal antibody to the p40 subunit of interleukin-12 and interleukin-23	Good safety profile. Also approved for psoriasis, so good option for IBD patients with psoriasis or psoriaform reactions to anti–TNF-α
Tofacitinib (Xeljanz)	5 mg or 10 mg oral twice a day	Janus kinase inhibitor	Risk of thromboembolic events; use with caution in patients with CV risk factors

5-ASA, 5-aminosalicylates; 6-MP, 6-mercaptopurine; anti–TNF-α, anti–tumor necrosis factor-α; CD, Crohn disease; CV, cardiovascular; GI, gastrointestinal; HBV, hepatitis B virus; IBD, inflammatory bowel disease; UC, ulcerative colitis.
aBrand name formulation of mesalamine.
bBrand name formulation of budesonide.

abdominal pain or tenderness, and intermittent nausea and vomiting without bowel obstruction. In UC, moderate to severe disease manifests with more than six bloody bowel movements daily, fever, mild anemia, and elevated ESR.[71] Risk factors for severe CD include age <30 years at initial diagnosis, extensive anatomic involvement, perianal and/or severe rectal disease, deep ulcers, prior surgical resection, and stricturing or penetrating behavior.[72] The goal of therapy is to induce remission rapidly with corticosteroids and to maintain remission with immunosuppressive agents and/or biologic agents as appropriate. Treatment is typically continued until the patient fails to respond to a particular agent or the agent is no longer tolerated. Glucocorticoids are often required to induce remission in patients with moderate to severe UC or CD; however, they carry significant side effects and should not be used to maintain remission. Azathioprine, 6-mercaptopurine, or methotrexate can be used to maintain remission but are not effective at inducing remission. **Anti–tumor necrosis factor-α (anti–TNF-α) monoclonal antibodies** are used to induce and maintain remission. Anti-TNF-α in combination with azathioprine is more effective at inducing remission than anti-TNF-α alone.[72] Other biologics are now available for inducing and maintaining remission, including vedolizumab, natalizumab, ustekinumab, and tofacitinib.

- **Severe or fulminant disease** patients are typically hospitalized because of the severity of their symptoms. Fulminant CD patients have persistent symptoms despite conventional glucocorticoids or anti–TNF-α therapy or have high fevers, persistent vomiting, intestinal obstruction, intra-abdominal abscess, peritoneal signs, or cachexia. Fulminant colitis (both CD and UC) can present with profuse bloody bowel movements, significant anemia, and systemic signs of toxicity (fever, sepsis, electrolyte disturbances, dehydration). **Toxic megacolon** occurs in 1%–2% of UC patients, wherein the colon becomes atonic and dilated, with significant systemic toxicity.
  - Supportive therapy consists of NPO status with NG suction if there is evidence of small bowel ileus or obstruction. Dehydration and electrolyte disturbances are treated vigorously. Anticholinergic and opioid medications should be discontinued.
  - Initial investigation includes cross-sectional imaging to evaluate for intra-abdominal abscess. Blood cultures and stool studies to exclude *C. difficile* colitis should be performed. Cautious flexible sigmoidoscopy with minimal insufflation and only with CO_2 may be done to determine severity of colonic inflammation and for biopsies to exclude CMV colitis.
  - Once infection is excluded, intensive medical therapy with IV **corticosteroids** (methylprednisolone 60 mg/day or hydrocortisone 100 mg three or 4 times per day).
  - Patients who fail to improve with 3–5 days of steroids should be treated with infliximab (5–10 mg/kg).[71] Cyclosporine infusion (2–4 mg/kg/d, to achieve blood levels of 200–400 ng/mL) is used in some centers.
  - Early surgical consultation for possible colectomy should be obtained in case medical therapy is unsuccessful.
  - Nutritional support is administered as appropriate after 5–7 days; TPN is often indicated if enteral nutrition is not tolerated.
  - Early surgical consultation should be obtained in case medical therapy is unsuccessful. Clinical deterioration/lack of improvement despite 7–10 days of intensive medical management, evidence of bowel perforation, and peritoneal signs are indications for urgent total colectomy.
  - Patients who respond to infliximab should continue it. Patients who respond to cyclosporine should transition to azathioprine or vedolizumab.[71]

Surgical Management

- Surgery in CD is generally reserved for fistulas, obstruction, abscess, perforation, or bleeding; medically refractory disease; and neoplastic transformation. Stricturoplasty is an option for focal tight strictures; biopsies should be obtained to rule out cancer at stricture sites.
- In CD, recurrence close to the resected margins is common after bowel resection. Efforts should be made to avoid multiple resections in CD because of the risk of short bowel syndrome.
- In UC, total colectomy is generally curative, though some patients may develop inflammation in the small intestinal pouch created after colectomy.

Lifestyle/Risk Modification

- CD patients with a stricture should consume a low-roughage diet to avoid precipitating a bowel obstruction.
- Patients with Crohn ileitis or ileocolonic resection may need vitamin B_{12} supplementation. Specific oral replacement of calcium, magnesium, folate, iron, vitamins A and D, and other micronutrients may be necessary in patients with small bowel CD.
- **TPN** may be necessary food intolerance for greater than 4 or 5 days or to improve nutrition prior to surgery.

SPECIAL CONSIDERATIONS

- Patients with both UC and Crohn colitis longer than 8 years should undergo annual or biennial colonoscopic surveillance for neoplasia, ideally using chromoendoscopy.[71]
- Consistent histopathologic evidence of any grade of dysplasia is an indication for total colectomy.
- **Smoking cessation** is warranted for all patients with IBD. There is epidemiologic evidence of a protective effect on a limited number of patients with UC, but the overall health risks of smoking outweigh the risks of disease exacerbation.
- **Venous thromboembolism:** Patients with IBD are at increased risk for venous thromboembolism and should treated with prophylaxis when admitted to the hospital.[71]
- **Family planning** is important in women with active disease as there is an increased risk of premature delivery, low birth weight, and congenital abnormalities. Active inflammation, rather than biologic medications, increase the risk of complications.[73] Thus, **biologics should NOT be discontinued.**
- **Symptom control** is an important adjunct to therapy but must be used cautiously.
  - **Antidiarrheal agents** may be useful as an adjunctive therapy in selected patients with mild exacerbations or postresection diarrhea. They are contraindicated in severe exacerbations and in toxic megacolon.
  - **Narcotics** should be used sparingly for pain control.

Functional Gastrointestinal Disorders

GENERAL PRINCIPLES

- Functional GI disorders are characterized by the presence of abdominal symptoms in the absence of a demonstrable organic disease process. Symptoms can arise from any part of the luminal gut.
- **Irritable bowel syndrome (IBS)**, primarily characterized by abdominal pain linked to altered bowel habits of at least 3 months in duration, is the best-recognized functional bowel disease.[74]

DIAGNOSIS

- Clinical evaluation should be directed toward excluding organic processes in the involved area of the gut while initiating therapeutic trials when functional symptoms are suspected.[74]

- **Serologic tests for celiac sprue** are recommended in IBS patients. The prevalence of celiac sprue in diarrhea-predominant IBS patients is estimated at 3.6% compared with 0.7% of the general population.[74]
- Patients >50 years old with new-onset bowel symptoms, patients with alarm symptoms (GI bleeding, anemia, weight loss, early satiety), and patients with symptoms not responding to empiric treatment need further workup with endoscopy. Routine cross-sectional imaging is not recommended with typical functional symptoms without alarm features.

TREATMENT

Nonpharmacologic Measures

Patient education, reassurance, and help with diet and lifestyle modification are keys to an effective physician–patient relationship. The psychosocial contribution to symptom exacerbation should be determined, and its management may be sufficient for many patients.

- **Diets** low in fermentable oligosaccharides, disaccharides, monosaccharides, and polyols (FODMAPs) appear to reduce functional GI symptoms in patients with IBS.[75] Food items that reliably trigger symptoms can also be avoided, for example, dairy products.
- **Peppermint oil** can improve symptoms in some patients with functional bowel disease. It can be administered either in capsule form or 6–8 drops in a glass of water taken daily.[76]
- **Adjunctive measures** useful in functional bowel disease include cognitive and behavioral therapy, hypnotherapy, mindfulness, acupuncture, and physical exercise.

Medications

- **Symptomatic management**
  - **Antiemetic agents** are useful in functional nausea and vomiting syndromes, in addition to neuromodulators.
  - When pain and bloating are the predominant symptoms, **antispasmodic** or **anticholinergic** medications (hyoscyamine, 0.125–0.25 mg PO/sublingual up to qid; dicyclomine, 10–20 mg PO qid) may provide short-term relief.
  - Stool frequency, but not abdominal pain, improves with increased dietary fiber (25 g/d) supplemented with PRN laxatives in constipation-predominant IBS.
  - **Loperamide** (2–4 mg, up to qid/PRN) can reduce stool frequency, urgency, and fecal incontinence.
  - Short-term nonabsorbable **antibiotic** therapy (particularly **rifaximin**) may improve bloating and diarrhea in IBS; long-term treatment has not been adequately studied.[77] **Probiotics** (e.g., bifidobacteria) are sometimes beneficial.
  - **Lubiprostone** (8 μg bid), a selective chloride channel activator, **linaclotide** (290 μg daily), and **plecanatide** (3 mg daily), guanylate cyclase C agonists, improve constipation-predominant IBS symptoms. Polyethylene glycol 3350 and electrolytes are suitable for use in constipation-predominant IBS.[74]
  - **Eluxadoline** (Viberzi, 75–100 mg bid), a μ- and κ-opioid receptor agonist, is approved for the management of diarrhea-predominant IBS.[78] Acute pancreatitis is a potentially serious side effect occurring in 0.4%; history of past pancreatitis, cholecystectomy, alcohol abuse, and hepatic impairment are contraindications.
  - **Alosetron** (Lotronex, 1 mg daily to bid), a 5-HT$_3$ antagonist, is useful in women with diarrhea-predominant IBS.[79] However, its use is restricted to refractory diarrhea because of the rare potential for ischemic colitis.

- **Neuromodulators**
  - Low-dose **TCAs** (e.g., amitriptyline, nortriptyline, imipramine, doxepin: 25–100 mg at bedtime) have neuromodulatory and analgesic properties that are independent of their psychotropic effects. These can be beneficial, especially in pain-predominant functional GI disorders.[74]
  - **Selective serotonin reuptake inhibitors (SSRIs)** (e.g., fluoxetine, 20 mg; paroxetine, 20 mg; sertraline, 50 mg; duloxetine, 20–60 mg) may also have efficacy, sometimes with better side effect profiles compared with TCAs.
  - **Cyclic vomiting syndrome (CVS)** is an increasingly recognized condition with stereotypic episodes of vigorous vomiting and asymptomatic intervals between episodes.[80] Treatment with low-dose TCAs or antiepileptic medications (zonisamide, levetiracetam) has prophylactic benefits. Sumatriptan (25–50 mg PO, 5–10 mg transnasally, or 6 mg SC) or other triptans may abort an episode, especially if administered during a prodrome or early in the episode. Established episodes may require IV hydration, scheduled IV antiemetics (ondansetron, prochlorperazine), benzodiazepines (lorazepam), and pain control with IV narcotics. Before the diagnosis of CVS is made, structural causes and cannabinoid hyperemesis syndrome need to be ruled out.[80]

Intestinal Pseudo-Obstruction (Ileus)

GENERAL PRINCIPLES

Definition

- **Acute intestinal pseudo-obstruction** or **ileus** consists of impaired transit of intestinal contents and obstructive symptoms (nausea, vomiting, abdominal distension, lack of bowel movements) without a mechanical explanation.
- **Acute colonic pseudo-obstruction** or **Ogilvie syndrome** describes massive colonic dilation without mechanical obstruction in the presence of a competent ileocecal valve, resulting from impaired colonic peristalsis.
- **Chronic intestinal pseudo-obstruction** is characterized by recurrent episodes of nausea, vomiting, and abdominal distention with bowel dilation without mechanical obstruction.[81] An exact cause is often not found. One well-described etiology is a paraneoplastic phenomenon from antineuronal antibodies (anti-Hu), most often seen with small cell lung cancer.

Etiology

Ileus is frequently seen in the postoperative period. Narcotic analgesics administered for postoperative pain control may contribute, as can other medications that slow down intestinal peristalsis (calcium channel blockers, anticholinergic medications, TCAs, antihistamines). Other predisposing causes include virtually any medical insult, particularly life-threatening systemic diseases, infection, vascular insufficiency, and electrolyte abnormalities. Similar factors predispose to acute colonic pseudo-obstruction.

DIAGNOSIS

- A careful history and physical examination is essential in the initial evaluation.
- Conventional laboratory studies (CBC, complete metabolic profile, amylase, lipase) help in assessing for a primary intra-abdominal inflammatory process.

- **Obstructive series** (supine and upright abdominal radiograph with a CXR) determines the distribution of intestinal gas and assesses for the presence of free intraperitoneal air.
- **Additional imaging studies** assess for mechanical obstruction and inflammatory processes and include CT, contrast enema, and small bowel series.

TREATMENT

- Basic **supportive measures** consist of NPO, fluid replacement, and correction of electrolyte imbalances. Medications that slow down GI motility (adrenergic agonists, TCAs, sedatives, narcotic analgesics) should be withdrawn or dose reduced. The ambulatory patient is encouraged to remain active.
- **Intermittent NG suction** prevents swallowed air from passing distally. In protracted cases, gastric decompression, either using an NG tube or a percutaneous endoscopic gastrostomy (PEG) tube, vents upper GI secretions and decreases vomiting and gastric distension.
- **Rectal tubes** help decompress the distal colon; more proximal colonic distension may necessitate **colonoscopic decompression**, especially when the cecal diameter approaches 12 cm. This should be performed carefully with minimal air insufflation. Turning the patient from side to side may potentiate the benefit of colonoscopic decompression.

Medications

- **Methylnaltrexone** (Relistor, 8–12 mg SC per dose every other day) can be administered in settings where opioid medication use is contributing.
- **Neostigmine** (2 mg IV administered slowly over 3–5 minutes) is beneficial in selected patients with acute colonic distension. This can induce rapid reestablishment of colonic tone. It is contraindicated if mechanical obstruction has not been ruled out. Side effects include abdominal pain, excessive salivation, symptomatic bradycardia, and syncope. A trial of neostigmine may be warranted before colonoscopic decompression in patients without contraindications.[82]
- **Erythromycin** (200 mg IV) acts as a motilin agonist and stimulates upper gut motility; it has been used with some success in refractory postoperative ileus.
- **Alvimopan** is a peripherally acting μ-opioid receptor antagonist that enhances return of bowel function after abdominal surgery but has not been shown to shorten hospital stay.[83]
- **Mosapride citrate** (15 mg PO tid), a 5-HT$_4$ receptor agonist, may reduce the duration of postoperative ileus when administered postoperatively.[84]
- **Prucalopride**, also a selective 5-HT$_4$ agonist, can relieve symptoms in patients with chronic intestinal pseudo-obstruction.[85]

Surgical Management

- **Surgical consultation** is required when the clinical picture is suggestive of mechanical obstruction or if peritoneal signs are present. Surgical exploration is reserved for acute cases with peritoneal signs, ischemic bowel, or other evidence of perforation.
- **Cecostomy** treats acute and chronic colonic distension when colonoscopic decompression fails.

CHAPTER 18

PANCREATICOBILIARY DISORDERS

Acute Pancreatitis

GENERAL PRINCIPLES

Definition

Acute pancreatitis consists of inflammation of the pancreas and peripancreatic tissue from activation of potent pancreatic enzymes within the pancreas, particularly trypsin.

Etiology

The most common causes are alcohol and gallstone disease, accounting for 75%–80% of all cases. Less common causes include abdominal trauma, hypercalcemia, hypertriglyceridemia, and a variety of drugs. Post–endoscopic retrograde cholangiopancreatography (ERCP) pancreatitis occurs in 5%–10% of patients undergoing ERCP; prophylaxis with rectal NSAIDs or placement of prophylactic pancreatic duct stents can help prevent post-ERCP pancreatitis.[86]

DIAGNOSIS

Clinical Presentation

Typical symptoms consist of acute onset of epigastric abdominal pain radiating to the back, nausea, and vomiting often exacerbated by food intake. Systemic manifestations can include fever, shortness of breath, altered mental status, anemia, electrolyte imbalances, and shock.

Diagnostic Testing

Laboratories
- Acute pancreatitis is diagnosed in the presence of two of the following three findings: (1) characteristic upper abdominal pain radiating to the back; (2) serum lipase or amylase greater than 3x the upper limit of normal; or (3) characteristic imaging findings. Serum **lipase** is more specific and sensitive than serum **amylase**, although both are usually elevated beyond 3× the upper limits of normal. These values do not correlate with severity or outcome of pancreatitis. Patients with renal insufficiency may have elevated enzymes at baseline from impaired clearance.[87] There is no utility in tracking serum levels over time.
- Hepatic function testing may identify biliary obstruction as a possible etiology, and a lipid panel may suggest hypertriglyceridemia as the cause of acute pancreatitis.

Imaging
- **Dual-phase (pancreas protocol) CT scan** is useful in the initial evaluation of severe acute pancreatitis but should be reserved for patients in whom the diagnosis is unclear, who fail to improve clinically within 48–72 hours, or in whom complications are suspected.[88] CT scan early in presentation may underestimate the severity of acute pancreatitis.
- **MRI with gadolinium** can also be used with at least similar efficacy, especially when CT is contraindicated. Magnetic resonance cholangiopancreatography (MRCP) is useful to detect a biliary source for pancreatitis before ERCP is performed.[88]

TREATMENT

- **Aggressive goal-directed volume repletion** with IV fluids must be undertaken, with careful monitoring of fluid balance, urine output, serum electrolytes (including calcium and glucose), and awareness of the potential for significant fluid sequestration within the abdomen. Intensive care unit monitoring may be necessary. The use of Ringer's lactate at a dose of 20 mL/kg bolus followed by 3 mL/kg/h has shown improved outcomes within 36 hours.[89] Ringer's lactate may be the preferred fluid, as it improved inflammatory markers compared to normal saline; however, no difference in outcomes has been demonstrated. Fluid status should be reassessed frequently, as overresuscitation may lead to poor outcomes.[89]
- Early **enteral nutrition** may improve clinical outcomes. In general, patients should be allowed to eat within 24 hours. If they are unable to meet their nutritional needs by 72 hours, an NG or nasoenteric feeding tube can be placed. A clinical trial showed no benefit to early (within 24 hours) tube feeding compared to on demand feeding.[90]

Medications

- **Narcotic analgesics** are usually necessary for pain relief.
- Routine use of antibiotics is not recommended in the absence of documented infection.[88]

Other Nonoperative Therapies

Urgent **ERCP and biliary sphincterotomy** within 72 hours of presentation can improve the outcome of severe gallstone pancreatitis in the presence of cholangitis.[88] There is no benefit to urgent ERCP in the absence of cholangitis.[91]

Surgical Management

Cholecystectomy is recommended during the index hospitalization in acute gallstone pancreatitis.[88]

COMPLICATIONS

- **Necrotizing pancreatitis** represents a severe form of acute pancreatitis, usually identified on dynamic dual-phase CT with IV contrast. Increasing abdominal pain, fever, marked leukocytosis, and bacteremia suggest infected pancreatic necrosis that requires broad-spectrum antibiotics and drainage. CT-guided percutaneous aspiration for Gram stain and culture can confirm the diagnosis of infected necrosis. **Carbapenems** or a combination of a **fluoroquinolone** and **metronidazole** has good penetration into necrotic tissue.
- The presence of **pseudocysts** is suggested by persistent pain or high amylase levels. Complications include infection, hemorrhage, rupture (pancreatic ascites), and obstruction of adjacent structures. Asymptomatic pseudocysts can be followed clinically with serial imaging studies to resolution. Decompression of symptomatic or infected pseudocysts can be performed by percutaneous, endoscopic, or surgical techniques. Noninvasive approaches should be used before surgery.[92]
- **Infection:** Potential sources of fever include pancreatic necrosis, abscess, infected pseudocysts, cholangitis, and aspiration pneumonia. Cultures should be obtained, and broad-spectrum antimicrobials appropriate for bowel flora should only be used when there is a high clinical suspicion for infection.

- **Pulmonary complications:** Atelectasis, pleural effusion, pneumonia, and acute respiratory distress syndrome can develop in severely ill patients (see Chapter 10, Pulmonary Diseases).
- **Renal failure** can result from intravascular volume depletion or acute tubular necrosis.
- **GI bleeding** can result from stress gastritis, pseudoaneurysm rupture, or gastric varices from splenic vein thrombosis.
- **Other complications:** Metabolic complications include hypocalcemia, hypomagnesemia, and hyperglycemia.

Chronic Pancreatitis

GENERAL PRINCIPLES

- Chronic pancreatitis represents inflammation, fibrosis, and atrophy of acinar cells resulting from recurrent acute or chronic inflammation of the pancreas.
- Most commonly seen with **chronic alcohol abuse**, it can also result from dyslipidemia, hypercalcemia, autoimmune disease, and exposure to various toxins. A rare inherited form (**hereditary pancreatitis**) can be associated with mutations in genes encoding cationic trypsinogen (*PRSS1*) or pancreatic secretory trypsin inhibitor (*SPINK1*).[93]
- **Autoimmune pancreatitis (AIP)** is an increasingly recognized subtype of chronic pancreatitis characterized by infiltration of IgG4-positive plasma cells in a classically sausage-shaped pancreas. AIP can be difficult to distinguish from pancreatic cancer on CT, but typically features diffuse narrowing of the main pancreatic duct without dilation.

DIAGNOSIS

Clinical Presentation

Chronic abdominal pain, exocrine insufficiency from acinar cell injury and fibrosis (manifesting as weight loss and steatorrhea), and **endocrine insufficiency** from destruction of islet cells (manifesting as brittle diabetes) are the main clinical manifestations.

Diagnostic Testing

Laboratory Tests
- Lipase and amylase may be elevated but are frequently normal. Bilirubin, alkaline phosphatase, and transaminases may be elevated if there is concomitant biliary obstruction.
- Indirect pancreatic function testing (such as secretin stimulation, fecal fat, and fecal elastase) can be obtained but are not widely available and difficult to perform.

Imaging
- **Calcification** of the pancreas can be seen on imaging. Contrast-enhanced CT has a sensitivity of 75%–90% and a specificity of 85% for the diagnosis of chronic pancreatitis; MRCP is equivalent and a suitable alternative.[93]

- **Endoscopic ultrasound (EUS)** has higher sensitivity for the diagnosis of chronic pancreatitis and is particularly useful for evaluating lesions concerning for neoplasia in the setting of chronic pancreatitis.

TREATMENT

Medications

- **Neuromodulators** (TCAs, SSRIs) and **pregabalin** may improve symptoms and decrease reliance on narcotics. Opioids should only be used when all other treatments have failed.[94]
- **Pancreatic enzyme supplements** are the mainstay of management of pancreatic exocrine insufficiency in conjunction with a low-fat diet (<50 g fat per day), facilitating weight gain and reduced stool frequency.[94] Enteric-coated preparations (Pancreaze, Zenpep, or Creon, one to two capsules with meals) are stable at an acidic pH.
- **Fat-soluble vitamin** supplementation may be necessary.
- **Insulin** therapy is generally required for endocrine insufficiency because the resultant diabetes mellitus is caused by insulin deficiency via beta cell loss rather than insulin resistance.
- When identified, treatment of the underlying disorder (e.g., hyperparathyroidism, dyslipidemia) is indicated.
- Alcohol and smoking cessation are essential. Performing procedures for pain relief in patients with chronic pancreatitis who are still smoking or consuming alcohol should be carefully considered.
- Steroids are used to treat autoimmune pancreatitis. Azathioprine can be considered to prevent relapse. Relapses may occur in the pancreas or biliary tree, although retreatment with steroids is effective at inducing remission.[95]

Other Nonoperative Therapies

- Patients with pancreatic duct obstruction from stones, strictures, or papillary stenosis may benefit from endoscopic therapies such as **ERCP with pancreatic sphincterotomy, stricture dilation, pancreatic duct stenting,** and/or **extracorporeal shock wave lithotripsy (ESWL).**
- **Celiac plexus block** can be used for short-term relief in selected patients with refractory pain.
- Surgery can be considered in selected patients who have a dilated pancreatic duct and fail medical and endoscopic treatment. Several surgical options for decompression exist (e.g., a lateral pancreaticojejunostomy if a dilated pancreatic duct is present). **Whipple procedure** is an option in rare cases.

Gallstone Disease

GENERAL PRINCIPLES

- **Asymptomatic gallstones (cholelithiasis)** are a common incidental finding for which no specific therapy is generally necessary. Cholesterol stones are the most common type, but pigmented stones can be seen with hemolysis or infection. Risk factors include obesity, female gender, parity, rapid weight loss, ileal disease, and maternal family history.
- **Symptomatic cholelithiasis**, when upper abdominal symptoms are linked to gallstones, is typically treated surgically with cholecystectomy.

CHAPTER 18

- **Acute cholecystitis** is caused most often by a gallstone obstructing the cystic duct, but acalculous cholecystitis can occur in critically ill patients.
- **Choledocholithiasis** refers to stones within the bile ducts.
- **Cholangitis** is infection of the bile ducts, usually caused by an impacted gallstone in the distal bile duct.

DIAGNOSIS

Clinical Presentation

- Cholelithiasis may present as **biliary colic**, a constant pain lasting for several hours, located in the right upper quadrant, radiating to the back or right shoulder, and sometimes associated with nausea or vomiting. Pain that lasts longer than several hours may suggest complications including choledocholithiasis or cholecystitis.
- Other presentations of gallstone disease include acute cholecystitis, acute pancreatitis, and cholangitis. Gallstone disease may rarely be associated with gallbladder cancer.
- Two-thirds of patients with **acute ascending cholangitis** present with right upper quadrant pain, fever with chills and/or rigors, and jaundice (**Charcot triad**), in the setting of biliary obstruction (choledocholithiasis, neoplasia, sclerosing cholangitis, biliary stent occlusion). The additional presence of hypotension and altered mentation defines the **Reynolds pentad.**

Diagnostic Testing

- **Ultrasound scans** have a high degree of accuracy in diagnosis (sensitivity and specificity >95%) and are the preferred initial test.
- **Hydroxy iminodiacetic acid (HIDA)** scan can demonstrate nonfilling of the gallbladder in patients with acute cholecystitis, although false-negative results may be seen in acalculous cholecystitis.
- **MRCP** is better than CT at visualizing the biliary tree. It can identify biliary ductal dilation and often the level of obstruction from a gallstone or mass. A pancreas protocol CT can be useful if a pancreatic mass is suspected as the cause of biliary obstruction.
- **EUS** is sensitive for detecting obstructing gallstones and allows for therapeutic ERCP to be done in the same setting.

TREATMENT

Medications

- **Supportive measures** include IV fluid resuscitation and broad-spectrum antimicrobial agents, especially in the event of complications such as acute cholecystitis with sepsis, perforation, peritonitis, abscess, or empyema formation.
- **Ursodeoxycholic acid** (8–10 mg/kg/d PO in two to three divided doses for prolonged periods) might be prudent in a select group of patients with small cholesterol stones in normally functioning gallbladders who are at high risk for complications from surgical therapy. Side effects include diarrhea and reversible elevation in serum transaminases.

Nonpharmacologic Therapies

Percutaneous cholecystostomy can be performed under fluoroscopy in severely ill patients with acute cholecystitis who are not surgical candidates, especially for acalculous cholecystitis.

Surgical Management

- **Cholecystectomy** is the therapy of choice for symptomatic gallstone disease and acute cholecystitis. Laparoscopic cholecystectomy is now standard of care. Open cholecystectomy is rarely performed.
- **ERCP** is now used primarily for therapeutic intervention, since MRCP and/or EUS are less invasive and provide enhanced diagnostic potential. Patients presenting with symptomatic cholelithiasis should be assessed as low or high risk of having choledocholithiasis based on laboratory evidence of biliary obstruction and biliary dilation on imaging. Patients at high risk for choledocholithiasis should undergo ERCP for stone removal prior to cholecystectomy. Patients at intermediate risk should either undergo further testing with EUS or MRCP, followed by ERCP if positive, or have an intraoperative cholangiogram during cholecystectomy.[96] An ERCP can be performed subsequently if choledocholithiasis is found.

COMPLICATIONS

- **Acute pancreatitis:** See Acute Pancreatitis section.
- **Choledocholithiasis:** Common bile duct obstruction, jaundice, biliary colic, cholangitis, or pancreatitis can result from stones retained in the common bile duct. The diagnosis can be made on ultrasonography, CT, or MRCP. ERCP with sphincterotomy and stone extraction is curative. The patient should be referred for cholecystectomy.
- **Acute ascending cholangitis** represents a medical emergency with high morbidity and mortality if biliary decompression is not performed urgently. The condition should be stabilized with IV fluids and broad-spectrum antibiotics. Drainage of the biliary tree can be performed through endoscopic (ERCP with sphincterotomy) or percutaneous approaches under fluoroscopic guidance.

OTHER GASTROINTESTINAL DISORDERS

Anorectal Disorders

- **Defecatory disorders** present with difficulty evacuating stool from the rectum or outlet constipation. The diagnosis is ideally made in the setting of compatible symptoms and abnormal testing, including DRE, balloon expulsion testing, barium defecography, MRI, anorectal manometry, and/or pelvic floor electromyography.[97] Management includes biofeedback therapy, laxatives, and suppositories/enemas.[52]
- **Thrombosed external hemorrhoids** present as acutely painful, tense, bluish lumps covered with skin in the anal area. The thrombosed hemorrhoid can be surgically excised under local anesthesia for relief of severe pain. In less severe cases, oral analgesics, sitz baths (sitting in a tub of warm water), stool softeners, and topical ointments may provide symptomatic relief.[98]
- **Internal hemorrhoids** commonly present with either bleeding or a prolapsing mass with straining. Bulk-forming agents such as fiber supplements are useful in preventing straining at defecation. Sitz baths and witch hazel pads may provide symptomatic relief. Ointments and suppositories that contain topical analgesics, emollients,

astringents, and hydrocortisone (e.g., Anusol HC Suppositories, one per rectum bid for 7–10 days) may decrease edema but do not reduce bleeding. Hemorrhoidectomy or band ligation can be curative and are indicated in patients with recurrent or constant bleeding.[98]

• **Anal fissures** present with acute onset of pain during defecation and are often caused by hard stool. Anoscopy reveals an elliptical tear in the skin of the anus, usually in the posterior midline. Acute fissures heal in 2–3 weeks with the use of stool softeners, oral or topical analgesics, and sitz baths. The addition of oral or topical nifedipine to these conservative measures can improve pain relief and healing rates.[99]

• **Perirectal abscess** commonly presents as a painful induration in the perianal area. Patients with IBD and immunocompromised states are particularly susceptible. Prompt drainage is essential to avoid the serious morbidity associated with delayed treatment. Antimicrobials directed against bowel flora (metronidazole, 500 mg PO tid, and ciprofloxacin, 500 mg PO bid) should be administered in patients with significant inflammation, systemic toxicity, or immunocompromised states.

Celiac Sprue

GENERAL PRINCIPLES

• Celiac sprue consists of chronic inflammation of proximal small bowel mucosa from an immunologic sensitivity to **gluten** (protein found in wheat, barley, and rye), resulting in malabsorption of dietary nutrients. The condition remains incompletely recognized and underdiagnosed.[100]

• Clinical presentation can vary greatly from asymptomatic iron deficiency anemia to significant diarrhea and weight loss. Other presenting features can include osteoporosis, dermatitis herpetiformis, abnormal liver enzymes, and abdominal pain; incidental recognition at endoscopy can also occur.[100]

• More than 7% of patients with nonconstipated IBS have celiac-associated antibodies, suggesting that gluten sensitivity may trigger symptoms resembling IBS.[101]

DIAGNOSIS

• Noninvasive serologic tests are highly sensitive and specific and should be checked while the patient is on a gluten-containing diet. Both **IgA anti-tissue transglutaminase (TTG) and antiendomysial antibodies** have accuracies close to 100%. Quantitative IgA levels should also be checked; IgG antibodies against TTG are checked if the patient is IgA deficient.[101]

• EGD with small bowel biopsies is performed to confirm diagnosis with positive serologic testing or if suspicion remains high despite negative noninvasive testing. Classic biopsy findings include blunting or absence of villi and prominent intraepithelial lymphocytosis.

• Almost all patients with celiac sprue carry HLA-DQ2 and HLA-DQ8, so absence of these alleles has high negative predictive value when the diagnosis is in question or if patients are on a gluten-free diet.

• Nonceliac gluten sensitivity should only be considered after exclusion of celiac disease with appropriate testing; differentiation is important for risk identification for nutrient deficiency, complications, and family member risk.

TREATMENT

Medications

- Patients may require iron, folate, vitamin D, and vitamin B_{12} supplements.
- **Corticosteroids** (prednisone, 10–20 mg/d) may be required in refractory cases once inadvertent gluten ingestion has been excluded; immunosuppressive drugs have also been used.[102]

Lifestyle/Risk Modification

- A **gluten-free diet** is first-line therapy and results in prompt improvement in symptoms. Dietary nonadherence is the most frequent cause for persistent symptoms.
- If symptoms persist despite a strict gluten-free diet, radiologic and endoscopic evaluation of the small bowel should be performed to rule out complications including collagenous colitis and **enteropathy-associated T cell lymphoma.** However, the prognosis of adults with unrecognized celiac disease is good despite positive celiac antibodies; therefore, mass screening appears unnecessary.[101]

Diverticular Disease

GENERAL PRINCIPLES

Definition

- **Diverticula** consist of outpouchings in the bowel, most commonly in the colon, but can also be seen elsewhere in the gut.
- **Diverticular bleeding** can occur from an artery at the mouth of the diverticulum.
- **Diverticulitis** results from microperforation of a diverticulum and resultant extracolonic or intramural inflammation.

DIAGNOSIS

Clinical Presentation

- Diverticulosis is usually asymptomatic. Although diverticulosis may be found in patients being investigated for symptoms of abdominal pain and altered bowel habits, a causal link is difficult to establish.
- Typical symptoms of diverticulitis include left lower quadrant abdominal pain, fevers and chills, and alteration of bowel habits. Localized left lower quadrant abdominal tenderness may be elicited on physical examination.

Diagnostic Testing

Laboratories

Diverticulitis may be associated with an elevated white blood cell count with a left shift.

Imaging

- Diverticula are frequently seen on screening colonoscopy.
- Imaging studies, most commonly CT scans, can be useful in the diagnosis of diverticulitis.
- **Colonoscopy is contraindicated for 4–6 weeks after an episode of acute diverticulitis**, but it should be performed after that interval to exclude a perforated neoplasm or IBD if a patient has not had a recent high-quality colonoscopy.[103]

TREATMENT

- Increased dietary fiber is generally recommended in patients with diverticulosis, although no conclusive data exist to support its benefit.
- A low-residue diet is recommended for mild diverticulitis, although no evidence exists to support this practice.[103]
- There is no evidence that patients with diverticulosis should avoid nuts or seeds.

Medications

- Oral **antibiotics** (e.g., ciprofloxacin, 500 mg PO bid, and metronidazole, 500 mg PO tid, for 10–14 days) may suffice for mild diverticulitis; spontaneous resolution has also been described in mild cases.[103]
- Hospital admission, bowel rest, IV fluids, and broad-spectrum IV antimicrobial agents are typically required in moderate to severe cases.

Surgical Management

- Surgical consultation should be obtained for perforation, abscess, fistula, or failure to improve with antibiotics.
- Abscesses may require percutaneous drainage in addition to antibiotics.
- Elective surgical resection is not recommended following acute uncomplicated diverticulitis, but may be necessary in recurrent diverticulitis; surgical decisions need to be individualized.[103]

COMPLICATIONS

- **Perforation:** Although microperforation is part of the pathogenesis of diverticulitis, frank perforation with peritonitis requires surgical consultation.
- **Abscess:** Large (>4 cm) abscesses may require percutaneous drainage. Small abscesses may resolve with antibiotics.
- **Fistula:** Inflammation from diverticulitis may lead to fistulization into adjacent organs, such as the bladder, vagina, or adjacent bowel. This typically requires surgery.
- **Segmental colitis associated with diverticulosis (SCAD)** is a rare entity where mucosal inflammation is seen in the sigmoid colon adjacent to diverticula, which is important to consider before diagnosing IBD in an elderly patient with diverticulosis.

Gastroparesis

GENERAL PRINCIPLES

Definition

Gastroparesis consists of abnormally delayed emptying of stomach contents into the small bowel in the absence of gastric outlet obstruction or ulceration, usually as a result of damage to the nerves or smooth muscle involved in gastric emptying. Symptoms significantly overlap with functional dyspepsia, which can also be associated with delay in gastric emptying on objective testing.[35]

Etiology

- **Mechanical obstruction should always be excluded.**
- In addition to evaluating for acute metabolic derangements and potential offending medications (e.g., narcotics, anticholinergic agents, chemotherapeutic agents, glucagon-like peptide 1 receptor agonists, and amylin analogs), patients with

gastroparesis should be screened for **diabetes mellitus**, thyroid dysfunction, neurologic disease, prior gastric or bariatric surgery, and autoimmune disorders (e.g., scleroderma).

• If no predisposing cause is identified, gastroparesis is designated **idiopathic.**

DIAGNOSIS

Clinical Presentation

Symptoms include nausea, bloating, and vomiting, usually hours after a meal.

Diagnostic Testing

A 4-hour **gastric-emptying study** (gamma camera scan after a radiolabeled meal) can quantify gastric emptying; medications that can delay gastric emptying (i.e., opioids and anticholinergics) should be stopped at least 48 hours prior to testing.[104] However, the finding of gastric emptying delay may not be consistent on repeat study.

TREATMENT

• First steps in management include fluid restoration, correction of electrolytes, nutritional support, and optimization of glucose control for diabetic patients. Indications for postpyloric enteral feeding include unintentional loss of >10% of usual body weight and/or refractory symptoms requiring repeated hospitalizations.

• Nutritional consultation can help address nutritional deficiencies and optimize diet, especially to decrease dietary fat and insoluble fiber. Small particle size diets reduce symptoms in patients with diabetic gastroparesis.[105]

Medications

• **Metoclopramide** (10 mg PO qid half an hour before meals) often represents the first line of prokinetic therapy but has variable efficacy, and side effects (drowsiness, tardive dyskinesia, parkinsonism) may limit chronic use as some are permanent.

• **Erythromycin** (125–250 mg PO tid or 200 mg IV) can improve gastric emptying in the short term, but tachyphylaxis is a significant limitation precluding chronic benefit.

• **Domperidone** (20 mg PO qid before meals and at bedtime) does not cross the blood–brain barrier, but hyperprolactinemia can result. ECGs should be checked at baseline and on follow-up given the risk of QT prolongation. Domperidone is not available in the United States.

• **Antiemetics** may improve associated nausea and vomiting but will not improve gastric emptying.

Surgical Management

• **Enteral feeding** through a jejunostomy feeding tube may be required for supplemental nutrition and is favored over TPN.

• **Gastric electrical stimulation** using a surgically implanted stimulator (Enterra) may reduce symptoms of nausea and vomiting in half of medically refractory patients, but gastric emptying is typically not enhanced by this approach.[106]

CHAPTER 18

Ischemic Intestinal Injury

GENERAL PRINCIPLES

- **Acute mesenteric ischemia** results from arterial (or rarely venous) compromise to the superior mesenteric circulation.
- Emboli and thrombus formation are the most common causes of acute mesenteric ischemia, although **nonocclusive mesenteric ischemia** from vasoconstriction can also give rise to the disorder.
- **Ischemic colitis** results from mucosal ischemia in the inferior mesenteric circulation during a low-flow state (hypotension, arrhythmias, sepsis, aortic vascular surgery), often in patients with atherosclerotic disease.[107] Vasculitis, sickle cell disease, vasospasm, and marathon running can also predispose to ischemic colitis.
- **Chronic mesenteric ischemia** is caused by atherosclerosis of all three major abdominal arteries leading to intermittent hypoperfusion.

DIAGNOSIS

Clinical Presentation

- Patients with acute mesenteric ischemia may present with abdominal pain, but physical examination and imaging studies can be unremarkable until infarction has occurred. As a result, diagnosis is often late and mortality is high.
- Ischemic colitis typically presents with sudden abdominal cramping with an urge to defecate, followed by passage of bright red blood per rectum in 24 hours. Severe insults can lead to gangrene, perforation, and stricture formation.
- Chronic mesenteric ischemia can present with abdominal pain after eating and weight loss from food avoidance.

Diagnostic Testing

- **Urgent angiography** is indicated if the suspicion for acute mesenteric ischemia is high.
- CT with IV contrast should be performed for suspected colonic ischemia, to evaluate for bowel wall thickening in watershed areas. Multiphasic CT angiography should be performed if acute mesenteric ischemia is suspected.[107] Pneumatosis or portal venous gas indicates transmural infarction and necessitates surgical consultation.
- In patients with ischemic colitis, characteristic "**thumb-printing**" of the involved colon may be seen on plain radiographs of the abdomen.
- Colonoscopy with minimal insufflation should be performed to confirm the diagnosis.[107] It may reveal mucosal erythema, edema, and ulceration, sometimes in a linear configuration; evidence of gangrene or necrosis is an indication for surgical intervention.
- CT angiography or Doppler ultrasound can show stenosis of the abdominal vasculature in suspected chronic mesenteric ischemia.

TREATMENT

- Treatment of acute mesenteric ischemia is essentially surgical and increasingly **endovascular.**[107]

- In patients with ischemic colitis, in the absence of peritoneal signs or evidence of gangrene or perforation, expectant management with fluid and electrolyte repletion and maintenance of stable hemodynamics usually suffices. Broad-spectrum antimicrobials should be used in moderate to severe cases. Evidence of gangrene or necrosis is an indication for surgery.
- Open and endovascular approaches are available for chronic mesenteric ischemia.[108] Atherosclerosis of the mesenteric vessels without symptoms should be treated with risk-factor modification (see Chapter 4, Ischemic Heart Disease).

REFERENCES

1. Hearnshaw SA, Logan RFA, Lowe D, et al. Acute upper gastrointestinal bleeding in the UK: patient characteristics, diagnoses and outcomes in the 2007 UK audit. *Gut.* 2011;60:1327-1335.
2. Raju GS, Gerson L, Das A, et al. American Gastroenterological Association (AGA) institute technical review on obscure gastrointestinal bleeding. *Gastroenterology.* 2007;133:1697-1717.
3. Aljebreen AM, Fallone CA, Barkun AN, et al. Nasogastric aspirate predicts high-risk endoscopic lesions in patients with acute upper-GI bleeding. *Gastrointest Endosc.* 2004;59:172-178.
4. Gralnek IM, Barkun AN, Bardou M. Management of acute bleeding from a peptic ulcer. *N Engl J Med.* 2008;359:928-937.
5. Lau JYW, Yu Y, Tang RSY, et al. Timing of endoscopy for acute upper gastrointestinal bleeding. *N Engl J Med.* 2020;382:1299-1308.
6. Altraif I, Handoo FA, Aljumah A, et al. Effect of erythromycin before endoscopy in patients presenting with variceal bleeding: a prospective, randomized, double-blind, placebo-controlled trial. *Gastrointest Endosc.* 2011;73:245-250.
7. Tsoi KK, Chan HC, Chiu PW, et al. Second-look endoscopy with thermal coagulation or injections for peptic ulcer bleeding: a meta-analysis. *J Gastroenterol Hepatol.* 2010;25:8-13.
8. Beck KR, Shergill AK. Colonoscopy in acute lower gastrointestinal bleeding: diagnosis, timing, and bowel preparation. *Gastrointest Endosc Clin N Am.* 2018;28:379-390.
9. Gerson LB, Fidler JL, Cave DR, et al. ACG clinical guideline: diagnosis and management of small bowel bleeding. *Am J Gastroenterol.* 2015;110:1265-1287.
10. Reddick AD, Ronald J, Morrison WG. Intravenous fluid resuscitation: was Poiseuille right? *Emerg Med J.* 2011;28:201-202.
11. Villanueva C, Colomo A, Bosch A, et al. Transfusion strategies for acute upper gastrointestinal bleeding. *N Engl J Med.* 2013;368:11-21.
12. Barkun AN, Almadi M, Kuipers EJ, et al. Management of nonvariceal upper gastrointestinal bleeding: guideline recommendations from the international consensus group. *Ann Intern Med.* 2019;171:805-822.
13. O'Leary JG, Greenberg CS, Patton HM, et al. AGA clinical practice update: coagulation in cirrhosis. *Gastroenterology.* 2019;157:34-43.e1.
14. Stanley AJ, Dalton HR, Blatchford O, et al. Multicentre comparison of the Glasgow Blatchford and Rockall Scores in the prediction of clinical end-points after upper gastrointestinal haemorrhage. *Aliment Pharmacol Ther.* 2011;34:470-475.
15. Lau JY, Sung JJ, Lee KK, et al. Effect of intravenous omeprazole on recurrent bleeding after endoscopic treatment of bleeding peptic ulcers. *N Engl J Med.* 2000;343:310-316.
16. Laine L, Jensen DM. Management of patients with ulcer bleeding. *Am J Gastroenterol.* 2012;107:345-360; quiz 361.
17. Wang CH, Ma MH, Chou HC, et al. High-dose vs non-high-dose proton pump inhibitors after endoscopic treatment in patients with bleeding peptic ulcer: a systematic review and meta-analysis of randomized controlled trials. *Arch Intern Med.* 2010;170:751-758.
18. Lau JY, Leung WK, Wu JC, et al. Omeprazole before endoscopy in patients with gastrointestinal bleeding. *N Engl J Med.* 2007;356:1631-1640.
19. Hwang JH, Shergill AK, Acosta RD, et al. The role of endoscopy in the management of variceal hemorrhage. *Gastrointest Endosc.* 2014;80:221-227.
20. Bernard B, Grangé JD, Khac EN, et al. Antibiotic prophylaxis for the prevention of bacterial infections in cirrhotic patients with gastrointestinal bleeding: a meta-analysis. *Hepatology.* 1999;29:1655-1661.
21. Ge ZZ, Chen HM, Gao YJ, et al. Efficacy of thalidomide for refractory gastrointestinal bleeding from vascular malformation. *Gastroenterology.* 2011;141:1629-1637.e1-4.
22. Garcia-Tsao G, Abraldes JG, Berzigotti A, et al. Portal hypertensive bleeding in cirrhosis – risk stratification, diagnosis, and management: 2016 practice guidance by the American Association for the study of liver diseases. *Hepatology.* 2017;65:310-335.

CHAPTER 18

23. García-Pagán JC, Caca K, Bureau C, et al. Early use of TIPS in patients with cirrhosis and variceal bleeding. *N Engl J Med*. 2010;362:2370-2379.

24. Hong CH, Kim HJ, Park JH, et al. Treatment of patients with gastric variceal hemorrhage: endoscopic N-butyl-2-cyanoacrylate injection versus balloon-occluded retrograde transvenous obliteration. *J Gastroenterol Hepatol*. 2009;24:372-378.

25. Sung JJ, Lau JY, Ching JY, et al. Continuation of low-dose aspirin therapy in peptic ulcer bleeding: a randomized trial. *Ann Intern Med*. 2010;152:1-9.

26. Bhatt DL, Cryer BL, Contant CF, et al. Clopidogrel with or without omeprazole in coronary artery disease. *N Engl J Med*. 2010;363:1909-1917.

27. Kushnir VM, Sharma S, Ewald GA, et al. Evaluation of GI bleeding after implantation of left ventricular assist device. *Gastrointest Endosc*. 2012;75:973-979.

28. Rommel N, Hamdy S. Oropharyngeal dysphagia: manifestations and diagnosis. *Nat Rev Gastroenterol Hepatol*. 2016;13:49-59.

29. Zerbib F, Omari T. Oesophageal dysphagia: manifestations and diagnosis. *Nat Rev Gastroenterol Hepatol*. 2015;12:322-331.

30. Shaheen NJ, Weinberg DS, Denberg TD, et al. Upper endoscopy for gastroesophageal reflux disease: best practice advice from the clinical guidelines committee of the American College of Physicians. *Ann Intern Med*. 2012;157:808-816.

31. Committee ASoP; Pasha SF, Acosta RD, Chandrasekhara V, et al. The role of endoscopy in the evaluation and management of dysphagia. *Gastrointest Endosc*. 2014;79:191-201.

32. Yadlapati R, Kahrilas PJ, Fox MR, et al. Esophageal motility disorders on high-resolution manometry: Chicago classification version 4.0((c)). *Neurogastroenterol Motil*. 2021;33:e14058.

33. Savarino E, di Pietro M, Bredenoord AJ, et al. Use of the functional lumen imaging probe in clinical esophagology. *Am J Gastroenterol*. 2020;115:1786-1796.

34. Gyawali CP, Carlson DA, Chen JW, et al. ACG clinical guidelines: clinical use of esophageal physiologic testing. *Am J Gastroenterol*. 2020;115:1412-1428.

35. Pasricha PJ, Grover M, Yates KP, et al. Functional dyspepsia and gastroparesis in tertiary care are interchangeable syndromes with common clinical and pathologic features. *Gastroenterology*. 2021;160:2006-2017.

36. Camilleri M, Parkman HP, Shafi MA, et al. Clinical guideline: management of gastroparesis. *Am J Gastroenterol*. 2013;108:18-37; quiz 38.

37. Riddle MS, DuPont HL, Connor BA. ACG clinical guideline: diagnosis, treatment, and prevention of acute diarrheal infections in adults. *Am J Gastroenterol*. 2016;111:602-622.

38. Thielman NM, Guerrant RL. Clinical practice. Acute infectious diarrhea. *N Engl J Med*. 2004;350:38-47.

39. Schiller LR, Pardi DS, Sellin JH. Chronic diarrhea: diagnosis and management. *Clin Gastroenterol Hepatol*. 2017;15:182-193.e3.

40. Surawicz CM, Brandt LJ, Binion DG, et al. Guidelines for diagnosis, treatment, and prevention of *Clostridium difficile* infections. *Am J Gastroenterol*. 2013;108:478-498; quiz 499.

41. Liu A, Meyer E, Johnston L, et al. Prevalence of graft versus host disease and cytomegalovirus infection in patients post-haematopoietic cell transplantation presenting with gastrointestinal symptoms. *Aliment Pharmacol Ther*. 2013;38:955-966.

42. Wong CS, Jelacic S, Habeeb RL, et al. The risk of the hemolytic-uremic syndrome after antibiotic treatment of *Escherichia coli* O157:H7 infections. *N Engl J Med*. 2000;342:1930-1936.

43. McDonald LC, Gerding DN, Johnson S, et al. Clinical practice guidelines for Clostridium difficile infection in adults and children: 2017 update by the Infectious Diseases Society of America (IDSA) and Society for Healthcare Epidemiology of America (SHEA). *Clin Infect Dis*. 2018;66:987-994.

44. Wilcox CM, Saag MS. Gastrointestinal complications of HIV infection: changing priorities in the HAART era. *Gut*. 2008;57:861-870.

45. Mounsey A, Raleigh M, Wilson A. Management of constipation in older adults. *Am Fam Physician*. 2015;92:500-504.

46. Nelson AD, Camilleri M, Chirapongsathorn S, et al. Comparison of efficacy of pharmacological treatments for chronic idiopathic constipation: a systematic review and network meta-analysis. *Gut*. 2017;66:1611-1622.

47. Lembo AJ, Schneier HA, Shiff SJ, et al. Two randomized trials of linaclotide for chronic constipation. *N Engl J Med*. 2011;365:527-536.

48. Brenner DM, Fogel R, Dorn SD, et al. Efficacy, safety, and tolerability of plecanatide in patients with irritable bowel syndrome with constipation: results of two phase 3 randomized clinical trials. *Am J Gastroenterol*. 2018;113:735-745.

49. Crockett S, Greer KB, Sultan S. Opioid-induced constipation (OIC) guideline. *Gastroenterology*. 2019;156:228.

50. Sharara AI, Abou Mrad RR. The modern bowel preparation in colonoscopy. *Gastroenterol Clin North Am*. 2013;42:577-598.

51. Perreault G, Goodman A, Larion S, et al. Split- versus single-dose preparation tolerability in a multiethnic population: decreased side effects but greater social barriers. *Ann Gastroenterol.* 2018;31:356-364.

52. Rao SS, Benninga MA, Bharucha AE, et al. ANMS-ESNM position paper and consensus guidelines on biofeedback therapy for anorectal disorders. *Neurogastroenterol Motil.* 2015;27:594-609.

53. Savarino E, Bredenoord AJ, Fox M, et al. Expert consensus document: advances in the physiological assessment and diagnosis of GERD. *Nat Rev Gastroenterol Hepatol.* 2017;14:665-676.

54. Gyawali CP, Fass R. Management of gastroesophageal reflux disease. *Gastroenterology.* 2018;154:302-318.

55. Dellon ES, Liacouras CA, Molina-Infante J, et al. Updated international consensus diagnostic Criteria for eosinophilic esophagitis: proceedings of the AGREE Conference. *Gastroenterology.* 2018;155:1022-1033 e10.

56. Hirano I, Chan ES, Rank MA, et al. AGA institute and the joint task force on allergy-immunology practice parameters clinical guidelines for the management of eosinophilic esophagitis. *Gastroenterology.* 2020;158:1776-1786.

57. Ahuja NK, Clarke JO. Evaluation and management of infectious esophagitis in immunocompromised and immunocompetent individuals. *Curr Treat Options Gastroenterol.* 2016;14:28-38.

58. Hoffman RS, Burns MM, Gosselin S. Ingestion of caustic substances. *N Engl J Med.* 2020;382:1739-1748.

59. Gyawali CP, Kahrilas PJ, Savarino E, et al. Modern diagnosis of GERD: the Lyon consensus. *Gut.* 2018;67:1351-1362.

60. Vaezi MF, Yang YX, Howden CW. Complications of proton pump inhibitor therapy. *Gastroenterology.* 2017;153(1):35-48.

61. Zerbib F, Bredenoord AJ, Fass R, et al. ESNM/ANMS consensus paper: diagnosis and management of refractory gastro-esophageal reflux disease. *Neurogastroenterol Motil.* 2021;33:e14075.

62. Spechler SJ, Hunter JG, Jones KM, et al. Randomized trial of medical versus surgical treatment for refractory heartburn. *N Engl J Med.* 2019;381:1513-1523.

63. Shaheen NJ, Falk GW, Iyer PG, et al. ACG clinical guideline: diagnosis and management of Barrett's esophagus. *Am J Gastroenterol.* 2016;111:30-50; quiz 51.

64. Vaezi MF, Pandolfino JE, Yadlapati RH, et al. ACG clinical guidelines: diagnosis and management of achalasia. *Am J Gastroenterol.* 2020;115:1393-1411.

65. Lanas A, Chan FKL. Peptic ulcer disease. *Lancet.* 2017;390:613-624.

66. Best LM, Takwoingi Y, Siddique S, et al. Non-invasive diagnostic tests for *Helicobacter pylori* infection. *Cochrane Database Syst Rev.* 2018;3:Cd012080.

67. Chey WD, Leontiadis GI, Howden CW, et al. ACG clinical guideline: treatment of Helicobacter pylori infection. *Am J Gastroenterol.* 2017;112:212-239.

68. Shah SC, Iyer PG, Moss SF. AGA clinical practice update on the management of refractory Helicobacter pylori infection: expert review. *Gastroenterology.* 2021;160:1831-1841.

69. Sugano K, Choi MG, Lin JT, et al. Multinational, double-blind, randomised, placebo-controlled, prospective study of esomeprazole in the prevention of recurrent peptic ulcer in low-dose acetylsalicylic acid users: the LAVENDER study. *Gut.* 2014;63:1061-1068.

70. Metz DC. Diagnosis of the Zollinger–ellison syndrome. *Clin Gastroenterol Hepatol.* 2012;10:126-130.

71. Rubin DT, Ananthakrishnan AN, Siegel CA, et al. ACG clinical guideline: ulcerative colitis in adults. *Am J Gastroenterol.* 2019;114:384-413.

72. Lichtenstein GR, Loftus EV, Isaacs KL, et al. ACG clinical guideline: management of Crohn's disease in adults. *Am J Gastroenterol.* 2018;113:481-517.

73. Mahadevan U, Long MD, Kane SV, et al. Pregnancy and neonatal outcomes after fetal exposure to biologics and thiopurines among women with inflammatory bowel disease. *Gastroenterology.* 2021;160:1131-1139.

74. Lacy BE, Pimentel M, Brenner DM, et al. ACG clinical guideline: management of irritable bowel syndrome. *Am J Gastroenterol.* 2021;116:17-44.

75. Halmos EP, Power VA, Shepherd SJ, et al. A diet low in FODMAPs reduces symptoms of irritable bowel syndrome. *Gastroenterology.* 2014;146:67-75 e5.

76. Chumpitazi BP, Kearns GL, Shulman RJ. Review article: the physiological effects and safety of peppermint oil and its efficacy in irritable bowel syndrome and other functional disorders. *Aliment Pharmacol Ther.* 2018;47:738-752.

77. Pimentel M, Saad RJ, Long MD, et al. ACG clinical guideline: small intestinal bacterial overgrowth. *Am J Gastroenterol.* 2020;115:165-178.

78. Dove LS, Lembo A, Randall CW, et al. Eluxadoline benefits patients with irritable bowel syndrome with diarrhea in a phase 2 study. *Gastroenterology.* 2013;145:329-338 e1.

79. Ford AC, Brandt LJ, Young C, et al. Efficacy of 5-HT3 antagonists and 5-HT4 agonists in irritable bowel syndrome: systematic review and meta-analysis. *Am J Gastroenterol.* 2009;104:1831-1843; quiz 1844.

80. Venkatesan T, Levinthal DJ, Tarbell SE, et al. Guidelines on management of cyclic vomiting syndrome in adults by the American neurogastroenterology and motility society and the cyclic vomiting syndrome association. *Neurogastroenterol Motil.* 2019;31(suppl 2):e13604.

81. Downes TJ, Cheruvu MS, Karunaratne TB, et al. Pathophysiology, diagnosis, and management of chronic intestinal pseudo-obstruction. *J Clin Gastroenterol.* 2018;52:477-489.

82. Kram B, Greenland M, Grant M, et al. Efficacy and safety of subcutaneous neostigmine for ileus, acute colonic pseudo-obstruction, or refractory constipation. *Ann Pharmacother.* 2018;52:505-512.

83. Abodeely A, Schechter S, Klipfel A, et al. Does alvimopan enhance return of bowel function in laparoscopic right colectomy? *Am Surg.* 2011;77:1460-1462.

84. Toyomasu Y, Mochiki E, Morita H, et al. Mosapride citrate improves postoperative ileus of patients with colectomy. *J Gastrointest Surg.* 2011;15:1361-1367.

85. Emmanuel AV, Kamm MA, Roy AJ, et al. Randomised clinical trial: the efficacy of prucalopride in patients with chronic intestinal pseudo-obstruction—a double-blind, placebo-controlled, cross-over, multiple n = 1 study. *Aliment Pharmacol Ther.* 2012;35:48-55.

86. Akshintala VS, Hutfless SM, Colantuoni E, et al. Systematic review with network meta-analysis: pharmacological prophylaxis against post-ERCP pancreatitis. *Aliment Pharmacol Ther.* 2013;38:1325-1337.

87. Banks PA, Bollen TL, Dervenis C, et al. Classification of acute pancreatitis--2012: revision of the Atlanta classification and definitions by international consensus. *Gut.* 2013;62:102-111.

88. Tenner S, Baillie J, DeWitt J, et al. American College of Gastroenterology guideline: management of acute pancreatitis. *Am J Gastroenterol.* 2013;108:1400-1415; 1416.

89. van Dijk SM, Hallensleben NDL, van Santvoort HC, et al. Acute pancreatitis: recent advances through randomised trials. *Gut.* 2017;66:2024-2032.

90. Bakker OJ, van Brunschot S, van Santvoort HC, et al. Early versus on-demand nasoenteric tube feeding in acute pancreatitis. *N Engl J Med.* 2014;371:1983-1993.

91. Schepers NJ, Hallensleben NDL, Besselink MG, et al. Urgent endoscopic retrograde cholangiopancreatography with sphincterotomy versus conservative treatment in predicted severe acute gallstone pancreatitis (APEC): a multicentre randomised controlled trial. *Lancet.* 2020;396:167-176.

92. van Santvoort HC, Besselink MG, Bakker OJ, et al. A step-up approach or open necrosectomy for necrotizing pancreatitis. *N Engl J Med.* 2010;362:1491-1502.

93. Witt H, Apte MV, Keim V, et al. Chronic pancreatitis: challenges and advances in pathogenesis, genetics, diagnosis, and therapy. *Gastroenterology.* 2007;132:1557-1573.

94. Gardner TB, Adler DG, Forsmark CE, et al. ACG clinical guideline: chronic pancreatitis. *Am J Gastroenterol.* 2020;115:322-339.

95. Hart PA, Kamisawa T, Brugge WR, et al. Long-term outcomes of autoimmune pancreatitis: a multicentre, international analysis. *Gut.* 2013;62:1771-1776.

96. Buxbaum JL, Abbas Fehmi SM, Sultan S, et al. ASGE guideline on the role of endoscopy in the evaluation and management of choledocholithiasis. *Gastrointest Endosc.* 2019;89:1075-1105.e15.

97. Rao SS, Bharucha AE, Chiarioni G, et al. Functional anorectal disorders. *Gastroenterology.* Published online 2016.

98. Davis BR, Lee-Kong SA, Migaly J, et al. The American society of colon and rectal surgeons clinical practice guidelines for the management of hemorrhoids. *Dis Colon Rectum.* 2018;61:284-292.

99. Stewart DB,Sr, Gaertner W, Glasgow S, et al. Clinical practice guideline for the management of anal fissures. *Dis Colon Rectum.* 2017;60:7-14.

100. Hujoel IA, Van Dyke CT, Brantner T, et al. Natural history and clinical detection of undiagnosed coeliac disease in a North American community. *Aliment Pharmacol Ther.* 2018;47:1358-1366.

101. Rubio-Tapia A, Hill ID, Kelly CP, et al. ACG clinical guidelines: diagnosis and management of celiac disease. *Am J Gastroenterol.* 2013;108:656-676; quiz 677.

102. Lebwohl B, Sanders DS, Green PHR. Coeliac disease. *Lancet.* 2018;391:70-81.

103. Peery AF, Shaukat A, Strate LL. AGA clinical practice update on medical management of colonic diverticulitis: expert review. *Gastroenterology.* 2021;160:906-911.e1.

104. Abell TL, Camilleri M, Donohoe K, et al. Consensus recommendations for gastric emptying scintigraphy: a joint report of the American neurogastroenterology and motility society and the society of nuclear medicine. *Am J Gastroenterol.* 2008;103:753-763.

105. Olausson EA, Storsrud S, Grundin H, et al. A small particle size diet reduces upper gastrointestinal symptoms in patients with diabetic gastroparesis: a randomized controlled trial. *Am J Gastroenterol.* 2014;109:375-385.

106. Lacy BE, Weiser K. Gastric motility, gastroparesis, and gastric stimulation. *Surg Clin North Am.* 2005;85:967-987, vi-vii.

107. Brandt LJ, Feuerstadt P, Longstreth GF, et al. ACG clinical guideline: epidemiology, risk factors, patterns of presentation, diagnosis, and management of colon ischemia (CI). *Am J Gastroenterol.* 2015;110:18-44; quiz 45.

108. Clair DG, Beach JM. Mesenteric ischemia. *N Engl J Med.* 2016;374:959-968.

Evaluation of Liver Disease

GENERAL PRINCIPLES

- Liver disease presents as a spectrum of clinical conditions that ranges from asymptomatic disease to end-stage liver disease (ESLD).
- A comprehensive investigation combining thorough history and physical examination with diagnostic tests, liver histology, and imaging can often establish a precise diagnosis.

DIAGNOSIS

Clinical Presentation

History

History taking should focus on the following:
- History of present illnesses
- Medication history: prescription, herbal medicine, and dietary supplements
- Toxin exposures: alcohol, illicit, and recreational drugs
- Common signs and symptoms of liver disease: icterus, jaundice, ascites and edema, pruritus, encephalopathy, and gastrointestinal (GI) bleeding
- Family history of liver disease
- Comorbid conditions: obesity, diabetes, hyperlipidemia, inflammatory bowel disease (IBD), systemic hypotension, and HIV
- Risk factors for infection: IV/intranasal drug use, body piercings, tattooing, high-risk sexual behavior, travel to foreign countries, and occupation

Physical Examination

A detailed physical examination is necessary. Physical stigmata of acute and chronic liver disease may include the following:
- Jaundice and icterus
- Ascites, peripheral edema, and pleural effusions
- Hepatomegaly and splenomegaly
- Gynecomastia and testicular atrophy
- Muscle wasting (temporal and/or proximal)
- Telangiectasias and palmar erythema
- Confusion and asterixis

Diagnostic Testing

Laboratories
- **Serum enzymes**
  - Elevations primarily in **aspartate aminotransferase (AST) and alanine aminotransferase (ALT)** suggest hepatocellular injury; however, AST elevations may be seen with muscle or red blood cell damage, for example, rhabdomyolysis, myocardial infarction, and hemolysis.

- **Alkaline phosphatase (ALP)** is an enzyme found in a variety of tissues (bone, intestine, kidney, leukocytes, liver, and placenta). The concomitant elevation of other hepatic enzymes (e.g., γ-glutamyl transpeptidase [GGT] or 5′-nucleotidase) confirms a hepatic process is causing the ALP elevation. ALP is often elevated in biliary obstruction, space-occupying lesions or infiltrative disorders of the liver, and conditions causing intrahepatic cholestasis (primary biliary cholangitis [PBC], primary sclerosing cholangitis [PSC], and drug-induced cholestasis).
- **Excretory products**
  - **Bilirubin** is a degradation product of hemoglobin and nonerythroid hemoproteins. Total serum bilirubin is composed of conjugated (direct) and unconjugated (indirect) fractions. Unconjugated hyperbilirubinemia occurs as a result of excessive bilirubin production (hemolysis, hemolytic anemias, ineffective erythropoiesis, and resorption of hematomas), reduced hepatic bilirubin uptake (Gilbert syndrome and drugs such as rifampin and probenecid), or impaired bilirubin conjugation (Gilbert and Crigler–Najjar syndrome). Elevation of conjugated and unconjugated fractions occurs in Dubin–Johnson and Rotor syndromes and in conditions associated with intrahepatic (i.e., hepatocellular, canalicular, or ductular damage) and extrahepatic (i.e., mechanical obstruction) cholestasis.
  - **α-Fetoprotein (AFP)** is normally produced by fetal liver cells. Its production falls to normal adult levels of <10 ng/mL within the first year of life. AFP is an insensitive and nonspecific biomarker for hepatocellular carcinoma (HCC), with a sensitivity and specificity of 61% and 81%, respectively, at a cutoff of 20 ng/mL and 22% and 100%, respectively, at a cutoff of 200 ng/mL.[1] Levels >400 ng/mL or a rapid doubling time are suggestive of HCC. Mild to moderate elevations can be seen in acute and chronic liver inflammation.

Imaging

- **Ultrasonography** is a relatively inexpensive, low-risk imaging test that can identify changes in the liver surface and parenchyma, biliary tree, and gallbladder. It is frequently used as a first-line imaging for the evaluation of right-sided abdominal pain, meal-related epigastric discomfort, and abnormal liver function tests (LFTs). It can reveal and characterize liver masses, abscesses, and cysts. Color flow Doppler ultrasonography assesses patency and direction of blood flow in the portal and hepatic veins and may be useful in the assessment of portal hypertension, a common finding in cirrhosis. Ultrasonography is recommended for HCC screening in patients with cirrhosis. However, ultrasonography is less sensitive for detecting small or infiltrative tumors in comparison to CT or MRI. Body habitus and central adiposity can limit the usefulness of ultrasound. Additionally, the sensitivity of this imaging modality is operator dependent.
- **CT scan** with IV contrast is useful to evaluate the liver parenchyma. This test can define space-occupying lesions (e.g., abscess or tumor) and calculate liver volume. Triple-phase CT or quadruple-phase CT is indicated for liver mass evaluation. A delayed phase is useful when HCC is suspected.
- **MRI** with contrast offers information similar to CT, with the additional advantage of better characterization of liver lesions, fatty infiltration, and iron deposition. It is the modality of choice in patients with an iodinated contrast allergy. However, MRI cannot be used in patients with renal failure (glomerular filtration rate [GFR] <30 mL/min/1.73 m²) because of the low risk of gadolinium-associated nephrogenic

systemic fibrosis. Of all the cross-sectional imaging techniques, MRI provides the highest tissue contrast. This, in conjunction with various contrast agents, allows for definitive noninvasive characterization of liver lesions.

- **Magnetic resonance cholangiopancreatography (MRCP)** is a specialized study that provides an alternative noninvasive diagnostic modality to visualize the intrahepatic and extrahepatic bile ducts. MRCP does not require contrast administration into the ductal system.
- **Elastography** is a method of measuring liver stiffness as a surrogate for fibrosis. Noninvasive tools for fibrosis staging are increasingly used in the evaluation of chronic liver disease, especially in chronic hepatitis C and nonalcoholic steatohepatitis (NASH). Vibration-controlled transient elastography (VCTE) was approved by the Food and Drug Administration (FDA) in 2013 and is the most extensively studied noninvasive tool. Other noninvasive tools for the evaluation of fibrosis include magnetic resonance elastography (MRE), two-dimensional and point shear wave elastography, or acoustic radiation force impulse elastography.

Diagnostic Procedures

- **Percutaneous transhepatic cholangiography (PTC) and endoscopic retrograde cholangiopancreatography (ERCP)** involve injection of contrast into the biliary tree. These invasive procedures are most effectively used to investigate abnormalities detected on ultrasonography, CT, or MRI/MRCP. PTC and ERCP allow for diagnostic and therapeutic maneuvers including biopsy, brushings, stenting, and drain placement.
- **Transjugular assessment of portal pressure** is an invasive procedure measuring the hepatic venous pressure gradient (HVPG): the difference between the wedged (representing the portal venous pressure) and the free hepatic venous pressures. The normal HVPG pressure is <6 mm Hg. HVPG >6 mm Hg is consistent with portal hypertension. Complications of portal hypertension, such as ascites and esophageal varices, usually occur with HVPG >12 mm Hg.[2]
- **Liver biopsy** is an invasive procedure that is typically performed percutaneously. Suspicious liver lesions are usually biopsied with ultrasound or CT guidance, although imaging is not absolutely required. If coagulopathy, thrombocytopenia, and/or ascites are of concern, a transjugular liver biopsy can be performed instead. Finally, surgical laparoscopy is also an alternative way to obtain liver tissue. Bleeding, pain, infection, injury to nearby organs, and (rarely) death are potential complications.
- Additional noninvasive tests to assess fibrosis and cirrhosis are available. These include serum direct and indirect biomarkers of fibrosis, proprietary and nonproprietary serum biomarkers, and other noninvasive imaging tools. They are considered as alternatives to biopsy, although precise guidelines for their use are not defined.

VIRAL HEPATITIS

The hepatotropic viruses include hepatitis A (HAV), hepatitis B (HBV), hepatitis C (HCV), hepatitis D (HDV), and hepatitis E (HEV) (Tables 19-1 and 19-2). Nonhepatotropic viruses, which indirectly affect the liver, include Epstein–Barr virus, cytomegalovirus, herpes simplex virus, measles, Ebola, and others. The novel coronavirus SARS-CoV-2 is also a cause of viral hepatitis. The pathogenesis is thought to be a direct virus-induced cytopathic effect versus immune response damage from the cytokine release syndrome.[3]

TABLE 19-1	Clinical and Epidemiologic Features of Hepatotropic Viruses				
Organism	Hepatitis A	Hepatitis B	Hepatitis C	Hepatitis D	Hepatitis E
Incubation	15–45 d	30–180 d	15–150 d	30–150 d	30–60 d
Transmission	Fecal–oral	Blood Sexual Perinatal	Blood Sexual (rare) Perinatal (rare)	Blood Sexual (rare)	Fecal–oral Organ transplantation
Risk groups	Residents of and travelers to endemic regions Children and caregivers in daycare centers	Injection drug users Multiple sexual partners Men who have sex with men Infants born to infected mothers Healthcare workers	Injection drug users Transfusion recipients	Any person with hepatitis B virus Injection drug users	Residents of and travelers to endemic regions Zoonosis: workers in pig farms
Fatality rate	1.0%	1.0%	<0.1%	2%–10%	1%
Carrier state	No	Yes	Yes	Yes	No
Chronic hepatitis	None	2%–10% in adults; 90% in children <5 y	70%–85%	Variable	Rare
Cirrhosis	No	Yes	Yes	Yes	No

Acute viral hepatitis is defined by an array of symptoms that may vary from mild, nonspecific symptoms to acute liver failure (ALF). This condition may resolve or progress to chronic hepatitis, in certain cases, or to liver failure as a consequence of diffuse necroinflammatory liver injury.

ALF is defined as the rapid development of severe liver injury with encephalopathy, jaundice, and coagulopathy in a patient without preexisting liver disease within <6 months from the onset of the acute illness.

Chronic viral hepatitis is defined as the presence of persistent (>6 months) virologic replication, as determined by serologic and molecular studies, with necroinflammatory and fibrotic injury. Symptoms and biochemical abnormalities may vary from none to moderate. Histopathologic classification of chronic viral hepatitis is based on etiology, grade, and stage. Grading and staging are measures of the severity of inflammation and fibrosis, respectively. Chronic viral hepatitis may lead to cirrhosis and HCC.

TABLE 19-2	Viral Hepatitis Serologies[a]			
Hepatitis	Acute	Chronic	Recovered/ Latent	Vaccinated
HAV	IgM anti-HAV+	NA	IgG anti-HAV+	IgG anti-HAV+
HCV	All tests possibly negative HCV NAT+ HCV RNA+ Anti-HCV Ab+	Anti-HCV Ab+ HCV RNA+	Anti-HCV Ab+ HCV RNA–[b]	NA
HDV	IgM anti-HDV+[c] HDV Ag+[c]	IgG anti-HDV+[c]	IgG anti-HDV+[c]	Vaccination against HBV
HEV	IgM anti-HEV	NA	IgG anti-HEV	NA

Ab, antibody; HAV, hepatitis A virus; HCV, hepatitis C virus; HDV, hepatitis D virus; HEV, hepatitis E virus; NA, not applicable.
[a]For hepatitis B virus serologies, see Table 19-3.
[b]Negative HCV RNA results should be interpreted with caution. Differences are found in thresholds for detection among assays and among laboratories.
[c]Markers of HBV infection are also present because HDV cannot replicate in the absence of HBV.

Hepatitis A Virus

GENERAL PRINCIPLES

- Transmitted via fecal–oral route and is the most common cause of acute viral hepatitis worldwide.
- Large-scale outbreaks can occur due to contamination of food and drinking water.
- A vaccine is available, with two doses given at least 6 months apart.
- The period of greatest infectivity is 2 weeks before the onset of clinical illness.
- Viral shedding in infected patients' feces continues for 2–3 weeks after the onset of symptoms.

DIAGNOSIS

- HAV can be silent (subclinical), especially in children and young adults. Symptoms vary from mild illness to ALF and commonly include malaise, fatigue, pruritus, headache, abdominal pain, myalgias, arthralgias, nausea, vomiting, anorexia, and fever.
- **Physical examination** may reveal jaundice, hepatomegaly, and, in rare cases, lymphadenopathy, splenomegaly, or a vascular rash.
- **Aminotransferase** elevations range from 10 to 100 times the upper limit of normal (ULN).
- The diagnosis of acute HAV is made by the detection of **IgM anti-HAV antibodies.**
- The recovery phase and immunity phase are characterized by the presence of IgG anti-HAV antibodies and the decline of IgM anti-HAV antibodies.
- Liver biopsy is rarely needed.
- **ALF** is rare. The risk increases with age: 0.1% in patients younger than 15 years to >1% in patients older than 40 years.

TREATMENT

- Supportive symptomatic treatment.
- Liver transplantation should be considered for ALF.

OUTCOME AND PROGNOSIS

- Symptoms of acute HAV hepatitis may last from weeks to months (median 8 weeks). HAV does not progress to chronic viral hepatitis.
- A prolonged cholestatic disease, characterized by persistent jaundice and waxing and waning of liver enzymes, is more frequently seen in adults.

Hepatitis B Virus

GENERAL PRINCIPLES

- The US is considered an area of low prevalence for the infection. Eight genotypes of HBV have been identified (A through H). The prevalence of HBV genotypes varies depending on the geographic location. Genotypes A, B, and C are the most prevalent in the US.
- Modes of transmission include vertical (mother to infant) and horizontal (person to person) via the following routes: parenteral or percutaneous (e.g., injection drug use, needlestick injuries), direct contact with the blood or open sores of an infected person, and sexual contact with an infected individual.
- The rate of progression from acute to chronic HBV is approximately 90% for a perinatal-acquired infection, 20%–50% for infections acquired between the age of 1 and 5 years, and <5% for an adult-acquired infection.

DIAGNOSIS

Clinical Presentation

- Four different **clinical phases** of chronic hepatitis B have been defined (Table 19-3). Most patients fit into one of the following phases:
  - Immune tolerant
  - Immune active (hepatitis B envelope antigen [HBeAg] positive)
  - Inactive phase
  - Immune reactivation phase (HBeAg negative)
- **Extrahepatic manifestations** include polyarteritis nodosa, glomerulonephritis, cryo-globulinemia, serum sickness–like illness, membranous nephropathy, membranopro-liferative glomerulonephritis, and papular acrodermatitis (predominantly in children).

Diagnostic Testing

- HBV antigens (hepatitis B surface antigen [HBsAg] and HBeAg) are identified in the serum.
- **HBV DNA** is the most accurate marker of viral replication. It is detected by poly-merase chain reaction (PCR).
- For use of HBV markers in clinical practice, see Table 19-3.
- **Liver biopsy** is useful to assess the degree of inflammation (grade) and fibrosis (stage) as well as other potential histologic abnormalities in patients with chronic hepatitis. Liver histology is an important adjuvant diagnostic test in guiding treat-ment decisions.

TABLE 19-3   Use of Hepatitis B Virus (HBV) Markers in Clinical Practice

Test	Acute HBV	Resolved Acute HBV	Immune-Tolerant Chronic HBV	Immune-Active Chronic HBV (Wild-Type)	Immune-Active Chronic HBV (Precore or Basal Core Promoter Mutant)	Low-Replication Chronic HBV	Vaccine Immunity
HBsAg	+	−	+	+	+	+	−
HBeAg	+	−	+	+	−	−	−
Anti-HBs	−	+	−	−	−	−	+
Anti-HBe	−	+	−	−	+	+	−
IgM anti-HBc	+	−	−	−	−	−	−
IgG anti-HBc	−	+	−	+	+	+	−
HBV DNA	>10^6 IU/mL	Neg	>10^{6-10} IU/mL	>10^6 IU/mL	>10^{3-4} IU/mL	<10^2 IU/mL	Neg
ALT/AST	++++	Normal	Normal	+++	++	Normal	Normal

ALT, alanine aminotransferase; AST, aspartate aminotransferase; HBc, hepatitis B core antigen; HBeAg, hepatitis B e antigen; HBsAg, hepatitis B surface antigen; Neg, negative.

CHAPTER 19

TREATMENT

The goal of treatment is viral eradication or suppression to prevent progression to ESLD and HCC. End points of treatment include the following (see Table 19-4):
• Normalization of serum ALT.
• Maintained suppression of serum HBV DNA levels to undetectable levels.
• HBeAg clearance and seroconversion to antibody anti-HBe.
• HBsAg clearance and seroconversion to antibody anti-HBs.
• Improvement in liver histology.

Medications

Medications for the treatment of hepatitis B are divided into three main groups: nucleoside analogs (entecavir, lamivudine [LAM], telbivudine), nucleotide analogs (tenofovir, adefovir), and the interferons (IFNs). Current practices recommend entecavir, tenofovir, and IFN.

• **Entecavir** is a potent anti-HBV oral nucleoside (guanosine) analog and is well tolerated. The dose is 0.5–1.0 mg daily in naïve and LAM-resistant patients. Entecavir has a high genetic barrier for resistance (1.2%) over several years. However, in patients resistant to LAM, the resistance to entecavir could be as high as 40%. In patients with renal impairment, dose adjustment is needed. Entecavir is pregnancy category C.
• **Tenofovir disoproxil fumarate (TDF)** is a potent anti-HBV oral nucleotide (acyclic) analog and is well tolerated. The dose is 300 mg daily. Tenofovir has a high genetic barrier for resistance; no clinical resistance has been identified thus far. It is rarely reported to induce renal failure and Fanconi syndrome and may also lead to decreased bone density. Tenofovir is pregnancy category B.
• **Tenofovir alafenamide (TAF)** is preferred over TDF for patients with renal or bone disease and appears to have comparable efficacy with TDF. Consider TAF for patients with GFR < 60, chronic steroid use, osteoporosis, or history of fragility fractures. For patients who cannot tolerate TDF and who have previously been exposed to LAM, switching to TAF is preferred over switching to entecavir.
• **Pegylated IFNs** (α2a and α2b, in their pegylated form) are antiviral, immunomodulatory, and antiproliferative glycoproteins that have been used in the treatment of chronic HBV for several years. IFNs are parenteral agents and associated with a poor tolerability profile, especially in patients with advanced liver disease. Long-term studies have shown a durable benefit in responders. Neither IFN nor pegylated IFN-α induces antiviral resistance. The IFNs are pregnancy category C.

PREVENTION

• **Preexposure prophylaxis**
  ○ **Consider HBV vaccination** in all patients, especially those from high-risk groups. HBV vaccines are made of inactivated viruses and are safe for immunocompromised patients.
  ○ The vaccination schedule is three IM injections at 0, 1, and 6 months in infants or healthy adults. Protective antibody response (anti-HBs positive) is achieved in >90% after the third dose.
• **Postexposure prophylaxis**
  ○ HBV positive mothers with viral load >200,000 should start antiviral therapy in the third trimester to decrease the risk of transmission.

TABLE 19-4	AASLD Treatment Guidelines for Chronic Hepatitis B			
	ALT	HBV DNA	Treatment?	Biopsy?[a]
HBeAg positive	<ULN	Any	No. If HBV DNA >20,000, monitor ALT and HBV DNA levels every 3–6 mo and HBeAg every 6–12 mo.	
	>ULN but <2× ULN	2000–20,000 IU/mL	Treat if lab abnormalities persist for >6 mo. Treat if ALT elevation persists and patient is older than 40 y or if there is at least F2 fibrosis or A3 inflammation.	Consider
		>20,000	Treat if ALT elevation persists and patient is older than 40 y or if there is at least F2 fibrosis or A3 inflammation.	Consider
	>2× ULN	2000–20,000 IU/mL	Treat if lab abnormalities persist for >6 mo. Treat if ALT elevation persists and patient is older than 40 y or if there is at least F2 fibrosis or A3 inflammation.	Consider
		>20,000	**Treat**	
HBeAg negative	<ULN	>2000 IU/mL	No. Monitor ALT and HBV DNA every 3 mo for 1 y and then every 6 mo.	
		<2000	No. Monitor ALT and HBV DNA levels every 3–6 mo and and HBsAg annually.	
	>ULN but <2× ULN	>2000 IU/mL	Treat if staging of liver disease is a least F2 fibrosis or A3 inflammation or age older than 40 y.	Consider
		<2000	Treat if staging of liver disease is a least F2 fibrosis or A3 inflammation or age older than 40 y.	Consider
	>2× ULN	>2000 IU/mL	**Treat**	
		<2000	Treat if staging of liver disease is a least F2 fibrosis or A3 inflammation or age older than 40 y.	Consider

AASLD, American Association for the Study of Liver Diseases; ALT, alanine aminotransferase; HBeAg, hepatitis B e antigen; HBV, hepatitis B virus; ULN, upper limit of normal (ULN for AASLD: 35 units/L for males, 25 units/L for females).
[a]Biopsy indicated for patients older than 40 years, ALT persistently 1–2× ULN, and family history of hepatocellular carcinoma. Alternative methods of noninvasive fibrosis testing may be used.

- Infants born to HBsAg-positive mothers should receive HBV vaccine and hepatitis B immunoglobulin (HBIg), 0.5 mL, within 12 hours of birth. Immunized infants should be tested at approximately 12 months of age for HBsAg, anti-HBs, and anti-HBc.
- Persons who are unvaccinated or do not demonstrate anti-HBs, and have had sexual contact or needlestick with an individual with HBV, should receive HBIg (0.04–0.07 mL/kg) and the first dose of HBV vaccine at different sites. This should be done as soon as possible, preferably within 48 hours, but no more than 7 days after exposure. A second dose of HBIg should be administered 30 days after exposure, and the vaccination series should be completed.
- Persons who have received all three doses of a hepatitis B vaccination series and have confirmed anti-HBs positivity require no further treatment.
- Postexposure prophylaxis with HBIg plus a nucleotide or nucleoside analog should be used initially after liver transplantation to prevent HBV recurrence in certain patients.

OUTCOME AND PROGNOSIS

Chronic hepatitis B
- Morbidity and mortality in chronic HBV are linked to the level and persistence of viral replication. Spontaneous clearance of HBsAg occurs in 0.5% of patients annually.
- For HCV/HBV-coinfected individuals, there is a risk of HBV reactivation during HCV treatment with direct-acting antivirals (DAAs).
- Once the diagnosis of chronic HBV is established, the 5-year cumulative incidence of developing cirrhosis ranges from 8% to 20%.
- About 5%–10% cases of chronic HBV progress to HCC regardless of preceding cirrhosis.

Hepatitis D (Delta) Virus

HDV is found throughout the world and is endemic to the Mediterranean basin, the Middle East, and the Amazon basin of South America. Outside of these areas, infections occur primarily in individuals who have received transfusions or inject drugs. HDV requires the presence of HBV for infection and replication. In countries such as the US where HDV infection is rare, testing for HDV coinfection is not necessary in all patients with HBV. In patients with coinfection (acute hepatitis B and D), the course is transient and self-limited. The rate of progression to chronicity is similar to that reported for acute HBV. IFN-α is the treatment of choice for chronic hepatitis D.

Hepatitis C Virus

GENERAL PRINCIPLES

- HCV is an RNA virus with six genotypes. Genotype 1 accounts for about 75% and genotypes 2 and 3 account for about 20% of HCV infections in the US.
- **HCV** is the most common chronic blood-borne infection and is a global health problem, with approximately **180 million carriers worldwide.**

- The most frequent mode of transmission is parenteral. Less common modes of transmission include high-risk sexual practices and perinatal transmission. Transmission by transfusion of blood products (and their derivatives) and organ transplantation has been reduced to near zero in developed countries due to screening.

DIAGNOSIS

Clinical Presentation

- The incubation period varies from 15 to 150 days.
- **Acute HCV hepatitis** is defined as presenting within 6 months of exposure to HCV. During this time, there is a 20%–50% chance of spontaneous resolution of infection.[4] Symptoms can be nonspecific and include malaise, fatigue, pruritus, headache, abdominal pain, myalgias, arthralgias, nausea, vomiting, anorexia, and fever.
- **Chronic HCV hepatitis** runs an indolent course, sometimes for decades, with fatigue often as the only symptom. It may only become clinically apparent late in the natural course, when symptoms associated with advanced liver disease develop.
- **Extrahepatic manifestations** include mixed cryoglobulinemia (10%–25% of patients with HCV), glomerular diseases (mixed cryoglobulinemia syndrome, membranous nephropathy, polyarteritis nodosa), porphyria cutanea tarda, cutaneous necrotizing vasculitis, lichen planus, lymphoma, diabetes mellitus, and other autoimmune disorders.

Diagnostic Testing

- **Antibodies against HCV (anti-HCV)** can be detectable within 2 weeks of infection with third-generation enzyme immunoassays, which have a sensitivity of 97% and specificity of 99%. Antibodies do not confer immunity. Anti-HCV testing is now available as point-of-care assay with equivalent performance as laboratory-based testing. A false-positive test (anti-HCV positive with HCV RNA negative) may be detected in the setting of autoimmune hepatitis (AIH) or hypergammaglobulinemia. A false-negative test (anti-HCV negative with HCV RNA positive) may be seen in HIV immunosuppressed individuals and in dialysis patients.
- **HCV RNA** detected by PCR is the gold standard for confirming the diagnosis of HCV infection and monitoring treatment response with detection limits of 12–43 IU/mL. HCV nucleic acid testing can detect infection in as early as 3–5 days and may be used as a confirmatory test.
  - **HCV genotypes and subtypes** can be detected by commercially available serologic and molecular assays. With the development of pangenotypic DAA regimens, pretreatment genotyping is only recommended for patients with previous HCV therapy failure.
- **Liver biopsy** is rarely used to guide HCV treatment because of the availability of highly effective DAAT.

TREATMENT

- Treatment should be considered for all patients with chronic HCV infection.
- Patients with limited life expectancy that cannot be remediated by HCV treatment, liver transplantation, or another directed therapy should not be treated.
- The goal of treatment is eradication of HCV, as determined by sustained virologic response (SVR). SVR is defined as the absence of detectable HCV RNA 12 weeks after completion of therapy. SVR reduces morbidity and end-stage complications of HCV infection including cirrhosis, HCC, and death.

CHAPTER 19

Medications

Current treatment regimens for chronic HCV are oral and IFN-free and may include the following:

- **Ribavirin** is a guanosine analog antiviral agent (nucleoside inhibitor). It is generally not effective when used alone but plays an important role in combination treatment.
- **DAAs** target specific nonstructural proteins of the virus, resulting in disruption of viral replication. Current treatment regimens for HCV include the combination of more than one DAA with or without ribavirin.
  - **Nonstructural protein 3/4A (NS3/4A) protease inhibitors (PIs)** include glecaprevir, asunaprevir, grazoprevir, voxilaprevir, and paritaprevir.
  - **NS5A inhibitors** include ledipasvir, daclatasvir, elbasvir, velpatasvir, pribrentasvir, and ombitasvir.
  - **NS5B polymerase inhibitors** include sofosbuvir and dasabuvir.
  - Pangenotypic regimens
    - Sofosbuvir (NS5B inhibitor) + velpatasvir (NS5A inhibitor) × 12 weeks. Ribavirin can be added for patients with decompensated cirrhosis or patients who have previously failed therapy.
    - Glecaprevir (NS3/4A PI) + pibrentasvir (NS5A inhibitor)—duration of therapy varies based on presence or absence of cirrhosis and history of therapy.
    - Sofosbuvir (NS5B inhibitor) + velpatasvir (NS5A inhibitor) + voxilaprevir (NS3/4A PI)—approved for patients who have previously received therapy with a standard DAA regimen.
- The selection of a particular treatment regimen is based on several factors, most notably:
  - Treatment-naïve (never-treated) or treatment-experienced (previously failed treatment)
  - HCV genotype and subtype
  - Cirrhosis
  - Decompensated cirrhosis
  - Potential drug interactions, especially the use of acid-blocking medications
  - Severe chronic renal disease or end-stage renal disease
  - Comorbid conditions (e.g., posttransplant state and HIV coinfection)
- For chronic infection, all treatment regimens have similar efficacy.

PREVENTION

No pre- or postexposure prophylaxis or vaccine exists. Prevention of high-risk behaviors and lifestyle modifications should be encouraged.

OUTCOME AND PROGNOSIS

HCC develops in approximately 2%–4% of patients with chronic hepatitis C–related cirrhosis per year.

Hepatitis E Virus

HEV is considered a zoonotic disease with reservoirs in pigs, wild boar, and deer. Transmission is fecal–oral, similar to HAV, and HEV can occur in outbreaks. Acute hepatitis E is clinically indistinguishable from other types of acute viral hepatitis and is usually self-limited, with the exception of cases during pregnancy (mortality can be as high as 10%–30% in the third trimester), preexisting chronic liver disease, and organ transplantation. Hepatitis E can rarely progress to chronic infection (HEV RNA for >6 months). Most chronic cases have occurred in solid organ transplant recipients or immunosuppressed individuals. In a retrospective multicenter study of 59 transplant recipients with chronic hepatitis E, ribavirin monotherapy for 3 months achieved an SVR of 78%.[5]

DRUG-INDUCED LIVER INJURY

GENERAL PRINCIPLES

- The National Institutes of Health maintains a searchable database of over 1000 drugs, herbal medications, and dietary supplements that have been associated with drug-induced liver injury (DILI) at http://livertox.nih.gov/.
- There are three major classifications of DILI that occur as a result of both intrinsic and idiosyncratic hepatotoxicity: hepatocellular, cholestatic, or mixed.
- DILI is responsible for approximately 50% of all cases of ALF in the US, with acetaminophen being the most common causative agent. Acute DILI (<3 months) progresses to chronic injury in 5%–10% of cases.[6]

DIAGNOSIS

Clinical Presentation

- The acute presentation can be clinically silent. Symptoms are nonspecific and include nausea/vomiting, malaise, fatigue, jaundice, pruritus, alcoholic stools, and abdominal pain. In the acute setting, the majority of patients will recover after cessation of the offending drug. Rare cases may progress to ALF.
- Fever and rash may also be seen in association with hypersensitivity reactions.

Diagnostic Criteria

- Clinical suspicion
- Temporal relation of liver injury to drug usage
- Resolution of liver injury after the suspected agent has been discontinued (except in cases of chronic DILI)

Diagnostic Testing

Biochemical Abnormalities

- **Hepatocellular injury:** AST and ALT elevation more than two times the ULN and disproportionately elevated when compared to ALP.
- **Cholestatic injury:** ALP and conjugated bilirubin elevation more than two times the ULN and disproportionately elevated when compared with AST and ALT.
- **Mixed injury:** Increases in all of the aforementioned biochemical abnormalities to more than two times the ULN.
- R ratio: ALT/ULN divided by ALP/ULN
  - R >5 suggests hepatocellular injury
  - R <2 suggests cholestatic injury
  - R >2 and <5 suggests mixed injury

Diagnostic Procedures

Liver biopsy may be indicated if the diagnosis is unclear.

TREATMENT

- Treatment includes cessation of offending drug and institution of supportive measures.
- An attempt to remove the agent from the GI tract should be made in most cases of acute toxic ingestion using lavage or cathartics (see Chapter 28, Toxicology).
  - Few specific therapies are beneficial. Two exceptions include N-acetylcysteine (NAC) for acetaminophen toxicity and L-carnitine for valproic acid overdose.
  - The effectiveness of NAC in nonacetaminophen DILI has not been well studied.
- Management of acetaminophen overdose is a medical emergency (see Chapter 28, Toxicology).

Surgical Management

Liver transplantation may be an option for patients with drug-induced ALF.

OUTCOME AND PROGNOSIS

Prognosis of DILI is often unique to the offending medication. Jaundice can take weeks to months to resolve.

ALCOHOLIC LIVER DISEASE

GENERAL PRINCIPLES

- Excessive alcohol intake can be defined as >30 g/d (one standard drink contains 14 g).
- The spectrum of alcoholic liver disease includes fatty liver, alcoholic steatohepatitis, severe alcoholic hepatitis, and cirrhosis. Fatty liver is the most common and occurs in up to 90% of alcoholics.
- Of all excessive alcohol users, between 10% and 20% will develop cirrhosis and 35% will develop alcoholic hepatitis. More than half of the latter will progress to cirrhosis.

DIAGNOSIS

Clinical Presentation

- **Hepatic steatosis**
  - Patients are usually asymptomatic.
  - Clinical findings may include hepatomegaly and liver enzyme abnormalities.
- **Alcoholic hepatitis**
  - Alcoholic hepatitis may be clinically silent or severe enough to lead to rapid development of hepatic failure and death.
  - Symptoms include fever, abdominal pain, anorexia, nausea, vomiting, weight loss, and jaundice.
  - In severe cases, patients may develop transient portal hypertension.
- **Alcoholic cirrhosis**
  - The presentation is variable, from clinically silent disease to stigmata of chronic liver disease to decompensated cirrhosis.

Diagnostic Testing

Laboratories
- In alcoholic hepatic steatosis, LFTs may be normal or demonstrate mild elevation in serum aminotransferases (AST >ALT) and ALP.
- In alcoholic hepatitis, LFTs typically demonstrate elevation in serum aminotransferases (AST >ALT with a 2:1 ratio) and ALP. Hyperbilirubinemia (conjugated) and elevated prothrombin time (PT)/international normalized ratio (INR) may also be observed.
- Laboratory abnormalities associated with a poor prognosis include renal failure, leukocytosis, a markedly elevated total bilirubin, and elevation of PT/INR that does not normalize with SC or IV vitamin K. Administration of oral vitamin K is not recommended because of poor gut absorption in patients with jaundice.
- A number of classification systems have been developed to risk-stratify patients with alcoholic hepatitis and assess response to treatment:
  - **Maddrey's discriminant function (DF)** = $4.6 \times (PT_{patient} - PT_{control}) +$ serum bilirubin. Scores <32 and >32 have 93% and 68% 1-month survival, respectively.
  - **The Glasgow Alcoholic Hepatitis Score (GAHS)** incorporates patient age, white blood cell count, blood urea, PT/INR, and serum bilirubin. A score <9 has no difference in survival between untreated and steroid-treated patients. A score >9 has a difference in short-term survival between untreated (52% 1-month survival) and steroid-treated (78% 1-month survival) patients.[7]
  - The **Lille model** incorporates age, renal insufficiency, albumin, PT, bilirubin, and the difference in bilirubin level (day 0 vs. day 7) to predict 6-month mortality in patients with severe alcoholic hepatitis who have received steroids. In a prospective study, a score of ≥0.45 was associated with a lower 6-month survival compared with a score <0.45 (25% vs. 85%). A score >0.45 suggests that a patient is not responding to steroid therapy.[8]

Diagnostic Procedures
- Liver biopsy may be indicated if the diagnosis of alcoholic hepatitis is unclear.
- Typical histopathologic findings in alcoholic liver disease include hepatocyte ballooning with or without Mallory–Denk bodies, lobular inflammation with neutrophilic infiltrates, hepatocyte necrosis, periportal fibrosis, perivenular and pericellular fibrosis, ductal proliferation, and fatty changes.

TREATMENT

- Encourage alcohol abstinence.
- Referral to programs or counselors for alcohol rehabilitation.
- Naltrexone is most strongly supported by placebo-controlled clinical trials for medication treatment in alcohol use disorder.
- Evaluate and correct nutrient deficiencies. Nutrition support can be given orally via a small-bore feeding tube or via peripheral parenteral nutrition or total parenteral nutrition. Good nutrition improves nitrogen balance, may improve LFTs, and may decrease hepatic fat accumulation, but it generally does not enhance survival.

CHAPTER 19

Medications

Treatment of acute alcoholic hepatitis with corticosteroids is controversial. However, there is evidence that patients with a DF >32 and GAHS >9 may have a short-term benefit from steroid therapy. An early decrease in bilirubin levels after 1 week of steroids portends a better prognosis (Lille score).

- **Oral prednisolone** (40 mg/d PO for 4 weeks, followed by a taper over 2–4 weeks) is a steroid treatment for patients with severe alcoholic hepatitis. Prednisolone is preferred over prednisone (but not proven to be better) as the latter requires conversion to its active form, prednisolone, within the liver. Prednisolone demonstrated a reduction in short-term mortality (28 days), though this did not reach significance. There was no benefit with regard to medium- or long-term mortality (90 days and 1 year, respectively).[9]
- **Pentoxifylline** (400 mg PO tid for 4 weeks) is a nonselective phosphodiesterase inhibitor that, in a previous randomized controlled trial, did not improve survival.

Surgical Management

Patients with cirrhosis and ESLD can be evaluated for liver transplantation but, historically, have been required to abstain from alcohol for 6 months prior to evaluation, maintain abstinence, and participate in a rehabilitation program. Recent data are emerging regarding the benefits and safety of early liver transplantation for highly selected patients with severe alcoholic hepatitis who have not attained 6 months of sobriety.

OUTCOME AND PROGNOSIS

- Hepatic steatosis (fatty liver) may be reversible with abstinence.
- In alcoholic hepatitis, prognosis depends on the severity of presentation and alcohol abstinence. The inhospital mortality for severe cases is high because of complications including sepsis and renal failure. Liver transplantation may be offered in highly selected patients with severe disease at initial presentation and excellent social support.[10]
- In alcoholic cirrhosis, prognosis is variable and depends on the degree of liver decompensation. Abstinence from alcohol may promote significant liver chemistry improvement.

IMMUNE-MEDIATED LIVER DISEASES

Autoimmune Hepatitis

GENERAL PRINCIPLES

Autoimmune hepatitis (AIH) is a chronic inflammation of the liver of unknown cause, associated with circulating autoantibodies and hyperglobulinemia.
- Women are affected more than men (gender ratio 4:1).
- Extrahepatic manifestations may be found in 30%–50% of patients and include synovitis, celiac disease, Coombs-positive hemolytic anemia, autoimmune thyroiditis, Graves disease, rheumatoid arthritis, ulcerative colitis (UC), and other immune-mediated processes.

Two types of AIH have been proposed based on differences in their immunologic markers. They have a good response to corticosteroid therapy.

- **Type I AIH** is the most common form of the disease and constitutes 80% of AIH cases. It is associated with antinuclear antibodies (ANA) and anti–smooth muscle antibodies.
- **Type 2 AIH** is characterized by antibodies to liver/kidney microsome type 1 and/or liver cytosol type 1. This type is predominately seen in children and young adults.

DIAGNOSIS

Clinical Presentation

- AST and ALT elevations are usually more marked than those of bilirubin and ALP, although a cholestatic pattern can occur.
- Elevated serum globulins, particularly γ-globulins (IgG), are characteristic of AIH. Hyperglobulinemia is generally associated with circulating autoantibodies, which are helpful in identifying AIH.
- In approximately 30%–40% of cases, the clinical presentation is similar to acute viral hepatitis. A smaller percentage of patients may present in ALF or with asymptomatic elevation of serum ALT. It presents with cirrhosis in at least 25% of patients.
- The most common symptoms at presentation include fatigue, jaundice, myalgias, anorexia, diarrhea, acne, abnormal menses, and right upper quadrant abdominal discomfort.
- Patients with AIH may overlap with clinical and histologic findings consistent with other liver diseases (e.g., PBC, PSC, Wilson disease [WD], and autoimmune cholangitis).
- The International Autoimmune Hepatitis Group developed a diagnostic scoring system. The scoring system accounts for sex, LFTs, elevated IgG, antibodies such as ANA/SMA, HLA genetic variants and history of other autoimmune disease, histologic features, treatment response, and likelihood of an etiology other than AIH.[11]

Diagnostic Testing

Liver biopsy is recommended for definitive diagnosis.

- **"Piecemeal necrosis" or interface hepatitis** with lobular or panacinar inflammation (lymphoplasmacytic infiltration) is the histologic hallmark of AIH.
- Histologic changes, such as ductopenia or destructive cholangitis, may indicate overlap syndromes with AIH and primary sclerosing cholangitis, PBC, or autoimmune cholangitis.

TREATMENT

Begin treatment in patients with serum AST and ALT levels > 10 times the ULN, IgG >2 times the ULN, and histologic features of interface hepatitis, bridging necrosis or multiacinar necrosis. Those with lower level transaminase elevations should be considered for treatment if the serum AST and ALT levels > two times the ULN along with symptoms, elevated IgG level, elevated conjugated bilirubin, and interface hepatitis on biopsy.

Medications

- Therapy consists of prednisone (50–60 mg/d PO) monotherapy or prednisone at a lower dose (30 mg/d PO) with azathioprine (AZA; 50 mg or up to 1–2 mg/kg).

CHAPTER 19

The dose of prednisone is tapered down over weeks to months. Tapering patients off corticosteroids within weeks to a few months is an option, especially if the liver tests normalize. The AZA dose can be increased if the liver tests fail to improve. AZA is usually continued long term. Some patients may achieve remission with cessation of AZA. However, stopping immunosuppressive therapy increases the risk of a disease flare, necessitating reinstitution of therapy.

- The combination of prednisone and AZA decreases corticosteroid-associated side effects; however, AZA should be used with caution in patients with pretreatment cytopenias or thiopurine methyltransferase (TPMT) deficiency.
- TPMT phenotyping should be obtained prior to initiating treatment.
- **Budesonide** (6–9 mg/d PO), in combination with AZA (1–2 mg/kg/d PO), may also result in normalization of AST and ALT, with fewer steroid-specific side effects, in **noncirrhotic** adults with AIH.[12]
- Second-line treatments for suboptimal response or treatment failures include mycophenolate mofetil, tacrolimus, cyclosporine, and budesonide.

Treatment Failure

- Consider liver transplantation in patients with ESLD and those with AIH-mediated fulminant hepatic failure (FHF).
- After transplantation, recurrent AIH is seen in approximately 15% of patients. De novo AIH or immunologically mediated hepatitis, defined as hepatitis with histologic features similar to AIH in patients transplanted for nonautoimmune diseases, has been described in about 5% of transplant recipients.[13]

MONITORING AND FOLLOW-UP

- About 90% of adults have improvements in the serum aminotransferase, bilirubin, and γ-globulin levels within the first 2 weeks of treatment.
- Histologic improvement lags behind clinical and laboratory improvement by 3–8 months.

OUTCOME AND PROGNOSIS

- The overall goal of treatment is normalization of aminotransferases, hyperglobulinemia (IgG), and liver histology.
- Remission is achieved in 65% and 80% of patients within 1.5–3 years of treatment, respectively.
- Relapses occur in at least 20%–50% of patients after cessation of therapy and require retreatment.

Primary Biliary Cholangitis

GENERAL PRINCIPLES

Primary biliary cholangitis (PBC) is a cholestatic hepatic disorder of unknown etiology with autoimmune features characterized by a T lymphocyte–mediated attack on small intralobular bile ducts.

- PBC most often affects middle-aged women (>90%) and is more commonly described in Caucasians. It is caused by granulomatous destruction of the interlobular bile ducts, which leads to progressive ductopenia and cholestasis.

- Cholestasis is generally slowly progressive but can lead to cirrhosis and liver failure.
- Extrahepatic manifestations include keratoconjunctivitis sicca (Sjögren), renal tubular acidosis, gallstones, thyroid disease, scleroderma, Raynaud phenomenon, CREST syndrome (calcinosis, Raynaud phenomenon, esophageal dysmotility, sclerodactyly, and telangiectasia), and celiac disease.

DIAGNOSIS

Clinical Presentation
- Fatigue, jaundice, and pruritus are often the most troublesome symptoms.
- Patients may present de novo with manifestations of ESLD.
- Although there are no examination findings that are specific for PBC, xanthomata and xanthelasma can be a clue to underlying cholestasis.

Diagnostic Testing
- Antimitochondrial (AMA) antibodies are present in >90% of patients.
- Typical features include elevated levels of ALP, total bilirubin, cholesterol, and IgM.
- To confirm the diagnosis, two out of three of the following are required: ALP at least >1.5 the ULN, positive AMA (1:40 or higher), and histologic evidence of PBC.

Diagnostic Procedures
Liver biopsy is helpful for both diagnosis and staging.

TREATMENT

Medications
- No curative therapy is available; treatment aims to slow down the progression of disease.
- **Ursodeoxycholic acid (UDCA)** (13–15 mg/kg/d PO) is a bile acid derivative with hepatocyte cytoprotective properties that stimulate hepatocellular and ductular secretions. Traditionally, UDCA has been suggested to reduce mortality when given over a long term.
- **Obeticholic acid** (OCA; 10–50 mg/d PO) is a derivative of the primary bile acid, chenodeoxycholic acid, and affects bile acid homeostasis. In a trial of patients with PBC with compensated liver disease who had an inadequate response to UDCA, 3-month treatment with OCA plus UDCA significantly reduced levels of ALP, GGT, and ALT when compared with UDCA plus placebo, but had a higher rate of pruritus.[14]

Surgical Management
- Liver transplantation is an option in advanced disease.
- Recurrent PBC after transplantation has been documented at a rate of 20% over 10 years.

PROGNOSIS AND OUTCOME

- PBC progresses along a path of increasingly severe histologic damage (florid bile duct lesions, ductular proliferation, fibrosis, and cirrhosis).
- Progression to cirrhosis and liver failure may occur years from diagnosis.

CHAPTER 19

Primary Sclerosing Cholangitis

GENERAL PRINCIPLES

Primary sclerosing cholangitis (PSC) is a cholestatic liver disorder characterized by inflammation, fibrosis, and obliteration of the extrahepatic and/or intrahepatic bile ducts.

- PSC can be subdivided into small duct and large duct disease. Small duct disease is defined as typical histologic features of PSC with a normal cholangiogram. In large duct disease or classic PSC, typical "beads on a string" strictures of the biliary tree can be detected by cholangiography. Small duct disease carries a more favorable prognosis.[15]
- The peak incidence is at about age 40 years. Most patients are middle-aged men, and the male-to-female ratio is 2:1.
- PSC is frequently associated with IBD (70% of patients have concomitant UC). The clinical course of these conditions is not correlated.
- PSC increases the risk of colon cancer, in addition to the risk conferred by IBD alone.

DIAGNOSIS

Clinical Presentation

- Clinical manifestations include intermittent episodes of jaundice, hepatomegaly, pruritus, weight loss, and fatigue. Patients may also present with acute cholangitis.
- Acute cholangitis is defined as an infection of the biliary ductal system usually caused by bacteria ascending from its junction with the duodenum and is a frequent complication in patients with strictures of the biliary ducts. Symptoms of acute cholangitis include fever, chills, rigors, jaundice, and right upper quadrant pain.
- Cholangiocarcinoma is the most frequent neoplasm associated with PSC. Patients with PSC have a 10%–15% lifetime risk of developing cholangiocarcinoma.
- Secondary causes of sclerosing cholangitis and IgG4 associated cholangitis/autoimmune pancreatitis must be ruled out.

Diagnostic Testing

- The diagnosis of PSC should be considered in individuals with IBD who have increased levels of ALP even in the absence of symptoms of hepatobiliary disease.
- ANA is positive in up to 50% of cases, and perinuclear antineutrophil cytoplasmic antibody is positive in 80% of cases.
- MRCP is the preferred diagnostic study of choice.

Diagnostic Procedures

- ERCP is a therapeutic procedure in patients with PSC when acute cholangitis is suspected. It is also performed when a dominant (severe) stricture is seen on MRCP to obtain duct brushings and biopsies to evaluate for cholangiocarcinoma. Sending brushings for fluorescence in situ hybridization may aid in the diagnosis of cholangiocarcinoma. Intraductal endoscopy, specifically cholangioscopy, can provide direct visualization of the biliary ducts with the advantage of direct tissue sampling.
- Liver biopsy is helpful in the diagnosis of small duct PSC, by excluding other diseases, and in staging. Characteristic histologic findings include concentric periductal fibrosis ("onion skinning"), degeneration of bile duct epithelium, ductular proliferation, ductopenia, and cholestasis.

TREATMENT

Medications

- At this time, there is no established medical treatment for PSC.
- Several randomized, placebo-controlled trials comparing the use of UDCA (13–23 mg/kg/d) to placebo showed improvement of LFTs in the UDCA group. However, there was no difference in long-term survival or time to liver transplantation. UDCA (>28 mg/kg/d) was associated with a higher risk of serious adverse events including death and transplantation and is not currently recommended for PSC.[16]
- Episodes of cholangitis should be managed with IV antibiotics and endoscopic therapy.

Nonpharmacologic Therapies

- ERCP can dilate and stent dominant strictures but does not mitigate disease progression.
- Surgical management
  - ○ Colectomy for UC does not affect the course of PSC.
  - ○ Patients with decompensated cirrhosis or recurrent cholangitis should be referred for liver transplantation. Recurrent PSC after liver transplantation has been documented.
  - ○ Selected hilar cholangiocarcinomas may be considered for liver transplantation.
  - ○ Gallbladder polyp follow-up should be comanaged with a liver or GI specialist.

COMPLICATIONS OF CHOLESTASIS

Nutritional Deficiencies

GENERAL PRINCIPLES

Any condition that blocks bile excretion (at the level of the liver cell or the biliary ducts) is defined as cholestasis. Laboratory evidence of cholestasis includes elevated ALP and bilirubin.

- Nutritional deficiencies result from fat malabsorption.
- Fat-soluble vitamin deficiency (vitamins A, D, E, and K) is often present in advanced cholestasis and is particularly common in patients with steatorrhea.

DIAGNOSIS

Clinical Presentation

- Characteristic manifestations of vitamin deficiencies are discussed in Chapter 2, Nutrition Support.
- Patients with steatorrhea may give a history of oily, foul-smelling diarrhea that sticks to the toilet bowl or is difficult to flush.

Diagnostic Testing

- 25-Hydroxyvitamin D serum concentrations reflect the total body stores of vitamin D. Vitamin D deficiency in the setting of malabsorption and steatorrhea is a good surrogate clinical marker for total body concentrations of other fat-soluble vitamins.
- Stool can be tested for fecal fat. Both spot tests and 24-hour collections can be done.

CHAPTER 19

TREATMENT

Medications
Vitamin supplements, given orally or parenterally, are given to correct deficiencies.

Osteoporosis

GENERAL PRINCIPLES

- **Osteoporosis** is defined as a decrease in the amount of bone (mainly trabecular bone), leading to a decrease in its structural integrity and increase in the risk of fractures.
- The relative risk of osteopenia in cholestasis is 4.4 times greater than the general population, matched for age and gender. It is particularly common in cholestasis caused by PBC.[17]

DIAGNOSIS

Bone mineral density should be measured by dual-energy x-ray absorptiometry in all patients at the time of diagnosis and during follow-up (every 1–2 years).

TREATMENT

Treatment of bone disease includes weight-bearing exercise, oral calcium supplementation (1.0–1.5 g/d), bisphosphonate therapy, and vitamin D supplementation.

Pruritus

GENERAL PRINCIPLES

The pathophysiology is debated and may be due to the accumulation of bile acid compounds or endogenous opioid agonists.

DIAGNOSIS

Patients with cholestasis can develop itching with either a normal or elevated bilirubin level. Serum bile acids level may aid the diagnosis when ALP or bilirubin is normal.

TREATMENT

Medications
First Line
Pruritus is best treated with cholestyramine, a basic anion exchange resin. It binds bile acids and other anionic compounds in the intestine and inhibits their absorption. The dose is 4 g mixed with water before and after the morning meal, with additional doses before lunch and dinner, up to a maximum of 16 g/d. Administer cholestyramine apart from other medicines or vitamins as cholestyramine will impair absorption. Colestipol, a similar resin, is also available.

Second Line
- Antihistamines (hydroxyzine, diphenhydramine, or doxepin, 25 mg PO at bedtime) and petrolatum may provide relief from pruritus.
- Rifampin (150–600 mg/d) and naltrexone (25–50 mg/d) are reserved for intractable pruritus. Long-term therapy with rifampin is associated with minor, transient elevations in serum aminotransferase levels in 10%–20% of patients—abnormalities that usually do not require dose adjustment or discontinuation. In rare instances, it can induce severe DILI.
- Ondansetron (Zofran) has demonstrated short-term efficacy in treating pruritus associated with cholestasis since it involves the serotonin system.
- Switching to sertraline (75–100 mg/d) or phenobarbital (90 mg QHS) can be tried if other measures fail.
- Some studies have demonstrated relief of pruritus with phototherapy or plasmapheresis, but clinical experience has been mixed.

METABOLIC LIVER DISEASES

Wilson Disease

GENERAL PRINCIPLES

Wilson disease (WD) is an autosomal recessive disorder (*ATP7B* gene on chromosome 13) that results in progressive copper overload.
- Female-to-male ratio is 2:1.
- Absent or reduced function of ATP7B protein leads to decreased hepatocellular excretion of copper into bile. This results in hepatic copper accumulation and injury. Eventually, copper is released into the bloodstream and deposited in other organs, notably the brain, kidneys, and cornea.
  - Extrahepatic manifestations include Kayser–Fleischer rings in the Descemet membrane in the periphery of the cornea due to copper deposition (diagnosed on slit-lamp examination), Coombs-negative hemolytic anemia, renal tubular acidosis, arthritis, osteopenia, and cardiomyopathy.

DIAGNOSIS

Clinical Presentation
- The average age at presentation of liver dysfunction is 6–20 years, but it can manifest later in life. Liver disease can be highly variable, ranging from asymptomatic with only mild biochemical abnormalities to ALF.
- Most patients who present with ALF resulting from WD have a characteristic pattern of clinical findings including Coombs-negative hemolytic anemia with features of acute intravascular hemolysis, rapid progression to renal failure, a rise in serum aminotransferases from the beginning of clinical illness (typically <2000 IU/L), and normal or markedly subnormal serum ALP (typically <40 IU/L).
- The diagnosis of WD should be considered in patients with unexplained liver disease with or without neuropsychiatric symptoms, first-degree relatives with WD, or individuals with ALF.
- Neuropsychiatric disorders usually occur later, most of the time in association with cirrhosis. The manifestations include asymmetric tremor, dysarthria, ataxia, and psychiatric features.

Diagnostic Testing

- Low serum ceruloplasmin level (<20 mg/dL), elevated serum free copper level (>25 μg/dL), and elevated 24-hour urinary copper level (>100 μg) are seen in patients with WD.
- Urinary copper excretion >1600 μg copper per 24 hours following the administration of 500 mg of D-penicillamine at the beginning and again 12 hours later during the 24-hour urine collection is seen in patients with WD.[18]
- Liver histology findings (massive necrosis, steatosis, glycogenated nuclei, chronic hepatitis, fibrosis, cirrhosis) are nonspecific and depend on the presentation and stage of the disease. Elevated hepatic copper levels of >250 μg/g dry weight (normal <40 μg/g) on biopsy are highly suggestive of WD.
- Mutation analysis by whole-gene sequencing is possible and should be performed on individuals in whom the diagnosis is not established by clinical and biochemical testing. Many patients are compound heterozygotes for mutations in the *ATP7B* gene, making identification of mutations difficult.

TREATMENT

Medications

Treatment is with copper-chelating agents penicillamine and trientine. Zinc salts that block intestinal absorption of copper are also used.

- **Penicillamine** 1–1.5 g/d (in divided doses bid or qid) and pyridoxine 25 mg/d (to avoid vitamin B_6 deficiency during treatment) are indicated in patients with hepatic failure. Use may be limited by side effects (e.g., hypersensitivity, bone marrow suppression, proteinuria, systemic lupus erythematosus, Goodpasture syndrome). Penicillamine should never be given as initial treatment to patients with neurologic symptoms, due to the risk of exacerbating neurologic manifestations.
- **Trientine** 1–1.5 g/d (in divided doses bid or qid) may also be used in hepatic failure. This has similar side effects as penicillamine but at a lower frequency. The risk of neurologic worsening with trientine is less than that with penicillamine.
- **Zinc salts** 50 mg tid are indicated in patients with chronic hepatitis and cirrhosis in the absence of hepatic failure. Other than gastric irritation, zinc has an excellent safety profile.

Surgical Management

Liver transplantation is the only therapeutic option in FHF or in patients with progressive dysfunction despite chelation therapy.

MONITORING AND FOLLOW-UP

- Serum copper and ceruloplasmin, liver biochemistries, INR, complete blood cell count, urinalysis (especially for those on chelation therapy), and physical examination should be performed regularly, at least twice annually.
- Annual measurement of 24-hour urinary excretion of copper may be needed if there is suspicion of noncompliance or if a dose adjustment is required. The estimated serum free copper may be elevated or low in situations of nonadherence and overtreatment, respectively.
- First-degree relatives of any newly diagnosed patient with WD should be screened for WD.
- After liver transplantation, in the absence of neurologic symptoms, patients require no further medical treatment.

Hereditary Hemochromatosis

GENERAL PRINCIPLES

Hereditary hemochromatosis (HH) is an autosomal recessive disorder of iron overload.
- This is the most common inherited form of iron overload affecting Caucasian populations. One in 200–400 Caucasian individuals is homozygous for hemochromatosis (*HFE*) gene mutations. It rarely manifests clinically before middle age (40–60 years).
- HH is most frequently caused by a missense mutation (C282Y) in the *HFE* gene located on chromosome 6. Approximately 90% of patients with HH are homozygote for the C282Y mutation. Less frequent mutations that lead to HH include H63D and S65C and the compound heterozygous C282Y/H63D and C282Y/S65C mutations.
- Secondary iron overload states include thalassemia major, sideroblastic anemia, chronic hemolytic anemias, iatrogenic parenteral iron overload, chronic hepatitis B and C, alcohol-induced liver disease, porphyria cutanea tarda, and aceruloplasminemia.

DIAGNOSIS

Clinical Presentation
- Presentation varies from asymptomatic disease to cirrhosis and HCC.
- Clinical findings include increased pigmentation, porphyria cutanea tarda, diabetes, cardiomyopathy, arthritis, hypogonadism, and hepatic dysfunction.

Diagnostic Testing
Diagnosis is based on laboratory testing, imaging, and liver biopsy.
- The diagnosis is suggested by high fasting transferrin saturation (>45%) (serum iron divided by the total iron-binding capacity). Other nonspecific laboratory tests include elevated serum iron and ferritin levels. Ferritin level >1000 ng/mL is an accurate predictor of the degree of fibrosis in patients with HH.
- If transferrin saturation is >45% and ferritin is elevated, check for HFE genotype homozygosity. If patient is a C282Y homozygote, then
  - If ferritin <1000 ng/mL and liver enzymes are normal, proceed to therapeutic phlebotomy.
  - If ferritin >1000 ng/mL or liver enzymes are elevated, proceed to liver biopsy for histology and hepatic iron concentration.
- In patients with elevated transferrin saturation and heterozygosity of the C282Y mutation, exclude other liver or hematologic diseases and consider liver biopsy.
- **MRI** is the modality of choice for noninvasive quantification of iron storage in the liver and for noninvasive surveillance of HCC. It allows for repeated measures and minimizes sampling error.

TREATMENT

- Therapy consists of **phlebotomy** every 7–14 days (500 mL blood) until iron depletion is confirmed by a ferritin level of 50–100 ng/mL and a transferrin saturation of <40%. Maintenance phlebotomy of one or two units of blood three to four times a year is continued for life, unless there are contraindications for rapid mobilization of iron stores (i.e., heart failure).
- Patients with HH should avoid excess alcohol consumption. Vitamin C and iron supplementation should be avoided.

CHAPTER 19

Medications

- Iron chelation with deferoxamine is an alternative to phlebotomy, but it is often more expensive and has side effects such as GI distress, visual and auditory impairments, and muscle cramps. Deferoxamine binds free iron, facilitates urinary excretion, and is recommended only when phlebotomy is contraindicated. Deferoxamine is only given IV, IM, or SC.
- Deferasirox is an oral iron chelator that selectively binds iron, forming a complex that is excreted through the feces.

Surgical Management

Liver transplantation may be considered in cases of HH with cirrhosis.

OUTCOME AND PROGNOSIS

- The survival rate in appropriately treated noncirrhotic patients is identical to that of the general population.
- The relative risk for HCC is approximately 20, with an annual incidence of 3%–4%. Patients with HH and advanced fibrosis or cirrhosis should be screened annually for HCC.[19]

α_1-Antitrypsin Deficiency

GENERAL PRINCIPLES

- α_1-Antitrypsin (α_1AT) deficiency is an autosomal recessive disease associated with accumulation of misfolded α_1AT in the endoplasmic reticulum of hepatocytes.
- The most common allele is protease inhibitor M (PiM—normal), followed by PiS and PiZ (deficient variants). African Americans have a lower frequency of these alleles.
- The most prevalent deficiency alleles Z and S are derived from European ancestry.[20]
- α_1AT deficiency can also be associated with emphysema in early adulthood, as well as other extrahepatic manifestations including panniculitis, pancreatic fibrosis, and membranoproliferative glomerulonephritis.

DIAGNOSIS

Clinical Presentation

- The disease may present as neonatal cholestasis or, later in life, as chronic hepatitis, cirrhosis, or HCC.
- The presence of significant pulmonary and hepatic disease in the same patient is rare (1%–2%).

Diagnostic Testing

- Low serum α_1AT level (10%–15% of normal) will flatten the α_1-globulin curve on serum electrophoresis.
- Deficient α_1AT phenotype (PiSS, PiSZ, and PiZZ).
- Elevated AST and ALT.

Diagnostic Procedures

Liver biopsy shows characteristic periodic acid–Schiff-positive diastase-resistant globules in the periportal hepatocytes.

TREATMENT

Currently, there is no specific medical treatment for liver disease associated with $\alpha_1 AT$ deficiency. Gene therapy for $\alpha_1 AT$ deficiency is a potential future alternative.

Surgical Management

Liver transplantation is an option for those with cirrhosis and is curative, with survival rates of 90% at 1 year and 80% at 5 years.

OUTCOME AND PROGNOSIS

- Chronic hepatitis, cirrhosis, or HCC may develop in 10%–15% of patients with the PiZZ phenotype during the first 20 years of life.
- Controversy exists as to whether liver disease develops in heterozygotes (PiMZ, PiSZ, PiFZ).

MISCELLANEOUS LIVER DISORDERS

Nonalcoholic Fatty Liver Disease

GENERAL PRINCIPLES

- Nonalcoholic fatty liver disease (NAFLD) is a clinicopathologic syndrome that encompasses several clinical entities that range from simple steatosis to steatohepatitis, fibrosis, ESLD, and HCC in the absence of significant alcohol consumption.
- NASH is part of the spectrum of NAFLD and is defined as the presence of hepatic steatosis and inflammation with hepatocyte injury (ballooning) with or without fibrosis.
- NAFLD is associated with an increasing prevalence of type 2 diabetes, obesity, and the metabolic syndrome in the US population.
- NAFLD has become one of the leading causes of liver transplantation in the US.

DIAGNOSIS

Clinical Presentation

The disease may vary from asymptomatic liver fatty infiltration to advanced fibrosis, cirrhosis, and HCC.

Diagnostic Testing

- When hepatic steatosis is detected on imaging and patients have symptoms or signs attributable to liver disease or have abnormal liver biochemistries, they should be evaluated for NAFLD and worked up accordingly.
- In patients with hepatic steatosis detected on imaging who lack any liver-related symptoms or signs and have normal liver biochemistries, it is reasonable to assess for metabolic risk factors (e.g., obesity, insulin resistance, dyslipidemia) and alternate causes for hepatic steatosis such as significant alcohol consumption or medications.
- Clinical diagnosis can be made based on adequate history, physical examination, laboratory tests, and typical imaging findings after excluding other causes of hepatic steatosis.

CHAPTER 19

- Noninvasive predictive models, serum biomarkers, and imaging studies are increasingly used as surrogate measures of liver fibrosis, inflammation, and steatosis, without replacing liver biopsy.
- VCTE or MRE are useful noninvasive tools to assess liver fibrosis in NAFLD patients. Liver biopsy should be considered in patients at high risk for steatohepatitis or advanced fibrosis or if the diagnosis remains unclear. It remains the gold standard test for the diagnosis of NASH, allowing assessment of the degree of inflammation and fibrosis.

TREATMENT

Nonpharmacologic Therapies

Therapies to correct or control associated conditions are warranted (weight loss through diet and exercise, tight control of diabetes and insulin resistance, appropriate treatment of hyperlipidemia, and discontinuation of possible offending agents).

All patients with NAFLD should be encouraged to lose at least 7%–10% of their body weight. Weight loss has been shown to improve liver enzymes and histology in clinical trials. Weight loss of 3% body weight can lead to improvement of steatosis. At least 7% weight loss can lead to resolution of NASH, while 10% or greater weight loss can lead to fibrosis regression. Weight loss is clearly effective; however, fewer than 20% of patients are able to maintain the lower body weight.

Medications

Medications with long-term efficacy and safety are lacking in NAFLD. Vitamin E and/or pioglitazone may be used but treatment should be given only in **biopsy-proven** NASH in patients without contraindications with ample discussions of risks and benefits.

Surgical Management

- Bariatric surgery should be considered for otherwise eligible obese patients with NASH. It is not yet considered a specific treatment for NASH, though prospective studies have shown significant improvement/resolution of NASH following bariatric surgery.
- Liver transplantation should be considered in patients with NASH-related ESLD.

OUTCOME AND PROGNOSIS

- Approximately 25% of patients with simple steatosis will progress to NASH.
- Progression to NASH cirrhosis has been reported at a rate of 11% over a 15-year period.
- Cardiovascular disease is the most common cause of death in NAFLD patients.[21]

Ischemic Hepatitis

GENERAL PRINCIPLES

Ischemic hepatitis results from acute liver hypoperfusion. Clinical circumstances associated with acute hypotension or hemodynamic instability include severe blood loss, substantial burns, cardiac failure, heat stroke, sepsis, sickle cell crisis, and others.

DIAGNOSIS

Clinical Presentation

Ischemic hepatitis presents with an acute, frequently transient, and severe rise of aminotransferases during or following an episode of liver hypoperfusion.

Diagnostic Testing

- Laboratory studies show a rapid rise in levels of serum AST, ALT (>1000 mg/dL), and lactate dehydrogenase (LDH) within 1–3 days of the insult.
- Total bilirubin, ALP, and INR may initially be normal but subsequently rise as a result of reperfusion injury.

Diagnostic Procedures

Liver biopsy is not routinely needed because the diagnosis can usually be made with clinical history. Classic histologic features include variable degrees of zone 3 (centrilobular) necrosis with collapse around the central vein. Coexistent features may include passive congestion, sinusoidal distortion, fatty change, and cholestasis. Inflammatory infiltrates are rare.

TREATMENT

Treatment consists of supportive care and correction of the underlying condition that caused the circulatory collapse.

OUTCOME AND PROGNOSIS

Prognosis is dependent on rapid and effective treatment of the underlying condition.

Hepatic Vein Thrombosis

GENERAL PRINCIPLES

Hepatic vein thrombosis (HVT), also known as Budd–Chiari syndrome, causes hepatic venous outflow obstruction. It has multiple etiologies and a variety of clinical consequences.
- Thrombosis is the main factor leading to obstruction of the hepatic venous system, frequently in association with myeloproliferative disorders (i.e., polycythemia vera), antiphospholipid antibody syndrome, paroxysmal nocturnal hemoglobinuria, factor V Leiden, protein C and S deficiency, Jak-2 mutation, and contraceptive use.
- Membranous obstruction of the inferior vena cava (IVC) and stenosis of the IVC anastomosis after liver transplantation are conditions that present clinically similar to HVT.
- Some cases are idiopathic.

DIAGNOSIS

Clinical Presentation

Patients may present with acute, subacute, or chronic illness characterized by ascites, hepatomegaly, and right upper quadrant abdominal pain. Other symptoms may include jaundice, encephalopathy, GI bleeding, and lower extremity edema.

Diagnostic Testing

- Serum-to-ascites albumin gradient (SAAG) is >1.1 g/dL. Serum albumin, bilirubin, AST, ALT, and PT/INR are usually abnormal.
- Laboratory evaluation to identify a hypercoagulable state should be performed (see Chapter 20, Disorders of Hemostasis and Thrombosis).
- The diagnosis can be established with Doppler ultrasound. Other diagnostic tools include magnetic resonance venography, hepatic venography, or cavography.
- Consider cross-sectional imaging to exclude space-occupying lesion leading to external compression and subsequently hepatic venous outflow obstruction.

TREATMENT

- Correct underlying cause when possible.
- To prevent propagation of the clot, initiate anticoagulation immediately, if there are no contraindications.
- Thrombolysis can be considered for well-defined clots and angioplasty if the venous obstruction is amenable to intervention for highly selected patients.
- Manage portal hypertension complications per guidelines.
- Consider transjugular intrahepatic portosystemic shunt (TIPS) if there is minimal improvement despite anticoagulation and maximal medical therapy.[22]

Surgical Management

Liver transplantation is an option in patients who develop cirrhosis or ALF.

Portal Vein Thrombosis

GENERAL PRINCIPLES

Portal vein thrombosis (PVT) is seen in a variety of clinical settings, including abdominal trauma, cirrhosis, malignancy, hypercoagulable states, intra-abdominal infections, pancreatitis, and after portocaval shunt surgery and splenectomy.

DIAGNOSIS

Clinical Presentation

- PVT can present as an acute or chronic condition.
- The acute phase may go unrecognized. Symptoms include abdominal pain/distension, nausea, anorexia, weight loss, diarrhea, or features of the underlying disorder. Bowel ischemia may result from extensive PVT with extension to the superior mesenteric vein.
- Chronic PVT may present with variceal hemorrhage or other manifestations of portal hypertension.

Diagnostic Testing

- In patients with no obvious etiology, a hypercoagulable workup should be performed.
- Doppler ultrasound examination is sensitive and specific for establishing the diagnosis. Portal venography, CT, or magnetic resonance venography can also be used.

TREATMENT

Medications

- In patients with acute PVT with or without cirrhosis, anticoagulation is recommended in the absence of any obvious contraindications. Treatment is aimed to prevent further thrombosis and recanalization, to treat complications and concurrent disease, and to mitigate underlying risk factors.
- In patients with chronic PVT, anticoagulation is recommended if they have hypercoagulable conditions without cirrhosis. Anticoagulation in cirrhotic patients with chronic PVT remains controversial, but should be considered in potential liver transplant candidates.[23,24]
- Optimal type of anticoagulant is not established, but recent meta-analysis suggests DOACs are most efficacious in recanalization compared to vitamin K antagonists and low-molecular-weight heparin with similar bleeding risk.[25]

Nonpharmacologic Therapies

In the setting of chronic PVT, treatment should focus on the complications of portal hypertension and include nonselective β-blockers, endoscopic band ligation, and diuretics for ascites.

Surgical Management

Portosystemic derivative surgery carries a high morbidity and mortality, especially in patients with cirrhosis. In some instances where surgery is precluded or the thrombus expands despite adequate anticoagulation, interventional radiology may be able to deploy TIPS. This may theoretically resolve symptomatic portal hypertension and prevent the thrombus recurrence or extension by the creation of a portosystemic shunt.[25]

ACUTE LIVER FAILURE

GENERAL PRINCIPLES

- ALF is a condition that includes evidence of a combination of coagulation abnormalities and any degree of mental alteration (encephalopathy) in a patient without preexisting liver disease and with an illness of <26 weeks in duration.
- In 20% of cases, no clear cause is identified. Acetaminophen hepatotoxicity and viral hepatitis are the most common causes of ALF. Other causes include AIH, drug and toxin exposure, ischemia, acute fatty liver of pregnancy, WD, and Budd–Chiari syndrome.
- Acute inflammation with varying degrees of necrosis and collapse of the liver's architectural framework are the typical histologic changes seen in ALF.

DIAGNOSIS

Clinical Presentation

- Patients often present with mild to severe mental status changes in the setting of moderate to severe acute hepatitis and coagulopathy.
- Patients may develop cardiovascular collapse, acute renal failure, cerebral edema, and sepsis.

CHAPTER 19

Diagnostic Testing

- Aminotransferases are typically elevated and, in many cases, are >1000 IU/L.
- INR >1.5 that does not correct with the administration of vitamin K is characteristic.
- Workup to determine the etiology of ALF should include acute viral hepatitis panel, serum drug screen (including acetaminophen level), ceruloplasmin, AIH serologies, and pregnancy test.
- Right upper quadrant ultrasound with Doppler should be obtained to evaluate obstruction of hepatic venous inflow or outflow.
- CT of the head may be obtained to evaluate and track progression of cerebral edema; however, the radiologic findings may lag behind its development and do not substitute for serial bedside assessments of neurologic status.
- Liver biopsy is seldom used to establish etiology or prognosis. Given the presence of coagulopathy, a transjugular approach to liver biopsy should be attempted if necessary.

TREATMENT

- Supportive therapy (quiet dark room, avoid patient stimulation, maintain head of bed elevation to 30 degrees) in the intensive care unit setting with liver transplant capabilities is essential.
- Precipitating factors, such as infection, should be identified and treated. Blood glucose, electrolytes, acid–base balance, coagulation parameters, and fluid status should be serially monitored.
- Sedatives should be avoided to appropriately gauge the patient's mental status.
- NAC may be used in cases of ALF in which acetaminophen ingestion is suspected or when circumstances surrounding admission is inadequate. NAC also appears to improve spontaneous survival when given during early hepatic encephalopathy stages (grades I and II), even in the setting of nonacetaminophen ALF.[27]
- Fresh frozen plasma and the use of recombinant activated factor VIIa should only be considered in the setting of active bleeding or when invasive procedures are required.
- Cerebral edema and intracranial hypertension are related to the severity of encephalopathy. In patients with grade III or IV encephalopathy, intracranial pressure monitoring may be considered if local expertise is available (intracranial pressure should be maintained below 20–25 mm Hg and cerebral perfusion pressure should be maintained above 50–60 mm Hg). Management of cerebral edema, when identified by CT imaging, includes intubation with sedation to avoid overstimulation, elevation of the head of the bed, use of mannitol (0.5–1 g/kg), and/or use of hypertonic saline (30% hypertonic saline at a rate of 5–20 mL/h to maintain a serum sodium of 145–155 mmol/L). Lactulose is not indicated for encephalopathy in this setting. Its use may result in increased bowel gas that can interfere with the surgical approach for liver transplantation.[28]
- Liver transplantation should be urgently considered in cases of severe ALF. Poor prognostic indicators in acetaminophen-induced ALF include arterial pH < 7.3, INR >6.5, creatinine >3.4 mg/dL, and encephalopathy grades III through IV (King's College Criteria).

OUTCOME AND PROGNOSIS

- In the US, 45% of adults with ALF have a spontaneous recovery, 25% undergo liver transplantation, and 30% die without liver transplantation.[29]
- Death often results from progressive liver failure, GI bleeding, cerebral edema, sepsis, or arrhythmia.
- A rapid decline in aminotransferases correlates poorly with prognosis and does not always indicate an improved response to therapy.

CIRRHOSIS

- **Cirrhosis** is a chronic condition characterized by diffuse replacement of liver cells by fibrotic tissue, which creates a nodular-appearing distortion of the normal liver architecture. Advanced fibrosis represents the end result of many etiologies of liver injury.
- Cirrhosis affects nearly 5.5 million Americans. In 2009, it was the 12th leading cause of death in the US.[30]
- The most common etiologies are alcohol-related liver disease, chronic viral infection, and NAFLD (diagnosis and treatment discussed earlier in respective sections).
- Main complications of cirrhosis include portal hypertension with various clinical manifestations (ascites, esophageal and gastric varices, portal hypertensive gastropathy (PHG) and colopathy, hypersplenism, gastric antral vascular ectasia, spontaneous bacterial peritonitis [SBP], hepatorenal syndrome [HRS], hepatic encephalopathy, and HCC). Frequent laboratory abnormalities encountered in a patient with cirrhosis include anemia, leukopenia, thrombocytopenia, hypoalbuminemia, coagulopathy, and hyperbilirubinemia.

Portal Hypertension

GENERAL PRINCIPLES

- Portal hypertension is the main complication of cirrhosis and is characterized by increased resistance to portal flow and increased portal venous inflow. Portal hypertension is established by measuring the pressure gradient between the hepatic vein and the portal vein (normal portosystemic pressure gradient is approximately <5 mm Hg).
- Direct and indirect clinical consequences of portal hypertension appear when the portosystemic pressure gradient exceeds 10 mm Hg.
- Causes of portal hypertension in patients without cirrhosis include idiopathic portal hypertension, schistosomiasis, congenital hepatic fibrosis, sarcoidosis, cystic fibrosis, arteriovenous fistulas, splenic and PVT, HVT (Budd–Chiari syndrome), myeloproliferative diseases, nodular regenerative hyperplasia, and focal nodular hyperplasia.

DIAGNOSIS

Portal hypertension frequently complicates cirrhosis and presents with ascites, splenomegaly, and GI bleeding from varices (esophageal or gastric), PHG, gastric antrum vascular ectasia (GAVE), or portal hypertensive colopathy.
- Ultrasonography, CT, and MRI showing cirrhosis, splenomegaly, collateral venous circulation, and ascites are suggestive of portal hypertension.
- Upper endoscopy may show varices (esophageal or gastric), PHG, or GAVE.
- Transjugular portal pressure measurements are uncommonly needed except when clinical diagnosis cannot be made.

TREATMENT

Treatment of GI bleeding because of portal hypertension is covered in Chapter 18, Gastrointestinal Diseases.

Ascites

GENERAL PRINCIPLES

Ascites is the abnormal (>25 mL) accumulation of fluid within the peritoneal cavity. Other causes of ascites, unrelated to portal hypertension, include cancer (peritoneal carcinomatosis), heart failure, TB, myxedema, pancreatic disease, nephrotic syndrome, surgery or trauma to the lymphatic system or ureters, and serositis.

DIAGNOSIS

- Presentation ranges from ascites detected only by imaging methods to a distended, bulging, and sometimes tender abdomen. Percussion of the abdomen may reveal shifting dullness.
- **SAAG** is calculated as serum albumin minus the ascites albumin; a gradient ≥1.1 indicates portal hypertension–related ascites (97% specificity).[31] A SAAG of <1.1 is found in nephrotic syndrome, peritoneal carcinomatosis, serositis, TB, and biliary or pancreatic ascites.
- Ultrasonography, CT, and MRI are sensitive methods to detect ascites.
- **Diagnostic paracentesis** (60 mL) should be performed in the setting of new-onset ascites, suspicion of malignant ascites, or to rule out SBP. **Therapeutic paracentesis** (large volume) should be performed when tense ascites causes significant discomfort or respiratory compromise or when suspecting abdominal compartment syndrome.
- Routine diagnostic testing should include SAAG calculation, red and white blood cell counts and differential, total protein, and culture. Amylase and triglyceride measurement, cytology, and mycobacterial smear/culture can be performed to confirm specific diagnoses.
- Bleeding, infection, persistent ascites leak, and intestinal perforation are possible complications.
- Large-volume paracentesis (>5 L) may lead to circulatory collapse, encephalopathy, and renal failure. Concomitant administration of IV albumin (6–8 g/L ascites removed) can be used to mitigate the risks of paracentesis-induced circulatory dysfunction and HRS.

TREATMENT

Medications

- **Diuretic therapy** is initiated along with **salt restriction** (<2 g sodium or 88 mmol Na⁺/d). Diuretics should be used with caution.
- **Spironolactone** 100 mg PO daily is a reasonable starting dose. The daily dose can be increased by 50–100 mg every 7–10 days to a maximum dose of 400 mg until satisfactory weight loss or side effects occur. Hyperkalemia and gynecomastia are common side effects. Other potassium-sparing diuretics such as amiloride, triamterene, or eplerenone are substitutes that can be used in patients in whom painful gynecomastia develops.

- **Loop diuretics**, such as furosemide (20–40 mg, increasing to a maximum dose of 160 mg PO daily), can be added to spironolactone. Torsemide or bumetanide may be considered in patients with unresponsiveness to furosemide.
- Patients should be observed closely for signs of dehydration, electrolyte disturbances, encephalopathy, muscle cramps, and renal insufficiency. NSAIDs may blunt the effect of diuretics and increase the risk of renal dysfunction.

Other Nonpharmacologic Therapies

- TIPS is effective in the management of recurrent or refractory ascites.
- Complications of TIPS include shunt occlusion, bleeding, infection, cardiopulmonary compromise, hepatic encephalopathy, hepatic failure, and death.

Spontaneous Bacterial Peritonitis

GENERAL PRINCIPLES

- Spontaneous bacterial peritonitis (SBP) is an infectious complication of portal hypertension–related ascites defined as >250 neutrophils/µL in the ascites fluid.
- Bacterascites is defined as culture-positive ascites in the presence of normal neutrophil counts (<250 neutrophils/µL) in the ascites fluid. This condition may be spontaneously reversible or the first step in the development of SBP. In the presence of signs or symptoms of infection, bacterascites should be treated like SBP.
- Risk factors for SBP include ascites fluid protein concentration <1 mg/dL, acute GI bleeding, and a prior episode of SBP.

DIAGNOSIS

Clinical Presentation

SBP may be asymptomatic. Clinical manifestations include abdominal pain and distention, fever, decreased bowel sounds, and worsening hepatic encephalopathy. Cirrhotic patients with ascites and evidence of any clinical deterioration should undergo diagnostic paracentesis to exclude SBP.

Diagnostic Testing

The diagnosis is confirmed when >250 neutrophils/µL are found in the ascites fluid. Gram stain reveals the organism in only 10%–20% of samples.
- Ascites cultures are more likely to be positive when 10 mL of the fluid is inoculated into two blood culture bottles at the bedside.
- The most common organisms are *Escherichia coli*, *Klebsiella*, and *Streptococcus pneumoniae*. Polymicrobial infection is uncommon and should lead to the suspicion of secondary bacterial peritonitis. Checking total protein, LDH, and glucose on ascites fluid is helpful in distinguishing secondary bacterial peritonitis from SBP.

TREATMENT

Medications

- Patients with SBP should receive empiric antibiotic therapy with IV third-generation cephalosporins (ceftriaxone, 2 g IV daily, or cefotaxime, 2 g IV q6–8h, depending on renal function). Therapy should be tailored based on culture results and antibiotic susceptibility. Paracentesis should be repeated if no clinical improvement occurs in 48–72 hours, especially if the initial fluid culture was negative.[32]

CHAPTER 19

- Oral quinolones can be considered a substitute for IV third-generation cephalosporins in the absence of vomiting, shock, grade II (or higher) hepatic encephalopathy, or serum creatinine >3 mg/dL.
- Patients with <250 neutrophils/μL in the ascites fluid and signs or symptoms of infection (fever or abdominal pain or tenderness) should also receive empiric antibiotic therapy.
- Concomitant use of albumin 1.5 g/kg body weight at the time of diagnosis and 1.0 g/kg body weight on day 3 improves survival and prevents renal failure in SBP.[32]

Primary Prophylaxis (No Prior History of SBP)
Patients with severe liver disease with ascitic fluid protein <1.5 mg/dL along with impaired renal function (creatinine ≥1.2, blood urea nitrogen ≥25, or serum Na ≤130) or liver failure (Child score ≥9 and bilirubin ≥3) should be treated with long-term norfloxacin 400 mg PO daily.

Secondary Prophylaxis (After the First Episode of SBP)
Ciprofloxacin 500 mg PO daily or trimethoprim–sulfamethoxazole single strength one tab PO daily is the treatment of choice for prevention of recurrent SBP.[33]

Acute Kidney Injury in Patients With Cirrhosis and HRS

GENERAL PRINCIPLES

Acute kidney injury (AKI) in decompensated cirrhosis is a common complication. Revised consensus recommendations define AKI as an increase in serum creatinine ≥0.3 mg/dL within 48 hours or a percentage increase of serum creatinine ≥50% from a known or presumed baseline within the prior 7 days. HRS results from severe peripheral vasodilatation, which leads to renal vasoconstriction. The definition of HRS–AKI (type I HRS) is provided in Table 19-5. Common precipitating factors include systemic bacterial infections, SBP, GI hemorrhage, and large-volume paracentesis without volume expansion. HRS is a diagnosis of exclusion.[34]

DIAGNOSIS

HRS is observed in cirrhotic patients with ascites, with and without hyponatremia. HRS has been divided into two types.
- **Type I** HRS is characterized by the acute onset of rapidly progressive renal failure (<2 weeks) unresponsive to volume expansion.
- **Type II** HRS progresses more slowly but relentlessly and often clinically manifests as diuretic-resistant ascites.

TREATMENT

Medications
Specific medical therapy is only recommended for type I HRS.
- 25% IV albumin at 1 g/kg body weight (max 100 g) for two consecutive days should be given if the cause of AKI is unidentifiable.
- Terlipressin (vasopressin analog) is not FDA approved for use in the US. In a placebo-controlled trial, 34% of patients who received terlipressin had a reversal of their HRS in comparison with 13% who received placebo.[35]

TABLE 19-5	Diagnostic Criteria of HRS–AKI

- Diagnosis of cirrhosis and ascites
- Diagnosis of AKI (an increase in serum creatinine ≥ 0.3 mg/dL within 48 h or a percentage increase of serum creatinine ≥ 50% from a known or presumed baseline within the prior 7 d)
  - Stage 1: Increase in serum creatinine ≥ 0.3 mg/dL or an increase ≥1.5- to 2-fold from baseline
  - Stage 2: Increase in serum creatinine >two- to threefold from baseline
  - Stage 3: increase in serum creatinine >threefold from baseline, >4 mg/dL with an acute increase ≥0.3 mg/dL, or initiation of renal replacement therapy
- No response after 2 consecutive days of diuretic withdrawal and plasma volume expansion with albumin 1 g/kg
- Absence of shock
- No current or recent use of nephrotoxic drugs (NSAIDs, aminoglycosides, iodinated contrast media, etc.)
- No macroscopic signs of structural kidney injury, defined as
  - Absence of proteinuria (>500 mg/d)
  - Absence of microhematuria (>50 RBCs per high-power field)
  - Normal findings on renal ultrasonography

AKI, acute kidney injury; HRS, hepatorenal syndrome; RBC, red blood cell.
Adapted from Angeli P, Gines P, Wong F, et al. Diagnosis and management of acute kidney injury in patients with cirrhosis: revised consensus recommendations of the International Club of Ascites. *J Hepatol.* 2015;62:968-974.

- SC somatostatin analogs (octreotide) and oral α-adrenergic agonist (midodrine) with IV albumin are commonly used regimens for the management of HRS in the US.
- Norepinephrine can be an alternative to terlipressin.
- Renal replacement therapy may be used when liver transplantation is an option.

Nonpharmacologic Therapies

Hemodialysis may be indicated in patients listed for liver transplantation.

Surgical Management

Liver transplantation may be curative. Patients receiving hemodialysis for more than 6 weeks should be considered for liver and kidney transplantation.

OUTCOME AND PROGNOSIS

Without treatment, patients with type I HRS have a poor prognosis, with death occurring within 1–3 months of onset. Patients with type II HRS have a longer median survival.

Hepatic Encephalopathy

GENERAL PRINCIPLES

- Hepatic encephalopathy is the syndrome of disordered consciousness and altered neuromuscular activity that is seen in patients with acute or chronic hepatocellular failure or portosystemic shunting.

CHAPTER 19

- Hepatic encephalopathy is classified according to the underlying disease into the following:
  - Type A: Resulting from ALF
  - Type B: Resulting from portosystemic bypass or shunting
  - Type C: Resulting from cirrhosis[36]
- The grades of hepatic encephalopathy are dynamic and can rapidly change.
  - Grade I: Sleep reversal pattern, mild confusion, irritability, tremor, asterixis
  - Grade II: Lethargy, disorientation, inappropriate behavior, asterixis
  - Grade III: Somnolence, severe confusion, aggressive behavior, asterixis
  - Grade IV: Coma
- **Precipitating factors** include medication noncompliance to lactulose, azotemia, FHF, opioids or sedative–hypnotic medications, acute GI bleeding, hypokalemia and alkalosis (diuretics and diarrhea), constipation, infection, high-protein diet, progressive hepatocellular dysfunction, and portosystemic shunts (surgical or TIPS).

DIAGNOSIS

- Asterixis (flapping tremor) is present in stage I through III encephalopathy. This motor disturbance is not specific to hepatic encephalopathy.
- The electroencephalogram shows slow, high-amplitude, and triphasic waves.
- Determination of blood ammonia level is not a sensitive or specific test for hepatic encephalopathy.

TREATMENT

Medications include nonabsorbable disaccharides (lactulose, lactitol, and lactose in lactase-deficient patients) and antibiotics (neomycin, metronidazole, and rifaximin).

- **Lactulose**, 15–45 mL PO (or via nasogastric tube) bid–qid, is the first choice for treatment of hepatic encephalopathy. Lactulose dosing should be adjusted to produce three to five soft stools per day. Oral lactulose should not be given to patients with ileus or possible bowel obstruction. In the acute phase, a starting dose of 30 mL every 1–2 hours is recommended. This can then be transitioned to every 4 hours, 6 hours, and then 8 hours once the patient starts having bowel movements.
- **Lactulose enemas** (prepared by the addition of 300 mL lactulose to 700 mL distilled water) may also be administered in patients who cannot tolerate oral intake.
- **Rifaximin** is an oral nonsystemic broad-spectrum antibiotic that is used at a dose of 550 mg PO bid with no serious adverse events. In a placebo-controlled trial, rifaximin reduced the risk of hepatic encephalopathy and the time to first hospitalization over a 6-month period.

Hepatocellular Carcinoma

GENERAL PRINCIPLES

HCC frequently occurs in patients with cirrhosis, especially when associated with viral hepatitis (HBV or HCV), alcoholic cirrhosis, α_1AT deficiency, and hemochromatosis.

DIAGNOSIS

Clinical Presentation
- Clinical presentation is directly proportional to the stage of disease. HCC may present with right upper quadrant abdominal pain, weight loss, and hepatomegaly.
- Suspect HCC in a cirrhotic patient who develops manifestations of liver decompensation.
- Surveillance for HCC should be performed every 6 months with a sensitive imaging study. The combination of imaging with AFP is not recommended because it is unlikely to provide a gain in the detection rate. In patients with hepatitis B, surveillance should begin after age 40 years even in the absence of cirrhosis.

Diagnostic Testing
- AFP (see section "Evaluation of Liver Disease").
- Liver ultrasound, triple-phase CT, and MRI with contrast are sensitive and often used for detection of HCC. Liver biopsy should be considered for patients at risk for HCC with suspicious liver lesions >1 cm with uncharacteristic imaging features (absence of arterial hypervascularity and venous or delayed phase washout).

TREATMENT

Surgical Management
- Hepatic resection is the treatment of choice in noncirrhotic patients.
- Liver transplantation is the treatment of choice for select cirrhotic patients who fall within Milan criteria (single HCC <5 cm or up to three nodules <3 cm).
- Milan criteria are used by the United Network for Organ Sharing for priority status (exception points) for liver transplantation candidacy in patients with HCC.

Locoregional Therapy
- Radiofrequency ablation (RFA) is a percutaneous ablation treatment using radiofrequency energy to produce a 3-cm area of necrosis. Sustained complete response and low complication rates were shown in very early HCC in patients with cirrhosis.
- Comparative effectiveness of other ablative techniques such as stereotactic body radiation and microwave ablation remains unclear.
- There are two transarterial embolization approaches available.
  - Transarterial chemoembolization with conventional approach or doxorubicin-eluting beads improves survival in selected nonsurgical patients with large or multifocal HCC who do not have vascular invasion or metastatic disease.
  - Transarterial radioembolization (TARE) with yttrium-90 may be considered in patients with HCC who are not candidates for resection or transplantation but data are still emerging.
- Selected patients with tumors beyond Milan criteria HCC can be bridged or downstaged to meet Milan criteria with TACE, RFA, and TARE prior to liver transplantation.
- The risk of hepatic decompensation because of locoregional therapy must be considered when selecting patients for bridging or downstaging.[37]

Medications
- **Sorafenib** is a small molecule that inhibits tumor cell proliferation and angiogenesis. In patients with advanced HCC and Child A cirrhosis, median survival and

radiologic progression were 3 months longer for patients treated with sorafenib compared with placebo. The benefits of sorafenib in Child B cirrhosis with advanced HCC have not been established.[38]

- Phase III trials comparing lenvatinib (multikinase inhibitor against VEGFR1, VEGFR2, and VEGFR3) or nivolumab (human IgG4 anti-PD-1 monoclonal Ab) with sorafenib in advanced HCC with metastatic disease are ongoing.

OUTCOME AND PROGNOSIS

Early diagnosis is essential because surgical resection and liver transplantation can improve long-term survival. Liver transplantation has demonstrated, in patients meeting Milan criteria, a recurrence-free survival of 80%–90% at 3–4 years. Advanced HCC that is beyond Milan criteria has a dismal prognosis, with a 5-year survival of approximately 10%.[37]

LIVER TRANSPLANTATION

GENERAL PRINCIPLES

- Liver transplantation is an effective therapeutic option for irreversible acute liver disease and ESLD for which available therapies have failed. Whole cadaveric livers and partial livers (split-liver, reduced-size, and living-related) are used in the US as sources for liver transplantation. There continues to be a disparity between supply and demand of suitable livers for transplantation.
- The Model for End-Stage Liver Disease (MELD) score allows for prioritization for liver transplantation. It is calculated by a formula that takes into account serum bilirubin, serum creatinine, and INR. Patients are regularly evaluated for a liver transplantation when they achieve a MELD of 15. Patients are considered for "exception MELD points" for conditions such as HCC within Milan criteria, hepatopulmonary syndrome, portopulmonary hypertension, polycystic liver disease, familial amyloidosis, small unresectable hilar cholangiocarcinoma, and unusual tumors.
- Sodium has been incorporated to MELD to increase priority for organ allocation.
- Patients with cirrhosis should be considered for transplant evaluation when they have a decline in hepatic synthetic or excretory functions, ascites, hepatic encephalopathy, or complications such as HRS, HCC, recurrent SBP, or variceal bleeding.
- Candidates for liver transplantation are evaluated by a multidisciplinary team that includes hepatologists, transplant surgeons, transplant nurse coordinators, social workers, psychologists, and financial coordinators.
- General **contraindications** to liver transplant include severe and uncontrolled extrahepatic infection, advanced cardiac or pulmonary disease, extrahepatic malignancy, multiorgan failure, unresolved psychosocial issues, medical noncompliance issues, and ongoing substance abuse (e.g., alcohol and illegal drugs).

TREATMENT

Immunosuppressive, infectious, and long-term complications are discussed in Chapter 17, Solid Organ Transplant Medicine.

REFERENCES

1. Lok AS, Sterling RK, Everhart JE, et al. Des-gamma-carboxy prothrombin and alpha-fetoprotein as biomarkers for the early detection of hepatocellular carcinoma. *Gastroenterology.* 2010;138:493-502.
2. Berzigotti A, Seijo S, Reverter E, Bosch J. Assessing portal hypertension in liver diseases. *Expert Rev Gastroenterol Hepatol.* 2013;7:141-155.
3. Fix OK, Hameed B, Fontana RJ, et al. Clinical best practice advice for hepatology and liver transplant providers during the COVID-19 pandemic: AASLD expert panel consensus statement. *Hepatology.* 2020;72:287-304.
4. Kamal SM. Acute hepatitis C: a systematic review. *Am J Gastroenterol.* 2008;103:1283-1297.
5. Kamar N, Izopet J, Tripon S, et al. Ribavirin for chronic hepatitis E virus infection in transplant recipients. *N Engl J Med.* 2014;370:1111-1120.
6. Andrade RJ, Lucena MI, Kaplowitz N, et al. Outcome of acute idiosyncratic drug-induced liver injury: long-term follow-up in a hepatotoxicity registry. *Hepatology.* 2006;44:1581-1588.
7. Forrest EH, Morris AJ, Stewart S, et al. The Glasgow alcoholic hepatitis score identifies patients who may benefit from corticosteroids. *Gut.* 2007;56:1743-1746.
8. Louvet A, Naveau S, Abdelnour M, et al. The Lille model: a new tool for therapeutic strategy in patients with severe alcoholic hepatitis treated with steroids. *Hepatology.* 2007;45:1348-1354.
9. Thursz MR, Richardson P, Allison M, et al. Prednisolone or pentoxifylline for alcoholic hepatitis. *N Engl J Med.* 2015;372:1619-1628.
10. Mathurin P, Moreno C, Samuel D, et al. Early liver transplantation for severe alcoholic hepatitis. *N Engl J Med.* 2011;365:1790-1800.
11. Manns MP, Czaja AJ, Gorham JD, et al. Practice guidelines of the American association for the study of liver diseases. Diagnosis and management of autoimmune hepatitis. *Hepatology.* 2010;51:2193-2213.
12. Manns MP, Woynarowski M, Kreisel W, et al. Budesonide induces remission more effectively than prednisone in a controlled trial of patients with autoimmune hepatitis. *Gastroenterology.* 2010;139:1198-1206.
13. Salcedo M, Rodríguez-Mahou M, Rodríguez-Sainz C, et al. Risk factors for developing de novo autoimmune hepatitis associated with anti-glutathione S-transferase T1 antibodies after liver transplantation. *Liver Transpl.* 2009;15:530-539.
14. Hirschfield GM, Mason A, Luketic V, et al. Efficacy of obeticholic acid in patients with primary biliary cirrhosis and inadequate response to ursodeoxycholic acid. *Gastroenterology.* 2015;148:751-761.
15. Chapman R, Fevery J, Kalloo A, et al. Diagnosis and management of primary sclerosing cholangitis. *Hepatology.* 2010;51:660-678.
16. Eaton JE, Talwalkar JA, Lazaridis KN, Gores GJ, Lindor KD. Pathogenesis of primary sclerosing cholangitis and advances in diagnosis and management. *Gastroenterology.* 2013;145(3):521-536.
17. Lindor KD, Gershwin ME, Poupon R, et al. American association for study of liver diseases. Primary biliary cirrhosis. *Hepatology.* 2009;50:291-308.
18. Roberts EA, Schilsky ML. Diagnosis and treatment of Wilson disease: an update. *Hepatology.* 2008;47:2089-2111.
19. Bacon BR, Adams PC, Kowdley KV, et al. Diagnosis and management of hemochromatosis: 2011 practice guideline by the American association for the study of liver diseases. *Hepatology.* 2011;54:328-343.
20. Fairbanks KD, Tavill AS. Liver disease in alpha 1-antitrypsin deficiency: a review. *Am J Gastroenterol.* 2008;103:2136-2142.
21. Chalasani N, Younossi Z, Lavine JE, et al. The diagnosis and management of nonalcoholic fatty liver disease: practice guidance from the American Association for the Study of Liver Diseases. *Hepatology.* 2018;67:328-357.
22. DeLeve LD, Valla DC, Garcia-Tsao G. Vascular disorders of the liver. *Hepatology.* 2009;49:1729-1764.
23. Rugivarodom M, Charatcharoenwitthaya P. Nontumoral portal vein thrombosis: a challenging consequence of liver cirrhosis. *J Clin Transl Hepatol.* 2020;8(4):432-444. doi:10.14218/JCTH.2020.00067.
24. Qi X, Han G, Fan D. Management of portal vein thrombosis in liver cirrhosis. *Nat Rev Gastroenterol Hepatol.* 2014;11:435-446.
25. Mohan BP, Veeraraghavan MA, Khan SR, et al. Treatment response and bleeding events associated with anticoagulant therapy of portal vein thrombosis in cirrhotic patients: systematic review and meta-analysis. *Ann Gastroenterol.* 2020; 33: 521-527.
26. European Association for the Study of the Liver. EASL Clinical Practice Guidelines: vascular diseases of the liver. *J Hepatol.* 2016;64:179-202.
27. Lee WM, Hynan LS, Rossaro L, et al. Intravenous N-acetylcysteine improves transplant-free survival in early stage non-acetaminophen acute liver failure. *Gastroenterology.* 2009;137:856-864.
28. Lee WM, Stravitz RT, Larson AM. Introduction to the revised American Association for the Study of Liver Diseases position paper on acute liver failure 2011. *Hepatology.* 2012;55:965-967.
29. Nguyen NT, Vierling JM. Acute liver failure. *Curr Opin Organ Transplant.* 2011;16:289-296.
30. Scaglione S, Kliethermes S, Cao G, et al. The epidemiology of cirrhosis in the United States: a population based study. *J Clin Gastroenterol.* 2015;49:690-696.

CHAPTER 19

31. Runyon BA, Montano AA, Akriviadis EA, et al. The serum-ascites albumin gradient is superior to the exudate-transudate concept in the differential diagnosis of ascites. *Ann Intern Med.* 1992;117:215-220.

32. Runyon BA. Introduction to the revised American Association for the Study of Liver Diseases Practice Guideline management of adult patients with ascites due to cirrhosis 2012. *Hepatology.* 2013;57:1651-1653.

33. Saab S, Hernandez JC, Chi AC, Tong MJ. Oral antibiotic prophylaxis reduces spontaneous bacterial peritonitis occurrence and improves short-term survival in cirrhosis: a meta-analysis. *Am J Gastroenterol.* 2009;104:993-1001.

34. Angeli P, Gines P, Wong F, et al. Diagnosis and management of acute kidney injury in patients with cirrhosis: revised consensus recommendations of the International Club of Ascites. *Gut.* 2015;64:531-537.

35. Sanyal AJ, Boyer T, Garcia-Tsao G, et al. A randomized prospective, double-blind, placebo-controlled trial of terlipressin for type 1 hepatorenal syndrome. *Gastroenterology.* 2008;134:1360-1368.

36. Vilstrup H, Amodio P, Bajaj J, et al. Hepatic encephalopathy in chronic liver disease: 2014 practice guideline by the American Association for the Study of Liver Diseases and the European Association for the study of the liver. *Hepatology.* 2014;60:715-735.

37. Heimbach JK, Kulik LM, Finn RS, et al. AASLD guidelines for the treatment of hepatocellular carcinoma. *Hepatology.* 2018;67:358-380.

38. Llovet JM, Ricci S, Mazzaferro V, et al.; SHARP Investigators Study Group. Sorafenib in advanced hepatocellular carcinoma. *N Engl J Med.* 2008;359(4):378-390.

20 Disorders of Hemostasis and Thrombosis

Kristen M. Sanfilippo, Brian F. Gage, Tzu-Fei Wang, and Roger D. Yusen

HEMOSTASIS DISORDERS

Hemostatic Disorders

GENERAL PRINCIPLES

- **Normal hemostasis** involves a sequence of interrelated reactions that lead to platelet aggregation (primary hemostasis) and activation of coagulation factors (secondary hemostasis) to produce a durable vascular seal.
  - **Primary hemostasis** consists of an immediate but temporary response to vessel injury, where platelets and von Willebrand factor (**vWF**) interact to form a primary hemostatic plug.
  - **Secondary hemostasis** results in formation of a fibrin clot (Figure 20-1). Injury exposes extravascular tissue factor to blood, which initiates activation of factors VII and X and prothrombin. Subsequent activation of factors XI, VIII, and V leads to generation of thrombin, conversion of fibrinogen to fibrin, and formation of a durable clot.[1]

DIAGNOSIS

Clinical Presentation

- A detailed history can assess bleeding risk or severity, determine congenital or acquired etiologies, and evaluate for primary or secondary hemostatic defects.
  - Prolonged bleeding after dental extractions, circumcision, menstruation, labor and delivery, trauma, or surgery may suggest an underlying bleeding disorder.
  - Family history may suggest an inherited bleeding disorder.

Physical Examination
- Primary hemostasis defects often cause mucosal bleeding and excessive bruising.
  - Petechiae: <2 mm subcutaneous lesions, do not blanch with pressure, typically present in areas subject to increased hydrostatic force (lower legs and periorbital area)
  - Ecchymoses: >3 mm black-and-blue patches due to rupture of small vessels from trauma
- Secondary hemostasis defects can result in hematomas, hemarthroses, or prolonged bleeding after trauma or surgery.

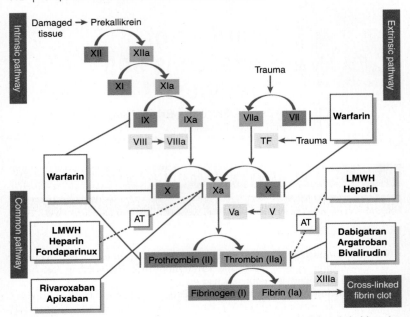

Figure 20-1. Coagulation cascade. *Solid arrows* indicate activation. *Solid* or *dashed lines* that run into a vertical line are associated with drugs represent a point of inhibition. Extrinsic pathway includes the right upper portion of cascade above factor X. Intrinsic pathway includes the left upper portion of the cascade above factor X. Common pathway includes the lower portion of the cascade from factor X and below. AT, antithrombin; LMWH, low-molecular-weight heparin; TF, tissue factor.

Diagnostic Testing

Laboratories

- Initial studies should include a complete blood count (**CBC**) with platelet count, as well as prothrombin time (**PT**), activated partial thromboplastin time (**aPTT**), and a peripheral blood smear.
- **Primary hemostasis tests**
  - A low **platelet count** requires review of the peripheral blood smear to rule out platelet clumping artifact or giant platelets as the cause of a falsely low platelet count.
  - The **platelet function assay-100 (PFA-100)** instrument assesses vWF-dependent platelet activation in flowing citrated whole blood. Patients with von Willebrand disease (**vWD**) and qualitative platelet disorders can have prolonged PFA-100 closure times, often with normal platelet counts. However, anemia (hematocrit < 30%) and/or thrombocytopenia (platelet < 100 × 10^9/L) can cause prolonged closure times without underlying bleeding disorders.
  - *In vitro* **platelet aggregation** studies measure platelet secretion and aggregation in response to platelet agonists (see Qualitative Platelet Disorders section).
  - Laboratory evaluation of vWD includes measurement of vWF antigen (**vWF:Ag**) and **vWF activity** and **vWF multimer analysis**.
- **Secondary hemostasis** (Figure 20-1)
  - **PT:** Measures time to form a fibrin clot after adding thromboplastin (tissue factor and phospholipid) and calcium to citrated plasma. An elevated PT is a sensitive

TABLE 20-1	Factor Deficiencies That Cause Prolonged Prothrombin Time and/or Activated Partial Thromboplastin Time and Correct With 50:50 Mix
Assay Result	**Suspected Factor Deficiencies**
↑ aPTT; normal PT	XII, XI, IX, VIII, HMWK, PK
↑ PT; normal aPTT	VII
↑ PT and ↑ aPTT	II, V, X, or fibrinogen

aPTT, activated partial thromboplastin time; HMWK, high-molecular weight kininogen; PK, prekallikrein; PT, prothrombin time.

test of deficiencies of **extrinsic pathway** (factor VII), **common pathway** (factors X and V and prothrombin), and **fibrinogen,** and to use of vitamin K antagonists. Reporting a PT ratio as an international normalized ratio (**INR**) reduces interlaboratory variation in monitoring warfarin use.[2]

○ **aPTT:** Measures the time to form a fibrin clot after activation of citrated plasma by calcium, phospholipid, and negatively charged particles. Unfractionated heparin, low-molecular weight heparin (**LMWH**), and fondaparinux prolong the aPTT. Deficiencies and inhibitors of coagulation factors of the **intrinsic pathway** (e.g., high-molecular weight kininogen, prekallikrein, factor XII, factor XI, factor IX, and factor VIII), **common pathway** (e.g., factors V and X, prothrombin), and **fibrinogen also cause aPTT** prolongation.

○ **Thrombin time:** Measures time to form a fibrin clot after addition of thrombin to citrated plasma. Unfractionated heparin, LMWH, fondaparinux, and direct thrombin (IIa) inhibitors prolong thrombin time, as do quantitative and qualitative deficiencies of fibrinogen and fibrin degradation products.

○ **Fibrinogen:** Measured by adding thrombin to dilute plasma and measuring clotting time. Conditions causing hypofibrinogenemia include decreased hepatic synthesis, massive hemorrhage, and disseminated intravascular coagulation (**DIC**).

○ D-**dimers** result from plasmin digestion of fibrin (i.e., fibrin degradation products). Elevated D-dimer concentrations occur in many disease states (i.e., venous thromboembolism [**VTE**], DIC, trauma, and cancer).

○ **Mixing studies** determine whether a factor deficiency or an inhibitor has prolonged the PT and/or aPTT. In a patient with factor deficiency, mixing patient plasma 1:1 with normal pooled plasma (all factor activities = 100%) restores deficient factors sufficiently to normalize or nearly normalize the PT or aPTT (Table 20-1). If mixing fails to correct the PT or aPTT, a specific factor inhibitor, a nonspecific inhibitor (e.g., lupus anticoagulant [**LA**]), or an anticoagulant drug may have caused the prolongation.

PLATELET DISORDERS

Thrombocytopenia

Thrombocytopenia, defined as a platelet count of $<150 \times 10^9/L$ (reference range varies depending on local laboratory standard), is caused by decreased production, increased destruction, or sequestration of platelets (Table 20-2).

TABLE 20-2	Classification of Thrombocytopenia	
Decreased Platelet Production	**Increased Platelet Clearance**	
Marrow failure syndromes	*Immune-mediated mechanisms*	
Congenital	Immune thrombocytopenic	
Acquired: Aplastic anemia, paroxysmal nocturnal hemoglobinuria	Thrombotic thrombocytopenic purpura/hemolytic-uremic syndrome	
Hematologic malignancies	Posttransfusion purpura	
Marrow infiltration: Cancer, granuloma	Heparin-induced thrombocytopenia	
Myelofibrosis: Primary or secondary	*Non–immune-mediated mechanisms*	
Nutritional: Vitamin B_{12} and folate deficiencies	DIC	
Physical damage to the bone marrow: Radiation, alcohol, chemotherapy	Local consumption (aortic aneurysm)	
	Acute hemorrhage	
Increased Splenic Sequestration	**Infections Associated With Thrombocytopenia**	
Portal hypertension	HIV, HHV-6, ehrlichia, rickettsia, malaria, hepatitis C, CMV, Epstein-Barr, *Helicobacter pylori*, *Escherichia coli* O157	
Felty syndrome		
Lysosomal storage disorders		
Infiltrative hematologic malignancies		
Extramedullary hematopoiesis		

CMV, cytomegalovirus; DIC, disseminated intravascular coagulation; HHV-6, human herpesvirus 6.

Immune Thrombocytopenia

GENERAL PRINCIPLES

Immune thrombocytopenia (ITP) is an acquired immune disorder in which antiplatelet antibodies cause shortened platelet survival and suppress megakaryopoiesis leading to thrombocytopenia and increased bleeding risk.[3] Etiologies of ITP include idiopathic (primary), associated with coexisting conditions (secondary), or drug induced.

Epidemiology
Adult primary **ITP** has an incidence of 3.3 cases per 10^5 persons.[4]

Etiology
- In **primary ITP**, autoantibodies bind to platelet surface antigens and cause premature clearance by the reticuloendothelial system in addition to immune-mediated suppression of platelet production.
- **Secondary ITP** occurs in the setting of systemic lupus erythematosus (**SLE**), antiphospholipid antibody syndrome (**APS**), HIV, hepatitis C virus (**HCV**), *Helicobacter pylori*, and lymphoproliferative disorders.[3]
- **Drug-dependent ITP** results from drug–platelet interactions prompting antibody binding.[5] Some common medications linked to thrombocytopenia include quinidine and quinine; platelet inhibitors abciximab, eptifibatide, tirofiban, and

ticlopidine; antibiotics linezolid, rifampin, sulfonamides, and vancomycin; the anticonvulsants phenytoin, valproic acid, and carbamazepine; analgesics acetaminophen, naproxen, and diclofenac; cimetidine; and chlorothiazide.

DIAGNOSIS

Clinical Presentation
ITP typically presents as mild mucocutaneous bleeding and petechiae or incidental thrombocytopenia. Occasionally, ITP can present as major bleeding. Risk of bleeding is highest with platelet counts <30 × 10^9/L.[6]

Diagnostic Testing
Normalization of platelet counts with discontinuation of suspected drug and confirmation if thrombocytopenia recurs when rechallenged support the diagnosis of **drug-induced ITP.**

Laboratories
- Review a peripheral blood smear to confirm automated platelet count, assess for platelet clumping and to determine platelet, red cell, and white cell morphologies.
- Laboratory tests do not confirm the diagnosis of primary ITP, although they help to exclude secondary causes. Primary **ITP** often has the scenario of isolated thrombocytopenia in the absence of a likely underlying causative disease or medication.
- Test for infection-associated causes (e.g., HIV, HCV).[6]
- Serologic tests for antiplatelet antibodies generally do not help diagnose **ITP** because of poor sensitivity and low negative predictive value (**NPV**).

Diagnostic Procedures
Diagnosis of ITP does not typically require bone marrow examination, although it can help to exclude other causes in select patients with additional CBC abnormalities, unresponsiveness to immune suppression therapy, or atypical signs or symptoms.[6]

TREATMENT

- The decision to treat **primary ITP** depends on the severity of thrombocytopenia and bleeding risk. The therapeutic goal is a safe platelet count to prevent major bleeding (typically ≥30 × 10^9/L) and minimization of treatment-related toxicities.
- Initial therapy, when indicated, consists of **glucocorticoids** (e.g., dexamethasone 40 mg orally for 4 days, followed by an additional 4 days in nonresponders or prednisone 1 mg/kg daily with prolonged taper).[7] Patients may also receive IV immunoglobulin (**IVIG**; 1 g/kg for one to two doses) to hasten response.
- Rh-positive patients may also receive anti-D immunoglobulin (**WinRho**) (ineffective postsplenectomy). WinRho may cause severe hemolysis and requires postinfusion monitoring (black box warning). Given effective therapies, WinRho is rarely used for ITP treatment at this time.
- Most primary ITP cases respond to therapy within 1–3 weeks; however, 30%–40% of patients will develop **relapsed/refractory ITP.**
- Choices for **second-line therapy of ITP** include **rituximab** (anti-CD20 monoclonal antibody), thrombopoietin receptor agonists (**TPO-RA**), and splenectomy.
  ○ There are three TPO-RA for treatment of refractory primary ITP patients: **romiplostim**,[8] dosed subcutaneously weekly; **eltrombopag**[9] and **avatrombopag**,[10]

taken orally once a day. TPO-RA produce durable platelet count improvements in >90% ITP patients beginning 5–7 days after initiation. Potential complications include thromboembolic events.

- ○ Rituximab is associated with a remission (platelet > $100 \times 10^9/L$ at 12 months) in ~25%.
- ○ Two-thirds of patients with refractory ITP will obtain a durable complete response following **splenectomy.** Administer pneumococcal, meningococcal, and *Haemophilus influenzae* type B vaccines before (preferred) or after splenectomy.

- **Fostamatinib**, a tyrosine kinase inhibitor (TKI) that inhibits the spleen tyrosine kinase Syk, increases platelet count by reducing platelet phagocytosis by macrophages. While response rates were low (18% achieved a stable platelet count > 50 $\times 10^9/L$) in trial, most patients had tried multiple prior therapies (median 3, range 1–13).[11]
- Additional treatment options for patients with relapsed/refractory disease include single or combined therapies with prednisone, IVIG, androgen therapy with danazol, other immunosuppressive agents.
- Management of **secondary ITP** may include a combination of treatment for the underlying disease and therapies similar to those used for primary ITP.
- Platelet transfusion for severe drug-induced thrombocytopenia may decrease risk of bleeding. IVIG, steroids, and plasmapheresis have uncertain benefit.

Thrombotic Thrombocytopenic Purpura and Hemolytic-Uremic Syndrome

GENERAL PRINCIPLES

Definition

Thrombotic thrombocytopenic purpura (TTP) and **hemolytic-uremic syndrome (HUS)** are thrombotic microangiopathies (**TMAs**) caused by platelet–vWF aggregates and platelet–fibrin aggregates, respectively, resulting in thrombocytopenia, microangiopathic hemolytic anemia (**MAHA**), and organ ischemia. Usually, clinical and laboratory features permit differentiation of TTP from HUS. TMA may also occur in association with DIC, HIV infection, malignant hypertension, vasculitis, organ and stem cell transplant–related toxicity, adverse drug reactions, and pregnancy-related complications of preeclampsia/eclampsia and **HELLP** (**h**emolysis, **e**levated **l**iver enzymes, **l**ow **p**latelets) syndrome.

Epidemiology

Acquired TTP has an incidence of approximately 11.3 cases per 10^6 persons, occurring more frequently in women and African Americans.[12] **Typical HUS** usually occurs in gastroenteritis outbreaks affecting children. Adults may present with both **typical** and **atypical** (non–gastroenteritis-associated) variants of **HUS**.

Etiology

- Autoantibody-mediated removal of plasma vWF-cleaving protease, A disintegrin and metalloproteinase with a thrombospondin type 1 motif, member 13 (ADAMTS13), leading to elevated levels of abnormally large vWF multimers, causes **acquired TTP.**[13] The abnormal vWF multimers spontaneously adhere to platelets and may produce occlusive vWF–platelet aggregates in the microcirculation and subsequent microangiopathy. Second-hit events may involve endothelial dysfunction or injury.

- **Typical or enteropathic HUS** has an association with *Escherichia coli* (O157:H7) production of Shiga-like toxins in Shiga toxigenic *E. coli* HUS (**STEC-HUS**).
- **HUS** can also be associated with transplant, endothelial-damaging drugs, and pregnancy.[14]
- Inherited or acquired defects in regulation of the alternative complement pathway are present in 30%–50% of **atypical HUS** cases.[14]

DIAGNOSIS

Clinical Presentation

- The complete clinical pentad of **TTP**, present in <30% of cases, includes **consumptive thrombocytopenia, MAHA, fever, renal dysfunction, and fluctuating neurologic deficits.**
- The findings of thrombocytopenia and MAHA should raise suspicion for **TTP-HUS** in the absence of other identifiable causes.
- Patients with autosomal recessive inherited ADAMTS13 deficiencies have relapsing TTP (Upshaw–Schulman syndrome).
- Diarrhea, usually bloody, and abdominal pain often precede STEC-HUS.
- Marked renal dysfunction usually occurs in atypical HUS.

Diagnostic Testing

- TMAs produce schistocytes (fragmented red cells) and thrombocytopenia on blood smears. The findings of anemia, elevated reticulocyte count, low or undetectable haptoglobin, and elevated lactate dehydrogenase (**LDH**) support the presence of hemolysis.
- Acquired TTP has TMA findings, normal PT/aPTT, very low or undetectable ADAMTS13 enzyme activity, and detectable ADAMTS13 inhibitory antibody.
- The PLASMIC score quantifies the pretest probability of **acquired TTP.** Each finding contributes one point: platelet < 30 × 10⁹/L, laboratory evidence of hemolysis, no cancer, no transplant, MCV < 90 fL, INR < 1.5, Creatinine < 2.0 mg/dL. Patients with 0–4 points have a low probability of acquired TTP whereas those with 6–7 points have a high probability.[15]
- Typical HUS has TMA and acute renal failure. *E. coli* O157 stool culture has a higher sensitivity than Shiga toxin assays.
- In the absence of precipitating risk factors, testing for **atypical HUS** should include molecular and serologic tests for complement regulator factor H and I mutations or autoantibodies through reference laboratories.

TREATMENT

- The mainstay of therapy for **TTP** consists of rapid treatment with plasma exchange (**PEX**) of 1.0–1.5 plasma volumes daily. PEX is continued for several days after normalization of platelet count and LDH.[16]
  - If PEX is unavailable or will be delayed, infuse **fresh frozen plasma (FFP)** immediately to replace ADAMTS13.
- Common practice includes the administration of **glucocorticoids**: prednisone 1 mg/kg orally per day. Consider a brief course of high-dose corticosteroids (methylprednisolone 0.5–1.0 g/d IV) in critically ill or in patients not responding to PEX.[17]
- In observational studies, **rituximab** (375 mg/m² IV) reduces the risk of relapse in patients with **acquired TTP** when added to initial therapy with PEX. Comparative

studies are needed to determine if low-dose rituximab (e.g., 100 mg/m^2 may induce a long-term response).[18,19]

- **Caplacizumab,** a humanized monoclonal antibody fragment that binds to vWF and blocks vWF-platelet glycoprotein Ib-IX-V interactions, reduces formation of microthrombi. It is approved for the initial treatment of acquired TTP in combination with PEX and immunosuppressive agents. In the phase III HERCULES trial, caplacizumab reduced mortality, normalized platelet count faster, resulting in fewer PEX days, and was associated with a decrease in relapse events within 30 days.[20]
- Avoid platelet transfusion in the absence of severe bleeding or an invasive procedure because of the potentially increased risk of additional microvascular occlusions in TTP.
- Ninety percent of treated patients have a remission; however, relapses may occur days to years later.
- **Immunosuppression** with cyclophosphamide, azathioprine, or vincristine and splenectomy may have success in the treatment of refractory or relapsing TTP.
- **STEC-HUS** does not usually improve with PEX, and treatment remains supportive. Antibiotic therapy does not hasten recovery or minimize toxicity for STEC-HUS.
- **TMA associated with calcineurin inhibitors** (cyclosporine, tacrolimus) usually responds to drug dose reduction or discontinuation of the offending agent.
- **Atypical HUS** often leads to chronic renal failure necessitating dialysis.
- **Eculizumab** is a humanized monoclonal antibody used to treat **atypical HUS** that binds to complement protein C5, which blocks its cleavage into C5a and the cytotoxic membrane attack complex C5b-9, thus inhibiting complement activation.[21]

Vaccinate for *Neisseria meningitides* 2 weeks before starting eculizumab; however, if not possible, administer prophylactic antibiotics against *N. meningitides* for 2 weeks after vaccination.

Heparin-Induced Thrombocytopenia

GENERAL PRINCIPLES

Definition

Heparin-induced thrombocytopenia (HIT) is an acquired hypercoagulable disorder associated with the use of heparin/heparin-like products due to autoantibodies that target platelet factor 4 (**PF4**) complexes. HIT typically presents with thrombocytopenia or a decrease in platelet count by at least 50% from preexposure baseline after exposure to heparin products. Major complications of HIT consist of arterial and venous thromboembolic events.

Epidemiology

The incidence of **HIT** ranges from 0.1% to 1.0% in medical and obstetric patients receiving prophylactic/therapeutic unfractionated heparin (**UFH**) to >1%–5% in patients receiving UFH after cardiothoracic surgery. Patients exposed only to LMWH have a low incidence of HIT. HIT rarely occurs in association with the synthetic pentasaccharide fondaparinux.[22]

Etiology

Autoantibodies that bind to PF4/heparin complexes can activate platelets causing thrombocytopenia and lead to clot formation through increased thrombin generation.

DIAGNOSIS

Clinical Presentation

- **HIT** usually develops within 5–14 days of heparin exposure (**typical-onset HIT**). Exceptions include **delayed-onset HIT**, which occurs after stopping heparin, and **early-onset HIT**, starts within 24 hours of heparin exposure in patients with recent exposure to heparin.
- The **4T scoring system** (Table 20-3) calculates HIT pretest probability (NPV > 95%).[23]
- HIT rarely causes severe thrombocytopenia (platelet count < 20 × 10^9/L) or bleeding.
- **Thromboembolic complications** occur in 30%–75% of HIT patients. Thrombosis can precede, be concurrent with, or follow thrombocytopenia.
  ○ HIT causing venous thrombi at heparin injection sites produces full-thickness skin infarctions, sometimes in the absence of thrombocytopenia.
- HIT can cause systemic allergic responses following an IV bolus of heparin characterized by fever, hypotension, dyspnea, and cardiac arrest.

Diagnostic Testing

- Obtain surveillance platelet counts every 2–3 days during heparin exposure in patients with >1% risk of HIT.
- For suspected HIT, laboratory tests for PF4 antibodies improve diagnostic accuracy.
  ○ PF4 antibody testing is a sensitive screening test but lacks specificity.
  ○ Specificity improves when a positive enzyme-linked immunosorbent assay (**ELISA**) is quantified in optical density (**OD**) units. The higher the OD, the more likely the patient has HIT.
  ○ Rapid tests for PF4 antibodies (i.e., latex immunoturbidimetric assays [**LIA**]) have a lower sensitivity than ELISA (96.8% vs. 100%).

TABLE 20-3	4T Scoring System for Pretest Probability of Heparin-Induced Thrombocytopenia		
T Category	**0 Points**	**1 Point**	**2 Points**
Thrombocytopenia	PLT fall <30% or nadir <10 × 10^9/L	PLT fall 30%–50% or nadir 10–19 × 10^9/L	PLT fall >50% and nadir ≥20 × 10^9/L
Timing of thrombocytopenia	≤4 d without prior exposure	Likely within 5–10 d, not clear; >10 d; ≤1 d (with exposure 31–100 d)	Within 5–10 d of exposure or ≤1 d (with exposure in last 30 d)
Thrombotic event	No thrombus	Thrombus recurrence or progression; erythematous skin lesion; suspected thrombus	Confirmed thrombus; skin necrosis; acute reaction after UFH bolus
Other causes for thrombocytopenia	Definite	Possible	None apparent

Sum the points for each of the four categories to determine the clinical probability: high (6–8 points), intermediate (4–5 points), low (0–3 points).
PLT, platelets; UFH, unfractionated heparin.
Data from Lo GK, Juhl D, Warkentin TE, Sigouin CS, Eichler P, Greinacher A. Evaluation of pretest clinical score (4 T's) for the diagnosis of heparin-induced thrombocytopenia in two clinical settings. *J Thromb Haemost.* 2006;4(4):759-765 and Warkentin TE, Linkins LA. Non-necrotizing heparin-induced skin lesions and the 4T's score. *J Thromb Haemost.* 2010;8(7):1483-1485.

- Two functional assays test for HIT: serotonin release assay (**SRA**) and heparin-induced platelet activation (**HIPA**).
  - Both detect PF4 antibodies in patients' serum that can activate control platelets in the presence of heparin.
  - Both tests have high specificity for HIT but lower sensitivity than PF4 antibody testing.
- For a low clinical probability of HIT, testing for HIT antibodies is *not* indicated.
- For a moderate to high clinical probability of HIT, PF4 ELISA testing is indicated. A negative PF4 antibody test effectively rules out HIT.
- A positive PF4 antibody test should lead to confirmatory functional testing (SRA or HIPA).

TREATMENT

- Because HIT test results are not often immediately available, clinical assessment should determine initial management.
- When HIT is strongly suspected, or confirmed, **eliminate all heparin/LMWH exposure.**
- Since patients with HIT have a high risk for VTE, they should undergo anticoagulation with a parenteral direct thrombin inhibitor (**DTI**)[24] (i.e., **argatroban or bivalirudin**), although fondaparinux also has been used.[25]
- Assess (e.g., venous compression ultrasound) for symptomatic and asymptomatic VTE because of the high risk for VTE and the subsequent indication for a full course of anticoagulation.[24]
- Start warfarin only after starting a DTI and when the platelet count normalizes to >150 × 10^9/L, at an initial dose no greater than 5 mg daily. Then, overlap warfarin with the DTI for 5 days to reduce the risk of limb gangrene due to ongoing hypercoagulable conditions and depletion of proteins C and S.
  DTIs prolong the INR and require careful monitoring when transitioning from DTI to warfarin (see Medications under Approach to Venous Thromboembolism).
- Evidence is increasing for the safety and efficacy of direct oral anticoagulant (DOACs) in HIT.[26]
- The recommended duration of anticoagulation therapy for HIT depends on the clinical scenario: 4–6 weeks for **isolated HIT** (without thrombosis) and 3 months for **HIT-associated thrombosis.**[24]

Posttransfusion Purpura

GENERAL PRINCIPLES

Definition

Posttransfusion purpura (PTP), a rare syndrome characterized by the formation of alloantibodies against platelet antigens, most commonly HPA-1a, follows blood component transfusion and causes severe thrombocytopenia.

Epidemiology

PTP has an incidence of 1 in 50,000–100,000 blood transfusions, although approximately 2% of the population has a potential risk for PTP based on the frequency of HPA-1b/1b.

Etiology

Glycoprotein (GP) IIIa has a polymorphic epitope called HPA-1a/b, the antigen most commonly involved in PTP. **PTP** typically occurs in HPA-1a/1b–negative multiparous women or previously transfused patients when re-exposed to HPA-1a by transfusion. An amnestic response produces alloantibodies to the HPA-1a, which appear to also recognize the patient's HPA-1a–negative platelets and cause thrombocytopenia via platelet destruction.

DIAGNOSIS

- In **PTP**, severe thrombocytopenia ($<15 \times 10^9$/L) usually occurs within 7–10 days of transfusion.
- Confirmation of suspected **PTP** requires detection of platelet alloantibodies.

TREATMENT

Although spontaneous platelet recovery eventually occurs, bleeding may require treatment. Effective therapies include IVIG and plasmapheresis. Transfusion with platelets from a donor who lacks the causative epitope (typically HPA-1a) does not clearly have higher efficacy than random platelet transfusion. Reserve transfusion for patients with PTP and severe bleeding.[27]

Gestational Thrombocytopenia

GENERAL PRINCIPLES

Definition

Gestational thrombocytopenia is a benign, mild thrombocytopenia (platelet count ≥ 70×10^9/L) that occurs in the third trimester of pregnancy and usually resolve promptly after delivery. The mother has no symptoms, and the fetus remains unaffected.

Epidemiology

Gestational thrombocytopenia occurs in 5%–7% of otherwise uncomplicated pregnancies.[28]

Differential Diagnosis

Other causes of thrombocytopenia during pregnancy include **ITP, preeclampsia, eclampsia, HELLP syndrome, TTP, and DIC**.

Diagnostic Testing

To distinguish between gestational thrombocytopenia and other syndromes, diagnostic testing includes an evaluation for infection, hypertension and laboratory testing for hemolysis and liver dysfunction.

Thrombocytosis

GENERAL PRINCIPLES

Definition

Thrombocytosis is defined as a platelet count of $>450 \times 10^9$/L by the World Health Organization (WHO).

Etiology

- Thrombocytosis has reactive and clonal etiologies that may coexist.
- **Reactive thrombocytosis** may occur during recovery from thrombocytopenia; after splenectomy; or in response to iron deficiency, acute infectious or chronic inflammatory states, trauma, and malignancies.
  - Low risks of thrombosis or bleeding.
  - Platelets normalize after improvement of the underlying disorder.
  - If accompanied by thrombotic complications, evaluate for an underlying myeloproliferative disorder.

DIAGNOSIS

Clinical Presentation

History

ET may present as an incidental discovery or present with thrombotic or hemorrhagic symptoms. The risk of thrombosis increases with age, prior thrombosis, duration of disease, and other comorbidities. Erythromelalgia, due to microvascular occlusive platelet thrombi, presents as intense burning or throbbing of the extremities, typically involving the feet. Cold exposure usually relieves symptoms. Hemorrhage can occur with platelet counts >1000 × 10^9/L due to acquired deficiencies of large vWF multimers.[29]

Physical Examination

Approximately 50% of ET patients develop mild splenomegaly. Typical signs of erythromelalgia include erythema and warmth of affected digits.

Diagnostic Criteria

The 2016 **WHO** revised criteria (requires all four) include[30]:
- Platelet count ≥ 450 × 10^9/L.
- Bone marrow biopsy showing increased mature megakaryocytes and no increase in erythropoiesis or granulopoiesis or reticulin fiber deposition greater than grade I.
- Exclusion of BCR-ABL1 positive chronic myelogenous leukemia (**CML**), polycythemia vera, primary myelofibrosis, myelodysplastic syndrome, or other myeloid neoplasm.
- Presence of *JAK2 V617F*, *CALR*, or *MPL* mutation **or**, if clonal marker not present, no evidence for reactive thrombocytosis.

TREATMENT

- Patients with high or intermediate risk of thrombosis based on the International Prognostic Score for Thrombosis in Essential Thrombocythemia (IPSET)[31] (high: age > 60 years with a *JAK2 V617F* mutation and/or a history of thrombosis at any age, intermediate: age > 60, no *JAK2* mutation, no history of thrombosis) require cytoreduction therapy.
  - Platelet-lowering drugs include **hydroxyurea** and **anagrelide** or **interferon-α** in pregnant patients or females in their childbearing years. The majority of thrombotic complications occur at modest platelet count elevations.
  - Hydroxyurea is superior that anagrelide to prevent thrombotic and hemorrhagic complications in the randomized controlled trial, so hydroxyurea and aspirin (ASA) is the standard first line therapy for patients with ET at high risk for vascular events.[32]
  - Treatment typically aims for a platelet count of ≤400 × 10^9/L.

- Patients age 60 or younger and no history of thrombosis can be managed without cytoreductive therapy; they are treated with aspirin or observation alone.
- Plateletpheresis rapidly lowers platelet counts, although it is reserved for patients who have acute arterial thromboses.

Qualitative Platelet Disorders

GENERAL PRINCIPLES

Qualitative platelet disorders present with mucocutaneous bleeding and excessive bruising with an adequate platelet count, PT, and aPTT and normal screening tests for vWD. Most potent platelet defects produce prolonged PFA-100 closure times. However, a normal PFA-100 does not exclude qualitative platelet disorders, and high clinical suspicion of a disorder should lead to further testing such as platelet aggregation.

Classification

- **Inherited disorders** of platelet function include receptor, signal transduction, cyclooxygenase (COX), secretory (e.g., storage pool disease), adhesion, or aggregation defects. *In vitro* platelet aggregation studies can identify patterns of agonist responses consistent with a particular defect, such as the rare autosomal recessive disorders of adhesion in **Bernard–Soulier syndrome** (lack of GP Ib/IX [vWF receptor]) and aggregation in **Glanzmann thrombasthenia** (lack of GP IIb/IIIa [fibrinogen receptor]).
- **Acquired** platelet defects are more common than hereditary platelet qualitative disorders.
  - Conditions associated with acquired qualitative defects include metabolic disorders (uremia, liver failure), myeloproliferative diseases, myelodysplasia, acute leukemia, monoclonal gammopathy, and cardiopulmonary bypass platelet trauma.
  - **Drug-induced** platelet dysfunction is a side effect of many drugs, including high-dose penicillin, ASA, and other **NSAIDs**, and ethanol. Other drug classes, such as β-lactam antibiotics, β-blockers, calcium channel blockers, nitrates, antihistamines, psychotropic drugs, tricyclic antidepressants, and selective serotonin reuptake inhibitors, cause platelet dysfunction *in vitro,* but they rarely cause bleeding.
  - Certain **foods and herbal products** may affect platelet function including omega-3 fatty acids, garlic and onion extracts, ginger, gingko, ginseng, and black tree fungus. Patients should stop using herbal medications and dietary supplements ≥1 week before major surgery.[33]

TREATMENT

- Treatment of **uremic platelet dysfunction** can include dialysis to improve uremia; desmopressin (**DDAVP**) 0.3 μg/kg IV to stimulate release of vWF from endothelial cells; or conjugated estrogens (0.6 mg/kg IV daily for 5 days) and platelet transfusions in actively bleeding patients, although transfused platelets rapidly acquire the uremic defect. Transfusion or give erythropoietin (**EPO**) to increase hematocrit toward 30% might assist in hemostasis.[34,35]

- Antifibrinolytic agents such as aminocaproic acid or tranexamic acid are commonly used as adjunct therapies with DDAVP for procedures or bleeding complications.
- Reserve platelet transfusions for major bleeding episodes. Anecdotal reports have described successful control of severe bleeding with recombinant factor VIIa (**rFVIIa**).
- **Reversal of drug-induced platelet dysfunction**
  - **NSAIDs** other than ASA reversibly inhibit **COX.** Their effects only last several days. **COX-2 inhibitors** have antiplatelet activity in large doses, but they have a minimal effect on platelets at therapeutic doses.
  - **ASA** irreversibly inhibits COX-1 and COX-2. Its effects diminish over 7–10 days because of new platelet production.
  - **Thienopyridines** inhibit platelet aggregation by irreversibly (clopidogrel and prasugrel) or reversibly (ticagrelor) blocking platelet adenosine diphosphate receptor P2Y12.
  - **Dipyridamole,** alone or in combination with ASA (Aggrenox), inhibits platelet function by increasing intracellular cyclic adenosine monophosphate (**cAMP**).
  - **Abciximab, eptifibatide, and tirofiban** block platelet IIb/IIIa–dependent aggregation (see Chapter 4, Ischemic Heart Disease).
  - Platelet transfusion compensates for drug-induced platelet dysfunction, except immediately following tirofiban and eptifibatide therapy.
  - Hold antiplatelet agents for 7 days before elective invasive procedures.

INHERITED BLEEDING DISORDERS

Hemophilia A

GENERAL PRINCIPLES

Definition

Hemophilia A is an X-linked recessive coagulation disorder due to mutations in the gene encoding factor VIII.

Epidemiology

Hemophilia A affects ~1 in 5000 live male births. Approximately 40% of cases occur in families with no prior history of hemophilia, reflecting the high rate of spontaneous germline mutations in the factor VIII gene.

DIAGNOSIS

Clinical Presentation

- Patients with severe hemophilia experience frequent spontaneous hemarthroses and hematomas, hematuria, and delayed posttraumatic and postoperative bleeding. Repeated bleeding into a "target" joint causes chronic synovitis and hemophilic arthropathy.
- Moderate hemophiliacs have fewer spontaneous bleeding episodes, and mild hemophiliacs may only bleed excessively after trauma or surgery.

Diagnostic Testing

The severity of hemophilia is based on baseline factor VIII activity: Severe (<1%), moderate (1%–5%), and mild (>5%–<40%). Mild hemophiliacs with factor VIII ≥30% may not have a prolonged aPTT.

TREATMENT

Medications

First Line

- Mild-to-moderate hemophilia A with minor bleeding: **DDAVP** (0.3 μg/kg IV infused over 30 minutes, or 150 μg intranasal) increases factor VIII activity three- to fivefold. Because not all patients have an expected response to DDAVP, they should undergo a DDAVP challenge to assess responsiveness before use. To avoid tachyphylaxis, no more than three consecutive doses should be given per week.
- Mild-to-moderate hemophilia A with major bleeding OR severe hemophilia A with any bleeding:
  - **Factor VIII replacement** is the mainstay of therapy with many hemophiliac patients able to do home infusion.
  - **Factor VIII concentrate** increases factor VIII activity by 2% for every 1 IU/kg infused, thus a 50 IU/kg IV bolus raises factor VIII activity by 100% over baseline. Extended treatment should follow with 25–30 IU/kg IV bolus q12h (products with normal half-life) and adjust dose based on peak and trough factor VIII levels to maintain sufficient levels.
  - One to three doses of **factor VIII** concentrates targeting peak plasma activities of 30%–50% typically stop mild hemorrhages.
  - Major traumas and surgery require maintenance of levels >80%.
  - Adjust doses based on peak and trough factor VIII levels to achieve individualized targets based on bleeding risk.
  - Continuous infusion of factor VIII provides a safe and effective alternative to intermittent infusion.[36]
  - Extended factor VIII concentrates extended half-lives 1.5–1.7-fold (to 15–19 hours) allow reduced frequency of factor infusion.[37]
- Emicizumab (Hemlibra), a bispecific humanized monoclonal antibody that bridges activated factor IX and X to restore the function of missing activated factor VIII. It had been approved for treatment in patients with congenital VIII deficiency with or without inhibitors, based on the remarkable results from HAVEN 1–4 studies, showing >90% reduction in annual bleed rate. It is given as subcutaneous injection once a week to once every 4 weeks (in contrast to frequent intravenous infusion needed for traditional factors), which led to a major change in the treatment of hemophilia patients.

Hemophilia B

GENERAL PRINCIPLES

Definition

Hemophilia B is an X-linked recessive coagulation disorder secondary to mutations in the gene encoding factor IX.

Epidemiology

Hemophilia B affects ~1 in 30,000 male births.

DIAGNOSIS

Clinical Presentation

Hemophilia B remains clinically indistinguishable from hemophilia A.

Diagnostic Testing

Factor IX activity. Hemophilia A (Factor VIII) and B (Factor IX) use the same severity scale based on degree of decreased factor activity.

TREATMENT

Therapy of hemophilia B consists of **factor IX replacement** with either **plasma-derived factor IX** or **recombinant factor IX** (BeneFIX).

- DDAVP lacks efficacy because it does **not** increase factor IX levels.
- Postinfusion peak targets, duration of therapy, and laboratory monitoring for treatment of hemophilia B–related bleeding are similar to those for hemophilia A.
- Every 1 IU/kg of factor IX replacement typically raises plasma factor IX activity by 1%. Standard Factor IX has a half-life of 18–24 hours.
- Extended factor IX products significantly prolonged the half-life by 4–6-fold, with half-life of 80–100 hours, allowing significant reduction of frequency in prophylactic factor infusion to 1–2 times a week.[37]
- Gene therapy for factor IX deficiency has been more successfully than for factor VIII deficiency but remains only available under clinical research setting.

COMPLICATIONS OF HEMOPHILIA A AND B THERAPY

Inhibitors

- Alloantibodies to factors VIII and IX in response to replacement therapy develop in approximately 20% and 12% of severe hemophilia A and B patients, respectively. These alloantibodies neutralize infused factor VIII or IX.
- Determining the titer of a factor VIII or IX inhibitor, using a laboratory assay that reports inhibitor strength in Bethesda units (**BUs**), predicts inhibitor behavior and guides therapy.
- Treatment options for factor VIII or IX inhibitors include[38]:
  - Large doses of factor VIII or IX concentrates overcome inhibitors for patients with low titer (BU < 5).
  - Because factor VIII or IX concentrates will not overcome inhibitors in patients with high titers (BU > 5), bypassing agents such as rFVIIa or activated prothrombin complex concentrate (aPCC) are used.[39]
    - **rFVIIa** (NovoSeven) is dosed at 90 μg/kg every 2 hours until hemostasis occurs.
    - **aPCC** (most commonly used-Factor Eight Inhibitor Bypassing Activity [FEIBA]), dosed at 75–100 IU/kg q12h. FEIBA contains activated factors VII, VIII, XI, X, and thrombin, and it can cause thrombosis or DIC.
- Emicizumab given as weekly subcutaneous injections and reduces annualized bleeding rate by 80%–90% in hemophilia A patients with inhibitors and is FDA-approved for this population.[40] Subsequently, emicizumab was studied in patients without inhibitors and now is FDA-approved for patients with and without factor VIII inhibitors.[41] Thrombotic microangiopathy is a rare complication in patients receiving concurrent aPCC.

von Willebrand Disease

GENERAL PRINCIPLES

Classification

- **vWD** has three main types[42]:
  - **Type 1 vWD,** due to a quantitative deficiency of vWF (70%–80% of cases)
  - **Type 2 vWD,** due to a qualitative defect of vWF, includes four subtypes (2A, 2B, 2M, 2N):
    - Type 2A: reduced vWF high molecular weight multimer
    - Type 2B: pathologically enhanced platelet affinity to vWF
    - Type 2M: reduced platelet affinity to vWF
    - Type 2N: defective FVIII binding to vWF
  - **Type 3 vWD,** due to a near complete lack of vWF.

Epidemiology

vWD, the most common inherited bleeding disorder, affects around 0.1%–1% of the population.

Etiology

Most forms of **vWD** have an autosomal dominant inheritance with variable penetrance, although autosomal recessive forms (types 2N and 3) exist. vWF circulates as multimers of variable size and facilitate adherence of platelets to injured vessel walls and stabilize FVIII in plasma.

DIAGNOSIS

Clinical Presentation

Clinical findings consist of mucocutaneous bleeding (epistaxis, menorrhagia, gastrointestinal bleeding), easy bruising, and bleeding from trauma or surgery.

Diagnostic Testing

Testing for suspected vWD should include vWF:Ag, vWF:RCo and FVIII activity. See American Society of Hematology pocket guide on vWD.

TREATMENT

- Goal of therapy is to raise vWF:RCo and factor VIII activity to ensure adequate hemostasis. vWF:RCo activities >50% control most hemorrhages.[43]
- **DDAVP** 0.3 μg/kg IV can be used to treat type 1 vWD. Because only two-thirds of patients will respond, a test dose should assess for a response. For responders undergoing **minor invasive procedures**, infuse 1 hour before, followed by q12–24h for three more doses postoperatively as needed, with or without oral antifibrinolytic drugs (i.e., aminocaproic acid or tranexamic acid).
  - DDAVP does not effectively treat most type 2 or type 3 vWD patients.
  - DDAVP is contraindicated in type 2B vWD because of the risk of thrombocytopenia.
  - Common side effects of DDAVP include hyponatremia, nausea, and flushing. Patients should limit fluid intake to 1200 mL/d within 24 hours of any dose.

- **vWF plasma-derived concentrate transfusions** (Alphanate, Humate-P, and Wilate) and **recombinant vWF** (Vonvendi) should aim to raise vWF:RCo activity to ~100% and maintain it between 50% and 100% until sufficient hemostasis occurs (typically 5–10 days).
- Recombinant vWF (Vonvendi) is now FDA-approved for control of bleeding episodes and perioperative management of bleeding in adults with von Willebrand disease.
- Indications for concentrate transfusions
  - Type 1 vWD-DDAVP nonresponders
  - Type 1 vWD-major bleeding or surgery
  - All other vWD types requiring hemostasis treatment

ACQUIRED COAGULATION DISORDERS

Vitamin K Deficiency

GENERAL PRINCIPLES

Vitamin K deficiency is usually caused by malabsorption states or poor dietary intake, often combined with antibiotic-associated loss of intestinal bacterial colonization. Hepatocytes require vitamin K to complete the γ-carboxylation-mediated synthesis of clotting factors (X, IX, VII, prothrombin) and the natural anticoagulant proteins C and S.

DIAGNOSIS

A **prolonged PT that corrects after a 1:1 mix with normal pooled plasma** suggests that a patient has vitamin K deficiency.

TREATMENT

Oral **vitamin K replacement** (e.g., phytonadione 5 mg PO daily) typically has good absorption in patients who have had poor dietary intake. In patients who have malabsorption, parental vitamin K should be given IV, rather than SC.

Liver Disease

GENERAL PRINCIPLES

Liver disease can impair hemostasis (**see** Figure 20-1) due to a reduction in synthesis of most coagulation factors. Cholestasis, which leads to impaired vitamin K absorption, can also impair hemostasis because of decreased production of Factors II, VII, IX, and X. Patients who have stable liver disease typically have a mild coagulopathy. Liver disease may produce other hemostatic complications that include thrombocytopenia due to splenic sequestration, DIC, and hyperfibrinolysis. Although PT/INR and aPTT prolongations imply an increased risk of bleeding, they do not reflect concurrent reductions in protein C and protein S nor compensatory increases in factor VIII and vWF.

TREATMENT OF BLEEDING IN PATIENTS WITH LIVER DISEASE

- **Vitamin K** replacement may shorten a prolonged PT/INR caused by a vitamin K antagonist (e.g., warfarin), dietary deficiency, or cholestasis, but it does not stop bleeding.
- **For patients who have an elevated INR or aPTT, FFP** may decrease bleeding, but it may cause volume overload and does not work immediately.
- **Prothrombin complex concentrate** (e.g., Kcentra 25 IU/kg IV) will work more rapidly than FFP in normalizing an elevated INR during bleeding and requires less volume administration, but it has not undergone extensive testing in patients who have liver disease.[44]
- **Cryoprecipitate,** 1.5 units/10 kg body weight, corrects hypofibrinogenemia (<100 mg/dL).
- **Recombinant factor VIIa** does not stop GI bleeding in liver disease and may cause thrombosis.[45]
- **Platelet transfusion or thrombopoietin** may decrease transfusion requirements in those with bleeding or undergoing an invasive procedure who have severe thrombocytopenia (<50 × 10^9/L).
- **Antifibrinolytic therapy** (e.g., tranexamic acid) can be used with persistent mucosal oozing or puncture wound bleeding.
- **Variceal bleeds** should be treated as in Chapter 18.

Disseminated Intravascular Coagulation

GENERAL PRINCIPLES

Etiology

DIC occurs in a variety of systemic illnesses that include sepsis, trauma, burns, shock, obstetric complications, and malignancies (notably, acute promyelocytic leukemia).

Pathophysiology

Exposure of tissue factor to the circulation generates excess thrombin, leading to platelet activation, consumption of coagulation factors (including fibrinogen) and regulators (antithrombin [**AT**] and proteins C and S), fibrin generation, generalized microthrombi, and reactive fibrinolysis.

DIAGNOSIS

Clinical Presentation

Consequences of **DIC** include bleeding, organ dysfunction secondary to microvascular thrombi and ischemia, and less often, large arterial and venous thrombosis.[46]

Diagnostic Testing

No test confirms diagnosis of DIC. The International Society on Thrombosis and Haemostasis (**ISTH**) devised a clinical scoring system for objective detection of DIC (Table 20-4). Serial "DIC panels" help assess clinical management and prognosis.

TABLE 20-4	International Society on Thrombosis and Haemostasis Disseminated Intravascular Coagulation Scoring System		
Use Only in Patients With an Underlying Condition Known to be Associated With DIC.			
	0 Points	1 Point	2 Points
Thrombocytopenia	>100 × 10⁹/L	≤100 × 10⁹/L	≤50 × 10⁹/L
D-dimer	Normal	<10 × upper limit of normal	≥10 × upper limit of normal
PT Prolongation	<3 s	3–6 s	>6 s
Fibrinogen	>100 mg/dL	≤100 mg/dL	

Sum the points for each of the four categories to determine the clinical probability of having DIC: compatible with overt DIC ≥5 points, and suggestive of nonovert DIC <5 points.
DIC, disseminated intravascular coagulation.
Data from Taylor FB Jr, Toh CH, Hoots WK, et al. Towards definition, clinical and laboratory criteria, and a scoring system for disseminated intravascular coagulation. *Thromb Haemost.* 2001;86(5):1327-1330 and Bakhtiari K, Meijers JC, de Jonge E, Levi M. Prospective validation of the International Society of Thrombosis and Haemostasis scoring system for disseminated intravascular coagulation. *Crit Care Med.* 2004;32(12):2416-2421.

TREATMENT

Treatment of DIC consists of supportive care and correction of the underlying disorder if possible. **FFP**, **cryoprecipitate**, and **platelets** can be administered when needed clinically (e.g., bleeding or surgery), rather than strictly based on a laboratory threshold. Despite the coagulopathy, patients who have large-vessel venous or arterial thrombi should undergo anticoagulation if they do not have other contraindications. Nonbleeding patients who have DIC should receive thromboprophylaxis with heparin.

Acquired Inhibitors of Coagulation Factors

GENERAL PRINCIPLES

Acquired inhibitors of coagulation factors may occur de novo (autoantibodies) or may develop in hemophiliacs (alloantibodies) following factor VIII or IX infusions. Of the acquired **inhibitors, those directed against factor VIII occur most commonly**. De novo inhibitors often arise in patients who have underlying lymphoproliferative or autoimmune disorders.

DIAGNOSIS

Patients who have a factor VIII inhibitor typically present with an abrupt onset of bleeding or bruising, a prolonged aPTT that does not correct after 1:1 mixing with normal plasma, a markedly decreased factor VIII activity, and a normal PT. Patients rarely develop autoantibodies that inhibit other factors (II, V, X) and subsequently prolong aPTT and PT, which do not correct after mixing studies.

TREATMENT

- **rFVIIa (NovoSeven) or aPCC,** used in a similar manner as for hemophiliacs who have alloantibodies to factor VIII (see Inherited Bleeding Disorders section), treats bleeding problems.
- **Recombinant porcine factor VIII (OBI-1)** lacks the B domain allowing low cross-reactivity to anti-Factor VIII antibodies. In addition, efficacy can be monitored with Factor VIII activity levels in conjunction with clinical evaluation. In an initial trial of patients with acquired hemophilia A, bleeding control was achieved in 86% of patients.[47]
- **Immunosuppression** with rituximab,[48] prednisone, or prednisolone ± cyclophosphamide[49] can eradicate inhibitors.

VENOUS THROMBOEMBOLIC DISORDERS

Approach to Venous Thromboembolism

GENERAL PRINCIPLES

Definition

- **Thrombosis** refers to a blood clot that occur in veins, arteries, or chambers of the heart.
- **VTE** refers to **deep vein thrombosis (DVT)** and/or **pulmonary embolism (PE).**
- **Thrombophlebitis** consists of inflammation in a vein due to a blood clot.
- **Superficial venous thrombophlebitis** refers to thrombosis in a nondeep vein.

Classification

- The anatomic location of DVT/PE, clot burden, and sequelae may affect prognosis and treatment recommendations.
- DVT can be **proximal** or **distal.**
  - **Proximal lower extremity DVTs** occur in the deep venous system at or more proximal to the popliteal vein (or the confluence of tibial and peroneal veins); **distal lower extremity DVTs** occur more distally in the tibial or peroneal veins.
  - **Proximal upper extremity DVTs** occur in the subclavian, brachiocephalic, axillary, and brachial veins, whereas **distal upper extremity DVTs** occur in the cephalic or basilic veins.
  - **Other** important venous thromboses sites include the vena cava (superior and inferior), abdominal veins (hepatic, portal, superior mesenteric, and splenic), pelvic veins (iliac, ovarian, penile), retinal veins, and cerebral veins, and cavernous sinus.
- The anatomic location of a **PE** in the pulmonary arterial system characterizes it as **central/proximal** (main, lobar, or segmental) or **distal** (subsegmental or smaller).
- **PE severity classification** may refer to **cardiovascular dysfunction** variables that define **submassive PE** (e.g., right ventricular [**RV**] strain, RV dysfunction, elevated troponin, elevated NT-proBNP) or **massive PE** (systemic hypotension). Severity classification may also include a risk (of short-term mortality or poor outcome) score that incorporates clinical variables (Table 20-5).

Epidemiology

- Without treatment, half of patients with proximal lower extremity DVT develop PE.
- DVTs in the upper extremities often occur with an indwelling catheter and may cause PE.
- Untreated acute symptomatic PE has a 10%–30% short-term mortality.[51]

TABLE 20-5	European Society of Cardiology Mortality Risk Classification of Patients Who Have Acute Pulmonary Embolism			
Risk Parameters and Scores				
Early Mortality Risk	Shock or Hypotension	PESI Class III–V or sPESI ≥1	Signs of RV Dysfunction on an Imaging Test[a]	Cardiac Laboratory Biomarkers[b]
High	+	(+)[c]	+	(+)[c]
Intermediate-high	–	+	Both positive	
Intermediate-low	–	+	Either one (or none) positive[d]	
Low	–	–	Assessment optional; if assessed, both negative[d]	

sPESI, Simplified Pulmonary Embolism Severity Index, which assigns 1 point each for: age > 80 years, cancer, chronic cardiopulmonary disease, HR ≥ 110, systolic BP < 100, and O_2 saturation < 90%.[50]

LV, left ventricle; RV, right ventricle.

[a]Echocardiographic criteria of RV dysfunction include RV dilation and/or an increased end-diastolic RV–LV diameter ratio (e.g., ≥1), hypokinesis of the free RV wall, or increased velocity of the tricuspid regurgitation jet. CT angiography criterion for RV dysfunction is an increased end-diastolic RV/LV diameter ratio (e.g., ≥1.0).

[b]Elevations in N-terminal pro-BNP or high-sensitivity troponin I or T.

[c]Classify shock or hypotension as high risk.

[d]Classify low-risk PESI (Class I–II) or sPESI patients (score of 0) who have elevated cardiac biomarkers or signs of RV dysfunction on imaging tests.

Adapted from Konstantinides SV, Meyer G, Becattini C, et al.; ESC Scientific Document Group. 2019 ESC Guidelines for the diagnosis and management of acute pulmonary embolism developed in collaboration with the European Respiratory Society (ERS). *Eur Heart J.* 2020;41(4):543-603. doi:10.1093/eurheartj/ehz405. PMID: 31504429.

- Patients who have hemodynamic instability associated with acute PE have a >15% risk of death in the subsequent 30 days, despite treatment.
- Patients who have acute PE without shock or hypotension but with signs of right ventricular dysfunction or myocardial injury have a 3%–15% 30-day mortality risk.
- Patients who have acute symptomatic PE with normal blood pressure and RV function have a 30-day mortality risk of <1%, low-risk.
- The 3-month mortality after the initiation of anticoagulant therapy in low-risk patients averages around 2%.[52]

Etiology

- Venous thromboemboli arise under conditions of **blood stasis**, **hypercoagulability** (changes in the soluble and formed elements of the blood), or venous **endothelial dysfunction/injury (Virchow's triad).**
- Hypercoagulable states may have an **inherited** or **acquired** etiology (see Risk Factors section).

- VTEs are classified as **provoked or unprovoked**, where provoked are attributed to an identifiable risk factor (e.g., surgery, oral contraception, pregnancy, immobility) and unprovoked have no identifiable cause.
- **Superficial thrombophlebitis** occurs in association with IVs, varicose veins, trauma, infection, and hypercoagulable disorders.

Risk Factors

- Risk factors for VTE can be categorized as **inherited, acquired, or unknown.**
- **Inherited thrombophilia** are suggested by spontaneous/unprovoked VTE at a young age (<50 years), recurrent (especially unprovoked) VTE, VTE in first-degree relatives, or thrombosis in unusual anatomic locations (i.e., abdominal).
- The most common inherited risk factors for VTE include gene mutations (**factor V Leiden and prothrombin gene G20210A**) and deficiencies of the natural anticoagulants **protein C, protein S, and AT.**
- **Homocystinuria**, a rare autosomal recessive disorder caused by deficiency of cystathionine-β-synthase, leads to extremely high plasma homocysteine and causes early-onset arterial and venous thromboembolic events. However, mild elevation of homocysteine may be caused by a mutation in methylenetetrahydrofolate reductase (**MTHFR**) but does not cause VTE. Therefore, thrombophilia testing should not include *MTHFR* mutation testing.
- **Spontaneous/unprovoked VTE in unusual locations**, such as cavernous sinus, mesenteric vein, or portal vein, may be the initial presentation of paroxysmal nocturnal hemoglobinuria (**PNH**) or myeloproliferative disorders (JAK2 mutation).
- **Spontaneous (unprovoked) VTEs** have a high risk of recurrence (8%–10% per year) after stopping anticoagulant therapy, regardless of the presence of an inherited thrombophilia.
- **Acquired hypercoagulable** states may arise secondary to malignancy, immobilization, infection, trauma, surgery, collagen vascular diseases, nephrotic syndrome, HIT, DIC, medications (e.g., estrogen), and pregnancy.
- Acquired **autoantibodies** associated with HIT and antiphospholipid syndrome (**APS**) can cause arterial or venous thrombi.
- **APS** is a hypercoagulable disorder that requires the presence of at least one clinical **and** one laboratory criterion.[53]
  - **APS clinical criteria:**
    - **Unprovoked** arterial or venous thrombosis in any tissue or organ *or*
    - **Pregnancy** morbidity of (1) unexplained late fetal death, (2) premature birth complicated by eclampsia, preeclampsia, placental insufficiency, or (3) ≥ three unexplained consecutive spontaneous abortions at <10 weeks of gestation or one at ≥10 weeks.
  - **APS laboratory criteria:** Presence of autoantibodies such as **lupus anticoagulant (LA)**, anticardiolipin, or β₂-glycoprotein-1 antibodies. Do not test for LA while the patient is on a DOAC because of the high risk of a false negative test result.[54]
    - LAs may prolong the aPTT or PT/INR without predisposing to bleeding.
    - Approximately 10% of patients with SLE have an LA; however, most patients with an LA do not have SLE.
    - Confirmation of positive autoantibody tests (must be done at least 12 weeks apart).
  - APS may include **other features**, such as thrombocytopenia, valvular heart disease, livedo reticularis, neurologic manifestations, and nephropathy.

Prevention

Identifying patients at high risk for VTE and instituting prophylactic measures should remain a high priority (see Chapter 1, Inpatient Care in Internal Medicine).

DIAGNOSIS

Clinical Presentation

- **Lower or upper extremity DVT symptoms** commonly include **pain, edema, redness, and warmth.**
- **Superficial thrombophlebitis** presents as a tender, warm, erythematous, and palpable thrombosed vein. An accompanying DVT may produce pain and swelling.
- **Likelihood of a PE** increases in a patient suspected of having it in the setting of: history of VTE, active cancer, surgery or immobility in the past 4 weeks, certain medications (e.g., estrogen), hemoptysis, older age, abnormal vital signs (tachycardia and hypoxia), signs and symptoms of DVT, or high suspicion of PE by the clinician (e.g., sudden onset of shortness of breath, hemoptysis, and pleuritic chest pain).[55,56]

Differential Diagnosis

- The **differential diagnoses of lower extremity DVT** include cellulitis, Baker cyst (behind knee), hematoma, venous insufficiency, postphlebitic syndrome, lymphedema, sarcoma, arterial aneurysm, myositis, rupture of the gastrocnemius, and abscess.
- **Symmetric, bilateral lower extremity edema** suggests heart, renal, or liver failure as the cause of the signs and symptoms, but it does not exclude the presence of DVT.
- The **differential diagnosis of PE** based on the presenting symptoms (e.g., chest pain, dyspnea, hemoptysis) or signs (e.g., hypoxemia, pleural effusion, pulmonary infiltrate) includes dissecting aortic aneurysm, pneumonia, acute bronchitis, pericardial or pleural disease, heart failure, costochondritis, rib fracture, and myocardial ischemia.

Diagnostic Testing

Clinical Probability Assessment

- **Clinical decision rules** help to exclude VTE when used in combination with other diagnostic tests (such as normal D-dimer).
  - **Clinical predictors of DVT** from **Wells criteria** include: history of DVT, paralysis/paresis/immobilization of the leg, recently bedridden, major surgery within 4 weeks, active cancer, leg vein tenderness, swelling of entire leg, calf diameter > 3 cm larger than other calf, pitting edema confined to symptomatic leg, dilated collateral superficial leg veins, and alternative diagnoses less likely than DVT. Outpatients who have one or fewer of these predictors (i.e., low Wells score) are unlikely to have a DVT.[57]
  - **Pretest assessment of the probability of a DVT** provides useful information when combined with the results of a **venous compression ultrasound, a D-dimer test**, or both, in determining whether to exclude or accept the diagnosis of DVT or to perform additional imaging studies.[57]
- **Validated clinical risk factors for a PE in outpatients who present to an emergency department** include signs and symptoms of DVT, high clinical suspicion of

PE (e.g., recent surgery or COVID-19 infection), tachycardia, immobility in the past 4 weeks, history of VTE, active cancer, hemoptysis,[58] and lack of an alternative diagnosis that is at least as likely as PE. Patients who have one or fewer of these predictors (i.e., a low **simplified Wells score**) are unlikely to have a PE.

- The combination of a **low (simplified) Wells score and a normal D-dimer** essentially rules out a PE.[59]
- A normal D-dimer and a negative chest CT essentially rule out PE, and a lower extremity compression ultrasound does not typically assist further with ruling in or out the presence of a PE.[60]

Laboratories
- **D-dimer** and fibrin degradation products may increase during VTE.
  - Since multiple conditions may elevate D-dimer, it has a low positive predictive value (**PPV**) and specificity for VTE; **patients with suspected VTE and an elevated D-dimer require further diagnostic testing.**
  - A **sensitive quantitative D-dimer assay** has a high enough NPV to exclude a **DVT** when the **objectively defined clinical probability** is low and/or a **noninvasive test** is negative.[61,62] In the setting of a moderate to high clinical pretest probability (e.g., patients with cancer or COVID-19), a negative D-dimer does not have sufficient NPV to exclude a DVT or PE,[63,64] so D-dimer testing is not useful in this setting.
  - Compared to a **fixed D-dimer cutoff of 500 µg/L**, an **upward age adjustment of the cutoff (age × 10 in patients at least age 50 years)** will increase the number of patients who can have PE excluded based on the combination of nonelevated D-dimer and objective clinical probability assessment (i.e., low-intermediate or unlikely pretest probability).[65]
- In the setting of **spontaneous VTE in unusual sites and hemolytic anemia**, use peripheral blood flow cytometry to assess for **PNH.**

Imaging
- **DVT-specific testing**
  - Initial diagnostic imaging for suspected acute DVT almost exclusively consists of **venous compression ultrasound (CUS),**[66] called **duplex examination** when performed with Doppler testing,[67] although some other diagnostic options include magnetic resonance venography, **CT** venography, and venography.
    - CUS has a high sensitivity in **symptomatic** patients and a low sensitivity in **asymptomatic** patients.
    - CUS has a low sensitivity for detecting **distal DVT,** and it may fail to visualize parts of the upper extremity venous system, iliac veins, or pelvic veins.
    - CUS may have difficulty distinguishing between acute and **chronic** DVT.
    - **Lower extremity venous CUS** may help diagnose or exclude VTE in patients who have suspected PE and a nondiagnostic ventilation/perfusion (**V/Q**) scan, a nondiagnostic or negative chest CT with high suspicion of PE, or a contraindication to or difficulty completing imaging for PE (see PE-specific testing section).
  - **Serial testing** can improve the diagnostic yield of CUS. If a patient with a clinically suspected lower extremity DVT has a negative initial ultrasound and no satisfactory alternative explanation, one can withhold anticoagulant therapy and **repeat testing** at least once 3–14 days later.
  - Patients who have **superficial venous thrombosis should undergo venous CUS testing** because of the high risk of having concomitant DVT.[68]

- **Acute PE-specific testing**
  - ○ **CT pulmonary angiogram**
    - Chest CT pulmonary angiography requires IV administration of iodinated contrast. Thus, contraindications to CT angiogram include renal dysfunction and dye allergy. For patients with a contraindication to CT, consider using MR pulmonary angiography or V/Q scan.[69]
    - The sensitivity of CT pulmonary angiography for PE improves by combining CT results with objective grading of clinical suspicion.
    - **Clinical suspicion discordant with the objective test finding** (e.g., high suspicion with a negative CT scan or low suspicion with a positive CT scan) **should lead to further testing.**
    - Advantages of CT scan over V/Q scan when assessing for PE include fewer indeterminate studies and the ability to assess for alternative or concomitant diagnoses, such as dissecting aortic aneurysm, pneumonia, and malignancy.[70]
    - For patients who have a contraindication to CT, a lower extremity venous compression ultrasound can be helpful, because proximal DVT may serve as a surrogate for the diagnosis of PE.
  - ○ **V/Q scan**
    - V/Q scans administer radioactive material (via inhaled and IV routes).
    - V/Q scans are classified as **normal, nondiagnostic** (i.e., very low probability, low probability, intermediate probability), or **high probability** for PE.
    - V/Q scans are most useful in patients who have a normal CXR because nondiagnostic V/Q scans commonly occur in the setting of an abnormal CXR.
    - Use of **clinical suspicion** improves the accuracy of V/Q scanning, resulting in a NPV of 96% for low pretest clinical suspicion of PE and a normal V/Q scan result, and a PPV of 96% for high pretest suspicion of PE and a high-probability V/Q scan result.[71]
  - ○ **Pulmonary angiography**
    - Angiography requires placement of a pulmonary artery catheter, infusion of IV contrast, and exposure to radiation.
    - Contraindications to angiography include renal dysfunction and dye allergy.
    - Less invasive tests (i.e., CT angiography) with similar or better diagnostic accuracy have mostly replaced pulmonary angiography for acute PE diagnostic testing.
    - **Electrocardiogram, troponin and brain natriuretic peptide (BNP) levels, arterial blood gas, CXR, and echocardiogram** may to help assess clinical probability of PE, cardiopulmonary reserve, and potential to benefit from thrombolysis (see thrombolytic therapy in Medications section), but these tests do not rule out or rule in PE, with the exception of seeing an intracardiac clot with echocardiography.
    - **Studies do not support extensive screening for an associated occult malignancy** in patients with a first, unprovoked VTE.[72] However, such patients should undergo a comprehensive history and physical examination, routine blood work, age- and gender-appropriate cancer screening, and specific cancer screening tests indicated for distinct populations (e.g., chest CT to search for lung cancer in those age 50 or older with a history of smoking).

TREATMENT

- **VTE therapy** should aim to prevent recurrent VTE, consequences of VTE (i.e., postphlebitic syndrome [i.e., pain, edema, and ulceration], pulmonary arterial hypertension, and death), and complications of therapy (e.g., bleeding).

- Clinicians should perform standard laboratory tests (i.e., CBC, PT/INR, and aPTT) and assess bleeding risk before starting an anticoagulant.
- Unless contraindications exist, **initial treatment of VTE should consist of anticoagulation** with IV UFH, SC LMWH, SC pentasaccharide (fondaparinux), or a rapid-onset DOAC (see **Medications**).

Medications

- **Anticoagulants, oral**
  - **Direct oral anticoagulants** (DOACs) (Table 20-6) have one of two primary mechanisms of action: **thrombin inhibition** (dabigatran) or **Xa inhibition** (rivaroxaban, apixaban, edoxaban, and betrixaban).
    - As compared to warfarin, DOACs have more rapid onset, wider therapeutic window, and more predictable pharmacokinetics. These features allow patients with a new VTE to begin apixaban or rivaroxaban immediately, without the need for an overlapping parenteral agent. In contrast, dabigatran and edoxaban require at least 5 days of initial parenteral anticoagulation if prescribed for a new VTE. None of the DOACs need INR monitoring or dose adjustments in patients with normal renal function, but the initial dose of some DOACs for a new VTE is higher than the maintenance dose (rivaroxaban 15 mg twice daily for 3 weeks then 20 mg daily, or apixaban 10 mg daily twice daily then 5 mg twice daily).

TABLE 20-6	Anticoagulants for Treatment of Venous Thromboembolism (VTE)			
Anticoagulant	Mechanism of Action	Initial Treatment Dose(s)	Extended Duration Dose	Contraindications[a]
Parental Agents				
Dalteparin[b]	FXa > FIIa inhibition	200 IU/kg SC daily	150 IU/kg SC daily	HIT; sensitivity to pork
Enoxaparin	FXa > FIIa inhibition	1 mg/kg SC q12h *or* 1.5 mg/kg SC q24h; lower dose if CrCl < 30 mL/min	1 mg/kg SC q12h *or* 1.5 mg/kg SC q24h; lower doses if CrCl <30 mL/min	HIT; sensitivity to pork
Fondaparinux	Binds to antithrombin, primarily inhibiting FXa	Weight < 50 kg: 5 mg SC daily Weight 50–100 kg: 7.5 mg SC daily Weight > 100 kg: 10 mg SC daily	NA	CrCl < 30 mL/min

(continued)

TABLE 20-6	Anticoagulants for Treatment of Venous Thromboembolism (VTE) *(continued)*			
Anticoagulant	Mechanism of Action	Initial Treatment Dose(s)	Extended Duration Dose	Contraindications[a]
Heparin (UFH)	Binds to antithrombin	Continuous IV: Goal aPTT 2.0–2.5× normal range	NA	HIT; sensitivity to pork
Tinzaparin[c]	FXa > FIIa inhibition	175 IU/kg SC daily	NA	HIT, not available in US
Oral Agents				
Apixaban	Direct FXa inhibitor	10 mg bid × 7 d, then 5 mg daily	2.5 or 5 mg bid	Pregnancy
Dabigatran	Direct thrombin (FIIa) inhibitor	Initially treat with parenteral anticoagulant for ≥5	150 mg bid (CrCl > 30 mL/min)	Pregnancy, CrCl < 30 mL/min
Edoxaban	Direct FXa inhibitor	Initially treat with parenteral anticoagulant for ≥5 d	30 or 60 mg daily (depending on CrCl, body weight, and use of P-gp inhibitor)	Pregnancy
Rivaroxaban	Direct FXa inhibitor	15 mg bid × 21 d, then 20 mg daily	10 or 20 mg daily;	Pregnancy, CrCl < 30 mL/min
Warfarin	Vitamin K antagonist	2–10 mg (see www.warfarin-dosing.org); overlapped for ≥5 d with a faster-acting anticoagulant	Adjusted per INR	1st trimester of pregnancy

aPTT, activated partial thromboplastin time; CrCl, creatinine clearance; FIIa, factor IIa; FXa, factor Xa; HIT, heparin-induced thrombocytopenia; INR, international normalized ratio; P-gp, P-glycoprotein.

[a]Invasive procedures (e.g., neuraxial anesthesia), bleeding, and bleeding diathesis (e.g., thrombocytopenia) are contraindications to all anticoagulants.
[b]FDA-approved only for VTE in cancer patients.
[c]Not available in the United States.

- Compared to warfarin, DOACs have a lower risk of intracranial hemrrhage.[73]
- Issues of concern include the risk of thrombosis due to missed doses and increased bleeding risk due to severe renal dysfunction. DOACs are not recommended in patients who have triple positive APS given their increased risk of arterial thromboses when compared to warfarin.
  - **Warfarin, an oral anticoagulant,** inhibits reduction of vitamin K to its active form, which leads to decreased synthesis of and subsequent depletion of the vitamin K–dependent clotting factors II, VII, IX, and X, and proteins C, S, and Z.
    - **Treatment of DVT/PE with warfarin requires overlap therapy with a parenteral anticoagulant** (UFH, LMWH, or pentasaccharide) for at least 4–5 days and until the INR reaches 2.0 or higher.[74] For DVT/PE, use a **target INR** range of 2–3.
    - The **starting dose** of warfarin depends on many factors and ranges from 2 to 4 mg in older or petite patients to 10 mg in young, robust patients (www.warfarindosing.org). Patients with known polymorphisms in genes for cytochrome P450 2C9 or vitamin K epoxide reductase (*VKORC1*) benefit from lower-dose warfarin initiation.[75]
    - Warfarin dosing adjustments depend on INR results.
    - Warfarin is teratogenic during the first trimester.
    - For outpatients **starting warfarin, INR monitoring** can be once or twice weekly initially with the interval between INRs gradually lengthening to monthly once the dose is stable.
    - **Warfarin dose adjustments** after the first few weeks of therapy typically change the weekly dose by 10%–25%.
    - Starting or discontinuing **medications that affect warfarin metabolism or binding**, especially amiodarone, certain antibiotics (e.g., rifampin, sulfamethoxazole), or antifungal drugs (e.g., fluconazole), should trigger more frequent INR monitoring and may require dose adjustments.
    - In eligible patients, home INR monitoring may improve INR control and patient satisfaction.[76]
- **Anticoagulants, parenteral**
  - **UFH** indirectly inactivates thrombin and factor Xa via AT.
    - At usual doses, UFH prolongs aPTT and thrombin time, and may mildly prolong the PT/INR.
    - Because the anticoagulant effects of UFH normalize within hours of discontinuation, and **protamine sulfate** reverses it even faster, UFH is the anticoagulant of choice during initial therapy for patients with a high risk of bleeding or those who will likely undergo an invasive procedure (e.g., **ICU patients**).
    - For **therapeutic anticoagulation for VTE**, UFH is usually administered IV with a bolus (e.g., 80 units/kg after a VTE) followed by continuous infusion (e.g., 18 units/kg/h) that has a dose titration based on standard protocols (i.e., heparin nomogram), usually to a goal aPTT of 2- to 2.5-fold of normal range (Table 20-6).
    - UFH is the anticoagulant of choice for inpatients with a mechanical heart valve who need **bridging** of anticoagulation.
  - **LMWHs,** produced by chemical or enzymatic cleavage of UFH, indirectly inactivate thrombin and factor Xa via AT.
    - LMWHs minimally prolong the aPTT.
    - LMWH treatment does not require Factor Xa monitoring, except in special circumstances: renal dysfunction, morbid obesity, or pregnancy.[77] Therapeutic

anticoagulation will have a peak factor Xa level, measured 4 hours after a dose, of 0.6–1.0 IU/mL for q12h dosing and 1–2 IU/mL for q24h dosing.[78]

- Different LMWH preparations have different dosing recommendations (Table 20-6). The usual prophylactic dose of enoxaparin is 40 mg SC daily. However, higher doses are more effective among inpatients with obesity such as BMI > 40 kg/m². Higher doses (e.g., enoxaparin 1 mg/kg twice daily) can be used for thromboprophylaxis among noncritically ill patients with COVID.[79]
- Given their **renal clearance**, LMWHs are generally avoided in patients with creatinine clearance (CrCl) <10 mL/min, and they should be dose-adjusted in patients who have a CrCl of 10–30 mL/min (e.g., enoxaparin 1 mg/kg daily instead of 1 mg/kg twice daily).
- **Pregnant** women (without artificial heart valves) who have VTE should be treated with LMWH.
- **Patients with cancer and VTE** should receive anticoagulation for more than 3 months and until cancer resolution or development of a contraindication.[80,81] They can be treated with **LMWHs** (e.g., with dalteparin (200 IU/kg SC daily × 1 month, then 150 IU/kg SC daily),[82] or a **DOAC**: apixaban (10 mg twice daily for the first 7 days, followed by 5 mg twice daily),[83] edoxaban (60 mg p.o. daily),[84] or rivaroxaban (15 mg twice daily for the first 21 days, then 20 mg daily).[85] Although warfarin (INR 2–3) has similar mortality to LMWHs and DOACs in patients with cancer and VTE, warfarin has higher rates of recurrent VTE.[86]

○ **Fondaparinux,** a synthetic pentasaccharide, indirectly inhibits factor Xa via AT.
  - The fondaparinux dose for VTE ranges from 5 to 10 mg SC daily.[87] (Table 20-6).
  - Similar to the LMWHs, factor Xa monitoring is not used routinely, and fondaparinux undergoes renal clearance.
  - Though not FDA-approved for use with suspected immunologic HIT, fondaparinux also is used in this setting.[88]

○ **Argatroban** is a synthetic direct thrombin inhibitor used for immunologic **HIT** therapy.
  - Argatroban has a half-life of <1 hour, and a reversal agent is not available.
  - Argatroban is infused IV at an initial rate of ≤2 μg/kg/min. Special populations require lower initial infusion rates: patients with recent cardiac surgery, heart failure, hepatic dysfunction, or anasarca.[89]
  - aPTT monitoring should occur 2 hours after beginning the infusion, and the infusion rate should undergo adjustment to achieve a therapeutic aPTT (1.5–3.0 times the baseline aPTT).
  - Once the platelet count has recovered, before conversion to warfarin, argatroban therapy should be overlapped with warfarin therapy for at least 5 days and until a therapeutic INR due to warfarin is achieved.
  - INR monitoring during argatroban and warfarin coadministration may cause confusion; for an INR > 4, discontinue argatroban, remeasure the INR within 4–6 hours, and then restart the argatroban (and adjust the warfarin dose).

○ **Bivalirudin** is a direct thrombin inhibitor with an indication for treatment of immunologic **HIT** in the setting of percutaneous coronary intervention in patients receiving ASA.
  - Bivalirudin has a half-life of 25 minutes in patients with normal renal function.
  - Bivalirudin requires reduction of the infusion rate in patients with renal insufficiency.
  - Bivalirudin dosing for HIT should start at a rate of 0.15–0.20 mg/kg/h IV with titration to a target aPTT 1.5–2.5 times baseline.[24,90]

- aPTT monitoring during bivalirudin therapy should occur 2 hours after a dose change.
- The interpretation of the INRs in patients receiving warfarin must consider the increased PT/INR caused by bivalirudin.

- **Thrombolytic therapy**
  - In the life-threatening situation of an acute PE associated with shock or persistent hypotension from RV overload, rapid reperfusion treatment and cardiorespiratory support relieves the RV overload and prevents hemodynamic deterioration.
  - Thrombolytic therapy (e.g., alteplase or recombinant tissue plasminogen activator [rtPA] as a 100-mg IV infusion over 2 hours) is indicated for patients who have **hemodynamically unstable ("massive") PE** who do not have a contraindication (e.g., a high risk of bleeding).[91-93]
  - Patients receiving anticoagulation for acute PE who subsequently have a **cardiac arrest from PE-associated RV failure or a suspected PE recurrence** may benefit from thrombolytic therapy,[92,93] such as a (non-FDA-approved) 50 mg IV bolus dose of rtPA[91] or a (non–FDA-approved) tPA dose of 10 mg IV bolus followed by drip of 40 mg IV over 15–30 minutes.
  - In patients who have **high intermediate-risk/submassive PE**, fibrinolytic therapy prevents hemodynamic decompensation but increases the risk of intracranial hemorrhage/stroke.[91,94,95]
  - **Thrombolytic therapy** (administered either IV or by catheter-directed thrombolysis) **for DVT** increases the risk of hemorrhage and does not prevent postthrombotic syndrome, with the possible exception of patients who have **massive iliofemoral DVT.**[96]

- **Duration of anticoagulation for DVT or PE**
  - An individual's risk of recurrent VTE, risk of hemorrhage, risk of adverse outcomes, and preferences should determine the duration of anticoagulation.
  - For treatment of provoked proximal DVT or provoked PE occurring in the setting of a surgical or nonsurgical (e.g., immobility, pregnancy) transient risk factor, 3 months of anticoagulation is sufficient because these events have low recurrence risk (≤2% per year).[93]
  - For **unprovoked PE**, we recommend anticoagulation for >3 months in patients with low to moderate risk of bleeding.[81,93,97]
  - Patients with **cancer and VTE** should continue anticoagulation until cancer resolution or development of a contraindication.[80,81]
  - For patients with a **first VTE and an inherited hypercoagulable risk factor**, consider an extended anticoagulation duration:
    - **Heterozygous factor V Leiden or heterozygous prothrombin 20210A** only modestly increases the odds of recurrence (relative risk, 1.6 and 1.4, respectively), so recommendation for anticoagulation duration should not change based on these.
    - **Deficiency of protein S, protein C, or AT** carries a high risk of recurrence; long-term anticoagulation is recommended.
    - **APS or two inherited risk factors** have a very high risk of recurrence, so indefinite anticoagulation is recommended.
  - Patients with **recurrent unprovoked VTE** should receive long-term anticoagulation, unless a contraindication develops.[81,97]
  - **Long-term anticoagulation after an unprovoked VTE** reduces the risk of recurrence but increases the risk hemorrhage in comparison to short-term anticoagulation.
    - The relative risk reduction of VTE depends on the secondary thromboprophylaxis: it is 32% with low-dose ASA.[98,99] More effective therapies are: rivaroxaban

20 mg or 10 mg daily,[100] apixaban 5 or 2.5 mg twice daily,[101] dabigatran 150 mg twice daily,[100,102] warfarin (target INR 2–3), or LMWH.
  ○ Effective LMWHs for extended secondary prophylaxis include **enoxaparin** (1.5 mg/kg daily or 1 mg/kg twice daily) and **dalteparin** 150 IU/kg daily.
• **Nonpharmacologic therapies**
  ○ **Leg elevation** reduces edema associated with DVT.
  ○ **Ambulation** is encouraged for patients with DVT, for improvement of pain and edema.
  ○ **Fitted below-the-knee graduated compression stockings** can reduce swelling after DVT, but do not prevent DVT recurrence, and the reduction of postthrombotic syndrome is controversial.[103]
  ○ **Inferior vena cava (IVC) filters** can be placed for acute VTEs when there are absolute contraindications to anticoagulation (e.g., bleeding). When transient contraindications resolve, patients should undergo full-dose anticoagulation.
  ○ Prophylactic IVC filters in patients with acute VTE reduce the short-term risk of nonfatal PE, but they do not decrease mortality, and they increase DVT recurrence.[104]
  If IVC filters are used, **temporary/retrievable IVC filters** should be used, and they should be removed when no longer indicated.

Surgical Management

Surgical Embolectomy
• Surgical embolectomy has a role in patients who have massive/high-risk PE and a contraindication to thrombolytic therapy or a failure to respond to thrombolytic therapy. Depending on center expertise, **catheter-based interventions** should be considered as a potential alternative option to surgical embolectomy.[98]
• Patients who have a **right heart thrombus that straddles the interatrial septum** via a patent foramen ovale/atrial septal defect should be considered for surgical embolectomy.[105]
• Embolectomy for **free-floating right heart thrombus** remains controversial.[106]

SPECIAL CONSIDERATIONS

Anticoagulant Bridging

• **Perioperative management of anticoagulation** requires coordination with the surgical service (see Perioperative Medicine in Chapter 1) to address timing of interventions and therapeutic changes with the aim of VTE and bleeding prevention.
• **Invasive procedures** usually require discontinuation of anticoagulation.
  ○ For patients receiving warfarin, stop the warfarin therapy 4–5 days before the invasive procedure.
  ○ BRIDGE study showed that in patients with atrial fibrillation who had warfarin treatment interrupted for an elective procedure, forgoing bridging anticoagulation was noninferior to perioperative bridging with LMWH for the prevention of arterial thromboembolism and decreased the risk of major bleeding.[107]
  ○ In situations where a clinician aims to minimize the patient's time off therapeutic anticoagulation (such as mechanical valve or APS), initiate parenteral anticoagulation (IV UFH or LMWH) when the INR becomes subtherapeutic, stop the parenteral anticoagulation 6–12 hours before the procedure, and resume anticoagulation as soon as hemostasis and bleeding risk reach an acceptable level, typically within 24 hours.[108]

- PAUSE regimen (including holding the DOAC 1 day before a low–bleeding-risk procedure and 2 days before a high–bleeding-risk procedure) is recommended for patients with AF on DOACs that requires interruption of anticoagulation.[109]
- Studies are needed to address the risks and benefits of anticoagulation for **isolated subsegmental PE.**
- **Upper extremity acute DVT** should receive standard-duration (e.g., 3 months) anticoagulation.[110] DVT associated with a functioning central venous catheter does not require catheter removal, but anticoagulation should continue as long as the catheter remains in place.
- **Isolated calf acute DVT** without symptoms or risk factors for extension may undergo serial imaging in 1–2 weeks instead of anticoagulation. Otherwise, treat with 6–12 weeks of anticoagulation.[111]
- **Superficial vein thrombophlebitis (SVT)**
  - **Small SVTs (<5 cm in length)** and SVT associated with IV infusion therapy do not require anticoagulation; treatment consists of oral NSAIDs and warm compresses.
  - Treatment of **extensive SVT (e.g., >5 cm in length)** with fondaparinux (2.5 mg SC daily for 45 days)[68] or rivaroxaban 10 mg daily[112] decreases the incidence of SVT recurrence, SVT extension, and VTE but increases the risk of bleeding.[113]
  - **Recurrent SVT** may be treated with anticoagulation or vein stripping.[113]
- **Chronic PE** occurs in 2%–4% of patients with PE,[114] and patients with this disorder should undergo evaluation for chronic thromboembolic pulmonary hypertension (**CTEPH**). Additionally, patients who have PH associated with acute PE should undergo evaluation for resolution of PH. Continued PH should lead to further testing (e.g., V/Q scan). Those diagnosed with CTEPH should undergo extended-duration anticoagulation, consideration of **riociguat** therapy,[115] and evaluation for possible pulmonary **thromboendarterectomy.**

COMPLICATIONS

- **Bleeding** is the major complication of anticoagulation.
  - Patients taking anticoagulants have a major bleeding rate of 1%–3% per year.
  - Concomitant use of **antiplatelet agents** increases the risk of bleeding. Major bleeding in patients taking antiplatelet agents can be treated with DDAVP (Desmopressin) 0.3–0.4 µg/kg IV.
  - Major bleeding after an acute VTE often leads to the discontinuation of anticoagulation and consideration of a temporary or permanent IVC filter. If the bleeding risk is resolved, the anticoagulant should be resumed and any temporary IVC filter can be retrieved.
- **Warfarin-associated INR elevation in asymptomatic patients**
  - For an asymptomatic minor INR elevation (INR < 5), hold or reduce the warfarin dose until the INR returns to a safe range, and then resume warfarin at a reduced dose.
  - For an asymptomatic moderate INR elevation 5 ≤ INR <10 in an asymptomatic patient, hold one or more warfarin doses. Oral vitamin K_1 is not needed for the INR to decline.[116]
  - For an asymptomatic severe INR elevation (INR ≥ 10), hold warfarin, consider checking for a spurious INR result, and consider treatment with vitamin K (e.g., oral vitamin K_1 2 mg).[117]

- **Bleeding with warfarin**
  - **For patients who have warfarin-associated bleeding and an elevated INR, give vitamin K replacement** PO or IV. IV vitamin K carries the risk of anaphylactoid reactions, so the oral route is preferred unless more rapid INR correction is necessary. With adequate replacement therapy, the INR will fall within 12 hours and normalize in 24–48 hours. Treat serious hemorrhage with IV vitamin K (10 mg) by slow infusion (over 30 minutes) and with IV 4-factor PCC (e.g., Kcentra 35 units of Factor IX/kg body weight [up to 3500 units]).[118] When 4-factor PCC is not available, use three-factor PCC and/or FFP (two or three units) Because of the long half-life of warfarin (approximately 36 hours), repeat the vitamin K treatment (e.g., oral vitamin K) every 8–12 hours to prevent INR rebound.
  - Although expensive and potentially thrombotic,[119] **rFVIIa** may stop life-threatening warfarin-associated (elevated INR) bleeding.
- **Bleeding with UFH, LMWH, and pentasaccharide**
  - Discontinuation usually sufficiently restores normal hemostasis.
  - With moderate to severe bleeding, **FFP** may reduce bleeding.
  - For patients receiving **UFH** who develop major bleeding, heparin can be completely reversed by infusion of **protamine sulfate** in situations where the potential benefits outweigh the risks (e.g., intracranial bleed, epidural hematoma, retinal bleed).
  - Approximately 1 mg of protamine sulfate IV neutralizes 100 units of heparin, up to a maximum dose of 250 mg. The dose can be given as a loading dose of 25–50 mg by slow IV injection over 10 minutes, with the rest of the dose over 12 hours.
  - For major bleeding associated with **LMWH**, protamine sulfate neutralizes only approximately 60% of LMWH.[120] Protamine does not reverse **pentasaccharide** (e.g., **fondaparinux**).
  - For patients with serious bleeding on fondaparinux, **aPCC** (20 IU/kg)[121] or **andexanet alfa** (see below) may be used.
- **Bleeding with direct oral anticoagulants (DOACs)**
  - **Reversal of dabigatran: Idarucizumab** (5 g IV) is a monoclonal antibody that binds to dabigatran with >350-fold affinity compared to thrombin and neutralizes its activity in minutes.[122] Because the majority of dabigatran remains unbound in plasma, hemodialysis can also decrease dabigatran concentration.
  - **Reversal of factor Xa inhibitors: Andexanet alfa (coagulation factor Xa inactivated-zhzo)** is a recombinant, modified human factor Xa decoy protein that binds and inactivates factor Xa inhibitors; it also inhibits tissue factor pathway inhibitor (TFPI), thus increasing tissue factor–associated thrombin generation.[123] Dosing includes a 400–800 mg bolus at 30 mg/min followed by followed by 4–8 mg/min for up to 120 min. Four-factor **PCC** (e.g., Kcentra 35 units of Factor IX/kg body weight [up to 3500 units]) can reverse bleeding from DOACs.[124]
- **Warfarin-induced skin necrosis**, associated with rapid depletion of protein C, may rarely occur (incidence <0.1%) during initiation of warfarin therapy.
  - Necrosis occurs most often in areas with a high percentage of adipose tissue, such as breast tissue, flank, hips, and thighs, and it can be life-threatening.
  - Therapeutic anticoagulation with an immediate-acting anticoagulant (e.g., UFH, LMWH) and/or avoiding "loading doses" of warfarin prevents warfarin-induced skin necrosis.

MONITORING/FOLLOW-UP

* For a suspicious clinical presentation, **testing for intrinsic hypercoagulable risk factors** should wait until the patient is in stable health and off anticoagulation therapy for at least 2 weeks (e.g., at the end of a standard course of treatment) **to avoid false-positive results** for nongenetic testing.
  ○ Although uncommon, if reasons exist to screen for hypercoagulable risk factors around the time of diagnosis, collect blood for **factor V Leiden and prothrombin gene mutations and LA.**
  ○ If done, blood collection for **protein C, protein S, and AT activity and antigen level** testing should occur while patients are not on anticoagulation and should be avoided in the setting of acute VTE. If testing occurs near the time of the acute VTE, normal protein C, protein S, and AT tests rule out congenital deficiencies, and abnormally low results require confirmation through repeat testing (or screening first-degree relatives).
  ○ Although **testing for PE in patients with DVT and testing for DVT in patients with PE** will produce many positive findings, such testing rarely affects therapy.
* **Outpatient therapy** is appropriate for most DVTs and for low-risk PEs.[125]

REFERENCES

1. Lippi G, Favaloro EJ, Franchini M, Guidi GC. Milestones and perspectives in coagulation and hemostasis. *Semin Thromb Hemost.* 2009;35(1):9-22. doi:10.1055/s-0029-1214144
2. Kirkwood TB. Calibration of reference thromboplastins and standardisation of the prothrombin time ratio. *Thromb Haemost.* 1983;49(3):238-244.
3. Cines DB, Bussel JB, Liebman HA, Luning Prak ET. The ITP syndrome: pathogenic and clinical diversity. *Blood.* 25 2009;113(26):6511-6521. doi:10.1182/blood-2009-01-129155
4. Terrell DR, Beebe LA, Vesely SK, Neas BR, Segal JB, George JN. The incidence of immune thrombocytopenic purpura in children and adults: a critical review of published reports. *American Journal of Hematology.* 2010;85(3):174-180. doi:10.1002/ajh.21616
5. Aster RH, Bougie DW. Drug-induced immune thrombocytopenia. *N Engl J Med.* 2007;357(6):580-587. doi:10.1056/NEJMra066469
6. Neunert C, Terrell DR, Arnold DM, et al. American Society of Hematology 2019 guidelines for immune thrombocytopenia. *Blood Adv.* 2019;3(23):3829-3866. doi:10.1182/bloodadvances.2019000966
7. Wei Y, Ji XB, Wang YW, et al. High-dose dexamethasone vs prednisone for treatment of adult immune thrombocytopenia: a prospective multicenter randomized trial. *Blood.* 2016;127(3):296-302; quiz 370. doi:10.1182/blood-2015-07-659656
8. Kuter DJ, Bussel JB, Lyons RM, et al. Efficacy of romiplostim in patients with chronic immune thrombocytopenic purpura: a double-blind randomised controlled trial. *Lancet.* 2008;371(9610):395-403. doi:10.1016/S0140-6736(08)60203-2
9. Cheng G, Saleh MN, Marcher C, et al. Eltrombopag for management of chronic immune thrombocytopenia (RAISE): a 6-month, randomised, phase 3 study. *Lancet.* 2011;377(9763):393-402. doi:10.1016/S0140-6736(10)60959-2
10. Jurczak W, Chojnowski K, Mayer J, et al. Phase 3 randomised study of avatrombopag, a novel thrombopoietin receptor agonist for the treatment of chronic immune thrombocytopenia. *Br J Haematol.* 2018;183(3):479-490. doi:10.1111/bjh.15573
11. Bussel J, Arnold DM, Grossbard E, et al. Fostamatinib for the treatment of adult persistent and chronic immune thrombocytopenia: results of two phase 3, randomized, placebo-controlled trials. *Am J Hematol.* 2018;93(7):921-930. doi:10.1002/ajh.25125
12. Terrell DR, Williams LA, Vesely SK, Lammle B, Hovinga JA, George JN. The incidence of thrombotic thrombocytopenic purpura-hemolytic uremic syndrome: all patients, idiopathic patients, and patients with severe ADAMTS-13 deficiency. *J Thromb Haemost.* 2005;3(7):1432-1436. doi:10.1111/j.1538-7836.2005.01436.x
13. Furlan M, Robles R, Galbusera M, et al. von Willebrand factor-cleaving protease in thrombotic thrombocytopenic purpura and the hemolytic-uremic syndrome. *N Engl J Med.* 1998;339(22):1578-1584. doi:10.1056/NEJM199811263392202
14. George JN. The thrombotic thrombocytopenic purpura and hemolytic uremic syndromes: overview of pathogenesis (Experience of the Oklahoma TTP-HUS Registry, 1989-2007). *Kidney Int Suppl.* 2009;2009(112):S8-S10. doi:10.1038/ki.2008.609

CHAPTER 20

15. Bendapudi PK, Hurwitz S, Fry A, et al. Derivation and external validation of the PLASMIC score for rapid assessment of adults with thrombotic microangiopathies: a cohort study. *Lancet Haematol.* 2017;4(4):e157-e164. doi:10.1016/S2352-3026(17)30026-1

16. Zheng XL, Vesely SK, Cataland SR, et al. ISTH guidelines for treatment of thrombotic thrombocytopenic purpura. *J Thromb Haemost.* 2020;18(10):2496-2502. doi:10.1111/jth.15010

17. Joly BS, Coppo P, Veyradier A. Thrombotic thrombocytopenic purpura. *Blood.* 2017;129(21):2836-2846. doi:10.1182/blood-2016-10-709857

18. Zwicker JI, Muia J, Dolatshahi L, et al. Adjuvant low-dose rituximab and plasma exchange for acquired TTP. *Blood.* 2019;134(13):1106-1109. doi:10.1182/blood.2019000795

19. Page EE, Kremer Hovinga JA, Terrell DR, Vesely SK, George JN. Rituximab reduces risk for relapse in patients with thrombotic thrombocytopenic purpura. *Blood.* 2016;127(24):3092-3094. doi:10.1182/blood-2016-03-703827

20. Scully M, Cataland SR, Peyvandi F, et al. Caplacizumab treatment for acquired thrombotic thrombocytopenic purpura. *N Engl J Med.* 2019;380(4):335-346. doi:10.1056/NEJMoa1806311

21. Licht C, Greenbaum LA, Muus P, et al. Efficacy and safety of eculizumab in atypical hemolytic uremic syndrome from 2-year extensions of phase 2 studies. *Kidney Int.* 2015;87(5):1061-1073. doi:10.1038/ki.2014.423

22. Shen YM, Wolfe H, Barman S. Evaluating thrombocytopenia during heparin therapy. *JAMA.* 2018;319(5):497-498. doi:10.1001/jama.2017.21898

23. Lo GK, Juhl D, Warkentin TE, Sigouin CS, Eichler P, Greinacher A. Evaluation of pretest clinical score (4 T's) for the diagnosis of heparin-induced thrombocytopenia in two clinical settings. *J Thromb Haemost.* 2006;4(4):759-765. doi:10.1111/j.1538-7836.2006.01787.x

24. Cuker A, Arepally GM, Chong BH, et al. American Society of Hematology 2018 guidelines for management of venous thromboembolism: heparin-induced thrombocytopenia. *Blood Adv.* 2018;2(22):3360-3392. doi:10.1182/bloodadvances.2018024489

25. Warkentin TE, Pai M, Sheppard JI, Schulman S, Spyropoulos AC, Eikelboom JW. Fondaparinux treatment of acute heparin-induced thrombocytopenia confirmed by the serotonin-release assay: a 30-month, 16-patient case series. *J Thromb Haemost.* 2011;9(12):2389-2396. doi:10.1111/j.1538-7836.2011.04487.x

26. Warkentin TE, Pai M, Linkins LA. Direct oral anticoagulants for treatment of HIT: update of Hamilton experience and literature review. *Blood.* 2017;130(9):1104-1113. doi:10.1182/blood-2017-04-778993

27. Loren AW, Abrams CS. Efficacy of HPA-1a (PlA1)-negative platelets in a patient with post-transfusion purpura. *Am J Hematol.* 2004;76(3):258-262. doi:10.1002/ajh.20093

28. George JN. Platelets. *Lancet.* 2000;355(9214):1531-1539. doi:10.1016/S0140-6736(00)02175-9

29. Budde U, Scharf RE, Franke P, Hartmann-Budde K, Dent J, Ruggeri ZM. Elevated platelet count as a cause of abnormal von Willebrand factor multimer distribution in plasma. *Blood.* 1993;82(6):1749-1757.

30. Barbui T, Thiele J, Gisslinger H, et al. The 2016 WHO classification and diagnostic criteria for myeloproliferative neoplasms: document summary and in-depth discussion. *Blood Cancer J.* 2018;8(2):15. doi:10.1038/s41408-018-0054-y

31. Barbui T, Finazzi G, Carobbio A, et al. Development and validation of an international prognostic score of thrombosis in World Health Organization-essential thrombocythemia (IPSET-thrombosis). *Blood.* 2012;120(26):5128-5133; quiz 5252. doi:10.1182/blood-2012-07-444067

32. Harrison CN, Campbell PJ, Buck G, et al. Hydroxyurea compared with anagrelide in high-risk essential thrombocythemia. *N Engl J Med.* 2005;353(1):33-45. doi:10.1056/NEJMoa043800

33. Basila D, Yuan CS. Effects of dietary supplements on coagulation and platelet function. *Thromb Res.* 2005;117(1-2):49-53; discussion 65-7. doi:10.1016/j.thromres.2005.04.017

34. Fernandez F, Goudable C, Sie P, et al. Low haematocrit and prolonged bleeding time in uraemic patients: effect of red cell transfusions. *Br J Haematol.* 1985;59(1):139-148. doi:10.1111/j.1365-2141.1985.tb02974.x

35. Vigano G, Benigni A, Mendogni D, Mingardi G, Mecca G, Remuzzi G. Recombinant human erythropoietin to correct uremic bleeding. *Am J Kidney Dis.* 1991;18(1):44-49. doi:10.1016/s0272-6386(12)80289-7

36. Bidlingmaier C, Deml MM, Kurnik K. Continuous infusion of factor concentrates in children with haemophilia A in comparison with bolus injections. *Haemophilia.* 2006;12(3):212-217. doi:10.1111/j.1365-2516.2006.01217.x

37. Mannucci PM. Hemophilia therapy: the future has begun. *Haematologica.* 2020;105(3):545-553. doi:10.3324/haematol.2019.232132

38. Berntorp E, Shapiro AD. Modern haemophilia care. *Lancet.* 2012;379(9824):1447-1456. doi:10.1016/S0140-6736(11)61139-2

39. Astermark J, Donfield SM, DiMichele DM, et al. A randomized comparison of bypassing agents in hemophilia complicated by an inhibitor: the FEIBA NovoSeven Comparative (FENOC) Study. *Blood.* 2007;109(2):546-551. doi:10.1182/blood-2006-04-017988

40. Oldenburg J, Mahlangu JN, Kim B, et al. Emicizumab prophylaxis in hemophilia A with inhibitors. *N Engl J Med.* 2017;377(9):809-818. doi:10.1056/NEJMoa1703068

41. Callaghan MU, Negrier C, Paz-Priel I, et al. Long-term outcomes with emicizumab prophylaxis for hemophilia A with or without FVIII inhibitors from the HAVEN 1-4 studies. *Blood.* 2021;137(16):2231-2242. doi:10.1182/blood.2020009217

42. James PD, Connell NT, Ameer B, et al. ASH ISTH NHF WFH 2021 guidelines on the diagnosis of von Willebrand disease. *Blood Adv.* 2021;5(1):280-300. doi:10.1182/bloodadvances.2020003265

43. Rodeghiero F, Castaman G, Tosetto A. How I treat von Willebrand disease. *Blood.* 2009;114(6):1158-1165. doi:10.1182/blood-2009-01-153296

44. Drebes A, de Vos M, Gill S, et al. Prothrombin complex concentrates for coagulopathy in liver disease: single-center, clinical experience in 105 patients. *Hepatol Commun.* 2019;3(4):513-524. doi:10.1002/hep4.1293

45. Bosch J, Thabut D, Albillos A, et al. Recombinant factor VIIa for variceal bleeding in patients with advanced cirrhosis: a randomized, controlled trial. *Hepatology.* 2008;47(5):1604-1614. doi:10.1002/hep.22216

46. Levi M, Toh CH, Thachil J, Watson HG. Guidelines for the diagnosis and management of disseminated intravascular coagulation. British Committee for Standards in Haematology. *Br J Haematol.* 2009;145(1):24-33. doi:10.1111/j.1365-2141.2009.07600.x

47. Kruse-Jarres R, St-Louis J, Greist A, et al. Efficacy and safety of OBI-1, an antihaemophilic factor VIII (recombinant), porcine sequence, in subjects with acquired haemophilia A. *Haemophilia.* 2015;21(2):162-170. doi:10.1111/hae.12627

48. Franchini M, Mannucci PM. Inhibitor eradication with rituximab in haemophilia: where do we stand? *Br J Haematol.* 2014;165(5):600-608. doi:10.1111/bjh.12829

49. Collins P, Baudo F, Knoebl P, et al. Immunosuppression for acquired hemophilia A: results from the European acquired haemophilia Registry (EACH2). *Blood.* 2012;120(1):47-55. doi:10.1182/blood-2012-02-409185

50. Jimenez D, Aujesky D, Moores L, et al. Simplification of the pulmonary embolism severity index for prognostication in patients with acute symptomatic pulmonary embolism. *Arch Intern Med.* 2010;170(15):1383-1389. doi:10.1001/archinternmed.2010.199

51. den Exter PL, van Es J, Klok FA, et al. Risk profile and clinical outcome of symptomatic subsegmental acute pulmonary embolism. *Blood.* 2013;122(7):1144-1149; quiz 1329. doi:10.1182/blood-2013-04-497545

52. Zondag W, Kooiman J, Klok FA, Dekkers OM, Huisman MV. Outpatient versus inpatient treatment in patients with pulmonary embolism: a meta-analysis. *Eur Respir J.* 2013;42(1):134-144. doi:10.1183/09031936.00093712

53. Garcia D, Erkan D. Diagnosis and management of the antiphospholipid syndrome. *N Engl J Med.* 2018;379(13):1290. doi:10.1056/NEJMc1808253

54. Favaloro EJ. Coagulation mixing studies: utility, algorithmic strategies and limitations for lupus anticoagulant testing or follow up of abnormal coagulation tests. *Am J Hematol.* 2020;95(1):117-128. doi:10.1002/ajh.25669

55. Freund Y, Cachanado M, Aubry A, et al. Effect of the pulmonary embolism rule-out criteria on subsequent thromboembolic events among low-risk emergency department patients: the PROPER randomized clinical trial. *JAMA.* 2018;319(6):559-566. doi:10.1001/jama.2017.21904

56. van der Hulle T, Cheung WY, Kooij S, et al. Simplified diagnostic management of suspected pulmonary embolism (the YEARS study): a prospective, multicentre, cohort study. *Lancet.* 2017;390(10091):289-297. doi:10.1016/S0140-6736(17)30885-1

57. Wells PS, Anderson DR, Bormanis J, et al. Value of assessment of pretest probability of deep-vein thrombosis in clinical management. *Lancet.* 1997;350(9094):1795-1798. doi:10.1016/S0140-6736(97)08140-3

58. Wells PS, Anderson DR, Rodger M, et al. Excluding pulmonary embolism at the bedside without diagnostic imaging: management of patients with suspected pulmonary embolism presenting to the emergency department by using a simple clinical model and d-dimer. *Ann Intern Med.* 2001;135(2):98-107. doi:10.7326/0003-4819-135-2-200107170-00010

59. Douma RA, Mos IC, Erkens PM, et al. Performance of 4 clinical decision rules in the diagnostic management of acute pulmonary embolism: a prospective cohort study. *Ann Intern Med.* 2011;154(11):709-718. doi:10.7326/0003-4819-154-11-201106070-00002

60. Righini M, Le Gal G, Aujesky D, et al. Diagnosis of pulmonary embolism by multidetector CT alone or combined with venous ultrasonography of the leg: a randomised non-inferiority trial. *Lancet.* 2008;371(9621):1343-1352. doi:10.1016/S0140-6736(08)60594-2

61. Stein PD, Hull RD, Patel KC, et al. D-dimer for the exclusion of acute venous thrombosis and pulmonary embolism: a systematic review. *Ann Intern Med.* 2004;140(8):589-602. doi:10.7326/0003-4819-140-8-200404200-00005

62. De Pooter N, Brionne-Francois M, Smahi M, Abecassis L, Toulon P. Age-adjusted D-dimer cut-off levels to rule out venous thromboembolism in patients with non-high pre-test probability: clinical performance and cost-effectiveness analysis. *J Thromb Haemos.* 2021;19(5):1271-1282. doi:10.1111/jth.15278

63. Lee AY, Julian JA, Levine MN, et al. Clinical utility of a rapid whole-blood D-dimer assay in patients with cancer who present with suspected acute deep venous thrombosis. *Ann Intern Med.* 1999;131(6):417-423. doi:10.7326/0003-4819-131-6-199909210-00004

64. Goldstein NM, Kollef MH, Ward S, Gage BF. The impact of the introduction of a rapid D-dimer assay on the diagnostic evaluation of suspected pulmonary embolism. *Arch Intern Med.* 2001;161(4):567-571. doi:10.1001/archinte.161.4.567

65. Righini M, Van Es J, Den Exter PL, et al. Age-adjusted D-dimer cutoff levels to rule out pulmonary embolism: the ADJUST-PE study. *JAMA.* 2014;311(11):1117-1124. doi:10.1001/jama.2014.2135

66. Bates SM, Jaeschke R, Stevens SM, et al. Diagnosis of DVT: antithrombotic therapy and prevention of thrombosis, 9th ed—American College of chest Physicians evidence-based clinical practice guidelines. *Chest.* 2012;141(2 suppl):e351S-e418S. doi:10.1378/chest.11-2299

67. Tapson VF, Carroll BA, Davidson BL, et al. The diagnostic approach to acute venous thromboembolism. Clinical practice guideline. American Thoracic Society. *Am J Respir Crit Care Med.* 1999;160(3):1043-1066. doi:10.1164/ajrccm.160.3.16030

68. Decousus H, Quere I, Presles E, et al. Superficial venous thrombosis and venous thromboembolism: a large, prospective epidemiologic study. *Ann Intern Med.* 2010;152(4):218-224. doi:10.7326/0003-4819-152-4-201002160-00006

69. Cronin P, Dwamena BA. A clinically Meaningful interpretation of the prospective investigation of pulmonary embolism diagnosis (PIOPED) II and III Data. *Acad Radiol.* 2018;25(5):561-572. doi:10.1016/j.acra.2017.11.014

70. Anderson DR, Kahn SR, Rodger MA, et al. Computed tomographic pulmonary angiography vs ventilation-perfusion lung scanning in patients with suspected pulmonary embolism: a randomized controlled trial. *JAMA.* 2007;298(23):2743-2753. doi:10.1001/jama.298.23.2743

71. Investigators P. Value of the ventilation/perfusion scan in acute pulmonary embolism. Results of the prospective investigation of pulmonary embolism diagnosis (PIOPED). *JAMA.* 1990;263(20):2753-2759. doi:10.1001/jama.1990.03440200057023

72. Carrier M, Lazo-Langner A, Shivakumar S, et al. Screening for occult cancer in unprovoked venous thromboembolism. *N Engl J Med.* 2015;373(8):697-704. doi:10.1056/NEJMoa1506623

73. van der Hulle T, Kooiman J, den Exter PL, Dekkers OM, Klok FA, Huisman MV. Effectiveness and safety of novel oral anticoagulants as compared with vitamin K antagonists in the treatment of acute symptomatic venous thromboembolism: a systematic review and meta-analysis. *J Thromb Haemost.* 2014;12(3):320-328. doi:10.1111/jth.12485

74. Duffett L, Castellucci LA, Forgie MA. Pulmonary embolism: update on management and controversies. *BMJ.* 2020;370:m2177. doi:10.1136/bmj.m2177

75. Gage BF, Bass AR, Lin H, et al. Effect of genotype-guided warfarin dosing on clinical events and anticoagulation control among patients undergoing hip or knee arthroplasty: the GIFT randomized clinical trial. *JAMA.* 2017;318(12):1115-1124. doi:10.1001/jama.2017.11469

76. Matchar DB, Jacobson A, Dolor R, et al. Effect of home testing of international normalized ratio on clinical events. *N Engl J Med.* 2010;363(17):1608-1620. doi:10.1056/NEJMoa1002617

77. Bates SM, Rajasekhar A, Middeldorp S, et al. American Society of Hematology 2018 guidelines for management of venous thromboembolism: venous thromboembolism in the context of pregnancy. *Blood Adv.* 2018;2(22):3317-3359. doi:10.1182/bloodadvances.2018024802

78. Garcia DA, Baglin TP, Weitz JI, Samama MM. Parenteral anticoagulants: antithrombotic therapy and prevention of thrombosis, 9th ed—American College of chest Physicians evidence-based clinical practice guidelines. *Chest.* 2012;141(2 suppl):e24S-e43S. doi:10.1378/chest.11-2291

79. ATTACC Investigators, ACTIV-4a Investigators, REMAP-CAP Investigators, et al. Therapeutic anticoagulation with heparin in noncritically ill patients with Covid-19. *N Engl J Med.* 2021;385(9):790-802. doi:10.1056/NEJMoa2105911

80. Lyman GH, Carrier M, Ay C, et al. American Society of Hematology 2021 guidelines for management of venous thromboembolism: prevention and treatment in patients with cancer. *Blood Adv.* 2021;5(4):927-974. doi:10.1182/bloodadvances.2020003442

81. Stevens SM, Woller SC, Kreuziger LB, et al. Antithrombotic therapy for VTE disease: second update of the CHEST guideline and expert panel report. *Chest.* 2021;160(6):e545-e608. doi:10.1016/j.chest.2021.07.055

82. Lee AY, Levine MN, Baker RI, et al. Low-molecular-weight heparin versus a coumarin for the prevention of recurrent venous thromboembolism in patients with cancer. *N Engl J Med.* 2003;349(2):146-153. doi:10.1056/NEJMoa025313

83. Agnelli G, Becattini C, Meyer G, et al. Apixaban for the treatment of venous thromboembolism associated with cancer. *N Engl J Med.* 2020;382(17):1599-1607. doi:10.1056/NEJMoa1915103

84. Raskob GE, van Es N, Verhamme P, et al. Edoxaban for the treatment of cancer-associated venous thromboembolism. *N Engl J Med.* 2018;378(7):615-624. doi:10.1056/NEJMoa1711948

85. Young AM, Marshall A, Thirlwall J, et al. Comparison of an oral factor Xa inhibitor with low molecular weight heparin in patients with cancer with venous thromboembolism: results of a randomized trial (SELECT-D). *J Clini Oncol.* 2018;36(20):2017-2023. doi:10.1200/JCO.2018.78.8034

86. Kahale LA, Hakoum MB, Tsolakian IG, et al. Anticoagulation for the long-term treatment of venous thromboembolism in people with cancer. *Cochrane Database Syst Rev.* 2018;6:CD006650. doi:10.1002/14651858.CD006650.pub5

87. Buller HR, Davidson BL, Decousus H, et al. Fondaparinux or enoxaparin for the initial treatment of symptomatic deep venous thrombosis: a randomized trial. *Ann Intern Med.* 2004;140(11):867-873. doi:10.7326/0003-4819-140-11-200406010-00007

88. Schindewolf M, Steindl J, Beyer-Westendorf J, et al. Use of fondaparinux off-label or approved anticoagulants for management of heparin-induced thrombocytopenia. *J Am Coll Cardiol.* 2017;70(21):2636-2648. doi:10.1016/j.jacc.2017.09.1099

89. Linkins LA, Dans AL, Moores LK, et al. Treatment and prevention of heparin-induced thrombocytopenia: antithrombotic therapy and prevention of thrombosis, 9th ed—American College of chest Physicians evidence-based clinical practice guidelines. *Chest.* 2012;141(2 suppl):e495S-e530S. doi:10.1378/chest.11-2303

90. Kiser TH, Burch JC, Klem PM, Hassell KL. Safety, efficacy, and dosing requirements of bivalirudin in patients with heparin-induced thrombocytopenia. *Pharmacotherapy.* 2008;28(9):1115-1124. doi:10.1592/phco.28.9.1115

91. Bottiger BW, Bode C, Kern S, et al. Efficacy and safety of thrombolytic therapy after initially unsuccessful cardiopulmonary resuscitation: a prospective clinical trial. *Lancet.* 2001;357(9268):1583-1585. doi:10.1016/S0140-6736(00)04726-7

92. Stevens SM, Woller SC, Baumann Kreuziger L, et al. Executive summary: antithrombotic therapy for VTE disease – second update of the CHEST guideline and expert panel report. *Chest.* 2021;160(6):2247-2259. doi:10.1016/j.chest.2021.07.056

93. Kearon C, Akl EA, Ornelas J, et al. Antithrombotic therapy for VTE disease: CHEST guideline and expert panel report. *Chest.* 2016;149(2):315-352. doi:10.1016/j.chest.2015.11.026

94. Chatterjee S, Chakraborty A, Weinberg I, et al. Thrombolysis for pulmonary embolism and risk of all-cause mortality, major bleeding, and intracranial hemorrhage: a meta-analysis. *JAMA.* 2014;311(23):2414-2421. doi:10.1001/jama.2014.5990

95. Meyer G, Vicaut E, Danays T, et al. Fibrinolysis for patients with intermediate-risk pulmonary embolism. *N Engl J Med.* 2014;370(15):1402-1411. doi:10.1056/NEJMoa1302097

96. Vedantham S, Goldhaber SZ, Julian JA, et al. Pharmacomechanical catheter-directed thrombolysis for deep-vein thrombosis. *N Engl J Med.* 2017;377(23):2240-2252. doi:10.1056/NEJMoa1615066

97. Ortel TL, Neumann I, Ageno W, et al. American Society of Hematology 2020 guidelines for management of venous thromboembolism: treatment of deep vein thrombosis and pulmonary embolism. *Blood Adv.* 2020;4(19):4693-4738. doi:10.1182/bloodadvances.2020001830

98. Simes J, Becattini C, Agnelli G, et al. Aspirin for the prevention of recurrent venous thromboembolism: the INSPIRE collaboration. *Circulation.* 2014;130(13):1062-1071. doi:10.1161/CIRCULATIONAHA.114.008828

99. Becattini C, Agnelli G. Aspirin for prevention and treatment of venous thromboembolism. *Blood Rev.* 2014;28(3):103-108. doi:10.1016/j.blre.2014.03.003

100. Weitz JI, Lensing AWA, Prins MH, et al. Rivaroxaban or aspirin for extended treatment of venous thromboembolism. *N Engl J Med.* 2017;376(13):1211-1222. doi:10.1056/NEJMoa1700518

101. Agnelli G, Buller HR, Cohen A, et al. Apixaban for extended treatment of venous thromboembolism. *N Engl J Med.* 2013;368(8):699-708. doi:10.1056/NEJMoa1207541

102. Schulman S, Kearon C, Kakkar AK, et al. Extended use of dabigatran, warfarin, or placebo in venous thromboembolism. *N Engl J Med.* 2013;368(8):709-718. doi:10.1056/NEJMoa1113697

103. Kahn SR, Shapiro S, Wells PS, et al. Compression stockings to prevent post-thrombotic syndrome: a randomised placebo-controlled trial. *Lancet.* 2014;383(9920):880-888. doi:10.1016/S0140-6736(13)61902-9

104. Klemen ND, Feingold PL, Hashimoto B, et al. Mortality risk associated with venous thromboembolism: a systematic review and Bayesian meta-analysis. *Lancet Haematol.* 2020;7(8):e583-e593. doi:10.1016/S2352-3026(20)30211-8

105. Mathew TC, Ramsaran EK, Aragam JR. Impending paradoxic embolism in acute pulmonary embolism: diagnosis by transesophageal echocardiography and treatment by emergent surgery. *Am Heart J.* 1995;129(4):826-827. doi:10.1016/0002-8703(95)90337-2

106. Chartier L, Bera J, Delomez M, et al. Free-floating thrombi in the right heart: diagnosis, management, and prognostic indexes in 38 consecutive patients. *Circulation.* 1999;99(21):2779-2783. doi:10.1161/01.cir.99.21.2779

107. Douketis JD, Spyropoulos AC, Kaatz S, et al. Perioperative bridging anticoagulation in patients with atrial fibrillation. *N Engl J Med.* 2015;373(9):823-833. doi:10.1056/NEJMoa1501035

108. Schulman S, Hwang HG, Eikelboom JW, Kearon C, Pai M, Delaney J. Loading dose vs. maintenance dose of warfarin for reinitiation after invasive procedures: a randomized trial. *J Thromb Haemost.* 2014;12(8):1254-1259. doi:10.1111/jth.12613

109. Douketis JD, Spyropoulos AC, Duncan J, et al. Perioperative management of patients with atrial fibrillation receiving a direct oral anticoagulant. *JAMA Intern Med.* 2019;179(11):1469-1478. doi:10.1001/jamainternmed.2019.2431

110. Kucher N. Clinical practice. Deep-vein thrombosis of the upper extremities. *N Engl J Med.* 2011;364(9):861-869. doi:10.1056/NEJMcp1008740

111. Chopard R, Albertsen IE, Piazza G. Diagnosis and treatment of lower extremity venous thromboembolism: a review. *JAMA.* 2020;324(17):1765-1776. doi:10.1001/jama.2020.17272

112. Beyer-Westendorf J, Schellong SM, Gerlach H, et al. Prevention of thromboembolic complications in patients with superficial-vein thrombosis given rivaroxaban or fondaparinux: the open-label, randomised, non-inferiority SURPRISE phase 3b trial. *Lancet Haematol.* 2017;4(3):e105-e113. doi:10.1016/S2352-3026(17)30014-5

113. Di Nisio M, Wichers I, Middeldorp S. Treatment of lower extremity superficial thrombophlebitis. *JAMA.* 2018;320(22):2367-2368. doi:10.1001/jama.2018.16623

114. Piazza G, Goldhaber SZ. Chronic thromboembolic pulmonary hypertension. *N Engl J Med.* 2011;364(4):351-360. doi:10.1056/NEJMra0910203

115. Ghofrani HA, Galie N, Grimminger F, et al. Riociguat for the treatment of pulmonary arterial hypertension. *N Engl J Med.* 2013;369(4):330-340. doi:10.1056/NEJMoa1209655

116. Crowther MA, Ageno W, Garcia D, et al. Oral vitamin K versus placebo to correct excessive anticoagulation in patients receiving warfarin: a randomized trial. *Ann Intern Med.* 2009;150(5):293-300. doi:10.7326/0003-4819-150-5-200903030-00005

117. Gunther KE, Conway G, Leibach L, Crowther MA. Low-dose oral vitamin K is safe and effective for outpatient management of patients with an INR>10. *Thromb Res.* 2004;113(3-4):205-209. doi:10.1016/j.thromres.2004.03.004

118. Sarode R, Milling TJ, Jr, Refaai MA, et al. Efficacy and safety of a 4-factor prothrombin complex concentrate in patients on vitamin K antagonists presenting with major bleeding: a randomized, plasma-controlled, phase IIIb study. *Circulation.* 2013;128(11):1234-1243. doi:10.1161/CIRCULATIONAHA.113.002283

119. Levi M, Levy JH, Andersen HF, Truloff D. Safety of recombinant activated factor VII in randomized clinical trials. *N Engl J Med.* 2010;363(19):1791-1800. doi:10.1056/NEJMoa1006221

120. Horlocker TT, Wedel DJ, Benzon H, et al. Regional anesthesia in the anticoagulated patient: defining the risks (the second ASRA Consensus Conference on Neuraxial Anesthesia and Anticoagulation). *Reg Anesth Pain Med.* 2003;28(3):172-197. doi:10.1053/rapm.2003.50046

121. Frontera JA, Lewin JJ, IIIrd, Rabinstein AA, et al. Guideline for reversal of antithrombotics in intracranial hemorrhage: executive summary. A statement for healthcare professionals from the neurocritical care society and the society of critical care medicine. *Crit Care Med.* 2016;44(12):2251-2257. doi:10.1097/CCM.0000000000002057

122. Pollack CV, Jr, Reilly PA, van Ryn J, et al. Idarucizumab for dabigatran reversal—full cohort analysis. *N Engl J Med.* 2017;377(5):431-441. doi:10.1056/NEJMoa1707278

123. Connolly SJ, Crowther M, Eikelboom JW, et al. Full study report of andexanet alfa for bleeding associated with factor Xa inhibitors. *N Engl J Med.* 2019;380(14):1326-1335. doi:10.1056/NEJMoa1814051

124. Eerenberg ES, Kamphuisen PW, Sijpkens MK, Meijers JC, Buller HR, Levi M. Reversal of rivaroxaban and dabigatran by prothrombin complex concentrate: a randomized, placebo-controlled, crossover study in healthy subjects. *Circulation.* 2011;124(14):1573-1579. doi:10.1161/CIRCULATIONAHA.111.029017

125. Aujesky D, Roy PM, Verschuren F, et al. Outpatient versus inpatient treatment for patients with acute pulmonary embolism: an international, open-label, randomised, non-inferiority trial. *Lancet.* 2011;378(9785):41-48. doi:10.1016/S0140-6736(11)60824-6

21 Hematologic Disorders and Transfusion Therapy

Bindiya G. Patel, Amy Zhou, Sana Saif Ur Rehman, and Ray Zhang

ANEMIA

GENERAL PRINCIPLES

Definition

Anemia is defined as a decrease in circulating red blood cell (RBC) mass, the usual criteria in adults being hemoglobin (Hgb) <12 g/dL or hematocrit (Hct) <36% for nonpregnant women and Hgb <13 g/dL or Hct <39% in men.

Classification

Anemia can be broadly classified into three etiologic groups: **blood loss (acute or chronic), decreased RBC production, and increased RBC destruction (hemolysis).** Anemia can also be categorized by RBC size as microcytic, normocytic, or macrocytic.

Clinical Presentation

Common signs and symptoms of anemia include pallor, tachycardia, hypotension, dizziness, tinnitus, headaches, decreased cognitive ability, fatigue, and weakness. Atrophic glossitis, angular cheilosis, koilonychia (spoon nails), and brittle nails are more common in severe, long-standing anemia. Patients may also experience reduced exercise tolerance, dyspnea on exertion, and heart failure. High-output heart failure and hypovolemic shock may be seen in acute, severe cases.

Diagnostic Testing

Laboratories

- The complete blood count (CBC), reticulocyte count, and inspection of the peripheral smear will guide further laboratory testing because they provide a morphologic classification and assessment of RBC production.
- The Hgb level is a measure of the concentration of Hgb in blood as expressed in grams per deciliter (g/dL), whereas the Hct is the percentage of the blood that is RBCs. Hgb and Hct are unreliable indicators of red cell mass in the setting of rapid shifts of intravascular volume (i.e., an acute bleed).
- The most useful red cell indices include the following:
  - Mean cellular volume (MCV): Measures the mean volume of the RBCs.
    - **Microcytic: MCV <80 fL**
    - **Normocytic: MCV 80–96 fL**
    - **Macrocytic: MCV >96 fL**
  - Red cell distribution width (RDW): Reflects the variability in the volume of the RBCs and is proportional to the standard deviation of the MCV. An elevated

RDW indicates an increased variability in RBC size, which is a nonspecific but important finding in anemic patients (i.e., increased reticulocytes can cause elevation in RDW as they are larger than mature RBCs).

○ Mean cellular Hgb: Defines the concentration of Hgb in each cell, and an elevated level is often indicative of spherocytes or a hemoglobinopathy.

• **The relative reticulocyte count** measures the percentage of immature red cells in the blood and reflects production of RBCs in the bone marrow (BM).

○ A normal RBC has a life span of approximately 120 days, and the reticulocytes circulate for about 1 day; therefore, the normal reticulocyte count is 0.4%–2.9%.

○ In the setting of anemia from blood loss, the BM should increase its production of RBCs in response to the blood loss, and thus a reticulocyte count of 1% in this setting is inappropriately low.

○ **The reticulocyte index** (RI) is a determination of the BM's ability to respond to anemia and is calculated by % reticulocytes/maturation correction × actual Hct/ normal Hct (normally 45). The maturation correction factor is 1.0 for Hct > 30%, 1.5 for 24%–30%, 2.0 for 20%–24%, and 2.5 for <20%. **RI <2 with anemia indicates decreased production of RBCs (hypoproliferative anemia). RI >2 with anemia may indicate a compensatory increase in RBC production caused by hemolysis or bleeding (hyperproliferative anemia).**

○ The absolute reticulocyte count (relative reticulocyte count × RBCs) may provide a more accurate reflection of a patient's response to anemia than the relative reticulocyte count.

• The **peripheral smear** should be reviewed to assess the morphologic characteristics of RBCs including the shape, size, presence of inclusions, and orientation of cells in relation to each other. RBCs assume many abnormal forms, such as acanthocytes, schistocytes, spherocytes, or tear drop cells, and abnormal orientation such as agglutination or rouleaux formation. Each is associated with several specific disease processes that may warrant additional evaluation.

Diagnostic Procedures

A **BM biopsy** may be indicated in cases of unexplained anemia with a low reticulocyte count or with anemia associated with other cytopenias. The severity of anemia that should trigger a BM biopsy is not well defined, but it should be strongly considered if the diagnosis is uncertain and RBC transfusions are required.

ANEMIAS ASSOCIATED WITH DECREASED RBC PRODUCTION

Iron Deficiency Anemia

GENERAL PRINCIPLES

• **Iron deficiency** is the most common cause of anemia in the ambulatory setting and is usually a chronic microcytic anemia with a low reticulocyte count.

• The most common causes of iron deficiency anemia are blood loss (e.g., menses, GI blood loss), decreased absorption (e.g., achlorhydria, celiac disease, bariatric surgery, *Helicobacter pylori* infection), and increased iron requirement (e.g., pregnancy).

• It is important to determine the cause of iron deficiency, and in the absence of menstrual bleeding, evaluation of the GI tract should be performed to identify a potential cause including the possibility of an occult malignancy.

DIAGNOSIS

Clinical Presentation

- Patients often present with cold intolerance along with fatigue or malaise that is typically worsened with activity. Pallor is also a common physical finding.
- Pica (consumption of substances of no nutritional value such as ice, starch, or clay) occurs in about 25% of patients with chronic iron deficiency anemia and rarely occurs in other clinical settings.
- Restless leg syndrome is a common but a nonspecific finding in patients with iron deficiency anemia.

Diagnostic Testing

- Peripheral blood smear may show hypochromia (increased central pallor of RBCs), microcytosis, and pencil-shaped cells (elliptocytes). The reticulocyte count is low in iron deficiency anemia.
- **Ferritin** is the primary storage form for iron in the liver and is a specific marker of an absolute iron deficiency. The reference range is 30–400 ng/mL.
  ○ A ferritin level of <10 ng/mL in women or <20 ng/mL in men almost always reflects low iron stores.
  ○ Ferritin is an acute-phase reactant, so normal levels may be seen in inflammatory states despite low iron stores. **A serum ferritin level of >200 ng/mL generally excludes an iron deficiency**; however, in renal dialysis patients, a functional iron deficiency may be seen with a ferritin up to 500 ng/mL.
- **Iron, total iron-binding capacity (TIBC), and transferrin saturation** are often used in combination with ferritin to diagnose iron deficiency anemia. Serum iron level alone is an unreliable indicator given its significant fluctuation after a meal.

Diagnostic Procedures

- A **BM biopsy** that shows absent staining for iron is the definitive test to diagnose iron deficiency anemia and is helpful when the serum tests do not clearly demonstrate the diagnosis.
- **An iron challenge** can be performed in the absence of response to oral iron replacement to differentiate poor absorption from other causes (e.g., nonadherence or occult blood loss). After an 8-hour fast, a baseline iron is measured immediately followed by oral intake of liquid ferrous sulfate 5 mg/kg given with orange juice or vitamin C–containing beverage. Serum iron is measured again after 90 minutes. Normal iron absorption will result in an increase of serum iron of at least 50 µg/dL and a lower level is indicative of poor absorption.

TREATMENT

- **Oral iron therapy.** Given in stable patients with mild symptoms. Several different preparations are available (Table 21-1).
  ○ Iron is best absorbed on an empty stomach, and 3–10 mg of elemental iron can be absorbed daily.
  ○ Oral iron ingestion may induce a number of GI side effects and as a result, nonadherence is a common problem. These side effects can be decreased by initially administering the drug with meals or every other day, which may be as effective as more frequent dosing.[1] Concomitant treatment with a stool softener can also alleviate constipation.

TABLE 21-1	Oral Iron Preparations	
Preparation	Common Dosing Regimen	Elemental Iron (mg per dose)
Ferrous sulfate	325 mg qd–tid	65
Ferrous gluconate	300 mg tid	36
Ferrous fumarate	100 mg tid	33
Iron polysaccharide complex	150 mg bid	150
Carbonyl iron	50 mg bid–tid	50

- ○ Ferrous sulfate is the most commonly prescribed formulation. If there are unacceptable side effects, consider using a lower dose or an alternative formulation such as ferrous gluconate or ferrous fumarate, which contains lower amounts of elemental iron.
- ○ In general, patients responding to oral iron therapy should see an increase in reticulocyte count within 1 week of therapy; an increase in Hgb of 2 g/dL every 3 weeks is expected. Treatment should be continued until the total iron deficit is replete.
- **Parenteral iron therapy** (Table 21-2). There are several formulations of IV iron, and indications for parenteral iron over oral iron include the following:
- ○ Poor absorption (e.g., inflammatory bowel disease, malabsorption).
- ○ Very high iron requirements that cannot be met with oral supplementation (e.g., ongoing bleeding).
- ○ Intolerance to oral preparations.
- ○ Functional iron deficiency in chronic kidney disease (CKD).

Specific Considerations

- IV iron infusion **should not be given** in patients with an active infection (i.e., fever) owing to concern for increased adverse reactions such as sepsis.
- The total iron replacement dose may be estimated using the patient's baseline Hgb and body weight with the Ganzoni formula:

$$\text{Total iron dose}(\text{mg}) = \Big[\text{actual body weight}(\text{kg}) \times \big(\text{target hemoglobin}(\text{g/dL})$$
$$- \text{actual hemoglobin}(\text{g/dL})\big)\Big] \times 2.4 + \text{iron stores}(\text{mg})$$

- Delayed reactions to IV iron, such as arthralgia, myalgia, fever, pruritus, and lymphadenopathy, may be seen within several days of therapy and usually resolve spontaneously or with NSAIDs.
- **Iron dextran** (INFeD) **is a less-expensive agent and allows for high-dose repletion in a single dose given over an hour**; however, infusion can be complicated by serious side effects including **anaphylaxis.**
- **Second-generation iron products** include **ferric gluconate** (Ferrlecit) and **iron sucrose** (Venofer) and can be given at a faster infusion rate than INFeD. Anaphylaxis is rare, and a test dose is not needed; however, a single infusion is typically insufficient to replenish the entire iron deficit, so multiple doses are required.
- **Third-generation iron products,** including **ferumoxytol** (Feraheme), **ferric carboxymaltose** (Injectafer), and **ferric derisomaltose** (Monoferric), allow for administration of a high dose with a rapid infusion. A rare complication is severe

TABLE 21-2	IV Iron Preparations	
Preparation	IV Administration	Caution
Iron dextran (INFeD)	The entire dose may be diluted and infused in one setting; 1000 mg can be given over 1 h	A 0.5-mL test dose should be given; observe patient for at least 1 h before full dose.
Iron sucrose (Venofer)	Administered undiluted as slow IV injection or infusion in diluted solution: Injection: 100 mg over 2–5 min 200 mg over 2–5 min Infusion: 100 mg/100 mL over 15 min 300 mg/250 mL over 1.5 h 400 mg/250 mL over 2.5 h >500 mg/250 mL over 3.5 h	
Ferric gluconate (Ferrlecit)	Injection: 125 mg over 10 min Infusion: 125 mg/100 mL over 1 h	
Ferumoxytol (Feraheme)	510 mg over 20 min; given as two doses 7 d apart	Observe patient for at least 30 min after administration. Serious hypersensitivity reactions have been observed with rapid IV injection (<1 min).
Ferric carboxymaltose (Injectafer)	750 mg over 15–30 min; given as two doses 7 d apart	
Ferric derisomaltose/ iron isomaltoside (Monoferric)	1000 mg as a single dose given over ≥20 min	Monitor for signs and symptoms of hypersensitivity reactions during and for ≥30 min and until clinically stable following infusion.

Chapter 21

hypotension, which can be related to the rapidity of the injection. Ferric carboxymaltose and ferric derisomaltose can be associated with hypophosphatemia.
- Of note, some IV irons can interfere with MRI results and **mimick hemosiderosis** on liver MRI. If MRI imaging is needed, it is recommended that a period of at least 1 week be given between the last IV iron sucrose and ferric gluconate infusion and MRI. Ferumoxytol is available as an MRI contrast agent and will transiently show a significant increase in iron stores in the liver, which can be seen for up to 3 months following infusion.

Thalassemia

GENERAL PRINCIPLES

Definition

The **thalassemia syndromes** are inherited disorders characterized by reduced Hgb synthesis associated with mutations in either the α- or β-gene of the molecule (Table 21-3).

Etiology

- **β-Thalassemia** results in a decreased production of β-globin and a resultant excess of α-globin, forming insoluble α-tetramers and leading to ineffective erythropoiesis.
  - **β-Thalassemia minor (trait)** occurs with one gene abnormality with underproduction of β-chain globin. Patients are asymptomatic and present with microcytic, hypochromic RBCs and Hgb levels >10 g/dL.
  - **β-Thalassemia intermedia** (non–transfusion-dependent) occurs with dysfunction in both β-globin genes so that anemia is more severe (Hgb 7–10 g/dL).
  - **β-Thalassemia major** (Cooley anemia or transfusion-dependent) is caused by mutations of both β globin genes that fail to produce significant amounts of β-globin and generally require lifelong RBC transfusion support.
- **α-Thalassemia** occurs with a deletion of one or more of the four α-globin genes, leading to a β-globin excess.
  - Mild microcytosis and mild hypochromic anemia (Hgb >10 g/dL) are seen with the loss of one or two α-globin genes (silent carrier and α-thal trait).
  - Deletion of three α-globin genes (Hgb H disease) results in splenomegaly and hemolytic anemia. In patients with Hgb H disease, transfusion or splenectomy

TABLE 21-3	Thalassemias			
	Genotype	Hemoglobin (g/dL)	Mean Cellular Volume (fL)	Transfusion Dependent
α-Thalassemia				
Silent carrier	αα/α–	Normal	None	No
Trait	α–/α– or αα/––	>10	<80	No
Hemoglobin H	α–/––	7–10	<70	±
Hydrops fetalis	––/––	Incompatible with life		
β-Thalassemia (Thal)				
Silent carrier	β/β+	>10	<80	No
β-Thal minor (trait)	β/β0	>10	<80	No
β-Thal intermedia	β+/β+	7–10	65–75	±
β-Thal major	β+/β0 or β0/β0	<7	<70	Yes

β+, β-thalassemia genes produce some β-globin chains but with impaired synthesis; β0, β-thalassemia genes produce no β-globin chains.

is often not necessary until after the second or third decade of life. In addition, oxidant drugs similar to those that exacerbate glucose-6-phosphate dehydrogenase (G6PD) deficiency should be avoided because increased hemolysis may occur.

- ○ Hydrops fetalis occurs with the loss of all four α-globin genes and is incompatible with life.

DIAGNOSIS

- Peripheral smear may show microcytic hypochromic RBCs, along with poikilocytosis and nucleated RBCs.
- Hgb electrophoresis is often diagnostic for β-thalassemia showing an increased percentage of Hgb A_2 and Hgb F.
- Silent carriers with a single α-chain loss generally have a normal electrophoresis. Adults with Hgb H disease demonstrate Hgb H (β-tetramers) on electrophoresis. The diagnosis of α-thalassemia is confirmed by α-globin gene analysis.

TREATMENT

- Patients with either α- or β-thalassemia trait require no specific treatment.
- In patients with more severe forms of the disease, chronic RBC transfusions to maintain an Hgb level of 9–10 g/dL are needed to prevent the skeletal deformities that result from accelerated erythropoiesis.
- In severe forms of thalassemia, repeated transfusions result in tissue iron overload, which may cause congestive heart failure (CHF), hepatic dysfunction, glucose intolerance, and secondary hypogonadism. **Iron chelation therapy** delays or prevents these complications. Once clinical organ deterioration has begun, it may not be reversible.
- **Chelation therapy** is indicated for transfusion-associated iron overload from any cause. It is indicated in patients with a ferritin consistently >1000 ng/mL, which may occur after a transfusion burden of >20 units of packed RBCs (pRBCs).[2]
  - ○ Deferoxamine, 40 mg/kg SC or IV over 8–12 hours of continuous infusion.
  - ○ Deferasirox dispersible tablet 20–40 mg/kg/d (Exjade) is an effective oral chelating agent, but GI disturbances often limit adherence to therapy. Deferasirox film-coated tablet (Jadenu) is available and dosed at 70% of Exjade (7–21 mg/kg/d). This formulation is often better tolerated. Dose can be titrated every 3–6 months based on ferritin level. Efficacy is similar to that of deferoxamine.
- Chelation therapy should be continued until ferritin levels of <1000 ng/mL are achieved and maintenance therapy is often needed when RBC transfusions are ongoing. **Luspatercept** (1 mg/kg every 3 weeks) is approved for transfusion-dependent β-thalassemia to reduce transfusion requirements with median time to response 12–24 days.[3]
- Stem cell transplantation (SCT) is the only curative therapy and should be considered in young patients with thalassemia major who have HLA-identical donors. Gene therapy is the subject of ongoing research and holds promise.[4]
- Splenectomy should be considered in patients with accelerated (more than two units/month) transfusion requirements. To decrease the risk of postsplenectomy sepsis, immunization against pneumococcus, *Haemophilus influenzae*, and *Neisseria meningitidis* should be administered at least 2 weeks before surgery if not previously vaccinated (see Appendix A, Immunizations and Postexposure Therapies). Splenectomy is rarely recommended in patients who are younger than 5–6 years because of the increased risk of sepsis.

Sideroblastic Anemias

GENERAL PRINCIPLES

Definition

Sideroblastic anemias are hereditary or acquired RBC disorders characterized by abnormal iron metabolism associated with the presence of ring sideroblasts (RS) in the developing RBCs in the BM.

Etiology

- Acquired
  - Primary sideroblastic anemia (myelodysplastic syndrome with ring sideroblasts [MDS-RS] or myelodysplastic/myeloproliferative neoplasms with ring sideroblasts [MDS/MPN-RS]).
  - Secondary sideroblastic anemia is caused by drugs (i.e., chloramphenicol, cycloserine, ethanol, isoniazid, pyrazinamide), lead or zinc toxicity, chronic alcohol use, or copper deficiency.
- Hereditary
  - X-linked
  - Autosomal
  - Mitochondrial

DIAGNOSIS

A BM examination including cytogenetics is needed to evaluate for the presence of RS or other abnormal marrow forms. MDS-RS and MDS/MPN-RS are often associated with mutations in *SF3B1*.

TREATMENT

- Remove any possible offending agent.
- Replete copper deficiency.
- Pyridoxine 50–200 mg daily may be effective to treat hereditary sideroblastic anemias.
- Luspatercept is approved for treatment of anemia in patients with MDS-RS or MDS/MPN-RS.[5]

Macrocytic/Megaloblastic Anemia

GENERAL PRINCIPLES

Definition

Megaloblastic anemia is a term used to describe disorders of impaired DNA synthesis in hematopoietic cells, but this also affects other normally proliferating cells such as in the GI tract.

Etiology

- **Vitamin B_{12}** (cobalamin) **deficiency** occurs insidiously over several years because daily vitamin B_{12} requirements are low compared to total body stores. Vitamin B_{12} is absorbed in the terminal ileum.

○ Most cases of megaloblastic anemia are due to vitamin B_{12} deficiency.
○ Vitamin B_{12} deficiency occurs in up to 20% of untreated patients within 8 years of partial gastrectomy and in almost all patients with total gastrectomy or pernicious anemia (PA). Older patients with gastric atrophy may develop a food-bound vitamin B_{12} deficiency in which vitamin B_{12} absorption is impaired. In nonvegan adults, vitamin B_{12} deficiency is almost always due to malabsorption.
○ PA usually occurs in individuals older than 40 years (mean age of onset, 60 years). Up to 30% of patients have a positive family history. PA is an immune-mediated disorder associated with other autoimmune disorders (Graves disease 30%, Hashimoto thyroiditis 11%, and Addison disease 5%–10%). In patients with PA, 90% have antiparietal cell antibodies, and 60% have anti-intrinsic factor antibodies.
○ Other etiologies of vitamin B_{12} deficiency include pancreatic insufficiency, bacterial overgrowth, celiac disease, medications (metformin, proton pump inhibitors, nitrous oxide), and intestinal parasites (*Diphyllobothrium latum*).
• **Folate deficiency** results from a negative folate balance arising from malnutrition, malabsorption, or increased requirement (pregnancy, hemolytic anemia). In contrast to B_{12} deficiency, it can develop more rapidly (weeks to months) given limited body stores. Folate is mainly absorbed in the upper third of small intestine.
○ Folate deficiency is now rare in the US because of fortification of grains with folic acid.
○ Patients on weight-losing diets, alcoholics, the elderly, and psychiatric patients are particularly at risk for nutritional folate deficiency.
○ Folate deficiency may be seen in several settings:
 ▪ **Pregnancy and lactation** in which there is a three- to fourfold increased daily folate requirements.
 ▪ Folate malabsorption can occur secondary to celiac disease or bariatric surgery.
 ▪ Drugs that can interfere with folate absorption include ethanol, trimethoprim, methotrexate, pyrimethamine, diphenylhydantoin, barbiturates, and sulfasalazine.
 ▪ Dialysis-dependent patients require more folate intake because of increased folate losses.
 ▪ Patients with hemolytic anemia, such as sickle cell anemia, require increased folate for accelerated erythropoiesis and can present with aplastic crisis (rapidly falling RBC counts) with folate deficiency.

DIAGNOSIS

Clinical Presentation
• In addition to symptoms of anemia, vitamin B_{12} deficiency may demonstrate neurologic symptoms, such as peripheral neuropathy, paresthesias, lethargy, hypotonia, and seizures.
• Important physical findings include signs of poor nutrition, pigmentation of skin creases and nail beds, or glossitis. Jaundice or splenomegaly may indicate ineffective and extramedullary hematopoiesis.
• Vitamin B_{12} deficiency may cause decreased vibratory and positional sense, ataxia, paresthesias, confusion, and dementia. Neurologic complications may occur in the absence of anemia and may not fully resolve despite adequate treatment. **Folic acid deficiency does not result in neurologic disease.**

Diagnostic Testing

- Macrocytic anemia is usually present unless there is also a coincident cause of microcytic anemia, and leukopenia and thrombocytopenia may occur.
- The peripheral smear may show macroovalocytes; hypersegmented neutrophils (containing six or more nuclear lobes) are common.
- Lactate dehydrogenase (LDH) and indirect bilirubin are typically elevated, reflecting ineffective erythropoiesis and premature destruction of RBCs (intramedullary hemolysis).
- Serum vitamin B_{12} and folate levels should be measured.
- **Serum methylmalonic acid (MMA) and homocysteine (HC)** may be useful when the vitamin B_{12} level is 100–400 pg/mL (or borderline low as defined by the laboratory reference range). MMA and HC are elevated in vitamin B_{12} deficiency; only HC is elevated in folate deficiency.
- Detecting **antibodies to intrinsic factor** is specific for the diagnosis of PA.

Diagnostic Procedures

BM biopsy may be necessary to rule out MDS or acute myeloid leukemia (AML) because these disorders may present with findings similar to those of megaloblastic anemia including a hypercellular marrow with an accumulation of immature cells.

TREATMENT

- Potassium supplementation may be necessary when treatment is initiated to avoid potentially serious arrhythmias due to transient hypokalemia induced by enhanced hematopoiesis.
- Reticulocytosis should begin within 1 week of therapy, followed by a rising of Hgb over 6–8 weeks.
- Coexisting iron deficiency is present in one-third of patients and is a common cause for an incomplete response to therapy.
- Folic acid 1 mg PO daily is given until the deficiency is corrected. High doses of folic acid (5 mg daily) may be needed in patients with malabsorption syndromes.
- Vitamin B_{12} deficiency is corrected by administering cyanocobalamin. Initial treatment (1 mg/d IM cyanocobalamin) is typically administered in the setting of severe anemia, neurologic dysfunction, or chronic malabsorption. After 1 week of daily therapy, a commonly employed regimen is 1 mg/wk given for 4 weeks and then 1 mg/mo for life.
- High-dose enteral therapy (1000–2000 μg/d PO) may be considered after initial repletion in those without neurologic involvement or for convenience or cost.[6]

Anemia of Chronic Renal Insufficiency

GENERAL PRINCIPLES

Anemia of chronic renal insufficiency is attributed primarily to decreased endogenous erythropoietin (EPO) production and may occur as the creatinine clearance declines to below 50 mL/min. Other causes including a functional iron deficiency may contribute to the etiology (see the previous description).

DIAGNOSIS

- RBCs are often normocytic and hypochromic, with the occasional presence of echinocytes (burr cells).

- Iron status should be evaluated in patients who are undergoing dialysis by obtaining levels of ferritin and transferrin saturation. Oral iron supplementation is not considered effective in CKD; therefore, parenteral iron to maintain a ferritin level of >500 ng/mL is recommended.

TREATMENT

- Treatment has been revolutionized by erythropoiesis-stimulating agents (ESAs) including EPO and darbepoetin alfa (Table 21-4).
- Therapy is initiated in predialysis patients who are symptomatic.
- Administration of ESAs can be IV (hemodialysis patients) or SC (predialysis or peritoneal dialysis patients). In dialysis and predialysis patients with CKD, **the target Hgb should not exceed 11 g/dL due to the increased risk for cardiovascular events, stroke, and venous thromboembolism.**[7] A rapid rise in Hb of > 1g/dL over 2 weeks may also be associated with these risks. Hgb and Hct should be measured at least monthly while receiving an ESA. Dose adjustments should be made to maintain the target Hgb.
- **Suboptimal responses to ESA therapy** are most often due to iron deficiency, inflammation, bleeding, infection, malignancy, malnutrition, and aluminum toxicity.
  - IV iron administration has become first-line therapy for individuals with transferrin saturation <20% and/or ferritin <500 ng/mL. It has also been shown to reduce the ESA dosage required to correct anemia.

TABLE 21-4	Erythropoietin Dosing	
	Agent and Initial Dose (SC or IV)	
Indication	**Erythropoietin[a] (Procrit, Epogen)**	**Darbepoetin[b] (Aranesp)**
Chemotherapy-induced anemia from nonmyeloid malignancy, multiple myeloma, or lymphoma; anemia secondary to malignancy or myelodysplastic syndrome	40,000 units/wk or 150 units/kg three times a week	2.25 µg/kg/wk or 100 µg/wk or 200 µg/2 wk or 500 µg/3 wk
Anemia associated with renal failure	50–150 units/kg three times a week	0.45 µg/kg/wk
Anemia associated with HIV infection	100–200 units/kg three times a week	Not approved
Anemia of chronic disease	150–300 units/kg three times a week	Not approved
Anemia in patients unwilling or unable to receive RBCs; anemic patients undergoing major surgery	600 units/kg/wk × 3 300 units/kg/d × 1–2 wk	Not recommended

RBC, red blood cell.
[a]Dose increase after 48 weeks up to 900 units/kg/wk or 60,000 units/wk; discontinue if hematocrit (Hct) is >40%; resume when Hct is <36% at 75% of previous dose.
[b]Dose increase after 6 weeks up to 4.5 mg/kg/wk or 150 mg/wk or 300 mg/2 weeks; hold dose if Hct is >36%, then resume when Hct is <36% at 75% of previous dose.

○ A ferritin level and transferrin saturation should be tested at least monthly during the initiation of ESA therapy with a goal ferritin level of >200 ng/mL and a transferrin saturation of >20% in dialysis-dependent patients and a ferritin level of >100 ng/mL and a transferrin saturation of >20% in predialysis or peritoneal dialysis patients.

○ Iron therapy is unlikely to be useful if the ferritin level is >500 ng/mL.

○ Secondary hyperparathyroidism that causes BM fibrosis and relative ESA resistance may also occur.

• Roxadustat, an oral hypoxia-inducible factor inhibitor, has been approved for the treatment of anemia in CKD in China and Japan.[8] It is currently undergoing evaluation by the Food and Drug Administration (FDA) for approval in the US.

Anemia of Chronic Disease/Inflammation

GENERAL PRINCIPLES

• Anemia of chronic disease (ACD) often develops in patients with long-standing inflammatory diseases, malignancy, autoimmune disorders, and chronic infection.

• Etiology is multifactorial, including defective iron mobilization during erythropoiesis, inflammatory cytokine-mediated suppression of erythropoiesis, and impaired EPO response to anemia. Hepcidin is a critical regulator of iron homeostasis and is normally low when iron is deficient, allowing for increased iron absorption and utilization. Chronic inflammation increases hepcidin levels and causes a functional iron deficiency due to impaired iron recycling and utilization. Hepcidin is renally cleared, suggesting a role in anemia of chronic renal disease.

DIAGNOSIS

• Anemia is normocytic in 75% of cases and microcytic in the remainder of cases.

• The soluble transferrin receptor level is helpful in differentiating ACD (normal) and iron deficiency (elevated) when the ferritin is indeterminate. Measurement of serum hepcidin may become part of the standard evaluation of anemia when the assay becomes widely available in the future, but currently is not utilized clinically.

• Iron studies may show low serum iron and TIBC.

TREATMENT

• Therapy for ACD is directed toward the underlying disease and eliminating exacerbating factors such as nutritional deficiencies and marrow-suppressive drugs.

• Ferritin level below 30 ng/mL suggests coexisting iron deficiency and should be treated with supplemental iron. Clinical responses to IV iron therapy may occur in patients with ferritin levels up to 100 ng/mL. Enteral iron is typically ineffective in ACD because of reduced intestinal absorption of iron.

Anemia in Cancer Patients

Although ESA therapy has been shown to reduce transfusion requirements in chemotherapy-related anemia, their use remains controversial because of evidence of increased mortality risk in cancer patients.[9] They confer an elevated risk of thrombosis regardless of baseline Hgb level. Current guidelines recommend ESA therapy should only be considered in transfusion-dependent cancer patients with Hgb level <10 g/dL who are receiving myelosuppressive **chemotherapy without a curative intent**, except in the case of patients with lower risk MDS. The goal of ESA therapy is to achieve the lowest Hgb concentration needed to reduce transfusion requirement. Iron replacement therapy can be used in conjunction to improve Hgb response in patients receiving ESA with or without iron deficiency.

Aplastic Anemia

GENERAL PRINCIPLES

- Aplastic anemia (AA) is a disorder of hematopoietic stem cells that usually presents with **pancytopenia.**
- Most cases are acquired and idiopathic, but AA can also arise from an inherited BM failure syndrome such as Fanconi anemia, dyskeratosis congenita, and Shwachman–Diamond syndrome.
- Approximately 20% of cases may be associated with drug or chemical exposure.
- Approximately 10% of cases are associated with viral illnesses (e.g., viral hepatitis, Epstein–Barr virus, parvovirus, cytomegalovirus [CMV]).
- Clonal hematopoiesis is a feature of AA, with MDS and AML developing in ~15% of patients.

DIAGNOSIS

Diagnostic Criteria
Prognosis in AA is dependent on disease severity and patient age:
- Moderate or nonsevere AA
  - BM cellularity <30%
  - Absence of criteria for severe AA
  - At least two of three blood lines are lower than normal
- Severe AA
  - BM cellularity <25% with normal cytogenetics, OR
  - BM cellularity <50% with normal cytogenetics, and <30% residual hematopoietic cells, AND two of three peripheral blood criteria:
    - Absolute neutrophil count (ANC) <500/μL
    - Platelet count <20,000/μL
    - Absolute reticulocyte count <20,000/μL
  - No other hematologic disease
- Very severe AA
  - The criteria of severe AA are met, AND
  - ANC <200/μL

Diagnostic Testing
BM biopsy is required for diagnosis. The BM results in a patient with AA may be difficult to distinguish from hypoplastic MDS; however, both may respond to immunosuppressive therapy (IST). Paroxysmal nocturnal hemoglobinuria clones can be detected by flow cytometry of the blood or BM.

TREATMENT

- Suspected offending drugs should be discontinued and exacerbating factors corrected. Rarely, spontaneous recovery of normal hematopoiesis can occur, usually within 1–2 months of discontinuing the offending drug.
- Once the diagnosis is established, care should be provided in a center experienced with AA.
- Therapy is optional in moderate AA unless there is transfusion dependence; however, severe or very severe AA requires urgent treatment given the high risk of infectious and hemorrhagic complications.
- Patients younger than 50 years with severe AA should be evaluated for eligibility for allogeneic SCT.
- Patients older than 50 years with severe AA or younger patients without SCT donor are treated with IST with eltrombopag 75–150 mg/d along with cyclosporine and antithymocyte globulin.[6] Overall response rates at 6 months were 94% and the 2-year survival rate was 97%.
- AA typically does not respond to ESAs. Granulocyte colony-stimulating factor may be effective in some patients and can be used while awaiting definitive therapy; however, there is no clear evidence of survival benefit with the use of these agents.
- Corticosteroids alone have not been shown to be effective and can increase the risk of infections and **should not** be used in the treatment of AA.
- **Transfusions in AA.** RBC transfusions should be kept to a minimum to avoid alloimmunization. Prophylactic platelet transfusions are generally recommended if the platelet count is <10,000/μL. Transfusion of irradiated, leukocyte-depleted blood products is preferred to decrease the risk of alloimmunization.

ANEMIAS ASSOCIATED WITH INCREASED RBC DESTRUCTION

Anemias Associated With Increased Erythropoiesis

GENERAL PRINCIPLES

Definition

Anemias associated with increased erythropoiesis (i.e., an elevated reticulocyte count) are caused by bleeding or hemolysis and may exceed the capacity of normal BM to correct the Hgb. Bleeding is much more common than hemolysis.

Etiology

- **Blood loss.** If no obvious source, suspect occult loss into GI tract, retroperitoneum, thorax, or deep compartments of thigh depending on history (recent instrumentation, trauma, hip fracture, coagulopathy).
- **Hemolysis** can be categorized into two broad groups based on the cause of destruction: intrinsic (caused by deficits inherit to the RBC) and extrinsic (caused by factors external to the RBC).
  ○ In general, intrinsic causes are inherited, whereas extrinsic causes tend to be acquired. Intrinsic disorders are a result of defects of the red cell membrane (i.e., hereditary spherocytosis), Hgb composition (i.e., sickle cell disease [SCD]), or enzyme deficiency (i.e., G6PD deficiency).

- Extrinsic disorders can result from antibodies (i.e., cold or warm reactive immunoglobulin), infectious agents (i.e., malaria), trauma, chemical agents (i.e., venom), or liver disease.
- Hemolytic disorders are also commonly categorized by the location of RBC destruction: intravascular (within the circulation) or extravascular (within the macrophage in the liver or spleen).

DIAGNOSIS

Laboratory findings of patients with suspected hemolysis typically include:
- **Normocytic or macrocytic anemia with an elevated reticulocyte count.**
- **Elevated LDH** and **indirect hyperbilirubinemia** reflect increased RBC turnover.
- **Decreased haptoglobin** due to binding of intravascular Hgb.
- The **direct Coombs test** (direct antiglobulin testing [DAT]) is an indicator of the presence of antibodies or complement bound to RBC.
- The **indirect Coombs test** indicates the presence of antibody in the plasma.
- A peripheral blood smear is essential and can aid in determining the etiology of hemolysis. Intravascular hemolysis may reveal red cell fragmentation (i.e., schistocytes, helmet cells), whereas spherocytes often occur in extravascular hemolysis. Polychromasia and nucleated RBCs are indicators of increased erythropoiesis.

Sickle Cell Disease

GENERAL PRINCIPLES

- SCD is a group of hereditary Hgb disorders in which Hgb undergoes a sickle shape transformation under conditions of deoxygenation.
- The most common are homozygous sickle cell anemia (Hgb SS) or other double-heterozygous conditions (Hgb SC, Hgb S–β^0, or Hgb S–β^+ thalassemia).
- Newborn screening programs for hemoglobinopathies are available throughout the US and identify most patients in infancy.
- In the US, the incidence of SCD is approximately 1 in 625 births.
- **Sickle cell trait** is present in 7%–8% of African Americans. It is generally considered to be a benign carrier state, but high-altitude hypoxia is associated with splenic infarction, whereas intense physical exertion has been associated with sudden death and rhabdomyolysis.
- Sickle cell trait has been associated with an increased risk of pulmonary embolism, proteinuria, and CKD. Minimizing other risk factors for kidney disease is likely to benefit patients at risk.

DIAGNOSIS

Diagnostic Testing

- Hgb analysis by high-pressure liquid chromatography is commonly used and distinguishes most hemoglobinopathies.
- Laboratory abnormalities include anemia (mean Hgb in SCD, 8 g/dL), reticulocytosis (3%–15%), indirect hyperbilirubinemia, elevated LDH, and decreased or absent haptoglobin. Leukocytosis (10,000–20,000/μL) and thrombocytosis (>450,000/μL) are common because of enhanced stimulation of the marrow compartment and autosplenectomy.

• Peripheral smear shows sickle-shaped RBCs, target cells (particularly in Hgb SC and Hgb S–β thalassemia), and Howell–Jolly bodies, indicative of functional asplenism.

Clinical Presentation

• Clinical presentation of SCD is heterogeneous and is dependent on the type and degree of hemoglobinopathy. The most common clinical manifestations of SCD result from hemolysis and/or vascular occlusions.
• **Vasoocclusive complications (VOCs)** result from polymerization of deoxygenated Hgb S. These polymerized RBCs assume the classic sickle shape and develop a marked loss of deformability, leading to vasoocclusion.
  ○ Acute painful episodes ("sickle cell pain crisis")
    ▪ Sickle cell pain crisis is the most common VOC and manifestation of SCD.
    ▪ Pain is typically in the long bones, back, chest, and abdomen.
    ▪ Precipitating factors can include stress, infection, dehydration, alcohol, and weather. However, a majority of cases have no identifiable trigger.
    ▪ Higher levels of Hgb F seem to be protective against VOC.
  ○ **Acute chest syndrome (ACS)** is a life-threatening emergency that occurs when there is irreversible occlusion of the pulmonary microvasculature. The diagnosis is based on a pulmonary infiltrate involving at least one complete segment and one of the following: fever, hypoxemia, tachypnea, respiratory failure, chest pain, or wheezing. ACS precipitated by pulmonary fat emboli as the inciting event may be more severe and associated with other organ dysfunction, including stroke.
  ○ **Priapism** often presents in adolescence and may result in impotence.
  ○ **Retinopathy** is caused by chronic vasoocclusion of the retina, which causes proliferative retinopathy and may lead to complications including vitreous hemorrhage and retinal detachment.
  ○ **Functional asplenia** results from recurrent splenic infarcts due to sickling and eventually results in the loss of splenic function. The majority of cases occur before the age of 1 year. Functional asplenia places patients at higher risk of infection, especially with encapsulated organisms.
  ○ **Avascular necrosis (AVN)** is the result of infarction of bone trabeculae and occurs most commonly in the femoral and humeral heads. Up to 50% of adults affected by SCD can manifest AVN, which is a leading cause of pain and disability.
• **Hemolytic complications**
  ○ **Cholelithiasis** is present in >80% of patients and is primarily due to bilirubin stones. It may lead to acute cholecystitis or biliary colic.
  ○ **Leg ulceration** occurring at the ankle is often chronic and recurring.
  ○ **Pulmonary hypertension** has been linked to several hemolytic disorders and can occur in up to 60% of patients with SCD. The American Society of Hematology 2019 evidence-based guidelines for SCD recommend considering screening echocardiography that symptomatic patients and those with tricuspid regurgitant jet velocity >2.5 m/s should proceed with a right-sided heart catheterization for confirmation of diagnosis.[10] The pathophysiology is unclear but may be the result of nitric oxide depletion.
• **Renal medulla infarction** is the result of repeated occlusion of renal medullary capillaries, resulting in CKD in many patients. This can lead to isosthenuria (inability to concentrate urine) and hematuria, predisposing patients to dehydration and thus increasing the risk of VOC.
• **Neurologic complications** occur in up to 25% of patients with SCD by the age of 45 years and include cerebrovascular events (transient ischemic attacks, ischemic stroke, cerebral hemorrhage), seizure, and sensory hearing loss.[11] Ischemic stroke

is felt to result from recurrent endothelial injury from hemolysis and vasoocclusion, resulting in intimal hyperplasia with large artery vasculopathy. High cerebral flow rate (>200 cm/s) detected by transcranial Doppler has been associated with increased risk of stroke in children. This risk is greatly reduced by routine transfusion or exchange therapy. "Silent strokes" are those without obvious neurological symptoms—affect one in three children and at least one in two adults with SCD. They cause cognitive impairment and are risk factors for future strokes. The American Society of Hematology recommends at least a one-time MRI screening to detect silent cerebral infarcts in adults with HbSS or HbSβ⁰ thalassemia.[12]

- **Infections** typically occur in tissues susceptible to vasoocclusive infarcts (i.e., lungs, bone, kidney). The most common infectious organisms include *Streptococcus pneumoniae*, *Staphylococcus aureus*, *Salmonella* spp., *Mycoplasma pneumoniae*, or *H. influenzae*. Vaccinations against encapsulated bacteria are key to prevention.
- **Aplastic "crisis"** occurs when there is a transient interruption of erythropoiesis due to an inciting event causing a sudden decrease in Hgb with a very low reticulocyte count. The most common etiology in children with SCD is parvovirus B19 infection. Folate deficiency has also been suspected in some cases.
- **Pregnancy** in a patient with sickle cell anemia should be considered high risk and is associated with an increase in both maternal and fetal complications. Maternal complications include an increased risk of VOC, ACS, and infections.[13] Fetal complications include preterm delivery, low birth weight, and increased risk of stillbirth.

TREATMENT

- **Acute painful episodes.** Management of **acute painful episodes** consists of rehydration, evaluation for and management of infections, analgesia, and if needed, antipyretic and empiric antibiotic therapy.
  - **Opioids** are typically used and are effectively administered by a **patient-controlled analgesia pump**, allowing the patient to self-administer medication within a set limit of infusions (lockout interval) and basal rate. Morphine or hydromorphone are the commonly used opioids for moderate or severe pain and the doses vary considerably from patient to patient.
  - Transfusion therapy has no proven role in the treatment of uncomplicated vasoocclusive crises unless a symptomatic anemia is present or other complications occur.
  - Supplemental oxygen does not benefit an acute pain crisis unless hypoxia is present.
- **ACS.** Multimodal treatment includes adequate analgesia, volume resuscitation, supplemental oxygen and incentive spirometry, and blood transfusion. It is unclear whether exchange transfusion is superior to simple RBC transfusion; however, it is standard practice to perform exchange transfusion for moderate to severe cases, whereas simple transfusion to >10 g/dL for mild cases may be sufficient. The presentation of ACS is clinically indistinguishable from pneumonia; thus, empiric broad-spectrum antibiotics should also be administered.
- **Priapism** is initially treated with hydration and analgesia. Persistent erections for more than 24 hours may require transfusion therapy or surgical drainage.
- **AVN** management consists of local heat, analgesics, and avoidance of weight bearing. Hip and shoulder arthroplasty are often effective at decreasing symptoms and improving function.
- **Cholelithiasis.** Induced acute cholecystitis should be treated medically with antibiotics followed by cholecystectomy when the attack subsides. Elective cholecystectomy for asymptomatic gallstones is controversial.

- **Leg ulcers** should be treated with rest, leg elevation, and intensive local care. Wet to dry dressings should be applied three to four times per day. A zinc oxide–impregnated bandage (Unna boot), changed weekly for 3–4 weeks, can be used for non-healing or more extensive ulcers.
- There is no standard therapy for treatment of **pulmonary hypertension** in SCD and clinically effective therapy remains elusive.[14]
- **Acute stroke** should be managed based on current standards. Long-term transfusions to maintain the Hgb S concentration to <30% for at least 5 years significantly reduce the incidence of recurrence.
- Patients with suspected **aplastic crisis** require hospitalization. Therapy includes folic acid, 5 mg/d, as well as RBC transfusions until recovery.
- **Iron chelation therapy** is used to treat iron overload in patients with transfusion-related iron overload similar to that described for thalassemia.
- Emerging therapies for potentially curative options for SCD include hematopoietic SCT, although its use is restricted by the high cost, toxicity, and limited availability of suitable donors. Less-toxic conditioning regimens and the use of alternative sources of donor cells have improved transplant success. However, SCT may be superseded by investigational gene therapy and gene editing approaches using either addition of a helpful gene encoding an antisickling β globin or a gene knockdown/editing of globin regulatory elements, to partially reverse the normal Hgb switching from fetal to adult Hgb. These approaches are currently being tested in phase II–III trials.

Risk Modification

- **Dehydration and hypoxia** should be avoided because they may precipitate or exacerbate irreversible sickling.
- **Folic acid** (1 mg PO daily) is administered to patients with SCD because of chronic hemolysis.
- **Hydroxyurea** (15–35 mg/kg PO daily) has been shown to increase levels of Hgb F and significantly decrease the frequency of VOC and ACS in adults with SCD.[15] In practice, the dose is increased until the ANCs are between 2000 and 4000/μL.
- **L-glutamine** (0.3 g/kg PO twice daily) recently became available for the prevention of VOC and may be incorporated into preventative care with or without concomitant hydroxyurea.[16]
- **Crizanlizumab**, a P-selectin inhibitor given as an infusion, was recently approved after showing significantly lower frequency of sickle cell–related pain crises in patients receiving this therapy, with or without hydroxyurea.[17]
- **Voxelotor,** an HbS polymerization inhibitor, is another recently approved agent shown to significantly increase Hgb levels and reduce markers of hemolysis in patients with SCD and anemia.[18]
- **Antimicrobial prophylaxis** with penicillin VK, 125 mg PO bid to age 3 years and then 250 mg PO bid until age 5 years, is effective at reducing risk of infection. Patients who are allergic to penicillin should receive erythromycin 10 mg/kg PO bid. Prophylaxis should be stopped at age 5 years to avoid development of resistant organisms.
- **Immunizations** against the usual childhood illnesses should be given to children with SCD, including hepatitis B vaccine. After 2 years of age, a polyvalent pneumococcal vaccine should be administered. Yearly influenza vaccine is recommended.
- **Ophthalmologic examinations** are recommended yearly in adults because of the high incidence of proliferative retinopathy.

- **Preoperative optimization.** Local and regional anesthesia can be used without special precautions. Care should be taken to avoid volume depletion, hypoxia, and hypernatremia. For surgery with general anesthesia, RBC transfusions to increase the Hgb to 10 g/dL is as effective as more aggressive thresholds to decrease postoperative complications and more effective than withholding preoperative transfusions.[19]

G6PD Deficiency

GENERAL PRINCIPLES

G6PD deficiency represents the most common disorder of RBC metabolism worldwide. Deficiency of G6PD renders RBCs more susceptible to oxidative damage through decreased glutathione reduction, leading to chronic or acute episodic hemolysis in the presence of oxidative stress.

Classification
More than 400 variants of G6PD are recognized. The severity of hemolysis depends on the degree of deficiency present.

Epidemiology
- X-linked inheritance; the degree of involvement in females is dependent on lyonization.
- G6PD is felt to be protective against malaria, accounting for its prevalence in malaria-endemic areas.
- Hemolysis is triggered by exposure to mediators of oxidative stress, infections, and fava beans. Patients being considered for medications that trigger G6PD-dependent hemolysis should be tested for a deficiency before starting the drug.

DIAGNOSIS

- Diagnosis is determined by measuring G6PD activity in RBCs from a peripheral blood sample. Peripheral smear may show bite cells and blister cells. Direct coombs test will be negative.
- **False-negative** results may occur in patients with a recent episode of hemolysis or in patients recently transfused because these cells have higher levels of G6PD.

TREATMENT

- In the most common form of G6PD deficiency, hemolytic episodes tend to be self-limiting; the mainstay of treatment is supportive. If acute hemolytic anemia is severe, blood transfusion may be needed.
- The underlying cause of oxidative stress should be addressed (i.e., treatment of infection, removal of drug).

Autoimmune Hemolytic Anemia

GENERAL PRINCIPLES

Definition
Autoimmune hemolytic anemia (AIHA) results from autoantibodies targeted to antigens on the patient's RBCs, resulting in either extravascular hemolysis (removal of

RBC by tissue macrophages in the liver or spleen) or complement-mediated intravascular hemolysis.

Classification

There are two main types of AIHA: warm and cold AIHA. Warm AIHA antibodies interact best with RBCs at 37°C, whereas cold antibodies (or cold agglutinins) are most active at temperatures below 37°C and almost always fix complement.

Etiology

- Warm AIHA is usually caused by an IgG autoantibody. It may be idiopathic or secondary to an underlying process (i.e., lymphoma, chronic lymphocytic leukemia [CLL], collagen vascular disorder, or drugs).
- Cold AIHA (or cold agglutinin disease [CAD]) is typically caused by an IgM autoantibody.
  - The acute form of CAD is often secondary to an infection (*Mycoplasma*, Epstein–Barr virus).
  - The chronic form is associated with an IgM paraprotein or lymphoproliferative disorder in approximately one-half of cases and is primary (idiopathic) in the others.

DIAGNOSIS

- Laboratory data usually identify hemolysis with anemia, reticulocytosis, elevated LDH, decreased haptoglobin, indirect hyperbilirubinemia, and hemoglobinuria (if intravascular hemolysis is present).
- Peripheral blood smear may show spherocytes, occasional fragmented RBCs in warm AIHA, and RBC agglutination in CAD. Polychromasia and nucleated RBCs may be seen in either form.
- The hallmark of diagnosis is by a positive **DAT (also known as a direct Coombs test).** The DAT detects the presence of IgG or complement in the form of C3 bound to the RBC surface. The typical results for the DAT are shown here:
  - Warm AIHA: IgG positive and C3 positive or negative
  - Cold AIHA: IgG negative and C3 positive
- The indirect antiglobulin test (indirect Coombs) detects the presence of autoantibodies in the serum but also detects alloantibodies in the serum from alternate causes, including from transfusion or maternal–fetal incompatibility.
- An elevated cold agglutinin titer is seen with cold AIHA.
- If secondary AIHA is suspected, a workup for the underlying cause should be performed.

TREATMENT

- Initial therapy should be aimed at correcting complications from the hemolytic anemia. Definitive therapy should include identification and treatment of any underlying cause.
- RBC transfusions may result in the hemolysis of transfused cells, but they are still indicated in severe or life-threatening anemia.
- **If a complete crossmatch cannot be completed in a timely manner, transfusion of universal donor (O-negative) or type-matched blood is appropriate.**
- **Warm AIHA.**

- First-line treatment involves **glucocorticoids**, such as oral prednisone 1–2 mg/kg/d, which is effective in 80%–90% of patients. Response is typically seen in 7–25 days. When hemolysis has abated, glucocorticoids can be tapered over 4–6 months. Rapid steroid taper can result in relapse.
- Second-line treatments include **rituximab**, a monoclonal antibody directed against CD20 antigen expressed on B cells. Rituximab 375 mg/m^2 weekly for four doses has been shown to be effective in 80% of cases with median response time of 3–6 weeks, and responses to treatment are observed with monotherapy or in combination with corticosteroids. Low-dose rituximab, 100 mg weekly for four doses, has also demonstrated efficacy in AIHA.[20] Splenectomy is as effective as rituximab with median response of 7–10 days but its use has declined due to increased risk of serious infections and thrombosis.
- Treatment for relapsed/refractory cases is not well defined and includes azathioprine, cyclophosphamide, cyclosporine, and mycophenolate mofetil.
- **Primary CAD**
  - Avoidance of cold exposure can minimize exacerbations. RBC transfusions at 37°C (blood warmer) and keeping the room warm can prevent exacerbation of hemolysis.
  - Glucocorticoids and splenectomy are not effective and should not be used.
  - Plasma exchange removes 60%–70% of IgM, thus offering effective, temporary control of the disease in severe hemolysis.
  - Rituximab as a single agent or in combination with other agents (i.e., bendamustine) has shown to be effective in some cases and may be used as first-line therapy.

Drug-Induced Hemolytic Anemia

GENERAL PRINCIPLES

- **Drug-induced hemolytic anemia** is anemia resulting from exposure to a medication. Hemolysis occurs by several mechanisms such as drug-induced antibodies, hapten formation, and immune complexes. The most commonly implicated agents are cephalosporins, penicillins, NSAIDs, and quinine or quinidines.
- Drug-dependent antibodies can be investigated by testing drug-treated RBCs or by testing RBCs in the presence of a solution of drug. This testing is offered at specialized hematology labs and may be useful in verifying the culprit drug.

TREATMENT

The initial treatment may be similar to treatment of warm AIHA with corticosteroids if the etiology is unclear, but if drug-induced hemolytic anemia is suspected, **the most important treatment is discontinuation of the offending agent**.

Microangiopathic Hemolytic Anemia

GENERAL PRINCIPLES

Definition

Microangiopathic hemolytic anemia (MAHA) is a syndrome of traumatic intravascular hemolysis causing fragmentation of the RBCs that are seen on peripheral blood smear (schistocytes). It is not a specific diagnosis but suggests a limited differential diagnosis.

Etiology

Possible causes of MAHA include **mechanical heart valve, malignant hypertension, vasculitis, adenocarcinoma, preeclampsia/eclampsia, disseminated intravascular coagulation (DIC), thrombotic thrombocytopenic purpura (TTP), and hemolytic uremic syndrome (HUS)/atypical HUS** (see Chapter 20, Disorders of Hemostasis and Thrombosis, for a discussion of DIC, TTP, and HUS/atypical HUS).

DIAGNOSIS

MAHA is established by confirming the presence of hemolysis with laboratory data (LDH, haptoglobin, indirect bilirubin) and identifying RBC fragments (schistocytes) on peripheral blood smear. Thrombocytopenia is also common.

TREATMENT

The treatment depends on the underlying etiology of microangiopathy (see Chapter 20, Disorders of Hemostasis and Thrombosis).

WHITE BLOOD CELL DISORDERS

Leukocytosis and Leukopenia

GENERAL PRINCIPLES

Definition

- Leukocytosis is an elevation in the absolute WBC count (>10,000 cells/μL).
- Leukopenia is a reduction in the WBC count (<3500 cells/μL).

Etiology

- **Leukocytosis**
  - An elevated WBC can be the normal BM response to an infectious or inflammatory process, corticosteroids, β-agonist or lithium therapy, or splenectomy and is usually associated with an **absolute neutrophilia**.
  - Occasionally, leukocytosis is due to a primary BM disorder with an increase in WBC production and/or delayed maturation. This may occur in the setting of hematologic malignancies such as leukemias and can affect any cell in the leukocyte lineage.
  - A "**leukemoid reaction**" is defined as an excessive WBC response usually reserved for neutrophilia (>50,000/μL) due to a reactive cause.
  - Lymphocytosis is less commonly encountered and is typically associated with atypical infections (i.e., viral), medication use, or leukemia/lymphoma.
- **Leukopenia**
  - Leukopenia can be classified as either congenital or acquired.
  - Acquired leukopenia can occur in response to infection (i.e., HIV), inflammation, primary BM disorders (i.e., malignancy), autoimmune disorders, medications, environmental exposure (i.e., heavy metals or radiation), and vitamin deficiencies. Many cases are medication induced (i.e., chemotherapeutic or immunosuppressive

drugs) and a careful history examining the timing of the onset of leukopenia/neutropenia and new medications is important.
- ○ Large granular lymphocytic leukemia can be a cause of neutropenia, especially in patients with rheumatoid arthritis.
- ○ Congenital neutropenias can include constitutional/ethnic neutropenia, severe congenital neutropenia, and cyclic neutropenia.

DIAGNOSIS

Diagnostic Testing
- Review of the peripheral smear is very helpful in the evaluation of WBC disorders. Predominant neutrophilia may suggest a reactive process. The presence of blasts is concerning for acute leukemia and warrants emergent evaluation.
- Flow cytometry of the blood may help determine if there is an underlying clonal process in lymphocytosis (i.e., CLL) or if an acute leukemia is suspected.
- A BCR–ABL molecular study may be warranted in cases of unexplained neutrophilia to diagnose chronic myeloid leukemia (CML), especially if there is associated eosinophilia or basophilia.

Diagnostic Procedures
A BM biopsy with ancillary studies such as cytogenetics, special stains, and flow cytometry may be required to establish the diagnosis.

TREATMENT

- The primary goal of therapy is identification and treatment of the underlying cause.
- See Chapter 22, Cancer, for the treatment of acute and chronic leukemia.
- Growth factor support should be considered in patients with chronic neutropenia and ongoing infections until the neutropenia resolves (see Oncologic Emergencies in Chapter 22, Cancer).

PLATELET DISORDERS

Discussed in Chapter 20, Disorders of Hemostasis and Thrombosis.

BM DISORDERS

Myelodysplastic Syndrome

Discussed in Chapter 22, Cancer.

Myeloproliferative Neoplasms

GENERAL PRINCIPLES

MPNs are a group of hematologic malignancies characterized by clonal expansion of a hematopoietic stem cell resulting in overproduction of mature, largely functional cells. The 2016 World Health Organization (WHO) designated seven conditions as MPNs, including polycythemia vera (PV), essential thrombocythemia (ET) (discussed in Chapter 22, Cancer), CML (discussed in Chapter 22, Cancer), primary myelofibrosis (PMF), chronic neutrophilic leukemia, chronic eosinophilic leukemia, and MPN unclassifiable.[21] The most common MPNs include PV, ET, CML, and PMF. This section will focus on PV and PMF.

DIAGNOSIS

Diagnostic Criteria

- **PV**
  Criteria for the diagnosis of PV have been updated in the WHO 2016. The diagnosis of PV requires meeting either all three major criteria, or the first two major criteria and the minor criterion[21] (Table 21-5).
- **PMF**
  The WHO 2016 diagnostic criteria for PMF are listed in Table 21-6.[21] The updated classification has divided PMF into pre-PMF and overt PMF. For both pre-PMF and overt PMF, all three major criteria and at least one minor criterion need to be met for the diagnosis.

Diagnostic Testing

- Patients with PV typically present with an elevated Hct but may also have elevations in WBC or platelet count. The *JAK2*V617F mutation is present in >95% of patients. A low EPO level is often present. PV patients who do not have a *JAK2*V617F mutation may have a *JAK2* exon 12 mutation.
- Patients with PMF may present with leukocytosis or cytopenias (i.e., anemia) and may have mutations in *JAK2* (50%), *MPL* (10%), or calreticulin (*CALR*) (40%). Immature granulocytes, tear drop cells, and nucleated RBCs may be seen on the peripheral blood smear (leukoerythroblastic smear).

TABLE 21-5	WHO 2016 Diagnostic Criteria for Polycythemia Vera

Major Criteria

1. Hgb >16.5 g/dL in men and Hgb >16.0 g/dL in women
   Or
   Hct >49% in men and Hct >48% in women
   Or
   Increased red cell mass more than 25% mean normal predicted value
2. BM biopsy showing hypercellularity for age with trilineage growth (panmyelosis) including prominent erythroid, granulocytic, and megakaryocytic proliferation with pleomorphic, mature megakaryocytes (differences in size)
3. Presence of *JAK2*V617F mutation or *JAK2* exon 12 mutation

Minor Criteria

Subnormal serum erythropoietin level

Diagnosis of PV requires meeting either all three major criteria or the first two major criteria and the minor criterion

BM, bone marrow; Hct, hematocrit; Hgb, hemoglobin; PV, polycythemia vera; WHO, World Health Organization.

Reprinted from Arber DA, Orazi A, Hasserjian R, et al. The 2016 revision to the World Health Organization classification of myeloid neoplasms and acute leukemia. *Blood*. 2016;127(20):2391-2405. Copyright © 2016 Elsevier. With permission.

TABLE 21-6	WHO 2016 Diagnostic Criteria for Primary Myelofibrosis (PMF)

Pre-PMF Criteria

Major Criteria

1. Megakaryocytic proliferation and atypia, without reticulin fibrosis >grade 1, accompanied by increased age-adjusted BM cellularity, granulocytic proliferation, and often decreased erythropoiesis
2. Not meeting the WHO criteria for *BCR–ABL1* CML, PV, ET, MDS, or other myeloid neoplasms
3. Presence of *JAK2*, *CALR*, or *MPL* mutation or in the absence of these mutations, presence of another clonal marker, or absence of minor reactive BM reticulin fibrosis

Minor Criteria

Presence of at least one of the following, confirmed in two consecutive determinations:

a. Anemia not attributed to a comorbid condition
b. Leukocytosis $\geq 11 \times 10^9$/L
c. Palpable splenomegaly
d. LDH increased to above upper normal limit of institutional reference range

Diagnosis of pre-PMF requires meeting all three major criteria and at least one minor criterion

Overt PMF criteria

Major Criteria

1. Presence of megakaryocytic proliferation and atypia, accompanied by either reticulin and/or collagen fibrosis grades 2 or 3
2. Not meeting WHO criteria for ET, PV, *BCR–ABL1* CML, MDS, or other myeloid neoplasms
3. Presence of *JAK2*, *CALR*, or *MPL* mutation or in the absence of these mutations, presence of another clonal marker, or absence of reactive myelofibrosis

Minor Criteria

Presence of at least one of the following, confirmed in two consecutive determinations:

a. Anemia not attributed to a comorbid condition
b. Leukocytosis $\geq 11 \times 10^9$/L
c. Palpable splenomegaly
d. LDH increased to above upper normal limit of institutional reference range
e. Leukoerythroblastosis

Diagnosis of overt PMF requires meeting all three major criteria and at least one minor criterion

BM, bone marrow; CML, chronic myelogenous leukemia; ET, essential thrombocythemia; LDH, lactate dehydrogenase; MDS, myelodysplastic syndrome; PV, polycythemia vera; WHO, World Health Organization.

Reprinted from Arber DA, Orazi A, Hasserjian R, et al. The 2016 revision to the World Health Organization classification of myeloid neoplasms and acute leukemia. *Blood.* 2016;127(20):2391-2405. Copyright © 2016 Elsevier. With permission.

Diagnostic Procedures

A BM biopsy should be included in the diagnostic workup of PMF, including reticulin stain, to evaluate for fibrosis. A BM biopsy may not be required for PV in cases with sustained absolute erythrocytosis defined as an Hgb >18.5 g/dL in men or >16.5 g/dL in women. Cytogenetic studies should be performed and have a significant impact on prognosis in PMF.[22]

TREATMENT

- **PV:** The main goal of treatment is to decrease the risk of thrombotic complications by maintaining the Hct <45.[23] All patients are recommended to be on aspirin 81 mg/d in the absence of bleeding contraindications.
  - In patients with low risk for thrombosis (age <60 years, no history of thrombosis): serial phlebotomy to keep goal Hct <45% in men and <42% in women.
  - Patients with high risk for thrombosis (age >60 years, prior thrombosis) should be treated initially with serial phlebotomy and hydroxyurea, with the ultimate goal of maintaining Hct <45% in men and <42% in women on hydroxyurea without the need for phlebotomy.
  - Ruxolitinib 10 mg twice a day, a JAK inhibitor first approved for treatment of myelofibrosis, is approved by the FDA for the treatment of PV in patients who fail hydroxyurea therapy. Ruxolitinib has been shown to improve pruritus.[24]
  - Ropeginterferon alfa-2b is an emerging therapy for patients with PV and demonstrated noninferiority to hydroxyurea in inducing hematological responses.[25]
- **PMF:** Patients are risk-stratified based on several prognostic scoring systems and treatment depends on the risk category.[22] Treatment may not be needed for low-risk patients.
  - Low-dose aspirin should be started to decrease the risk of thrombosis in the absence of significant thrombocytopenia.
  - Cytoreductive agents such as hydroxyurea have been used historically to improve leukocytosis but do not significantly improve constitutional symptoms or splenomegaly and can cause myelosuppression.
  - Allogeneic hematopoietic SCT is the only curative therapy and should be considered for high-risk patients.
  - JAK inhibitors such as ruxolitinib and fedratinib are approved for the treatment of patients with intermediate- and high-risk myelofibrosis. They are effective in improving constitutional symptoms and splenomegaly.[26,27]
  - Splenectomy may be considered for painful splenomegaly in patients intolerant to or not responsive to the JAK inhibitor; however, it is associated with an increased risk for thrombosis and infections.
  - Involved-field radiotherapy may also offer symptomatic relief for drug-refractory splenomegaly or sites of extramedullary hematopoiesis; however, the effects are usually transient.

MONOCLONAL GAMMOPATHIES

Monoclonal Gammopathy of Unknown Significance

GENERAL PRINCIPLES

Definition

Monoclonal gammopathy of unknown significance (MGUS) is a commonly occurring premalignant condition characterized by the presence of a small (<10%) population of neoplastic, clonal plasma cells or lymphoplasmacytic cells in the BM that occurs in the absence of any end-organ damage.

DIAGNOSIS

- Patients with MGUS are asymptomatic and diagnosed when a monoclonal protein is detected on serum protein electrophoresis (SPEP) during workup of an elevated serum protein or other unrelated clinical finding.
- Serum free light chain assay is used in both the prognosis of MGUS and in the diagnosis of multiple myeloma.
- The Multiple Myeloma International Working Group diagnostic criteria for non-IgM MGUS requires all three of the following criteria[28,29]:
  ○ Presence of a serum monoclonal protein (non-IgM type) <3 g/dL
  ○ Presence of clonal BM plasma cells comprising <10% of the marrow
  ○ Absence of end-organ damage attributed to the underlying plasma cell disorder, such as hypercalcemia, renal insufficiency, anemia, or lytic bone lesions
- The Multiple Myeloma International Working Group diagnostic criteria for IgM MGUS requires the following diagnostic criteria[28,29]:
  ○ Serum IgM monoclonal protein <3 g/dL
  ○ BM lymphoplasmacytic infiltration <10%
  ○ No evidence of anemia, constitutional symptoms, hyperviscosity, lymphadenopathy, hepatosplenomegaly, or other end-organ damage that can be attributed to the underlying lymphoproliferative disorder

TREATMENT

There is no treatment recommended for MGUS. The vast majority of patients will not progress to myeloma. Yearly surveillance with a CBC, serum creatinine and calcium, SPEP, urine protein electrophoresis (UPEP), and serum free light chains is recommended. If a patient develops an anemia, hypercalcemia, renal dysfunction, or bone pain, additional evaluation including a BM biopsy and imaging (i.e., skeletal survey, positron emission tomography, CT scan, or MRI) is recommended.

PROGNOSIS

For non-IgM MGUS, progression to a more serious disorder including multiple myeloma, Waldenström macroglobulinemia (WM), or primary amyloidosis (AL) occurs at a rate of approximately 1% per year. For IgM MGUS, progression to WM or primary AL amyloidosis occurs at a rate of 1%–5% per year.

Factors for higher risk of progression include an M protein >1.5 g/dL, non-IgG monoclonal gammopathy, and abnormal serum free light chain ratio (<0.26 or >1.65).

Multiple Myeloma

Discussed in Chapter 22, Cancer.

Waldenström Macroglobulinemia

WM is an uncommon IgM monoclonal disorder also known as lymphoplasmacytic lymphoma, characterized by mild hematologic abnormalities, and accompanied by tissue infiltration including lymphadenopathy, splenomegaly, or hepatomegaly.

Because of its high molecular weight and concentration, IgM gammopathy can lead to hyperviscosity (central nervous system, visual, cardiac) manifestations. In these cases, emergent plasmapheresis to decrease IgM concentration is indicated. The *MYD88* L265P mutation is a commonly recurring mutation in patients with WM and can be useful in differentiating WM from B-cell disorders that have similar features. Asymptomatic patients may be observed initially, whereas durable responses have been observed in those requiring chemotherapy. The Bruton tyrosine kinase inhibitor ibrutinib is also approved for treatment of WM with an overall response rate of 62%.

Amyloidosis

GENERAL PRINCIPLES

Primary (AL) amyloidosis is an infiltrative disorder due to monoclonal, light chain deposition in various tissues most often involving the kidney (renal failure, nephrotic syndrome), heart (nonischemic cardiomyopathy), peripheral nervous system (neuropathy), and GI tract/liver (macroglossia, diarrhea, nausea, vomiting). Unexplained findings in any of these organ systems should prompt evaluation for amyloidosis. Primary AL amyloidosis must be distinguished from nonclonal secondary systemic amyloidosis.

DIAGNOSIS AND TREATMENT

- SPEP, UPEP, and serum free light chains may detect an M protein or an abnormal free light chain ratio that is found in >90% of patients with AL amyloidosis. In the absence of a measurable M protein, consider other types of secondary systemic amyloidosis. In addition to Congo red staining for amyloid in the BM or other affected tissue, mass spectroscopy to identify the presence of light chains establishes the diagnosis of AL amyloidosis. An NT-proBNP, troponin T or I, and 24-hour urinary protein are important in assessing organ involvement and staging.
- Several effective chemotherapy regimens have been developed during the last decade, including bortezomib-based regimens such as **CyBorD** (cyclophosphamide, bortezomib, dexamethasone).[30] Additionally, those with adequate organ function and a good performance status should be considered for autologous stem cell transplant (auto-SCT).
- **Daratumumab**, an anti-CD38 monoclonal antibody approved for the treatment of multiple myeloma, has demonstrated efficacy in AL amyloid and has been used off label for relapsed systemic AL amyloidosis.[31]
- Treatment of amyloidosis remains difficult, and progressive organ failure is frequent. Cardiac involvement generally portends the worst prognosis.

TRANSFUSION MEDICINE

GENERAL PRINCIPLES

Transfusion is a therapy for several hematologic and hemostatic aberrations but its benefits must be weighed carefully against its risks as blood products are a limited resource with potentially life-threatening side effects.

TREATMENT

- **pRBCs.** RBC transfusion is indicated to increase the oxygen-carrying capacity of blood in anemic or bleeding patients.
  - Current practice guidelines use the following Hgb thresholds[32]:
    - Hemodynamically stable adult inpatients, including critically ill patients: ≤7 g/dL.
    - Patients undergoing orthopedic surgery, cardiac surgery, or those with preexisting cardiovascular disease: ≤8 g/dL.
    - Patients with acute coronary syndrome, severe thrombocytopenia, or chronic transfusion–dependent anemia: not established (consider 8–10 g/dL).
  - One unit of pRBCs increases the Hgb level by approximately 1 g/dL or Hct by 3% in an average 70 kg adult.
  - In the absence of cerebrovascular or cardiovascular injury, transfusions should be avoided for easily treatable anemias such as from iron or vitamin B_{12} deficiencies.
- **Fresh frozen plasma (FFP):** Plasma transfusion is indicated to replace coagulation factors to treat bleeding patients, or as bleeding prophylaxis for certain invasive procedures.
  - Common indications include the following:
    - Acquired coagulopathy in the setting of major bleeding.
    - Warfarin overdose with major bleeding. However, four-factor (II, VII, IX, X) prothrombin complex concentrates are generally preferred over FFP.
    - Factor deficiencies for which specific factor concentrates are unavailable.
  - The usual dose of FFP is 10–20 mL/kg. One unit of FFP contains approximately 250 mL of plasma and 250 units of factor activity for each factor.
  - FFP should not be used as a volume expander. FFP is usually not indicated for patients who are not actively bleeding, even when the PT or activated PTT is abnormal. In the case of warfarin overdose with a prolonged PT but no bleeding, vitamin K is preferred.
  - FFP has been used in patients undergoing high-risk surgery (e.g., neurosurgery) with international normalized ratio (INR) >1.5. However, there is no evidence supporting this practice. FFP is typically ineffective for decreasing mildly elevated INR values.
- **Platelets:** Platelet transfusion is indicated to prevent or treat bleeding in thrombocytopenic patients or patients with dysfunctional platelets (e.g., due to aspirin).
  - Current practice guidelines use the following platelet count thresholds[33]:
    - Nonbleeding, stable inpatients: ≤10 × 10^9/L.
    - Nonbleeding, stable outpatients: ≤20 × 10^9/L.
    - Central venous catheter placement: ≤20 × 10^9/L.
    - Major surgery or lumbar puncture: ≤50 × 10^9/L.
    - High-risk surgery (e.g., neurosurgery) or life-threatening bleeding: not established (consider 50–100 × 10^9/L).
  - Pooled platelets from multiple donors were historically used. However, most platelet products in the US today are from single donors collected by platelet apheresis.
  - Platelets have a short shelf life (<5 days) and are stored at room temperature; they should not be placed on ice or refrigerated, which can cause platelet activation.
  - One unit of single-donor platelets increases the platelet count by 30–50 × 10^9/L in an average 70 kg patient, but this response may be blunted in patients with platelet refractoriness.
  - **Platelet refractoriness** (poor platelet count increment after transfusion) may be due to immunologic causes (anti-ABO, anti-HLA, or antiplatelet antibodies) or

nonimmunologic causes (e.g., sepsis, DIC, fever, active bleeding, splenic sequestration, certain drugs). A general rule of thumb is immunologic causes are likely when a 10- to 60-minute posttransfusion platelet count shows $<15 \times 10^9/L$ increment, indicating a potential need for ABO- and/or HLA-compatible platelets.

- **Cryoprecipitate**
  - Cryoprecipitate contains the cold-precipitated portion of plasma enriched in the following factors:
    - Fibrinogen
    - von Willebrand factor (vWF)
    - Factor VIII
    - Factor XIII
  - Cryoprecipitate was used historically to replace vWF and factor VIII; however, specific replacement of these factors is now preferred. The main indication for cryoprecipitate today is to replace **fibrinogen** in patients with hypofibrinogenemia or DIC.
  - One unit increases fibrinogen concentration by approximately 7–8 mg/dL. Doses are typically ordered in pools of 5 or 10 units.

SPECIAL CONSIDERATIONS

- **Pretransfusion testing**
  - The **type and screen** procedure tests the recipient's RBCs for the A, B, and D (Rh) antigens and also screens the recipient's serum for antibodies against other RBC antigens.
  - The **crossmatch** tests the recipient's serum for antibodies against antigens on a specific donor's RBCs and is performed for each unit of blood that is dispensed for a patient. If a patient has no history of RBC antibodies, the serologic crossmatch may be replaced by an instantaneous computer crossmatch. Plasma and platelets do not require a crossmatch.
- **Modifications of blood products**
  - **Leukoreduction** is performed by the use of filters to eliminate WBC contamination before storage or at the bedside. It is indicated for all patients to reduce the risk of the following transfusion complications:
    - Nonhemolytic febrile transfusion reactions
    - Transfusion-transmitted CMV infection
    - Formation of HLA alloantibodies
  - **CMV-seronegative** blood products may be indicated for immunocompromised patients who are CMV-seronegative to reduce the risk of CMV transmission. However, prestorage leukoreduced products are considered equivalently "CMV-reduced risk" and can be used in place of CMV-seronegative products.
  - **Irradiation** eliminates immunologically competent lymphocytes to prevent transfusion-associated graft-versus-host disease and is indicated for certain immunocompromised patients, SCT recipients, and patients who receive directed donations from HLA-matched donors or relatives.
  - **Washing** of pRBCs is rarely indicated but should be considered for patients in whom plasma proteins may cause a serious reaction (e.g., recipients with IgA deficiency or a history of anaphylactic reactions).
  - **Pathogen reduction** uses UV light to inactivate replicating pathogens such as bacteria and most viruses, as well as donor leukocytes, replacing CMV reduced risk blood and irradiation. It is currently only approved for platelets and plasma and is not in widespread use.

- **Blood administration**
  - Patient and blood product identification procedures must be carefully followed to avoid any transfusion-related errors including ABO-incompatible transfusion.
  - The IV catheter should be at least 18 gauge to allow adequate flow.
  - All blood products should be administered through a 170- to 260-μm "standard" filter to prevent infusion of macroaggregates, fibrin, and debris.
  - No fluids other than saline may be infused into the same line during transfusion.
  - Patients should be observed with vital signs for the first 10–15 minutes of each transfusion for adverse effects and at regular intervals thereafter.
  - RBC infusion is typically administered over 1–2 hours, with a maximum of 4 hours.
- **Emergency transfusion** may be considered in situations in which massive blood loss has resulted in cardiovascular compromise.
  - Before the patient's ABO type can be confirmed, "emergency release" blood may be used, consisting of uncrossmatched group O pRBCs and group AB or A plasma.
  - If **massive transfusion** (replacement of ≥10 units of pRBCs in <24 hours) is indicated, hemostatic components (plasma, platelets, and cryoprecipitate) should be included to correct the loss and dilution of hemostatic factors. In addition, care must be taken to manage the potential iatrogenic complications of massive transfusion, such as hypothermia, hypocalcemia (due to the citrated preservative solution), and hyperkalemia.

COMPLICATIONS

- **Transfusion-transmitted infections**
  - Donors and blood products are screened for HIV-1/2, human T-lymphotropic virus 1/2, hepatitis B, hepatitis C, West Nile virus, Zika virus, COVID-19, syphilis, *Trypanosoma cruzi* (Chagas), and bacteremia (platelets only).
  - Viral transmission may occur when donors are in the "window period" (i.e., undetectable to testing).
    - The risk of hepatitis B transmission is approximately 1 in 1,000,000; other tested viruses have a transmission risk of <1 in 1,000,000.
    - CMV transmission risk may be reduced in immunocompromised patients by the use of CMV-seronegative or prestorage leukoreduced products, as well as pathogen reduction.
  - Bacterial transmission may occur from either a donor infection or a contaminant at the time of collection or processing.
    - Platelet transfusions are more likely than RBCs to have bacterial contamination because they are stored at room temperature. This risk may be mitigated by pathogen reduction.
    - The most common organisms identified are *Yersinia enterocolitica* in RBCs and *Staphylococcus* spp. in platelets.
  - Blood donors are also screened for COVID-19 antibodies. However, as of 2021, this screen is only used to identify eligibility of a blood donation for convalescent plasma and is not used to prevent the release of a blood product for the purpose of transfusion-transmitted infection prevention.
- **Noninfectious hazards of transfusion**
  - **Acute hemolytic transfusion reactions** are usually caused by **preformed antibodies** in the recipient and are characterized by intravascular hemolysis of the transfused RBCs soon after the administration of ABO-incompatible blood.

- **Fever, chills, back pain, chest pain, nausea, vomiting, anxiety, and hypotension** may develop. Acute renal failure with hemoglobinuria may occur. In the unconscious patient, hypotension or hemoglobinuria may be the only manifestation.
- If a hemolytic transfusion reaction is suspected, **the transfusion should be stopped immediately and all IV tubing should be replaced.** Samples of the patient's blood should be delivered to the blood bank along with the remainder of the suspected unit for repeat of the crossmatch. Direct and indirect Coombs tests should be performed, and the plasma and freshly voided urine should be examined for free Hgb.
- Management includes preservation of intravascular volume and protection of renal function. Urine output should be maintained at ≥100 mL/h with the use of IV fluids and diuretics or mannitol, if necessary. The excretion of free Hgb can be aided by alkalinization of the urine. Sodium bicarbonate can be added to IV fluids to increase the urinary pH to ≥7.5.
  - **Delayed hemolytic transfusion reactions** typically occur 3–10 days after transfusion and are caused by either a primary or an anamnestic antibody response to specific RBC antigens on donor RBCs.
    - Hgb and Hct levels may fall.
    - The DAT is usually positive, depending on when the follow-up testing is conducted.
    - Reactions may at times be severe; these cases should be treated similarly to acute hemolytic reactions.
  - **Nonhemolytic febrile transfusion reactions** are characterized by fevers and chills.
    - Cytokines released from white cells are thought to be the cause.
    - Treatment and future prophylaxis may include acetaminophen and prestorage leukoreduced blood products.
  - **Allergic reactions** are characterized by urticaria and, in severe cases, bronchospasm and hypotension.
    - The reactions are due to plasma proteins that elicit an IgE-mediated response. The reaction may be specific to the plasma proteins of a particular donor and therefore may occur infrequently or never again.
    - Treatment and future prophylaxis may include antihistamines such as diphenhydramine or corticosteroids.
    - **Anaphylactic reactions** may require the addition of corticosteroids and washed or plasma-reduced products. Additionally, check serum immunoglobulins because patients with IgA deficiency who receive IgA-containing blood products may experience anaphylaxis with small exposure to donor plasma.
  - **Transfusion-associated circulatory overload** (TACO) is a relatively common yet underrecognized complication of blood transfusion. Volume overload with pulmonary edema and signs of CHF may be seen when patients with cardiovascular compromise are transfused. The clinical and radiographic features may be difficult to distinguish from that of transfusion-related acute lung injury (TRALI). Slowing the rate of transfusion and judicious use of diuretics help prevent this complication, as well as avoidance of unnecessary transfusion.
  - **TRALI** is indistinguishable from acute respiratory distress syndrome and occurs within 6 hours of a transfusion.
    - Symptoms include dyspnea, hypoxemia, and possibly fever.
    - New or worsening pulmonary edema is typically seen on CXR, as with TACO, but without evidence of volume overload.

- Anti-HLA or antineutrophil antibodies in the donor's serum directed against the recipient's WBCs are thought to cause the disorder.
- On recognition, transfusions must be stopped and the blood bank notified so that other products from the donor(s) in question may be quarantined.
- Hypoxemia resolves rapidly, typically in about 24 hours, but ventilatory assistance may be required during that time.
- Despite clinical or radiographic findings that suggest pulmonary edema, data indicate that diuretics have no role and may be detrimental.[34]

○ **Transfusion-associated graft-versus-host disease** is a rare but serious complication usually seen in immunocompromised patients (and immunocompetent patients receiving blood from a relative) and is thought to result from the infusion of immunocompetent donor T lymphocytes.
- Symptoms include rash, elevated liver function tests, and severe pancytopenia.
- Mortality is >80%.
- **Irradiation** or pathogen reduction of blood products for at-risk patients prevents this disease.

○ **Posttransfusion purpura** is a rare syndrome of severe thrombocytopenia and purpura or bleeding that starts 7–10 days after exposure to blood products. This disorder is described in Chapter 20, Disorders of Hemostasis and Thrombosis, in the "Platelet Disorders" section.

REFERENCES

1. Stoffel NU, Cercamondi CI, Brittenham G, et al. Iron absorption from oral iron supplements given on consecutive versus alternate days and as single morning doses versus twice-daily split dosing in iron-depleted women: two open-label, randomised controlled trials. *Lancet Haematol.* 2017;4(11):e524-e533.
2. Brittenham GM. Iron-chelating therapy for transfusional iron overload. *N Engl J Med.* 2011;364(2):146-156.
3. Cappellini MD, Viprakasit V, Phil D, et al. A phase 3 trial of luspatercept in patients with transfusion-dependent β thalassemia. *N Engl J Med.* 2020;382:1219-1231.
4. Frangoul H, Altshuler D, Cappellini D, et al. CRISPR-Cas9 gene editing for sickle cell disease and β-thalassemia. *N Engl J Med.* 2021;384:252-260.
5. Fenaux P, Platzbecker U, Mufti GJ, et al. Luspatercept in patients with lower-risk myelodysplastic syndrome. *N Engl J Med.* 2020;382:140-151.
6. Townsley DM, Scheinberg P, Winkler T, et al. Eltrombopag added to standard immunosuppression for aplastic anemia. *N Engl J Med.* 2017;376(16):1540-1550.
7. Singh AK, Szczech L, Tang KL, et al. Correction of anemia with epoetin alfa in chronic kidney disease. *N Engl J Med.* 2006;355(20):2085-2098.
8. Chen N, Chuanming H, Peng X, et al. Roxadustat for anemia in patients with kidney disease not receiving dialysis. *N Engl J Med.* 2019;381:1001-1010.
9. Tonia T, Mettler A, Robert N, et al. Erythropoietin or darbepoetin for patients with cancer. *Cochrane Database Syst Rev.* 2012;12:CD003407.
10. Liem RI, Lanzkron S, Coates T, et al. American Society of Hematology 2019 guidelines for sickle cell disease: cardiopulmonary and kidney disease. *Blood Adv.* 2019;3(23):3867-3897.
11. Powars D, Wilson B, Imbus C, Pegelow C, Allen J. The natural history of stroke in sickle cell disease. *Am J Med.* 1978;65(3):461-471.
12. DeBaun MR, Jordan LC, King AA, et al. American Society of Hematology 2020 guidelines for sickle cell disease: prevention, diagnosis, and treatment of cerebrovascular disease in children and adults. *Blood Adv.* 2020;4(8):1554-1588.
13. Boga C, Ozdogu H. Pregnancy and sickle cell disease: a review of the current literature. *Crit Rev Oncol Hematol.* 2016;98:364-374.
14. Shilo NR, Morris CR. Pathways to pulmonary hypertension in sickle cell disease: the search for prevention and early intervention. *Expert Rev Hematol.* 2017;10(10):875-890.
15. Steinberg MH, Barton F, Castro O, et al. Effect of hydroxyurea on mortality and morbidity in adult sickle cell anemia: risks and benefits up to 9 years of treatment. *JAMA.* 2003;289(13):1645-1651.
16. Niihara Y, Miller ST, Kanter J, et al. A phase 3 trial of l-glutamine in sickle cell disease. *N Engl J Med.* 2018;379(3):226-235.

17. Ataga KI, Kutlar A, Kanter J, et al. Crizanlizumab for the prevention of pain crises in sickle cell disease. *N Engl J Med* 2017;376(5):429-439.
18. Vichinsky E, Hoppe CC, Ataga KI, et al. HOPE Trial Investigators. A phase 3 randomized trial of voxelotor in sickle cell disease. *N Engl J Med*. 2019;381(6):509-519.
19. Howard J, Malfroy M, Llewelyn C, et al. The Transfusion Alternatives Preoperatively in Sickle Cell Disease (TAPS) study: a randomised, controlled, multicentre clinical trial. *Lancet*. 2013;381(9870):930-938.
20. Barcellini W, Zaja F, Zaninoni A, et al. Low-dose rituximab in adult patients with idiopathic autoimmune hemolytic anemia: clinical efficacy and biologic studies. *Blood*. 2012;119(16):3691-3697.
21. Arber DA, Orazi A, Hasserjian R, et al. The 2016 revision to the World Health Organization classification of myeloid neoplasms and acute leukemia. *Blood*. 2016;127(20):2391-2405.
22. Gangat N, Caramazza D, Vaidya R, et al. DIPSS plus: a refined Dynamic International Prognostic Scoring System for primary myelofibrosis that incorporates prognostic information from karyotype, platelet count, and transfusion status. *J Clin Oncol*. 2011;29(4):392-397.
23. Marchioli R, Finazzi G, Specchia G, et al. Cardiovascular events and intensity of treatment in polycythemia vera. *N Engl J Med*. 2013;368:22-33.
24. Vannucchi AM, Kiladjian JJ, Griesshammer M, et al. Ruxolitinib versus standard therapy for the treatment of polycythemia vera. *N Engl J Med*. 2015;372(5):426-435.
25. Gisslinger H, Klade C, Georgiev P, et al. Ropeginterferon alfa-2b versus standard therapy for polycythaemia vera (PROUD-PV and CONTINUATION-PV): a randomized, non-inferiority, phase 3 trial and extension study. *Lancet Haematol*. 2020;7:e196-e208.
26. Verstovsek S, Mesa RA, Gotlib J, et al. A double-blind, placebo-controlled trial of ruxolitinib for myelofibrosis. *N Engl J Med*. 2012;366(9):799-807.
27. Pardanani A, Harrison C, Cortes JE, et al. Safety and efficacy of fedratinib in patients with primary and secondary myelofibrosis: a randomized clinical trial. *JAMA Oncol*. 2015;1:643-651.
28. Rajkumar SV, Dimopoulos MA, Palumbo A, et al. International myeloma working group updated criteria for the diagnosis of multiple myeloma. *Lancet Oncol*. 2014; 15:e538-e548.
29. Rajkumar SV. Updated diagnostic criteria and staging system for multiple myeloma. *Am Soc Clin Oncol Educ Book*. 2016;35:e418-e423.
30. Venner CP, Lane T, Foard D, et al. Cyclophosphamide, bortezomib, and dexamethasone therapy in AL amyloidosis is associated with high clonal response rates and prolonged progression-free survival. *Blood*. 2012;119(19):4387-4390.
31. Roussel M, Merlini G, Chevret S, et al. A prospective phase II of daratumumab in previously treated systemic light chain amyloidosis (AL) patients. *Blood*. 2020;135(18):1531-1540.
32. Carson JL, Guyatt G, Heddle NM, et al. Clinical practice guidelines from the AABB: red blood cell transfusion thresholds and storage. *JAMA*. 2016;316(19):2025-2035.
33. Kaufman RM, Djulbegovic B, Gernsheimer T, et al. Platelet transfusion: a clinical practice guideline from the AABB. *Ann Intern Med*. 2015;162(3):205-213.
34. Silliman CC, Ambruso DR, Boshkov LK. Transfusion-related acute lung injury. *Blood*. 2005;105(6):2266-2273.

22 Cancer

Zachary D. Crees, Siddhartha Devarakonda,
Amanda Cashen, Ramaswamy Govindan, and
Daniel Morgensztern

GENERAL PRINCIPLES

BACKGROUND

Cancer is one of the leading causes of mortality both worldwide and in the US, accounting for approximately 608,000 deaths in the US in 2020.[1] The most common malignancies in the US are lung cancer, prostate cancer, breast cancer, and colon cancer (Table 22-1). Cancer death rates have declined by an estimated 29% over the past 3 decades owing to better uptake of screening strategies, advances in drug development, and the availability of better supportive care. Improved understanding of the molecular pathways operative in cancer cells and their complex interactions with the immune system and the tumor microenvironment has also led to the development of targeted agents, immunotherapies, and personalized treatment approaches associated with significant clinical benefit.

Risk Factors

- Tobacco use is the most common cause of cancer and is associated with lung, head and neck, esophageal, gastric, pancreatic, kidney, and bladder cancers.
- Diet, obesity, inactivity, and alcohol abuse have been associated with increased risk of developing certain cancers.
- Chronic inflammatory states such as ulcerative colitis and infections including HIV, hepatitis, Epstein–Barr virus (EBV), human papillomavirus (HPV) and *Helicobacter pylori* are associated with increased cancer risk.
- Numerous familial cancer syndromes have been described and have important implications for cancer risk and screening (Table 22-2).
- Prior exposure to cytotoxic chemotherapy or radiation therapy is associated with an increased risk of secondary cancers. For example, exposure to alkylating agents or topoisomerase II inhibitors increases the risk of treatment-related leukemia, and exposure to radiation therapy increases risk for cancers such as breast cancer, angiosarcoma, and osteosarcoma.

DIAGNOSIS

- Obtaining tissue is crucial for obtaining a definitive diagnosis, examining molecular features of the cancer, and planning treatment.
- Cytology specimens often consist of only a few malignant cells that are obtained either invasively through fine-needle aspiration (FNA), brushings (Pap smear or endoscopic), or aspiration of body fluids (blood, cerebrospinal fluid [CSF], pleural, pericardial, or peritoneal) or noninvasively through collection of fluids such as sputum and urine. Although these approaches are relatively less invasive compared to surgical biopsies, cytologic samples may be inadequate for molecular testing.

TABLE 22-1	Estimated New Cancer Cases and Rates of Death for Most Common Cancer Diagnoses in the US for 2020			
	New Cases			Deaths
Sites	Both Sexes	Male	Female	Total
Lung	228,820	116,300	112,520	135,720
Prostate	191,930	191,930	–	33,330
Breast	279,100	2,620	276,480	42,690
Colon/rectal	147,950	78,300	69,650	53,200

Furthermore, the absence of information about tissue architecture may prevent a final diagnosis in certain malignancies, such as lymphomas.
• Histology specimens are obtained through core-needle biopsies, excisional biopsies, or surgical resection. These specimens are ideal for diagnosing most malignancies and provide sufficient tissue for molecular testing, although they are more invasive.

STAGING

• Once a tissue diagnosis is obtained, most cancer patients require additional imaging, procedures, and laboratory testing to determine the extent of disease and stage.
• Cancer stage provides an assessment of the extent of tumor dissemination, which is crucial for determining prognosis and treatment planning.
• The staging workup is cancer and patient specific and also varies by local and institutional patterns of practice. Organizations such as the American Society of Clinical Oncology, American Society of Hematology, National Comprehensive Cancer Network, and European Society of Medical Oncology review the available evidence and issue periodic recommendations to guide appropriate staging and management.
  ○ Most solid malignancies are staged according to the tumor, lymph node, and metastasis (TNM) system with stages I to IV. The T classification is based on the size and extent of local invasion. The N classification describes the extent of lymph node involvement and the M classification is based on the presence or absence of distant metastases.
  ○ Most hematologic malignancies do not use TNM staging, but rather use disease-specific staging and risk criteria, which are frequently based on a combination of relevant clinical cytogenetic and molecular features.
  ○ Performance status provides a quantitative measure of a patient's functional capacity and quality of life, with important implications for treatment planning (Table 22-3).

TREATMENT

Surgical Therapy

• Surgical resection is often performed with curative intent, although select patients may benefit from palliative surgery performed to debulk large tumor masses (ovarian cancer), increase the efficacy of immunotherapy (renal cell carcinoma [RCC]), or relieve local symptoms (mastectomy in a patient with metastatic disease breast cancer).

TABLE 22-2	List of Selected Familial Cancer Syndromes With High Penetrance	
Syndrome	**Defect**	**Associated Cancer Type**
Ataxia–telangiectasia	*ATM*	Multiple; predominantly leukemia and lymphoma
Birt–Hogg–Dube	*BHD*	Chromophobe RCC
Bloom syndrome	*BLM*	Multiple
Cowden syndrome	*PTEN*	Multiple; predominantly breast, thyroid, RCC, endometrial
Familial adenomatous polyposis	*APC*	Colorectal, desmoid
Fanconi anemia	*DNA* repair complex	Multiple; predominantly MDS and AML
Hereditary breast–ovarian cancer	*BRCA1* and *BRCA2*	Multiple; predominantly breast, ovarian
Hereditary diffuse gastric cancer	*CDH1*	Gastric, lobular breast cancer
Hereditary leiomyomatosis and RCC	*FH*	Papillary RCC
Lynch syndrome (HNPCC)	Mismatch repair	Multiple; predominantly colorectal
Hereditary papillary RCC	*MET*	Papillary RCC
Juvenile polyposis syndrome	*MADH4 (SMAD4), BMPR1A*	Digestive tract and pancreas
Li-Fraumeni syndrome	*TP53*	Multiple
MEN type 1	*MEN1*	Islet cell tumors
MEN type 2	*RET*	Medullary thyroid cancer
Neurofibromatosis type 1	*NF1*	MPNST, glioma
Neurofibromatosis type 2	*NF2*	Meningioma, glioma, schwannoma
Nijmegen breakage syndrome	*NBS1*	Predominantly lymphoma
Peutz–Jeghers syndrome	*LKB1 (STK11)*	Multiple; predominantly breast, GI, pancreas
Retinoblastoma, hereditary	*RB*	Retinoblastoma, primitive neuroectodermal tumor
Rothmund–Thomson syndrome	*RECQL4*	Osteosarcoma
Tuberous sclerosis (TS)	*TSC1, TSC2*	RCC, giant cell astrocytoma
von Hippel-Lindau	*VHL*	Clear cell RCC
Xeroderma pigmentosum	Nucleotide excision repair	Multiple, cutaneous

AML, acute myeloid leukemia; GI, gastrointestinal; HNPCC, hereditary nonpolyposis colorectal cancer; MDS, myelodysplastic syndrome; MEN, multiple endocrine neoplasia; MPNST, malignant peripheral nerve sheath tumor; RCC, renal cell carcinoma.

CHAPTER 22

TABLE 22-3   **Eastern Cooperative Oncology Group (ECOG) and Karnofsky Score**

ECOG	Karnofsky Score Correlate	Description
0	100	Fully active, able to carry on all predisease performance without restriction.
1	80–90	Restricted in physically strenuous activity but ambulatory and able to carry out work of a light or sedentary nature (e.g., light housework, office work).
2	60–70	Ambulatory and capable of all self-care but unable to carry out any work activities. Up and about >50% of waking hours.
3	40–50	Capable of only limited self-care, confined to bed or chair >50% of waking hours.
4	20–30	Completely disabled. Cannot carry on any self-care. Totally confined to bed or chair.
5	0	Dead.

Reprinted with permission from Oken MM, Creech RH, Tormey DC, et al. Toxicity and response criteria of the Eastern Cooperative Oncology Group. *Am J Clin Oncol.* 1982;5(6):649-655.

- Surgery can facilitate staging and guide subsequent therapeutic decisions including the need for adjuvant treatment.
- Surgical resection of isolated or oligometastatic sites in select patients may improve survival. Some examples include solitary brain metastases, pulmonary metastases in sarcoma, and liver metastases in colorectal cancer.

Radiation Therapy

- Commonly used forms of radiation include external-beam photons, electrons, and protons.
- Brachytherapy is an alternative delivery method, where radioactive sources are placed close to or in contact with the target tissue. Brachytherapy sources can be temporary or permanent.
- Radioactive therapy can also be administered systemically (oral iodine-131 in thyroid cancer, injection of yttrium-90 microspheres into liver vasculature in hepatocellular cancer, and intravenous radium-223 for prostate cancer with skeletal metastases).
- Radiation therapy planning is designed to optimize precision doses of radiation to a tumor while minimizing radiation to surrounding tissues.
- Curative intent radiotherapy is used in several settings.
  - Neoadjuvant: Preoperative therapy intended to reduce both the extent of surgery and the risk of local relapse. Radiation in this setting is commonly administered in combination with chemotherapy.
  - Adjuvant: Postoperative therapy intended to reduce the risk of local relapse.
  - Definitive: High dose with curative intent.

○ Concurrent chemoradiation: Chemotherapy combined with definitive radiation is associated with increased efficacy but also increased toxicity compared to chemotherapy or radiation alone.
- Palliative radiotherapy is used to reduce cancer-related symptoms, such as bone pain, bleeding, and neurologic symptoms.
- The total dose of radiation administered is usually divided over multiple days (fractionated), which allows normal tissue to repair and increases the probability of delivering radiation to tumor cells in a radiosensitive phase of the cell cycle. Radiation treatments are typically delivered on conventional fractionation, hypofractionation, hyperfractionation, or accelerated fractionation schedules, as detailed below.
  ○ Conventional fractionation consists of daily fractions typically of 1.8–2.0 Gy, 5 days per week.
  ○ Hypofractionation consists of delivering radiation divided into larger doses, with treatment once a day or less often.
  ○ Hyperfractionation refers to delivering radiation in smaller doses per fraction, with treatments more than once per day.

Additional Local Therapies

Local ablative therapy with modalities such as lasers, cryoablation, microwave, radiofrequency, and high intensity-focused ultrasound is increasingly used in cancer patients for pain palliation, for attempting local disease control or in treating oligometastatic disease in certain types of cancer.

Chemotherapy

- Cytotoxic chemotherapy targets all dividing cells and has a broad spectrum of toxicities, which can be life-threatening.
- In patients with resectable disease, chemotherapy may be used before (neoadjuvant) or following surgery (adjuvant).
- Chemotherapy is typically given in cycles of 1–4 weeks. In most regimens, IV treatment is given on the first few days of the cycle, with no further treatment until the next cycle. In other regimens, treatments are administered weekly for 2–3 weeks, with 1 week off between cycles.
- Curative intent chemotherapy often includes neoadjuvant, adjuvant, and chemoradiation regimens in solid tumors. Chemotherapy alone or in combination with immunotherapy or stem cell transplantation may be curative in many lymphomas, leukemias, and germ cell tumors (GCTs).
- Palliative chemotherapy is used in advanced solid tumors and relapsed hematologic malignancies, with a focus on prolonging survival and improving the quality of life.
- Most agents have a narrow therapeutic index and dosing is based on weight (mg/kg) or body surface area (mg/m^2), with close attention to renal, hepatic, and bone marrow function.

Targeted Therapy

- The use of molecularly targeted agents has led to improved outcomes in many cancer-types.
- The most common classes of drugs are monoclonal antibodies and receptor tyrosine kinase inhibitors (TKIs). Monoclonal antibodies (mAbs) are administered IV and by standard nomenclature have names that end with the stem -mab. Substems indicate the source and target of the antibody. The most common source substems in oncology include -xi- indicating a chimeric antibody (cetuximab), -zu- indicating humanized antibody (bevacizumab), and -u- indicating fully human antibodies

(ipilimumab). The most common target substems include -ci- indicating circulatory system (bevacizumab), -tu- indicating tumor (cetuximab), and -li- indicating immune system modulating (ipilimumab).

- TKIs are administered orally and have names that end with -ib.
- Most monoclonal antibodies are used in combination with chemotherapy or radiation, whereas TKIs are commonly used as single agents or in combination with other TKIs.
- Toxicities of targeted therapies are unique to each agent, although specific classes of drugs can be associated with characteristic side effects.
  ○ Inhibitors of the epidermal growth factor receptor (EGFR) frequently cause an acne-like rash on the face and upper chest, which can be severe. Treatment is typically with topical corticosteroids or oral tetracyclines (minocycline, doxycycline).
  ○ Inhibitors of human epidermal growth factor receptor 2 (HER2) are associated with a reversible decline in cardiac systolic function, which should be monitored closely.
  ○ Inhibitors of angiogenesis are associated with endothelial toxicity, leading to hypertension, proteinuria, delayed wound healing, cardiac toxicity, bleeding, thromboembolism, and gastrointestinal (GI) perforation or fistula. All antiangiogenics should be held in the perioperative period due to impaired wound healing.

Immunotherapy

Under normal physiological conditions, the innate and adaptive immune system perform surveillance for and elimination of cancer cells within the body. In addition, the immune system maintains self-tolerance via checkpoint molecules to prevent autoimmunity and limit collateral inflammatory damage to normal tissues during response to infections. However, tumor cells may co-opt this pathway to escape T cell–induced antitumor activity.

- Programmed cell death 1 (PD-1) is one such immune checkpoint and is a receptor expressed primarily on the surface of activated T cells. Binding of PD-1 to one of its ligands, PD-L1 or PD-L2, inhibits the cytotoxic T cell response. PD-1 and PD-L1 interactions may be blocked by monoclonal antibodies against PD-1 (nivolumab, pembrolizumab) or PD-L1 (atezolizumab, durvalumab, avelumab). These immune checkpoint inhibitors (ICIs) have been approved for the treatment of numerous solid and hematologic malignancies. In addition, PD-L1 expression by immunohistochemistry (IHC) has been associated with response to anti-PD-1 or PD-L1 antibodies in some, but not all cancers.
- Chimeric antigen receptor T cells (CAR-Ts) are genetically engineered T cells with specialized receptors which target antigens expressed on tumor cells, such as CD19 or BCMA, to promote an anticancer immune response. Currently, five CAR-Ts have been approved by the Food and Drug Administration (FDA) in the US for certain hematologic malignancies, with many more in clinical development for both solid and hematologic malignancies.
- Other modalities of immunotherapy include engineered, antibody-based bispecific T cell–engaging therapies such as blinatumomab (CD3 × CD19), which engage T cells and cancer cells to promote an anticancer immune response.

Response to Therapy

Objective assessment of changes in tumor burden is crucial for planning cancer treatment and evaluating treatment efficacy. Criteria such as the Response Evaluation Criteria in Solid Tumors (RECIST) are commonly used for this purpose (Table 22-4). Whereas response assessments for hematologic malignancies often use disease-specific

TABLE 22-4	Summary of Selected Response Evaluation Criteria in Solid Tumors (RECIST) 1.1 Criteria
Measurable lesions	Tumor: >10 mm in longest diameter (LD) on axial CT or MRI
	Lymph node: >15 mm in short axis on CT
Method	Sum of longest diameter (SLD) of the lesions in axial plane. Up to five target lesions (two per organ).
Response	
Complete response (CR)	Disappearance of all non-nodal target lesions. All target lymph nodes must be <10 mm in short axis.
Partial response (PR)	At least 30% decrease in the SLD of target lesions, with baseline sum of diameters as reference.
Progressive disease (PD)	New lesions or SLD increased by ≥20%.
Stable disease (SD)	Neither PR nor PD.

CHAPTER 22

criteria such as Lugano classification and Deauville five-point scale for lymphoma, International Working Group (IWG) Criteria for leukemia, International Myeloma Working Group (IMWG) Criteria for multiple myeloma, and others.

SOLID MALIGNANCIES

Lung Cancer

EPIDEMIOLOGY AND ETIOLOGY

Lung cancer is the most common cause of cancer death in the US, with an estimated 135,720 deaths in 2020.[1] Smoking is the strongest risk factor for lung cancer, with over 90% of cases being tobacco-related. Other environmental risks include exposure to asbestos and possibly gases, such as radon.

PATHOLOGY

Non–small-cell lung cancer (NSCLC) accounts for >85% of cases. The most common histologic subtypes are adenocarcinoma and squamous cell carcinoma. Small-cell lung cancer (SCLC) is associated with rapid tumor growth and early development of metastases compared to NSCLC.

SCREENING

Lung cancer screening with low-dose computed tomography (LDCT) reduces lung cancer mortality and the U.S. Preventive Services Task Force (USPSTF) currently recommends annual screening for lung cancer with LDCT in current smokers or former smokers who quit within the past 15 years, are between 50 and 80 years old, and have a ≥20-pack-year smoking history.

CLINICAL PRESENTATION

- Patients with early-stage disease are often asymptomatic. However, when present, symptoms may be related to local disease (cough, dyspnea, hemoptysis), intrathoracic extension (hoarseness from recurrent laryngeal nerve involvement, dysphagia, chest wall pain, Horner syndrome, brachial plexus involvement, superior vena cava [SVC] syndrome), systemic metastases (fever, jaundice, bone pain, headaches), or paraneoplastic syndromes.
- Paraneoplastic syndromes in lung cancer typically include hypercalcemia (humoral or osteolytic), hyponatremia from syndrome of inappropriate antidiuretic hormone, and hypertrophic pulmonary osteoarthropathy.

DIAGNOSTIC TESTING

- Any patient with a smoking history and concerning pulmonary symptoms should undergo a CT scan of the chest. A normal chest radiograph (CXR) does not exclude lung cancer. Diagnosis can be made from bronchoscopy with biopsy, brushings or washings, ultrasound- or CT-guided needle biopsy, and pleural fluid cytology if an effusion is present. Core-needle biopsy is preferable to FNA for molecular testing, which plays an important role in treatment planning.
- Staging evaluation in all patients should include a CT scan of the chest and abdomen. Additional imaging depends on the initial findings. In potentially curable patients, the evaluation also typically includes a brain magnetic resonance imaging (MRI), positron emission tomography (PET) CT scan, and mediastinoscopy.

STAGING

TNM: T1 (tumors ≤3 cm), T2a (>3 but ≤4 cm), T2b (>4 but ≤5 cm), T3 (>5 but ≤7 cm or separate nodules in the same lobe, or invasion of chest wall, pericardium, or phrenic nerve), T4 (>7 cm or tumor nodules in an ipsilateral different lobe or invasion of other structures including mediastinum, heart, trachea, spine, esophagus, recurrent laryngeal nerve), N0 (no lymph node involvement), N1 (ipsilateral pulmonary or hilar lymph nodes), N2 (ipsilateral mediastinal lymph nodes), N3 (supraclavicular or contralateral lymph nodes), M0 (no metastases), M1a (pleural or pericardial nodules or effusion, separate nodule(s) in the contralateral lung), M1b (single extrathoracic metastasis), M1c (multiple extrathoracic metastases). Stage: I (T1-T2aN0M0), IIA (T2bN0M0), IIB (T3N0M0 or T1-2N1M0), IIIA (T1-2N2M0, T3N1M0, or T4N0-1M0), IIIC (T3-4N3M0), IVA (T1-4N1-3M1a-M1b), IVB (T1-4N1-3M1c).

TREATMENT

Non–Small-Cell Lung Cancer

- Stages I, II, and selected IIIA: Surgery is the preferred therapy. Adjuvant platinum doublet chemotherapy improves overall survival in patients with surgically resected stage II and III NSCLC. Adjuvant therapy with osimertinib for 3 years is approved for patients with EGFR-mutated NSCLC.[2] Radiation therapy, with or without chemotherapy, is an option for those who decline or are not candidates for surgical resection.

- Stage III: The standard therapy is with concurrent chemoradiation followed by consolidation durvalumab for 1 year. Surgery is indicated in select patients.
- Stage IV (metastatic): Therapy is administered with palliative intent, and choice of therapy is guided by presence of targetable alterations (*EGFR, ALK, ROS1, ERBB2, BRAF, KRAS, MET, RET*, and *NTRK*), PD-L1 expression of the tumor as measured by IHC, histology, and patient performance status.[3,4]
  - Several ICIs have been approved for the treatment of NSCLC, in the first-line setting alone or in combination with chemotherapy, including nivolumab with or without ipilimumab, pembrolizumab, or atezolizumab.
    - Pembrolizumab or atezolizumab monotherapy has been shown to be superior to chemotherapy alone in patients whose tumors show >50% PD-L1 expression.
    - Combining pembrolizumab with platinum doublet chemotherapy (pemetrexed for nonsquamous, paclitaxel or albumin-bound paclitaxel [nab-paclitaxel] for squamous) has been shown to be superior to chemotherapy alone, regardless of tumor PD-L1 status.
  - There are several effective medications for patients with specific genomic alterations:
    - *EGFR* mutation: Osimertinib, gefitinib, erlotinib, afatinib, dacomitinib
    - *ALK* rearrangements: Alectinib, crizotinib, ceritinib, lorlatinib, and brigatinib
    - *KRAS* G12C mutation: Sotorasib
    - *ROS1* rearrangements: Crizotinib, entrectinib, and lorlatinib
    - *MET* exon 14 mutation: Crizotinib, capmatinib, and tepotinib
    - *BRAF* V600E mutation: Dabrafenib alone or in combination with trametinib
    - *RET* rearrangements: Selpercatinib, pralsetinib, and cabozantinib
    - *NTRK* gene fusions: Larotrectinib and entrectinib

Small-Cell Lung Cancer

- Stages I to III (limited stage): The standard therapy includes concurrent chemoradiation with a platinum agent (carboplatin or cisplatin) plus etoposide followed by prophylactic cranial irradiation (PCI).
- Stage IV (extensive stage): Chemotherapy is the preferred therapy, usually with a platinum agent (cisplatin or carboplatin) plus etoposide and a PD-L1 inhibitor (atezolizumab or durvalumab). The role for PCI in patients with stage IV disease is not clearly defined.
- Second-line therapies for recurrent disease may include topotecan, lurbinectedin, irinotecan, paclitaxel, docetaxel, and temozolomide.

Breast Cancer

EPIDEMIOLOGY AND ETIOLOGY

Breast cancer is the most common cancer in women in developed countries and the second leading cause of cancer death.[1] Less than 1% of cases are reported in men. The lifetime risk of breast cancer among women in the US is 12%. *BRCA1* and *BRCA2* mutations are associated with significantly increased lifetime risk of breast cancer. However, less than 10% of all breast cancers are attributable to mutations involving susceptibility genes.[5] Other risk factors include alcohol consumption, early menarche, late menopause, nulliparity, postmenopausal obesity, hormone replacement therapy, delayed first pregnancy, and prior mantle field radiation for Hodgkin lymphoma.

CHAPTER 22

PATHOLOGY

- Noninvasive tumors include ductal carcinoma in situ (DCIS) and lobular carcinoma in situ (LCIS). The most common types of epithelial invasive breast carcinoma are ductal carcinoma (50%–75%) and lobular carcinoma (5%–15%).
- Estrogen receptor (ER) is expressed in approximately 75% of cases. ER positivity (ER+) is associated with better prognosis and responsiveness to endocrine therapies. Progesterone receptor (PR) expression usually correlates with ER expression. Approximately 20% of tumors are HER2 (ERBB2) positive (HER2+) by IHC or fluorescent in situ hybridization (FISH). HER2 positivity is associated with higher grade cancers and patients may benefit from HER2-targeted therapies. Approximately 15% of breast cancers lack ER, PR, and HER2 expression (triple negative). These cancers are more aggressive and do not benefit from hormone receptor or HER2-targeted therapies.

SCREENING AND PREVENTION

- The American Cancer Society recommends annual mammography from age 45, for as long as the person does not have serious illnesses that may shorten life expectancy. The USPSTF recommends biennial mammography from age 50 to 74. MRI along with mammography may be indicated in select individuals with a strong family history of breast cancer or a high-risk cancer predisposition syndrome.
- Prophylactic mastectomy and oophorectomy are offered to carriers of *BRCA1* or *BRCA2* mutations with consideration of individual reproductive wishes. Chemoprevention with tamoxifen or raloxifene is an option in women who are at high risk for developing breast cancer including those with strong family history or LCIS.

CLINICAL PRESENTATION

Most breast cancers are identified by screening tests, but patients may present with a palpable mass in the breast or axilla. Some patients may have nipple discharge, pain, nipple retraction, or skin changes associated with the mass. Patients with inflammatory breast cancer may complain of a "heavy" warm breast with an associated erythematous rash.

DIAGNOSTIC TESTING

Patients with palpable breast masses require diagnostic mammograms. Ultrasound may help differentiate between solid and cystic lesions. Patients with an axillary mass and no detectable breast mass by routine imaging and examination should have MRI to identify occult cancer. Any clinically concerning nodule should be biopsied irrespective of its radiographic appearance. CT of the chest and abdomen is indicated in patients with stage T3N1 disease or higher, localizing symptoms, or abnormal liver enzymes. Bone scan is also recommended in patients with T3N1 disease or higher, localizing symptoms, or increased alkaline phosphatase.

STAGING

TNM: T1 (tumor <2 cm), T2 (2–5 cm), T3 (>5 cm), T4 (any size with extension to the chest wall or skin, T4d is inflammatory carcinoma), clinical cN1 (mobile ipsilateral axillary lymph nodes), cN2 (fixed or matted axillary or ipsilateral internal mammary lymph nodes), cN3 (infraclavicular, supraclavicular, or combined ipsilateral and internal mammary lymph nodes), pathological pN1 (1–3 axillary lymph nodes), pN1 mi (micro-metastases larger than 0.2 mm but not larger than 2 mm), pN2 (4–9 axillary lymph or ipsilateral internal mammary lymph nodes), pN3 (10 or more axillary, supraclavicular, or internal mammary plus more than 3 axillary), M0 (no metastases), M1 (metastases larger than 0.2 mm in distant organs or nonregional lymph nodes). Stage: IA (T1N0M0), IB (T0N1M0), IIA (T2N1M0 or T3N0M0), IIIA (T3N1M0 or T0-3N2M0), IIIB (T4N0-2M0), IIIC (T0-4N3M0), IV (M1).

TREATMENT

- Stage 0 (DCIS and LCIS): Treatment options include mastectomy (with or without sentinel lymph node biopsy) or lumpectomy with negative margins followed by adjuvant radiation. Repeat resections for positive margins may be necessary. Endocrine therapy is typically used if the tumor is ER+.
- Stages I–III (resectable)
  - The surgical approach depends on the size of the tumor, patient preference, and the presence or absence of contraindications to breast conservation surgery (BCS). Contraindications for BCS include multicentric disease, extensive microcalcifications, and previous irradiation. Neoadjuvant chemotherapy, with or without immunotherapy or hormonal therapy, may be used to shrink larger tumors to facilitate BCS. Sentinel lymph node biopsy is done to pathologically stage the axilla unless there are clinical or radiologic signs of lymph node involvement. In the case of clinically positive lymph nodes, an axillary lymph node dissection is done at the time of surgery.
  - Adjuvant radiation therapy is indicated for patients undergoing BCS and after mastectomy with T3 or T4 disease, positive margins, or more than three positive lymph nodes. BCS with adjuvant radiation is equivalent to mastectomy. For ER/PR+ cancers, adjuvant endocrine therapy with tamoxifen or a combination of aromatase inhibitor (AI) and ovarian suppression is recommended in premenopausal women. AI with ovarian suppression is the preferred adjuvant endocrine therapy for women ≤35 years old and women at higher risk of recurrence. For postmenopausal women, an AI is standard of care. The standard treatment duration is 5–10 years. Adjuvant chemotherapy may be recommended based on biomarkers (ER, PR, HER2 status), stage, node positivity, and prognostic multigene assay results (Oncotype Dx or Mammaprint) in ER/PR positive stage I/II cancers.[6] Adjuvant treatment with the HER2 monoclonal antibody trastuzumab reduces rate of relapse and improves survival in HER2+ breast cancer. The addition of pertuzumab (an additional HER2 monoclonal antibody) to trastuzumab may be considered in the neoadjuvant, adjuvant, and metastatic settings. Adjuvant treatment with the antibody–drug conjugate (ADC) Ado-trastuzumab emtansine may also be considered in those with residual invasive HER2+ disease following neoadjuvant taxane-based chemotherapy and trastuzumab.
- Stage IV
  - Most patients with ER+ tumors are treated with a combination of endocrine therapy and a CDK4/6 inhibitor (palbociclib, ribociclib, or abemaciclib). Everolimus (a mammalian target of rapamycin inhibitor) in combination with endocrine therapy may be considered in the second-line setting. Chemotherapy is used in patients with negative hormone receptors and high visceral tumor burden or when endocrine therapy is no longer effective. The treatment of triple negative metastatic

breast cancer includes chemotherapy alone in patients with PD-L1 <1% and the combination of nab-paclitaxel with atezolizumab if PD-L1 ≥1%.[7] Patients with a *BRCA* mutation may be treated with a poly-ADP-ribose phosphorylase (PARP) inhibitor such as olaparib or talazoparib. HER2+ relapsed and metastatic breast cancer may be treated with a number of HER2 targeting therapies including monoclonal antibodies (trastuzumab, pertuzumab, and margetuximab), TKIs (lapatinib, neratinib, or tucatinib) usually in combination with chemotherapy and HER2 targeting ADCs (Ado-trastuzumab emtansine and fam-trastuzumab deruxtecan). Sacituzumab govitecan, which is an ADC targeting the protein TROP-2, is also approved for use in patients with triple-negative disease.[5]

- ○ Bone-protecting agents, such as bisphosphonates or denosumab (an anti-RANKL antibody), are recommended for patients with bone metastases to reduce risk of fracture or other skeletal complications.

Head and Neck Cancer

EPIDEMIOLOGY AND ETIOLOGY

Head and neck squamous cell cancer (HNSCC) includes carcinoma of the lip, oral cavity, oropharynx, nasopharynx, and larynx. It is estimated that approximately 53,260 patients in the US will be diagnosed with HNSCC in the year 2020.[1] Tobacco use and alcohol consumption are associated with increased risk of developing HNSCC. HPV infection is implicated in oropharyngeal squamous cell carcinomas, and the incidence of HPV-associated HNSCC is increasing. EBV infection is associated with nasopharyngeal cancers. Given the diffuse nature of mucosal exposure to tobacco smoke or smokeless tobacco, the primary cancer site is often surrounded by areas of premalignant lesions such as carcinoma in situ and dysplasia. For this reason, patients with tobacco-associated HNSCC are at increased risk for secondary HNSCCs.

CLINICAL PRESENTATION

Patients with HNSCC can present with a variety of symptoms depending on the primary tumor site including an oral mass, nonhealing ulcers, trismus from invasion of pterygoid muscles, dysphagia, odynophagia, otitis media from eustachian tube blockage, hoarseness, a neck mass, weight loss, and cranial nerve palsies. Nasopharyngeal tumors can invade the cavernous sinus and frequently affect the abducens and trigeminal nerves. Salivary gland tumors may invade the facial nerve.

DIAGNOSTIC TESTING

- Comprehensive ear, nose, and throat evaluation with fiberoptic endoscopy or mirror examination is required. Particular attention should be paid to dentition. Functional evaluation that includes assessment of swallowing, biting, chewing, and speech should be performed.
- Examination under anesthesia is a critical component of staging. Imaging should include a panoramic dental radiograph to evaluate dentition and mandibular involvement. A CT of the neck and chest should be obtained to evaluate lymph node involvement and rule out pulmonary metastases, respectively. Whole-body PET can be considered in select patients.

- Positivity of p16 on IHC is used as a surrogate for HPV infection and is an independent favorable prognostic factor for survival. PD-L1 status may help guide therapy in the recurrent, unresectable, and metastatic settings.

STAGING

The TNM classification and staging is specific to each site of disease and HPV status. However, in general, stage I to II disease indicates the absence of lymph node involvement. Stage III tumors are larger (defined as >4 cm for most sites) or have isolated or regional lymph node involvement. Unlike most other malignancies, stage IVA and IVB HNSCC are locally advanced tumors and only stage IVC tumors are defined by distant metastases.

TREATMENT

- Stage I–II (local): Patients may be treated with either surgery or definitive radiation with a 70%–90% long-term survival.[8]
- Stage III–IVB (locally advanced): Treatment options include surgical resection followed by adjuvant radiation with or without chemotherapy; concurrent chemoradiotherapy; induction chemotherapy followed by concurrent chemotherapy and radiation; or radiation alone. Chemoradiation or induction chemotherapy followed by radiation can potentially spare patients from undergoing a total laryngectomy and improve quality of life. Surgery is most commonly used for tumors of the oral cavity. Nodal neck dissection is an important part of surgical management. Radical neck dissection refers to surgical removal of lymph nodes from all five neck stations unilaterally, along with excision of the internal jugular vein, spinal accessory nerve, and sternocleidomastoid. Modified neck dissections spare some of these structures. Cisplatin is the chemotherapy agent most commonly used in combination with radiation for definitive treatment.
- Stage IVC (metastatic): Treatment options include chemotherapy, ICIs, or combination chemoimmunotherapy. Cisplatin is often combined with 5-fluorouracil (5-FU) or a taxane (paclitaxel or docetaxel). The role of pembrolizumab depends on the clinical setting and composite or combined PD-L1 score (CPS). Patients with CPS >20 and without rapidly progressing tumors may be treated with pembrolizumab alone, whereas those with CPS between 1 and 20 may be treated with pembrolizumab alone or in combination with platinum-based chemotherapy. Patients with CPS <1 may be treated with chemotherapy alone or in combination with cetuximab, an EGFR mAb.[9]

GASTROINTESTINAL MALIGNANCIES

Esophageal Cancer

EPIDEMIOLOGY AND ETIOLOGY

Esophageal cancer is estimated to account for approximately 18,440 deaths in the US in 2020.[1] Esophageal cancer is 3–4 times more common in men. The main risk factors for squamous cell carcinoma include tobacco and alcohol use, while less common risk factors include achalasia and thermal injury from high-temperature foods/beverages. Risk factors for adenocarcinoma include tobacco, obesity, gastroesophageal reflux disease, and Barrett esophagus.

PATHOLOGY

Adenocarcinomas are most common in the lower third of the esophagus and at the gastroesophageal junction, with incidence rising sharply over the last few decades in the US. Squamous cell carcinomas are more common in the upper and mid-esophagus.

CLINICAL PRESENTATION

A small percentage of patients have asymptomatic tumors detected during endoscopy for unrelated causes or surveillance for Barrett esophagus. However, most patients present with dysphagia, initially to solids when the esophageal lumen is 13 mm or less, but progressing to liquids as the tumor grows and the lumen narrows. The diagnosis may be delayed because patients adjust the dietary intake to avoid foods that cause dysphagia. Other less common presentations include cough, hoarseness due to recurrent laryngeal nerve involvement, palpable cervical lymph nodes, and iron deficiency anemia from chronic gastrointestinal blood loss.

DIAGNOSTIC TESTING

- The diagnosis is usually established through upper endoscopy with biopsy. Staging workup includes CT of the chest and abdomen, with or without the addition of PET scan, to determine the presence of distant metastases. For patients without distant metastases, endoscopic ultrasonography (EUS) is required to define tumor depth and lymph node status for staging and treatment planning.
- Tumors located above the carina increase the risk of tracheoesophageal (TE) fistula formation and should be evaluated with bronchoscopy. Patients with TE fistulas often present with postprandial cough and aspiration pneumonia.

STAGING

The TNM classification is similar between squamous and adenocarcinoma histologies, including Tis (carcinoma *in situ*), T1 (invades lamina propria, muscularis mucosa or submucosa), T2 (invades muscularis propria), T3 (invades adventitia), T4 (invades adjacent structures), N0 (no lymph node involvement), N1 (1–2 regional lymph nodes), N2 (3–6 regional lymph nodes), N3 (7 or more lymph nodes), M0 (no metastases), M1 (distant metastases). Stage: staging varies slightly by histology, but in general: I (T1N0), II–III (T2-3 and/or N1), IVA (T4 or N2-3), IVB (M1).

TREATMENT

- Stage I (local): Endomucosal or surgical resection.
- Stage II–III (locally advanced, resectable): The standard therapy typically includes concurrent neoadjuvant chemoradiation with a platinum-based regimen followed by surgical resection. Patients who have residual disease on postoperative pathology may benefit from adjuvant nivolumab.[10]
- Stage IVA (locally advanced, unresectable): Standard therapy typically includes definitive concurrent chemoradiation with a platinum-based regimen.[11]
- Stage IVB (metastatic): Patients with metastatic disease may be treated with combination chemotherapy regimens including fluoropyrimidines (5-FU or capecitabine),

platinum agents (cisplatin or oxaliplatin), taxanes (docetaxel or paclitaxel), and irinotecan. Commonly used regimens include leucovorin, 5-FU and oxaliplatin (FOLFOX), capecitabine and oxaliplatin (CAPEOX or XELOX), and cisplatin and 5-FU. Patients with adenocarcinoma and HER2+ tumors should receive trastuzumab in combination with first-line chemotherapy. Patients with PD-L1 CPS ≥5 may benefit from the addition of pembrolizumab to initial chemotherapy. Options for previously treated patients with recurrent disease include use of a regimen not used previously, including taxanes, irinotecan, ramucirumab, and pembrolizumab (if PD-L1 CPS ≥1, deficient mismatch repair (dMMR), or micro-satellite instability (MSI-high) is present).

Gastric Cancer

EPIDEMIOLOGY AND ETIOLOGY

The highest incidence rates for gastric cancer are in eastern Asia, Eastern Europe, and South America, whereas the lowest incidence is in North America and Africa. Gastric cancer is estimated to account for 27,600 cases and 11,010 deaths in the US in 2020.[1] Gastric cancer occurs more frequently in males. Risk factors include *H. pylori* infection, high salt intake, diets low in fruits and vegetables, previous partial gastrectomy for benign ulcer, achlorhydria associated with pernicious anemia, cigarette smoking, alcohol consumption, and blood group A. Hereditary diffuse gastric cancer (HDGC) is an inherited type of gastric cancer in families with germline *CDH1* (E-cadherin) mutations and any patient presenting with HDGC under the age of 40 or with a known *CDH1* mutation should be offered genetic counseling and prophylactic total gastrectomy. A number of additional hereditary cancer syndromes are also associated with gastric cancers.[12]

PATHOLOGY

More than 90% of gastric cancers are adenocarcinomas and nearly 15%–20% of patients with gastric cancer may have *HER2* amplification or overexpression.

CLINICAL PRESENTATION

The most common symptoms are weight loss, decreased appetite or early satiety, and abdominal discomfort. Dysphagia or regurgitation may occur with gastroesophageal junction tumors and refractory vomiting may occur with pyloric obstruction. Physical examination may show metastases to the left supraclavicular node (Virchow node) or periumbilical node (Sister Mary Joseph node). Iron deficiency anemia may develop from chronic gastrointestinal blood loss.

DIAGNOSTIC TESTING

Diagnosis is established by upper endoscopy. CT of the chest and abdomen should be obtained in all patients, and CT of the pelvis should be performed in women to exclude ovarian involvement (Krukenberg tumor). Additional tests include *H. pylori* testing, EUS, and PET scan. Staging laparoscopy may be indicated before surgery to assess for peritoneal involvement in some cases.

STAGING

The TNM classification is generally similar to that of esophageal cancer. Clinical stage: 0 (TisN0M0), I (T1-2N0M0), IIA (T1-2N1-3M0), IIB (T3-4N0M0), III (T3-4aN1-3M0), IVA (T4bN1-3M0), IVB (M1).

TREATMENT

- Stage I–IVA: Medically fit patients with resectable disease should undergo surgery. Perioperative chemotherapy with a fluoropyrimidine-based regimen is frequently included, except in patients with T1 disease (submucosal invasion or less) who may be treated with surgery alone. Medically unfit patients or those with unresectable disease may be treated with chemoradiation or chemotherapy alone.
- Stage IVB (metastatic): Treatment options for metastatic gastric cancer are similar to those used in esophageal cancer, with combination regimens including fluoropyrimidines, platinum drugs, taxanes, irinotecan, trastuzumab, and ICIs.[12]

Colorectal Cancer

EPIDEMIOLOGY AND ETIOLOGY

Colorectal cancer is the third most common malignancy worldwide. The incidence is higher in Western industrialized countries, with an estimated 147,950 new cases in the US in 2020.[1] Risk factors include age >50, physical inactivity, obesity, type 2 diabetes, diet with increased red meat and decreased fiber, alcohol consumption, personal history of polyps or colorectal cancer, inflammatory bowel disease, positive family history, and hereditary cancer syndromes such as Lynch syndrome and familial adenomatous polyposis.

SCREENING AND PREVENTION

The USPSTF and American College of Gastroenterology recommend screening for all average-risk adults aged 45–75, as well as selected individuals aged 76–85.[13,14] Screening methods include high-sensitivity fecal occult blood tests or fecal immunochemical testing (FIT) every year, stool DNA-FIT every 1–3 years, CT colonography every 5 years, flexible sigmoidoscopy every 5 years, flexible sigmoidoscopy every 5 years plus annual FIT, and colonoscopy every 10 years. Abnormal stool-based tests should be evaluated with colonoscopy.

CLINICAL PRESENTATION

The most common symptoms include rectal bleeding, microcytic anemia, abdominal pain, change in bowel habits, and obstruction. Patients can also rarely present with perforation, peritonitis, and fever. Colorectal carcinomas may also be identified through screening colonoscopies.

DIAGNOSTIC TESTING

A thorough family history should be obtained to assess for hereditary cancer syndromes, especially in patients younger than 50 years. The diagnosis is typically made via colonoscopy with biopsy. Imaging studies include CT scan of the chest, abdomen, and pelvis. PET scan is not routinely indicated but is useful in patients being considered for definitive resection of oligometastatic disease.

STAGING

TNM: Tis (carcinoma *in situ*), T1 (invades submucosa), T2 (invades muscularis propria), T3 (invades through the muscularis propria), T4 (invades adjacent structures), N0 (no lymph node involvement), N1 (1–3 regional lymph nodes), N2 (>4 regional lymph nodes), M1 (distant metastases). Stage: 0 (Tis), I–II (T1-4N0), III (T1-4N1-2), IV (M1).

TREATMENT

- Stage I–III (local): Localized colon cancer should be treated with surgical resection. Adjuvant chemotherapy is indicated in patients with stage III disease (defined by the presence of regional lymph node involvement) and may also be beneficial in select patients with high-risk stage II disease. The preferred regimens in the adjuvant setting are FOLFOX and CAPEOX for 3–6 months. Patients with early stage rectal cancer should be treated with surgical resection including either low anterior resection (LAR) for tumors located in the middle and upper third of the rectum or abdominoperineal resection (APR). Patients with locally advanced rectal tumors are usually treated with neoadjuvant chemoradiotherapy followed by surgical resection and adjuvant chemotherapy.[15]
- Stage IV (metastatic): Patients with metastatic colorectal cancer are treated with a combination of fluoropyrimidines (5-FU/leucovorin or capecitabine) plus either oxaliplatin (FOLFOX) or irinotecan (FOLFIRI). The survival is improved with the addition of the vascular endothelial growth factor (VEGF) mAb bevacizumab or one of the EGFR mAbs, cetuximab or panitumumab. Anti-EGFR mAbs are not used in patients with *KRAS* mutant tumors and are less effective than bevacizumab in right-sided tumors (cecum to hepatic flexure), while the efficacy is increased in left-sided tumors (splenic flexure to rectum).[16]
- Selected patients with synchronous hepatic or pulmonary metastases may be treated with neoadjuvant chemotherapy followed by colectomy and metastasectomy with curative intent.
- Second-line therapy options include a switch from an oxaliplatin-based therapy to irinotecan-based therapy or vice-versa. Other options for select patients include the combination of cetuximab or panitumumab with the BRAF inhibitor encorafenib for patients with *BRAF* V600E mutation, ICI therapy with pembrolizumab, nivolumab alone or nivolumab plus ipilimumab in patients with dMMR or MSI-high tumors. Other approved treatments include the multityrosine kinase inhibitor regorafenib or trifluridine-tipiracil (TAS-102).

Pancreatic Cancer

EPIDEMIOLOGY AND ETIOLOGY

Pancreatic cancer is the fourth most common cause of cancer-related death in the US, with an estimated 47,050 deaths in 2020.[1] Incidence increases with age, with median age at diagnosis between 60 and 80 years. Risk factors include cigarette smoking, obesity, chemical exposure, and certain genetic predisposition syndromes.

CHAPTER 22

PATHOLOGY

Pancreatic adenocarcinoma is the most common subtype. Pancreatic neuroendocrine tumors are less common, associated with a better prognosis, and are managed differently.

CLINICAL PRESENTATION

Most patients present with nonspecific symptoms including asthenia, anorexia, weight loss, epigastric pain, and back pain. Tumors of the pancreatic head may present with painless jaundice. Pancreatic cancer should be considered in patients >50 years with abrupt-onset diabetes mellitus.

DIAGNOSTIC TESTING

Patients with a suspected pancreatic tumor should undergo initial imaging with CT scan or abdominal ultrasound. However, additional imaging with a pancreatic protocol CT is often necessary to define extent of tumor involvement. Metastatic disease, if present, should be biopsied when feasible. If there is still suspicion for pancreatic cancer but the CT or ultrasound do not show a suspicious lesion, endoscopic retrograde cholangiopancreatography (ERCP) or magnetic resonance cholangiopancreatography (MRCP) may be indicated. MRI of the liver and PET CT may also be performed for further evaluation of indeterminate liver lesions. Staging laparoscopy may be indicated in select patients with tumors in the body or tail, large tumors, or severe abdominal pain. CA19-9 levels have an 80% sensitivity and 80%–90% specificity in symptomatic patients.

STAGING

Although TNM classification is used in pancreatic cancer, clinical management is often guided by resectability of the disease. Resectability is defined by the absence of distant metastases; no tumor contact with the superior mesenteric artery, celiac axis, or hepatic artery; and no tumor contact with the superior mesenteric vein or portal vein or ≤180° vein contact without vein contour irregularity.

TREATMENT

- Surgical resection is the only treatment with curative potential. The most commonly performed surgery is pancreaticoduodenectomy (Whipple procedure), which is indicated for tumors of the pancreatic head. Patients may also receive perioperative neoadjuvant or adjuvant chemotherapy. Commonly used regimens include FOLFORINOX (leucovorin, 5-FU, irinotecan, and oxaliplatin) or gemcitabine plus capecitabine.
- Patients with unresectable locally advanced or metastatic disease are treated with combination chemotherapy including FOLFORINOX, and gemcitabine plus nab-paclitaxel. Patients with germline *BRCA1* or *BRCA2* mutations and no progression after at least 16 weeks of platinum-based chemotherapy may benefit from maintenance therapy with the PARP inhibitor, olaparib. Pembrolizumab is effective in patients with dMMR or MSI-high. Patients with *NTRK* fusion positive tumors may be treated with entrectinib or larotrectinib.[17]

Hepatocellular Carcinoma

EPIDEMIOLOGY AND ETIOLOGY

An estimated 42,810 patients will be diagnosed with liver and intrahepatic bile duct tumors in 2020 in the US.[1] The main risk factors include chronic viral hepatitis B or C and alcohol abuse. With the increased use of hepatitis B vaccination and effective antiviral therapy against hepatitis C, it is possible that nonalcoholic fatty liver disease may become the leading cause of liver cancer in the Western industrialized countries.[18] Patients with hepatitis C typically develop HCC in the presence of cirrhosis, whereas patients with hepatitis B may develop HCC without cirrhosis. However, hepatic cirrhosis from any cause increases risk of hepatocellular carcinoma (HCC).

SCREENING

Patients at high-risk for developing HCC are candidates for screening, including those with cirrhosis, chronic hepatitis B, or a family history of HCC. Screening is performed most commonly using abdominal ultrasonography every 6 months with or without α-fetoprotein (AFP). However, the use of AFP alone is not recommended owing to poor sensitivity and specificity.

CLINICAL PRESENTATION

Patients may be asymptomatic at presentation. Those with more advanced disease may have abdominal pain, early satiety, weight loss, hepatomegaly, ascites, and jaundice. Several paraneoplastic syndromes may occur, including hypoglycemia, erythrocytosis, or hypercalcemia. HCC should also be suspected in patients with stable cirrhosis who decompensate rapidly.

DIAGNOSTIC TESTING

Lesions <1 cm should be followed with repeated abdominal ultrasound in 3–4 months. For lesions ≥1 cm, workup includes contrast-enhanced CT or MRI. Since the malignant lesions are supplied by the hepatic artery, whereas the benign nodules are supplied by branches of the portal system, the pattern of hyperenhancement during the arterial phase of contrast administration with washout in the venous or delayed phases (malignant lesion brighter than the surrounding parenchyma in the arterial phase and less bright in the venous phase) is considered the radiologic hallmark of HCC, with a sensitivity of approximately 70% and specificity of more than 90% in patients with cirrhosis. Patients with this radiological finding do not need a biopsy to confirm the diagnosis.

STAGING

The most commonly used staging system is the Barcelona Clinic Liver Clinic algorithm, which classifies HCC into one of five stages based on liver function, Eastern Cooperative Oncology Group (ECOG) performance status (PS), and tumor burden, which is often used in combination with the Child-Pugh score to define the optimal treatment plan.[18]

TREATMENT

- Treatment options include surgery in patients with early stage disease (single nodule <2 cm), good performance status (ECOG 0), and preserved liver function (Child-Pugh A). Patients with cirrhosis and limited tumor burden, defined by the Milan criteria as the presence of single lesion ≤5 cm or up to three lesions ≤3 cm without vascular invasion, may be candidates for liver transplant. Tumor ablation or transarterial therapy, mostly with transarterial chemoembolization may be used to downstage the tumor or prevent tumor progression while on the waiting list.
- Cytotoxic chemotherapy has limited efficacy in HCC. The main systemic therapy options include multitarget TKIs (sorafenib, lenvatinib, regorafenib, or cabozantinib), ramucirumab, or ICIs plus bevacizumab or ramucirumab, with the latter indicated for AFP ≥400 ng/mL. Nivolumab alone is approved for patients with HCC progressing on sorafenib.[18,19]

GENITOURINARY MALIGNANCIES

Renal Cancer

EPIDEMIOLOGY AND ETIOLOGY

RCC is estimated to result in approximately 74,750 cases and 14,830 deaths in the US in 2020.[1] It is more commonly diagnosed in men and the risk increases with age. Other established risk factors include tobacco smoking, obesity, and hypertension.

PATHOLOGY

RCC is a malignancy of the renal parenchyma. Clear cell RCC is the most common subtype (80%–85%), followed by papillary types 1 and 2 (15%) and chromophobe (5%).

CLINICAL PRESENTATION

Most patients in the US are diagnosed by incidental findings on CT scan. Symptoms may occur due to local tumor growth, metastatic disease, or paraneoplastic syndrome. The most common symptoms include anemia, hematuria, cachexia, and fever. The classic triad of flank pain, hematuria, and a palpable mass is uncommonly seen. Paraneoplastic syndromes include hypercalcemia, erythrocytosis, and Stauffer syndrome, which is defined by the presence of nonmetastatic hepatic dysfunction with elevated alkaline phosphatase, serum bilirubin and transaminases, and a prolonged prothrombin time.

DIAGNOSTIC TESTING

The initial workup should include CT of the abdomen and pelvis, but ideally will also include CT of the chest. MRI may be used to evaluate for involvement of the inferior vena cava or in patients that cannot receive contrast due to allergy or moderate renal insufficiency. The probability of RCC increases with the diameter of the lesion and with enhancement greater than 15 Hounsfield units by CT scan. The role of PET imaging is limited due to the high background activity from the normal renal excretion of fluorodeoxyglucose (FDG). Since most brain and bone metastases are symptomatic, bone scan and brain MRI are performed only when clinically indicated rather than routinely. Centrally located lesions may represent urothelial carcinoma, with further evaluation indicated as this is treated as bladder cancer. For patients that are not surgical candidates, a biopsy of the renal lesion or metastatic site may be used to confirm the diagnosis. Otherwise, patients with suspicious lesions by imaging should be evaluated for surgical resection which can be both diagnostic and therapeutic.

STAGING

TNM: T1 (<7 cm), T2 (7–10 cm), T3 (extends into veins or perinephric tissues), T4 (extends beyond Gerota fascia), N0 (no lymph node involvement), N1 (involved lymph nodes), M1 (distant metastasis). Stage: I (T1N0M0), II (T2N0M0), III (T1-2N1M0 or T3N0-1M0), IV (T4 or M1).

TREATMENT

- Stage I (local): The treatment of choice for patients with localized disease is surgical resection including either radical or partial (nephron-sparing) nephrectomy.
- Stage II–III (locally advanced): The treatment of choice is radical nephrectomy, which involves removal of the Gerota fascia, perirenal fat, regional lymph nodes, and ipsilateral adrenal gland, although select patients may be considered for partial nephrectomy.
- Stage IV (metastatic): The choice of therapy typically depends on the histology, patient risk stratification, and disease burden. One such risk stratification tool is the International Metastatic Renal Cell Carcinoma Database Consortium (IMDC) model which stratifies RCC into low-, intermediate-, or high-risk categories, based on the presence of 0, 1–3, or >3 of the following risk factors: (1) Karnofsky performance status (KPS) <80%, (2) time from diagnosis to treatment <1 year, (3) hemoglobin concentration less than the lower limit of normal (LLN), (4) serum calcium greater than the upper limit of normal (ULN), (5) neutrophil count greater than the ULN, and (6) platelet count greater than the ULN. Treatment options for patients with clear cell histology include pembrolizumab in combination with axitinib or lenvatinib and the combination of nivolumab with cabozantinib. Additional options or patients with intermediate or poor risk include nivolumab plus ipilimumab and single-agent cabozantinib. Subsequent treatments depend on prior regimens used and include ICIs, multitargeted TKIs, and everolimus. Select patients may benefit from cytoreductive nephrectomy.[20]

Bladder Cancer

EPIDEMIOLOGY AND ETIOLOGY

Bladder cancer is one of the most commonly diagnosed malignancies in the US, with 81,400 estimated cases in 2020.[1] Bladder cancer is three times more common in men with a median age of 65 at diagnosis. Common risk factors include advanced age, male sex, and cigarette smoking. Additional risk factors include pelvic radiation, prolonged use of cyclophosphamide, chronic indwelling Foley catheter, and chronic bacterial or *Schistosoma haematobium* infections.

PATHOLOGY

Transitional cell or urothelial carcinoma is the most common histology.

CLINICAL PRESENTATION

Most patients present with painless gross hematuria. Other presentations may include isolated microscopic hematuria and lower urinary tract symptoms such as frequency, urgency, and dysuria.

DIAGNOSTIC TESTING

Patients with macroscopic hematuria should be evaluated with cystoscopy and CT urogram, whereas in those with asymptomatic microscopic hematuria, defined as ≥3 red blood cells (RBCs) per high power field (HPF), the indication for cystoscopy is defined by the following risk stratification system. Patients with high risk, defined by the presence of age >60, >30 pack-year smoking history, or >25 RBCs per HPF on a single urinalysis should undergo cystoscopy and CT urogram. Patients with intermediate risk, defined by age 50–59 in women or 40–59 in men, 10–30 pack-year smoking history, or 11–25 RBCs per HPF should undergo cystoscopy and renal ultrasound. Patients with low risk may repeat a urinalysis in 6 months or undergo cystoscopy plus renal ultrasound. During the cystoscopy, newly identified tumors should be treated with transurethral resection of bladder tumor (TURBT), which provides diagnostic, staging and therapeutic results. An adequate TURBT should include sampling of the muscularis propria.[21]

STAGING

In addition to TNM staging classification, bladder cancers can be broadly divided into non-muscle-invasive, muscle-invasive, and metastatic cancers, which impacts management. For nonmetastatic tumors, the TURBT should define the depth of invasion and differentiate between non-muscle-invasive and muscle-invasive based on the invasion of the muscularis propria.

TREATMENT

• Non-muscle-invasive tumors (stages 0–I) are treated with TURBT with subsequent treatment based on the risk stratification. Patients with low-risk disease, defined as a low-grade, noninvasive (Ta), ≤3 cm solitary lesion should undergo surveillance. Patients with intermediate-risk disease may be considered for intravesical bacille Calmette-Guérin (BCG), whereas those with high-risk, defined as high-grade, carcinoma in situ with invasion of the lamina propria (T1), >3 cm lesion or multifocal lesions, should undergo intravesical BCG. Patients that are not candidates for cystectomy may be treated with chemoradiotherapy, radiation therapy alone, or TURBT.

- The standard treatment options for patients with metastatic disease include cisplatin plus gemcitabine (or cisplatin plus methotrexate) with vinblastine and doxorubicin (MCAV). Other options include single-agent gemcitabine, ICIs, erdafitinib for patients with *FGFR2* or *FGFR3* alterations, as well as two ADCs, sacituzumab govitecan which targets TROP-2 and enfotumab vedotin which targets nectin-4.[21]

Prostate Cancer

EPIDEMIOLOGY AND ETIOLOGY

Prostate cancer is the most common cancer in men in the US, with an estimated 191,330 new cases and 33,330 deaths in 2020.[1] Common risk factors include advanced age, family history, and ethnicity, with higher incidences in African-Americans and lower incidence in Asians. In the US, the lifetime risk of being diagnosed with prostate cancer is approximately 11%, whereas the risk of dying from prostate cancer is 2.5%.

PATHOLOGY

Adenocarcinoma is the most common histology.

SCREENING

Although screening may be associated with a modest decrease in the probability of death from prostate cancer, it may be also be associated with harms including false-positive tests leading to prostate biopsy with its associated complications, overdiagnosis, and overtreatment. Therefore, the 2018 USPSTF guidelines recommend that the decision regarding PSA-based screening for prostate cancer in men aged 55–69 years should be individualized after an informed discussion with the patient regarding the potential benefits and harms.[22]

CLINICAL PRESENTATION

The most common presentation in the US is asymptomatic elevation in PSA. Digital rectal examination (DRE) of the prostate may demonstrate asymmetric induration or nodules. Obstructive symptoms, new-onset erectile dysfunction, hematuria, or hematospermia are less common. Bone is the most common site of metastatic involvement, and patients with skeletal metastases can present with pain, fractures, or nerve root compression.

DIAGNOSTIC TESTING

The diagnosis of prostate cancer is usually made through transrectal ultrasonography-guided biopsy, although MRI-guided biopsies may also be used. PSA levels should be obtained. Bone scan and CT of the abdomen and pelvis are recommended for patients with high-risk disease and select patients with intermediate-risk disease. PSMA PET CT imaging increases the rate of detection of metastases to pelvic lymph nodes or occult distant sites.

STAGING

Based on TNM classification, early stage disease (T1–T2) is confined to the prostate, locally advanced disease (T3–T4) is defined by local invasion outside the prostate, and stage IV disease is defined by nodal involvement (N1) and/or metastatic
disease (M1). Further risk classification of prostate cancer is based on PSA, stage,
and Gleason score (GS), with the latter representing the summation of the most
prominent and second most prominent Gleason patterns, each ranging from 1 to
5 and added together to give a GS of low (≤6), intermediate (7), or high (>7).
This classification may be converted into the International Society of Urological
Pathology (ISUP) groups which include group 1 (GS ≤6), group 2 (GS 3 + 4 = 7),
group 3 (GS 4 + 3 = 7), group 4 (GS 8), and group 5 (GS ≥9). Patients are then
classified as very low risk (PSA<10 ng/mL, group 1, nonpalpable tumor identified
on biopsy alone [T1c or less], and <3 biopsy cores positive and <50% cancer/core),
low risk (PSA <10, group 1, and tumor involving no more than one half of one
side of the prostate [T2a]), intermediate risk (PSA 10–20, group 2 or 3, or tumor
involving up to both sides of prostate [T2c or less]), high risk (PSA >20, group
>3 or extraprostatic spread [T3a]), and very high risk (primary Gleason pattern 5,
>4 cores of group 4 or 5, invades seminal vesicles and/or other adjacent structures
[T3b–T4], multiple high-risk features).[23]

TREATMENT

• Patients with clinically localized disease (stage T1 or T2) may be managed with
  surveillance, radiation therapy (external beam radiation or brachytherapy), or surgery. Specifically, for patients with very-low-risk disease and expected survival >10
  years, active surveillance is the preferred option. Patients with low-risk disease and
  >10 years life-expectancy may be considered for active surveillance, radiation therapy, or surgery. Patients with intermediate- or high-risk disease should be treated
  with radical prostatectomy plus pelvic lymph node dissection or radiation therapy
  (external beam radiation or brachytherapy) with or without androgen deprivation
  therapy (ADT). Docetaxel may be added to radiotherapy plus ADT in patients
  with high-risk disease. ADT includes surgical orchiectomy or medical castration
  with a gonadotropin-releasing hormone (GnRH) agonist (leuprolide or goserelin)
  or antagonist (degarelix).
• Metastatic disease may be treated with ADT in combination with docetaxel or an
  AR signaling inhibitor (abiraterone/prednisone, enzalutamide, or apalutamide).
  Patients with castration-resistant disease may be treated with docetaxel or cabazi-
  taxel. Other options for subsequent therapy include ICIs, the autologous cellular
  therapy sipuleucel-T, Radium-223, and PARP inhibitors for patients with *BRCA1*,
  BRCA2, or *ATM* mutations.[23]

Testicular Cancer and Germ Cell Tumors

EPIDEMIOLOGY AND ETIOLOGY

Testicular cancers are uncommon tumors with an estimated 9610 new cases and 440
deaths in the US in 2020.[1] However, they are the most common tumors diagnosed in
men aged 15–35. Risk factors include cryptorchidism, contralateral testicular cancer,
and Klinefelter syndrome.

PATHOLOGY

GCTs account for approximately 95% of all testicular tumors and may be divided into pure seminomas and nonseminomas, with the latter subdivided into embryonal carcinoma, choriocarcinoma, yolk sac tumor, teratoma, and mixed GCTs including seminoma and nonseminoma components. Sex cord tumors account for approximately 5% of the testicular cancers, including Sertoli cell tumor, Leydig cell tumor, granulosa cell tumor, mixed and unclassified tumors. GCTs may rarely originate in extragonadal sites including the retroperitoneum and mediastinum.[24]

CLINICAL PRESENTATION

The most common presentation is that of a painless testicular mass, but patients may also present with testicular pain, hydrocele, or gynecomastia. Advanced testicular cancer may present with back or flank pain, fevers, night sweats, and weight loss.

DIAGNOSTIC TESTING

Patients with a palpable testicular mass should be evaluated for testicular cancer, initially with a testicular ultrasound and tumor markers (AFP, LDH [lactic dehydrogenase], and beta-hCG [human chorionic gonadotropin]). Testicular GCTs are usually heterogeneous, hypoechoic, and vascular. Patients with a heterogeneous, hypoechoic intratesticular lesion on ultrasound should undergo unilateral radical orchiectomy as the next evaluation step. Trans-scrotal biopsies should not be performed due to the increased risk of local or atypical recurrences. Patients with metastatic disease may undergo biopsy of the metastatic site rather than orchiectomy for diagnosis. Postdiagnostic workup includes CT of the abdomen and pelvis, chest radiograph, and repeat tumor markers. In the case of pure seminomas, which do not produce AFP, CT of the chest is indicated in case of abdominal lymph node enlargement or abnormal chest radiograph.

STAGING

Staging is based on TNM status and serum markers (S). In general, stage I represents disease confined to the scrotum (T1-4), stage II indicates lymph node involvement (N1-3), and stage III is defined by the presence of visceral/distant metastases (M1). There is no stage IV category for testicular cancers. The serum marker classification includes: S0 (normal markers), S1 (LDH <1.5 ULN and hCG <5000 [mIU/mL] and AFP <1000 [ng/mL]), S2 (LDH 1.5–10× ULN or hCG 5000–50,000 or AFP 1000–10,000), and S3 (LDH >10× ULN or hCG >50,000 or AFP >10,000).

TREATMENT

- Prior to starting treatment, patients should be offered sperm banking for fertility preservation.
- Seminomas: Patients with stage I seminomas are treated with orchiectomy followed by surveillance, single-agent carboplatin, or radiation. Patients with stages IIA or IIB (no lymph node larger than 5 cm) may be treated with chemotherapy

or radiation therapy, whereas those with stage IIC (lymph node larger than 5 cm) or III with good risk (normal AFP, no nonpulmonary visceral metastases) are treated with chemotherapy including three cycles of bleomycin, etoposide, and cisplatin (BEP) or four cycles of EP. Patients with stage III and intermediate risk (normal AFP, nonpulmonary visceral metastases) are treated with four cycles of BEP or etoposide, ifosfamide, and cisplatin (VIP). No patient with pure seminoma is classified as poor risk.

- Nonseminomas: Patients with stage I are treated with orchiectomy and then surveillance, one cycle of BEP, or retroperitoneal lymph node dissection (RPLND). Patients with stage II are treated with nerve-sparing RPLND, three cycles of BEP, or four cycles of EP. Patients with stage IIC or good risk IIIA (no nonpulmonary visceral metastases and post-orchiectomy S1) are treated with three cycles of BEP or four cycles of EP. Patients with intermediate (no nonpulmonary visceral metastases, S2) or poor risk (nonpulmonary visceral metastases, mediastinal primary tumor, or S3) are treated with four cycles of BEP or VIP.

- Subsequent therapies: Treatment options for patients with GCTs who relapse after the initial treatment include alternative cisplatin-based regimens such as VeIP (vinblastine, ifosfamide, cisplatin) and TIP (paclitaxel, ifosfamide, cisplatin), pembrolizumab for MSI-high tumors and high-dose chemotherapy with autologous stem cell transplant.[24]

GYNECOLOGIC MALIGNANCIES

Cervical Cancer

EPIDEMIOLOGY AND ETIOLOGY

Cervical cancer death rates have declined by approximately 80% since 1930 because of the widespread implementation of screening programs, accounting for an estimated 13,800 new cases and 4290 deaths in the US in 2020.[1] In countries that lack screening and prevention programs, cervical cancer is the second most common cancer in women. HPV infection is detected in >99% of tumors, most commonly HPV-16 and -18. Other risk factors include early onset of sexual activity, multiple sexual partners, high-risk partners, history of sexually transmitted illness, and chronic immunosuppression.

SCREENING AND PREVENTION

The 2018 USPSTF recommends screening for cervical cancer with cervical cytology every 3 years for women aged 21–29. For women aged 30–65, screening options include cervical cytology alone every 3 years, high-risk HPV (hrHPV) testing alone every 5 years, or combined cytology and hrHPV every 5 years. Women younger than 21 or older than 65 with adequate prior screening and women who have undergone hysterectomy do not need screening.[25] HPV vaccines include the bivalent vaccine (Cervarix) which targets HPV 16 and 18; the quadrivalent vaccine (Gardasil) which targets HPV 16, 18, 6, and 11; and the 9-valent vaccine (Gardasil-9) which targets HPV 16, 18, 6, 11, 31, 33, 45, 52, and 58. Vaccination should ideally start before the onset of sexual activity and is recommended for both sexes by 11–12 years old.

PATHOLOGY

The most common histologies are squamous cell carcinoma (75%–85%) and adeno-carcinoma (15%–25%).

CLINICAL PRESENTATION

Patients with early stage lesions are commonly asymptomatic and diagnosed incidentally on Pap smear, which underscores the importance of screening. Symptoms observed at presentation may include irregular or heavy vaginal bleeding or postcoital bleeding, usually occurring in patients without Pap smear for several years. Patients with advanced disease may present with back pain, hematochezia, or vaginal passage of urine or stool due to fistula formation from invasive cancer.

DIAGNOSTIC TESTING

Diagnosis is obtained through colposcopy with cervical cytology and biopsy. A cone biopsy is recommended in women without gross cervical lesions or with microinvasive disease to define the depth of the lesion. Clinical examination in conjunction with imaging, such as chest radiograph, CT, PET CT, and pelvic MRI, may be used to assess International Federation of Gynecology and Obstetrics (FIGO) stage, as indicated.

STAGING

Staging is based on the FIGO system. In general, stage I disease is confined to the cervix. Stage II disease invades beyond the uterus but does not extend into the lower third of the vagina or the pelvic wall. Stage III involves the lower third of the vagina, the pelvic wall, the pelvic/para-aortic lymph nodes and/or causes hydroureter. Stage IV disease extends beyond the pelvis.

TREATMENT

Patients with early stage disease may be treated with fertility sparing resection, hysterectomy, or radiation therapy. Chemoradiation can be used in locally advanced tumors and as adjuvant therapy in high-risk patients following hysterectomy. Metastatic disease is treated with chemotherapy, most commonly a platinum (cisplatin or carboplatin) alone or in combination with paclitaxel with or without bevacizumab. Immunotherapy may be considered in those with PD-L1 positive or with MSI-high tumors who progress after platinum-based chemotherapy.[26]

Uterine Cancer

EPIDEMIOLOGY AND ETIOLOGY

Uterine cancer is the most common gynecologic cancer in the US, with an increasing incidence estimated to account for 65,620 new cases and 12,590 deaths in 2020.[1] Risk factors include obesity, early menarche, late menopause, nulliparity, diabetes mellitus, use of tamoxifen, and hereditary disorders such as Lynch syndrome. The risk is reduced with parity and the use of oral contraceptives. Most patients are perimenopausal or postmenopausal.

CHAPTER 22

PATHOLOGY

Approximately 95% of uterine tumors arise in the lining of the uterus and are termed endometrial carcinomas. Endometrial carcinomas may be subdivided into endometrioid and nonendometrioid, with the former accounting for approximately 80% of cases and related to relative estrogen excess, whereas the latter are hormone-independent and usually occur in older postmenopausal women. Nonendometrioid endometrial carcinoma includes serous carcinoma, clear-cell carcinoma, and carcinosarcoma. Nonendometrial uterine tumors may include sarcomas and lymphomas.

CLINICAL PRESENTATION

The most common presentation is vaginal bleeding, usually occurring in postmenopausal women. Of note, the severity of the bleeding does not correlate with the risk of malignancy.

DIAGNOSTIC TESTING

Premenopausal women with irregular vaginal bleeding and risk factors for endometrial cancer and all postmenopausal women with any vaginal bleeding should be evaluated for endometrial cancer with pelvic examination, transvaginal ultrasound, and endometrial biopsy. Patients with endometrial thickness less than 4 mm on transvaginal ultrasound may not need endometrial biopsy in the absence of additional bleeding episodes.

STAGING

The TNM and FIGO staging systems are both used in uterine cancer. In general, FIGO stage I is similar to T1 disease, with tumor confined to the uterus. FIGO stage II is similar to T2 disease, with tumor invading the cervix but not otherwise extending beyond the uterus. FIGO stage IIIA/B is similar to T3 disease, with tumor involving serosa, adnexa, vagina, or parametrium. FIGO stage IIIC is similar to N1-2 disease. FIGO stage IVA is similar to T4 disease, with tumor involving bladder or bowel. FIGO stage IVB is similar to M1 disease, with distant metastatic disease.

TREATMENT

- The primary treatment modality is surgery with additional therapy depending on the surgical staging. Patients with stage IA (limited to the endometrium or invading less than half of the myometrium) usually do not require additional therapy, although select patients with higher risk disease may be treated with vaginal brachytherapy. Patients with surgically staged IB-IV disease are treated with radiation therapy, primarily vaginal brachytherapy in stage IB and external beam radiation in stages II to IV (with or without the addition of brachytherapy). Patients with stage III or IV disease should also receive systemic therapy.
- The most commonly used chemotherapy regimen carboplatin plus paclitaxel. Trastuzumab may be added to chemotherapy in patients with HER2+ tumors. Patients with ER+ tumors and an indolent course may be treated with endocrine therapy, such as AIs or tamoxifen. Additional treatment options may include pembrolizumab with or without lenvatinib, as well as several other chemotherapeutic and/or targeted agents.[27]

Ovarian Cancer

EPIDEMIOLOGY AND ETIOLOGY

Ovarian cancer is the leading cause of gynecologic mortality in the US, with an estimated 21,750 new cases and 13,940 deaths estimated in 2020.[1] Common risk factors include older age, early menarche, late menopause, nulliparity, infertility, endometriosis, and genetic factors including *BRCA 1/2* mutations and Lynch syndrome. The risk is reduced by oral contraceptives, breast feeding, and parity.

PATHOLOGY

The most common ovarian tumors are epithelial, GCTs, and sex cord-stromal tumors. Epithelial tumors represent 65%–70% of cases and are subdivided into serous (70%), mucinous, endometrioid, clear cell, and transitional.

CLINICAL PRESENTATION

Patients with early-stage disease have nonspecific symptoms including bloating or pelvic and abdominal discomfort. In patients with more advanced disease, the symptoms often reflect the intra-abdominal spreading of the disease causing ascites, abdominal pain, and constipation.

DIAGNOSTIC TESTING

Women suspected to have ovarian cancer should undergo additional evaluation including a physical examination, serum CA 125, and transvaginal ultrasound. The diagnosis is usually made through surgical resection with the exploratory laparotomy providing diagnostic, staging, and potentially therapeutic results.

STAGING

The TNM and FIGO staging systems are both used in ovarian cancer. In general, FIGO stage I is similar to T1 disease, with tumor confined to the ovaries or fallopian tubes. FIGO stage II is similar to T2 disease, with tumor extending below the pelvic brim or the presence of primary peritoneal disease. FIGO stage III is similar to T3 and/or N positive disease, defined by the presence of peritoneal metastasis outside the pelvis and/or metastasis to the retroperitoneal lymph nodes. FIGO stage IV is similar to M1 disease, with metastasis beyond the peritoneal cavity and/or the retroperitoneal lymph nodes.

TREATMENT

- Since epithelial ovarian cancers disseminate predominantly through the abdominal cavity, cytoreductive surgery (also known as debulking) is the optimal initial therapy. Optimal debulking is defined by the presence of no residual tumor nodules >1 cm, although an R0 resection should be the therapeutic goal.
- Adjuvant therapy is defined by the surgical stage and histology. Patients with stage IA or IB disease (tumor limited to the ovaries and fallopian tubes) are usually treated with surgery alone, whereas those with stage II disease and select patients with stage IC disease (surgical spill or malignant ascites) are treated with adjuvant

chemotherapy (usually carboplatin plus paclitaxel). Patients with stage III or IV disease are treated with chemotherapy.

- The most commonly used systemic chemotherapy is carboplatin plus paclitaxel with or without bevacizumab. Patients with tumor relapse >6 months after the first-line therapy are considered platinum-sensitive and may benefit from repeating the original chemotherapy regimen. Several other chemotherapeutic agents may be considered for previously treated patients, as well as pembrolizumab in patients with MSI-high disease, PARP inhibitors, or hormonal therapy.[28]

Melanoma

EPIDEMIOLOGY AND ETIOLOGY

It is estimated that nearly 100,350 new cases of cutaneous melanoma were diagnosed in 2020 in the US.[1] The main risk factors include exposure to ultraviolet (UV) radiation (particularly UVB), light skin, tendency to freckle, presence of dysplastic nevi, personal history, and family history.

PATHOLOGY

Melanoma is usually recognized using the ABCDE criteria which includes **a**symmetry, **b**order irregularity, **c**olor variegation, **d**iameter >6 mm, and **e**volving characteristics such as change in size, shape, or color. In patients with multiple pigmented lesions, the detection of melanoma may be improved with intra-patient comparison and search for the "ugly duckling sign," which is represented by a nevus with different color or size compared to other lesions.

DIAGNOSTIC TESTING

The workup often involves adequate sampling of the lesion, IHC for markers of melanocytic origin (S100, MART1, HMB45), and molecular profiling for detection of mutations in the *BRAF* gene and overall tumor mutational burden. Primary lesions >0.75 mm in Breslow thickness, with ulceration, ≥ 1 mitoses/mm^2, or lymphovascular invasion require a sentinel lymph node biopsy. In the presence of positive lymph nodes, whether if clinically palpable or after SLNB, patients should undergo imaging studies including CT scans or PET CT and brain MRI.

STAGING

Stages I and II are based on tumor thickness (T1 up to 1 mm, T2 >1–2 mm, T3 >2–4 mm, T4 >4 mm) and absence (T1a, T2a, T3a, or T4a) or presence (T1b, T2b, T3b, or T4b) of ulceration. Whereas regional lymph node involvement and distant metastases characterizing stage III and IV respectively.

TREATMENT

- Patients with resected stage I or II melanoma do not require adjuvant therapy. Patients with stage III disease may be treated with adjuvant nivolumab or pembrolizumab, or dabrafenib plus trametinib if *BRAF* V600E mutated.[29]
- Patients with metastatic melanoma may be treated with pembrolizumab, nivolumab, or one of the combinations of BRAF and MEK inhibitors including vemurafenib

plus cobimetinib, dabrafenib plus trametinib, and encorafenib plus binimetinib if *BRAF* V600E mutated. Treatment options after the first-line therapy include combination ICI and ipilimumab, interleukin-2, and talimogene laherparepvec (T-VEC), which is a genetically modified HSV-1 virus with decreased virulence and selective intratumoral replication injected into the tumor which may induce an immune response to the malignancy.[29]

Central Nervous System Tumors

EPIDEMIOLOGY AND ETIOLOGY

Brain and other central nervous system (CNS) tumors are estimated to account for 23,890 new cancer diagnoses and 18,020 deaths in 2020.[1] Risk factors include ionizing radiation and familial cancer syndromes including neurofibromatosis, tuberous sclerosis, Li-Fraumeni, and others.

PATHOLOGY

Glioblastoma is the most common subtype of primary brain tumors. Meanwhile, the World Health Organization classification further classifies CNS tumors based on histology and grade (I–IV).

CLINICAL PRESENTATION

Patients with glioblastomas usually present with symptoms caused by rapid tumor expansion leading to displacement or infiltrative destruction of brain structures, progressive headaches, seizures, focal neurologic signs, and changes in mental status.

DIAGNOSTIC TESTING

Workup includes MRI of the brain and molecular testing of a surgical biopsy or resected tumor specimen for methylguanine-DNA methyltransferase (*MGMT*) methylation, 1p/19q codeletion, *IDH1* mutations, and BRAF V600E activating mutations, which may help guide therapy.

TREATMENT

- The current treatment paradigm for glioblastoma is surgery with maximal safe resection followed by concurrent radiation therapy and temozolomide followed by temozolomide alone for 6 months. *MGMT* is a DNA repair enzyme that reverses the DNA damage caused by alkylating agents resulting in resistance to these drugs, including temozolomide. Methylation of the *MGMT* promoter silences the enzyme, increasing the sensitivity to alkylating drugs. The benefit from temozolomide in patients with glioblastoma is observed predominately in those with *MGMT* promoter methylation.[30] Patients with recurrent *MGMT*-methylated glioblastoma may be retreated with temozolomide depending on the interval from the previous treatment.
- Other treatment options include glucocorticoids, lomustine, bevacizumab, regorafenib, and use of tumor treating fields, which employ noninvasive alternating electrical fields to disrupt tumor cell division.

Sarcoma

EPIDEMIOLOGY AND ETIOLOGY

Sarcomas of the soft tissues, bones, and joints are estimated to account for 16,730 new cases and 16,830 deaths in the year 2020.[1] Predisposing factors include age, prior radiation, chemical and chemotherapy exposure, genetic/hereditary syndromes, Paget disease of the bone, HIV/human herpesvirus 8 (HHV8) infection (Kaposi sarcoma), and chronic lymphedema (lymphangiosarcoma [Stewart–Treves syndrome]).

PATHOLOGY

Soft tissue sarcomas consist of at least 70 different types of histologies. Review by a pathologist who has expertise in the diagnosis of sarcoma is recommended.

CLINICAL PRESENTATION

Symptoms depend on the site of disease. Sarcomas arising in extremities can present as a painless soft tissue mass. Visceral sarcomas can be associated with GI bleeding, early satiety, dysphagia, dyspepsia, or vaginal bleeding depending on the organs involved. Retroperitoneal tumors may result in early satiety, nausea, paresthesias, or an abdominal mass.

DIAGNOSTIC TESTING

Initial imaging studies include MRI for sarcomas involving the extremities or pelvis, and CT for retroperitoneal or visceral sarcomas. PET CT may be useful in staging high-grade sarcomas. Chest imaging with CT is important to rule out pulmonary metastases, which is the most common site of distant disease in sarcomas.

STAGING

TNM staging is specific to the sarcoma histology and sites of disease. Additionally, the tumor grade (taking into account the degree of differentiation, mitotic count, and necrosis score) factors into the stage of disease.

TREATMENT

- Early stage, nonvisceral soft tissue sarcomas (stages I–III): Surgical excision is the mainstay of therapy. Adjuvant radiotherapy is often indicated in patients with large tumors and positive or equivocal margins when re-excision is not feasible. Neoadjuvant and adjuvant chemotherapy may be considered in select cases.[31]
- Metastatic soft tissue sarcoma: Palliative chemotherapy is the primary mode of treatment. Doxorubicin, ifosfamide, gemcitabine, docetaxel, dacarbazine, eribulin, and trabectedin are commonly used. Targeted agents may also include crizotinib, ceritinib, or brigatinib (if *ALK* translocation present); larotrectinib and entrectinib (if NTRK gene fusion present); as well as pazopanib, sorafenib, sunitinib, bevacizumab, pexidartinib, imatinib, palbociclib, sirolimus, ripretinib, avapritib, everolimus, and temsirolimus in certain subtypes of sarcoma.[31] Metastasectomy can be considered in patients with oligometastatic disease.

- GI stromal tumors (GIST) commonly harbor mutations in *KIT* and are highly responsive to imatinib. Adjuvant and/or neoadjuvant imatinib may be considered in select patients.
- Ewing sarcoma differs from many soft tissue sarcomas in that it has a high cure rate and highly responsive to chemotherapy and radiation. Metastatic disease can be potentially cured with chemotherapy in some cases.

Cancer of Unknown Primary

Cancer of unknown primary is defined as biopsy-proven malignancy for which the primary site of origin cannot be identified.

PATHOLOGY

These malignancies may include adenocarcinoma (60%), poorly differentiated carcinoma/poorly differentiated adenocarcinoma (29%), squamous cell carcinoma (5%), poorly differentiated malignant neoplasm (5%), and neuroendocrine carcinoma (1%). Further identification may require specialized IHC staining, electron microscopy, and molecular/genetic analysis.

DIAGNOSTIC TESTING

In most cases, several studies are needed to facilitate a diagnosis, including comprehensive examination, urine/stool occult blood testing, and tumor marker testing in select patients (e.g., PSA in older men, β-hCG/AFP in younger men). CT of the chest, abdomen, and pelvis; PET CT; and symptom-oriented endoscopy may be useful in select patients.

TREATMENT

- Treatment for favorable subgroups of patients with cancer of unknown primary is tailored to the most likely primary site of origin. For instance, adenocarcinoma of unknown primary in women involving the axillary nodes is typically managed like stage II or III breast carcinoma. Papillary serous adenocarcinoma of unknown primary within the peritoneal cavity in women is typically managed as stage III ovarian carcinoma. The presence of blastic bone metastases and an elevated PSA in men is suggestive of stage IV prostate cancer and thus typically managed as such. Poorly differentiated midline carcinomas of unknown primary in men should be managed as extragonadal GCTs. Squamous cell carcinoma involving the cervical lymph nodes is typically managed as a locally advanced head and neck cancer, whereas squamous cell carcinoma involving isolated inguinal lymph nodes is typically managed with inguinal lymph node dissection with or without adjuvant radiation therapy.
- Poorly differentiated neuroendocrine carcinomas are typically managed with platinum-based chemotherapy regimens. A single, localized mass of unknown primary can be managed with definitive local treatment with either surgery or radiation, based on the location of the mass. Empiric combination chemotherapy regimen, such as carboplatin and paclitaxel, is typically considered in patients whose disease cannot be categorized into any of the favorable subgroups.

HEMATOLOGIC MALIGNANCIES

Myelodysplastic Syndrome

EPIDEMIOLOGY AND ETIOLOGY

Myelodysplastic syndromes (MDS) comprise a heterogeneous group of myeloid neoplasms that are broadly characterized by ineffective clonal hematopoiesis, cytopenias and an increased risk of leukemic transformation. Age-related clonal hematopoiesis and clonal cytopenias of undetermined significance commonly precede development of MDS by years, with age being one of the strongest risk factors for MDS (median age at diagnosis 65 years). Environmental factors, prior radiation and/or chemotherapy, as well as certain genetic syndromes and benign hematologic disorders (paroxysmal nocturnal hemoglobinuria) have been associated with increased risk of MDS.

PATHOLOGY

Bone marrow biopsy is characterized by dysplasia in at least one hematopoietic cell line, with or without increased blasts. Chromosome abnormalities occur in up to 80% of cases, often resulting from the accumulation of multiple genetic lesions related to RNA splicing, DNA methylation, histone modification, transcription regulation, DNA repair, and intracellular signaling. Numerous cytogenetic abnormalities occur in MDS, but commonly include del(5q) (15%), monosomy 7 or del(7q) (10%), and trisomy 8. The most common recurrently mutated genes include *ASXL1, DNMT3A, RUNX1, SF3B1, SRSF2,* and *TET2.*

CLINICAL PRESENTATION

Symptoms are typically related to bone marrow failure and cytopenias, including fatigue and dyspnea due to anemia, fever/infection due to leukopenia, and/or easy bruising/bleeding due to thrombocytopenia. Macrocytosis is common.

DIAGNOSTIC TESTING

Complete blood counts with cytopenias in at least one cell one must be present. Obtaining a bone marrow aspirate and core biopsy is necessary and will frequently reveal a dysplastic and hypercellular bone marrow. Cytogenetics and FISH are required to identify chromosomal abnormalities. Further molecular profiling, typically with next generation sequencing, is increasingly used to aid in risk stratification, prognostication, and treatment planning.

RISK CLASSIFICATION

The current WHO classification system includes MDS with unilineage dysplasia (anemia, neutropenia, or thrombocytopenia); MDS with multilineage dysplasia; MDS with ring sideroblasts; MDS with excess blasts (5%–19%); MDS with isolated deletion of 5q; and MDS unclassifiable.[32] The Revised International Prognostic Scoring System (IPSS-R) assigns points for patients' cytogenetics, bone marrow blast %, hemoglobin level, neutrophil count, and platelet count, with the total score used to determine patient risk category and treatment approach (Table 22-5).

TABLE 22-5	Revised International Prognostic Scoring System (IPSS-R) for Myelodysplastic Syndromes				
Score	Cytogenetics	Marrow Blasts (%)	Hemoglobin (g/dL)	Neutrophils ($\times10^9$/L)	Platelets ($\times10^9$/L)
0	Very good: −Y, del(11q)	≤2	≥10	≥0.8	≥100
0.5	–	–	–	<0.8	50–99
1	Good: normal, del(5q), del(12p), del(20q), double including del(5q)	2.1–4.9	8–9.9	–	<50
1.5	–	–	<8	–	–
2	Intermediate: del(7q), +8, +19, i(17q), any other single or double independent clones	5–10	–	–	–
3	Poor: −7, inv(3)/ t(3q)/del(3q), double including −7/del(7q), complex with 3 abnormalities	>10	–	–	–
4	Very poor: complex with >3 abnormalities	–	–	–	–

Total Score	Risk Category	Median Overall Survival (y)	Median Time to 25% Acute Myeloid Leukemia Risk (years)
≤1.5	Very low	8.8	NR
2.0–3.0	Low	5.3	10.8
3.5–4.5	Intermediate	3	3.2
5.0–6.0	High	1.6	1.4
>6.0	Very high	0.8	0.73

TREATMENT

Asymptomatic patients with IPSS-R low-risk disease can be followed with support-ive care (transfusions, iron chelation, etc.) but otherwise without specific therapy. Patients with very-low-risk or low-risk MDS and symptomatic anemia with a low erythropoietin level (<500 mU/mL) can be treated with erythropoiesis-stimulating agents. Treatment with immunosuppressive agents such as antithymocyte globulin and cyclosporine can be considered in patients who have hypoplastic MDS and/or demonstrate a concomitant paroxysmal nocturnal hemoglobinuria clone. Treatment with hypomethylating agents such as 5-azacytidine or decitabine should be considered in patients with intermediate- or high-risk MDS. Additionally, patients with high- and very-high-risk MDS may be considered for allogeneic stem cell transplantation. MDS with del(5q) is associated with a good prognosis and higher probability of response to treatment with lenalidomide. Patients with MDS with ring sideroblasts may benefit from treatment with luspatercept. Patients with an *IDH 1/2* mutation may benefit from treatment with an IDH inhibitor (ivosidenib or enasidenib).[32]

Acute Myeloid Leukemia

EPIDEMIOLOGY AND ETIOLOGY

AML is the most common type of acute leukemia in adults with an estimated 19,940 new cases in 2020.[1] Median age at presentation is around 65 years. Risk factors are similar to those of MDS. Antecedent MDS or myeloproliferative neoplasms, as well as certain bone-marrow failure syndromes and familial cancer syndromes increase the risk of AML.

PATHOLOGY

The WHO classification includes six categories for AML: AML with recurrent genetic abnormalities (Table 22-6); AML with MDS-related changes; therapy-related AML; AML, not otherwise specified (NOS); myeloid sarcoma, and myeloid proliferations related to Down syndrome. The AML NOS category includes the traditional French–American–British (FAB) subtypes M0 (AML minimally differentiated), M1 (AML without maturation), M2 (AML with maturation), M4 (acute myelomonocytic leukemia), M5 (acute monocytic leukemia), M6 (acute erythroleukemia), and M7 (acute megakaryoblastic leukemia). The FAB subtype M3 (acute promyelocytic leukemia [APL]) is classified as AML with recurrent genetic abnormalities due to the presence of t(15;17).

TABLE 22-6	Acute Leukemias With Recurrent Genetic Abnormalities
Acute Myeloid Leukemia	**Acute Lymphoblastic Leukemia (ALL)**
Recurrent genetic abnormalities	Recurrent genetic abnormalities
t(8;21); *RUNX1-RUNX1T1*	t(9;22); *BCR1-ABL*
inv(16) or t(16;16); *CEFB-MYH11*	t(variable;11q23); *MLL* (*KMT2A*) rearranged
t(15;17); *PML-RARA*	t(12;21); *TEL/AML1* (*ETV6-RUNX1*)
t(9;11); *MLLT3-KMT2A*	t(1;19); *TCF3-PBX1*
t(6;9); *DEK-NUP214*	t(5;14); *IL3-IGH*
inv(3) or t(3;3); *GATA2, MECOM*	ALL with hyperdiploidy
t(1;22); *RBM15-MKL1*	ALL with hypodiploid
NPM1 mutated	Provisional entities: BCR-ABL-like, iAMP21
CEBPA biallelic mutations	–

CLINICAL PRESENTATION

Most patients present with pancytopenia, circulating blasts, and symptoms related to cytopenias, including fatigue and dyspnea due to anemia, fever/infection due to leukopenia, and easy bruising/bleeding due to thrombocytopenia. Leukostasis is a medical emergency and may be manifested by dyspnea, chest pain, headache, confusion, or neurologic deficits. Extramedullary tissue invasion by leukemic cells (most commonly with AML-M5) can result in hepatomegaly, splenomegaly, lymphadenopathy, rashes (leukemia cutis), gingival hypertrophy, CNS dysfunction, cranial neuropathies, or infiltrative masses (granulocytic sarcomas or chloromas).

DIAGNOSTIC TESTING

AML is defined by the presence of ≥20% blasts in the bone marrow or in the peripheral blood. AML with t(8;21), inv(16) and t(15;17) can be diagnosed irrespective of the blast percentage. Bone marrow specimens should be submitted for routine pathology, IHC, flow cytometry, cytogenetics, FISH, and molecular testing/sequencing. This information is used to classify AML into prognostic groups and to guide treatment.[33]

TREATMENT

- Induction: standard intensive induction chemotherapy for AML typically consists of the "7 + 3" regimen which includes cytarabine over 7 days given concurrently with an anthracycline (daunorubicin or idarubicin) for 3 days. Approximately 60%–80% of AML patients achieve a remission with induction chemotherapy. However, nearly all patients achieving a remission will eventually relapse without additional consolidation therapy. The addition of targeted agents to 7 + 3 induction may include midostaurin (multikinase FLT3 inhibitor) in *FLT3* mutated AML and gemtuzumab ozogamicin (CD33 ADC) typically used in younger CD33 positive AML patients with favorable risk disease. In patients who are ineligible for intensive induction chemotherapy, venetoclax (*BCL2* inhibitor) in combination with a hypomethylating agent (azacitidine or decitabine) or the combination of glasdegib (hedgehog pathway inhibitor) with low-dose cytarabine may be considered. In patients with therapy-related AML and AML with MDS-related changes, CPX-351 (liposomal cytarabine and daunorubicin) may be considered. Additional targeted therapies for patients with AML harboring specific mutations may include decitabine for *TP53*, ivosidenib for *IDH1*, enasidenib for *IDH2*, and gilteritinib for *FLT3* mutated AML.[34]
- Consolidation: intensive consolidation typically includes high-dose cytarabine (HiDAC) with or without subsequent allogeneic stem cell transplantation depending on risk group (Table 22-7). Also see section "Principles of Stem Cell Transplantation."
- Relapsed/refractory AML is associated with very poor prognosis and may be managed with salvage chemotherapy, targeted therapies, tapering of immunosuppression with donor lymphocyte infusion if relapsing after allo-transplant, or enrollment in clinical trials.
- APL (AML-M3) represents a unique subset of AML which is characterized by high cure rates. Treatment includes the use of all-*trans*-retinoic acid (ATRA) and arsenic trioxide (ATO) for low–intermediate-risk patients (WBC ≤10 × 10^9/L at

TABLE 22-7	Cytogenetic Abnormalities in Acute Myeloid Leukemia and Associated Prognosis	
Risk Group	Cytogenetic and Molecular Features	Preferred Consolidation Strategy
Favorable	t(15;17), t(8;21), inv(16) or t(16;16), mutated *NPM1* without *FLT3*-ITD, or biallelic mutated *CEBPA*	Chemotherapy
Intermediate	Normal cytogenetics, mutated *NPM1* and *FLT3*-ITD, wt*NPM1* without *FLT3*-ITD, t(9;11)	Allogeneic hematopoietic cell transplantation
Unfavorable	Complex karyotype (defined as ≥3 abnormalities, excluding the favorable-risk cytogenetics), monosomal karyotype, inv(3), t(6;9), t(9;22) KMT2A rearranged, mutated RUNX1, ASXL1 or TP53 and MDS or therapy-related	Allogeneic hematopoietic cell transplantation

presentation) and ATRA, ATO, and the addition of an anthracycline for high-risk patients (WBC >10 × 10⁹/L at presentation). Glucocorticoids may also be added to the induction regimen for APL as prophylaxis for or treatment of differentiation syndrome.

Acute Lymphoblastic Leukemia

EPIDEMIOLOGY AND ETIOLOGY

Acute lymphoblastic leukemia (ALL) is the most common childhood leukemia with an estimated 6150 new cases in the US in 2020.[1] The median age at presentation is 35 years with a bimodal distribution including a peak at 4–5 years and a second gradual peak after the age of 50.

PATHOLOGY

ALL can arise from B- or T-lymphocyte progenitors, with B cell ALL comprising more than two-thirds of cases. The WHO classifies ALL into three categories: B cell with recurrent genetic abnormalities (see Table 22-6), T cell, and B cell NOS.

CLINICAL PRESENTATION

Symptoms may include fatigue, fever, and bleeding. Leukostasis is uncommon, even with high white blood cell counts. Lymphadenopathy and splenomegaly are present in approximately 20% of cases. CNS may be involved at presentation, manifesting as headache or cranial nerve palsies.

DIAGNOSTIC TESTING

Basic workup is similar to that required in AML. Immunophenotyping by flow cytometry is often necessary to distinguish ALL from AML. CSF sampling for CNS involvement should be assessed.

TREATMENT

Several complex regimens such as the Berlin–Frankfurt–Munster; hyperfractionated cyclophosphamide, vincristine, doxorubicin, and dexamethasone (hyper-CVAD); Cancer and Leukemia Group B 8811; and the German Multicenter ALL regimen have been used for the treatment of ALL. Treatment is subdivided into induction, consolidation, and maintenance phases, usually administered over a course of 2–3 years. Due to the high risk of CNS relapse, prophylactic intrathecal therapy is administered during the induction and consolidation phases. Adolescents and young adults (AYA) may benefit from pediatric-inspired treatment regimens similar to those used for the treatment of pediatric ALL, which often contain more CNS prophylaxis and asparaginase.[35]

Additional therapies may include the following:
- Rituximab added to the regimen in those with CD20+ ALL.
- A *BCR-ABL1* TKI (imatinib, dasatinib, etc.) to the regimen for those with *BCR-ABL1*+ ALL.
- Blinatumomab (CD3 × CD19 BiTE) for patients in an MRD positive remission or those with CD19 positive relapsed/refractory disease.
- Inotuzumab ozogamicin (CD22 ADC) for CD22 positive relapsed/refractory disease.
- Tisagenlecleucel (CD19 CAR-T therapy) for patients up to age 25 years with B-cell precursor ALL that is refractory or in second or later relapse.
- Allogeneic stem cell transplantation may be considered in relapsed ALL and for those with high-risk disease. High-risk genetic features include hypodiploidy, t(9;22) *BCR-ABL1*, *KMT2A* (*MLL*) rearrangement, and *BCR-ABL1*-like genotype based on gene expression profiling. Age ≤1 year or ≥10 years old and WBC ≥50 × 10⁹/L are also poor prognostic factors.[35]

Chronic Myeloid Leukemia

EPIDEMIOLOGY AND ETIOLOGY

Chronic myeloid leukemia (CML) accounts for 14% of leukemias diagnosed in the US, with an estimated 8450 new cases in 2020 and a median age at diagnosis of 65 years[1]

PATHOLOGY

The characteristic peripheral blood smear of patients with CML demonstrates basophilia and granulocytosis with neutrophils and immature granulocytes, while the bone marrow aspirate commonly reveals hyperplasia of the granulocytic series (promyelocytes, myelocytes, metamyelocytes, band forms, and mature granulocytes). The hallmark of CML is the fusion of two genes, *BCR* on chromosome 22 and *ABL1* on chromosome 9, resulting in the *BCR-ABL1* fusion gene t(9;22) also known as the Philadelphia chromosome.

CHAPTER 22

CLINICAL PRESENTATION

The natural history of CML is a triphasic process with a chronic phase, an accelerated phase, and a blast phase. Chronic phase is associated with an asymptomatic accumulation of differentiated myeloid cells in the marrow, spleen, and peripheral circulation. CML patients will invariably progress to accelerated and blast phases without treatment. The majority of patients present in chronic phase CML identified incidentally by routine CBC. Symptoms may be related to splenomegaly (left-sided abdominal pain, early satiety) or anemia. Peripheral blood counts show increased white blood cells with all levels of granulocytic differentiation, from myeloblasts to segmented neutrophils. Transformation from chronic to blast phase may be insidious or abrupt.

DIAGNOSTIC TESTING

The presence of the *BCR-ABL1* rearrangement by cytogenetics, FISH, or polymerase chain reaction (PCR) along with the characteristic blood or bone marrow findings confirms the diagnosis of CML.

TREATMENT

- Patients in chronic and accelerated phase are treated with oral TKIs such as imatinib, dasatinib, nilotinib, bosutinib, or ponatinib. The choice of agent typically depends on treatment-related adverse effects and patient preference. Ponatinib is typically reserved for those who have failed two prior TKIs or who develop tyrosine kinase domain resistance mutations, such as T315I.[36] Quantitative PCR (qPCR) for *BCR-ABL1* is performed every 3 months to monitor response to treatment. Complete hematologic remission (CHR) is defined as normalization of peripheral blood counts and absence of splenomegaly, whereas complete cytogenetic response (CCyR) is defined by the absence of Philadelphia chromosome metaphases on bone marrow cytogenetic analysis; major molecular remission is defined by qPCR when *BCR-ABL1* transcripts in the peripheral blood are ≤0.1% on the International Scale (IS). Treatment milestones: CHR and/or *BCR-ABL1* transcripts in the marrow ≤10% (IS) by 3 months, CCyR and/or *BCR-ABL1* transcripts in the marrow ≤1% (IS) by 6 months, and *BCR-ABL1* transcripts in the marrow ≤0.1% (IS) by 12 months after starting a TKI constitute an optimal response to therapy. Failure to achieve treatment milestones may warrant switching TKIs and assessment for acquired mutations within the tyrosine kinase domain which confer resistance to TKIs. For patients who develop TKI resistance, ponatinib, asciminib (STAMP [specifically targeting ABL myristoyl pocket] inhibitor), and omacetaxine may be considered.[36]
- Blast crises are more challenging to manage and the treatment often involves TKIs, chemotherapy, and stem cell transplantation. In addition, stem cell transplantation can be considered in patients who relapse after initial response to TKIs and/or who develop resistance to TKIs.

Chronic Lymphocytic Leukemia

EPIDEMIOLOGY AND ETIOLOGY

Chronic lymphocytic leukemia (CLL) is the most common leukemia in the US, with an estimated 21,040 new cases in 2020 and a median age at diagnosis of 72 years.[1]

PATHOLOGY

CLL is typically positive for the B cell antigens CD19, CD20 (dim), and CD23, as well as aberrant expression of the T cell antigen, CD5. CLL is typically negative for cyclin D1 and CD10.

STAGING

The traditional classification of CLL is based on the Rai and Binet staging systems (Table 22-8). Molecular and cytogenetic markers have become increasingly useful for prognostication, including high-risk markers: del(17p) or *TP53*, del(11q) or unmutated IGHV; and the low-risk markers: del(13q), trisomy 12 or mutated IGHV.[37]

CLINICAL PRESENTATION

Most patients are diagnosed while asymptomatic, often presenting with lymphocytosis on routine laboratory evaluation. When present, symptoms may include fatigue, weight loss, lymphadenopathy, symptoms of anemia or thrombocytopenia, and infections. Patients may also present with an autoimmune hemolytic anemia, immune thrombocytopenia, or Richter transformation of CLL to a more aggressive diffuse large B cell lymphoma.

DIAGNOSTIC TESTING

The diagnosis of CLL requires a peripheral blood absolute lymphocyte count of >5 × 10^9/L and characteristic cell surface markers on peripheral blood flow cytometry. Patients should also have peripheral blood FISH for prognostic markers.

TREATMENT

Many patients do not require treatment at the time of initial diagnosis. The indication for treatment is based on the presence of active disease, defined by the International Workshop on CLL by at least one of the following: progressive marrow failure, massive or symptomatic splenomegaly (>6 cm below costal margin), lymphadenopathy (>10 cm in longest diameter), progressive lymphocytosis (>50% increase in 2 months or doubling time of <6 months), autoimmune hemolytic anemia or thrombocytopenia that is poorly responsive to standard therapy, and/or the

TABLE 22-8	Chronic Lymphocytic Leukemia Clinical Staging
Rai	**Binet**
Stage 0: Lymphocytosis	Stage A: Lymphocytosis
Stage 1: Lymphadenopathy	Stage B: Lymphadenopathy in ≥3 areas
Stage 2: Splenomegaly	Stage C: Hgb <10 g/dL or platelets <100,000/µL
Stage 3: Hgb <11 g/dL	
Stage 4: Platelets <100,000/µL	

Hgb, hemoglobin.

CHAPTER 22

presence of constitutional symptoms.[37] Chemotherapeutic options traditionally include alkylating agents (chlorambucil, cyclophosphamide, bendamustine), purine analogues (fludarabine), and anti-CD20 monoclonal antibodies such as rituximab, ofatumumab, or obinutuzumab. Oral targeted agents have shown significant efficacy in CLL and are particularly effective in patients with high-risk cytogenetics, such as 17p and 11q deletions, leading to a significant shift from chemotherapy-based regimens to molecularly targeted agents in the treatment of CLL, including ibrutinib or acalibrutinib (BTK inhibitors), idelalisib (PI3K inhibitor), and venetoclax.[37]

Hairy Cell Leukemia

EPIDEMIOLOGY AND ETIOLOGY

Hairy cell leukemia is a rare disorder, most commonly seen in elderly men.

PATHOLOGY

Peripheral blood leukocytes have the characteristic "hairy" appearance and are tartrate-resistant acid phosphatase positive. Flow cytometry is positive for CD20, CD11c, CD103, CD123, cyclin D1, and annexin A1. Genetic sequencing commonly reveals *BRAF* V600E mutation.

CLINICAL PRESENTATION

Most patients present with malaise and fatigue. Splenomegaly and hepatomegaly may be evident on examination. Patients with advanced disease may experience pancytopenia leading to symptomatic anemia, easy bruising/bleeding, or recurrent infections.

DIAGNOSTIC TESTING

In addition to routine labs, bone marrow assessment with flow cytometry, cytogenetics, FISH, and molecular testing/sequencing may be obtained.

TREATMENT

The decision to treat is based on the development of cytopenias, symptomatic splenomegaly, constitutional symptoms, and recurrent infections. The treatment options include cladribine and pentostatin. The addition of rituximab may deepen responses and lengthens remission but is also associated with increased immunosuppression.

Hodgkin Lymphoma

EPIDEMIOLOGY AND ETIOLOGY

The incidence of Hodgkin lymphoma (HL) follows a bimodal distribution with a peak at age 25 and second peak at age 50 years, with an estimated 8480 new cases in the US in 2020.[1] EBV and HIV infections, autoimmune conditions, and immunosuppressant use have been described as risk factors for HL.

PATHOLOGY

HL is subdivided into nodular lymphocyte predominant (NLPHL) and classical HL subtypes based on the pathologic appearance. The Reed–Sternberg (RS) cells consistently express CD30 and CD15. In contrast to the other histologic subtypes, RS cells are infrequent in NLPHL. Instead, "popcorn cells" are seen within a background of inflammatory cells in NLPHL.

CLINICAL PRESENTATION

Most patients present with painless lymphadenopathy. Presence of B symptoms including fevers, significant weight loss, and drenching night sweats are more common in advanced stages.

DIAGNOSTIC TESTING

FNA is often inadequate to make a diagnosis and therefore a minimum of a core-needle biopsy is necessary. If initial biopsy is nondiagnostic, excisional biopsy may be required. Additional workup includes routine labs, LDH, erythrocyte sedimentation rate (ESR), CT, FDG PET CT, and bone marrow examination.

STAGING

The traditional Ann Arbor staging system has since been replaced by the Lugano classification (Table 22-9). Patients with early-stage disease (stages I–II) may be further stratified into favorable- and unfavorable-risk categories. Favorable risk is defined by the presence of ≤2 sites of disease, mediastinal width less than one-third of maximal thoracic diameter, ESR <50 mm/h (<30 mm/h with B symptoms), and absence of extranodal extension.[38]

TABLE 22-9	Lugano Staging of Lymphomas[a]
Stage	Description
I	Involvement of a single lymph node region (I) or single extralymphatic organ (IE).
II	Involvement of ≥2 lymph node regions in the same side of the diaphragm.
III	Involvement of lymph node regions in both sides of the diaphragm.
IV	Diffuse or disseminated involvement of one or more extralymphatic organs, including any involvement of the CSF, bone marrow, liver, or multiple lung lesions (unless considered stage IIE).

[a]Modifying features: HL, A: absence of B features; B: presence of B features. NHL no longer uses A and B modifiers. Both HL and NHL, E, involvement of a single extranodal site contiguous or proximal to the involved nodal site; S, spleen involvement; X, bulky disease definition varies by histology (HL: lymph node ≥10 cm or than ≥one-third of thoracic diameter; FL: ≥6 cm; DLBCL: ≥10 cm).

TREATMENT

- The treatment of choice for early stage HL (stages I–II) is chemotherapy with ABVD (doxorubicin, bleomycin, vinblastine, dacarbazine) for 2–4 cycles, with or without involved field radiotherapy (IFRT), depending on favorable versus unfavorable risk and interim PET response (Deauville 5-point scale).
- The treatment of choice for advanced stage HL (stages III-IV, as well as stage II with bulky nodal disease) is chemotherapy with ABVD, BV+AVD (brentuximab vedotin. a CD30-directed ADC, plus doxorubicin, vinblastine, and dacarbazine), or escalated BEACOPP (bleomycin, etoposide, doxorubicin, cyclophosphamide, vincristine, procarbazine, and prednisone). BV+AVD and BEACOPP have been associated with improved PFS, but not OS, compared to ABVD.
- Relapsed disease is treated with salvage chemotherapy with or without stem cell transplantation. The PD-1 inhibitors pembrolizumab or nivolumab are effective treatments for relapsed HL.[38]

Non-Hodgkin Lymphoma

EPIDEMIOLOGY AND ETIOLOGY

Non-Hodgkin lymphoma (NHL) is the fifth most common malignancy in the US, with an estimated 77,240 new cases in 2020.[1] Risk factors include immuno-deficiency, autoimmune disorders, bacterial infections (*H. pylori, Borrelia burg-dorferi,* and *Chlamydia psittaci*), viral infections (HIV, EBV, HHV8, and human T-lymphotropic virus-1), and immunosuppression in the setting of previous solid organ transplantation.

PATHOLOGY

NHL represents a diverse group of hematologic malignancies derived from B cells, T cells, and rarely NK cells which exist at various stages of differentiation. NHL may be broadly divided into indolent (e.g., follicular, marginal zone, small lymphocytic), aggressive (e.g., diffuse large B cell, mantle cell, peripheral T cell, anaplastic large cell lymphoma), and very aggressive (e.g., Burkitt, precursor B and T lymphoblastic leu-kemias/lymphomas, adult T cell leukemia–lymphoma) subtypes.[39] Several recurrent chromosomal abnormalities have been described in patients with NHL (Table 22-10).

CLINICAL PRESENTATION

Clinical manifestations depend on the histologic subtype and can be characteristic in some rare subtypes of NHL. For instance, pruritic plaques can be seen in mycosis fungoides (a primary cutaneous T cell NHL) and isolated splenomegaly may occur in splenic marginal zone lymphomas. Occasionally, patients with aggressive lymphomas can present with a spontaneous tumor lysis syndrome (TLS).

DIAGNOSTIC TESTING

Essential workup often includes history, physical examination, complete blood cell count, chemistry, PET/CT, lymph node biopsy, and in certain cases, bone marrow biopsy. The CSF evaluation is indicated in patients with high-grade lymphomas,

TABLE 22-10	Select Chromosomal Abnormalities in B-Cell Non-Hodgkin Lymphomas	
Cytogenetic Abnormality	Histology	Oncogene
t(14;18)	Follicular, DLBCL	BCL2
t(11;14)	Mantle cell	Cyclin D1
t(1;14)	MALT lymphoma	BCL10
t(11;18)	Marginal zone/extranodal marginal zone	MALT1
t(2;5)	ALK-positive anaplastic large-cell lymphoma	ALK
t(9;14)	Lymphoplasmacytic lymphoma	–
8q24 translocations	Burkitt lymphoma	MYC

DLBCL, diffuse large B-cell lymphoma; MALT, mucosa-associated lymphoid tissue.

CHAPTER 22

HIV-related lymphomas, and involvement of the epidural space, testes, nasopharynx, or paranasal sinuses. Patients suspected to have primary CNS lymphomas require an ophthalmologic examination.

STAGING

Patients are staged by the Lugano classification (Table 22-9). Patients with aggressive lymphoma are usually stratified according to the International Prognostic Index, which uses five adverse prognostic factors: age >60 years, stage III or IV, serum LDH >ULN, ≥2 extranodal sites involved, and ECOG PS ≥2. Each is assigned 1-point and higher scores predict a worse overall prognosis.

TREATMENT

Indolent Lymphomas

• Stage I–II: Observation, IFRT, single-agent rituximab, rituximab with chemotherapy, and combined-modality therapy using rituximab, chemotherapy, and IFRT are all options. Gastric mucosa-associated lymphoid tissue (MALT) lymphomas are related to *H. pylori* infection and respond well to *H. pylori*–directed therapy. Gastric MALT lymphomas that do not respond to or relapse after *H. pylori* therapy, and other isolated extranodal lymphomas (salivary gland, breast, conjunctiva) may be treated with IFRT, rituximab, surgery, chemotherapy, or a combination of these modalities.[39]

• Stage III–IV: There is no convincing evidence to support early intervention compared to "watchful waiting" in asymptomatic patients. A combination of an anti-CD20 antibody (rituximab or obinutuzumab) and chemotherapy or single-agent rituximab can be used for treatment.

• Relapsed disease: First-line therapy can be repeated in patients who were in first remission for >2 years. Lenalidomide, PI3 kinase inhibitors (e.g., idelalisib, duvelisib, copanlisib), CD19 CAR-T therapy, and stem cell transplant are all effective options. Tazemetostat is approved for use in patients with relapsed follicular lymphoma that is *EZH2* mutated.

Aggressive Lymphomas

- Diffuse Large B-Cell Lymphoma:
  - Stage I–II: Limited-stage disease is managed with chemotherapy (rituximab, cyclophosphamide, doxorubicin, vincristine, and prednisone [R-CHOP]) with or without IFRT.
  - Stage III–IV: Patients beginning therapy for aggressive lymphomas should be monitored closely for signs of TLS and should receive adequate IV hydration and appropriate prophylaxis with allopurinol and/or rasburicase. Chemotherapy with R-CHOP is standard. Patients with *MYC* translocations, especially those with "double-hit" lymphomas (combined translocations of *MYC* and either *BCL2* or *BCL6*), have significantly worse outcomes and are often treated with regimen dose-adjusted R-EPOCH.[39] CNS prophylaxis with intrathecal chemotherapy or high-dose methotrexate should be considered for patients with testicular, orbital, epidural, paranasal sinus or extensive bone marrow involvement, or a combination of elevated LDH, serum albumin <3.5 g/L, >60 years of age, retroperitoneal lymph node involvement, and involvement of >1 extranodal site resulting in a high CNS International Prognostic Index (IPI) score. Primary CNS lymphoma is treated with complex regimens that usually incorporate high-dose methotrexate, cytarabine, and rituximab, often with consolidation stem cell transplantation. Whole-brain radiation is an effective therapy but should be avoided if possible, because of the high rate of late neurotoxicity.
- Burkitt lymphoma: Burkitt lymphomas are a highly aggressive form of B-cell lymphoma usually treated with complex multidrug protocols and CNS prophylaxis.
- Aggressive peripheral T-cell lymphomas are generally treated with CHOP or CHOEP-regimens. If CD30 expressing, brentuximab-vedotin may be considered. Relapsed and refractory disease may be treated using a number of agents, such as pralatrexate, romidepsin, belinostat, and alisertib.[39]
- Mantle cell lymphoma (MCL): Chemoimmunotherapy regimens incorporating rituximab, cytarabine, bendamustine, or anthracyclines are often used. Consolidation with autologous stem cell transplantation can be considered in first remission. Maintenance rituximab is considered in select patients. Relapses may be treated with BTK inhibitors or a number of other agents. Brexucabtagene autoleucel is a US FDA-approved CD19 CAR-T therapy for patients with relapsed or refractory mantle cell lymphoma.
- Relapsed/refractory non-Hodgkin lymphoma: Several effective salvage regimens such as ICE (ifosfamide, carboplatin, etoposide), DHAP (dexamethasone, cisplatin, cytarabine), and ESHAP (etoposide, methylprednisone, cytarabine, cisplatin) are available. Rituximab is added to the salvage regimens for B cell lymphomas. Younger, medically fit patients with chemotherapy sensitive disease are candidates for autologous stem cell transplantation at relapse. Allogeneic transplantation can be considered in patients with relapsed Burkitt or lymphoblastic lymphoma, chemotherapy refractory disease at relapse or a duration of remission of <1 year after initial therapy. Additionally, CD19 targeting CAR-T therapies, such as axicabtagene ciloleucel, tisagenlecleucel, brexucabtagene autoleucel, and lisocabtagene maraleucel, are highly effective and are US FDA-approved for use in patients with certain categories of refractory B-cell lymphoma, including DLBCL, primary mediastinal LBCL, DLBCL arising from follicular lymphoma, follicular lymphoma, and MCL.

Multiple Myeloma

EPIDEMIOLOGY AND ETIOLOGY

Multiple myeloma (MM) is the second most frequent hematologic malignancy after NHL with an estimated 32,270 new cases in the US in 2020.[1] The median age at diagnosis is 66 years.

CLINICAL PRESENTATION

The most common presentation is anemia. Patients can also have bone pain, renal failure, fatigue, weight loss, hypercalcemia, and recurrent infections. Patients with extramedullary plasmacytomas can present with radiculopathy, cord compression, or CNS involvement.

DIAGNOSTIC TESTING

Initial evaluation includes routine blood work, β_2-microglobulin (B2M), serum and urine protein electrophoresis, serum free light chain assessment, bone marrow examination, and cross-sectional imaging with either whole body LDCT, PET CT, or whole body MRI. Of note, cross-sectional imaging is preferred over skeletal survey with plain radiographs due to increased sensitivity for bone lesions. The diagnosis of MM is confirmed by the presence of 10% or more clonal plasma cells in the bone marrow or a biopsy-proven plasmacytoma, with evidence of end-organ damage (CRAB Criteria: hypercalcemia, renal dysfunction, anemia, or bone lesions). A clonal marrow plasma cell percentage of ≥60%, κ or λ free light chain ratio of ≥100, and the presence of one or more focal lesions on MRI are also criteria (SLiM Criteria) for diagnosis of MM because they are associated with a high risk of progression to end-organ damage.[40]

STAGING AND RISK STRATIFICATION

The Revised-International Staging System (R-ISS) for MM uses B2M, albumin, LDH, and the presence/absence of high-risk cytogenetic abnormalities to stratify patients (Table 22-11).

TREATMENT

- Transplant-eligible patients are typically offered 4–6 cycles of induction therapy with a four-drug regimen including an anti-CD38 mAb (daratumumab), a proteasome inhibitor (bortezomib), an immunomodulatory agent (lenalidomide), and dexamethasone followed by a melphalan-conditioned autologous stem cell transplantation. In transplant-ineligible patients who are otherwise fit, the induction regimen may be continued for 12–18 months, whereas in frail patients an immunomodulatory agent (e.g., lenalidomide) and dexamethasone alone may be considered.
- Maintenance therapy (lenalidomide or bortezomib) is often considered following initial therapy, with selection of agent typically based on the patient's risk category.
- For relapsed and refractory disease, various combinations of several classes of drugs including chemotherapy (cyclophosphamide, melphalan, melflufen), additional

TABLE 22-11	Revised-International Staging System and Risk Stratification in Myeloma
R-ISS Stage I	B2M <3.5 mg/dL, albumin >3.5 g/dL, normal LDH, and absence of del(17p), t(4;14), or t(14;16) by FISH
R-ISS Stage II	Neither stage I nor stage III R-ISS
R-ISS Stage III	B2M >5.5 mg/dL plus LDH elevation and/or presence of del(17p), t(4;14), or t(14;16) by FISH
Standard Risk Cytogenetics	Trisomies (hyperdiploidy), t(11;14), and t(6;14)
High Risk Cytogenetics	Del(17p) or TP53 deletion, t(4;14), t(14;16), t(14;20), gain 1q

B2M, β_2-microglobulin; LDH, lactic dehydrogenase.

immunomodulatory agents (pomalidomide) and proteosome inhibitors (carfilzomib, ixazomib), monoclonal antibodies targeting CD38 (daratumumab, isatuximab) and SLAMF7 (elotuzumab), histone deacetylase inhibitors (e.g., panobinostat), nuclear export inhibitors (selinexor), BCMA targeted ADCs (belantamab-mafodotin), and a BCMA CAR-T therapy (idecabtagene vicleucel) are now FDA approved.[40]

Principles of Stem Cell Transplantation

BACKGROUND

- Hematopoietic stem cell transplantation involves the infusion of either allogeneic or autologous stem cells, which is typically preceded by conditioning chemotherapy and sometimes total-body irradiation to clear residual disease and immunosuppress the recipient. Depending on the extent of myelosuppression achieved as a result of this conditioning, the regimens are classified as myeloablative, reduced intensity, or nonmyeloablative.
- Autologous transplantation involves collection, cryopreservation, and reinfusion of a patient's own stem cells. This allows administration of myeloablative doses of chemotherapy with the intent of maximizing the efficacy of chemotherapy while rescuing hematopoiesis using stem cell re-infusion after chemotherapy.
- Allogeneic transplantation refers to the infusion of stem cells collected from either HLA-matched or mismatched donors. In addition to facilitating the administration of high doses of chemotherapy, allogeneic transplantation also allows for an immunologic effect mediated by donor T and natural killer cells on the tumor (graft-versus-tumor effect).

INDICATIONS

- Stem cell transplantation can be considered for patients with high-risk or relapsed malignancy that is thought to be chemosensitive or susceptible to graft-versus-tumor effect. MM and lymphoma are the most common indications for autologous transplantation, whereas MDS and acute leukemia are the most common indications for allogeneic transplantation.
- Stem cell transplantations may also be also considered in certain nonmalignant disorders.

DONOR SELECTION

Appropriate donor selection is crucial and is based on the following factors:
- HLA typing: Major histocompatibility class I and II alleles code for HLA proteins that are expressed on the cell surface and play a major role in immune recognition. High-resolution typing of 10 HLA alleles (e.g., HLA-A, HLA-B, HLA-C, HLA-DRB1, and HLA-DQB1) is the current standard.
- The chance of any given sibling being a full HLA match is only 25%. Patients who lack HLA-identical siblings should have a search for HLA-matched unrelated donors through the National Marrow Donation Program (NMDP), although chances of finding an HLA-matched unrelated donor is significantly influenced by the patient's ethnicity due to disparities in NMDP participation.
- Partial HLA-mismatched transplantations, umbilical cord blood, and haploidentical transplantations (3/6 match) are alternate sources of stem cells for patients without matched sibling or matched unrelated donors.
- Cytomegalovirus (CMV)-negative donors are preferred for CMV-negative patients.
- Younger donors are preferred over older donors.

SOURCE OF STEM CELLS

- Bone marrow can be obtained under general anesthesia via repeated bone marrow aspiration.
- Peripheral blood stem cells can be collected by leukapheresis after mobilization with use of granulocyte colony-stimulating factor (G-CSF) and plerixafor (CXCR4 antagonist), or chemotherapy (e.g., cyclophosphamide). Peripheral blood stem cells are the most common source stem cells for clinical use currently.
- Umbilical cord blood stem cells can be collected by umbilical cord venipuncture after delivery.

COMPLICATIONS

- Graft-versus-host disease (GVHD): GVHD occurs when the donor T cells react with recipient tissues, leading to acute and/or chronic inflammation in recipient tissues. The most common tissues affected are the skin, liver, and GI tract. Acute and chronic GVHD are associated with significant morbidity and mortality in allogeneic transplantation patients. Chronic GVHD can result in sclerodermatous-type skin changes. The prophylaxis and treatment of GVHD includes the use of posttransplant cyclophosphamide, glucocorticoids, tacrolimus, cyclosporine, ruxolitinib, methotrexate, sirolimus, and mycophenolate.
- Infections: Owing to the conditioning chemotherapy and prolonged immunosuppression, transplant patients are susceptible to a variety of infections in the peritransplant setting. The postengraftment period is complicated by susceptibility to a broad range of bacterial, viral, and fungal infections, such as gram-negative bacilli, CMV, BK virus, *Pneumocystis jirovecii* pneumonia, *Aspergillus*, and other opportunistic infections. Given the significantly increased risk of opportunistic infections, prophylactic antimicrobial regimens (acyclovir, trimethoprim/sulfamethoxazole, fluconazole, ciprofloxacin, etc.) are frequently used. The choice of agent and duration of use vary, depending on the type of transplant, the immunosuppression regimen used, and the type of anticancer treatments used.

CHAPTER 22

ONCOLOGIC EMERGENCIES AND SUPPORTIVE CARE

Oncologic Emergencies

The most common oncology emergencies are febrile neutropenia (FN), TLS, malignant hypercalcemia, spinal cord compression, SVC syndrome, hyperleukocytosis, and brain metastases with increased intracranial pressure (Table 22-12).

TABLE 22-12	Oncologic Emergencies		
Emergency	Etiology	Presentation	Management
Neutropenic fever	Infectious	ANC <500/ μL and Temp >38.3°C or >38°C twice (1 h apart), may present with sepsis and/ or hypotensive shock	• Infectious workup with complete physical exam, BCx (bacterial and fungal), UCx, CXR, RVP, and stool studies (if diarrhea) • Antibiotics: gram-negative anti-pseudomonal coverage; add gram-positive anti-MRSA coverage if: catheters, pneumonia, mucositis, *Staphylococcus* colonization, sepsis; add fungal coverage if clinically warranted • IV hydration, G-CSF and supportive care, as indicated
Tumor lysis syndrome (TLS)	Massive lysis of cancer cells High risk: leukemia, lymphoma, or bulky tumors	High LDH, uric acid, K and PO_4, low Ca, AKI, cardiac arrhythmia, and/or seizures	• Prevention: IV fluids and prophylactic allopurinol or rasburicase based on estimated risk of TLS • Treatment: IV fluids, allopurinol, rasburicase, dialysis if indicated
Malignant hyper-calcemia	PTH, PTHrP, calcitriol-mediated, osteolytic metastasis	Polyuria/ polydipsia, dehydration, confusion, constipation, weakness, cardiac arrhythmias	• IV fluids • Bisphosphonates or denosumab (if low creatinine clearance) • Calcitonin (if severe, symptomatic) • Steroids can be useful in some cases

TABLE 22-12	Oncologic Emergencies (continued)		
Emergency	Etiology	Presentation	Management
Spinal cord compression	Compression of spinal cord due to malignant involvement	Back pain (most common), weakness, sensory loss, incontinence, ataxia	• Total spine MRI • Glucocorticoids • Neurosurgery and Radiation Oncology consultation • Chemotherapy for chemosensitive tumors
Superior vena cava (SVC) syndrome	Obstruction of SVC by primary or metastatic cancer	Dyspnea, stridor (laryngeal edema), facial and upper extremity swelling, risk of respiratory failure, cerebral edema, and herniation	• CT head, neck, and chest • Airway support, as indicated • Endovascular stent if comatose • Intubation if airway compromise • Treatment depends on tumor type: SCLC, lymphoma, germ cell: chemotherapy; NSCLC: RT; thymic tumors: surgery, etc.
Hyperleukocytosis with leukostasis	Intravascular accumulation of blasts, with or without TLS/DIC	Chest pain, respiratory distress, altered mental status, bleeding and/or clotting (if DIC is present)	• Leukapheresis: symptomatic patients (count threshold AML >50 × 10³/µL, ALL and CML >150 × 10³/µL, CLL >500 × 10³/µL); asymptomatic patients (AML >100 × 10³/µL, ALL >200 × 10³/µL) • Hydroxyurea, glucocorticoids, empiric antibiotics, TLS/DIC management if present
Intracranial mass	Increased intracranial pressure, cerebral edema	Headache, altered mental status, focal neurologic deficits, potentially asymptomatic	• CT head and/or MRI brain • Glucocorticoids • Neurosurgery and Radiation Oncology consultation • Consider antiepileptics, if indicated

AKI, acute kidney injury; ALL, acute lymphoblastic leukemia; AML, acute myeloid leukemia; CLL, chronic lymphocytic leukemia; CML, chronic myeloid leukemia; CNS, central nervous system; DIC, disseminated intravascular coagulation; G-CSF, granulocyte colony-stimulating factor; LDH, lactic dehydrogenase; MRSA, methicillin-resistant *Staphylococcus aureus*; NSCLC, non–small-cell lung cancer; PTHrP, parathyroid hormone-related protein; RT, radiotherapy; RVP, respiratory viral panel; SCLC, small-cell lung cancer.

Supportive Care

NAUSEA AND VOMITING

- If nausea/vomiting occurs, chemotherapy-induced nausea and vomiting (CINV), as well as alternative etiologies such as bowel obstruction, brain metastasis, constipation and gastroenteritis, should be considered.
- CINV can be categorized as acute (<24 hours) or delayed (>24 hours). Acute CINV is an important predictor of delayed CINV.
- Commonly used antiemetic medications for prevention and management of CINV include dexamethasone, 5-hydroxytryptamine-3 (5-HT$_3$) receptor antagonists (ondansetron, granisetron, dolasetron, palonosetron), neurokinin-1 receptor antagonists (aprepitant, fosaprepitant, etc.), prochlorperazine, anxiolytics (lorazepam), and olanzapine (atypical antipsychotic).

DIARRHEA

- Diarrhea can be a common complication of chemotherapy (irinotecan, 5FU, capecitabine), targeted therapy (erlotinib, cetuximab, sunitinib, lapatinib), immunotherapy (ipilimumab, nivolumab, pembrolizumab), and stem cell transplantation (GI GVHD, CMV colitis) or may be a manifestation of cancer itself (carcinoid syndrome in neuroendocrine tumors).
- Treatment should be tailored to the underlying etiology. Supportive care with IV fluids and antidiarrheal medications (loperamide, diphenoxylate, atropine), antibiotics for infectious etiologies (oral vancomycin or IV metronidazole for *Clostridioides difficile*), and glucocorticoids for immune-related etiologies (ICIs or GI GVHD) may all be considered in the appropriate clinical context. Interruption of treatment with the causative agent (until resolution of symptoms) and/or dose reduction may be considered, as indicated.

IMMUNE-CHECKPOINT INHIBITOR–RELATED ADVERSE EVENTS

- ICI-related adverse events (AEs) are due to activation of a patient's immune system toward self-antigens leading to autoimmune mediated toxicities, which can sometimes be permanent and life-threatening. ICI-related AEs may include but are not limited to: rash, gastroenteritis/colitis, hepatitis, endocrinopathies, arthritis, pneumonitis, myocarditis, and cytopenias.
- The treatment of choice for ICI-mediated AEs is largely driven by the severity of the AE (grade) and usually involves prompt discontinuation of the ICI and initiation of glucocorticoids, such as prednisone (doses ranging from 0.5 to 1 mg/kg daily). Depending on the type of ICI-related AE, prolonged treatment with steroids followed by a long and gradual taper may be necessary. "Flare" of the ICI-related AE may be observed with weaning of steroids, even in the absence of re-exposure to the immunotherapy.
- Additional supportive care for ICI-related AEs may include supplementation of hormones such as insulin for new-onset type-1 diabetes, thyroid replacement (levothyroxine) for hypothyroidism, and supportive care with hydration and antidiarrheal medications for colitis, and transfusions and growth factors as necessary for cytopenias.

CYTOKINE RELEASE SYNDROME AND IMMUNE EFFECTOR CELL-ASSOCIATED NEUROTOXICITY SYNDROME

- Cellular and cell-engaging therapies, such as CAR-Ts, are associated with unique toxicities including cytokine release syndrome (CRS) and immune effector cell–associated neurotoxicity syndrome (ICANS). CRS is characterized by the systemic release of supraphysiologic proinflammatory cytokines (e.g., IL-2, IL-6, IFN-gamma, TNF-alpha) by immune effector cells characterized by systemic inflammation, fevers, hypotension, and hypoxemia. ICANS is an incompletely understood syndrome characterized clinically by the presence of tremor, dysgraphia, expressive speech impairment (particularly naming objects), decreased level of consciousness, and when severe, coma, cerebral edema, and seizures.
- Grading and treatment: The American Society of Transplantation and Cellular Therapy (ASTCT) has published guidelines for the grading and management of CRS and ICANS.[41]
- CRS is graded on a scale of 0–4, with Grade 0 representing no CRS up to Grade 4 representing severe CRS characterized by fevers, hypotension requiring multiple vasopressors, and/or respiratory failure requiring mechanical ventilation. In general, CRS is managed with supportive care including empiric antibiotics, IV fluids, antipyretics, blood pressure support, and O_2 support adjusted to the associated CRS Grade. In addition, tocilizumab (an IL-6 receptor monoclonal antibody), siltuximab (an IL-6 monoclonal antibody), and glucocorticoids are frequently used in the management of Grade 2–4 CRS.
- The ICANS Grade is determined by combining the Immune Effector Cell-Associated Encephalopathy (ICE) Score with the presence of additional clinical findings. The ICE score ranges from 10 representing a normal score to 0 representing a severely impaired score. The clinical findings impacting ICANS include level of consciousness, seizures, cerebral edema, and other neurologic deficits. ICANS is graded on a scale of 0–4, with Grade 0 representing no ICANS up to Grade 4 representing severe ICANS characterized by complete obtundation, ICE score of 0, cerebral edema, and the potential for focal neurologic deficits and/or seizures. In general, ICANS is managed with supportive care, seizure prophylaxis (levetiracetam), close neurologic monitoring, glucocorticoids, and intensive management of seizures and/or cerebral edema if they occur.

CANCER PAIN

- Cancer patients frequently experience pain due to multiple etiologies, including somatic pain (bone metastases, musculoskeletal inflammation, surgery/procedures), visceral pain (tumor infiltration/compression/distention of viscera), and neuropathic pain (tumor infiltration of nervous tissue, nerve injury due to chemotherapy, radiotherapy, or surgery).
- Cancer pain is usually managed through a rational, stepwise approach to target the underlying cause of pain as well as the symptoms of pain. Common pain medications include non-opioid analgesics (NSAIDs, acetaminophen, and/or topical agents), opioids (tramadol, hydrocodone, oxycodone, morphine, hydromorphone, methadone, transdermal fentanyl, etc.), systemic glucocorticoids in certain circumstances, (bone metastases, spinal cord or nerve compression), antidepressants (nortriptyline, etc.), gabapentin, or pregablin. In addition, bisphosphonates and radiolabeled agents (strontium-89 and samarium-153) may help in treating bone

metastases–related pain. Patients who experience inadequate pain control despite aggressive medical therapy may benefit from interventional therapies, such as regional infusion of analgesics and neuroablative or neurostimulatory procedures.
• Common side effects of opioid therapy include constipation, nausea, respiratory depression, and sedation. Constipation prophylaxis with stimulant laxatives (senna) and stool softeners (docusate) is frequently used. Constipation, if it occurs, can be managed with lactulose, magnesium citrate, polyethylene glycol, enemas, and/or mu opioid receptor antagonists.

FATIGUE

Fatigue occurs in an estimated 80% of patients with advanced cancer, often with multiple contributing factors such as pain, poor nutrition, emotional distress, sleep disturbance, and medical comorbidities (anemia, infection, organ dysfunction). Appropriate pain management, nutrition support, sleep therapy, exercise, and necessary supportive care can help address some of these issues. Transfusion support and erythrocyte stimulating agents may be helpful in select patients with anemia. Psychostimulants such as methylphenidate or modafinil can prove helpful in some patients with severe symptoms. Antidepressants may be useful if concurrent depression is present.

ANOREXIA AND CACHEXIA

Decreased appetite and weight loss are common. In addition to caloric supplementation orally, enterally (nasogastric or gastric tube), or parenterally (total parenteral nutrition), patients may benefit from pharmacologic therapy to increase appetite, including megestrol acetate, glucocorticoids, or dronabinol.

REFERENCES

1. Siegel RL, Miller KD, Jemal A. Cancer statistics, 2020. *CA Cancer J Clin.* 2020;70(1):7-30.
2. Wu Y-L, Tsuboi M, He J, et al. Osimertinib in resected EGFR-mutated non–small-cell lung cancer. *N Engl J Med.* 2020;383(18):1711-1723.
3. Herbst RS, Morgensztern D, Boshoff C. The biology and management of non-small cell lung cancer. *Nature.* 2018;553:446-454.
4. Hanna NH, Robinson AG, Temin S, et al. Therapy for stage IV non-small cell lung cancer with driver alterations: ASCO and OH (CCC) joint guideline update. *J Clin Oncol.* 2021;39(9):1040-1091.
5. Waks AG, Winer EP. Breast cancer treatment: a review. *J Am Med Assoc.* 2019;321(3):288.
6. Sparano JA, Gray RJ, Makower DF, et al. Adjuvant chemotherapy guided by a 21-gene expression assay in breast cancer. *N Engl J Med.* 2018;379:111-121.
7. Schmid P, Adams S, Rugo HS, et al. Atezolizumab and nab-paclitaxel in advanced triple-negative breast cancer. *N Engl J Med.* 2018;379(22):2108-2121.
8. Chow LQM. Head and neck cancer. *N Engl J Med.* 2020;382(1):60-72.
9. Johnson DE, Burtness B, Leemans CR, et al. Head and neck squamous cell carcinoma. *Nat Rev Dis Primers.* 2020;6(1):92.
10. Kelly RJ, Ajani JA, Kuzdzal J, et al. Adjuvant nivolumab in resected esophageal or gastroesophageal junction cancer. *N Engl J Med.* 2021;384(13):1191-1203.
11. Shah MA, Kennedy EB, Catenacci DV, et al. Treatment of locally advanced esophageal carcinoma: ASCO guideline. *J Clin Oncol.* 2020;38(23):2677-2694.
12. Smyth EC, Nilsson M, Grabsch HI, et al. Gastric cancer. *Lancet.* 2020;396(10251):635-648.
13. US Preventive Services Task Force, Davidson KW, Barry MJ, et al. Screening for colorectal cancer: US Preventive Services Task Force recommendation statement. *J Am Med Assoc.* 2021;325(19):1965-1977.
14. Shaukat A, Kahi CJ, Burke CA, et al. ACG clinical guidelines: colorectal cancer screening 2021. *Am J Gastroenterol.* 2021;116(3):458-479.
15. Dekker E, Tanis PJ, Vleugels JLA, et al. Colorectal cancer. *Lancet.* 2019;394(10207):1467-1480.
16. Biller LH, Schrag D. Diagnosis and treatment of metastatic colorectal cancer: a review. *J Am Med Assoc.* 2021;325(7):669-685.

17. Mizrahi JD, Surana R, Valle JW, et al. Pancreatic cancer. *Lancet*. 2020;395(10242):2008-2020.
18. Villanueva A. Hepatocellular carcinoma. *N Engl J Med*. 2019;380(15):1450-1462.
19. Llovet JM, Kelley RK, Villanueva A, et al. Hepatocellular carcinoma. *Nat Rev Dis Primers*. 2021;7(1):6.
20. Roberto M, Botticelli A, Panebianco M, et al. Metastatic renal cell carcinoma management: from molecular mechanism to clinical practice. *Front Oncol*. 2021;11:657639.
21. Lenis AT, Lec PM, Chamie K. Bladder cancer: a review. *J Am Med Assoc*. 2020;324(19):1980.
22. US Preventive Services Task Force, Grossman DC, Curry SJ, et al. Screening for prostate cancer: US Preventive Services Task Force recommendation statement. *J Am Med Assoc*. 2018;319(18):1901.
23. Rebello RJ, Oing C, Knudsen KE, et al. Prostate cancer. *Nat Rev Dis Primers*. 2021;7(1):9.
24. Hanna NH, Einhorn LH. Testicular cancer—discoveries and updates. *N Engl J Med*. 2014;371(21):2005-2016.
25. US Preventive Services Task Force, Curry SJ, Krist AH, et al. Screening for cervical cancer: US preventive Services Task Force recommendation statement. *J Am Med Assoc*. 2018;320(7):674.
26. Cohen PA, Jhingran A, Oaknin A, et al. Cervical cancer. *Lancet*. 2019;393(10167):169-182.
27. Lu KH, Broaddus RR. Endometrial cancer. *N Engl J Med*. 2020;383(21):2053-2064.
28. Matulonis UA, Sood AK, Fallowfield L, et al. Ovarian cancer. *Nat Rev Dis Primers*. 2016;2(1):16061.
29. Curti BD, Faries MB. Recent advances in the treatment of melanoma. *N Engl J Med*. 2021;384(23):2229-2240.
30. Wen PY, Weller M, Lee EQ, et al. Glioblastoma in adults: a Society for Neuro-Oncology (SNO) and European Society of Neuro-Oncology (EANO) consensus review on current management and future directions. *Neuro Oncol*. 2020;22(8):1073-1113.
31. Gamboa AC, Gronchi A, Cardona K. Soft-tissue sarcoma in adults: an update on the current state of histiotype-specific management in an era of personalized medicine. *CA Cancer J Clin*. 2020;70(3):200-229.
32. Cazzola M. Myelodysplastic syndromes. *N Engl J Med*. 2020;383(14):1358-1374.
33. Döhner H, Estey E, Grimwade D, et al. Diagnosis and management of AML in adults: 2017 ELN recommendations from an international expert panel. *Blood*. 2017;129:424-447.
34. Kantarjian H, Kadia T, DiNardo C, et al. Acute myeloid leukemia: current progress and future directions. *Blood Cancer J*. 2021;11(2):41.
35. Malard F, Mohty M. Acute lymphoblastic leukaemia. *Lancet*. 2020;395(10230):1146-1162.
36. Hochhaus A, Baccarani M, Silver RT, et al. European LeukemiaNet 2020 recommendations for treating chronic myeloid leukemia. *Leukemia*. 2020;34(4):966-984.
37. Burger JA. Treatment of chronic lymphocytic leukemia. *N Engl J Med*. 2020;383(5):460-473.
38. Connors JM, Cozen W, Steidl C, et al. Hodgkin lymphoma. *Nat Rev Dis Primers*. 2020;6(1):61.
39. Armitage JO, Gascoyne RD, Lunning MA, et al. Non-Hodgkin lymphoma. *Lancet*. 2017;390(10091):298-310.
40. Rajkumar SV. Multiple myeloma: 2020 update on diagnosis, risk-stratification and management. *Am J Hematol*. 2020;95(5):548-567.
41. Lee DW, Santomasso BD, Locke FL, et al. ASTCT consensus grading for cytokine release syndrome and neurologic toxicity associated with immune effector cells. *Biol Blood Marrow Transplant*. 2019;25(4):625-638

CHAPTER 22

23 Diabetes Mellitus and Related Disorders

Cynthia J. Herrick and Janet B. McGill

DIABETES MELLITUS

GENERAL PRINCIPLES

- **Diabetes mellitus** is a group of metabolic diseases characterized by hyperglycemia resulting from defects in insulin secretion, insulin action, or both. In 2018, diabetes was present in 13.0% of persons age ≥18 years in the United States and 26.8% of those age 65 and older. A substantial percentage of affected persons are not diagnosed. Type 2 diabetes mellitus (T2DM) represents 90%–95% of all cases of diabetes, with type 1 diabetes mellitus (T1DM) and other causes representing the remaining 5%–10%.[1,2]
- Patients with diabetes are at risk for microvascular complications, including retinopathy, nephropathy, and neuropathy, and are at increased risk for macrovascular disease.
- T2DM is accompanied by hypertension (approximately 75%) and hyperlipidemia (>50%) in adult patients and is considered a "cardiac risk equivalent" because of the excess risk for macrovascular disease, cardiovascular disease (CVD) events, and mortality.[3]

Classification

Diabetes mellitus is classified into four clinical classes

- **T1DM** accounts for <10% of all cases of diabetes and results from a cellular-mediated autoimmune destruction of the beta (β) cells of the pancreas.
- **T2DM** accounts for >90% of all cases of diabetes. T2DM is characterized by insulin resistance followed by reduced insulin secretion from β cells that are unable to compensate for the increased insulin requirements.
- **Other specific types of diabetes** include those that result from genetic defects in insulin secretion or action (known as monogenic diabetes), pancreatic surgery or disease of the exocrine pancreas (cystic fibrosis), endocrinopathies (e.g., Cushing syndrome, acromegaly), or drugs (corticosteroids, antiretroviral, atypical antipsychotics), and diabetes associated with other syndromes. Pancreatic diabetes is now commonly referred to as type 3c diabetes.
- **Gestational diabetes** (GDM) is glucose intolerance with onset or diagnosis during pregnancy. The prevalence of GDM depends on the criteria used for diagnosis and varies by age and ethnic group (generally from 5% to 6% of pregnancies to 15%–20% of pregnancies). Diagnostic criteria for GDM vary based on practice location with a two-step method (50-g, 1-hour screen followed by 100-g, 3-hour oral glucose tolerance test [OGTT]) used in the United States and a one-step method (75-g, 2-hour OGTT) more common internationally.[4] About 50% of women with GDM will develop T2DM in the ensuing 5–10 years, and all remain at an increased risk for the development of T2DM later in life.

○ All patients with GDM should undergo diagnostic testing 4–12 weeks postpartum with a 2-hour OGTT or fasting plasma glucose and every 1–3 years thereafter with either test or an A1C to determine whether abnormal carbohydrate metabolism has persisted or is recurrent.

○ Weight loss, exercise, and breastfeeding are encouraged to decrease the risk of persistent prediabetes or T2DM after delivery.

DIAGNOSIS

• Progression from impaired fasting glucose or impaired glucose tolerance to T2DM occurs at the rate of 2%–22% (average, about 12%) per year depending on the population studied.

• Lifestyle modification, including a balanced hypocaloric diet to achieve 7% weight loss in overweight patients and regular exercise of ≥150 min/wk, is recommended for persons with prediabetes to prevent progression to T2DM.[5]

• Metformin may be considered in patients with prior GDM, those with body mass index (BMI) ≥35, age <60 years, or those with progressive hyperglycemia.

• Diagnostic criteria for prediabetes and diabetes are listed in Table 23-1.

TREATMENT

• **Goals of therapy** are alleviation of symptoms, achievement of glycemic control, blood pressure and lipid targets, and prevention of acute and chronic complications of diabetes.

CHAPTER 23

TABLE 23-1	Diagnosis of Diabetes		
	Prediabetes	Diabetes[a]	Gestational Diabetes[b]
FPG	100–125 mg/dL (5.6–6.9 mmol/L) (IFG)	≥126 mg/dL (7.0 mmol/L)	≥92 mg/dL (5.1 mmol/L)
2-h 75-g oGTT	140–199 mg/dL (7.8–11.0 mmol/L) (IGT)	≥200 mg/dL (11.1 mmol/L)	≥153 mg/dL (8.5 mmol/L)
HbA1C	5.7%–6.4% (39–46 mmol/mol)	≥6.5% (48 mmol/mol)	N/A

FPG, fasting plasma glucose; IFG, impaired fasting glucose; IGT, impaired glucose tolerance; HbA1C, hemoglobin A1C; oGTT, oral glucose tolerance test.

[a]Requires two tests to confirm diagnosis unless random glucose ≥200 mg/dL (11.1 mmol/mol) with polyuria, polydipsia.

[b]These are IADPSG guidelines used internationally. A single abnormal value is considered diagnostic of gestational diabetes on these guidelines. 1-h post 75-g glucose load ≥180 mg/dL (10 mmol/L) can be used for diagnosis of GDM on these guidelines as well. In the United States, a two-step method is still most common: nonfasting 1-h post 50-g glucose challenge ≥140 mg/dL (7.8 mmol/L) (some centers use 130 mg/dL [7.2 mmol/L] or 135 mg/dL [7.5 mmol/L]) necessitates a 3-h 100-g oGTT and Carpenter and Coustan Criteria are used for diagnosis (exceeding 2+ of the following thresholds: fasting ≥95 mg/dL [5.3 mmol/L], 1-hour ≥180 mg/dL [10 mmol/L], 2-hour ≥155 mg/dL [8.6 mmol/L], 3-hour ≥ 140 mg/dL [7.8 mmol/L]).

- Glycemic control recommendations are the same for T1DM and T2DM outside of pregnancy: Fasting and preprandial capillary blood glucose (BG) 80–130 mg/dL (4.4–7.2 mmol/L) and postprandial capillary BG <180 mg/dL (<10 mmol/L). The American Diabetes Association and American Association of Clinical Endocrinologists now recommend a customized A1C goal based upon an individual's age and comorbidities. Goals for younger individuals without comorbidities can be <6.5% (48 mmol/mol) while individuals who are over 65 and have cardiovascular comorbidities or with limited life expectancy may reasonably aim for A1C < 8% (64 mmol/mol).[6,7] A1C <6.5%–7% (<48–53 mmol/mol) has been associated with the lowest risk for microvascular complications in patients with T1DM and T2DM.[8,9] However, the customized goals recognize that it is also important to avoid frequent hypoglycemia.
- To minimize the risk of fetal macrosomia and neonatal hypoglycemia, glycemic goals in pregnancy are fasting BG 70–95 mg/dL (3.9–5.3 mmol/L), 1 hour postprandial ≤ 140 mg/dL (7.8 mmol/L), 2-hour postprandial ≤120 mg/dL (6.7 mmol/L).
- Consensus on continuous glucose monitoring goals for type 1 and 2 diabetes include >70% time in range (70–180 mg/dL; 3.9–10.0 mmol/L) with <4% below 70 mg/dL (3.9 mmol/L), <1% below 54 mg/dL (3.0 mmol/L), <25% above 180 mg/dL (10 mmol/L), and <5% above 250 mg/dL (13.9 mmol/L). In pregnancy, goal time in range for type 1 diabetes is >70% (63–140 mg/dL; 3.5–7.8 mmol/L).[10]
- Intensive diabetes therapy leading to very tight glycemic control in patients with risk factors for CVD has been associated with increased mortality in two studies,[11,12] but not in others.[13] Hypoglycemia was implicated as the cause of higher mortality in one of the studies.
- The blood pressure target for patients with diabetes is <140/90 mm Hg, but a lower goal of <130/80 mm Hg may be considered for younger patients or those at high risk of CVD (ASCVD 10 years risk ≥ 15%). The use of either an angiotensin-converting enzyme (ACE) inhibitor or an angiotensin receptor blocker (ARB) is recommended as first-line therapy. Thiazide diuretics and calcium channel blockers are reasonable second-line agents. Two agents should be started in individuals with blood pressure ≥ 160/100 or not at goal on one agent.
- High-intensity statin therapy (atorvastatin 40–80 mg daily or rosuvastatin 20–40 mg daily) is recommended in patients with diabetes age 40–75 with CVD risk factors. Moderate-intensity statin therapy can be considered in patients age 40–75 with no other CVD risk factors and in patients with age <40 or >75 with CVD risk factors.
- The low-density lipoprotein (LDL) goal for patients with diabetes and CVD is <70 mg/dL (3.9 mmol/L). If that goal is not achieved with statin therapy, the addition of either ezetimibe or a PCSK9 inhibitor is advised.
- Aspirin therapy should be recommended in patients with diabetes and cardiovascular disease. Low doses (75–162 mg) are appropriate. Aspirin may be considered for primary prevention in individuals with diabetes after considering potential benefit and risk of bleeding. Clopidogrel (75 mg/d) may be used for secondary prevention in individuals with aspirin allergy.
- Individuals with diabetes are at high risk for nonalcoholic fatty liver disease. Weight loss is recommended as first-line therapy for treating this comorbidity (see Chapter 19, Liver Diseases).
- **Assessment of glycemic control** consists of the following:
  - **Self-monitoring of blood glucose (SMBG)** is recommended for all patients who take insulin and provides useful information for those on noninsulin therapies. Patients using multiple daily injections or insulin pumps should test their blood

glucose three or more times daily. Less frequent testing may be appropriate for those on noninsulin therapies. Although most SMBG is done before meals and at bedtime, periodic testing 1–2 hours after eating may be necessary to achieve postprandial glucose targets.

○ **Continuous glucose monitoring (CGM)** has been shown to reduce A1C in adults older than 25 years and reduce hypoglycemia in patients of all ages on intensive insulin therapy. CGM measures interstitial glucose, which provides a close approximation of BG values. Hypoglycemia and hyperglycemia alarms may help patients with widely fluctuating BG levels or hypoglycemia unawareness. Some of the CGM devices are approved for insulin dosing and may supplant the need for SMBG.[14]

○ **A1C** provides an integrated measure of BG values over the preceding 2–3 months. A1C should be obtained every 3 months in patients not at goal, when either diabetes therapy or clinical condition changes, or twice yearly in well-controlled patients. A1C should confirm results of SMBG or CGM, and discordant values should be investigated. An A1C level that is higher than expected should be evaluated by a diabetes educator to ensure meter accuracy, appropriate technique, and frequency of testing. When the A1C is lower than expected, blood loss, transfusion, hemolysis, and hemoglobin variants should be considered. The correlation between A1C and mean plasma glucose is sufficiently strong that laboratory reports may include both the A1C result and the estimated average glucose.

○ **Ketones** can be detected in a fingerstick blood sample by measuring β-hydroxybutyrate with a handheld meter. Urine ketones can be qualitatively identified, using Ketostix or Acetest tablets. Patients with T1DM should test for ketones during febrile illness, for persistent elevation of glucose (>300 mg/dL [16.7 mmol/L]), or if signs of impending diabetic ketoacidosis (e.g., nausea, vomiting, abdominal pain) develop.

MANAGEMENT

Comprehensive diabetes management includes coordinated diet, exercise, and medication plans. **Patient education** in medical nutrition therapy, exercise, SMBG, medication use, and insulin dosing and administration is integral to the successful management of diabetes.

Medical Nutrition Therapy

• Medical nutrition therapy includes dietary recommendations for a healthy, balanced diet to achieve adequate nutrition and maintain an ideal body weight.[15]

• Caloric restriction is recommended for overweight individuals, with individualized targets that may be as low as 1000–1500 kcal/d for women and 1200–1800 kcal/d for men depending on activity level and starting body weight, and goal weight loss of at least 5%.

• No ideal distribution of calories from fat, protein, and carbohydrate has been defined. Multiple eating patterns such as Mediterranean, plant-based, DASH diet, or low-carbohydrate diet may be used to meet dietary goals for individuals with diabetes.

• A focus on avoiding sugar-sweetened beverages and optimizing nonstarchy vegetable and whole grain intake is appropriate.

• "Carbohydrate counting" is a useful skill for patients on intensified insulin therapy who adjust insulin doses based on the carbohydrate content of meals and snacks.

Exercise

Exercise improves insulin sensitivity, reduces fasting and postprandial BG levels, and offers numerous metabolic, CV, and psychological benefits in patients with diabetes.

- In general, 150 min/wk of moderate to vigorous aerobic activity is recommended as part of a healthy lifestyle and has been shown to assist with the prevention and management of T2DM in adults. Resistance exercise 2–3 times/wk is also important.
- Patients may need individualized guidance regarding exercise, and they are more likely to exercise when counseled by their physician to do so.
- Prolonged sitting over 30 minutes at a time should be avoided.

Diabetes Mellitus in Hospitalized Patients

GENERAL PRINCIPLES

Diabetes-specific Indications for Hospitalization

- **Diabetic ketoacidosis (DKA)** is characterized by a plasma glucose level of >250 mg/dL (13.9 mmol/L) in association with an arterial pH <7.30 or serum bicarbonate level of <15 mEq/L and moderate ketonemia or ketonuria; however, patients may present with ketoacidosis and lower glucose levels.
- **Hyperosmolar hyperglycemic state (HHS)** includes marked hyperglycemia (≥600 mg/dL [33.3 mmol/L]) and elevated serum osmolality (>320 mOsm/kg), often accompanied by impaired mental status.[16]
- **Hypoglycemia** is an indication for hospitalization if it is induced by a sulfonylurea (SFU) medication, is due to a deliberate drug overdose, or results in coma, seizure, injury, or persistent neurologic change.
- **Newly diagnosed T1DM** or newly recognized GDM can be indications for hospitalization, even in the absence of ketoacidosis.
- **Patients with T2DM** are rarely admitted to the hospital for initiation or change in insulin therapy unless hyperglycemia is severe and associated with mental status change or other organ dysfunction.

MANAGEMENT

Management of Diabetes in Hospitalized Patients

Hyperglycemia (BG ≥140 mg/dL [7.8 mmol/L]) is a common finding in hospitalized patients and may be due to previously diagnosed diabetes, undiagnosed diabetes, medications, or stress-induced hyperglycemia. Up to 40% of general medical and surgical patients exhibit hyperglycemia, and approximately 80% of intensive care unit (ICU) patients will demonstrate transient or persistent hyperglycemia.[17]

- Patients with T1DM should be clearly identified as such at the time of admission.
- A1C can help identify previously undiagnosed diabetes in hospitalized patients and may assist with the evaluation of prior glucose control. A1C is not accurate in patients who are severely anemic, bleeding, hemolyzing, or who have been transfused.
- Data regarding use of noninsulin therapies in inpatients are increasing. Dipeptidyl peptidase 4 inhibitor and glucagon-like peptide-1 (GLP-1) receptor agonists alone or with basal insulin may provide adequate glucose control with less hypoglycemia than basal-bolus insulin regimens.

- **SGLT2 inhibitors should generally not be used in the hospital setting as they should be avoided in individuals with severe illness, ketonemia, prolonged fasting, and surgical procedures.**
- Medication reconciliation on admission should include a careful assessment of home diabetes medications, level of glucose control, kidney function, expected diagnostic studies and treatments, and the possible need for insulin treatment.
- Patients who are required to fast for diagnostic testing or treatments should have all noninsulin therapies stopped.
- **Patients hospitalized for reasons other than diabetes and who are eating normally** may continue or restart outpatient diabetes treatments, unless specifically contraindicated.
- Use of noninsulin therapies may be appropriate in psychiatric units, rehabilitation settings, or stable patients preparing for discharge.
- **Glucose targets for inpatients** aim to reduce morbidity and mortality, while minimizing hypoglycemia.
  - In critical care settings, the glucose target is 140–180 mg/dL (7.8–10.0 mmol/L) with frequent monitoring recommended to avoid hypoglycemia.
  - In non–critical care settings, the glucose target is <140 mg/dL (7.8 mmol/L) fasting and premeal and <180 mg/dL (10.0 mmol/L) postmeal or on a random glucose check with reassessment of the insulin regimen if glucose falls below 100 mg/dL (5.6 mmol/L).

Management of Hyperglycemia in Critical Care Settings

- Variable IV insulin infusion is recommended for critical illness, emergency surgery, or major surgery. Numerous algorithms have been published that direct insulin dose adjustments based on capillary BG values performed hourly at the bedside.
- An IV infusion of a dextrose-containing solution or other caloric source should be provided to prevent hypoglycemia and ketosis. For fluid-restricted patients, 10% dextrose in water (D10W) can be infused at a rate of 10–25 mL/h to provide a steady, consistent source of calories.
- An intermediate- or long-acting insulin should be given 2 hours prior to insulin infusion discontinuation.

Management of Hyperglycemia in Non–critical Care Hospital Settings

- BG should be checked on admission in all patients and monitored four times per day in hyperglycemic patients, especially in patients treated with insulin.
- Scheduled insulin with basal, nutritional, and correction components provides superior glycemic control compared to correction or "sliding scale" insulin alone.
- For patients who are naïve to insulin, the starting dose of basal insulin should equal 0.1–0.2 units/kg. Scheduled premeal insulin should be 0.1–0.2 units/kg divided by three meals.
  Example: Your patient weighs 80 kg. The starting insulin dose should be 8–16 units of long-acting insulin plus 3–5 units of rapid-acting insulin before each meal. A correction dose of 1–2 units per 50 mg/dL (2.8 mmol/L) of BG, beginning at 140 mg/dL (7.8 mmol/L), can be added to the premeal doses.
- Patients with T1DM should continue their home insulin doses. These patients may continue the use of an insulin pump if there is a hospital policy in place to do so and the patient is alert and capable of managing their pump. Insulin doses in patients with T2DM should be reduced by 20% on admission. If their home insulin dose is excessive compared with a weight-based dose of 0.4–0.5 units/kg or distribution between basal and premeal insulin is uneven, further reductions and adjustments may be necessary.

- Meal-time insulin doses should be given shortly before or immediately after meals, and the correction factor or sliding scale dose should be added to the premeal dose.
- The glucose threshold for sliding scale (corrective) insulin should be higher at bedtime, or corrective insulin should not be given at bedtime. Adjustments in the next-day basal or premeal insulin doses are indicated if correction doses of insulin are frequently required or if clinical status or medications change.
- Extreme hyperglycemia (≥300 mg/dL [16.7 mmol/L]) on one or more consecutive tests should prompt testing for ketoacidosis with electrolytes and ketone measurements.
- Hypoglycemia should be treated promptly with oral or IV glucose, and the capillary BG should be repeated every 10 minutes until >100 mg/dL (5.5 mmol/L) and stable. Reevaluation of scheduled doses and assessment of risk factors for hypoglycemia (declining renal function, hepatic impairment, poor intake) should be undertaken for any BG <70 mg/dL (3.9 mmol/L).
- **Enteral nutrition:** Intermittent tube feeds should be matched by either short-acting (human regular) insulin or intermediate-acting (human NPH [neutral protamine Hagedorn]) insulin. Patients with baseline hyperglycemia may need a basal insulin dose in addition to the doses given to cover tube feeds. For example, nighttime enteral feeding lasting 6–8 hours should be managed with NPH, with or without a basal insulin dose. Rapid-acting insulin can be given 6 times daily for continuous tube feeds, allowing a rapid change in insulin dose if feeding is interrupted.
- **Total parenteral nutrition (TPN):** Patients supported with TPN are likely to develop hyperglycemia, and some require large amounts of insulin. See Chapter 2, Nutrition Support, for insulin management of patients on TPN.

Diabetic Ketoacidosis

GENERAL PRINCIPLES

Epidemiology

DKA, a potentially fatal complication of diabetes, occurs in up to 5% of patients with T1DM annually and can occur in insulin-deficient patients with T2DM. It occurs less often in individuals with pancreatic diabetes due to deficient alpha and beta cell function.

Pathophysiology

DKA is a catabolic condition that results from severe insulin deficiency, often in association with stress and activation of counterregulatory hormones (e.g., catecholamines, glucagon).

Risk Factors

Precipitating factors for DKA include inadvertent or deliberate interruption of insulin therapy, sepsis, trauma, myocardial infarction (MI), and pregnancy. DKA may be the first presentation of T1DM and, rarely, T2DM. DKA with euglycemia or lower-than-expected glucoses can occur with use of the sodium–glucose cotransporter-2 (SGLT2) inhibitor drugs, atypical antipsychotic agents, and some chemotherapy agents.

Prevention

DKA can be prevented in many cases, and its occurrence often suggests a breakdown in patient education and communication. Therefore, diabetes education should be reinforced at every opportunity, with special emphasis on (1) self-management skills during sick days; (2) the body's need for more, rather than less, insulin during illness; (3) testing of blood or urine for ketones; and (4) procedures for obtaining timely and preventive medical advice.

DIAGNOSIS

History

- Patients may describe a variety of symptoms including polyuria, polydipsia, weight loss, nausea, vomiting, and vaguely localized abdominal pain generally in the setting of persistent hyperglycemia. A high index of suspicion is warranted because clinical presentation may be nonspecific.
- Tachycardia; prolonged capillary refill; rapid, deep, and labored breathing (Kussmaul respiration); and fruity breath odor are common physical findings.
- Prominent gastrointestinal (GI) symptoms and abdominal tenderness on examination should raise suspicion for intra-abdominal pathology.
- Dehydration is invariable and respiratory distress, shock, and coma can occur.

Diagnostic Testing

- Metabolic panel revealing anion gap metabolic acidosis.
- Positive serum β-hydroxybutyrate or ketones (a semiquantitative measurement of acetone, acetoacetate, and β-hydroxybutyrate) and positive urine ketones.
- Plasma glucose ≥250 mg/dL (13.9 mmol/L). Euglycemic DKA (plasma glucose <200 mg/dL [11.1 mmol/L]) has been described in pregnancy, alcohol ingestion, fasting or starvation, during hospitalization, and in patients with both T1DM and T2DM treated with SGLT2 inhibitors.[18]
- Hyponatremia, hyperkalemia, azotemia, and hyperosmolality are other possible findings.
- A focused search for a precipitating infection is recommended if clinically indicated.
- An ECG should be obtained to evaluate electrolyte abnormalities and for unsuspected myocardial ischemia.

TREATMENT

Management of DKA should preferably be conducted in an ICU (Table 23-2). **If treatment is conducted in a non-ICU setting, close monitoring is mandatory until ketoacidosis resolves and the patient's condition is stabilized.** Mild to moderate DKA may be managed with subcutaneous insulin protocols in non-ICU settings.[19] The therapeutic priorities are fluid replacement, adequate insulin administration, and potassium repletion. Administration of bicarbonate, phosphate, or magnesium, or other therapies are not routinely advised but may be appropriate in selected patients.

- **Monitoring of therapy**
  - BG levels should be monitored hourly, serum electrolyte levels every 2–4 hours, and arterial blood gas values as often as necessary for a severely acidotic or hypoxic patient.
  - Serum sodium tends to rise as hyperglycemia is corrected; failure to observe this trend suggests that the patient is being overhydrated with free water.
  - Dextrose should be initiated when the blood glucose is <250 mg/dL (13.9 mmol/L) or is predicted to fall to <200 mg/dL (11.1 mmol/L) in 1 hour. Use of a separate dextrose-containing fluid bag allows fluid resuscitation and glucose infusion to be titrated separately (two-bag approach) and has been shown to result in shorter duration of treatment.[20]

CHAPTER 23

TABLE 23-2	Treatment of Diabetic Ketoacidosis
Medication	**Dosing**
IV fluids Goals: First, replete circulating volume and then replenish total-body water deficit Estimate fluid deficit by subtracting current weight from recent dry weight Usually 7%–9% of body weight Hypotension → >10% loss of body fluids (Diabetes Care. 2004;27:S94)	**Replete circulating volume** 0.9% saline: 1 L bolus and then 500–1000 mL/h if cardiac and renal function normal **Replenish total-body water deficit** 0.45% saline (0.9% saline if hyponatremic): 150–500 mL/h Adjust repletion according to BP and UOP examinations; no faster than 3 mOsm/kg/h; aim for positive fluid balance over 12–24 h
Insulin Goals: Turn off ketogenesis; correct hyperglycemia	**Do not start until K >3.5 mmol/L** **Bolus: 0.1 units/kg** **Infusion: 0.1 units/kg/h** (Regular insulin 100 units in 100 mL 0.9% saline at 10 mL/h = 10 units/h) Goal decrease in BG = 50–75 mg/dL/h (2.8–4.2 mmol/L/h) Avoid correcting >100 mg/dL/h (5.6 mmol/L/h) to reduce risk of osmotic encephalopathy **Continue at 1–2 units/h until HCO_3 >15 mEq/L, clinical improvement, and anion gap closed** **Administer SC basal insulin 2 h prior to stopping insulin infusion**
Dextrose (5%) Goal: Prevent hypoglycemia	Add when BG <250 mg/dL (13.9 mmol/L) Consider giving glucose as a separate infusion of 50–100 mL/h (two-bag approach). Concurrently reduce insulin infusion to 0.05 units/kg/h
Potassium as KCl Goal: Prevent hypokalemia as insulin shifts potassium into the cell	Add to fluids at 10–20 mEq/h
Bicarbonate	Not routinely recommended May consider if (1) shock/coma; (2) pH <6.9; (3) HCO_3 <5 mEq/L; (4) cardiac/respiratory dysfunction; or (5) severe hyperkalemia 50–100 mEq in 1 L 0.45% saline over 30–60 min; follow arterial pH Avoid hypokalemia by adding 10 mEq KCl

TABLE 23-2	Treatment of Diabetic Ketoacidosis *(continued)*
Medication	**Dosing**
Phosphate and magnesium	Not routinely recommended
	May give KPhos IV fluids if not eating
	May give 10–20 mEq of magnesium sulfate IV with ventricular arrhythmias

BG, blood glucose; BP, blood pressure; HCO₃, bicarbonate; K, potassium; KCl, potassium chloride; KPhos, potassium phosphate; UOP, urine output.

- ○ Serial measurements of β-hydroxybutyrate in addition to electrolytes may provide additional information about recovery. Restoration of renal buffering capacity by normalization of the serum bicarbonate level is the most reliable index of metabolic recovery. Note that hyperchloremia may cause closure of the anion gap before the serum bicarbonate level has normalized, making anion gap closure a less reliable indicator of recovery of DKA than serum bicarbonate.
  - ○ Telemetry is recommended given the propensity for electrolyte abnormalities.
- • **IV antimicrobial therapy** should be started promptly for documented or suspected bacterial, fungal, and other treatable infections. Empiric broad-spectrum antibiotics can be started in septic patients pending results of blood cultures. Note that DKA is not typically accompanied by fever, so infection must be considered in a febrile patient.

COMPLICATIONS

Complications of DKA include life-threatening conditions that must be recognized and treated promptly.
- • **Lactic acidosis** may result from prolonged dehydration, shock, infection, and tissue hypoxia in DKA patients. Lactic acidosis should be suspected in patients with refractory metabolic acidosis and a persistent anion gap despite optimal therapy for DKA. Management includes adequate volume replacement, control of sepsis, and judicious use of bicarbonate.
- • **Arterial thrombosis** manifesting as stroke, MI, or an ischemic limb occurs with increased frequency in DKA. However, anticoagulation only indicated as specific therapy for a thrombotic event.
- • **Cerebral edema** is observed more frequently in children than adults.
  - ○ Symptoms of increased intracranial pressure (e.g., headache, altered mental status, papilledema) or a sudden deterioration in mental status after initial improvement in a patient with DKA should raise suspicion for cerebral edema.
  - ○ Overhydration with free water and excessively rapid correction of hyperglycemia are known risk factors. Watch for a decrease in serum sodium level or failure to rise during therapy.
  - ○ Neuroimaging with a CT scan can establish the diagnosis. Prompt recognition and treatment with IV mannitol is essential and may prevent neurologic sequelae in patients who survive cerebral edema.
- • **Rebound ketoacidosis** can occur because of premature cessation of IV insulin infusion or inadequate doses of subcutaneous (SC) insulin after the insulin infusion has been discontinued. All patients with T1DM and patients with T2DM

who develop DKA (indicating severe insulin deficiency) require both basal and premeal insulin in adequate doses to avoid recurrence of metabolic decompensation. **Basal insulin should be administered 2 hours prior to discontinuation of IV insulin.**

Hyperosmolar Hyperglycemic State

GENERAL PRINCIPLES

HHS is one of the most serious life-threatening complications of T2DM.

Epidemiology

• HHS occurs primarily in patients with T2DM. In 30%–40% of cases, it is the initial presentation of a patient's diabetes.
• HHS is significantly less common than DKA, with an incidence of <1 case per 1000 person-years.[21]

Pathophysiology

• Ketoacidosis is absent because the ambient insulin level may effectively prevent lipolysis and subsequent ketogenesis while being inadequate to facilitate peripheral glucose uptake and to prevent hepatic residual gluconeogenesis and glucose output.
• Precipitating factors for HHS include dehydration, stress, infection, stroke, noncompliance with medications, dietary indiscretion, and alcohol and cocaine abuse. Impaired glucose excretion is a contributory factor in patients with renal insufficiency or prerenal azotemia.

DIAGNOSIS

Clinical Presentation

In contrast to DKA, the onset of HHS is usually insidious. Several days of deteriorating glycemic control are followed by increasing lethargy. Clinical evidence of severe dehydration is the rule. Some alterations in consciousness and focal neurologic deficits may be found at presentation or may develop during therapy. Therefore, repeated neurologic assessment is recommended.

Differential Diagnosis

The differential diagnosis of HHS includes any cause of altered level of consciousness, including hypoglycemia, hyponatremia, severe dehydration, uremia, hyperammonemia, drug overdose, and sepsis. Seizures and acute stroke-like syndromes are common presentations.

Diagnostic Testing

Clinical findings include (1) hyperglycemia, often >600 mg/dL (33.3 mmol/L); (2) plasma osmolality >320 mOsm/L; (3) absence of ketonemia; and (4) pH > 7.3 and serum bicarbonate level of >20 mEq/L (>15 mmol/L in UK guidelines). Prerenal azotemia and lactic acidosis can develop. Although some patients will have detectable urine ketones, most patients do not have a metabolic acidosis. Lactic acidosis may develop from an underlying ischemia, infection, or other cause.

TREATMENT

- See Table 23-3 for detailed treatment recommendations.
- **Underlying illness:** Detection and treatment of any underlying predisposing illness are critical in the treatment of HHS. Antibiotics should be administered early, after appropriate cultures, in patients in whom infection is known or suspected as a precipitant to HHS. A high index of suspicion should be maintained for underlying pancreatitis, GI bleeding, renal failure, and thromboembolic events, especially acute MI.

COMPLICATIONS

Complications of HHS include thromboembolic events (cerebral and MI, mesenteric thrombosis, pulmonary embolism, and disseminated intravascular coagulation), cerebral edema, acute respiratory distress syndrome, and rhabdomyolysis.

TABLE 23-3	Treatment of Hyperosmolar Hyperglycemic State
IV Fluids Goals: Restore Hemodynamic stability and intravascular volume by fluid replacement; this is the primary treatment and supersedes insulin; patients often require much more fluid than with diabetic ketoacidosis	**Replete Circulating Volume** 0.9% saline × 1–1.5 L **Replenish total-body water deficit** 0.45% saline if Na is elevated Aim for positive fluid balance over 24–72 h; may require 10–12 L
Potassium as KCl Goal: Prevent hypokalemia as insulin shifts potassium into the cell	Add to fluids at 10–20 mEq/h; begin as soon as urine output confirmed **Do not start until K >3.5 mmol/L**
Insulin Goals: Plays a secondary role; slowly corrects hyperglycemia	**Bolus: 5–10 units (if BG >600 mg/dL); smaller bolus if BG <600 mg/dL (33.3 mmol/L)** **Infusion: 0.10–0.15 units/kg/h** Avoid correcting >100 mg/dL/h (5.6 mmol/L/h) to reduce risk of osmotic encephalopathy **Administer SC basal insulin 2 h prior to stopping insulin infusion**
Dextrose (5%) Goal: Prevent hypoglycemia	Add when BG 250–300 mg/dL (13.9–16.7 mmol/L) Can give as a separate infusion of 50–100 mL/h (two-bag approach) Concurrently reduce insulin infusion to 1–2 units/h
Bicarbonate	Not routinely recommended May be required if concurrent lactic acidosis

BG, blood glucose; K, potassium; KCl, potassium chloride.

MONITORING/FOLLOW-UP

- **Monitoring of therapy:** Use of a flowchart is helpful for tracking clinical data and laboratory results.
- Initially, BG levels should be monitored every 30–60 minutes and serum electrolyte levels every 2–4 hours; frequency of monitoring can be decreased during recovery.
- Neurologic status must be reassessed frequently; persistent lethargy or altered mentation indicates inadequate therapy. On the other hand, relapse after initial improvement in mental status suggests too rapid correction of serum osmolarity.

Type 1 Diabetes

GENERAL PRINCIPLES

A comprehensive approach is necessary for successful management of T1DM. A team approach that includes the expertise of physicians, diabetes educators, dietitians, and other members of the diabetes care team offers the best chance of success.

DIAGNOSIS

T1DM can present at any age, and because of the variable time course and severity of hyperglycemia, the diagnosis can be challenging in adults.

- The rate of destruction of β cells is rapid in infants and children and slower in adults. Therefore, ketoacidosis as an initial presentation is more common in young patients.
- T1DM is characterized by severe insulin deficiency. Exogenous insulin is required to control BGs, prevent DKA, and preserve life. Ketosis develops in 8–16 hours and ketoacidosis in 12–24 hours without insulin.
- Early in the course of T1DM, some insulin secretory capacity remains, and the insulin requirement may be lower than expected (0.3–0.4 units/kg). Tight control of BG level from the onset has been shown to preserve the residual β-cell function and prevent or delay later complications.
- Latent autoimmune diabetes in adults (LADA) is characterized by mild to moderate hyperglycemia at presentation that often responds to noninsulin therapies initially. Adults with LADA will have one or more β cell–specific autoantibodies and tend to require insulin therapy sooner than patients with classic T2DM (months to years).
- T1DM should be suspected when there is a family history of T1DM, thyroid disease, celiac disease or other autoimmune disease. Presentation with ketoacidosis suggests T1DM, but confirmatory tests may be useful to guide therapy.
- Autoantibodies include islet cell autoantibodies, antibodies to insulin, antibodies to glutamic acid decarboxylase (anti-GAD), antibodies to zinc transporter 8 (ZnT8), and antibodies to tyrosine phosphatases IA-2 and IA-2β. Measuring one or more of these autoantibodies along with a C-peptide can help to confirm the diagnosis of T1DM; however, 20% of insulin-deficient adults are antibody negative.

TREATMENT

Treatment of T1DM requires lifelong insulin replacement and careful coordination of insulin doses with food intake and activity.[22]
- A regimen of **multiple daily insulin injections** that include basal, premeal, and correction doses is preferred to obtain optimal control in both hospitalized patients

and outpatients. This regimen implies that capillary glucose monitoring will occur four times daily, 10–30 minutes before meals and at bedtime or that a patient is using a CGM device.

○ The **insulin requirement** for optimal glycemic control is approximately 0.5–0.8 units/kg/d for the average nonobese patient. A conservative total daily dose (TDD) of 0.4 units/kg/d is given initially to a newly diagnosed patient; the dose is then adjusted, using SMBG values. Higher doses may be required in obese or insulin-resistant patients, in adolescents, and in the latter part of pregnancy.

○ **Basal insulin** (administered as NPH twice daily, detemir once or twice daily, glargine once or twice daily, or insulin degludec once daily) should provide 40%–50% of the TDD of insulin and should be adjusted by 5%–10% daily until the fasting glucose is consistently <130 mg/dL (7.2 mmol/L). In general, basal insulin is given regardless of nothing by mouth (NPO) or dietary status and should not be held without a direct order.

○ **Premeal insulin** doses of insulin are given to cover caloric intake at meals or with snacks. Bolus doses are adjusted according to the BG, the anticipated carbohydrate intake, and the anticipated activity level. The total premeal complement should roughly equal the total basal dose, with one-third given before or after each meal. Rapid-acting insulins (lispro, aspart, glulisine, or inhaled technosphere insulin) are preferred, but regular human insulin can be used. There are now ultrarapid forms of lispro and aspart with a faster onset of action and earlier peak action.[23]

○ The third component of a comprehensive insulin regimen is "**correction factor**" insulin, which is similar to sliding scale. This category of insulin therapy is adjusted according to the premeal fingerstick glucose testing (or CGM reading) and the patient's estimated insulin sensitivity. In general, patients with lower BMI should use a less aggressive scale than patients with higher BMI or more insulin-resistant patients. Correction factor and premeal doses should use the same insulin and be given together in the same syringe. At times, a correction dose of rapid-acting insulin may be needed to treat hyperglycemia in the absence of food intake.

• **Insulin preparations:** After SC injection, there is individual variability in the duration and peak activity of insulin preparations and day-to-day variability in the same subject (Table 23-4).

• **SC insulin administration:** The abdomen, thighs, buttocks, and upper arms are the preferred sites for SC insulin injection. Absorption is fastest from the abdomen, followed by the arm, buttocks, and thigh, probably as a result of differences in blood flow. Injection sites should be rotated within the regions, rather than randomly across separate regions, to minimize erratic absorption. Exercise or massage over the injection site may accelerate insulin absorption.

• Regular human insulin is available in an **inhaled form as technosphere insulin.** This comes in 4-, 8-, and 12-unit cartridges for bolus dose insulin administration. Onset occurs at 0.2–0.25 hour with peak effect within the first hour and a duration of action of 3 hours. It is contraindicated in patients with asthma or chronic obstructive pulmonary disease because of risk of bronchospasm. Pulmonary function tests are required prior to starting and at regular intervals during therapy.

• **Continuous SC insulin infusion** with an insulin pump is widely used for insulin delivery in patients with T1DM, and increasingly in T2DM. Use of an insulin pump integrated with CGM adds additional features. Sensor augmented pump (SAP) therapy allows automated suspension of insulin delivery on reaching a preset low threshold, or above the threshold if glucose is declining and predicted to reach a hypoglycemic value within a specified period. Hybrid closed loop (HCL) systems allow the basal rate to automatically adjust according to CGM data while the patient continues to input bolus dosing information.

TABLE 23-4	Approximate Kinetics of Insulin Preparations		
Insulin Type	Onset of Action (h)	Peak Effect (h)	Duration of Activity (h)
Ultrarapid-acting			
Lispro-aabc, aspart	<0.25	1.0	5
Rapid-acting			
Lispro, aspart, glulisine	0.25–0.50	0.50–1.50	3–5
Regular	0.50–1.00	2–4	6–8
Technosphere insulin	0.25–0.5	1.0–1.5	2–3
Intermediate-acting			
NPH	1–2	6–12	16–20
Lente[a]	1–2	6–12	16–20
Long-acting[b]			
Detemir	3–4	8–12	18–24
Glargine	4–6	Possible[c]	20–24
Ultralente[a]	3–4	Variable	18–24
PZI[a]	3–4	Unclear	18–24
Degludec	3–4	Flat	24–40

NPH, neutral protamine Hagedorn; PZI, protamine zinc insulin.

[a]Not available in the United States; possibly generic manufacturers.

[b]Some patients with type 1 diabetes have improved control when the long-acting basal insulin is given twice a day rather than once daily.

[c]Insulin dosage and individual variability in absorption and clearance rates affect pharmacokinetic data. Duration of insulin activity is prolonged in renal failure. After a lag time of approximately 5 hours, insulin glargine generally has a mostly flat peakless effect over a 22- to 24-hour period; however, broad peaks can occur. Insulin degludec has the longest duration of action, allowing administration at any time of the day.

○ A typical regimen provides 50% of total daily insulin as basal insulin and the remainder as multiple preprandial bolus doses of insulin. A rapid-acting insulin (aspart, lispro, or glulisine) is used to fill the pump and is infused continuously to provide basal insulin.

○ Insulin pumps have advanced features that allow patients to fine-tune their basal and bolus doses but require diabetes education to use the pump to its full potential. Patients must check their blood sugars regularly because DKA can occur rapidly if the insulin infusion is disrupted (i.e., faulty infusion set).

○ SAP and HCL systems are currently available. Fully closed loop systems, whereby the patient will not manually enter information, are being developed.

Type 2 Diabetes

GENERAL PRINCIPLES

• T2DM results from defective insulin secretion followed by loss of β-cell mass in response to increased demand as a result of insulin resistance.[24]

- T2DM is usually diagnosed in adults, with both incidence and prevalence increasing with age. However, type 2 diabetes prevalence has increased substantially since 2001 in youth aged 10–19, comprising about 20% of cases of diabetes in that age group in 2017.[25]
- T2DM is associated with obesity, family history of diabetes, history of GDM or prediabetes, hypertension, physical inactivity, race/ethnicity, and other social determinants of health (socioeconomic status, food insecurity). African Americans, Latinos, Asian Indians, Native Americans, Pacific Islanders, and some groups of Asians have a greater risk of developing T2DM than Caucasians.
- T2DM may be asymptomatic and, therefore, can remain undiagnosed for months to years.
- The loss of pancreatic β cells is progressive. Insulin secretion is usually sufficient to prevent ketosis, but DKA or HHS can develop during severe stress. T2DM in patients who present with or later develop ketosis or DKA, but who do not require insulin between episodes, is termed ketosis-prone T2DM.
- The mechanisms underlying the β-cell loss and defective insulin secretory dysfunction in T2DM are not clear, but cell death, transdifferentiation, and dedifferentiation in response to oxidative stress and endoplasmic reticulum stress in the setting of environmental exposure and genetic predisposition have been proposed. Glycemic state may also affect the beta cell over prolonged periods of time.[26]

TREATMENT

- The achievement of glycemic control requires individualized therapy and a comprehensive approach that incorporates lifestyle and pharmacologic interventions. Guidelines have been published by several professional organizations regarding the choice and sequence of antidiabetic therapy.[27]
- Considerations for selecting noninsulin therapy (Table 23-5) in patients with T2DM include the following:
  ○ Pharmacologic therapy should be initiated early in conjunction with diet and exercise.
  ○ Metformin is the recommended first-line therapy if tolerated.
  ○ Based upon results of the cardiovascular outcome trials, GLP-1 receptor agonists should be considered first-line in individuals with cardiovascular disease or stroke. SGLT2 inhibitors should be considered first-line in individuals with heart failure or diabetic kidney disease.
  ○ The glucose-lowering effects of metformin, insulin secretagogues, DPP-4 inhibitors GLP-1 receptor analogs, and SGLT2 inhibitors are observed within days to weeks, whereas the maximum effect of thiazolidinediones may not be observed for several weeks to months.
  ○ Combination therapy with two or more oral or injectable agents may be needed at the time of diagnosis to achieve A1C and glucose targets in patients presenting with significant hyperglycemia (A1C >9%; 75 mmol/mol) and will likely be needed as β-cell function deteriorates over time.
  ○ Insulin therapy should be considered for patients presenting in DKA or with very high glucose levels (A1C >10%; 86 mmol/mol). Insulin therapy can sometimes be stopped after glucose toxicity is corrected but may need to be continued in patients with persistent insulin deficiency.

TABLE 23-5	Noninsulin Medications for Diabetes	
	Renal Dosing Necessary?	Main Adverse Effects

Oral therapies

Biguanide: Inhibits hepatic glucose output and stimulates glucose uptake by peripheral tissues. Weight neutral. Hold for 48 h after radiographic contrast procedure. Avoid in patients with cardiogenic or septic shock, moderate or severe CHF, severe liver disease, hypoxemia, and tissue hypoperfusion.

Metformin (available in liquid and long-acting formulations)	Reduce dose to 500 mg 2× daily if eGFR <45 mL/min/1.73 m^2; stop if eGFR <30 mL/min/1.73 m^2	GI symptoms (20%–30%); lactic acidosis (3/100,000 patient-years)

Sulfonylureas (SFU): Increase insulin secretion by binding specific β-cell receptors. Give 30–60 min before food. *Never* give if fasting. Start with lowest dose and increase over days to weeks to optimal dose (usually half the maximum approved dose).

Glyburide (glibenclamide)	Avoid if CrCl <50 mL/min	Hypoglycemia, weight gain; avoid with renal insufficiency; caution in elderly
Glipizide	Yes, if CrCl <50 mL/min	Same; fewer problems in kidney disease
Glimepiride	Start lowest dose and titrate slowly	Same; fewer problems in kidney disease
Gliclazide[a]		Same; fewer problems in kidney disease

Meglitinides: Increase insulin secretion; much shorter onset and half-life than SFUs. Dose before each meal. *Never* give if fasting.

Nateglinide	No	Hypoglycemia, weight gain; not as severe as SFUs
• Give 10 min before meal • Metabolized by cytochrome P450		
Repaglinide	Yes, if CrCl ≤40 mL/min	Same
• Give 30 min before meal		
Mitiglinide[a]		Same

α-Glucosidase inhibitors: Block polysaccharide and disaccharide breakdown and decrease postprandial hyperglycemia. Give with food. Start with low dose and increase weekly. Do not use in patients with intestinal disease.

Acarbose	Avoid if serum Cr >2.0 mg/dL (176.8 μmol/L)	Gas, bloating, diarrhea, abdominal pain (25%–50%); transaminase elevations

TABLE 23-5	Noninsulin Medications for Diabetes (*continued*)	
	Renal Dosing Necessary?	Main Adverse Effects
Miglitol	Avoid if serum Cr >2.0 mg/dL (176.8 µmol/L)	Gas, bloating, diarrhea, abdominal pain (25%–50%)
Voglibose[a]	No; not renally excreted; not studied in CKD	Same

Thiazolidinediones: Increase insulin sensitivity in muscle, adipose tissue, and liver. Start with low dose and increase after several weeks. Avoid in patients with New York Heart Association class III/IV heart failure. Caution in patients with coronary artery disease, hypertension, long-standing diabetes, left ventricular hypertrophy, preexisting edema or edema on therapy, insulin use, advanced age, renal failure, and aortic or mitral valve disease (Diabetes Care. 2004;27:256).

| Pioglitazone • Alters levels of medicines metabolized by CYP3A4 | No | Edema, heart failure, fractures in women, possible increased risk of bladder cancer, mild pancytopenia |

DPP-4 inhibitors: Inhibit enzyme that breaks down endogenous GLP (incretin secreted from intestinal L cells). Increased GLP reduces blood glucose by inhibiting glucagon release and stimulating insulin secretion. Avoid in patients with a history of pancreatitis.

Alogliptin	Yes, if eGFR <60 mL/min	Anaphylaxis, angioedema, skin reactions, liver injury, URI
Linagliptin	No	Anaphylaxis, angioedema, exfoliative skin reactions, URI
Saxagliptin	Yes, if eGFR ≤50 mL/min/1.73 m^2	Urticaria, facial edema, URI
Sitagliptin	Yes, if eGFR <50 mL/min/1.73 m^2	AKI, ESRD, anaphylaxis, angioedema, exfoliative skin reactions, URI
Vildagliptin[a] (not indicated in severe hepatic impairment, LFT >3× upper limit of normal)	Yes, if eGFR <50 mL/min/1.73 m^2; not indicated in severe renal impairment	Blistering skin lesions in animals, increased LFTs

SGLT2 inhibitors: Inhibit sodium glucose cotransporter-2 in the proximal renal tubule, decreasing glucose reabsorption by the kidney.

| Canagliflozin | Yes, if eGFR 30–<60 mL/min/1.73 m^2 use the lower dose, stop if eGFR <30 mL/min/1.73 m^2 | Female genital mycotic infections, urinary tract infections, polyuria; hypotension, volume depletion, renal failure; increased LDL-C |

(continued)

CHAPTER 23

TABLE 23-5	Noninsulin Medications for Diabetes (*continued*)	
	Renal Dosing Necessary?	Main Adverse Effects
Dapagliflozin	Not indicated for eGFR <45 mL/min/1.73 m^2	Same; possible increased risk for bladder cancer
Empagliflozin	Not indicated for eGFR <30 mL/min/1.73 m^2	Same
Ertugliflozin	Not indicated for eGFR <45 mL/min/1.73 m^2	Same
Bile acid sequestrants		
Colesevelam hydrochloride (contraindicated in bowel obstruction or GI motility disorders; pregnancy class B; can be used in renal and hepatic disease; take on an empty stomach)	No	Constipation, reduced absorption of some medications; raises triglycerides
Dopamine agonists		
Bromocriptine mesylate (do not use with other dopamine agonists or antagonists)	No	Nausea, asthenia, dizziness, headache, constipation, diarrhea
SC injectable therapies		
GLP-1 receptor agonists: Structurally similar to endogenous GLP-1 but resist breakdown by DPP-4. They have a longer half-life and reach higher levels in blood and tissues. They are given by injection and can improve satiety and result in weight loss. Avoid in patients with history of pancreatitis. Avoid in patients with history of medullary thyroid cancer or MEN2 given increased C-cell tumors in rodents (all except immediate-release exenatide).		
Dulaglutide (dosed weekly)	No; monitor for GI side effects in patients with renal impairment	Diarrhea, nausea, vomiting, abdominal pain, decreased appetite
Exenatide (dosed twice daily)	Do not use in severe renal impairment or ESRD; caution with moderate renal impairment or history of renal transplant	Nausea, vomiting, GI distress, reported cases of pancreatitis
Exenatide extended release (dosed weekly)	Do not use in severe renal impairment or ESRD; caution with moderate renal impairment or history of renal transplant	Nausea, vomiting, injection site reaction, headache, diarrhea, dyspepsia
Liraglutide (dosed once daily)	Caution when initiating or escalating dose in patients with renal impairment	Headache, nausea, vomiting, diarrhea, urticaria

TABLE 23-5	Noninsulin Medications for Diabetes (*continued*)	
	Renal Dosing Necessary?	**Main Adverse Effects**
Lixisentatide (dosed once daily)	Do not use if eGFR is <30 mL/min/1.73m²	Diarrhea, nausea, vomiting, abdominal pain, decreased appetite
Semaglutide Injectable (dosed once weekly) Oral (dosed daily)	No renal adjustment	Diarrhea, nausea, vomiting, constipation, abdominal pain, decreased appetite
Amylin analogs: Blunt postprandial blood glucose response		
Pramlintide acetate (given as a separate injection with meals; insulin dose reduction is required when starting)	Not defined with CrCl <20 mL/min	Nausea, vomiting, diarrhea, headache, hypoglycemia

AKI, acute kidney injury; CKD, chronic kidney disease; CHF, congestive heart failure; Cr, creatinine; CrCl, creatinine clearance; DPP-4, dipeptidyl peptidase 4; eGFR, estimated glomerular filtration rate; ESRD, end-stage renal disease; GI, gastrointestinal; GLP, glucagon-like peptide; LDL-C, low-density lipoprotein cholesterol; LFT, liver function test; MEN2, multiple endocrine neoplasia type 2; URI, upper respiratory infection.
Please refer to country-specific prescribing information before using any of the antidiabetes therapies.
[a]Not available in the United States.

- Because pancreatic β-cell function is required for the glucose-lowering effects of all noninsulin therapies, many patients will require insulin replacement therapy at some point. Insulin therapy can be initiated with basal insulin in addition to other therapies.
- The toxicity profile of some oral and injectable antidiabetic agents may preclude their use in patients with preexisting illnesses.
- Doses of noninsulin therapies may need to be reduced for declining kidney function (Table 23-5).
- Cardiovascular outcome trials (CVOTs) comparing anti-hyperglycemic medications versus placebo have shown that none increase the risk of CVD. Studies with DPP-4 inhibitors have shown CVD safety but no benefit.
- In a meta-analysis of CVOTs, GLP-1 receptor agonists reduced major adverse cardiovascular events, all-cause mortality, composite kidney outcomes, and heart failure.[28]
- In meta-analysis of CVOTs, SGLT2 inhibitors reduced the risk of hospitalization for heart failure and cardiovascular death and reduced progression of renal disease. Major adverse cardiovascular events were reduced in those with preexisting cardiovascular disease.[29]
- **Insulin therapy** in T2DM is indicated in the following:
  - Patients in whom oral or injectable agents have failed to achieve or sustain glycemic control
  - Metabolic decompensation: DKA, HHS

- Newly diagnosed patients with severe hyperglycemia
- Patients with chronic kidney disease that precludes use of noninsulin therapies
- Pregnancy and other situations in which oral agents are contraindicated

- **The success of insulin therapy** depends on both the adequacy of the insulin TDD (0.6 to >1.0 units/kg of body weight per day) and the appropriateness of the insulin regimen for a given patient to achieve target glucose and A1C values.
  - A once-daily injection of intermediate- or long-acting insulin at bedtime or before breakfast (basal insulin) added to oral or injectable agents may achieve the target A1C goal.
  - Premeal insulin may be required if basal insulin plus other agents are not adequate. Short- or rapid-acting insulin administered before meals can be added to basal insulin. Alternatively, a premixed insulin can be given twice daily before breakfast and dinner. In general, the secretagogues are discontinued when premeal insulin is added, but sensitizing and other agents are continued based on individual patient needs.
  - The TDD of insulin required to achieve glycemic targets varies widely in patients with T2DM and is based on BMI, the continuation of oral agents, and the presence of comorbid conditions. Large doses of insulin (>100 units/d) may be required for optimal glycemic control. Weight gain with insulin use is a concern.
  - Insulin-induced hypoglycemia, the most dangerous side effect, may increase CV event rates and death. Avoidance of hypoglycemia while achieving an A1C as low as can be safely achieved requires close collaboration between physician, patient, and diabetes educators. The frequency of hypoglycemia increases as patients approach normal A1C levels or when kidney function declines.
- **Concentration:** The standard insulin concentration is 100 units/mL (U-100), with vials containing 1000 units in 10 mL. A highly concentrated form of regular insulin containing 500 units/mL (Humulin U-500) is available for patients with severe insulin resistance (usually T2DM) requiring more than 200 units per day. The vial size for U-500 insulin is 20 mL. Pens containing 3 mL are also available for U-100 and U-500 insulins. Concentrated forms of insulin glargine, a formulation that is 300 units/mL (U-300), insulin degludec, and insulin lispro formulated with 200 units/mL (U-200), are available in pens.
- **Mixed insulin therapy:** Short- and rapid-acting insulins (regular, lispro, aspart, and glulisine) can be mixed with NPH insulin in the same syringe for convenience. The rapid-acting insulin should be drawn first, cross-contamination should be avoided, and the mixed insulin should be injected immediately. Commercial premixed insulin preparations do not allow dose adjustment of individual components but are convenient for patients who are unable or unwilling to do the mixing themselves. Premixed insulins are an option for patients with T2DM who have a regular eating and activity schedule and, in general, should not be used in T1DM. Premixed insulins are not advised for use in hospitalized patients.

CHRONIC COMPLICATIONS OF DIABETES MELLITUS

- Prevention of long-term complications is one of the main goals of diabetes management. Appropriate treatment of established complications may delay their progression and improve quality of life.
- **Microvascular complications** include diabetic retinopathy (DR), nephropathy, and neuropathy. These complications are directly related to hyperglycemia. Tight glycemic control has been shown to reduce the development and progression of these complications.

Diabetic Retinopathy

GENERAL PRINCIPLES

Classification

- DR is classified as preproliferative retinopathy (microaneurysms, retinal infarcts, lipid exudates, cotton wool spots, and/or microhemorrhages) with or without macular edema, and proliferative retinopathy.
- Other ocular abnormalities associated with diabetes include cataract formation, dyskinetic pupils, glaucoma, optic neuropathy, extraocular muscle paresis, floaters, and fluctuating visual acuity. The latter may be related to changes in BG levels.
- The presence of floaters may be indicative of preretinal or vitreous hemorrhage, and immediate referral for ophthalmologic evaluation is warranted.

Epidemiology

The incidence of DR and vision impairment has dropped significantly with improved management of glycemia, blood pressure, and lipids in patients with both T1DM and T2DM. Early identification and treatment of DR have further reduced vision impairment once it is diagnosed. DR is less frequent in T2DM, but maculopathy may be more severe. It is the fifth leading cause of severe vision loss or blindness worldwide.[30]

DIAGNOSIS

Annual examination by an ophthalmologist is recommended at the time of diagnosis of all T2DM patients and at the beginning of puberty or 3–5 years after diagnosis for patients with T1DM. Dilated eye examination should be repeated annually by an optometrist or ophthalmologist because progressive DR can be completely asymptomatic until sudden loss of vision occurs. Early detection of DR is critical because therapy is more effective before severe maculopathy or proliferation develops. Any patient with diabetes and visual symptoms should be referred for ophthalmologic evaluation.[31]

TREATMENT

Glycemic control is first-line therapy to prevent DR progression. Blood pressure management, using ACE inhibitors or ARBs, and addition of fenofibrate in individuals with hyperlipidemia can also benefit DR. Preproliferative retinopathy is not usually associated with loss of vision unless macular edema is present (25% of cases). The development of macular edema or proliferative retinopathy (particularly new vessels near the optic disk) requires elective laser photocoagulation therapy or intra-ocular injections of vascular endothelial growth factor (VEGF)-neutralizing antibodies. For macular edema, anti-VEGF therapies have better outcomes than laser therapy to preserve vision, and anti-VEGF therapies are also a reasonable alternative to laser photocoagulation for proliferative retinopathy. Vitrectomy is indicated for patients with vitreous hemorrhage or retinal detachment.

Diabetic Nephropathy

GENERAL PRINCIPLES

Epidemiology

Approximately 20%–40% of patients with either type of diabetes develop clinically evident diabetic nephropathy during their lifetime. Diabetic nephropathy is the leading cause of end-stage renal disease (ESRD) in the United States and a major cause of morbidity and mortality in patients with diabetes.

Risk Factors

Albuminuria is defined as an urinary albumin-to-creatinine ratio ≥30 mg/g. Poor glycemic control is the major risk factor for diabetic nephropathy, but hypertension and smoking are contributors. Obesity may contribute to kidney damage in T2DM.

Prevention

Prevention of diabetic nephropathy starts at the time of diagnosis with achievement of glycemic, blood pressure, and lipid targets and smoking cessation. **Patients with CKD are at higher risk for CVD and mortality,** so management of other CV risk factors is particularly important.

DIAGNOSIS

- Measurement of the albumin-to-creatinine ratio (normal, <30 mg of albumin/g of creatinine) in a random urine sample is recommended for screening annually for individuals with T1DM >5 years and T2DM beginning at diagnosis. At least two to three measurements within a 6-month period should be performed to establish the diagnosis of diabetic nephropathy.
- Measurement of serum creatinine and serum urea nitrogen should be performed annually, along with calculation of the estimated GFR. Patients with diabetes may have reduced kidney function without manifesting albumin in their urine. Testing and treatment of associated disorders such as anemia, secondary hyperparathyroidism, hyperkalemia, and acid–base disturbances should begin when the estimated GFR is <60 mL/min/1.73 m^2 or during stage 3 CKD (see Chapter 13, Renal Diseases).

TREATMENT

Intensive control of both diabetes and hypertension is important to reduce the rate of progression of CKD due to diabetes. Lower blood pressure targets, less than 130/80 mm Hg, are recommended for persons with diabetes and evidence of kidney damage or dysfunction.

Medications

- Antihypertensive treatment with ACE inhibitor or ARB drugs is recommended as first-line therapy for all patients with diabetes and hypertension and may be considered in patients with normal blood pressure or prehypertension.

- SGLT2 inhibitors have demonstrated benefit in reducing risk of progression of kidney disease and should be used regardless of A1C or concomitant therapy. Empagliflozin and canagliflozin can be initiated at eGFR of 30 mL/min/1.73 m^2 and continued until renal replacement is planned.
- Diuretics and dihydropyridine calcium channel blockers can be added. Mineralocorticoid receptor antagonist can be added if not at goal on above agents; however, hyperkalemia is common. The nonsteroidal mineralocorticoid receptor antagonist, finerenone, has been shown to reduce progression of CKD and provide CV benefit with less hyperkalemia in persons with T2DM and CKD.[32]

Lifestyle/Risk Modification

- Dietary protein intake of 0.8 g/kg/d (based on ideal body weight) is recommended. Further reduction does not alter glycemic control, CVD risk, or kidney function decline.
- Avoidance of renal toxins is important for preservation of kidney function.

Diabetic Neuropathy

GENERAL PRINCIPLES

Classification

Diabetic neuropathy can be classified as (1) subclinical neuropathy, determined by abnormalities in electrodiagnostic and quantitative sensory testing; (2) diffuse symmetrical polyneuropathy with distal symmetric sensorimotor losses ± autonomic syndromes; and (3) focal syndromes.[33]

Epidemiology

Distal symmetric polyneuropathy (DPN) is the most common neuropathy in developed countries and accounts for more hospitalizations than all the other diabetic complications combined. Sensorimotor DPN is a major risk factor for foot trauma, ulceration, and Charcot arthropathy and is responsible for 50%–75% of nontraumatic amputations.

Prevention

- Sensation in the lower extremities should be documented at least annually, using a combination of modalities such as 10 g monofilament, tuning fork (frequency of 128 Hz) or pinprick, and temperature.
- Foot examination should be conducted at least annually to evaluate the presence of musculoskeletal deformities, skin changes, and pulses, in addition to the sensory examination.

TREATMENT

- **Painful peripheral neuropathy** responds variably to treatment with tricyclic antidepressants (e.g., amitriptyline 10–150 mg PO at bedtime), topical capsaicin (0.075% cream), or anticonvulsants (e.g., carbamazepine 100–400 mg PO bid, gabapentin 900–3600 mg/d, or pregabalin 150–300 mg/d). Patients should be warned about adverse effects, including sedation and anticholinergic symptoms (tricyclics), burning sensation (capsaicin), and blood dyscrasias (carbamazepine). α-Lipoic acid (600 mg bid) and high-dose thiamine (50–100 mg tid) have been tested in early DPN. Vitamin B$_{12}$ should be checked and replaced if low.

- **Orthostatic hypotension**: Treatment is symptomatic and includes postural maneuvers, use of compressive garments (e.g., Jobst stockings), and intravascular expansion using sodium chloride 1–4 g PO qid and fludrocortisone 0.1–0.3 mg PO daily. Causes of orthostatic hypotension (other than diabetic autonomic neuropathy) should be excluded.
- **Intractable nausea and vomiting** may be manifestations of impaired GI motility from autonomic neuropathy. **DKA** should be ruled out when nausea and vomiting are acute and adrenal insufficiency should be excluded. Frequent, small meals (six to eight per day) of soft consistency that are low in fat and fiber provide intermittent relief. Parenteral nutrition may become necessary in refractory cases.

  Pharmacologic therapy includes the prokinetic agent metoclopramide, 10–20 mg PO (or as a suppository) before meals and at bedtime, and erythromycin, 125–500 mg PO qid for short-term therapy. Extrapyramidal side effects (tremor and tardive dyskinesia) from the antidopaminergic actions of metoclopramide may limit therapy. Cyclical vomiting unrelated to a GI motility disorder appears to respond to amitriptyline 25–50 mg PO at bedtime.
- **Diabetic cystopathy,** or bladder dysfunction, results from impaired autonomic control of detrusor muscle and sphincteric function. Manifestations include urgency, dribbling, incomplete emptying, overflow incontinence, and urinary retention. Recurrent urinary tract infections are common in patients with residual urine. Treatment with bethanechol 10 mg tid or intermittent self-catheterization may be required to relieve retention.
- **Chronic, persistent diarrhea** in patients with diabetes is probably multifactorial. Celiac disease and inflammatory bowel diseases should be ruled out, particularly in patients with T1DM. Exocrine pancreatic dysfunction should be considered. Bacterial overgrowth has been considered as an etiology but is difficult to diagnose. Empiric treatment with broad-spectrum antibiotics (e.g., azithromycin, tetracycline, cephalosporins) along with metronidazole may be beneficial. Antifungal agents and probiotic replacement can be tried. If diarrhea persists, loperamide or octreotide 50–75 mg SC bid can be effective in patients with intractable diarrhea.

MACROVASCULAR COMPLICATIONS OF DIABETES MELLITUS

Coronary Heart Disease

GENERAL PRINCIPLES

- Coronary heart disease (CHD), stroke, and peripheral vascular disease (PVD) are responsible for 80% of deaths in persons with diabetes (see Chapter 4, Ischemic Heart Disease).
- **Coronary artery disease (CAD)** occurs at a younger age and may have atypical clinical presentations in patients with diabetes.
- MI carries a worse prognosis, and angioplasty gives less satisfactory results in patients with diabetes.
- Persons with diabetes have an increased risk of ischemic and nonischemic heart failure (HF) and sudden death.[34]

Risk Factors

Risk factors for macrovascular disease that are common in persons with diabetes include insulin resistance, hyperglycemia, albuminuria, hypertension, hyperlipidemia, cigarette smoking, and obesity.

Prevention

- CV risk factors should be assessed at least annually and treated aggressively.
- Screening asymptomatic persons with cardiac stress test has not been shown to reduce mortality or events in asymptomatic patients with T2DM.[35]
- Aspirin 81–325 mg/d has proven beneficial in secondary prevention of MI or stroke in patients with diabetes and may be considered for persons over age 40 years with diabetes.

TREATMENT

- Glycemic control should be optimized to A1C <7% (<53 mmol/mol) and as close to normal as possible in the first few years after diagnosis. Hypoglycemia should be avoided.
- Hypertension should be controlled to a target blood pressure of <140/90 mm Hg (or <130/80 mm Hg if this can be achieved without adverse effects).
- Hyperlipidemia should be treated appropriately, with a high-intensity statin in patients with known CVD.
- Cigarette smoking should be actively discouraged, and weight loss should be promoted in obese patients.

Heart Failure

GENERAL PRINCIPLES

HF is more common and carries a worse prognosis in persons with diabetes than in persons without diabetes. The hazard ratio for HF among those with prediabetes is 1.2–1.7 in different populations; while in persons with diabetes, the HR is about 2.5. The prognosis for survival is much worse in persons with diabetes and HF compared with those without diabetes.[36]

DIAGNOSIS

HF is suspected after an ischemic event, confirmed by echocardiography or during cardiac catheterization. Diabetes affects both the structure and function of the myocardium, leading to left ventricular concentric remodeling, hypertrophy, and impaired myocardial energetics. Symptoms include reduced exercise tolerance, shortness of breath, and edema.

TREATMENT

Guidelines do not recommend a different approach to the management of HF in persons with diabetes. Metformin is considered safe in mild to moderate HF and may be associated with better outcomes. Observational trial data and post hoc analyses of randomized clinical trials testing sulfonylureas and insulin have provided conflicting results. Thiazolidinediones are known to cause fluid retention and increase the risk of HF events. The DPP-4 inhibitors have neutral CV effects overall. Saxagliptin and alogliptin had increased risk of HF in large CVOTs; however, these effects have not been seen in retrospective analyses or observational cohorts. The GLP-1 receptor agonists have had neutral to positive effects on MACE endpoints but have had neutral effects in HF patients. The SGLT2 inhibitors have had consistently positive effects on HF hospitalization, including populations with HFrEF and HFpEF. The newest

CHAPTER 23

consensus statement from the European Association for the Study of Diabetes and the ADA recommends the preferential use of a GLP-1-RA (liraglutide, semaglutide, dulaglutide) or SGLT2 inhibitor (empagliflozin, canagliflozin) with proven CV benefit in individuals with atherosclerotic CVD. If HF and CKD are prominent in individuals with or without CVD, then SGLT2 inhibitors are the recommended agents.[37]

Peripheral Vascular Disease

GENERAL PRINCIPLES

Diabetes and smoking are the strongest risk factors for PVD. In patients with diabetes, the risk of PVD is increased by age, duration of diabetes, and presence of peripheral neuropathy. PVD is a marker for systemic vascular disease involving coronary, cerebral, and renal vessels. Persons with diabetes and PVD have increased risk for subsequent MI or stroke regardless of PVD symptoms.

DIAGNOSIS

Clinical Presentation
Symptoms of PVD include intermittent claudication, rest pain, tissue loss, and gangrene, but patients with diabetes may have fewer symptoms because of concomitant neuropathy.

Physical Examination
Physical examination findings include diminished pulses, dependent rubor, pallor on elevation, absence of hair growth, dystrophic toenails, and cool, dry, fissured skin.

Diagnostic Testing
• The ankle-to-brachial index (ABI), defined as the ratio of the systolic blood pressure in the ankle divided by the systolic blood pressure at the arm, is the best initial diagnostic test. An ABI <0.9 by a handheld 5- to 10-MHz Doppler probe has a 95% sensitivity for detecting angiogram-positive PVD.
• ABI should be performed in patients with diabetes with signs or symptoms of PVD.

TREATMENT

• Risk factors should be controlled, with similar goals described for CAD.
• Antiplatelet agents such as clopidogrel (75 mg/d) have additional benefits when compared with aspirin in patients with diabetes and PVD.
• Patients with intermittent claudication could also benefit from exercise rehabilitation and cilostazol (100 mg bid). This medication is contraindicated in patients with CHF.

MISCELLANEOUS COMPLICATIONS

Erectile Dysfunction

GENERAL PRINCIPLES

Epidemiology
It is estimated that 40%–60% of men with diabetes have erectile dysfunction (ED), and the prevalence varies depending on the age of the patient and duration of diabetes.

In addition to increasing age, ED is associated with smoking, poor glycemic control, low high-density lipoprotein, neuropathy, and retinopathy.

Etiology

ED can result from nerve damage, impaired blood flow (vascular insufficiency), adverse drug effects, low testosterone, psychological factors, or a combination of these etiologies.

DIAGNOSIS

Evaluation should include assessment for hypogonadism (see Chapter 24 Endocrinology).

TREATMENT

If testosterone is low, and both PSA and prostate examination are normal, then testosterone replacement may be beneficial, and a trial of phosphodiesterase type 5 inhibitors (sildenafil, tadalafil, vardenafil) is often warranted. Macular edema should be ruled out before starting these agents.

Hypoglycemia

GENERAL PRINCIPLES

Classification

Iatrogenic factors usually account for hypoglycemia in the setting of diabetes, complicating therapy with insulin or SFUs and limiting achievement of glycemic control during intensive therapy in patients with diabetes.[38] Hypoglycemia is uncommon in patients not treated for diabetes and can be classified as fasting or postprandial hypoglycemia.

Risk Factors

Hypoglycemia resulting from too intensive diabetes management with insulin or SFU may increase the risk of mortality in older patients with CV risk factors and should be avoided.
- Risk factors for hypoglycemia during insulin or SFU treatment include skipped or insufficient meals, unaccustomed physical exertion, misguided therapy, alcohol ingestion, and drug overdose.
- Recurrent episodes of hypoglycemia impair recognition of hypoglycemic symptoms, thereby increasing the risk for severe hypoglycemia (hypoglycemia unawareness).
- Hypoglycemia unawareness results from defective glucose counterregulation with blunting of autonomic symptoms and counterregulatory hormone secretion during hypoglycemia. Seizures or coma may develop in such patients without the usual warning symptoms of hypoglycemia.

DIAGNOSIS

Clinical Presentation
- Hypoglycemia is a clinical syndrome in which low serum (or plasma) glucose levels lead to symptoms of sympathetic–adrenal activation (sweating, anxiety, tremor,

CHAPTER 23

nausea, palpitations, and tachycardia) from increased secretion of counterregulatory hormones (e.g., epinephrine).

- Neuroglycopenia occurs as the glucose levels decrease further (fatigue, dizziness, headache, visual disturbances, drowsiness, difficulty speaking, inability to concentrate, abnormal behavior, confusion, and ultimately loss of consciousness or seizures).

Differential Diagnosis

Plasma or capillary BG values should be obtained, whenever feasible, to confirm hypoglycemia.

- **Hypoglycemia in persons with diabetes**
  - Classified as level 1 (BG <70 mg/dL or 3.9 mmol/L), level 2 (BG <54 mg/dL or 3 mmol/L), or severe hypoglycemia (altered mental status, needing assistance for recovery).
  - Mitigation strategies for iatrogenic hypoglycemia include diabetes education to determine the cause of mismatched insulin doses with food intake; reduction in insulin or SFU doses; increased monitoring using SMBG; or use of CGM with alarms.
- **Evaluation of hypoglycemia in persons without diabetes**
  - In persons without diabetes, a serum glucose concentration of <60 mg/dL (3.3 mmol/L) is concerning for a hypoglycemic disorder, and further evaluation is required if the value is <55 mg/dL (3.0 mmol/L).
  - These levels are usually accompanied by symptoms of hypoglycemia. Absence of symptoms suggests the possibility of artifactual hypoglycemia. Whipple's triad includes symptoms and/or signs of hypoglycemia, a documented low plasma glucose, and resolution of symptoms with an increase in plasma glucose.
  - Detailed evaluation is usually required in a healthy appearing patient without diabetes, whereas hypoglycemia may be readily recognized as part of the underlying illness in a sick patient.
  - **Fasting hypoglycemia** in persons without diabetes can be caused by inappropriate insulin secretion (e.g., insulinoma), alcohol abuse, severe hepatic or renal insufficiency, hypopituitarism, glucocorticoid deficiency, or surreptitious injection of insulin or ingestion of an SFU.
  - These patients present with neuroglycopenic symptoms, but episodic autonomic symptoms may be present.
  - Definitive diagnosis of fasting hypoglycemia requires hourly BG monitoring during a supervised fast lasting up to 72 hours, and measurement of plasma insulin, C-peptide, proinsulin, beta-hydroxybutyrate, and SFU metabolites if hypoglycemia (<55 mg/dL [3.0 mmol/L]) is documented on a plasma glucose sample. Patients who develop hypoglycemia and have measurable plasma insulin and C-peptide levels without SFU metabolites require further evaluation for an insulinoma.
  - **Postprandial hypoglycemia** occurs 1 or more hours after meals.
  - This should be considered in patients with a history of partial gastrectomy or intestinal resection in whom recurrent symptoms develop 1–2 hours after eating. The mechanism is thought to be related to too rapid glucose absorption, resulting in a robust insulin response and altered incretin response. These symptoms should be distinguished from dumping syndrome, which is not associated with hypoglycemia and occurs in the first hour after food intake. Frequent small meals with reduced carbohydrate content may ameliorate symptoms.

TREATMENT

Isolated episodes of mild hypoglycemia may not require specific intervention in persons with diabetes. Recurrent episodes require a review of lifestyle factors; adjustments may be indicated in the content, timing, and distribution of meals, as well as medication dosage and timing. Severe hypoglycemia is an indication for supervised treatment.

- **Readily absorbable carbohydrates** (e.g., glucose and sugar-containing beverages) can be administered orally to conscious patients for rapid effect. Alternatively, milk, candy bars, fruit, cheese, and crackers may be used in some patients with mild hypoglycemia. Glucose tablets and carbohydrate supplies should be readily available to patients with DM at all times.
- **IV dextrose** is indicated for severe hypoglycemia, in patients with altered consciousness, and during restriction of oral intake. An initial bolus, 20–50 mL of 50% dextrose, should be given immediately, followed by infusion of 5% dextrose in water (D5W) (or D10W) to maintain BG levels above 100 mg/dL (5.6 mmol/L). Prolonged IV dextrose infusion and close observation are warranted in SFU overdose, in the elderly, and in patients with defective counterregulation.
- **Glucagon**, 1 mg IM (or SC), is an effective initial therapy for severe hypoglycemia in patients unable to receive oral intake or in whom an IV access cannot be secured immediately. Vomiting is a frequent side effect, and therefore, care should be taken to prevent the risk of aspiration. A glucagon kit should be available to patients with a history of severe hypoglycemia; family members and roommates should be instructed in its proper use. Glucagon is now available in an autoinjector and a nasal spray.

CHAPTER 23

PATIENT EDUCATION

- **Education** regarding etiologies of hypoglycemia, preventive measures, and appropriate adjustments to medication, diet, and exercise regimens is an essential task to be addressed during hospitalization for severe hypoglycemia.
- **Hypoglycemia unawareness** can develop in patients who are undergoing intensive diabetes therapy. These patients should be encouraged to monitor their BG levels frequently and take timely measures to correct low values (<70 mg/dL [3.9 mmol/L]). Continuous glucose monitor technology with low alert alarms helps prevent severe hypoglycemia. In patients with very tightly controlled diabetes, slight relaxation in glycemic control and scrupulous avoidance of hypoglycemia may restore the lost warning symptoms.

REFERENCES

1. Centers for Disease Control and Prevention. *National Diabetes Statistics Report.* 2020 [article online], Available from https://www.cdc.gov/diabetes/pdfs/data/statistics/national-diabetes-statistics-report.pdf:https://www.cdc.gov/diabetes/pdfs/data/statistics/national-diabetes-statistics-report.pdf
2. American Diabetes Association. 2. Classification and diagnosis of diabetes: standards of medical care in diabetes-2021. *Diabetes Care.* 2021;44:S15-S33.
3. American Diabetes Association. 10. Cardiovascular disease and risk management: standards of medical care in diabetes-2021. *Diabetes Care.* 2021;44:S125-S150.
4. American Diabetes Association. 14. Management of diabetes in pregnancy: standards of medical care in diabetes-2021. *Diabetes Care.* 2021;44:S200-S210.
5. American Diabetes Association. 3. Prevention or delay of type 2 diabetes: standards of medical care in diabetes-2021. *Diabetes Care.* 2021;44:S34-S39.
6. American Diabetes Association. 6. Glycemic targets: standards of medical care in diabetes-2021. *Diabetes Care.* 2021;44:S73-S84.

7. Garber AJ, Abrahamson MJ, Barzilay JI, et al. Consensus statement by the American Association of Clinical Endocrinologists and American College of Endocrinology on the comprehensive type 2 diabetes management algorithm - 2018 executive summary. *Endocr Pract*. 2018;24:91-120.

8. Diabetes Control and Complications Trial Research Group; Nathan DM, Genuth S, Lachin J, et al. The effect of intensive treatment of diabetes on the development and progression of long-term complications in insulin-dependent diabetes mellitus. *N Engl J Med*. 1993;329:977-986.

9. Holman RR, Paul SK, Bethel MA, et al. 10-year follow-up of intensive glucose control in type 2 diabetes. *N Engl J Med*. 2008;359:1577-1589.

10. Battelino T, Danne T, Bergenstal RM, et al. Clinical targets for continuous glucose monitoring data Interpretation: recommendations from the international consensus on time in range. *Diabetes Care*. 2019;42:1593-1603.

11. Action to Control Cardiovascular Risk in Diabetes Study Group; Gerstein HC, Miller ME, Byington RP, et al. Effects of intensive glucose lowering in type 2 diabetes. *N Engl J Med*. 2008;358:2545-2559.

12. Duckworth W, Abraira C, Moritz T, et al. Glucose control and vascular complications in veterans with type 2 diabetes. *N Engl J Med* 2009;360:129-139.

13. ACCORD Group; Patel A, MacMahon S, Chalmers J, et al. Intensive blood glucose control and vascular outcomes in patients with type 2 diabetes. *N Engl J Med*. 2008;358:2560-2572.

14. American Diabetes Association. 7. Diabetes technology: standards of medical Care in diabetes-2021. *Diabetes Care*. 2021;44:S85-S99.

15. American Diabetes Association. 5. Facilitating behavior change and well-being to improve health outcomes: standards of medical care in diabetes-2021. *Diabetes Care*. 2021;44:S53-S72.

16. Umpierrez G, Korytkowski M. Diabetic emergencies - ketoacidosis, hyperglycaemic hyperosmolar state and hypoglycaemia. *Nat Rev Endocrinol*. 2016;12:222-232.

17. American Diabetes Association. 15. Diabetes care in the hospital: standards of medical care in diabetes-2021. *Diabetes Care*. 2021;44:S211-S220.

18. Blau JE, Tella SH, Taylor SI, Rother KI. Ketoacidosis associated with SGLT2 inhibitor treatment: analysis of FAERS data. *Diabetes Metab Res Rev*. 2017;2017:33:doi:10.1002/dmrr.2924

19. Andrade-Castellanos CA, Colunga-Lozano LE, Delgado-Figueroa N, Gonzalez-Padilla DA. Subcutaneous rapid-acting insulin analogues for diabetic ketoacidosis. *Cochrane Database Syst Rev*. 2016;2016:CD011281.

20. Haas NL, Gianchandani RY, Gunnerson KJ, et al. The two-bag method for Treatment of diabetic ketoacidosis in adults. *J Emerg Med*. 2018;54:593-599.

21. Dhatariya KK, Vellanki P. Treatment of diabetic ketoacidosis (DKA)/Hyperglycemic hyperosmolar state (HHS): novel advances in the management of hyperglycemic crises (UK versus USA). *Curr Diab Rep*. 2017;17:33.

22. Diabetes Canada Clinical Practice Guidelines Expert Committee; McGibbon A, Adams L, et al. Glycemic management in adults with type 1 diabetes. *Can J Diabetes*. 2018;42(suppl 1):S80-S87.

23. Heise T, Linnebjerg H, Coutant D, et al. Ultra rapid lispro lowers postprandial glucose and more closely matches normal physiological glucose response compared to other rapid insulin analogues: a phase 1 randomized, crossover study. *Diabetes Obes Metab*. 2020;22:1789-1798

24. Weyer C, Bogardus C, Mott DM, Pratley RE. The natural history of insulin secretory dysfunction and insulin resistance in the pathogenesis of type 2 diabetes mellitus. *J Clin Invest*. 1999;104:787-794.

25. Lawrence JM, Divers J, Isom S, et al. Trends in prevalence of type 1 and type 2 diabetes in children and adolescents in the US, 2001-2017. *JAMA* 2021;326:717-727.

26. Mizukami H, Kudoh K. Diversity of pathophysiology in type 2 diabetes shown by islet pathology. *J Diabetes Investig*. Published online 2021.doi:10.1111/jdi.13679

27. American Diabetes Association. 9. Pharmacologic approaches to glycemic treatment: standards of medical care in diabetes-2021. *Diabetes Care* 2021;44:S111-S124.

28. Sattar N, Lee MMY, Kristensen SL, et al. Cardiovascular, mortality, and kidney outcomes with GLP-1 receptor agonists in patients with type 2 diabetes: a systematic review and meta-analysis of randomised trials. *Lancet Diabetes Endocrinol*. 2021;9:653-662.

29. Zelniker TA, Wiviott SD, Raz I, et al. SGLT2 inhibitors for primary and secondary prevention of cardiovascular and renal outcomes in type 2 diabetes: a systematic review and meta-analysis of cardiovascular outcome trials. *Lancet*. 2019;393:31-39.

30. Jampol LM, Glassman AR, Sun J. Evaluation and care of patients with diabetic retinopathy. *N Engl J Med*. 2020;382:1629-1637.

31. American Diabetes Association. 11. Microvascular complications and foot care: standards of medical care in diabetes-2021. *Diabetes Care*. 2021;44:S151-S167.

32. Bakris GL, Agarwal R, Anker SD, et al. Effect of finerenone on chronic kidney disease outcomes in type 2 diabetes. *N Engl J Med*. 2020;383:2219-2229.

33. Vinik AI. Clinical practice: diabetic sensory and motor neuropathy. *N Engl J Med*. 2016;374:1455-1464

34. Rawshani A, Rawshani A, Franzen S, et al. Mortality and cardiovascular disease in type 1 and type 2 diabetes. *N Engl J Med*. 2017;376:1407-1418.

35. Young LH, Wackers FJ, Chyun DA, et al. Cardiac outcomes after screening for asymptomatic coronary artery disease in patients with type 2 diabetes—the DIAD study: a randomized controlled trial. *JAMA*. 2009;301:1547-1555.
36. Lehrke M, Marx N. Diabetes mellitus and heart failure. *Am J Cardiol*. 2017;120:S37-S47.
37. Davies MJ, D'Alessio DA, Fradkin J, et al. Management of hyperglycaemia in type 2 diabetes, 2018. A consensus report by the American Diabetes Association (ADA) and the European Association for the Study of Diabetes (EASD). *Diabetologia*. 2018;61:2461-2498.
38. Seaquist ER, Anderson J, Childs B, et al. Hypoglycemia and diabetes: a report of a workgroup of the American diabetes association and the endocrine society. *Diabetes Care*. 2013;36:1384-1395.

24 Endocrine

Samantha E. Adamson, Cynthia J. Herrick,
Amy E. Riek, and William E. Clutter

Evaluation of Thyroid Function[1]

GENERAL PRINCIPLES

The major hormone secreted by the thyroid is **thyroxine (T_4),** which is converted by deiodinases in many tissues to the more potent **triiodothyronine (T_3).** Both are bound reversibly to plasma proteins, primarily **thyroxine-binding globulin.** Only the free (unbound) fraction enters cells and produces biologic effects. T_4 secretion is stimulated by **thyroid-stimulating hormone (TSH)** from the pituitary gland. In turn, TSH secretion is inhibited by T_4, forming a negative feedback loop that keeps free T_4 levels within a narrow normal range. Diagnosis of thyroid disease is based on clinical findings, palpation of the thyroid, and measurement of plasma TSH and thyroid hormones.

DIAGNOSIS

Clinical Presentation

Thyroid palpation determines the size and consistency of the thyroid and the presence of nodules, tenderness, or a thrill.

Diagnostic Testing

- **Plasma TSH** is the best initial test in most patients with suspected thyroid disease. TSH levels are elevated in very mild primary hypothyroidism and are suppressed in very mild hyperthyroidism. Thus, **a normal plasma TSH level excludes nearly all causes of hyperthyroidism,** as well as primary hypothyroidism. Because even slight changes in thyroid hormone levels affect TSH secretion, **abnormal TSH levels are not specific for clinically important thyroid disease.** Changes in plasma TSH lag behind changes in plasma T_4, and TSH levels may be misleading when plasma T_4 levels are changing rapidly, as during treatment of hyperthyroidism.
  - TSH levels may be suppressed in severe nonthyroidal illness, in mild (or subclinical) hyperthyroidism, and during treatment with dopamine or high doses of glucocorticoids. In addition, TSH levels remain suppressed for 6–8 weeks after hyperthyroidism is corrected.
  - Plasma TSH is mildly elevated (up to 20 μU/mL) in some euthyroid patients recovering from nonthyroidal illnesses and in mild (or subclinical) hypothyroidism.
  - TSH levels are usually within the reference range in secondary hypothyroidism and thus cannot be used to diagnose this rare form of hypothyroidism.
- **Plasma-free T_4** confirms the diagnosis and assesses the severity of hyperthyroidism when plasma TSH is low. It is also used to diagnose secondary hypothyroidism and adjust thyroxine therapy in patients with pituitary disease. Most laboratories measure free T_4 by immunoassay.
- **Free T_4 measured by equilibrium dialysis** is the most reliable measure of unbound T_4, but results are seldom rapidly available. It is needed only in rare cases in which the diagnosis is not clear from measurement of plasma TSH and free T_4 by immunoassay.

- **Effect of nonthyroidal illness on thyroid function tests:** Many illnesses alter thyroid tests without causing true thyroid dysfunction (the nonthyroidal illness or euthyroid sick syndrome). These changes must be recognized to avoid mistaken diagnosis.
  - **Low T_3** occurs in many illnesses, during starvation, and after trauma or surgery. Conversion of T_4 to T_3 is decreased, and plasma T_3 levels are low. Plasma-free T_4 and TSH levels are normal. This may be an adaptive response to illness, and thyroid hormone therapy is not beneficial.
  - **Low T_4** occurs in severe illness. TSH levels decrease early in severe illness, sometimes to <0.1 μU/mL. In prolonged illness, free T_4 may also fall below normal. During recovery, TSH rises, sometimes to levels slightly above the normal range (rarely >20 μU/mL).
  - Some drugs affect thyroid function tests (see Table 24-1). Iodine-containing drugs (**amiodarone** and radiographic contrast media) and immune modulators

TABLE 24-1	Effects of Drugs on Thyroid Function Tests
Effect	**Drug**
Decreased free and total T_4	
True hypothyroidism (TSH elevated)	Iodine (amiodarone, radiographic contrast)
	Lithium
	Some tyrosine kinase inhibitors
	Some immune modulators (e.g., interferon-α, checkpoint inhibitors)
Inhibition of TSH secretion	Glucocorticoids
	Dopamine
Multiple mechanisms (TSH normal)	Phenytoin
Decreased total T_4 only	
Decreased TBG (TSH normal)	Androgens
Inhibition of T_4 binding to TBG (TSH normal)	Furosemide (high doses)
	Salicylates
Increased free and total T_4	
True hyperthyroidism (TSH <0.1 μU/mL)	Iodine (amiodarone, radiographic contrast)
	Some immune modulators (e.g., interferon-α, checkpoint inhibitors)
Inhibited T_4 to T_3 conversion (TSH normal)	Amiodarone
Increased free T_4 only	
Displacement of T_4 from TBG in vitro (TSH normal)	Heparin, low-molecular-weight heparin
Increased total T_4 only	
Increased TBG (TSH normal)	Estrogens, tamoxifen, raloxifene
Variable effect	
Interferes with immunoassays causing lab artifact (no effect on actual thyroid levels)	Biotin

T_3, triiodothyronine; T_4, thyroxine; TBG, thyroxine-binding globulin; TSH, thyroid-stimulating hormone.

CHAPTER 24

may cause hyperthyroidism or hypothyroidism in susceptible patients. In general, plasma TSH levels are a reliable guide to whether true hyperthyroidism or hypothyroidism is present.

- Biotin, commonly taken as an over-the-counter supplement, can interfere with immunoassays for TSH, free T4, and/or free T3 at high concentrations. It has a short half-life and should be held for 1–2 days before laboratory testing.

Hypothyroidism[2-4]

GENERAL PRINCIPLES

- **Primary hypothyroidism** (due to disease of the thyroid itself) accounts for >90% of cases.
- **Chronic lymphocytic thyroiditis (Hashimoto disease)** is the most common cause in developed nations and may be associated with Addison disease and other endocrine deficits. Its prevalence is greater in women and increases with age.
- **Iatrogenic hypothyroidism** due to thyroidectomy or radioactive iodine (RAI; iodine-131) therapy is also common.
- Transient hypothyroidism occurs in postpartum (painless) thyroiditis and subacute thyroiditis, usually after a period of hyperthyroidism.
- **Drugs that may cause hypothyroidism** include iodine-containing drugs, lithium, interferon (IFN)-α, IFN-β, interleukin-2, thalidomide, bexarotene, sunitinib, amiodarone, and checkpoint inhibitors.
- Secondary hypothyroidism due to TSH deficiency is uncommon but may occur in any disorder of the pituitary or hypothalamus. However, it rarely occurs without other evidence of pituitary disease.

DIAGNOSIS

Clinical Presentation

History

Most symptoms of hypothyroidism are nonspecific and develop gradually. They include cold intolerance, fatigue, somnolence, poor memory, constipation, menorrhagia, myalgias, and hoarseness. Hypothyroidism is readily treatable and should be suspected in any patient with compatible symptoms.

Physical Examination

Signs include slow tendon reflex relaxation, bradycardia, facial and periorbital edema, dry skin, and nonpitting edema (myxedema). Mild weight gain may occur, but hypothyroidism does not cause marked obesity. Rare manifestations include hypoventilation, pericardial or pleural effusions, deafness, and carpal tunnel syndrome.

Diagnostic Testing

- Laboratory findings may include hyponatremia and elevated plasma levels of cholesterol, triglycerides, and creatine kinase.
- In suspected primary hypothyroidism, plasma TSH is the best initial test.
  - A normal value excludes primary hypothyroidism, and a markedly elevated value (>20 μU/mL) confirms the diagnosis.

○ Mild elevation of plasma TSH (<20 μU/mL) may be because of recovery from nonthyroidal illness, but it usually indicates mild (or subclinical) primary hypothyroidism, in which thyroid function is impaired but increased secretion of TSH maintains normal plasma-free T_4 levels. These patients may have nonspecific symptoms that are compatible with hypothyroidism and a mild increase in serum cholesterol and low-density lipoprotein cholesterol. They develop clinical hypothyroidism at a rate of 2.5% per year.

• Antibodies against thyroid peroxidase and thyroglobulin are very common and should prompt evaluation for hypothyroidism. However, they do not change the management of hypothyroidism and therefore need not be typically measured.

• If secondary hypothyroidism is suspected because of evidence of pituitary disease, plasma-free T_4 should be measured. Plasma TSH levels are usually within the reference range in secondary hypothyroidism and cannot be used alone to make this diagnosis. Patients with secondary hypothyroidism should be evaluated for other pituitary hormone deficits and for a mass lesion of the pituitary or hypothalamus (see "Pituitary Adenomas and Hypopituitarism" section).

• **In severe nonthyroidal illness,** the diagnosis of hypothyroidism can be difficult. Plasma-free T_4 measured by routine assays may be low.

○ **Plasma TSH is the best initial diagnostic test.** A normal TSH value is strong evidence that the patient is euthyroid, except when there is evidence of pituitary or hypothalamic disease or in patients treated with dopamine or high doses of glucocorticoids. Marked elevation of plasma TSH (>20 μU/mL) establishes the diagnosis of primary hypothyroidism.

○ Moderate elevations of plasma TSH (<20 μU/mL) may occur in euthyroid patients recovering from nonthyroidal illness and are not specific for hypothyroidism. Plasma-free T_4 should be measured if TSH is moderately elevated or if secondary hypothyroidism is suspected, and patients should be treated for hypothyroidism if plasma-free T_4 is low. Thyroid function in these patients should be reevaluated after recovery from illness.

TREATMENT

• **Thyroxine** is the drug of choice. The average replacement dose is 1.6 μg/kg PO daily, and most patients require doses between 75 and 150 μg/d. In elderly patients, the average replacement dose is lower. The need for lifelong treatment should be emphasized. Thyroxine should be taken 30 minutes before a meal, because some foods interfere with its absorption, and should not be taken with other medications.

• **Initiation of therapy:** Young and middle-aged adults should be started on 1.6 μg/kg/d. This regimen gradually corrects hypothyroidism because several weeks are required to reach steady-state plasma levels of T_4. In otherwise healthy elderly patients, the initial dose should be 50 μg/d. Patients with cardiac disease should be started on 25 μg/d and monitored carefully for exacerbation of cardiac symptoms.

• **Dose adjustment and follow-up**

○ **In primary hypothyroidism, the goal of therapy is to maintain plasma TSH within the normal range.** Plasma TSH should be measured 6–8 weeks after initiation of therapy. The dose of thyroxine should then be adjusted in 12- to 25-μg increments at intervals of 6–8 weeks until plasma TSH is normal. Thereafter, annual TSH measurement is adequate to monitor therapy. TSH should also be measured in the first trimester of pregnancy because the thyroxine dose requirement often increases at this time (see "Special Considerations" section, below). Overtreatment, indicated by a subnormal TSH, should be avoided because it increases the risk of osteoporosis and atrial fibrillation.

○ **In secondary hypothyroidism, plasma TSH cannot be used to adjust therapy.** The goal of therapy is to maintain the **plasma-free T$_4$** in the upper half of the reference range. The dose of thyroxine should be adjusted at 6- to 8-week intervals until this goal is achieved. Thereafter, annual measurement of plasma-free T$_4$ is adequate to monitor therapy.

SPECIAL CONSIDERATIONS

- **Situations in which thyroxine dose requirements change:** Difficulty in controlling hypothyroidism is most often because of **poor compliance** with therapy. Other causes of increasing thyroxine requirement include the following:
  ○ Malabsorption because of intestinal disease or drugs that interfere with thyroxine absorption (e.g., calcium carbonate, ferrous sulfate, cholestyramine, sucralfate, aluminum hydroxide)
  ○ Drug interactions that increase thyroxine clearance (e.g., estrogen, rifampin, carbamazepine, phenytoin) or block conversion of T$_4$ to T$_3$ (amiodarone)
  ○ Gradual failure of remaining endogenous thyroid function after RAI treatment of hyperthyroidism
- **Pregnancy:** Thyroxine dose increases by an average of 40%–50% in the first half of pregnancy. In women with primary hypothyroidism, plasma TSH should be measured as soon as pregnancy is confirmed and monthly thereafter through the second trimester. The thyroxine dose should be increased as needed to maintain plasma TSH < 2.5 μU/mL to avoid fetal hypothyroidism.
- **Subclinical hypothyroidism** should be treated if any of the following are present: (1) symptoms compatible with hypothyroidism, (2) goiter, (3) hypercholesterolemia that warrants treatment, or (4) plasma TSH >10 μU/mL. Untreated patients should be monitored annually, and thyroxine should be started if symptoms develop or serum TSH increases to >10 μU/mL.
- **Urgent therapy** for hypothyroidism is rarely necessary. Most patients with hypothyroidism and concomitant illness can be treated in the usual manner. However, hypothyroidism may impair survival in critical illness by contributing to hypoventilation, hypotension, hypothermia, bradycardia, or hyponatremia.
  ○ Hypoventilation and hypotension should be treated intensively, along with any concomitant diseases. Confirmatory tests (plasma TSH and free T$_4$) should be obtained before thyroid hormone therapy is started.
  ○ **Thyroxine, 50–100 μg IV, can be given q6–8h for 24 hours**, followed by 75–100 μg IV daily until oral intake is possible. No clinical trials have determined the optimum method of thyroid hormone replacement, but this method rapidly alleviates hypothyroidism while minimizing the risk of exacerbating underlying coronary disease or heart failure. **Rapid correction is warranted only in extremely ill patients.** Vital signs and cardiac rhythm should be monitored carefully to detect early signs of exacerbation of heart disease. Hydrocortisone, 50 mg IV q8h, is recommended during rapid replacement of thyroid hormone because this therapy may precipitate adrenal crisis in patients with adrenal failure.

Hyperthyroidism[4,5]

GENERAL PRINCIPLES

- **Graves disease** causes most cases of hyperthyroidism, especially in young patients. This **autoimmune** disorder may also cause **proptosis** (Graves orbitopathy) and pretibial myxedema, neither of which is found in other causes of hyperthyroidism.
- **Toxic multinodular goiter (MNG)** may cause hyperthyroidism, more commonly in older patients.
- Unusual causes include **iodine-induced hyperthyroidism** (precipitated by drugs such as **amiodarone** or radiographic contrast media), thyroid adenomas, subacute thyroiditis (painful tender goiter with transient hyperthyroidism), painless thyroiditis (nontender goiter with transient hyperthyroidism, most often seen in the postpartum period), and surreptitious ingestion of thyroid hormone. TSH-induced hyperthyroidism is extremely rare.

DIAGNOSIS

Clinical Presentation

History
- Symptoms include heat intolerance, weight loss, weakness, palpitations, oligomenorrhea, and anxiety.
- **In the elderly,** hyperthyroidism may present with only atrial fibrillation, heart failure, weakness, or weight loss, and a high index of suspicion is needed to make the diagnosis.

Physical Examination
- Signs include brisk tendon reflexes, fine tremor, proximal weakness, stare (related to eyelid retraction), and eyelid lag. Cardiac abnormalities may be prominent, including sinus tachycardia, atrial fibrillation, and exacerbation of coronary artery disease or heart failure.
- Key differentiating physical examination findings (Table 24-2) include the following:
  ○ The presence of proptosis or pretibial myxedema, seen only in Graves disease (although many patients with Graves disease lack these signs)
  ○ A diffuse nontender goiter, consistent with Graves disease or painless thyroiditis
  ○ Recent pregnancy, neck pain, or recent iodine administration, suggesting causes other than Graves disease.

TABLE 24-2	Differential Diagnosis of Hyperthyroidism
Type of Goiter	**Diagnosis**
Diffuse, nontender goiter	Graves disease or painless thyroiditis
Multiple thyroid nodules	Toxic multinodular goiter
Single thyroid nodule	Thyroid adenoma
Tender painful goiter	Subacute thyroiditis
Normal thyroid gland	Graves disease, painless thyroiditis, or factitious hyperthyroidism

CHAPTER 24

Diagnostic Testing

* In suspected hyperthyroidism, plasma TSH is the best initial diagnostic test.
  * A normal TSH level virtually excludes clinical hyperthyroidism. If plasma TSH is low, **plasma-free T$_4$** should be measured to determine the severity of hyperthyroidism and as a baseline for therapy. If plasma-free T$_4$ is elevated, the diagnosis of clinical hyperthyroidism is established.
  * **If plasma TSH is <0.1 µU/mL but free T$_4$ is normal,** the patient may have clinical hyperthyroidism because of elevation of plasma T$_3$ alone, and plasma-free T$_3$ should be measured in this case.
  * **Mild (or subclinical) hyperthyroidism** may suppress TSH to <0.1 µU/mL, and thus suppression of TSH alone does not confirm that symptoms are due to hyperthyroidism.
  * TSH may also be suppressed by **severe nonthyroidal illness** (see "Evaluation of Thyroid Function" section).
  * In rare cases, **24-hour radioactive iodine uptake (RAIU)** is needed to distinguish Graves disease or toxic nodules (in which RAIU is elevated) from postpartum thyroiditis, iodine-induced hyperthyroidism, or factitious hyperthyroidism (in which RAIU is very low).

TREATMENT

* Some forms of hyperthyroidism (subacute or postpartum thyroiditis) are transient and require only **symptomatic therapy**. A **β-adrenergic antagonist** (such as **atenolol** 25–100 mg daily) relieves symptoms of hyperthyroidism, such as palpitations, tremor, and anxiety, until hyperthyroidism is controlled by definitive therapy or until transient forms of hyperthyroidism subside. The dose is adjusted to alleviate symptoms and tachycardia and then reduced gradually as hyperthyroidism is controlled.
* Three methods are available for definitive therapy (none of which control hyperthyroidism rapidly): RAI, thionamides, and thyroidectomy.
  * During treatment, patients are followed by clinical evaluation and measurement of plasma-free T$_4$. Plasma TSH is not helpful in assessing the initial response to therapy because it remains suppressed until after the patient becomes euthyroid.
  * Regardless of the therapy used, all patients with Graves disease require lifelong follow-up for recurrent hyperthyroidism or development of hypothyroidism.
* **Choice of definitive therapy**
  * **In Graves disease, RAI therapy is our preferred treatment for almost all patients.** It is simple and highly effective but **cannot be used in pregnancy** (see "Hyperthyroidism" section). Thionamides achieve long-term control in fewer than half of patients with Graves disease, and they carry a small risk of life-threatening side effects (agranulocytosis, liver dysfunction). Thyroidectomy may be used in patients who refuse RAI therapy, have significant Graves ophthalmopathy, or who relapse or develop side effects with thionamide therapy.
  * **Other causes of hyperthyroidism:** We prefer to treat toxic nodules with RAI (except in pregnancy or during breastfeeding), though thionamides or partial thyroidectomy can also be used. Transient forms of hyperthyroidism because of thyroiditis should be treated symptomatically with atenolol. Iodine-induced hyperthyroidism is treated with thionamides and atenolol until the patient is euthyroid. Although treatment of some patients with amiodarone-induced hyperthyroidism with glucocorticoids has been advocated, **nearly all patients with amiodarone-induced hyperthyroidism respond well to thionamide therapy.**

- **RAI therapy**
  - A single dose permanently controls hyperthyroidism in 90% of patients, and further doses can be given if necessary.
  - A **pregnancy test** is done immediately before therapy in potentially fertile women.
  - A 24-hour RAIU is usually measured and used to calculate the dose.
  - Thionamides interfere with RAI therapy and should be stopped at least 3 days before treatment. If iodine treatment has been given, it should be stopped at least 2 weeks before RAI therapy.
  - **Follow-up:** Usually, several months are needed to restore euthyroidism. Patients are evaluated at 4- to 6-week intervals, with assessment of clinical findings and plasma-free T_4.
    - If thyroid function stabilizes within the normal range, the interval between follow-up visits is gradually increased to annual intervals.
    - If symptomatic hypothyroidism develops, thyroxine therapy is started (see "Hypothyroidism" section).
    - If symptomatic hyperthyroidism persists after 6 months, RAI treatment can be repeated.
  - Side effects
    - **Hypothyroidism** occurs in most patients within the first year and thereafter continues to develop at a rate of approximately 3% per year.
    - Because of the release of stored hormone, a slight rise in plasma T_4 may occur in the first 2 weeks after therapy. This development is important only in **patients with severe cardiac disease**, which may worsen as a result. Such patients should be treated with thionamides to restore euthyroidism and to deplete stored hormone before treatment with RAI.
    - There have been mixed results as to whether RAI has a clinically important effect on the course of Graves eye disease, but early treatment to prevent hypothyroidism after RAI seems to be beneficial. Patients should also be counseled to stop smoking, as this is a known contributor to worsening of the eye disease. Patients with clinical evidence of Graves orbitopathy should be evaluated by an ophthalmologist before treatment with RAI. Sometimes glucocorticoids or teprotumumab, an insulin-like growth factor 1 receptor antibody, is utilized in the treatment of Graves orbitopathy.
    - This treatment does not increase the risk of malignancy or cause congenital abnormalities in the offspring of women who conceive after RAI therapy.
- **Thionamides:** Methimazole and propylthiouracil (PTU) inhibit thyroid hormone synthesis. PTU also inhibits extrathyroidal deiodination of T_4 to T_3. Once thyroid hormone stores are depleted (after several weeks to months), T_4 levels decrease. These drugs have no permanent effect on thyroid function. **In the majority of patients with Graves disease, hyperthyroidism recurs within 6 months after therapy is stopped.** Spontaneous remission of Graves disease occurs in approximately one-third of patients during thionamide therapy, and in this minority, no other treatment may be needed. Remission is more likely in mild, recent onset hyperthyroidism and if the goiter is small. Because of a better safety profile, **methimazole should be used instead of PTU** except in specific situations (see the following text).
  - **Initiation of therapy:** Before starting therapy, patients must be warned of side effects and precautions. Usual starting doses are methimazole, 10–40 mg PO daily, or PTU, 100–200 mg PO tid; higher initial doses can be used in severe hyperthyroidism.

CHAPTER 24

- ○ **Follow-up:** Restoration of euthyroidism takes up to several months.
  - Patients are evaluated at 4-week intervals with assessment of clinical findings and plasma-free T_4. If plasma-free T_4 levels do not fall after 4–8 weeks, the dose should be increased. Doses as high as methimazole, 60 mg PO daily, or PTU, 300 mg PO qid, may be required.
  - Once the plasma-free T_4 level falls to normal, the dose is adjusted to maintain plasma-free T_4 within the normal range.
  - No consensus exists on the optimal duration of therapy, but periods of 6 months to 2 years are usually used. Patients must be monitored carefully for recurrence of hyperthyroidism after the drug is stopped.
- ○ **Side effects** are most likely to occur within the first few months of therapy.
  - Minor side effects include rash, urticaria, fever, arthralgias, and transient leukopenia.
  - **Agranulocytosis** occurs in 0.3% of patients treated with thionamides. Other life-threatening side effects include **hepatitis**, vasculitis, and drug-induced lupus erythematosus. These complications usually resolve if the drug is stopped promptly.
  - **Patients must be warned to stop the drug immediately if jaundice or symptoms suggestive of agranulocytosis develop (e.g., fever, chills, sore throat)** and to contact their physician promptly for evaluation. Routine monitoring of the white blood cell count is not useful for detecting agranulocytosis, which develops suddenly.
- **Thyroidectomy:** This procedure provides long-term control of hyperthyroidism in most patients.
  - ○ Surgery may trigger a perioperative exacerbation of hyperthyroidism, and patients should be prepared for surgery by one of two methods.
  - ○ **A thionamide** is given until the patient is nearly euthyroid. **Supersaturated potassium iodide (SSKI)**, 40–80 mg (one to two drops) PO bid, is then added 1–2 weeks before surgery. Both drugs are stopped postoperatively.
  - ○ **Atenolol** (50–100 mg daily) is started 1–2 weeks before surgery. The dose of atenolol is increased, if necessary, to reduce the resting heart rate below 90 bpm and is continued for 5–7 days postoperatively. SSKI is given as mentioned earlier.
  - ○ Patients should be started on thyroxine replacement after surgery, and plasma TSH and free T4 should be measured 6 weeks later.
  - ○ **Complications** of thyroidectomy include **hypothyroidism** and **hypoparathyroidism.** Rare complications include permanent vocal cord paralysis, due to recurrent laryngeal nerve injury, and perioperative death.

SPECIAL CONSIDERATIONS

- **Subclinical hyperthyroidism** is present when the plasma TSH is below normal but the patient has no symptoms that are definitely caused by hyperthyroidism, and plasma levels of free T_4 and T_3 are normal.
  - ○ Subclinical hyperthyroidism increases the risk of **atrial fibrillation** in patients older than 65 years and those with heart disease and predisposes to **osteoporosis** in postmenopausal women; it should be treated in these patients. Treatment should also be considered in asymptomatic individuals without risk factors but with TSH persistently <0.1 µU/mL.
  - ○ Asymptomatic young patients with mild Graves disease can be observed for spontaneous resolution of hyperthyroidism or the development of symptoms or increasing free T_4 levels that warrant treatment.

- **Urgent therapy** is warranted when hyperthyroidism exacerbates heart failure or acute coronary syndromes and in rare patients with severe hyperthyroidism complicated by fever and delirium (thyroid storm). Concomitant diseases should be treated intensively, and confirmatory tests (serum TSH and free T_4) should be obtained before therapy is started.
  - **PTU 300 mg PO q6h or methimazole 60 mg/d PO** should be started immediately.
  - **Iodide (SSKI**, two drops PO q12h) should be started to inhibit thyroid hormone secretion rapidly.
  - **Propranolol**, 40 mg PO q6h (or an equivalent dose IV), should be given to patients with angina or myocardial infarction, and the dose should be adjusted to prevent tachycardia. β-Adrenergic antagonists may benefit some patients with heart failure and marked tachycardia but can further impair left ventricular systolic function. In patients with clinical heart failure, it should be given only with careful monitoring of left ventricular function.
  - Plasma-free T_4 is measured every 4–6 days. When free T_4 approaches the normal range, the doses of methimazole and iodine are gradually decreased. RAI therapy can be scheduled 2–4 weeks after iodine is stopped.
- **Hyperthyroidism in pregnancy:** If hyperthyroidism is suspected, plasma TSH should be measured. Plasma TSH declines in early pregnancy but rarely to <0.1 µU/mL due to the stimulatory effect of human chorionic gonadotropin on TSH receptors.
  - If TSH is <0.1 µU/mL, the diagnosis should be confirmed by measurement of plasma-free T_4.
  - RAI is contraindicated in pregnancy, and therefore, patients should be treated with **PTU in the first trimester** because of its lower risk of severe congenital defects, whereas **methimazole can be used in later pregnancy.** The dose should be adjusted at 4-week intervals to maintain the plasma-free T_4 near the upper limit of the normal range to avoid fetal hypothyroidism. The dose required often decreases in the later stages of pregnancy.
  - **Atenolol, 25–50 mg PO daily,** can be used to relieve symptoms while awaiting the effects of PTU.
  - The fetus and neonate should be monitored for hyperthyroidism. The **maternal plasma level of thyroid receptor antibodies** should be assessed in early pregnancy, and if elevated or if the patient requires thionamide treatment during pregnancy, it should be repeated at weeks 18–22 and again at weeks 30–34 to assess this risk.

Goiter, Thyroid Nodules, and Thyroid Carcinoma[6,7]

GENERAL PRINCIPLES

- The evaluation of goiter is based on palpation of the thyroid and evaluation of thyroid function. If the thyroid is enlarged, the examiner should determine whether the enlargement is **diffuse or nodular.** Both forms of goiter are common, especially in women.
- Thyroid scans and ultrasonography do not provide additional useful information about goiters that are diffuse by palpation and should not be performed in these patients. In contrast, all palpable thyroid nodules should be evaluated by ultrasonography.

CHAPTER 24

- In rare patients, more commonly in those with MNG, the gland compresses the trachea or esophagus and causes dyspnea or dysphagia, necessitating treatment. Thyroxine treatment has little, if any, effect on the size of MNGs. Subtotal thyroidectomy is most commonly used to relieve compressive symptoms. RAI therapy will reduce gland size and relieve symptoms in most patients if surgery is not an option, though much higher doses are necessary if the patient is euthyroid.
- **Diffuse goiter**
  - Almost all euthyroid diffuse goiters in the US are due to **chronic lymphocytic thyroiditis (Hashimoto thyroiditis).** This diagnosis can be confirmed by measurement of antithyroid peroxidase antibodies. Because Hashimoto thyroiditis may also cause hypothyroidism, plasma TSH should be measured.
  - Diffuse euthyroid goiters are usually asymptomatic, and therapy is seldom required. Patients should be monitored regularly for the development of hypothyroidism.
  - Diffuse hyperthyroid goiter is most commonly because of Graves disease, and treatment of the hyperthyroidism usually improves the goiter (see "Hyperthyroidism" section).
- **Nodular goiter**
  - Between 30% and 50% of people have nonpalpable thyroid nodules that are detectable by ultrasound. These nodules rarely have any clinical importance, but their incidental discovery may lead to unnecessary diagnostic testing and treatment.
  - Nodules are more common in older patients, especially women, and 5%–10% of thyroid nodules are thyroid carcinomas.

DIAGNOSIS

Clinical Presentation
History
Clinical findings that increase the risk of carcinoma include the presence of cervical lymphadenopathy, a history of radiation to the head or neck, and a family history of medullary thyroid carcinoma or multiple endocrine neoplasia syndromes type 2A or 2B.

Physical Examination
A hard, fixed nodule, recent nodule growth, or hoarseness due to vocal cord paralysis suggests malignancy.

Diagnostic Testing
- All patients with one or more palpable thyroid nodules on examination or thyroid nodules identified by other imaging modality should undergo a dedicated **thyroid ultrasound** as this is the most informative imaging for malignancy risk in thyroid nodules.
- Guidelines from the American Thyroid Association classify malignancy risk and biopsy recommendations based on nodule characteristics and size.
  - Nodules are characterized into the following risk classes based on their ultrasound appearance: high suspicion (>70%–90% malignancy risk), intermediate suspicion (10%–20% malignancy risk), low suspicion (5%–10% malignancy risk), very low suspicion (<3% malignancy risk), and benign (<1% malignancy risk).
  - High and intermediate suspicion nodules warrant evaluation by fine needle aspiration (FNA) when they are >1 cm. Low suspicion nodules should be evaluated at >1.5 cm and very low risk nodules at 2 cm. Benign nodules require no further follow-up.

○ In a few patients, **hyperthyroidism** develops as a result of "toxic" nodules that overproduce thyroid hormone (see "Hyperthyroidism" section). These nodules can be identified with a radionuclide scan and do not require FNA evaluation as the malignancy risk is only 1%–2%.

TREATMENT

Patients with thyroid carcinoma or suspicion for thyroid carcinoma by FNA cytology typically initially undergo surgical resection with either **hemi- or total thyroidectomy**, sometimes followed by **adjuvant therapy with RAI,** and should be managed in consultation with an endocrinologist.

FOLLOW-UP

- **Further follow-up depends on FNA results.** Benign nodules should undergo repeat ultrasound depending on initial ultrasound risk: high risk in 6–12 months and low intermediate in 12–24 months. The utility of following very low-risk nodules is unclear. Nodules with benign cytology should also be reevaluated periodically by palpation. Thyroxine therapy has little or no effect on the size of thyroid nodules and is not indicated.
- Nodules with **nondiagnostic cytology** because of insufficient sampling should undergo **repeat biopsy.**
- The management of thyroid nodules with **indeterminate cytology** is less clear. Nodules with atypia of undetermined significance or follicular lesion by cytology can be further evaluated with **molecular diagnostic testing** to estimate risk and guide surgical decision-making.

Adrenal Failure[8,9]

GENERAL PRINCIPLES

- Adrenal failure may be due to disease of the adrenal glands **(primary adrenal failure, Addison disease)**, with deficiency of both cortisol and aldosterone and elevated plasma adrenocorticotropic hormone (ACTH), or due to ACTH deficiency caused by disorders of the pituitary or hypothalamus **(secondary adrenal failure)**, with deficiency of cortisol alone.
- **Primary adrenal failure** is most often due to **autoimmune adrenalitis**, which may be associated with other endocrine deficits (e.g., hypothyroidism).
- Adrenal failure may also develop in patients with infiltrative or infectious diseases of the adrenal glands, such as adrenal lymphoma, metastases, disseminated cytomegalovirus, mycobacterial infection, or fungal infection. Some of the causative infections are more common in immunosuppressed individuals.
- **Hemorrhagic adrenal infarction** may occur in the postoperative period, in coagulation disorders and hypercoagulable states, and in sepsis. Adrenal hemorrhage often causes abdominal or flank pain and fever; CT scan of the abdomen reveals high-density bilateral adrenal masses.
- Less common etiologies include adrenoleukodystrophy that causes adrenal failure in young men and drugs such as ketoconazole and etomidate that inhibit steroid hormone synthesis.

CHAPTER 24

- **Secondary adrenal failure** is most often due to **glucocorticoid therapy.** Any patient who has been treated with greater than physiologic replacement doses of glucocorticoids for more than a few months should be considered to have secondary adrenal failure until proven otherwise. This can be investigated by tapering to a physiologic steroid dose and then performing a cosyntropin stimulation test. ACTH suppression may persist for a year after therapy is stopped. Any disorder of the pituitary or hypothalamus can cause ACTH deficiency, but other evidence of these disorders is usually obvious.
- **Checkpoint inhibitors** commonly used for immunotherapy to treat various cancers can cause hypophysitis or, less commonly, adrenalitis, potentially leading to secondary or primary adrenal failure, respectively.

DIAGNOSIS

Clinical Presentation

- Adrenal failure should be suspected in patients with otherwise unexplained hypotension, weight loss, persistent nausea, hyponatremia, hyperkalemia, or hypoglycemia.
- **Clinical findings** in adrenal failure are nonspecific, and without a high index of suspicion, the diagnosis of this potentially lethal but readily treatable disease is easily missed.
  - Symptoms include anorexia, nausea, vomiting, weight loss, weakness, and fatigue. Orthostatic hypotension and hyponatremia are common.
  - Symptoms are usually chronic, but **shock** may develop suddenly and is fatal unless promptly treated. Often, this adrenal crisis is triggered by illness, injury, or surgery. All these symptoms are due to cortisol deficiency and occur in both primary and secondary adrenal failure.
- Hyperpigmentation (because of marked ACTH excess) and hyperkalemia and volume depletion (because of aldosterone deficiency) occur only in primary adrenal failure.

Diagnostic Testing

- The **cosyntropin (Cortrosyn) stimulation test** is used for diagnosis. Cosyntropin, 250 μg, is given IV or IM, and **plasma cortisol is measured 30 and 60 minutes later.** The normal response is a stimulated plasma cortisol >18 μg/dL. Newer monoclonal antibody immune assays or liquid chromatography–mass spectrometry (LC-MS)/MS assays are more specific for cortisol, so a stimulated cortisol of 14–15 mg/dL is normal with these assays. This test detects primary and secondary adrenal failure, except within a few weeks of onset of pituitary dysfunction (e.g., shortly after pituitary surgery; see "Pituitary Adenomas and Hypopituitarism" section). Note that plasma cortisol is protein bound, and in situations where patients have very low albumin levels, cortisol levels may appear falsely low; thus, cosyntropin stimulation tests in these patients should be interpreted with caution.
- The clinical presentation usually helps to distinguish between primary and secondary adrenal failure. Hyperkalemia, hyperpigmentation, or other autoimmune endocrine deficits are more suggestive of primary adrenal failure, whereas deficits of other pituitary hormones, symptoms of a pituitary mass (e.g., headache, visual field loss), or known pituitary or hypothalamic disease are more suggestive secondary adrenal failure.

- If the cause is unclear, the **plasma ACTH** level distinguishes primary adrenal failure (in which it is markedly elevated) from secondary adrenal failure. **High renin and low aldosterone levels** are suggestive of primary adrenal insufficiency.
- Most cases of primary adrenal failure are due to autoimmune adrenalitis, but other causes should be considered. Radiographic evidence of adrenal enlargement or calcification indicates that the cause is infection or hemorrhage.
- Patients with secondary adrenal failure should be tested for other pituitary hormone deficiencies and should be evaluated for a pituitary or hypothalamic tumor (see "Pituitary Adenomas and Hypopituitarism" section).

TREATMENT

- **Adrenal crisis** with hypotension must be treated immediately. Patients should be evaluated for an underlying illness that precipitated the crisis.
- **If the diagnosis of adrenal failure is known, hydrocortisone, 100 mg IV q8h,** should be given, and **0.9% saline with 5% dextrose** should be infused rapidly until hypotension is corrected. The dose of hydrocortisone is decreased gradually over several days as symptoms and any precipitating illness resolve and then changed to oral maintenance therapy. Mineralocorticoid replacement is not needed until the dose of hydrocortisone is <100 mg/d.
- **If the diagnosis of adrenal failure has not been established,** a single dose of **dexamethasone**, 10 mg IV, should be given, and a rapid infusion of 0.9% saline with 5% dextrose should be started. A **Cortrosyn stimulation test** should be performed, regardless of the time of day. Dexamethasone is used because it does not interfere with measurement of plasma cortisol. After the Cortrosyn stimulation test is complete, hydrocortisone, 100 mg IV q8h, should be given until the test result is known.
- High-dose hydrocortisone provides sufficient mineralocorticoid activity to cover for suspected primary adrenal insufficiency until diagnosis is clarified.
- **Maintenance therapy** in all patients requires cortisol replacement with prednisone or hydrocortisone. Most patients with primary adrenal failure also require replacement of aldosterone with fludrocortisone.
  - **Prednisone,** 5 mg PO every morning, or hydrocortisone 10 mg Qam and 5 mg Qpm should be started. The dose is then adjusted with the goal being the lowest dose that relieves the patient's symptoms, to prevent osteoporosis and other signs of Cushing syndrome. Most patients require doses between 4.0 and 7.5 mg PO daily. Concomitant therapy with rifampin, phenytoin, or phenobarbital accelerates glucocorticoid metabolism and increases the dose requirement.
  - **During illness, injury, or the perioperative period, the dose of glucocorticoid must be increased.** For minor illnesses, the patient should double the dose of prednisone for 2–3 days. If the illness resolves, the maintenance dose is resumed.
  - **Vomiting requires immediate medical attention,** with IV glucocorticoid therapy and IV fluid. Patients can be given a 4-mg vial of dexamethasone to be self-administered IM for vomiting or severe illness if medical care is not immediately available.
  - **For severe illness or injury,** hydrocortisone, 50 mg IV q8h, should be given, with the dose tapered as severity of illness wanes. The same regimen is used in patients undergoing surgery, with the first dose of hydrocortisone given preoperatively. The dose can be tapered to maintenance therapy by 2–3 days after uncomplicated surgery.

CHAPTER 24

- **In primary adrenal failure, fludrocortisone, 0.1 mg PO daily,** should be given. The dose is adjusted to maintain blood pressure (supine and standing) and serum potassium within the normal range; the usual dosage is 0.05–0.20 mg PO daily.
- Patients should be educated in management of their disease, including adjustment of prednisone dose during illness. They should also wear a medical identification tag or bracelet.

Cushing Syndrome[10]

GENERAL PRINCIPLES

- Cushing syndrome is most often **iatrogenic** because of glucocorticoid therapy.
- **ACTH-secreting pituitary microadenomas (Cushing disease)** account for 80% of cases of endogenous Cushing syndrome.
- Adrenal tumors and ectopic ACTH secretion account for the remainder.

DIAGNOSIS

Clinical Presentation

- Findings include truncal obesity, rounded face, fat deposits in the supraclavicular fossae and over the posterior neck, hypertension, hirsutism, amenorrhea, and depression. More specific findings include thin skin, easy bruising, reddish striae, proximal muscle weakness, and osteoporosis.
- Hyperpigmentation or hypokalemic alkalosis suggests Cushing syndrome due to ectopic ACTH secretion.
- Diabetes mellitus develops in some patients.

Diagnostic Testing

- **Diagnosis** requires the establishment of hypercortisolism due to increased cortisol excretion, lack of normal feedback inhibition of ACTH and cortisol secretion, or loss of the normal diurnal rhythm of cortisol secretion. Three initial tests are available:
  - The best initial test is the **24-hour urine cortisol** measurement;
  - Alternatively, an **overnight dexamethasone suppression test** may be performed (1 mg dexamethasone given PO at 11:00 PM; plasma cortisol measured at 8:00 AM. the next day; normal range: plasma cortisol <1.8 µg/dL); reflex dexamethasone levels can be obtained to ensure the test was performed appropriately; or
  - **Salivary cortisol** may be measured at home during the nadir of normal plasma cortisol at 11:00 PM.
- All these tests are very sensitive, and a normal value virtually excludes the diagnosis. If the overnight dexamethasone suppression test or 11:00 PM. salivary cortisol is abnormal, 24-hour urine cortisol should be measured.
  - If the 24-hour urine cortisol excretion is more than 3–4 times the upper limit of the reference range in a patient with compatible clinical findings, the diagnosis of Cushing syndrome is established.
  - Testing should not be done during severe illness or depression, which may cause false-positive results. Phenytoin therapy also causes a false-positive test by accelerating metabolism of dexamethasone.
- After the diagnosis of Cushing syndrome is made, tests to determine the cause and appropriate treatment are best done in consultation with an endocrinologist.

Incidental Adrenal Nodules[11]

GENERAL PRINCIPLES

- Adrenal nodules are a common incidental finding on abdominal imaging studies.
- Most incidentally discovered nodules are benign adrenocortical tumors that do not secrete excess hormone.

DIAGNOSIS

Clinical Presentation

Patients should be evaluated for hypertension, symptoms suggestive of pheochromocytoma (episodic headache, palpitations, and sweating), and signs of Cushing syndrome (see "Cushing Syndrome" section).

Differential Diagnosis

- In patients without a known malignancy elsewhere, the diagnostic issues are whether a syndrome of hormone excess or an adrenocortical carcinoma is present.
- The differential diagnosis includes adrenal adenomas causing Cushing syndrome or primary hyperaldosteronism, pheochromocytoma, adrenocortical carcinoma, and metastatic cancer.
- The imaging characteristics of the nodule may suggest a diagnosis but are not specific enough to obviate further evaluation.

Diagnostic Testing

- Plasma potassium, metanephrines, and dehydroepiandrosterone sulfate should be measured, and an overnight dexamethasone suppression test should be performed.
- Patients who have potentially resectable cancer elsewhere and in whom an adrenal metastasis must be excluded may require fluorodeoxyglucose–positron emission tomography.
- Patients with hypertension (especially if they have hypokalemia) should be evaluated for primary hyperaldosteronism by measuring the ratio of plasma aldosterone (in nanograms per deciliter [ng/dL]) to plasma renin activity (in ng/mL/h). If the ratio is <20, the diagnosis of primary hyperaldosteronism is excluded, whereas a ratio >50 makes the diagnosis very likely. Patients with an intermediate ratio should be further evaluated in consultation with an endocrinologist.
- An abnormal overnight dexamethasone suppression test should be evaluated further (see "Cushing Syndrome" section).
- Elevation of plasma dehydroepiandrosterone sulfate or a large nodule (>4 cm in diameter) suggests adrenocortical carcinoma.

TREATMENT

- Most incidental nodules are <4 cm in diameter, do not produce excess hormone, and do not require therapy. A measurement of <10 Hounsfield units on CT is reassuring for adrenal adenoma. One repeat imaging procedure 3–6 months later is recommended to ensure that the nodule is not enlarging rapidly (which would suggest an adrenal carcinoma).

CHAPTER 24

- A policy of resecting all nodules >4 cm in diameter appropriately treats the great majority of adrenal carcinomas while minimizing the number of benign nodules that are removed unnecessarily.
- If clinical or biochemical evidence of a pheochromocytoma is found, the nodule should be resected after appropriate α-adrenergic blockade.

Pituitary Adenomas and Hypopituitarism[9,12]

GENERAL PRINCIPLES

- The anterior pituitary gland secretes **prolactin**, **growth hormone**, and four **trophic hormones**, including corticotropin (ACTH), thyrotropin (TSH), and the gonadotropins, luteinizing hormone and follicle-stimulating hormone. Each trophic hormone stimulates a specific target gland.
- Anterior pituitary function is regulated by hypothalamic hormones that reach the pituitary via portal veins in the pituitary stalk. The predominant effect of hypothalamic regulation is to stimulate secretion of pituitary hormones, except for prolactin, which is inhibited by hypothalamic dopamine secretion.
- Secretion of trophic hormones is also regulated by negative feedback by their target gland hormone, and the normal pituitary response to target hormone deficiency is increased secretion of the appropriate trophic hormone.
- **Anterior pituitary dysfunction** can be caused by disorders of either the pituitary or hypothalamus.
- **Pituitary adenomas** are the most common pituitary disorder. They are classified by size and function.
  - **Microadenomas** are <10 mm in diameter and cause clinical manifestations only if they produce excess hormone. They are too small to produce hypopituitarism or mass effects.
  - **Macroadenomas** are >10 mm in diameter and may produce any combination of pituitary hormone excess, hypopituitarism, and mass effects (headache, visual field loss).
  - **Secretory adenomas** produce prolactin, growth hormone, or ACTH.
  - **Nonsecretory macroadenomas** may cause hypopituitarism or mass effects.
  - **Nonsecretory microadenomas** are common incidental radiographic findings, seen in approximately 10%–20% of the normal population, and do not require therapy.
- **Other pituitary or hypothalamic disorders,** such as head trauma, pituitary surgery or radiation, and postpartum pituitary infarction (Sheehan syndrome), may cause hypopituitarism. Other tumors of the pituitary or hypothalamus (e.g., craniopharyngioma, metastases) and inflammatory disorders (e.g., sarcoidosis, Langerhans cell histiocytosis, lymphocytic hypophysitis) may cause hypopituitarism or mass effects. Some immunomodulatory medications, most notably checkpoint inhibitors used for cancer treatment, can cause hypophysitis and hypopituitarism.

DIAGNOSIS

Clinical Presentation

- Hypopituitarism may be suspected in the presence of clinical signs of target hormone deficiency (e.g., hypothyroidism) or pituitary mass effects.
- In **hypopituitarism** (deficiency of one or more pituitary hormones), gonadotropin deficiency is most common, causing amenorrhea in women and androgen

deficiency in men. Secondary hypothyroidism or adrenal failure rarely occurs alone. Secondary adrenal failure causes cortisol deficiency but does not affect aldosterone; hyperkalemia and hyperpigmentation do not occur, although life-threatening adrenal crisis may develop.

- **Hormone excess** most commonly results in **hyperprolactinemia**, which can be due to a secretory adenoma or due to nonsecretory lesions that damage the hypothalamus or pituitary stalk. Growth hormone excess **(acromegaly)** and ACTH and cortisol excess **(Cushing disease)** are caused by secretory adenomas. Hormone excess can be present concurrently with other hormone deficiencies.
- **Mass effects** because of pressure on adjacent structures, such as the optic chiasm, include headaches and loss of visual fields or acuity. Hyperprolactinemia may also be due to mass effect. **Pituitary apoplexy** is sudden enlargement of a pituitary tumor due to hemorrhagic necrosis.
- Asymptomatic pituitary adenomas are commonly incidentally discovered on imaging.

Diagnostic Testing

- **Incidental adenoma**
  - If an incidental microadenoma is found on imaging done for another purpose, the patient should be evaluated for clinical evidence of hyperprolactinemia, Cushing disease, or acromegaly.
  - Plasma **prolactin and insulin-like growth factor 1** (IGF-1) should be measured, and tests for Cushing syndrome should be performed if symptoms or signs of this disorder are evident.
  - If no pituitary hormone excess exists, therapy is not required. Whether such patients need repeat imaging is not established, but the risk of enlargement is clearly small.
  - Incidental discovery of a macroadenoma is unusual. Patients should be evaluated for hormone excess and hypopituitarism. Most macroadenomas should be treated because they are likely to grow further.
- **Hypopituitarism**
  - Laboratory evaluation begins with evaluation of **target hormone function**, including **plasma-free T_4** and a **Cortrosyn stimulation test** (see "Adrenal Failure" section).
  - If recent onset of secondary adrenal failure is suspected (within a few weeks of evaluation), the patient should be treated empirically with glucocorticoids and should be tested 4–8 weeks later because the Cortrosyn stimulation test cannot detect secondary adrenal failure of recent onset.
  - In men, plasma testosterone should be measured. The best evaluation of gonadal function in women is the menstrual history.
  - **If a target hormone is deficient,** its trophic hormone is measured to determine whether target gland dysfunction is secondary to hypopituitarism. An elevated trophic hormone level indicates primary target gland dysfunction. In hypopituitarism, trophic hormone levels are not elevated and are usually within (not below) the reference range. Thus, pituitary trophic hormone levels can be interpreted only with knowledge of target hormone levels, and **measurement of trophic hormone levels alone is useless in the diagnosis of hypopituitarism.** If pituitary disease is obvious, target hormone deficiencies may be assumed to be secondary, and trophic hormones need not be measured.
- Anatomic evaluation of the pituitary gland and hypothalamus is best done by MRI and should be performed to evaluate any pituitary hormone excess or deficiency.

However, hyperprolactinemia and Cushing disease may be caused by microadenomas too small to be seen. The prevalence of incidental microadenomas should be kept in mind when interpreting MRIs. Visual acuity and visual fields should be tested when imaging suggests compression of the optic chiasm.

TREATMENT

- Secondary adrenal failure should be treated immediately, especially if patients are to undergo surgery (see "Adrenal Failure" section).
- Treatment of secondary hypothyroidism should be monitored by measurement of **plasma-free T_4** (see "Hypothyroidism" section).
- Infertility due to gonadotropin deficiency may be correctable, and patients who wish to conceive should be referred to an endocrinologist.
- Treatment of hypogonadism in premenopausal women requires replacement of estrogen and progesterone. This can be conveniently done with combination oral contraceptives.
- Treatment of hypogonadism in men requires testosterone replacement, with either topical testosterone gel, 40–50 mg applied daily, or by injection of testosterone enanthate or testosterone cypionate, 100–200 mg IM every 2 weeks. Testosterone replacement therapy disrupts spermatogenesis; men who are concerned about fertility should be seen by an endocrinologist.
- Treatment of growth hormone deficiency in adults has been advocated by some, but the long-term benefits, risks, and cost-effectiveness of this therapy are not established.
- Treatment of pituitary macroadenomas generally requires transsphenoidal surgical resection, except for prolactin-secreting tumors.

Hyperprolactinemia[13,14]

GENERAL PRINCIPLES

- In women, the most common causes of pathologic hyperprolactinemia are prolactin-secreting pituitary **microadenomas** and **idiopathic hyperprolactinemia** (Table 24-3).
- In men, the most common cause is a prolactin-secreting **macroadenoma.**
- Hypothalamic or pituitary lesions that cause deficiency of other pituitary hormones often cause hyperprolactinemia.
- **Medications** are an important cause to consider in all patients.

DIAGNOSIS

Clinical Presentation

- In women, hyperprolactinemia causes amenorrhea or irregular menses and infertility. Only approximately half of these women have galactorrhea. Prolonged estrogen deficiency increases the risk of osteoporosis. Plasma prolactin should be measured in women with amenorrhea, whether or not galactorrhea is present. Mild elevations should be confirmed by repeat measurements.
- In men, hyperprolactinemia causes androgen deficiency and infertility but not gynecomastia; mass effects and hypopituitarism are common.
- The history should include medications and symptoms of pituitary mass effects or hypothyroidism.

TABLE 24-3	Major Causes of Hyperprolactinemia
Pregnancy and lactation	
Prolactin-secreting pituitary adenoma (prolactinoma)	
Idiopathic hyperprolactinemia	
Drugs (e.g., phenothiazines, atypical antipsychotic medications, metoclopramide, verapamil)	
Interference with synthesis or transport of hypothalamic dopamine	
Hypothalamic lesions	
Nonsecretory pituitary macroadenomas	
Primary hypothyroidism	
Chronic renal failure	

Diagnostic Testing

Pituitary imaging should be performed in most cases because large nonfunctional pituitary or hypothalamic tumors may present with hyperprolactinemia. Testing for hypopituitarism is needed only in patients with a macroadenoma or hypothalamic lesion (see "Pituitary Adenomas and Hypopituitarism" section).

TREATMENT

- For **microadenomas and idiopathic hyperprolactinemia**, most patients are treated because of infertility or to prevent estrogen deficiency and osteoporosis. Indications for treatment include adenoma >1 cm, bothersome symptomatic galactorrhea, or hypogonadism.
- Some women may be observed without therapy by periodic follow-up of prolactin levels and symptoms. In most patients, hyperprolactinemia does not worsen, and prolactin levels sometimes return to normal. Enlargement of microadenomas is rare.
- **Dopamine agonists: cabergoline and bromocriptine** suppress plasma prolactin and restore normal menses and fertility in most women.
  - Initial dosages are bromocriptine, 1.25–2.50 mg PO at bedtime, or cabergoline, 0.25 mg twice a week.
  - Plasma prolactin levels are initially obtained at 2- to 4-week intervals, and doses are adjusted to the lowest dose required to maintain prolactin in the normal range. In general, the maximally effective doses are bromocriptine 2.5 mg tid and cabergoline 1.5 mg twice a week.
  - **Side effects** include nausea and orthostatic hypotension, which can be minimized by increasing the dose gradually and usually resolve with continued therapy. Side effects are less severe with cabergoline.
  - Women should consider barrier contraception because fertility may be restored quickly.
  - **Women who want to become pregnant** should be managed in consultation with an endocrinologist.
  - **Women who do not want to become pregnant** should be followed with clinical evaluation and plasma prolactin levels every 6–12 months. Every few years, plasma prolactin may be measured after the dopamine agonist has been withdrawn for several weeks to determine whether the drug is still needed. Follow-up imaging studies are not warranted unless prolactin levels increase substantially.

- **Prolactin-secreting macroadenomas** should be treated with a dopamine agonist, which usually suppresses prolactin levels to normal, reduces tumor size, and improves or corrects abnormal visual fields in 90% of cases.
  - If mass effects are present, the dose should be increased to maximally effective levels over a period of several weeks. Visual field tests, if initially abnormal, should be repeated 4–6 weeks after therapy is started.
  - Pituitary imaging should be repeated 3–6 months after initiation of therapy. If tumor shrinkage and correction of visual abnormalities are satisfactory, therapy can be continued indefinitely, with periodic monitoring of plasma prolactin levels.
  - The full effect on tumor size may take more than 6 months. Further pituitary imaging is probably not warranted unless prolactin levels rise despite therapy.
  - **Transsphenoidal surgery** is indicated to relieve mass effects if the tumor does not shrink or if visual field abnormalities do not resolve quickly with dopamine agonist therapy. However, the likelihood of surgical cure of a prolactin-secreting macroadenoma is low, and most patients require further therapy with a dopamine agonist.
  - **Women with prolactin-secreting macroadenomas should not become pregnant** unless the tumor has been resected surgically or has decreased markedly in size with dopamine agonist therapy because the risk of symptomatic enlargement during pregnancy is 15%–35%. Contraception is essential during dopamine agonist treatment for macroadenoma.

Acromegaly[15]

GENERAL PRINCIPLES

Acromegaly is the syndrome caused by growth hormone excess in adults and is due to a growth hormone–secreting pituitary adenoma in the vast majority of cases.

DIAGNOSIS

Clinical Presentation
Clinical findings include thickened skin and enlargement of hands, feet, jaw, and forehead. Arthritis or carpal tunnel syndrome may develop, and the pituitary adenoma may cause headaches and vision loss. Obstructive sleep apnea and diabetes mellitus can develop. Mortality from cardiovascular disease is increased.

Diagnostic Testing
- **Plasma IGF-1,** which mediates most effects of growth hormone, is the best diagnostic test. Marked elevations establish the diagnosis.
- If IGF-1 levels are only moderately elevated, the diagnosis can be confirmed by giving 75 mg glucose orally and measuring serum growth hormone every 30 minutes for 2 hours. Failure to suppress growth hormone to <1 ng/mL confirms the diagnosis of acromegaly. Once the diagnosis is made, the pituitary should be imaged.

TREATMENT

- The treatment of choice is transsphenoidal resection of the pituitary adenoma. Most patients have macroadenomas, and complete tumor resection with cure of acromegaly is often impossible. If IGF-1 levels remain elevated after surgery, radiotherapy is used to prevent regrowth of the tumor and to control acromegaly.

- The somatostatin analog **octreotide** in depot form can be used to suppress growth hormone secretion while awaiting the effect of radiation. A dose of 10–40 mg IM monthly suppresses IGF-1 to normal in about 60% of patients. Side effects include cholelithiasis, diarrhea, and mild abdominal discomfort.
- **Pegvisomant** is a growth hormone antagonist that lowers IGF-1 to normal in almost all patients. The dose is 10–30 mg SC daily. Few side effects have been reported, but patients should be monitored for pituitary adenoma enlargement and transaminase elevation.

Osteomalacia[16,17]

GENERAL PRINCIPLES

- Osteomalacia is characterized by defective mineralization of osteoid. Bone biopsy reveals increased thickness of osteoid seams and decreased mineralization rate, assessed by tetracycline labeling.
- Suboptimal vitamin D nutrition, indicated by plasma 25-hydroxy vitamin D (25[OH]D) levels <30 ng/mL, is very common and contributes to the development of osteoporosis.
- Etiology
  - Dietary vitamin D deficiency
  - Malabsorption of vitamin D and calcium because of intestinal, hepatic, or biliary disease
  - Disorders of vitamin D metabolism (e.g., renal disease, vitamin D–dependent rickets)
  - Vitamin D resistance
  - Chronic hypophosphatemia
  - Renal tubular acidosis
  - Hypophosphatasia

DIAGNOSIS

Clinical Presentation

- Clinical findings include diffuse skeletal pain, proximal muscle weakness, waddling gait, and propensity to fractures.
- Osteomalacia should be suspected in a patient with osteopenia, elevated serum alkaline phosphatase, and either hypophosphatemia or hypocalcemia.

Diagnostic Testing

- Serum alkaline phosphatase is elevated. Serum phosphorus, calcium, or both may be low.
- **Serum 25(OH)D** levels may be low, establishing the diagnosis of vitamin D deficiency or malabsorption.
- Radiographic findings include osteopenia and radiolucent bands perpendicular to bone surfaces (pseudofractures or Looser zones). Bone density is decreased.

TREATMENT

- **Dietary vitamin D deficiency** can initially be treated with ergocalciferol 50,000 international units (IU) PO weekly for 8 weeks to replete body stores, followed by long-term therapy with cholecalciferol 2000 IU/d.

- **Malabsorption of vitamin D** may require continued therapy with high doses such as 50,000 IU PO per week. The dose should be adjusted to maintain serum 25(OH) D levels above 30 ng/mL. Calcium supplements, 1 g PO daily, tid, may also be required. Serum 25(OH)D and serum calcium should be monitored every 6–12 months to avoid hypercalcemia.

Paget Disease[18]

GENERAL PRINCIPLES

Paget disease of bone is a focal skeletal disorder characterized by rapid, disorganized bone remodeling. It usually occurs after the age of 40 years and most often affects the pelvis, femur, spine, and skull.

DIAGNOSIS

Clinical Presentation

- Clinical manifestations include bone pain and deformity, degenerative arthritis, pathologic fractures, neurologic deficits because of nerve root or cranial nerve compression (including deafness), and, rarely, high-output heart failure and osteosarcoma.
- Most patients are asymptomatic, with disease discovered incidentally because of elevated serum alkaline phosphatase or a radiograph taken for other reasons.

Diagnostic Testing

- **Serum alkaline phosphatase** is elevated, reflecting the activity and extent of disease. Serum and urine calcium are usually normal but may increase with immobilization, as after a fracture.
- The **radiographic appearance is usually diagnostic.** A bone scan will reveal areas of skeletal involvement, which can be confirmed by radiography.

TREATMENT

- **Indications for therapy** include (1) bone pain because of Paget disease, (2) nerve compression syndromes, (3) pathologic fracture, (4) elective skeletal surgery, (5) progressive skeletal deformity, (6) immobilization hypercalcemia, and (7) asymptomatic involvement of weight-bearing bones or the skull.
- **Bisphosphonates** inhibit excessive bone resorption, relieve symptoms, and restore serum alkaline phosphatase to normal in most patients. **Zoledronic acid,** 5 mg IV by a single infusion, is the drug of choice. The effectiveness of therapy is monitored by measuring serum alkaline phosphatase annually. Therapy can be repeated if serum alkaline phosphatase rises above normal. Bisphosphonates are not recommended in patients with renal insufficiency.

Transgender Medicine[19]

GENERAL PRINCIPLES

Care of transgender patients is multifaceted and can include gender-affirming hormone therapy, surgical interventions, and assistance with other ancillary support such as speech therapy, dermatologic therapy, or assistance in navigating legal processes such as for name change.

DIAGNOSIS

- Diagnosis of gender dysphoria is guided by DSM-5 criteria, which includes (1) a marked incongruence between one's experienced/expressed gender and natal gender of at least 6 months in duration and (2) the condition is associated with clinically significant distress due to impairment in social, occupational, or other important areas of functioning. It can be important to involve mental health professionals in situations where patients may be experiencing conditions that have similar features such as body dysmorphic disorder or in situations where abuse or other psychiatric illness such as depression or anxiety may coexist and impact treatment.
- Patients seeking gender-affirming hormone therapy should have persistent, well-documented gender dysphoria/gender incongruence, the capacity to make a fully informed decision and to consent for treatment, and mental health concerns, if present, must be reasonably well controlled.
- The World Professional Association for Transgender Health and Endocrine Society recommends an **"informed consent" model** for gender-affirming hormone therapy in individuals aged 18 years and older, which does not require a specific mental health evaluation or diagnosis prior to treatment. Informed consent includes a discussion of risks and benefits of gender-affirming hormone therapy, reversible and nonreversible effects, and time course of anticipated changes.
- Individuals should be counseled about options for **fertility preservation** prior to initiating treatment with gender-affirming hormone therapy. It is important to set realistic expectations about the timing of effects of hormone therapy including timing of onset and time to maximum effect. Individuals must be informed about potential risks of gender-affirming hormone therapy.

Clinical Presentation

- Understanding each individual's journey is important in order to build rapport and trust in the patient–physician relationship. **Goals of therapy should be discussed and revisited as they may change over time.** Understanding social context is also important such as whether patient has supportive friends and family and whether the patient is presenting as transgender in all private and public situations including the workplace. Knowing these details of a patient's life can help clinicians offer specific support and keep them attuned to patients' struggles and challenges.
- **A sexual history should be obtained from transgender patients**, as with all sexually active patients, in order to screen for high-risk behaviors, assess for sexually transmitted infections, and potentially offer PrEP (pre-exposure prophylaxis for HIV) therapy if desired by the patient.
- Screening for **depression and abuse** is also paramount.

TREATMENT

Gender-Affirming Hormone Therapy
Transgender Men (Female-to-Male)

- **Testosterone therapy** is the mainstay of gender-affirming hormone therapy for transgender men. Testosterone is available in IM or SC injections, transdermal gel preparations, or transdermal patches. Testosterone enanthate or cypionate can be given at a starting does of 50 mg IM or SC weekly or 100 mg IM or SC every 2 weeks. A 21–23 gauge 1" needle is used for IM injection and 25 gauge 5/8" needle is used for SC injection. An autoinjector for SC testosterone is now available for individuals with significant needle phobia. Topical testosterone gel can be applied daily. The starting dose is 50 mg daily. Care should be taken to prevent transfer of the gel to another person. Patches may be started at 2–4 mg daily but may cause skin irritation. Patient preference and insurance coverage may guide selection of route of administration.

- Testosterone therapy results in increased muscle mass, decreased fat mass, increased facial hair and acne, male pattern baldness in those genetically predisposed, increased sexual desire, clitoromegaly, temporary or permanent decreased fertility, deepening of the voice, cessation of menses, and increased body hair.
- Side effects of testosterone therapy can include erythrocytosis, sleep apnea, hypertension, excessive weight gain, lipid changes, excessive or cystic acne, hypertension, and breast or uterine cancer.
- Adverse events are more likely if testosterone levels are supraphysiologic. **Testosterone levels within the normal male range are the goal of therapy.**
- Hemoglobin and hematocrit should be monitored in patients on testosterone. Lipid panel should also be measured annually.

Transgender Women (Male-to-Female)

- **Estrogen therapy** is used to produce secondary sexual characteristics and to suppress testosterone production in transgender women. Oral estradiol, 2–8 mg/d in divided doses, is most often used. Allowing estradiol tablets to dissolve sublingually as opposed to swallowing tablets may improve efficacy and reduce side effect profiles by bypassing first-pass liver metabolism. Transdermal estradiol (typical starting dose of 0.1 mg with uptitration to 0.4 mg) or IM or SC estradiol (starting dose may vary: 2–3 mg weekly or 4–6 mg every other week estradiol valerate, 0.5–1 mg weekly or 1–2 mg estradiol cypionate every other week) can also be prescribed.
- As with testosterone, administration route is guided by patient preference. Estrogen effects include breast tissue development, softening of the skin, and redistribution of adipose tissue. Some patients may also note estrogen alone is insufficient to suppress testosterone levels. A common adjunctive medication is **spironolactone,** which directly blocks androgen receptor activation. Other adjunctive medications include GnRH agonists and antiandrogenic progestins.
- 5α-reductase inhibitors do not reduce testosterone levels and have adverse effects so should not be used.
- Side effects of estrogen therapy include thromboembolic disease, breast cancer, coronary or cerebrovascular disease, cholelithiasis, and hypertriglyceridemia. **Thromboembolic risk is high with ethinyl estradiol, which is typically avoided.** Individuals are strongly encouraged to avoid tobacco use in order to minimize risk of venous thromboembolism and cardiovascular complications.
- It is important to monitor cardiovascular risk factors by screening for lipid abnormalities and diabetes.
- Clinicians should measure serum estradiol and serum testosterone and maintain them **at the level for premenopausal females** (100–200 pg/mL and 50 ng/dL, respectively). Creatinine and potassium levels should also be monitored on spironolactone. Prolactin should also be checked annually.
- Treatment should be tailored to patient goals. For example, hormone therapy in transgender females can result in loss of spontaneous erections and this should be discussed as some patients may wish to be able to continue to have erections while other patients do not. Phosphodiesterase-5 inhibitors may be used in transgender women who are experiencing erectile dysfunction.

Nonbinary Patients

- Individuals who identify as **genderqueer or nonbinary** (do not identify as specifically male or female) may or may not seek gender-affirming hormone therapy or gender-affirming surgery. When they do, they may be seeking different clinical outcomes than their binary transgender peers.
- Doses of gender-affirming hormones may be started at lower doses with goal hormone levels that are lower to try to achieve a more androgynous appearance; however, part of the informed consent process should stress that this goal cannot be guaranteed.
- Additional research is needed to guide care for nonbinary patients and help them meet their specific goals.

Monitoring

Sex steroid hormone levels should be monitored **every 3 months** during the first year of hormone therapy and then once or twice yearly thereafter. Individuals on injectable therapy should have levels measured in the middle of the injection interval.

Gender-Affirming Surgery

- Individuals desiring genital gender-affirming surgery are recommended to have completed at least **1 year of consistent and compliant hormone therapy.**
- Transgender males may seek mastectomy, hysterectomy, phalloplasty or metoidioplasty, and/or facial masculinization surgery.
- Transgender females may seek facial feminization, breast augmentation, body feminization surgery which typically includes trunk liposuction and buttocks augmentation, orchiectomy, and vaginoplasty. Typically breast augmentation surgery is delayed until at least 2 years of estrogen therapy as breast tissue can continue to grow during that time.

Other Ancillary Treatments

- **Speech therapy** can be an important aspect of treatment for transgender individuals as modifying speech patterns can improve patient confidence. Transgender women often work with speech therapists to modulate vocal pitch because this cannot be achieved with estradiol therapy. Transgender men who do not achieve sufficient voice deepening with testosterone may also access these services. Vocal cord surgery is also an option for patients.
- Transfeminine individuals may also seek laser hair removal or electrolysis as estradiol and antiandrogen therapy alone often does not eliminate terminal hair growth on the face and other areas of the body. Hair removal is part of the preparation process for both transmasculine and transfeminine gender-affirming genital surgeries and may take up to 1 year.

SPECIAL CONSIDERATIONS

- Interpreting labs or bone mineral densities for transgender patients can be challenging as the reference range may be given for patients' assigned sex at birth and not their affirmed gender. Clinicians must always be vigilant to **utilize appropriate reference ranges** to interpret test results.
- Transgender persons who have undergone gonadectomy may choose not to continue consistent sex steroid treatment after hormonal and surgical sex reassignment, thereby becoming **at risk for bone loss.**

CHAPTER 24

- **Routine care and cancer screening are still necessary** for transgender persons with relevant anatomy. Transgender males should continue cervical cancer screening per guidelines. Discussion of prostate cancer screening with transgender women should continue.

REFERENCES

1. Baloch Z, Carayon P, Conte-Devolx B, et al. Laboratory medicine practice guidelines. Laboratory support for the diagnosis and monitoring of thyroid disease. *Thyroid.* 2003;13:3-126.
2. McDermott M. Hypothyroidism. *Ann Intern Med.* 2009;151:ITC6.
3. Jonklaas J, Bianco AC, Bauer AJ, et al. Guidelines for the treatment of hypothyroidism: prepared by the American Thyroid Association task force on thyroid hormone replacement. *Thyroid.* 2014;24:1670-1751.
4. Alexander EK, Pearce EN, Brent GA, et al. 2017 Guidelines of the American Thyroid Association for the diagnosis and management of thyroid disease during pregnancy and the postpartum. *Thyroid.* 2017;27:315-389.
5. Ross DS, Burch HB, Cooper DS, et al. 2016 American Thyroid Association guidelines for diagnosis and management of hyperthyroidism and other causes of thyrotoxicosis. *Thyroid.* 2016;26:1343-1421.
6. Chen AY, Bernet VJ, Carty SE, et al. American Thyroid Association statement on optimal surgical management of goiter. *Thyroid.* 2013;24:181-189.
7. Haugen BR, Alexander EK, Bible KC, et al. 2015 American Thyroid Association management guidelines for adult patients with thyroid nodules and differentiated thyroid cancer: the American Thyroid Association guidelines task force on thyroid nodules and differentiated thyroid cancer. *Thyroid.* 2016;26:1-133.
8. Bornstein SR, Allolio B, Arlt W, et al. Diagnosis and treatment of primary adrenal insufficiency: an endocrine society clinical practice guideline. *J Clin Endocrinol Metab.* 2016;101:364-389.
9. Fleseriu M, Hashim IA, Karavitaki N, et al. Hormonal replacement in hypopituitarism in adults: an endocrine society clinical practice guideline. *J Clin Endocrinol Metab.* 2016;101:3888-3921.
10. Nieman LK, Biller BMK, Findling JW, et al. The diagnosis of Cushing's syndrome: an endocrine society clinical practice guideline. *J Clin Endocrinol Metab.* 2008;93:1526-1540.
11. Young WF. The incidentally discovered adrenal mass. *N Engl J Med.* 2007;356:601-610.
12. Freda PU, Beckers AM, Katznelson L, et al. Pituitary incidentaloma: an endocrine society clinical practice guideline. *J Clin Endocrinol Metab.* 2011;96:894-904.
13. Melmed S, Casanueva FF, Hoffman AR, et al. Diagnosis and treatment of hyperprolactinemia: an endocrine society clinical practice guideline. *J Clin Endocrinol Metab.* 2011;96:273-288.
14. Molitch ME. Drugs and prolactin. *Pituitary.* 2008;11:209-218.
15. Katznelson L, Laws ER, Melmed S, et al. Acromegaly: an endocrine society clinical practice guideline. *J Clin Endocrinol Metab.* 2014;99:3933-3951.
16. Holick MF, Binkley NC, Bischoff-Ferrari HA, et al. Evaluation, treatment, and prevention of vitamin D deficiency: an endocrine society clinical practice guideline. *J Clin Endocrinol Metab.* 2011;96:1911-1930.
17. Munns CF, Shaw N, Kiely M, et al. Global consensus recommendations on prevention and management of nutritional rickets. *J Clin Endocrinol Metab.* 2016;101:394-415.
18. Singer FR, Bone HG, Hosking DJ, et al. Paget's disease of bone: an endocrine society clinical practice guideline. *J Clin Endocrinol Metab.* 2014;99:4408-4422.
19. Hembree WC, Cohen-Kettenis PT, Gooren L, et al. Endocrine treatment of gender-dysphoric/gender-incongruent persons: an endocrine society clinical practice guideline. *J Clin Endocrinol Metab.* 2017;102(11):3869-3903.

25 Arthritis and Rheumatologic Diseases

Andrea Ramirez Gomez and Deepali Sen

Basic Approach to Joint Pain

GENERAL PRINCIPLES

- **The first step** is to differentiate between arthritis versus periarthritis. **Arthritis** is any process affecting a joint or joints, causing pain, swelling, and stiffness. **Periarthritis**, which mimics arthritis, involves the soft tissues surrounding the joint like tendons and bursal structures. Pain from arthritis is usually present in all directions of motion, whereas pain from periarthritis is usually evident at a single point or direction in the range of motion. In addition, pain occurs primarily with active movement in periarthritis, while it can occur with active and passive movements in arthritis.
- **The second step** is to categorize arthritis as **inflammatory or noninflammatory.** This will depend on the pattern of joint involvement and the evidence of inflammatory findings on joint exam. Features of inflammatory arthritis include swelling, erythema, warmth over the joint, as well as the presence of prolonged morning stiffness of more than 1 hour that worsens with inactivity. Associated symptoms such as fever, weight loss, skin rashes, uveitis, scleritis, mouth ulcers, and serositis, among others, may give clues to an underlying systemic connective tissue disease (CTD).

DIAGNOSIS

Arthritis can be approached by the number, pattern, and acuity of joint involvement (Figure 25-1).

Ancillary Tests

- Laboratory tests and imaging are helpful in supporting a diagnosis if their use is directed by the specific findings on the history and physical examination. Laboratory evidence of inflammation may be helpful although not specific. These include erythrocyte sedimentation rate (ESR), C-reactive protein (CRP), and synovial fluid analysis.
- Arthrocentesis should be performed in all patients with acute monoarthritis. Synovial fluid analysis should be sent for cell count, microscopic examination for crystals, Gram stain, and cultures (Table 25-1). Normal joints contain a small volume of synovial fluid that is highly viscous, clear, and essentially acellular.

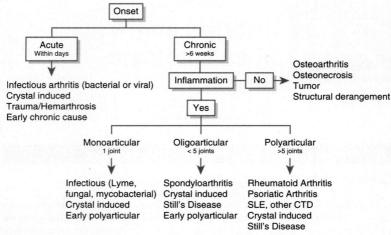

Figure 25-1. Approach to joint pain. CTD, connective tissue disease.

TABLE 25-1	Synovial Fluid Analysis				
Measure	Normal	Noninflammatory	Inflammatory	Septic	Hemorrhagic
Appearance	Clear	Clear, yellow	Clear to opaque	Opaque	Bloody
WBC/mm³	<200	0–2000	>2000	>20,000	Variable
Polymorphonuclear leukocytes %	<25	<25	≥50	≥75	50–75
Culture	(−)	(−)	(−)	(+)	(−)

Important Factors for Synovial Fluid Interpretation

- Septic arthritis is associated with white blood cell counts >20,000 and frequently >50,000. The cutoff is no longer 50,000 due to lowered sensitivity, 50%–70%, although the specificity is high, 80%–90%.[1] The chances of septic arthritis increase as counts increase. Counts of <20,000 may be observed in disseminated gonococcal infection.
- Monosodium urate: sensitivity 63%–78%, specificity 93%–100%. Calcium pyrophosphate dihydrate crystals: sensitivity 12%–83%, specificity 78%–96%. **The presence of crystals does not exclude infection.**
- Gram stain should be performed but sensitivity is low. A negative Gram stain does not rule out an infection.

TREATMENT

Therapeutic approaches involve either local or systemic administration of analgesic, anti-inflammatory, immunomodulatory, or immunosuppressive drugs. This will be reviewed in each section.

RHEUMATOID ARTHRITIS

GENERAL PRINCIPLES

Rheumatoid arthritis (RA) is a systemic disease of unknown etiology that is characterized by a symmetric inflammatory polyarthritis, extra-articular manifestations (rheumatoid nodules, pulmonary fibrosis, serositis, scleritis, vasculitis), and serum rheumatoid factor (RF). The course of RA is variable but tends to be chronic and progressive.

DIAGNOSIS

Clinical Presentation

- Most patients describe the insidious onset of pain, swelling, and morning stiffness in the hands and/or wrists or feet. Synovitis may be evident on examination of the metacarpophalangeal (MCP), proximal interphalangeal (PIP), wrist, or other joints. Suspect the diagnosis in patients presenting with symmetric arthritis in three or more joints, especially involving small joints and associated with morning stiffness lasting more than 30 minutes.
- Joint deformities include ulnar deviation, swan neck (MCP flexion, PIP hyperextension, and DIP [distal interphalangeal] flexion), boutonniere (PIP flexion, DIP hyperextension), and cock-up deformities in feet.
- Less commonly affects C1-C2, but it is important to recognize since it can lead to myelopathy.
- Extra-articular manifestations occur in up to 40% of the patients, especially if they are seropositive.[2] Some of these include rheumatoid nodules (most commonly on extensor surfaces), Raynaud phenomenon (RP), cutaneous vasculitis, interstitial lung disease (ILD), pericarditis, mononeuritis multiplex, CNS (central nervous system) vasculitis, scleritis, episcleritis, keratoconjunctivitis sicca (secondary Sjogren syndrome), neutropenia (1% develop Felty syndrome), among others. Gastrointestinal or renal manifestations are exceedingly rare.

Diagnostic Testing

RF may be positive in 80% of patients. Cyclic citrullinated peptide (CCP) antibodies may be detected in 50%–60% of patients with early RA.[3]

- CCP antibodies are more specific (>90%) for RA than RF.[3] RF can be positive in other conditions, which can be remembered by the mnemonic **CHRONIC**. It stands for **CH**ronic disease (primary biliary cirrhosis, silicosis, asbestosis), **R**heumatoid arthritis, **O**ther CTDs (systemic lupus erythematosus [SLE], Sjogren syndrome, systemic sclerosis, etc.), **N**eoplasms (lymphoma), **I**nfections (hepatitis C, subacute bacterial endocarditis, tuberculosis), and **C**ryoglobulinemia. RF can also be positive in healthy population.[4]
- Hand and wrist radiographs may show early changes of erosions or periarticular osteopenia.
- Musculoskeletal MRI and ultrasonography are more sensitive than plain radiographs and may be used in equivocal cases to demonstrate clinically inapparent synovitis or erosions.

TREATMENT

- The treatment strategy for RA is based on a treat-to-target approach, the target being remission or low disease activity at the least. This translates into pain control, suppression of inflammation, prevention of progressive joint destruction, and maintenance of joint and muscle function.

- **Disease-Modifying Anti-Rheumatic Drugs (DMARDs)** appear to alter the natural history of RA by retarding the progression of bony erosions and cartilage loss. Because RA may lead to substantial long-term disability (and is associated with increased mortality), the standard of care is to **initiate therapy with such agents early in the course of RA**.
- Symptomatic treatment alone with NSAIDs is not appropriate since it does not modify the course of the disease.
- Glucocorticoids have some disease-modifying activity, but their toxicity precludes the long-term use.
- Since DMARDs typically take 1–3 months to have their maximal effect, NSAIDs or glucocorticoids can be given as "bridging" therapy while allowing enough time to DMARDs to achieve their maximal effect.

Disease-Modifying Anti-Rheumatic Drugs

- Multiple synthetic and biologic DMARDs are approved for the treatment of RA, but they also have significant potential toxicities. Selection of DMARDs should be based on patient comorbidities, and careful monitoring for side effects is imperative.
  ○ Typically, **methotrexate** is the initial choice for moderate to severe RA.
  ○ **Leflunomide** is also an alternative.
  ○ **Hydroxychloroquine** or **sulfasalazine** can be used as the initial choice in mild RA.
  ○ **Combinations of DMARDs** can be used if the patient has a partial response to the initial agent. Combination therapy with methotrexate, hydroxychloroquine, and sulfasalazine, known as **triple therapy**, is felt to have efficacy similar to biologics in the treatment of RA.[5] Methotrexate and leflunomide may have additive hepatotoxicity, and this combination should be used cautiously.
- If response to monotherapy or combination of conventional DMARD agents is unsatisfactory after an adequate trial (or if limiting toxicity supervenes), addition of a biologic DMARD should be considered.
- Available biologic DMARDs for RA include:
  ○ Anti-TNF: adalimumab, etanercept, infliximab, golimumab, certolizumab pegol
  ○ JAK inhibitors (technically molecule-targeted DMARD): tofacitinib, baricitinib, upadacitinib
  ○ Anti-IL-1: anakinra
  ○ Anti-IL-6: tocilizumab, sarilumab
  ○ Costimulation inhibitor: abatacept
  ○ B cell–depleting therapy (anti-CD20): rituximab
- Combinations of synthetic DMARDs plus targeted or biologic DMARDs are increasingly used treatment regimens. Methotrexate is commonly combined with tumor necrosis factor (TNF) antagonists because there is evidence for additive efficacy and for a decrease in the formation of human antichimeric antibodies against the TNF blocker. Methotrexate is often used in combination with rituximab or abatacept. But it is important to note that **combination therapy with two biologic DMARDs is contraindicated because of increased infectious complications.**
- **For dosing, side effects, and contraindications please see the "Medications in Rheumatology" section at the end of the chapter.**

NSAIDs and Glucocorticoids

- **NSAIDs or glucocorticoids** may be used as an adjunct to DMARD therapy. Indications for glucocorticoids include symptomatic relief while awaiting response to a slow-acting immunosuppressive or immunomodulatory agent, persistent synovitis despite adequate trials of DMARDs and NSAIDs, severe constitutional symptoms (e.g., fever and weight loss), or extra-articular disease (vasculitis, episcleritis, or pleurisy).

- **Oral administration** of prednisone 5–20 mg daily usually is sufficient for the treatment of synovitis, whereas severe constitutional symptoms or extra-articular disease may require up to 1 mg/kg PO daily.
- **Intra-articular administration** may provide temporary symptomatic relief when only a few joints are inflamed. The beneficial effects of intra-articular steroids may persist for days to months and may delay or negate the need for systemic glucocorticoid therapy.

COMPLICATIONS

- **Patients with RA and a single joint inflamed out of proportion to the rest of the joints must be evaluated for coexistent septic arthritis.**
- **Felty syndrome:** The triad of RA, splenomegaly, and granulocytopenia also occurs in a small subset of patients, and these patients are at risk for recurrent bacterial infections and nonhealing leg ulcers.
- Approximately 70% of patients show irreversible joint damage on radiography within the first 3 years of disease.[6] Work disability is common, and life span may be shortened.

Cardiovascular Risk

Cardiovascular disease (CVD) is accelerated in patients with RA and is the most common cause of death. CVD risk in RA is similar to that in diabetes. Traditional CAD risk factors do not explain this increased risk which is felt to be due to underlying chronic inflammation, and side effects from medications like NSAIDs and glucocorticoids. EULAR recommends calculating cardiovascular risk every 5 years, but it should be noted that traditional risk calculators are not accurate to predict cardiovascular risk in RA.[7,8] Aggressive primary prevention, minimizing exposure to glucocorticoids and NSAIDs, and control of RA disease activity are recommended to reduce cardiovascular risk.

CRYSTALLINE ARTHRITIS

GENERAL PRINCIPLES

Definition

Crystalline arthritis is caused by deposition of microcrystals in joints and periarticular tissues. Common types of crystalline arthritis are **gout**, **pseudogout**, and **apatite disease**.

Gout

Gout is a monosodium urate crystal deposition disease. This can occur in joints (inflammatory arthritis), soft tissues (tophi), and kidneys. Is the most common form of inflammatory disease in men. Gout is uncommon in premenopausal women due to the uricosuric effect of estrogens.

GENERAL PRINCIPLES

Etiology

Gout is characterized by hyperuricemia that can be due to underexcretion or overproduction of uric acid.

* **Overproduction:** Primary: due to genetic polymorphisms associated with changes in uric acid excretion. Secondary: patients with psoriasis, myeloproliferative disorders, multiple myeloma, hemolytic anemia, and cytotoxic drugs. May also occur because of intake of purine-rich diet, alcohol, or fructose.
* **Underexcretion:** chronic kidney disease (CKD), lead nephropathy, hyperparathyroidism, hypothyroidism. Medications such as loop diuretics, thiazides, low-dose aspirin, cyclosporine, tacrolimus, niacin, and ethambutol all interfere with renal excretion of uric acid.

DIAGNOSIS

Clinical Phases

Natural disease history is divided into three phases.

* Asymptomatic hyperuricemia: defined as uric acid levels >6.8 mg/dL without arthritis or urate nephropathy. Usually present for many years prior to the first attack. The majority of the patients with asymptomatic hyperuricemia do not develop gout.
* Acute intermittent gout: acute attacks of arthritis followed by symptom-free intercritical periods.
* Chronic gouty arthritis: may occur in untreated patients. They experience pain during the intercritical periods between the attacks. Tophi, urate nephropathy, or uric acid stones may occur.

Clinical Presentation

* **Acute gouty arthritis** presents as an excruciating attack of pain. Characterized by sudden onset of pain, erythema, and swelling. Usually in a single joint of the foot or ankle although other joints may be affected. Inflammation of the first metatarsophalangeal joint called as podagra is a classic presenting feature of gout. Acute gouty arthritis attacks can be precipitated by surgery, dehydration, diuretics, fasting, binge eating, or heavy ingestion of alcohol.
* **Chronic gouty arthritis:** When left untreated the disease can progress to chronic gouty arthritis. It may cause a symmetric large and small joint involvement known as a pseudorheumatoid arthritis pattern.

Diagnostic Testing

* Hyperuricemia alone is not diagnostic.
* Serum uric acid level is normal in 30% of patients with acute gout.[9]
* Increased ESR and CRP.
* Synovial fluid analysis of the affected joint or bursa is the gold standard for diagnosing gout. A definitive diagnosis of gout is made by finding **intracellular crystals** in synovial fluid examined with a compensated polarized light microscope. Crystals can also be identified during the intercritical period in asymptomatic patients but are usually not intracellular. **Urate crystals** are needle-shaped and strongly negatively birefringent. Leukocyte counts are elevated, usually >15,000/μL with neutrophilic predominance.

Imaging
- Joint x-rays are normal early in the disease course. Later they may show punched-out joint erosions with overhanging borders. Tophaceous deposits may be visible in the soft tissues on x-rays.
- Ultrasonography can detect joint effusions, erosions, crystal deposition on the cartilage surface (double-contour sign), crystal aggregates in synovial fluid (snowstorm appearance), and tophaceous deposits.
- Dual-energy computed tomography (DECT) enables visualization and volume assessment of tophi.

TREATMENT

- **Asymptomatic hyperuricemia** is not routinely treated. However, patients should be monitored closely for the development of complications if the serum uric acid level is at least 12 mg/dL in men or 10 mg/dL in women. Lifestyle measures such as avoidance of alcohol and limiting intake of sugar and foods rich in purines should be discussed with all patients.
- **Management of gout** includes symptom control with anti-inflammatories in acute gout flares, urate-lowering therapy (ULT), prophylaxis of mobilization flares, and management of risk factors.

Acute Gout Treatment
Although the acute gouty attack will subside spontaneously over several days, prompt treatment can abort the attack within hours (Table 25-2).

Urate-Lowering Therapy
- **Indications**: Indicated in patients with two or more acute gout flares a year, presence of tophi, urate nephropathy, or radiographic damage. In patients experiencing their first gout attack, ULT should be considered if uric acid is greater than 9 mg/dl, presence of nephrolithiasis, or if the patient has CKD ≥ stage 3.
- **Uric acid level goal** will depend on the presence or absence of tophi. If tophi are present, uric acid goal is <5 mg/dL, but if tophi are not present, uric acid goal is <6 mg/dL.
- **Timing**: ULT can be initiated at least 2 weeks after the attack subsides and while the patient has had at least 1 week of prophylactic therapy (reviewed below). If the patient is on ULT, **do not discontinue it during an attack** because any alteration in uric acid levels may worsen or prolong an attack. Once you reach uric acid level goals, ULT should be continued indefinitely (Table 25-3).

Prophylaxis of Mobilization Flares
Patients who are started on ULT will have uric acid mobilization which can precipitate acute gout flares. Prophylactic therapy should be given in patients starting ULT to prevent this. Options include colchicine 0.6 mg PO daily (consider every other day dosing in CKD and elderly) and low-dose NSAIDs. Low-dose steroids (i.e., prednisone 5–10 mg) can be used if the above are contraindicated.

Management of Risk Factors
- Dietary recommendations include weight loss, avoiding organ meats and food and beverages containing high fructose, and limiting the intake of beef, lamb, pork, shellfish, and alcoholic beverages (especially beer).
- Aspirin (uricoretentive) and diuretics should be avoided if possible.

TABLE 25-2	**Acute Gout Treatment**		
Treatment Option	**Dosage**	**Indications**	**Contraindications**
NSAIDs	Commonly used include: Indomethacin: 50 mg PO tid. Ibuprofen: 800 mg PO tid. Naproxen: 500 mg bid. Meloxicam: 15 mg daily.	Considered first-line therapy	CKD, history of peptic ulcer disease or on anticoagulation
Colchicine	1.2 mg PO followed by 0.6 mg PO 1 h later	Consider in patients who cannot take NSAIDs. Most effective within the first 24 h of attack onset	CKD. Avoid concomitant use with carvedilol or drinking grapefruit juice (both can raise blood levels of colchicine)
Intra-articular steroids (triamcinolone or methylprednisolone)	40 mg intra-articularly for large joints, 10–20 mg for small joints or bursae	Consider in patients with contraindications to NSAIDs and CKD who have a monoarticular attack Effective within the first 24 h of an attack in 90% of patients	Septic arthritis should be ruled out
Oral steroids	Prednisone 40–60 mg once daily until flare resolution begins and then taper the dose over 7–10 d	For patients that failed or have contraindications to NSAIDs and colchicine and are not appropriate for intra-articular steroids	Caution in patients with poorly controlled diabetes
IL-1 inhibitor (anakinra)	100 mg SQ once daily for 3 d If CKD (<30 CrCl) dose it every other day	When standard therapy is contraindicated or ineffective	Active infection

CKD, chronic kidney disease.

TABLE 25-3	Urate-Lowering Therapies			
Medication	**Dosage**	**Comments**	**Side Effects**	**Contraindications**
Xanthine Oxidase inhibitors				
Allopurinol	Starting dose is 100 mg PO daily. Start at 50 mg PO daily in patients with CKD stage 4 or higher. Titrate to uric acid goal in 100 mg increments (or 50 mg in CKD) every 2–5 wk. Doses up to 800 mg may be required	This is the first-line agent Screen for HLA-B*5801 in African Americans and Southeast Asians	Diarrhea Nausea Transaminitis Rash Severe rash-1%–5% develop allopurinol hypersensitive syndrome which carries 25% mortality	Avoid in positive HLA-B*5801 to prevent severe cutaneous reaction Blocks metabolism of azathioprine and 6-mercaptopurine, reduce 60%–75% the dose of these cytotoxic drugs
Febuxostat	40–80 mg daily 40 mg is roughly equivalent to 300 mg of allopurinol	Second-line agent More expensive than allopurinol	Transaminitis Higher rate cardiovascular events	
Uricosuric				
Probenecid	Initial dose 500 mg PO daily. Titrate in 500 mg increments weekly to reach uric acid goal Maximum dose 3000 mg/d Most patients require 1–1.5 g/d in two to three divided doses	First choice among uricosurics for ULT monotherapy	Rash Bone marrow suppression	Uric acid nephrolithiasis 24-h urine levels of uric acid >800 mg/24 h Ineffective in patients with renal impairment. Not recommended if CrCl is <50 mL/min Avoid salicylates

(continued)

CHAPTER 25

TABLE 25-3		Urate-Lowering Therapies	(continued)	
Medication	Dosage	Comments	Side Effects	Contraindications
Lesinurad	200 mg PO daily	Used in combination with xanthine oxidase inhibitors	Headache Acute renal injury	Same as probenecid
Uricase				
Pegloticase	8 mg IV every 2 wk	Consider it in patients refractory or intolerant to conventional ULT Monitor uric acid prior to each infusion	Nausea Vomiting Antidrug antibodies Anaphylaxis	G6PD Discontinue it if uric acid rises above 6 mg/dL before the next infusion as this may increase risk of anaphylactic reaction

CKD, chronic kidney disease; ULT, urate-lowering therapy.

Pseudogout/Calcium Pyrophosphate Deposition Disease

GENERAL PRINCIPLES

Etiology

Pseudogout results when calcium pyrophosphate dihydrate crystals deposited in bone and cartilage are released into synovial fluid and induce acute inflammation. It can present in various ways that mimic other rheumatologic diseases.

Classification

- Asymptomatic calcium pyrophosphate dihydrate deposition (CPPD) disease
- Osteoarthritis (OA) with CPPD, also known as "pseudo-OA," refers to patients who have chondrocalcinosis or CPP crystals in a joint affected by OA
- Acute CPP crystal arthritis, also known as "pseudo-gout"
- Chronic CPP crystal inflammatory polyarthropathy, also known as "pseudo-RA"
  - **CPPD** is primarily a disease of the elderly and the majority of these cases are idiopathic. Risk factors include older age, advanced OA, neuropathic joint, diabetes mellitus, joint trauma, or surgery.
  - Early onset of CPPD can be due to an underlying condition such as hypophosphatasia (low alkaline phosphatase activity), hyperparathyroidism, hemochromatosis, hypomagnesemia, or familial CPPD disease due to genetic mutations.

DIAGNOSIS

Clinical Presentation

Pseudogout may present as an **acute monoarthritis or oligoarthritis**, mimicking gout, or as a **chronic polyarthritis** resembling RA or OA. Usually, the knee or wrist is affected, although any synovial joint can be involved.

Diagnostic Testing

- These can be useful if an underlying metabolic disease associated with CPPD is suspected, particularly in young patients or patients with severe arthritis. Workup should include calcium, phosphorous, PTH (hyperparathyroidism), iron, total iron-binding capacity, ferritin (hemochromatosis), alkaline phosphatase (hypophosphatasia), and magnesium (hypomagnesemia).
- Synovial fluid analysis
  ○ **Definitive diagnosis of CPPD is by identification of calcium pyrophosphate dihydrate crystals** in synovial fluid or tissue biopsy. CPP crystals are pleomorphic and weakly positively birefringent, which makes it more difficult to detect than urate crystals. Presence of crystals does not exclude coincident infection.
  ○ **Leukocyte counts** during an acute attack usually ranges between 15,000 and 30,000 cells/mm³ with neutrophilic predominance.

Imaging

Calcium deposition in the cartilage or chondrocalcinosis is a finding that is supportive of (but not diagnostic for) pseudogout and its absence does not exclude it. Hook-like osteophytes can be seen, especially in MCPs, but unlike RA, CPPD does not have typical bony erosions. If pseudogout is suspected, films of the wrists, knees, and pubic symphysis may be ordered, as these are the most common sites for chondrocalcinosis.

TREATMENT

- Treatment is targeted at symptom control. Treatment of associated conditions should be considered, although its beneficial effect on CPPD arthritis is unknown.
- **Acute symptomatic treatment:** As in gout, the therapy of choice for most patients is a brief high-dose course of an NSAID. Oral corticosteroids, intra-articular corticosteroids, and colchicine may also relieve symptoms promptly.
- **Treatment of chronic or recurrent symptoms:** Different medications can be used including the following:
  ○ NSAIDs
  ○ Colchicine 0.6 mg PO daily or twice a day
  ○ Methotrexate 5–20 mg PO weekly or hydroxychloroquine 200–400 mg PO daily can be considered in resistant cases

Other Crystalline Arthritis

Besides monosodium urate and calcium pyrophosphate crystals, other crystals can deposit in the joints and cause arthritis. These include basic calcium phosphate (BCP) and calcium oxalate crystals.
- Apatite/BCP crystals may cause periarthritis, tendonitis, or a destructive arthritis. Shoulders are the most affected joint, either in the form of calcific periarthritis or with true joint arthritis, which is called Milwaukee shoulder.

- Hydroxyapatite complexes and BCP complexes can be identified only by electron microscopy and mass spectroscopy. Therefore, apatite disease should be suspected when no crystals are present in the synovial fluid.
- Treatment of apatite disease is similar to that for pseudogout.

SPONDYLOARTHRITIS

GENERAL PRINCIPLES

- The **spondyloarthritides** (SpAs) are an interrelated group of disorders characterized by one or more of the following features: spondylitis, sacroiliitis, enthesopathy (inflammation at sites of tendon insertion), and asymmetric oligoarthritis. The majority of the patients present before the age of 45. SpAs have an association with HLA-B27. These diseases are classified by their location (peripheral or axial) and by the subtype.
  - ○ Ankylosing spondylitis (AS)
  - ○ Psoriatic arthritis (PsA)
  - ○ Reactive arthritis (ReA)
  - ○ Inflammatory bowel disease (IBD) or enteropathic arthritis
  - ○ Undifferentiated spondyloarthritis (USpA)
- In clinical practice, SpAs overlap significantly. USpA refers to patients with features of SpA without AS, psoriasis, IBD, or a prodromal infection that could account for ReA. Of the subtypes, AS and PsA are the most prevalent.

DIAGNOSIS

Clinical Presentation
- Shared clinical manifestations include inflammatory back pain, peripheral arthritis, enthesitis, and dactylitis. Extra-articular features of this group of disorders may include inflammatory eye disease, urethritis, and mucocutaneous lesions.
- Inflammatory back pain characteristics include onset at <45 years of age, morning stiffness longer than 60 minutes, frequent nocturnal pain, and improvement with exercise. Patients may also describe alternating buttock pain.
- Peripheral inflammatory arthritis is usually asymmetric, commonly involves the lower extremities, and usually affects less than five joints (oligoarthritis).
- Enthesitis refers to the inflammation at the site of tendon or ligament insertion. Common sites include Achilles tendon, plantar fascia, elbow epicondyles, iliac crests, and tibial tuberosities.
- Dactylitis, also known as "sausage digit," is the result of tenosynovitis of the flexor tendons of the digits and synovitis of the joint spaces. It can affect fingers and toes.
- Uveitis is the most common extra-articular manifestation. It can occur in any of the SpAs but is most commonly associated with AS. Uveitis tends to be anterior and unilateral.
- Uncommon manifestations include oral ulcers, aortitis, aortic regurgitation, pericarditis, conduction defects, immunoglobulin A nephropathy, and amyloidosis (Table 25-4).

Physical Examination
A thorough exam should be performed to evaluate for axial and peripheral involvement as well as extra-articular manifestations.

TABLE 25-4	Distinguishing Manifestations			
Finding	Ankylosing Spondylitis	IBD-Associated Arthritis	Psoriatic Arthritis	Reactive Arthritis
Axial involvement	Bilateral sacroiliitis, spinal fusion, bamboo spine	Symmetric sacroiliitis	Asymmetric sacroiliitis	Less prominent than peripheral
Peripheral involvement	Commonly hips, knees, and ankles	Frequent. Lower extremities more than upper	Frequent. Upper extremities more commonly. Can be asymmetric oligoarthritis or symmetric polyarthritis	Frequent. Asymmetric oligoarthritis (knees predominantly)
Enthesitis	Frequent	Uncommon	Frequent	Frequent
Dactylitis	Uncommon	Uncommon	Frequent	Frequent
Ocular manifestations	Uveitis	Uveitis	Uveitis also conjunctivitis and episcleritis	Predominantly conjunctivitis. Less commonly uveitis and keratitis
Skin manifestations	None	Pyoderma gangrenosum, erythema nodosum	Psoriasis, nail pitting, onycholysis	Keratoderma blennorrhagica, circinate balanitis

IBD, inflammatory bowel disease.

- Axial skeleton evaluation should include spinal forward flexion using modified Schober's test (normal is >5 cm), lateral flexion (distance from the middle fingertip to the floor), cervical motion measuring the occiput to wall distance (normal distance is zero), and chest expansion by measuring circumference of the chest in inspiration and expiration (normal >2.5 cm).
- Peripheral joints should be evaluated for swelling, erythema, warmth, tenderness at the site of tendon insertion, joint effusions, and dactylitis.
- The skin should be thoroughly evaluated for evidence of rashes, with special attention to the scalp, gluteal fold, and umbilical areas since these are commonly affected areas by psoriasis and are often overlooked.

Diagnostic Testing
- Inflammatory markers such as ESR and CRP lack sensitivity and specificity and are not diagnostic.
- HLA-B27 test is nonspecific since it is present in up to 8% of the general healthy population. It is estimated that only 5% of the general population with HLA-B27 will develop SpA. The prevalence of HLA-B27 varies across the SpAs, ranging from

30% to 90%.[10] Therefore, its positive predictive value is low in the absence of high clinical suspicion.

- If ReA is suspected, infectious workup should be considered. The triggering infection may have been asymptomatic. Testing for stool pathogens is low yield if the diarrheal illness has resolved. However, in patients with ongoing diarrhea, stool cultures to test for *Salmonella, Shigella, Campylobacter,* and *Yersinia* are recommended. In patients with neither gastrointestinal nor genitourinary symptoms or in patients with suspected *Chlamydia trachomatis* infection, urine testing for chlamydia using nucleic acid amplification techniques may be helpful if the clinical syndrome is consistent with ReA.

Imaging

- X-rays usually detect late changes including sacroiliac erosions or sclerosis or calcification of the spinal ligaments with bridging syndesmophytes (bamboo spine). Peripheral joint x-rays should also be obtained to evaluate for erosions, entheseal calcifications, and osteitis.
- MRI is preferred for early detection of inflammation like sacroiliitis. Typically ordered if there is a high clinical suspicion for SpA and x-rays are negative or equivocal. Supportive findings of sacroiliitis include bone marrow edema (although low specificity), erosions, synovitis, and ankylosis.
- CT is also sensitive for detection of sacroiliitis but involves more radiation.

TREATMENT

Behavioral

- Physical therapy emphasizing extension exercises and posture is recommended to minimize possible late postural defects and respiratory compromise.
- Patients should be instructed to sleep supine on a firm bed without a pillow and to practice postural and deep-breathing exercises regularly.
- Cigarette smoking should be strongly discouraged.

Medications

- **NSAIDs,** such as indomethacin and **selective COX-2 inhibitors**, are used to provide symptomatic relief in all SpAs.
- **Conventional DMARDs like methotrexate and sulfasalazine** provide benefit for peripheral involvement in SpAs.
- **Other conventional DMARDs and biologics have been specifically approved for different SpAs.**
  - AS approved treatments include anti-TNF (inflximab, adalimumab, golimumab, certolizumab pegol), and anti-IL-17 (secukinumab, ixekizumab).
  - PsA approved treatments include apremilast, anti-TNF, anti-IL-17, anti-IL-12/23 (ustekinumab, guselkumab), anti CTLA-4 (abatacept), and JAK inhibitors (tofacitinib).
  - IBD-associated arthritis approved treatments include anti-TNF (except etanercept since it is ineffective for the treatment of IBD, and it is associated with a higher risk of uveitis in SpA patients). NSAIDs should be used with caution because they may trigger IBD flares. Anti-IL-17 should be avoided as they increase the rate of IBD flares and other adverse events. Use of non-TNF inhibitor biologics for IBD-related arthritis should be a shared decision between the patient, rheumatologist, and gastroenterologist.

- ○ ReA: in patients who fail NSAIDs and conventional DMARDs, anti-TNFs have shown some benefit although they are not FDA-approved for this indication. Treatment for chlamydia infection, if detected, is appropriate. Prolonged empiric antibiotic therapy has not been shown to be beneficial.
- ○ Local **injection of glucocorticoids** is a useful adjunctive measure.

Surgical Management

Many patients develop osteoporosis in the fused spondylitic spine and are at risk of spinal fracture. Surgical procedures to correct some spine and hip deformities may result in significant rehabilitation in carefully selected patients.

SYSTEMIC LUPUS ERYTHEMATOSUS

GENERAL PRINCIPLES

Definition

SLE is a multisystem disease of unknown etiology that primarily affects women of childbearing age. The female-to-male ratio is 9:1. It is most common in African Americans and typically occurs in the second and third decades of life.

Pathophysiology

Pathophysiology is multifactorial and incompletely understood, with interplay of genetic predisposition and environmental factors.

DIAGNOSIS

Clinical Presentation

- Disease manifestations are protean, ranging in severity from fatigue, malaise, weight loss, and fever to potentially life-threatening cytopenias, nephritis, cerebritis, vasculitis, pneumonitis, myositis, and myocarditis.
- Photosensitivity is considered a hallmark. Patients often get the "butterfly" rash in the malar area with nasolabial sparing; rash can be seen in all sun-exposed areas. Other symptoms like joint pain, fatigue, and mucosal ulcers can also be triggered by sun exposure.
- Skin involvement is classified as acute, subacute, or chronic. Subacute lupus can present with annular or psoriasiform lesions. Discoid lupus can occur alone or with systemic disease and can cause long-term scaring and pigmentation changes.
- Renal involvement is common and can sometimes be the only or presenting manifestation. It can present with proteinuria >500 mg/d, hematuria, pyuria, or elevated creatinine. There are several types of renal disease associated with SLE which can affect the glomerular, tubular, and vascular compartments of the kidney.
- Classification criteria are used primarily for research purposes, but are helpful to review when suspicion arises. Most recent 2019 EULAR/ACR criteria were updated from 2012 SLICC to improve sensitivity and specificity as well as to improve early detection. If ANA (antinuclear antibody) is not present, the patient does not classify as having SLE. Patients are classified as having SLE with a score of 10 or more points. 2019 EULAR/ACR criteria have a sensitivity of 96.1% and a specificity of 93.4%.[11]

CHAPTER 25

Diagnostic Testing

- Workup should include routine laboratory testing more specific tests as well like antibody and complements levels.
- General tests should include complete blood count (CBC) to look for anemia, leukopenia, or thrombocytopenia; basic metabolic panel for renal dysfunction; urinalysis for hematuria, proteinuria, pyuria, or cellular casts, and urine protein-creatinine ratio. Specific tests include ANA by indirect immunofluorescence, ESR, CRP, and C3 and C4 complement levels.
- It should be noted that up to 15% of the general healthy population have a positive ANA at 1:80.[12] Patients with SLE typically have ANA at significant titers (>1:320). If ANA is positive, more specific antibodies should be ordered, which include:
  - Anti-double-stranded DNA is highly specific for SLE and seen in approximately 70%.
  - Anti-Smith is highly specific for SLE as well, but less sensitive and seen in 30%.[13,14]
  - Ro/SSA, La/SSB: these are more commonly associated with Sjogren syndrome but can be seen in with SLE.
  - U1 ribonucleoprotein (RNP): always present in patients with mixed connective tissue disease (MCTD) but can be present in 25% of patients with SLE.[14]
  - Antiphospholipid antibodies: lupus anticoagulant, anticardiolipin antibodies, and anti-beta2-glycoprotein can also be present in patients with SLE.

TREATMENT

Medications

- Treatment varies according to disease severity. Patients with only mucocutaneous, musculoskeletal, leukopenia, mild thrombocytopenia, and serositis are considered to have mild disease. Moderate disease is considered in patients who have symptoms that are unresponsive to standard treatment, especially if low C3/C4 and high dsDNA. Severe disease includes lupus nephritis, CNS involvement, pneumonitis, vasculitis, and severe cytopenias.
- **NSAIDs** usually help SLE-associated arthritis, arthralgias, fever, and mild serositis but not fatigue, malaise, or major organ system involvement. The response to **selective COX-2 inhibitors** is similar. Hepatic and renal toxicities of NSAIDs appear to be increased in SLE.
- **Glucocorticoid therapy**
  - **Indications** for systemic glucocorticoids at high doses include life-threatening manifestations of SLE, such as glomerulonephritis, CNS involvement, thrombocytopenia, and hemolytic anemia. Steroids can also be used as initial therapy for skin rashes, serositis, and joint symptoms for immediate relief of flares.
  - **Dosage:** Patients with severe or potentially life-threatening complications of SLE should be treated with high-dose prednisone (1–2 mg/kg PO daily) which can be given in divided doses. After disease is controlled, prednisone should be tapered slowly, with the dosage being reduced by 10% every 7–10 days. More rapid reduction may result in relapse. **IV pulse therapy** in the form of methylprednisolone, 500–1000 mg IV daily for 3–5 days, has been used in SLE in such life-threatening situations as rapidly progressive renal failure, active CNS disease, and severe thrombocytopenia. Patients who do not show improvement with this regimen are probably unresponsive to steroids, and other therapeutic alternatives must be considered. A course of oral prednisone should follow completion of pulse therapy.

- **Hydroxychloroquine** 5 mg/kg is recommended for all patients with SLE. It is effective in the treatment of rash, photosensitivity, arthralgias, arthritis, alopecia, and malaise associated with SLE and in the treatment of **discoid and subacute cutaneous lupus erythematosus.** The drug is not effective for treating major organ manifestations, but long-term usage reduces disease progression number of flares and long-term damage from the disease. Hydroxychloroquine also reduces incidence of thrombosis in lupus patients with antiphospholipid antibody syndrome.
- **Immunosuppressive therapy**
  - Indications for immunosuppressive therapy in SLE include life-threatening manifestations of SLE such as glomerulonephritis, CNS involvement, thrombocytopenia, hemolytic anemia, and the inability to reduce corticosteroid dosage or severe corticosteroid side effects.
  - Choice of an immunosuppressive therapy is individualized to the clinical situation. **Cyclophosphamide** is reserved for life-threatening manifestations of SLE. **Azathioprine** and **mycophenolate mofetil** are also used as steroid-sparing agents for serious lupus manifestations. There is increasing evidence that mycophenolate mofetil may be as effective as cyclophosphamide in certain classes of lupus nephritis due to fewer side effects and is particularly preferred in the younger population where fertility maintenance is a concern.[15]
  - **Methotrexate** is often used for musculoskeletal and skin manifestations. **Rituximab** has been shown in uncontrolled observational studies to be effective in cases of severe SLE not responding to conventional treatment; however, placebo-controlled studies have been disappointing. **Belimumab** was approved by the FDA in 2012 for the treatment of adult autoantibody-positive lupus patients who are receiving standard,[16] and in 2020, the FDA approved it for lupus nephritis. The addition of belimumab to standard therapy increased the response rate and prevented worsening of renal disease. **Voclosporin** is a calcineurin inhibitor which does not require monitoring of drug levels. It was approved by the FDA in 2021 for lupus nephritis in combination with standard-of-care therapy. Studies showed marked reduction of proteinuria and higher rates of complete renal response.[17] **For dosing, side effects, and contraindications of individual medications, please refer to** Table 25-5.

Nonpharmacologic Therapies

- **General supportive measures** include adequate sleep and fatigue avoidance.
- All patients, not just those with photosensitive rashes, are advised on use of sunscreens with sun protection factor (SPF) of 30 or greater, protective clothing, and sun avoidance. Isolated skin lesions may respond to **topical steroids.**
- Consider prophylaxis against *Pneumocystis* pneumonia in patients treated with cyclophosphamide. Also consider adding prophylaxis for the prevention of bladder and gonadal toxicity from this agent. Appropriate immunizations should be considered prior to initiation of immunosuppressive therapy, especially against influenza and pneumococcus. Immunization with live vaccines is contraindicated in immunosuppressed patients.

SPECIAL CONSIDERATIONS

- Patients with lupus have accelerated **coronary and peripheral vascular disease**, especially with high disease activity and chronic steroid use, and cardiovascular risk factors should be managed aggressively.

TABLE 25-5 Synthetic DMARDs

Medication	Dosage	Indications	Mechanism	Side Effects (Aside From Infections)	Contraindications
Hydroxychloroquine	5 mg/kg/d of real body weight PO	RA SLE Sjogren syndrome	Inhibits neutrophil trafficking, complement-dependent antigen–antibody responses and interferes with lysosomal enzymes	Retinopathy Bone marrow suppression Myocardial toxicity	G6PD Macular degeneration Porphyria Severe renal or liver impairment
Methotrexate	Start at 10–15 mg/wk (PO or SC) Max 25 mg/wk	RA SLE GCA Sjogren syndrome DM AAV Sarcoidosis Systemic sclerosis Spondyloarthropathies Uveitis	Inhibits dihydrofolate reductase. Acts as a folate antimetabolite inhibiting DNA synthesis and repair	Anorexia Nausea Diarrhea Stomatitis Alopecia Transaminitis Bone marrow suppression Pneumonitis * Incidence reduced by intake of folic acid 1 mg daily	Pregnancy Alcoholism Chronic liver disease Severe renal impairment Preexisting bone marrow suppression

Leflunomide	10–20 mg/d PO	RA	Inhibits dihydroorotate dehydrogenase causing pyrimidine inhibitor	Diarrhea Weight loss Alopecia Transaminitis Rash Hypertension Headache Neuropathy	Pregnancy Severe hepatic dysfunction combination with rifampin Alcoholism Preexisting bone marrow suppression
Sulfasalazine	Start 500–1000 mg daily PO Can increase to 3 g divided into two doses	RA Spondyloarthropathies	Exact mechanism unknown. Felt to have anti-inflammatory and immunomodulatory effects	Headache Rash Nausea Vomiting Diarrhea Reversible oligospermia Bone marrow suppression Transaminitis Interstitial nephritis	G6PD Sulfa allergy Severe hepatic or renal impairment

(continued)

TABLE 25-5   Synthetic DMARDs (continued)

Medication	Dosage	Indications	Mechanism	Side Effects (Aside From Infections)	Contraindications
Azathioprine	Start with 1 mg/kg/d PO. Can increase to a max of 2.5 mg/kg/d	SLE DM AAV RA Uveitis	Inhibits purine metabolism	Nausea Vomiting Diarrhea Leukopenia Transaminitis	Dosage reduction or selection of alternative therapy is recommended in patients with TPMT deficiency
Mycophenolate mofetil	Start with 500 mg bid PO. Can increase to a max of 1500 mg bid	SLE AAV DM Systemic sclerosis Uveitis	Inhibits the novo guanosine nucleotide synthesis by blocking IMPDH	Nausea Vomiting Diarrhea Hypertension Bone marrow suppression	Pregnancy Severe renal impairment
Cyclosporine	Start with 2.5 mg/kg/d PO divided into two doses. Can increase to a max of 4 mg/kg/d	SLE RA	Blocks interleukin (IL)-2 production and release from T cell lymphocytes	Hypertension Edema Hypertriglyceridemia Nausea/vomiting Diarrhea Renal failure	Pregnancy Severe renal impairment

Drug	Dosing	Indications	Mechanism	Side effects	Contraindications
Cyclophosphamide	Dosing depends on the disease severity. If PO 1–2 mg/kg/d, if IV 0.25–1 g/m² monthly	SLE AAV Systemic sclerosis ILD	Alkylating agent, interferes with DNA synthesis	Nausea/vomiting Diarrhea Stomatitis Alopecia Sterility Acute hemorrhagic cystitis (*prevention with Mesna) Bone marrow suppression Bladder transitional cell carcinoma	Pregnancy Bone marrow suppression Severe renal or hepatic impairment
Apremilast	30 mg PO bid	Psoriasis Psoriatic arthritis Behcet disease Recurrent aphthous stomatitis	Phosphodiesterase 4 inhibitor	Diarrhea Nausea Headache	Severe depression

AAV, ANCA-associated vasculitis; DM, dermatomyositis; GCA, giant cell arteritis; ILD, interstitial lung disease; IMPDH, inosine monophosphate dehydrogenase; RA, rheumatoid arthritis; SLE, systemic lupus erythematosus; TPMT, thiopurine S-methyltransferase.

- **Transplantation and chronic hemodialysis** have been used successfully in SLE patients with renal failure. Clinical and serologic evidence of disease activity often remits when renal failure ensues.
- **Pregnancy in SLE:** An increased incidence of second-trimester spontaneous miscarriages and stillbirths has been reported in women with antibodies to cardiolipin or lupus anticoagulant. SLE patients may experience flares during pregnancy if the lupus is active at the time of conception. Differentiation between active SLE and preeclampsia is often difficult. Women in whom SLE is well controlled are less likely to have a flare of disease during pregnancy.
- **Neonatal lupus** may occur in offspring of anti-SSA- or anti-SSB-positive mothers, with skin rash and heart block being the most common manifestations. **Drug-induced lupus** typically has a sudden onset and is associated with serositis and musculoskeletal manifestations. Renal and CNS manifestations are rare. Serology includes positive ANA and **antihistone antibodies**, negative anti-SM, and anti–double-stranded DNA antibodies along with normal complement levels. The disease usually resolves with drug discontinuation. Offending drugs include procainamide, hydralazine, minocycline, diltiazem, isoniazid, chlorpromazine, quinidine, methyldopa, and anti-TNF biologics.

SYSTEMIC SCLEROSIS

GENERAL PRINCIPLES

Definition

Systemic sclerosis (scleroderma) is a systemic illness characterized by progressive fibrosis of the skin and visceral organs. The etiology is unknown, but immune dysregulation, vasculopathy, and fibrosis are implicated in disease pathogenesis.

Classification

- Scleroderma can be subdivided based on anatomic skin distribution into **localized scleroderma** (morphea and linear scleroderma) and **systemic sclerosis** (diffuse cutaneous, limited cutaneous, and systemic sclerosis sine scleroderma). The limited cutaneous form involves the extremities distal to the knees and elbows as well as the face. Diffuse cutaneous scleroderma involves the skin of the proximal extremities and the trunk. Systemic sclerosis sine scleroderma affects the internal organs without skin involvement. The **CREST syndrome** is **c**alcinosis, **R**aynaud phenomenon, **e**sophageal dysmotility, **s**clerodactyly, and **t**elangiectasias.
- **Overlap syndrome** is the term used to describe patients who have overlapping clinical or serologic features of two or more CTDs. Arguably, the most well-defined of these overlap syndromes is MCTD which encompasses features of SLE, systemic sclerosis, and inflammatory myopathies. Therefore, it is important to recognize that the features of systemic sclerosis that will be reviewed here can be present along with features of other CTDs.

DIAGNOSIS

Clinical Presentation

- Nearly all patients with systemic sclerosis have **RP**. It is typically the presenting feature. Nail fold capillary changes are also common. Digital ischemia can result in

digital pitting or ulcers and in some cases digital resorption. Ulcerations can also occur over DIP and PIP joint contractures.
- **Diffuse scleroderma** is associated with scleroderma "renal crisis," and multiple internal organs are affected. Long-term survival is poor.
  - **Skin involvement:** presents initially with edematous skin, erythema may be present reflecting active inflammation. Pruritus is often present in early stages. Pigment changes with the classic "salt and pepper" appearance can be seen. Eventually the skin tightens and becomes hide bound. Some patients may experience loosening of skin over time either spontaneously or with treatment. Calcium deposition can also occur in the skin often in areas subject to pressure.
  - **GI involvement:** Decreased gut motility can occur, leading to bacterial overgrowth, malabsorption, diarrhea, and weight loss. Occasionally, severe constipation and intestinal pseudo-obstruction occur. Classic endoscopic findings include colonic wide-mouth diverticula, patulous esophagus, esophageal strictures, and gastric antral vascular ectasia (GAVE), also known as watermelon stomach.
  - **Renal involvement:** The appearance of sudden hypertension and renal insufficiency indicates potential scleroderma renal crisis. It is associated with a microangiopathic hemolytic anemia and carries a poor prognosis.
  - **Cardiac involvement:** Patchy myocardial fibrosis can result in heart failure or arrhythmias.
  - **Pulmonary involvement** includes pleural effusions and ILD. Predominantly nonspecific interstitial pneumonia pattern although one-third develop usual interstitial pneumonia pattern.
  - **Musculoskeletal involvement:** manifestations range from arthralgias to arthritis with joint contractures because of the regional skin involvement. Myositis can be seen especially in patients with overlap syndrome. Tendon friction rubs are very typical of this diagnosis, often heard over the tendons of the hands.
- **Limited scleroderma** is more often associated with primary pulmonary hypertension in the absence of ILD, telangiectasias, and calcinosis. There is a strong association with primary biliary cirrhosis.

Diagnostic Testing
- More than 95% of scleroderma patients are ANA positive.[18] Well-known antibodies associated with scleroderma are anticentromere antibodies (ACA) and anti-DNA topoisomerase I (Scl-70), but many others have been described. These tend to correlate with the scleroderma subtype and specific manifestations.[19]
- Antibodies associated with **limited scleroderma:**
  - ACA: pulmonary arterial hypertension (PAH), ILD, digital ulcerations, and calcinosis
  - Th/To: ILD and PAH
  - U11/U12 RNP: severe ILD
- Antibodies associated with **diffuse scleroderma:**
  - Scl-70: ILD, digital ulcerations and myopathy
  - RNA polymerase III: renal crisis, severe skin involvement, and GAVE
  - U3-RNP: PAH, myositis, cardiomyopathy, severe GI involvement
- Antibodies associated with **overlap syndromes:**
  - U1-RNP (MCTD): ILD, myositis, and arthritis
  - PmScl: ILD and myositis
  - Ku: myositis
- Common disease-antibody scenarios include
  - Limited scleroderma + ACA: highest risk PAH. Lower risk ILD or renal crisis

- Limited scleroderma + Scl-70: higher risk ILD. Lower risk renal crisis
- Diffuse scleroderma + RNA III: highest of renal crisis and higher risk of malignancy

TREATMENT

- Therapeutic options for scleroderma are limited. Treatment focuses on organ involvement and symptoms. In general, the indications for immunosuppressive therapy include progressive skin thickening, ILD, inflammatory myopathy, and inflammatory arthritis. Other manifestations require symptomatic treatment but not immunosuppression.
- **Skin:** Methotrexate and mycophenolate mofetil (MMF) are commonly used and can prevent progression. **Physical therapy** is important to retard and reduce joint contractures.
- **GI involvement**
  - Reflux esophagitis generally responds to standard therapy (e.g., H^2-receptor antagonists, proton pump inhibitors, and promotility agents).
  - For dysmotility, short courses of prokinetic drugs like domperidone, metoclopramide, or erythromycin can be considered. Injectable octreotide has been used in severe or refractory cases.
  - For symptomatic small intestine bacterial overgrowth, intermittent or rotating antibiotics like rifaximin, ciprofloxacin, amoxicllin-clavulanic acid, or metronidazole can be used.
  - Occasionally, esophageal strictures require mechanical **esophageal dilation**.
- **Renal involvement:** Aggressive blood pressure control with **ACE inhibitors** is indicated in scleroderma renal crisis. ARBs do not appear to be as effective. Blood pressure and renal function should be carefully monitored if the patient is receiving glucocorticoids since it is known that use of glucocorticoids can precipitate scleroderma renal crisis.
- **Cardiac involvement:** Coronary artery vasospasm can cause angina pectoris and may respond to calcium channel antagonists.
- **Pulmonary involvement,** such as pulmonary hypertension, is treated with standard therapies for these conditions. For patients with ILD, MMF is considered first-line treatment. Cyclophosphamide is viewed as a second-line agent due to the increased risk of adverse effects when compared to MMF.[20] Refractory cases may benefit from the addition of nintedanib, an antifibrotic agent.[21]

RAYNAUD PHENOMENON

GENERAL PRINCIPLES

Raynaud phenomenon (RP) is a vasospasm of the digital arteries and can result in ischemia of the digits. It manifests as repeated episodes of color changes in the finger, toes, and less commonly ears and nose after cold exposure or emotional stress. The sequential color changes are white to blue to red, but this triad may not be seen in all patients. Well-demarcated pallor (white phase) is the most definitive phase. Patients may also experience numbness during the ischemic phase and pain during the rewarming phase.

Classification

- RP can be classified as primary (idiopathic) or secondary if an underlying condition is present. Secondary RP is associated with multiple conditions and can be divided into different categories.

- Systemic rheumatic disease: systemic sclerosis, MCTD, SLE, inflammatory myopathies, Sjogren syndrome, Burger disease, RA, vasculitis
- Drugs or chemical induced: ergots, beta-blockers, bromocriptine, interferon-alfa, chemotherapeutic agents (vinblastine, bleomycin, cisplatin), vinyl chloride
- Traumatic: pneumatic hammer operators, rock drillers, lumberjacks, etc.
- Hyperviscosity syndrome: myeloproliferative disorders, paraproteinemia, leukemia, cryoglobulinemia, and cold agglutinins
- Occlusive arterial disease: thrombotic/embolic arterial occlusion, thoracic outlet syndrome
- Endocrinopathies: hypothyroidism, pheochromocytoma, carcinoid
- Other: infections, complex regional pain syndrome, peripheral arteriovenous fistula
- A thorough review of systems and physical examination is critical to differentiate between primary and secondary RP. Some of the other differences include:
  - **Primary RP** is more common in women and onset is typically between the ages of 15–30 years. These patients do not develop complications like ulceration, pitting, or gangrene. Nailfold capillary examination is normal and serologies are negative (although up to one-third may have low titer positive ANA).
  - **Secondary RP** may affect men or women. Onset tends to be in the third or fourth decade. Review of systems and physical examination may reveal signs or symptoms of an underlying condition. These patients are more prone to develop complications, nailfold capillary examination is abnormal, and serologies may be positive.

DIAGNOSIS

- **Nailfold capillary microscopy (NCM)** can be done by placing a drop of surgical lubricant on the cuticle of the finger and visualizing the capillaries with an ophthalmoscope set at 40 diopters.
- Abnormal NCM may show tortuous capillary loops, microhemorrhages, and avascular areas ("dropout"). **No laboratory test is pathognomonic of RP**. In patients with clinical suspicion of an underlying disease, studies to evaluate for CTD (ANA, extractable nuclear antigens, ACA), hypothyroidism (thyroid stimulating hormone), hypercoagulable state (CBC, serum protein electrophoresis, urine protein electrophoresis, free light chains), or cryoglobulinemia should be considered.

TREATMENT

Preventive Measures
Patients should be instructed to avoid exposure to cold, protect the hands and feet from trauma, limit caffeine intake, and discontinue cigarette smoking.

Medications
- **Calcium channel antagonists** (of the dihydropyridine group) are the preferred initial agents, although they may exacerbate gastroesophageal reflux and constipation.
- Alternative vasodilators such as prazosin are occasionally helpful but can have limiting side effects, including orthostatic hypotension.
- Other agents that might improve vasospasm include **topical nitroglycerin** applied to the dorsum of the hands.
- Phosphodiesterase inhibitor (e.g., **sildenafil**) and endothelin receptor antagonist (e.g., **bosentan**) can be used for secondary RP and are effective at controlling symptoms and prevention of ulcer formation.
- Daily low-dose aspirin therapy is often prescribed for its antiplatelet effects.

- Patients with severe ischemic digits should be hospitalized, and conditions such as macrovascular disease, vasculitis, or a hypercoagulable state should be ruled out. An IV infusion of a prostaglandin or prostaglandin analog may be considered.

Surgical Management
- **Sympathetic ganglion blockade** with a long-acting anesthetic agent may be useful when a patient has progressive digital ulceration that fails to improve with medical therapy.
- Surgical digital sympathectomy may be beneficial.

IDIOPATHIC INFLAMMATORY MYOPATHIES

GENERAL PRINCIPLES

Idiopathic inflammatory myopathies are a group of heterogeneous disorders characterized by inflammation of the skeletal muscle. These can be differentiated by the pattern of muscle involvement, extramuscular manifestations, specific serologies, and findings on muscle biopsy.

Classification
- **Dermatomyositis (DM):** inflammatory myopathy associated with proximal muscle weakness and a characteristic skin rash. DM includes clinically amyopathic dermatomyositis (CADM) and juvenile-onset DM.
- **Polymyositis (PM):** inflammatory myopathy that presents as proximal weakness and occasionally tenderness of the proximal musculature but lacks characteristic rash.
- **Overlap syndromes:** Inflammatory myopathy that occurs in the setting of another systemic rheumatic disease (i.e., SLE, systemic sclerosis, etc.).
- **Anti-synthetase syndrome** is a spectrum of inflammatory myopathies defined by the presence of an antibody directed against one of several aminoacyl-transfer RNA (tRNA) synthetases.
- **Inclusion body myositis (IBM):** inflammatory myopathy that commonly involves distal musculature and has specific muscle biopsy findings.
- **Immune-mediated necrotizing myositis (IMNM):** this inflammatory myopathy resembles PM, but muscle necrosis and minimal inflammatory infiltrate seen on muscle biopsy distinguish it from PM.

DIAGNOSIS

Clinical Presentation
- Muscle weakness: insidious onset of weakness over 3–6 months. If onset occurs in less than 2 months, suspect IMNM. All with the exception of IBM affect proximal musculature in a symmetric fashion. IBM can present with distal and asymmetric muscle involvement. A small proportion of patients can have bulbar muscle involvement. In general, muscle pain is absent or minimal.
- Cutaneous: present in DM and may precede the onset of myopathy. The most specific finding is Gottron papules, which are violaceous papules over the dorsum of MCP and PIP joints, wrists, elbows, and knees. Other findings include a photosensitive erythematous rash on the face, scalp, anterior chest (V sign), and back and shoulders (shawl sign) and a purplish discoloration over the upper eyelids called heliotrope rash. Calcinosis is common in juvenile DM and sometimes occurs in adult DM. Patients with antisynthetase syndrome may develop hyperkeratotic, fissured skin on the palmar and lateral aspects of the fingers, called "mechanic's hands."

- Arthritis: mild joint pain and swelling of small joints can be seen in DM and anti-synthetase syndrome.
- Pulmonary: ILD is often found in DM. Other less common manifestations include diffuse alveolar hemorrhage or restrictive lung disease secondary to muscle weakness.
- Cardiac: can develop myo/pericarditis, conduction abnormalities. Heart failure is uncommon.
- Gastrointestinal: dysphagia and aspiration pneumonia can be seen in DM.

Diagnostic Testing

- Elevated muscle enzyme levels: creatine kinase (CK), aldolase, transaminases, and lactate dehydrogenase (LDH). CK can be normal or only slightly (up to 10 times upper limit of normal) elevated in IBM, moderately elevated in DM and PM and can be very high in IMNM (>50 times upper limit of normal).
- Autoantibodies: these are generally divided into two: **myositis-specific antibodies (MSAs)** and **myositis-associated antibodies (MAAs).** MSAs are detected primarily in patients with inflammatory myopathies and MAAs are detected in patients with other autoimmune diseases that can be associated with myositis. Different antibodies are associated with different clinical manifestations and have therapeutic and prognostic implications (Table 25-6).

TABLE 25-6	Myositis-Specific Antibodies (MSA)
Antibody	**Clinical Presentation**
Dermatomyositis	
Mi-2	Classic DM rash. Excellent prognosis
MDA-5	Clinically amyopathic DM, rapidly progressive ILD, cutaneous ulcers, arthritis. High morbidity and mortality
TIF-1(p155/140)	Classic DM rash, usually severe. Strong association with malignancy
NXP2	Classic DM rash, subcutaneous calcifications (especially juvenile DM). Associated with malignancy
SAE	Classic DM rash
Anti-synthetase syndrome	
Anti-synthetase antibodies: Jo-1(the most common), PL-7, PL-12, EJ, OJ, KS, Zo, Ha	Myositis, rash, ILD, Raynaud phenomenon, mechanic hands, arthritis
Immune-mediated necrotizing myositis	
SRP	Severe weakness, very high levels of CK, myocarditis, and dysphagia
HMGCR	High levels of CK, associated with statin use (up to 50% are statin naïve)
Inclusion body myositis	
cN1A	The most common IIM in patients older than 50 years. Asymmetric insidious muscle weakness

DM, dermatomyositis, IIM, idiopathic inflammatory myopathy; ILD, interstitial lung disease.

- **Myositis-associated antibodies (MAAs)** and their associations include the following:
  - PM/Scl—overlap PM and systemic sclerosis
  - U1-RNP—MCTD
  - U3-snRNP (fibrillarin)—systemic sclerosis
  - Ku—overlap PM and systemic sclerosis
  - Ro52—frequently coupled with other MSAs. Associated with ILD
  - Ro60/SSA—Sjogren syndrome, SLE
  - LA/SSB—Sjogren syndrome, SLE

Other Diagnostic Procedures
- Characteristic findings can be seen on electromyogram; these include insertional activity, but these changes are not specific and can be seen in infectious or metabolic myopathies.
- A muscle biopsy can establish the diagnosis but may not be required if myositis-related antibodies are present in the right clinical setting.
- MRI is useful for the detection of muscle inflammation and necrosis and can aid in identifying a biopsy location.
- Screening for common neoplasms, such as colon, lung, breast, and prostate cancer, should be considered in these patients as well as individual risk-based assessment. Risk factors for malignancy in the setting of myositis include the presence of DM, cutaneous vasculitis, male sex, advanced age and TIF-1(p155/140) or NXP-2 antibodies.

TREATMENT

- When PM or DM occurs without associated disease, it usually responds well to **prednisone**, 1–2 mg/kg PO daily. Systemic complaints, such as fever and malaise, respond first, followed by muscle enzymes, and finally, muscle strength. Once serum enzyme levels normalize, the prednisone dosage should be reduced slowly to maintenance levels of 10–20 mg PO daily. Appearance of steroid-induced myopathy and hypokalemia may complicate therapeutic assessment.
- Patients often need early initiation of steroid-sparing treatment and **methotrexate, mycophenolate mofetil**, and **azathioprine** are used as first-line agents.
- IV infusion of **immunoglobulin** are useful in patients who do not respond to steroids or have severe manifestations like truncal weakness or severe dysphagia.
- Severe cases are typically treated with **rituximab**, effective in patients with antisynthetase syndrome especially those that are Jo-1 positive, or intravenous immunoglobulin (IVIG).
- PM or DM associated with neoplasia tends to be less responsive to glucocorticoid therapy but may improve after removal of the malignant tumor.
- **Physical therapy** is essential in the management of myositis.

VASCULITIS

GENERAL PRINCIPLES

- **Vasculitis** is characterized by inflammation of blood vessels, leading to tissue damage and necrosis. This diagnosis includes a broad spectrum of disorders with various causes that involve vessels of different types, sizes, and locations. The immunopathologic process may involve immune complexes.

- Although in most cases the inciting agent has not been identified, some are associated with chronic hepatitis B and C.
- Vasculitis "mimics" should be considered, including bacterial endocarditis, HIV infection, atrial myxoma, paraneoplastic syndromes, cholesterol emboli, and cocaine and amphetamine use.
- Vasculitides are classified by vessel sizes (Table 25-7).
- Vasculitis should be suspected whenever a patient with systemic symptoms has organ dysfunction. Symptoms are associated with the size of the affected vessel (Table 25-8).
- We will review some of the most common vasculitis in the following sections.

TABLE 25-7	Vasculitis Classification	
Vessel Size	Types of Vessel	Types of Vasculitis
Large vessel	Aorta and main branches	• Takayasu arteritis • Giant cell arteritis
Medium vessel	Main visceral arteries and veins and their initial branches	• Polyarteritis nodosa • Kawasaki disease
Small vessel	Arterioles, venules, and capillaries	ANCA-associated vasculitis: • Granulomatosis with polyangiitis • Eosinophilic granulomatosis with polyangiitis • Microscopic polyangiitis Immune complex mediated: • Cryoglobulinemic vasculitis • Henoch-Schönlein purpura (HSP) • Hypocomplementemic urticarial vasculitis
Variable vessel	Can involve any vessel size	• Behcet disease • Cogan syndrome

TABLE 25-8	Vasculitis Features by Vessel Size		
Organ System	Small Vessel	Medium Vessel	Large Vessel
Dermatologic	Palpable purpura	Livedo reticularis	Cyanosis
Renal	Hematuria with RBC casts, proteinuria	Hematuria, flank pain	Hypertension
Gastrointestinal	GI bleeding	Bowel perforation	Bowel infarction
Neurologic	Polyneuropathy	Polyneuropathy, strokes	Strokes

LARGE VESSEL VASCULITIS

Takayasu Arteritis

GENERAL PRINCIPLES

Epidemiology

Also known as the "pulseless disease." It is most common in individuals of Asian descent and affects women more than men; the peak onset is in the third decade.

DIAGNOSIS

Clinical Presentation

- Clinical presentation is divided into three phases, but disease presentation is variable. Only half of the patients have constitutional symptoms and monophasic disease can also occur.
- Prepulseless phase is manifested by constitutional symptoms like fever, weight loss, generalized malaise, myalgias, and arthralgias.
- Second phase is characterized by vessel pain and tenderness, like carotidynia, due to vessel inflammation.
- Burned-out or fibrotic phase is characterized by ischemic symptoms due to arterial stenoses. Some of the symptoms include limb claudication secondary to subclavian stenosis, chest pain secondary to aortitis, and less commonly coronary arteries involvement, hypertension secondary to aortic or renal arteries involvement, strokes or transient ischemic attack (TIA) due to common carotid stenosis or dizziness, and visual impairment due to vertebral artery involvement.

Diagnostic Testing

- There are no specific tests for the diagnosis of Takayasu arteritis. Some of the laboratory abnormalities are the reflection of inflammation like anemia of chronic disease, thrombocytosis, elevated ESR, and CRP.
- Imaging studies include:
- MRI and CT angiography for the identification of wall edema, vessel thickness, and areas of stenosis. However, there is no good correlation between the wall changes and disease activity.
- Intra-arterial angiography is the gold standard to detect the involved vessels. It is important to note that it only provides information about the vessel lumen but no details about the vessel walls.
- PET scan technology is useful to detect areas of active arteritis. This can help differentiate between the inflammatory versus burned-out phases.

TREATMENT

Medications

- Patients in the inflammatory phases (phase one and two) are started on pharmacologic therapy to prevent further development of stenosis or aneurysms. Patients are initially treated with oral glucocorticoids (prednisone 1 mg/kg) and then started on a steroid-sparing agent. Options include methotrexate, azathioprine, leflunomide, mycophenolate mofetil, cyclophosphamide, anti-TNF agents, and tocilizumab.

Selection of steroid-sparing agent will depend on disease severity and medication tolerance. Hypertension should also be aggressively treated to prevent ischemia.
• Surgical management is also available for amenable stenosis. These include angioplasty, endovascular stenting, and bypass surgery.

Giant Cell Arteritis

GENERAL PRINCIPLES

Epidemiology

Giant cell arteritis (GCA) is the most common systemic vasculitis in people older than 50 years. The median age of onset is 75 years, and it is four times more common in women than men. Patients of Northern European descent are more likely to develop GCA compared to Southern European, Hispanics, and African Americans.

DIAGNOSIS

Clinical Presentation
• Symptom onset tends to be gradual rather than abrupt. Patients can present with systemic, cranial, and/or large vessel manifestations. In addition, 40%–50% will have overlapping polymyalgia rheumatica (PMR) symptoms.
• Systemic symptoms include fatigue, fever, weight loss, night sweats, and generalized malaise. Cranial symptoms are various. Headache, which is typically in the temporal lobes, can also be seen over the parietal or occipital lobes. Temporal tenderness, jaw claudication (one of the most specific symptoms), and TIA or strokes which result from the involvement of internal carotid or vertebral artery. There are also multiple different visual manifestations including:
  ○ Amaurosis fugax: temporary vision loss due to focal ophthalmic artery lesions. Patients may also report diplopia or blurry vision.
  ○ Anterior ischemic optic neuropathy (AION) is the most common visual manifestation in GCA. It is a permanent monocular vision loss due to lack of blood flow to the posterior ciliary artery leading to the ischemia of the optic nerve.
  ○ Posterior ischemic optic neuropathy is uncommon; also leads to permanent monocular vision loss but it is due to the interruption of blood flow to the retrobulbar portion of the optic nerve.
  ○ Homonymous hemianopia is rarely seen in patients with GCA; it is a consequence of the involvement of the vertebrobasilar circulation leading to occipital lobe infarction.
• Large vessel symptoms can present in combination with cranial and systemic symptoms or can be isolated. Some symptoms include arm claudication, asymmetric pulses, paresthesias secondary to subclavian or axillary artery involvement, chest pain, aortic aneurysms, or dissection secondary to aortitis.
• PMR symptoms include symmetric morning stiffness and achiness of shoulder and hip girdles, neck, and torso. Peripheral synovitis, mimicking RA or remitting seronegative symmetrical synovitis with pitting edema, can occur in some patients.

Diagnostic Testing
• Laboratories may show anemia of chronic disease, thrombocytosis, and significant elevations of ESR and CRP. A normal ESR reduces the probability of a positive temporal artery biopsy by fivefold.[22]

CHAPTER 25

- Imaging: Different imaging modalities have been studied in GCA. These include ultrasound with Doppler, magnetic resonance angiography, and PET scan, but the best imaging method for the investigation of GCA is yet to be defined.
- Temporal artery biopsy: It is considered the gold standard for the diagnosis of GCA. The mean sensitivity for a unilateral temporal artery biopsy is 86.9%.[23] Sensitivity is lower in patients with isolated large vessel involvement, in which case diagnosis is based on imaging findings. Given the segmental nature of arterial involvement by GCA, at least 2 cm should be obtained to avoid false negative result.

TREATMENT

- High-dose systemic glucocorticoids are the mainstay of therapy and should be started as soon as there is high diagnostic suspicion of GCA, especially in patients with threatened visual loss.
  - ○ Treatment should not be withheld while awaiting the performance temporal artery biopsy or imaging studies.
  - ○ Resolution of the inflammatory infiltrate of GCA occurs slowly, and histologic evidence will be evident for at least a month after glucocorticoid therapy has been instituted.
  - ○ Dose will depend on the presence or absence of visual manifestations.
  - ○ Given the prolonged course of high doses of steroids, osteoporosis prevention with calcium and vitamin D supplementation and PCP prophylaxis should be pursued in all patients.
- In patients with visual loss (or threatened) intravenous pulses of methylprednisolone are recommended. 500–1000 mg IV daily for three doses followed by oral prednisone at 1 mg/kg/d. Patients without visual loss oral steroids are recommended, prednisone 1 mg/kg (maximum 60 mg/d) or its equivalent administered daily. Taper schedule will depend on the treatment response. Dose is reduced by 10 mg every 2 weeks until 40 mg is reached. Subsequently decreased by 5 mg every 2 weeks and once 10 mg is reached, if the patient does not develop a flare, taper is usually slowed to 1 mg decrements monthly.
- Tocilizumab is the **first-line steroid-sparing agent** approved for GCA.[24] It is an anti-IL-6 receptor monoclonal antibody; given that IL-6 plays an important role in the acute phase response, ESR and CRP measurement become unreliable to monitor disease activity.
- Methotrexate is sometimes used with moderate efficacy controlling the disease, but the three randomized controlled trials showed conflicting results.

MEDIUM VESSEL VASCULITIS

Polyarteritis Nodosa

GENERAL PRINCIPLES

Epidemiology

Polyarteritis nodosa (PAN) affects men more than women, typically between the ages of 40 and 60 years. Most of the cases are idiopathic and a minority are caused by hepatitis B virus infection.

DIAGNOSIS

Clinical Presentation

* Most of the patients will have systemic symptoms such as fever, malaise, weight loss, arthralgias, and myalgias. Presentation may be nonspecific; it will depend on the organ systems affected. Some of the manifestations include the following:
  * Skin: erythematous nodules, purpura, livedo reticularis, ulcers
  * Renal: hypertension, perirenal hematomas, renal infarctions
  * Neurologic: typically, mononeuritis multiples. CNS involvement is exceedingly rare
  * Gastrointestinal: mesenteric arteritis leading to abdominal pain, melena, bloody or nonbloody diarrhea, and life-threatening gastrointestinal bleeding
  * Cardiac: narrowing or occlusion of coronary arteries leading to myocardial ischemia and heart failure
  * Musculoskeletal: myalgias and muscle weakness
  * Reproductive: orchitis, testicular tenderness
  * Ocular: ischemic retinopathy or optic neuropathy
* Limited cutaneous PAN is a term used for isolated skin involvement which rarely converts into systemic PAN. Isolated single-organ PAN can also occur; it is considered a monocyclic disease that rarely relapses.

Diagnostic Testing

* Laboratory findings, just like in other vasculitis, include anemia of chronic disease, and elevated ESR and CRP. A small percentage of patients may have eosinophilia. Hematuria may be present, but no active urine sediment and hepatitis serologies should be checked as well.
* Angiography, typically mesenteric, renal, or coronary, is often diagnostic. These demonstrate microaneurysms and/or stenoses in small to medium size vessels.
* Biopsy should be pursued whenever possible. Skin, nerve, muscle, or testicle biopsies may be easily accessible and provide diagnosis.

TREATMENT

* Glucocorticoids are considered first-line treatment. In patients with severe, life-threatening manifestations (creatinine > 1.5 mg/dL, cardiomyopathy, GI or CNS involvement), pulse intravenous methylprednisolone 1000 mg daily for 3–5 days is recommended. In patients without these manifestations, oral prednisone at 1 mg/kg is commonly started.
* Patients with severe manifestations or those with mild disease but unable to be tapered off steroids should be started on additional treatment. Cyclophosphamide is considered first line; if not tolerated or disease is resistant, other medications should be considered including rituximab, methotrexate, azathioprine, or mycophenolate mofetil.
* Hepatitis B–associated PAN treatment is based on the treatment of the infection with antivirals. Patients with severe manifestations can be started on glucocorticoids and plasma exchange until antiviral therapy becomes effective.

CHAPTER 25

SMALL VESSEL VASCULITIS

ANCA-Associated Vasculitis

- ANCA (antineutrophil cytoplasmic antibody)-associated vasculitis (AAV) are subclassified as:
  - ○ Granulomatosis with polyangiitis (GPA)
  - ○ Microscopic polyangiitis (MPA)
  - ○ Eosinophilic granulomatosis with polyangiitis (EGPA)
  - ○ Renal limited vasculitis with pauci-immune necrotizing glomerulonephritis (RLV)
- ANCA antibody association (Table 25-9):
- Brief review of each of the ANCA-associated vasculitis (AAV) is presented below.

Granulomatosis with Polyangiitis

Granulomatosis with polyangiitis is a necrotizing granulomatous vasculitis of small vessels. It affects men and women equally, and the peak age of onset is between the age of 60 and 70. It most commonly affects respiratory tract and kidneys, but many other organs can be involved. Clinical manifestations by organ system include the following:

- Upper respiratory tract: rhinitis, sinusitis, oral/nasal ulcers, nasal septum perforation, saddle nose deformity, recurrent otitis, sensorineural hearing loss, subglottic stenosis
- Lower respiratory tract: cough, hemoptysis, pulmonary infiltrates, nodules, diffuse pulmonary hemorrhage, pleurisy
- Renal: rapidly progressive glomerulonephritis
- Ocular: scleritis, episcleritis, orbital pseudotumor, uveitis
- Musculoskeletal: arthralgias or migratory arthritis
- Neurologic: mononeuritis multiplex, symmetric polyneuropathy and less commonly cranial neuropathies
- Cutaneous: palpable purpura, ulcers, subcutaneous nodules, livedo reticularis
- Abdominal vasculitis can manifest with abdominal pain, gut ulceration, or infarction

TABLE 25-9	Sensitivity of ANCA Antibodies		
Disease	PR3 (%)	MPO (%)	Negative ANCA (%)
GPA	66	24	10
MPA	26	58	10–15
RLV	20	64	15–20
EGPA	10	50	35–50

Atypical ANCA pattern is associated with drug-induced vasculitis, nonvasculitic rheumatic diseases, primary sclerosing cholangitis, ulcerative colitis, cystic fibrosis, and endocarditis. ANCA, antineutrophil cytoplasmic antibodies; EGPA, eosinophilic granulomatosis with polyangiitis; GPA, granulomatosis with polyangiitis; MPA, microscopic polyangiitis; MPO, myeloperoxidase; RLV, renal limited vasculitis.
Modified from Mark M. Antineutrophil cytoplasmic antibody-associated vasculitis. In: West S, Kolfenbach J. *Rheumatology Secrets*. 4th ed. Elsevier; 2020:224-235. Copyright © 2020 Elsevier. With permission.

DIAGNOSIS

- Laboratory findings include anemia of chronic disease, elevated ESR/CRP, elevated creatinine, hematuria, proteinuria, and positive ANCA (commonly PR3).
- Imaging studies may show lung nodules, infiltrates, or cavities. Biopsy of kidney, lung, or skin can be done if affected.
- Nasal biopsies usually have low specificity. Kidney biopsy often shows pauci-immune glomerulonephritis. Lung biopsies may show capillaritis or necrotizing granulomatosis.

TREATMENT

- Treatment includes induction therapy followed by maintenance therapy. The use of glucocorticoid alone is inadequate and should always be used in combination with a DMARD.
  - Induction therapy is usually the combination of IV methylprednisolone 1 g for 3 days followed by oral prednisone 1 mg/kg daily plus rituximab or cyclophosphamide or both. Based on the RAVE study, rituximab is as effective as cyclophosphamide and favored in relapsing disease.[25]
  - Maintenance treatment options, once remission is achieved, include azathioprine, methotrexate, and mycophenolate mofetil. Low-dose rituximab can also be used for maintenance. For patients with limited GPA, only upper airway involvement, induction, and maintenance therapy with oral DMARDs alone can be considered.
  - PEXIVAS trial showed that plasmapheresis does not reduce the risk of end-stage renal disease or death in patients with ANCA vasculitis, but it demonstrated that a rapid steroid taper was equally effective, and patients had less side effects.[26] Thus, steroid taper protocol used in the trial is recommended. TMP/SMX should be considered for all patients for PCP prophylaxis.

Microscopic Polyangiitis

- Clinically similar to GPA but not granulomatous and without upper airway involvement. The majority of the patients have renal involvement (rapidly progressive glomerulonephritis) and some pulmonary, neurologic or cutaneous manifestations.
- Diagnosis is based on similar laboratory findings, positive ANCA (commonly MPO) and biopsy shows necrotizing non-granulomatous vessel inflammation.
- Treatment approach for MPA is similar as GPA.

Eosinophilic Granulomatosis With Polyangiitis

- This is a rare disease that affects men and women equally. Clinical presentation can be divided into three phases. First is a prodromal phase characterized by allergic rhinitis, sinusitis, nasal polyposis, and asthma. Second phase is characterized by peripheral blood and tissue eosinophilia and the third phase consists of small vessel vasculitis manifestations similar to GPA with a higher rate of cardiac involvement.
- Diagnostic approach is similar to GPA and MPA; 50% will be ANCA positive (commonly MPO). In addition, patients will have eosinophilia (usually 5000–9000 eosinophil/uL) and elevated immunoglobulin E levels. Tissue biopsies show microgranulomas, fibrinoid necrosis, and thrombosis of small vessels with eosinophilic infiltrates.

• Treatment for EGPA has some similarities to GPA, but additional treatments targeting IL-5 and IgE are used. Treatment approach includes glucocorticoids at the same dose as GPA ± cyclophosphamide if severe life-threatening manifestations are present. Maintenance treatment options are the same as GPA. Anti-IL-5 therapy with mepolizumab at the dose of 300 mg every 4 weeks has been recently approved for treatment of EGPA. IL-anti-IgE therapy with omalizumab is also beneficial for EGPA with primarily asthma and sinonasal disease.[27]

MEDICATIONS IN RHEUMATOLOGY

GLUCOCORTICOIDS

• **Mechanism of action:** corticosteroids exert a pluripotent anti-inflammatory effect via the inhibition of inflammatory mediator gene transcription but significant toxicity with prolonged use.
• **Indication:** Anti-inflammatory, the goal of therapy is to suppress disease activity with the minimum effective dosage.
• **Dosage:** highly dependent on disease and clinical situation.
• **Medications:** Prednisone (PO), prednisolone (PO), hydrocortisone (PO, IM, IV), methylprednisolone (PO, IV, intra-articular), dexamethasone (PO, IM, IV), and triamcinolone (intra-articular). The following are relative anti-inflammatory potencies of common glucocorticoid preparations: cortisone, 0.8; hydrocortisone, 1; prednisone, 4; methylprednisolone, 5; dexamethasone, 25. Prednisone (PO) and methylprednisolone (IV) are generally the preferred drugs because of cost and half-life considerations.
• **Side effects:** Adverse effects are related to dosage and duration of administration. Usually seen with doses >10 mg/d of prednisone (or equivalent). It may affect the following systems:
  ○ **Endocrine:** Hyperglycemia, weight gain, iatrogenic Cushing syndrome, osteoporosis. Adrenal suppression can be assumed in patients receiving more than 20 mg of prednisone (or equivalent) for more than 3 weeks. The risk can be minimized by using a single daily dose of a short-acting preparation like prednisone. Adrenal crisis can develop in the setting of severe stress like major surgery or infection and should be treated with "stress-dose" glucocorticoids. For osteoporosis prevention, supplemental calcium, 1–1.5 g/d PO, should be given along with vitamin D, 1000 units daily PO, as soon as steroid therapy is begun. Bisphosphonates are most often used for prophylactic prevention of bone loss. A weight-bearing exercise program and avoidance of alcohol and tobacco are recommended.
  ○ **Cardiovascular:** dyslipidemia, hypertension.
  ○ **Ophthalmologic:** cataracts, glaucoma.
  ○ **Immunologic:** Glucocorticoid therapy reduces resistance to infections which is the major cause of morbidity and mortality in these patients. Minor infections may become systemic, quiescent infections may be activated, and organisms that usually are nonpathogenic may cause disease. Local and systemic signs of infection may be partially masked, although fever associated with infection generally is not suppressed. Consider *Pneumocystis jirovecii* prophylaxis in patients on prednisone ≥20 mg for more than 1 month.
  ○ **Dermatologic:** Acne, purpura, and cutaneous atrophy.
  ○ **Psychiatric:** Changes in mental status ranging from mild nervousness, euphoria, and insomnia to severe depression or psychosis may occur.
  ○ **Musculoskeletal:** Glucocorticoid can induce myopathy. Generally, affects proximal musculature, muscles are not tender, and generally CK, aldolase, and

TABLE 25-10	Nomenclature
Drug Suffix	**Nomenclature**
Mab	Monoclonal Ab
Cept	Soluble receptor
Xi	Chimeric
Zu	Humanized
U	Human
Pegol	Pegylated—decreased immunogenicity

electromyography are normal. Myopathy resolves slowly after discontinuation. Ischemic bone necrosis can also occur; most commonly affects femoral head, humeral head, and tibial plateau.

DISEASE-MODIFYING ANTIRHEUMATIC DRUGS

Immunomodulatory and immunosuppressive drugs, also known as **disease-modifying antirheumatic drugs (DMARDs)**, include a number of pharmacologically diverse agents that exert anti-inflammatory or immunosuppressive effects. They are characterized by a delayed onset of action and the potential for serious toxicity. Consequently, they should be prescribed with the guidance of a rheumatologist and in cooperative patients who are willing to comply with meticulous follow-up.

Classification of DMARDs

- DMARDs are classified as synthetic and biologic DMARDs. Synthetic DMARDs are subclassified as conventional synthetic DMARDs (csDMARD) and targeted synthetic DMARDs (tsDMARDs). The latter category corresponds to small molecules targeting intracellular transduction pathways (Table 25-5). Biologic DMARDs are a novel class of medications that has revolutionized the treatment of rheumatologic conditions (Table 25-10). These selectively block important pathways in immunity that interfere with cytokine function, signal transduction or production, T cell costimulation, or B cell depletion.
- Shared side effects:
  - Injection site/infusion reaction
  - Increased risk of infections (including reactivation of hepatitis B, hepatitis C, tuberculosis)
  - Increased risk of malignancy
- Screen all the patients for hepatitis B, hepatitis C, and tuberculosis before starting a biologic DMARD. Ideally, all patients should be up to date with vaccinations prior to initiation. With the exception of rituximab, biologic DMARDs should be avoided in patients with active malignancy (Table 25-11).
- **Combinations of DMARDs** can be used if the patient has a partial response to the initial agent. Methotrexate and leflunomide may have additive hepatotoxicity, and this combination should be used cautiously. **Combination therapy with two biologic DMARDs is contraindicated because of increased infectious complications.**

TABLE 25-11	Biologic DMARDs				
Category	Medication	Dosage	Indications	Side Effects	Contraindications
Cytokine inhibitors					
TNF inhibition	Certolizumab pegol	200 mg q2weeks or 400 mg monthly	RA	Headache	Heart Failure NYHA III/IV
	Adalimumab	40 mg SC q1 to 2 wk	JIA Spondyloarthropathies	Nausea	Demyelinating disease
	Etanercept	50 mg SC weekly	Uveitis (except etanercept)	Rash	Optic neuritis
	Infliximab	3–10 mg/kg IV q4 to q8 weeks	Off label uses: Behcet disease, sarcoidosis, RP, AOSD, TRAPS, pyoderma gangrenosum, SAPHO, hidradenitis suppurativa	Transaminitis Demyelinating disease Palmo-plantar psoriasis Drug-induced lupus Cutaneous vasculitis Nonmelanoma skin cancer	Seizure disorder Pregnancy (except certolizumab)
	Golimumab	50 mg SC monthly or 2 mg/kg IV q8weeks			
IL-1 Inhibition	Anakinra	100 mg SC daily	RA	Urticaria	Pregnancy
	Canakinumab	150 mg SC q8 weeks	Gout JIA	Flu-like symptoms	Use with caution in patients with asthma or renal impairment
	Rilonacept	160 mg SC weekly	NMOID Mediterranean fever CAPS TRAPS Muckle-Wells syndrome Hyper-IgD periodic fever syndrome Mevalonate kinase deficiency Familial cold urticaria	Neutropenia	

IL-6 inhibition	Tocilizumab	4–8 mg/kg IV q4 weeks or 162 mg SC q1-2 weeks	RA JIA Giant cell arteritis	Nausea/vomiting Diarrhea Intestinal perforation Transaminitis Rash Hypertriglyceridemia Bone marrow suppression	History of peptic ulcer disease or diverticulitis Hepatic impairment
	Sarilumab	200 mg SC q2 weeks			
IL-17 inhibition	Secukinumab	150–300 mg SC q4 weeks	Psoriasis Psoriatic arthritis Ankylosing spondylitis	Nasopharyngitis Diarrhea Neutropenia Higher risk of fungal infections	Inflammatory bowel disease
	Ixekinumab	80 mg SC monthly			
IL-12/23 inhibition	Ustekinumab	90 mg SC q12 weeks	Psoriasis Psoriatic arthritis	Nasopharyngitis Reversible posterior leuko-encephalopathy syndrome	-
	Guselkumab	100 mg SC q8 weeks			
Costimulation blockade					
CTLA4-Ig	Abatacept	500–1000mg IV q4 weeks or 125 mg SC weekly	RA Psoriatic arthritis JIA	Headache Nausea Hypertension COPD exacerbation	COPD

(continued)

TABLE 25-11	Biologic DMARDs	(continued)			
Category	Medication	Dosage	Indications	Side Effects	Contraindications
B cell directed					
Depletion (anti CD-20)	Rituximab	RA: 1 gr IV at 0 and 2 wk, then repeat q6 to 12 months AAV: 375 mg/m² weekly for four doses followed by 500 mg at 0 and 2 wk every 6 mo	RA AAV Off label SLE	Rash Nausea Bone marrow suppression Hypogammaglobulinemia JC virus reactivation (rare) leading to PML	-
Inhibition (anti BLyS)	Belimumab	10 mg/kg IV q4 wk or 200 mg SC weekly	SLE	Nausea/vomiting Diarrhea Depression/anxiety Migraine Leukopenia Few cases of PML	Caution in patients with severe depression
Kinase inhibition					
JAK-1 and JAK-3	Tofacitinib	IR: 5 mg PO bid ER: 11 mg PO daily	RA JIA Psoriatic arthritis	Bone marrow suppression Dyslipidemia Transaminitis	History of diverticulitis
JAK-1 and JAK-2	Baricitinib	2 mg PO daily	RA	Increased risk of varicella Zoster reactivation (provide Shingrix vaccine prior to initiation)	
JAK-1 selective	Upadacitinib	15 mg PO daily	RA	Intestinal perforation Increased risk of venous thromboembolism	

Complement targeted

Anti C5 protein	Eculizumab	1200 mg IV q2 weeks	AHUS PNH NMO Off label use: SLE and systemic sclerosis-associated TMA, CAPS	Headache Hypertension Diarrhea Leukopenia Meningococcemia	Patients not vaccinated against *Neisseria meningitidis*
C5a receptor inhibitor	Avacopan	30 mg PO bid	AAV	Transaminitis	-

AAV, ANCA-associated vasculitis; AHUS, atypical hemolytic uremic syndrome; AOSD, adult-onset Still disease; COPD, chronic obstructive pulmonary disease; CAPS, catastrophic antiphospholipid syndrome; CAPS, cryopyrin-associated periodic syndromes; DM, dermatomyositis; ER, extended release; IR, immediate release; JIA, juvenile idiopathic arthritis; NMO, neuromyelitis optica; NMOID, neonatal-onset multisystem inflammatory disease; PML, progressive multifocal leukoencephalopathy; PNH, paroxysmal nocturnal hemoglobinuria; RA, rheumatoid arthritis; RP, relapsing polychondritis; SLE, systemic lupus erythematosus; TMA, thrombotic microangiopathy; TRAPS, TNF receptor-associated fever syndrome.

CHAPTER 25

REFERENCES

1. Margaretten ME, Kohlwes J, Moore D, et al. Does this adult patient have septic arthritis? *JAMA.* 2007;297(13):1478.
2. Turesson C, O'Fallon WM, Crowson CS, et al. Extra-articular disease manifestations in rheumatoid arthritis: incidence trends and risk factors over 46 years. *Ann Rheum Dis.* 2003;62(8):722.
3. Lee DM, Schur PH. Clinical utility of the anti-CCP assay in patients with rheumatic diseases. *Ann Rheum Dis.* 2003;62(9):870.
4. Nielsen SF, Bojeson SE, Schnohr P, et al. Elevated rheumatoid factor and long term risk of rheumatoid arthritis: a prospective cohort study. *BMJ* 2012;345:e5244.
5. van der Heijde DM, van Leeuwen MA, van Riel PL, et al. Biannual radiographic assessments of hands and feet in a three-year prospective followup of patients with early rheumatoid arthritis. *Arthritis Rheum.* 1992; 35(1):26.
6. van Vollenhoven RF, Geborek P, Forslind K, et al. Swefot trial. *Lancet.* 2009;374(9688):459-466.
7. Rowson CS, Matteson EL, Roger VL, et al. Usefulness of risk scores to estimate the risk of cardiovascular disease in patients with rheumatoid arthritis. *Am J Cardiol.* 2012;110(3):420-424.
8. Agca R, Heslinga SC, Rollefstad S, et al. EULAR recommendations for cardiovascular disease risk management in patients with rheumatoid arthritis and other forms of inflammatory joint disorders: 2015/2016 update. *Ann Rheum Dis.* 2017;76:17-28.
9. Schlesinger N, Norquist JM, Watson DJ. Serum urate during acute gout. *J Rheumatol.* 2009;36(6):1287. Epub 2009 Apr 15.
10. Brown MA. Human leucocyte antigen-B27 and ankylosing spondylitis. *Intern Med J.* 2007;37(11):739.
11. Aringer M, Costenbader K, Daikh D, et al. 2019 European League against Rheumatism/American College of Rheumatology classification criteria for systemic lupus erythematosus. *Arthritis Rheumatol.* 2019;71(9):1400-1412.
12. Tan EM, Feltkamp TE, Smolen JS, et al. Range of antinuclear antibodies in "healthy" individuals. *Arthritis Rheum.* 1997;40(9):1601-1611.
13. Haugbro K, Nossent JC, Winkler T, et al. Anti-dsDNA antibodies and disease classification in antinuclear antibody positive patients: the role of analytical diversity. *Ann Rheum Dis.* 2004;63(4):386.
14. Migliorini P, Baldini C, Rocchi V, et al. Anti-Sm and anti-RNP antibodies. *Autoimmunity.* 2005;38(1):47-54.
15. Appel GB, Contreras G, Dooley MA, et al. Mycophenolate mofetil versus cyclophosphamide for induction treatment of lupus nephritis. *J Am Soc Nephrol.* 2009;20(5):1103. Epub 2009 Apr 15.
16. Navarra SV, Guzmán RM, Gallacher AE, et al. Efficacy and safety of belimumab in patients with active systemic lupus erythematosus: randomized, placebo-controlled, phase 3 trial. *Lancet.* 2011;377(9767):721. Epub 2011 Feb 4.
17. Arriens C, Polyakova S, Adzerikho I, et al. AURORA phase 3 study demonstrates voclosporin statistical superiority over standard of care in lupus nephritis. *Ann Rheum Dis.* 2020;79:2.
18. Kavanaugh A, Tomar R, Reveille J, et al. Guidelines for clinical use of the antinuclear antibody test and tests for specific autoantibodies to nuclear antigens. American College of Pathologists. *Arch Pathol Lab Med.* 2000;124(1):71.
19. Nihtyanova SI, Denton CP. Autoantibodies as predictive tools in systemic sclerosis. *Nat Rev Rheumatol.* 2010;6:112.
20. Tashkin DP, Roth MD, Clements PJ, et al. Mycophenolate mofetil versus oral cyclophosphamide in scleroderma-related interstitial lung disease (SLS II): a randomised controlled, double-blind, parallel group trial. *Lancet Respir Med.* 2016;4:708.
21. Seibold JR, Maher TM, Highland KB, et al. Safety and tolerability of nintedanib in patients with systemic sclerosis-associated interstitial lung disease: data from the SENSCIS trial. *Ann Rheum Dis.* 2020;79:1478.
22. Smetana GW, Shmerling RH. Does this patient have temporal arteritis? *JAMA.* 2002;287(1):92-101.
23. Niederkohr RD, Levin LA. Management of the patient with suspected temporal arteritis a decision-analytic approach. *Ophthalmology.* 2005;112(5):744-756.
24. Stone JH, Tuckwell K, Dimonaco S, et al. Trial of tocilizumab in giant-cell arteritis. *N Engl J Med.* 2017;377(4):317.
25. Stone JH, Merkel PA, Spiera R, et al. Rituximab versus cyclophosphamide for ANCA-associated vasculitis. *N Engl J Med.* 2010;363(3):22.
26. Walsh M, Merkel PA, Peh CA, et al. Plasma exchange and glucocorticoids in severe ANCA-associated vasculitis. *N Engl J Med.* 2020;382(7):622.
27. Wechsler ME, Akuthota P, Jayne D, et al. Mepolizumab or placebo for eosinophilic granulomatosis with polyangiitis. *N Engl J Med.* 2017;376(20):1921.

26 Medical Emergencies

SueLin Hilbert, Mark D. Levine, and Evan S. Schwarz

AIRWAY EMERGENCIES

Emergent Airway Management

GENERAL PRINCIPLES

Recognition of the need to manage a patient's airway must be made in a timely and rapid fashion. Respiratory failure can occur suddenly and without obvious signs and symptoms. Increasing evidence shows that to prevent poor outcomes, the most experienced provider should perform the intubation.

Etiology

The need to emergently manage an airway typically arises because of:
• Loss of airway protective reflexes
• Respiratory failure
• Cardiopulmonary arrest

TREATMENT

• If the provider is not prepared to provide a definitive airway, temporary support of the airway should be performed.
• Basic maintenance of airway and/or ventilation is performed with:
  ○ High-flow nasal cannula oxygen at 15 L/min
  ○ Nonrebreather (NRB) oxygen mask at 15 L/min
  ○ Bag valve mask (BVM)
• While preparing for definitive airway control/endotracheal intubation, the following steps should be performed:
  ○ Place the patient upright to decrease dependent lung volume before intubation.
  ○ Place the patient on NRB mask for 3 minutes if possible.
  ○ If the patient needs ventilator assistance, deliver eight vital capacity breaths via BVM.
  ○ Place a positive end expiratory pressure valve set to 5–20 cm H_2O on the BVM, which adds positive pressure to both bagging and passive oxygenation.

Emergent Airway Adjuncts

• **Laryngeal mask airway (LMA)** is an easy-to-use rescue device for nearly all airway events. It is a tube with a cup-shaped diaphragm at the end that is inflated to cover the trachea and allow passage of air. It does not occlude the esophagus or protect against aspiration. It should not be used in patients with an upper airway obstruction that cannot be cleared or patients with excessive airway pressures such as with chronic obstructive pulmonary disease (COPD), asthma, or pregnancy. There are models of LMAs (which are preferred) that allow an endotracheal tube (ETT) to be passed through them when a definitive airway is desired. Excessive bagging through an LMA can lead to emesis.

- **Fiber-optic/digital airway devices** are considered by many to be the new standard of care. These devices allow the person intubating to get a view of the vocal cords via a camera or fiber-optic scope without direct oropharyngeal visualization, making intubation much easier. Excessive secretions or blood can obstruct the camera, so the operator needs to be capable of direct laryngoscopy as well as indirect fiber-optic laryngoscopy.
- **Gum elastic bougie** is a flexible rubbery stick with a "hockey stick" tip. The bougie can be used blindly but is better suited for direct laryngoscopy where the person intubating cannot visualize the cords. The goal is to obtain the best view possible and for the coude tip of the bougie to be distal and anterior. When the bougie is in the trachea, the tracheal rings are felt as the bougie is slid back and forth. Alternatively, the bougie can be advanced down the oropharynx as deep as possible without losing control of it. If in the esophagus, the bougie will slide all the way down past the stomach with minimal resistance. If in the trachea, the bougie will quickly hit a bronchus and meet resistance. Once in the trachea, one can simply slide an ETT over the bougie and verify placement as usual.

Pneumothorax

GENERAL PRINCIPLES

- Pneumothorax may occur spontaneously or as a result of trauma.
- **Primary spontaneous pneumothorax** occurs without obvious underlying lung disease.
- **Secondary spontaneous pneumothorax** results from underlying parenchymal lung disease including COPD and emphysema, interstitial lung disease, necrotizing lung infections, *Pneumocystis jirovecii* pneumonia, tuberculosis, and cystic fibrosis.
- **Traumatic pneumothorax** occurs as a result of penetrating or blunt chest trauma.
- **Iatrogenic pneumothorax** occurs after thoracentesis, central line placement, transbronchial biopsy, transthoracic needle biopsy, or barotrauma from mechanical ventilation.
- **Tension pneumothorax** results from continued accumulation of air in the chest that is sufficient to shift mediastinal structures and impede venous return to the heart. This results in abnormal gas exchange, hypotension, and ultimately, cardiovascular collapse.
  - The causes include barotrauma due to mechanical ventilation, a chest wound that allows ingress but not egress of air, or a defect in the visceral pleura that behaves in the same way ("ball valve" effect).
  - Suspect tension pneumothorax when a patient experiences hypotension and respiratory distress on mechanical ventilation or after any procedure in which the thorax is violated.

DIAGNOSIS

Clinical Presentation
History
- Patients commonly complain of acute onset ipsilateral chest or shoulder pain. A history of recent chest trauma or medical procedure can suggest the diagnosis.
- Dyspnea is usually present.

Physical Examination

- Although examination of the patient with a small pneumothorax may be normal, classic findings include decreased breath sounds and more resonance to percussion on the ipsilateral side.
- With a larger pneumothorax or with underlying lung disease, tachypnea and respiratory distress may be present. The affected hemithorax may be noticeably larger (due to decreased elastic recoil of the collapsed lung) and relatively immobile during respiration.
- If the pneumothorax is very large, and particularly if it is under tension, the patient may exhibit severe distress, diaphoresis, cyanosis, and hypotension. In addition, the patient's trachea may be shifted to the contralateral side.
- If the pneumothorax is the result of penetrating trauma or pneumomediastinum, subcutaneous emphysema may be felt.
- Clinical features alone do not predict the relative size of a pneumothorax, and in a stable patient, further diagnostic studies must be used to guide treatment strategy. However, tension pneumothorax remains a clinical diagnosis, and if suspected in the appropriate clinical scenario, immediate intervention should be undertaken before further evaluation.

Diagnostic Testing

Electrocardiography

An **ECG** may reveal diminished anterior QRS amplitude and an anterior axis shift. In extreme cases, tension pneumothorax may cause electromechanical dissociation.

Imaging

- A **CXR** will reveal a separation of the pleural shadow from the chest wall. If the posteroanterior radiograph is normal and pneumothorax is suspected, a lateral or decubitus film may aid in diagnosis.[1] Air travels to the highest point in a body cavity; thus, a pneumothorax in a supine patient may be detected as an unusually deep costophrenic sulcus and excessive lucency over the upper abdomen caused by the anterior thoracic air. This observation is particularly important in the critical care unit, where radiographs of the mechanically ventilated patient are often obtained with the patient in supine position.
- Although tension pneumothorax is a clinical diagnosis, radiographic correlates include mediastinal and tracheal shift toward contralateral side and depression of the ipsilateral diaphragm.
- **Ultrasonography** is a useful tool for bedside diagnosis of pneumothorax, especially on patients who must remain supine or who are too unstable to undergo CT scanning. Placement of the probe in the intercostal spaces provides information regarding the pleura and underlying lung parenchyma. During normal inspiration, the visceral and parietal pleura move along one another and produce a "sliding sign" phenomenon. In addition, the air-filled lung parenchyma below the pleura produces raylike opacities known as "comet tails." Presence of the sliding sign and comet tails on ultrasound during inspiration rule out a pneumothorax with high reliability at the point of probe placement. Conversely, absence of these signs is a highly reliable predictor for the presence of pneumothorax. Several places on the chest should be evaluated, including places that air is most likely to accumulate such as the anterior and lateral chest.[2] Studies have shown that in the hands of an experienced clinician with ultrasound training, chest ultrasound is more sensitive than CXR.[3]
- Chest CT is the gold standard for diagnosis and determining the size of pneumothorax. Although not always necessary, it may be particularly useful for differentiating pneumothorax from bullous disease in patients with underlying lung conditions.[4]

TREATMENT

Treatment depends on cause, size, and degree of physiologic derangement.

- **Primary pneumothorax**
  - A small, primary, spontaneous pneumothorax without a continued pleural air leak may resolve spontaneously. Air is resorbed from the pleural space at roughly 1.5% daily, and therefore, a small (approximately 15%) pneumothorax is expected to resolve without intervention in approximately 10 days.
  - If the pneumothorax has not increased in size upon evaluation with a 6-hour repeat CXR and symptoms have not changed, the patient may be discharged if they are asymptomatic (apart from mild pleurisy). Obtain follow-up radiographs to confirm resolution of the pneumothorax in 7–10 days. Air travel is discouraged during the follow-up period because a decrease in ambient barometric pressure may cause a larger pneumothorax.
  - If the pneumothorax is **small but the patient is mildly symptomatic**, far from home, or has barriers with follow-up, admit the patient and administer high-flow oxygen; the resulting nitrogen gradient will speed resorption.
  - If the patient is **more than mildly symptomatic or has a larger pneumothorax**, simple aspiration is a reasonable initial management strategy. However, aspiration may not be successful for very large pneumothoraces. In patients in whom aspiration fails, proceed with thoracostomy tube insertion.[1]
  - **Pleural sclerosis** to prevent recurrence is recommended by some experts but, in most cases, is not used after a first episode unless a persistent air leak is present.
- **Secondary pneumothorax**
  - Individuals with a secondary spontaneous pneumothorax are usually symptomatic and require lung reexpansion.
  - Often, a bronchopleural fistula persists and a larger thoracostomy tube and suction are required.
  - **Consult a pulmonologist** about pleural sclerosis for persistent air leak and to prevent recurrence.
  - **Surgery** may be required for persistent air leak and should be considered for high-risk patients for prevention of recurrence.
- **Iatrogenic pneumothorax**
  - If the pneumothorax is small and the patient is minimally symptomatic, they can be managed conservatively. If the procedure that caused the pneumothorax required sedation, admit the patient, administer oxygen, and repeat the CXR in 6 hours to ensure the patient's stability. If the patient is completely alert and the CXR shows no change, the patient can be discharged.
  - If the patient is symptomatic or if the pneumothorax is too large for expectant care, a pneumothorax catheter with aspiration or a one-way valve is usually adequate and can often be removed the following day.
  - Iatrogenic pneumothorax due to barotrauma from mechanical ventilation almost always has a persistent air leak and should be managed with a chest tube and suction.
- **Tension pneumothorax**
  - When the clinical situation and physical examination strongly suggest this diagnosis, decompress the affected hemithorax immediately with a 14-gauge needle. Place the needle in the second intercostal space, midclavicular line, just superior to the rib. Release of air with clinical improvement confirms the diagnosis. An alternative placement of the needle is in the fourth intercostal space in the anterior-lateral midaxillary line.

○ Recognize that a patient with obesity or a patient with a large amount of breast tissue may not have resolution of tension with a standard angiocatheter because of the inability to reach the chest wall or weight of the tissue kinking off the catheter. These patients may require a longer needle to reach the intrathoracic space for decompression or require insertion of a larger gauge reinforced catheter to stent open the pathway for air release.

○ If long-needle decompression or reinforced catheter insertion is unsuccessful, and the diagnosis is highly probable in an unstable patient, surgical decompression can be performed by incision of the pleura in the fourth to fifth anterior axillary line above the rib in the same space in which thoracostomy tubes are inserted. This technique has been shown to be effective; however, safety and complication rates are not able to be determined because of lack of studies.[5]

○ Seal any chest wound with an occlusive dressing and arrange for placement of a thoracostomy tube.

HEAT-INDUCED ILLNESS

Exertion, environmental exposure, or a combination of both can lead to an elevation of core temperature and the subsequent continuum of pathologies that comprise heat-induced injuries. There are no strict diagnostic criteria for heat-induced injuries, except the general assertion that heat stroke should include a core temperature >40°C and central nervous system (CNS) dysfunction. Diagnosis and treatment are based primarily on exposure history, potential predisposing factors, and clinical presentation.

Heat Exhaustion

GENERAL PRINCIPLES

Heat exhaustion often results from a combination of water and sodium depletion. Water depletion is the result of either overwhelming losses, such as profuse sweating or vomiting, or inadequate replacement. Persons at risk include the elderly, patients taking diuretics, and those working in hot environments with limited water replacement. Salt depletion occurs in unacclimatized individuals who replace fluid losses with large amounts of hypotonic solution.

DIAGNOSIS

• The patient presents with headache, nausea, vomiting, dizziness, weakness, irritability, and/or cramps.
• The patient may have postural hypotension, diaphoresis, and normal or minimally increased core temperature.

TREATMENT

• Treatment consists of removing excess or restrictive clothing, resting the patient in a cool environment, accelerating heat loss by fan evaporation, and using salt-containing solutions for fluid repletion.
• If the patient is not vomiting and has stable blood pressure, an oral, commercial, balanced salt solution is adequate.

- If the patient is vomiting or hemodynamically unstable, check electrolytes and give 1–2 L of 0.9% isotonic crystalloid IV.
- The patient should avoid exertion in a hot environment for 2–3 additional days.

Heat Syncope

GENERAL PRINCIPLES

- Heat syncope is a variant of postural hypotension.
- Exertion in a hot environment results in peripheral vasodilation and pooling of blood, with subsequent loss of consciousness. The affected individual has normal body temperature and regains consciousness promptly when supine, which separates this syndrome from heat stroke.

TREATMENT

Treatment is the same as for heat exhaustion.

Heat Stroke

GENERAL PRINCIPLES

- Heat stroke occurs in two varieties: classic and exertional. Both are present with high core temperatures that result in direct thermal tissue injury. Secondary effects include acute renal failure from rhabdomyolysis. Even with rapid therapy, mortality rates can be very high for body temperatures above 41.1°C (106°F). The distinction between classic and exertional heat stroke is not important because the therapeutic goals are similar in both and a delay in cooling increases mortality rate.
- The cardinal features of heat stroke are **hyperthermia (>40°C [104°F]) and altered mental status.** Although patients presenting with classic heat stroke may have anhidrosis, this is not considered a diagnostic criterion because 50% of patients are still diaphoretic at presentation.
- The CNS is very vulnerable to heat stroke with the cerebellum being highly sensitive. Ataxia may be an early sign. Seizures are common. Neurologic injury is a function of maximum temperature and duration of exposure.[6]

DIAGNOSIS

Diagnosis is based on the history of exposure or exercise, a core temperature usually of 40.6°C (105°F) or higher, and changes in mental status ranging from confusion to delirium and coma.

Differential Diagnosis

- Drug associated
  - Toxicity
    - Anticholinergic
    - Stimulant toxicity
    - Salicylate toxicity
  - Neuroleptic malignant syndrome (NMS) is associated with antipsychotic drugs. It is worth noting that NMS and malignant hyperthermia are both accompanied by severe muscle rigidity.

- ○ Serotonin syndrome
- ○ Malignant hyperthermia
- ○ Drug withdrawal syndrome (ethanol withdrawal)
- ○ Drug fever
- Infections
  - ○ Generalized infections (sepsis, malaria, etc.)
  - ○ CNS infections (meningitis, encephalitis, brain abscess)
- Endocrine
  - ○ Thyroid storm
  - ○ Pheochromocytoma
- Hypothalamic dysfunction due to stroke or hemorrhage
  - ○ Status epilepticus
  - ○ Cerebral hemorrhage[7]

Diagnostic Testing
Laboratories
- Laboratory studies should be directed toward identifying potential end organ damage or other underlying etiology and may include complete blood count (CBC); partial thromboplastin time; prothrombin time; electrolytes; blood urea nitrogen (BUN); creatinine, glucose, calcium, and creatine kinase levels; liver function tests (LFTs); and urinalysis.
- If an infectious etiology is suspected, obtain appropriate cultures.
- If there is a concern for cardiac ischemia, obtain an ECG and troponin.

Imaging
If a CNS etiology is considered likely, CT imaging followed by spinal fluid examination is appropriate.

TREATMENT

- If the patient is obtunded or hemodynamically unstable, acute life support measures should be initiated, such as intubation or central venous access.
- **Immediate cooling** should be started within 30 minutes of illness recognition.[7]
  - ○ For most young, athletic, or otherwise healthy patients, cold water immersion therapy is considered the most efficient cooling method in both the field and hospital settings.[8] Ideally, this consists of immersing the patient up to the neck in a slurry of ice and water but may be impractical in many settings and can interfere in other resuscitative efforts.
  - ○ Evaporative measures are also very effective and often more feasible. In this case, remove the patient's clothing to achieve maximum body surface exposure. Mist the patient continuously with tepid water (20–25°C [68–77°F]) and cool the patient with a large electric fan.
  - ○ Ice packs should be placed at points of major heat transfer, such as the groin, axillae, and chest, to further speed cooling, but there is no evidence to suggest they be used as a primary cooling method.
  - ○ Neither antipyretics nor dantrolene sodium are indicated.[8]
- Monitor core temperatures continuously by rectal probe or Foley catheter. Oral and tympanic membrane temperatures may be inaccurate.
- Discontinue cooling measures when the core temperature reaches 39°C (102.2°F), which should ideally be achieved within 30 minutes. A temperature rebound may occur in 3–6 hours and should be retreated.

- **For hypotension, administer crystalloids:** If refractory, treat with vasopressors and monitor hemodynamics. Avoid pure α-adrenergic agents because they cause vasoconstriction and impair cooling. Administer crystalloids cautiously to normotensive patients.

COLD-INDUCED ILLNESS

Exposure to the cold may result in several different forms of injury. A risk factor is accelerated heat loss, which is promoted by exposure to high wind or by immersion. Extended cold exposure may result from alcohol or drug abuse, injury or immobilization, and mental impairment.

Chilblains

GENERAL PRINCIPLES

- Chilblains are among the mildest form of cold injury and result from exposure of bare skin to a cold, windy environment (0.6–15.6°C [33–60°F]).
- The ears, fingers, and tip of the nose typically are injured, with itchy, painful erythema on rewarming.

TREATMENT

Treatment involves rapid rewarming (see Frostnip section), moisturizing lotions, analgesics, and instructing the patient to avoid reexposure.

Immersion Injury (Trench Foot)

GENERAL PRINCIPLES

Immersion injury is caused by prolonged immersion (longer than 10–12 hours) at a temperature <10°C (<50°F).

TREATMENT

Treat by rewarming followed by dry dressings. Treat secondary infections with antibiotics.

Frostnip (Superficial Frostbite)

GENERAL PRINCIPLES

Superficial frostbite involves the skin and subcutaneous tissues.

DIAGNOSIS

Areas with first-degree involvement are white, waxy, and anesthetic; have poor capillary refill; and are painful on thawing. Second-degree involvement is manifested by clear or milky bullae.

TREATMENT

The **treatment of choice** is rapid rewarming. Immerse the affected body part for 15–30 minutes; hexachlorophene or povidone iodine can be added to the water bath. Narcotic analgesics may be necessary for rewarming pain. Typically, no deep injury ensues and healing occurs in 3–4 weeks.

Deep Frostbite

GENERAL PRINCIPLES

- Deep frostbite involves death of skin, subcutaneous tissue, and muscle (third degree) or deep tendons and bones (fourth degree).
- Diabetes mellitus, peripheral vascular disease, an outdoor lifestyle, and high altitude are additional risk factors.

DIAGNOSIS

- The tissue appears frozen and hard.
- On rewarming, there is no capillary filling.
- Hemorrhagic blisters form, followed by eschars. Healing is very slow, and demarcation of tissue with autoamputation may occur.
- The majority of deep frostbite occurs at temperatures <6.7°C (44°F) with exposures longer than 7–10 hours.

TREATMENT

- The treatment is rapid rewarming as described earlier. **Rewarming should not be started until there is no chance of refreezing.**
- Administer analgesics (IV opioids) as needed.
- Early surgical intervention is not indicated.
- **Elevate** the affected extremity, prevent weight-bearing, separate the affected digits with cotton wool, prevent tissue maceration by using a blanket cradle, and prohibit smoking.
- Update tetanus immunization.
- Intra-arterial vasodilators, heparin, dextran, prostaglandin inhibitors, thrombolytics, and sympathectomy are not routinely justified.
- Role of antibiotics is unclear.[9]
- Amputation is undertaken only after full demarcation has occurred.

Hypothermia

GENERAL PRINCIPLES

Definition

Hypothermia is defined as a core temperature of <35°C (95°F).

Classification

Classification of severity by temperature is not universal. One scheme defines hypothermia as mild at 34–35°C (93.2–95°F), moderate at 30–34°C (86–93.2°F), and severe at <30°C (86°F).

Etiology

- The most common cause of hypothermia in the United States is cold exposure due to alcohol intoxication.
- Another common cause is cold water immersion.

DIAGNOSIS

Clinical Presentation

Presentation varies with the temperature of the patient on arrival. All organ systems can be involved.

- **CNS effects**
  - At **32.2°C (90°F)**, the ability to shiver is lost and deep tendon reflexes are diminished.
  - At temperatures **below 32°C (89.6°F)**, mental processes are slowed and affect is flattened.
  - At **28°C (82.4°F)**, coma often occurs.
  - **Below 18°C (64.4°F)**, the electroencephalogram is flat. On rewarming from severe hypothermia, central pontine myelinolysis may develop.
- **Cardiovascular effects**
  - After an initial increased release of catecholamines, there is a decrease in cardiac output and heart rate with relatively preserved mean arterial pressure. ECG changes manifest initially as sinus bradycardia with T-wave inversion and QT interval prolongation and may manifest as atrial fibrillation at temperatures of <32°C (<89.6°F).
  - Osborne waves (J-point elevation) may be visible, particularly in leads II and V_6.
  - An increased susceptibility to ventricular arrhythmias occurs at temperatures **below 32°C (89.6°F).**
  - At temperatures of **30°C (86°F)**, the susceptibility to ventricular fibrillation is increased significantly, and unnecessary manipulation or jostling of the patient should be avoided.
  - A decrease in mean arterial pressure may also occur, and at temperatures of **28°C (82.4°F)**, progressive bradycardia supervenes.
- **Respiratory effects**
  - After an initial increase in minute ventilation, respiratory rate and tidal volume decrease progressively with decreasing temperature.
  - Arterial blood gases (ABGs) measured with the machine set at 37°C (98.6°F) should serve as the basis for therapy without correction of pH and carbon dioxide tension (PCO_2).[10]
- **Renal manifestations:** Cold-induced diuresis and tubular concentrating defects may be seen.

Differential Diagnosis

- Cerebrovascular accident
- Drug overdose
- Diabetic ketoacidosis
- Hypoglycemia
- Uremia
- Adrenal insufficiency
- Myxedema

Diagnostic Testing

Laboratories
- Basic laboratory studies should include CBC, coagulation studies, LFTs, BUN, electrolytes, creatinine, glucose, creatine kinase, calcium, magnesium, amylase levels, urinalysis, ABG, and ECG.
- Serum potassium is often increased.
- Elevated serum amylase may reflect underlying pancreatitis.
- Hyperglycemia may be noted but should not be treated because rebound hypoglycemia may occur with rewarming.
- Disseminated intravascular coagulation may also occur.

Imaging
Obtain chest, abdominal, and cervical spine radiographs to evaluate all patients with a history of trauma or immersion injury.

TREATMENT

Medications
- Administer supplemental oxygen.
- Supplement **thiamine** to most patients with cold exposure because exposure due to alcohol intoxication is common.
- Administration of **antibiotics** is a controversial issue. Although some recommend antibiotic administration for 72 hours (pending cultures), antibiotics should be reserved for when an infection is suspected. In general, the patients with hypothermia due to exposure and alcohol intoxication are less likely to have a serious underlying infection than those who are elderly or who have an underlying medical illness.

Nonpharmacologic Therapies
- **Rewarming:** The patient should be rewarmed with the goal of increasing the temperature by 0.5–2.0°C/h (32.9–35.6°F/h), although the rate of rewarming has not been shown to be associated with improved outcomes.
- **Passive external rewarming**
  ○ This method depends on the patient's ability to shiver.
  ○ It is effective only at core temperatures of **32°C (89.6°F) or higher.** Patients cannot shiver below 32°C.
  ○ Remove wet clothing, cover the patient with blankets in a warm environment, and monitor.
- **Active external rewarming**
  ○ It is indicated for patients with hypothermia and stable circulation.[11]
- **Active core rewarming is preferred for treatment of severe hypothermia**, although there are minimal data on outcomes.[12]
  ○ **Heated oxygen** is the initial therapy of choice for the patient whose cardiovascular status is stable. This therapeutic maneuver can be expected to raise core temperatures by 0.5–1.2°C/h (32.9–34.2°F/h).[13] Administration through an ETT results in more rapid rewarming than delivery via face mask. Administer heated oxygen through a cascade humidifier at a temperature of 45°C (113°F) or lower.
  ○ **IV fluids** can be warmed or delivered through a blood warmer.
  ○ **Heated nasogastric or bladder lavage** is of limited efficacy because of low-exposed surface area and is reserved for the patient with cardiovascular instability.

- ○ **Heated peritoneal lavage** with fluid warmed to 40–45°C (104–113°F) is more effective than heated aerosol inhalation, but it should be reserved for patients with cardiovascular instability. Only those who are experienced in its use should perform heated peritoneal lavage, in combination with other modes of rewarming.
- ○ **Closed thoracic lavage** with heated fluid by thoracostomy tube has been recommended but is unproven.[14] It can be considered in patients where extracorporeal circulation is not an option.
- ○ **Hemodialysis** can be used for the severely hypothermic, particularly when due to an overdose that is amenable to treatment in this way.
- ○ **Extracorporeal circulation** (cardiac bypass and extracorporeal membrane oxygenation [ECMO]) is used only in hypothermic individuals who are in cardiac arrest; in these cases, it may be dramatically effective.[15] Extracorporeal circulation may raise the temperature as rapidly as 10–25°C/h (50–77°F/h). Although bypass must be performed in an operating room, ECMO can be initiated in the emergency department. In patients treated with extracorporeal methods, survival without neurologic impairment is reported to range from 47% to 63%.[11]

Resuscitation

- Maintain the airway and administer oxygen. Patients <32°C (89.6°F) should be moved gently owing to the risk of triggering ventricular fibrillation.
- If intubation is required, the most experienced operator should perform it.
- Conduct **cardiopulmonary resuscitation (CPR).** Perform simultaneous vigorous core rewarming; as long as the core temperature is severely decreased, it should be assumed that the patient can be resuscitated. Although reliable defibrillation requires a core temperature of 32°C (89.6°F) or higher, patients with temperatures below 32°C (89.6°F) can be defibrillated. Administration of vasopressors is controversial. Standard teaching was to withhold vasopressors in patients with temperatures <30°C (86°F), but some research indicates an increased rate of return of spontaneous circulation with vasopressors.[16] However, patients may be resistant to most treatment modalities until their core temperature is >32°C (89.6°F). Prolonged efforts (to a core temperature >32°C [89.6°F]) may be justified because of the neuroprotective effects of hypothermia.
- If ventricular fibrillation occurs, begin CPR as per the advanced cardiac life support protocol.
- Monitor ECG rhythm, urine output, and if possible central venous pressure in all patients with an intact circulation.

Disposition

- Admit patients with an underlying disease, physiologic derangement, or core temperature <32°C (<89.6°F), preferably to an ICU.
- Consider discharge for individuals with mild hypothermia (32–35°C [89.6–95°F]) and no predisposing medical conditions or complications when they are normothermic, and an adequate home environment can be ensured.

MONITORING/FOLLOW-UP

- Monitor core temperature.
- A standard oral thermometer registers only to a lower limit of 35°C (95°F). Monitor the patient continuously with a Foley catheter thermometer with a full range of 20–40°C (68–104°F).

REFERENCES

1. Henry M, Arnold T, Harvey J. BTS guidelines for the management of spontaneous pneumothorax. *Thorax.* 2003;58(suppl 2):ii39.
2. Alrajhi K, Woo MY, Vaillancourt C. Test characteristics of ultrasonography for the detection of pneumothorax: a systematic review and meta-analysis. *Chest.* 2012;141(3):703-708.
3. Jalli R, Sefidbakht S, Jafari SH. Value of ultrasound in diagnosis of pneumothorax: a prospective study. *Emerg Radiol.* 2013;20(2):131-134.
4. Maskell N, Butland R. BTS guidelines for the investigation of a unilateral pleural effusion in adults. *Thorax.* 2003;58(suppl 2):ii8.
5. Waydhas C, Sauerland S. Pre-hospital pleural decompression and chest tube placement after blunt trauma: a systematic review. *Resuscitation.* 2007;72(1):11-25.
6. Bouchama A, Knochel JP. Heat stroke. *N Engl J Med.* 2002;346(25):1978-1988.
7. Atha WF. Heat-related illness. *Emerg Med Clin North Am.* 2013;31(4):1097-1108.
8. Gaudio FG, Grissom CK. Cooling methods in heat stroke. *J Emerg Med.* 2016;50(4):607-616.
9. Ikäheimo TM, Junila J, Hirvonen J, et al. Chapter 202. Frostbite and other localized cold injuries. In: Tintinalli JE, Stapczynski J, Ma O, Cline DM, Cydulka RK, Meckler GD, eds. *Tintinalli's Emergency Medicine: A Comprehensive Study Guide.* 7th ed. McGraw-Hill; 2011.
10. Delaney KA, Howland MA, Vassallo S, et al. Assessment of acid-base disturbances in hypothermia and their physiologic consequences. *Ann Emerg Med.* 1989;18(1):72-82.
11. Brown DJ, Brugger H, Boyd J, et al. Accidental hypothermia. *N Engl J Med.* 2012;367(20):1930-1938.
12. Weinberg AD. The role of inhalation rewarming in the early management of hypothermia. *Resuscitation.* 1998;36(2):101-104.
13. Miller JW, Danzl DF, Thomas DM. Urban accidental hypothermia: 135 cases. *Ann Emerg Med.* 1980;9(9):456-461.
14. Hall KN, Syverud SA. Closed thoracic cavity lavage in the treatment of severe hypothermia in human beings. *Ann Emerg Med.* 1990;19(2):204-206.
15. Walpoth BH, Walpoth-Aslan BN, Mattle HP, et al. Outcome of survivors of accidental deep hypothermia and circulatory arrest treated with extracorporeal blood warming. *N Engl J Med.* 1997;337(21):1500-1505.
16. Wira CR, Becker JU, Martin G, et al. Anti-arrhythmic and vasopressor medications for the treatment of ventricular fibrillation in severe hypothermia: a systematic review of the literature. *Resuscitation.* 2008;78(1):21-29.

CHAPTER 26

Alterations in Consciousness

GENERAL PRINCIPLES

Definition

- **Coma:** A state of complete behavioral unresponsiveness to external stimulation. Evaluation and treatment should be performed concurrently and expeditiously as multiple etiologies can lead to irreversible brain damage.
- **Delirium:** An acute state of confusion that can result from diffuse or multifocal cerebral dysfunction and is characterized by relatively rapid reduction in the ability to focus, sustain, or shift attention. Changes in cognition, fluctuations in consciousness, disorientation, and even hallucinations are common.

Epidemiology

- Between 14% and 56% of all hospitalized patients and as high as 82% of mechanically ventilated patients develop delirium.[1]
- Delirious patients often have prolonged stays and are at greater risk for subsequent cognitive decline.

Etiology

- Coma results from diffuse or multifocal dysfunction that involves both cerebral hemispheres or the reticular activating system in the brainstem.
- Etiologies of altered mental status are listed in Table 27-1.
- Mild systemic illness (e.g., urinary tract infections), introduction of new medications, fever, and/or sleep deprivation are common causes of delirium in the elderly and patients with chronic central nervous system (CNS) dysfunction of any etiology.

DIAGNOSIS

- Initial assessment should focus on recognizing the development and progression of altered consciousness. Query for history of trauma, seizures, stroke, medication changes, and alcohol or drug use as possible etiologies. A collateral source is often necessary.
- The AWOL tool is a quick bedside measure that can be used to assess patients' risk of delirium at the time of admission.[2] The AWOL score is derived from assigning one point for each of the following variables (**a**ge ≥80, inability to spell the word "**w**orld" backward, disorientation to location, and nurse-rated illness severity [with a point given for patients considered to be at least moderately ill]). In the pilot study describing this tool, 2% of patients with a score of 0 went on to develop delirium, whereas 64% of patients with a score of 4 went on to develop delirium.

TABLE 27-1	Causes of Altered Mental Status

Metabolic derangements/diffuse etiologies
- Hypernatremia/hyponatremia
- Hypercalcemia
- Hyperglycemia/hypoglycemia
- Hyperthyroidism/hypothyroidism
- Acute intermittent porphyria
- Hypertensive encephalopathy/reversible posterior leukoencephalopathy
- Hypoxia/hypercapnia
- Global cerebral ischemia from hypotension

Infections
- Meningitis/encephalitis
- Sepsis
- Systemic infectious with spread to CNS

Drugs/toxins/poisons
- Prescription medications and side effects of medications
- Drugs of abuse
- Withdrawal situations
- Medication side effects
- Inhaled toxins

Inborn errors of metabolism

Nutritional deficiency (i.e., thiamine)

Seizures
- Subclinical seizures
- Postictal state

Head trauma

Vascular
- Ischemic stroke (only certain stroke locations cause altered mental status)
- Hemorrhage

Structural
- Hydrocephalus
- Tumor

Systemic organ failure
- Hepatic failure
- Renal failure

Psychiatric

Autoimmune/inflammatory
- Vasculitis (primary CNS or systemic)
- Encephalitis
- Autoantibody-mediated encephalopathies (e.g., anti–voltage-gated potassium channel complex antibodies like anti-LGI1 and anti-Caspr2)

CNS, central nervous system.

Clinical Presentation
- Search for signs of systemic illness associated with coma (e.g., cirrhosis, hemodialysis fistula/graft, rash of meningococcemia) or signs of head trauma (e.g., lacerations,

periorbital or mastoid ecchymosis, hemotympanum). The physical and neurologic examination may reveal systemic illness (e.g., pneumonia or elevated temperature) or neurologic signs (meningismus or paralysis) that can help narrow the differential diagnosis.

- **Herniation** occurs when mass lesions or edema cause shifts in brain tissue. The diagnosis of brain herniation **requires immediate recognition and treatment.** If a risk of herniation is present, the patient should be monitored in a neurosurgical/neurologic critical care unit, and frequent (q1-2 hour) "neuro checks" should be performed to evaluate for signs of impending herniation.
  - ○ **Nonspecific signs and symptoms of increased intracranial pressure** include headache, nausea, vomiting, hypertension, bradycardia, papilledema, and sixth nerve palsy. Alteration in consciousness is a late finding.
  - ○ **Uncal herniation** is caused by unilateral supratentorial lesions. The earliest sign is diminished consciousness, followed by a dilated pupil ipsilateral to the mass, then hemiparesis, first contralateral to the mass and later ipsilateral to the mass (Kernohan notch syndrome).
  - ○ **Central herniation** is caused by medial or bilateral supratentorial lesions. Signs include progressive alteration of consciousness, Cheyne–Stokes or normal respirations followed by central hyperventilation, midposition and unreactive pupils, loss of upward gaze, and posturing of the extremities.
  - ○ **Tonsillar herniation** occurs when pressure in the posterior fossa forces the cerebellar tonsils through the foramen magnum, compressing the medulla. Signs include altered level of consciousness and respiratory irregularity or apnea.
- In general, the neurologic assessment should ascertain the patient's ability to focus, sustain, and shift attention appropriately. Due to fluctuations, repeated examinations are often necessary.
- **Level of consciousness** can be semiquantitatively assessed and followed by using the Glasgow coma scale (GCS). Scores range from 3 (unresponsive) to 15 (normal).
- **Respiratory rate and pattern**
  - ○ Cheyne–Stokes respirations (rhythmic crescendo–decrescendo hyperpnea alternating with periods of apnea) are seen in metabolic coma, supratentorial lesions, chronic pulmonary disease, and congestive heart failure (CHF).
  - ○ Hyperventilation is seen in metabolic acidosis, hypoxemia, pneumonia, or other pulmonary diseases but can also occur with an upper brainstem injury.
  - ○ Apneustic breathing (long pauses after inspiration), cluster breathing (breathing in short bursts), and ataxic breathing (irregular breaths without pattern) are signs of brainstem injury and are commonly associated with impending respiratory arrest.
- **Pupil size and light reactivity**
  - ○ Anisocoria (asymmetric pupils) in a patient with altered mental status requires immediate diagnosis (i.e., stat head CT) for exclusion and treatment of possible herniation.
  - ○ Anisocoria may be physiologic or produced by mydriatics (e.g., scopolamine, atropine) and therefore requires well-documented serial examinations.
  - ○ Small but reactive pupils are seen in narcotic overdose, metabolic encephalopathy, and pontine lesions.
  - ○ Fixed midposition pupils imply midbrain lesions or transtentorial herniation.
  - ○ Bilaterally fixed and dilated pupils occur with severe anoxic encephalopathy or drug intoxication (e.g., scopolamine, atropine, glutethimide, or methanol).
- **Eye movements**
  - ○ To test the oculocephalic reflex ("doll's eyes" maneuver, assuming no cervical injury is present), the examiner quickly turns the head laterally or vertically (head

impulse test). Intact brainstem oculomotor function, in the setting of coma, will result in conjugate eye movements opposite to the direction of head movement (back to the examiner).
- ○ In the absence of a history to suggest a drug-induced cause (e.g., barbiturates, phenytoin, paralytics) or a preexisting disorder such as progressive external ophthalmoplegia, absence of all eye movements indicates a bilateral pontine lesion.
- ○ A conjugate gaze preference to one side suggests a unilateral pontine or frontal lobe lesion.
- ○ Impaired vertical eye movement occurs in midbrain lesions and central herniation. Conjugate depression and impaired elevation suggest a tectal lesion (e.g., pinealoma) or hydrocephalus.
- **Motor responses** also help with localization. Asymmetric motor responses (spontaneous or stimulus induced, including noxious stimuli if necessary) also have localizing value.

Diagnostic Testing

Laboratory Studies

Obtain serum electrolytes, creatinine, glucose, calcium, complete blood count (CBC), and urinalysis. Drug levels should be ordered if appropriate. An accurate medication list and any history to suggest intoxication are critical features of the evaluation. Toxicology screen of blood and urine should be considered.

Imaging

A head CT should be obtained to evaluate for structural abnormalities. Brain MRI can be useful if head CT is nondiagnostic and there is suspicion for an ischemic or parenchymal lesion (especially of the posterior fossa).

Diagnostic Procedures

- Lumbar puncture (LP) should be considered in patients with fever and/or new headache or those with high risk of infection. A funduscopic examination and/or head imaging should be performed prior to performing the LP to assess risk of herniation. Patients with focal neurologic symptoms, altered mental status, a history of CNS disease (e.g., stroke or tumor), or recent seizures should undergo head CT prior to LP. Basic cerebrospinal fluid (CSF) studies include protein, glucose (with concurrent serum glucose), cell count, Gram stain, and aerobic culture. Additional studies should be obtained depending on the possible etiology (e.g., viral polymerase chain reactions, immune markers).
- Electroencephalography (EEG) can be considered to rule out seizures. Nonconvulsive status epilepticus (NCSE) is a common cause of unexplained encephalopathy in the critically ill population. Interictal abnormalities can be suggestive of specific etiologies (e.g., periodic lateralized epileptiform discharges in herpes simplex virus [HSV] encephalitis, triphasic waves in hepatic or uremic encephalopathy, and β activity or voltage suppression in barbiturate or other sedative intoxications).

TREATMENT

Delirium

- Repeated attempts should be made to reorient the patient and possibly have a sitter present if necessary.
- A quiet room with close observation is necessary. Patients should have a well-lit environment with familiar objects during the day and dark, quiet (minimize stimulation if possible) environments at night.

- Physical and pharmacologic restraints should be used only as a last resort and with appropriate documentation in the medical record. If restraints are needed, they should be carefully adjusted and checked periodically to prevent excessive constriction.
- Ramelteon may be used in patients at risk for delirium.[3]

Coma

- Ensure adequate airway and ventilation, administer oxygen as needed, and maintain normal body temperature.
- Establish secure IV access and adequate circulation.
- Neurosurgical consult may need to be obtained for intracranial pressure monitoring and treatment, if applicable.

Medications

- IV thiamine (100–500 mg), followed by dextrose (50 mL of 50% dextrose in water = 25 g dextrose), should be administered. **Thiamine is administered first because dextrose administration in thiamine-deficient patients may precipitate Wernicke encephalopathy.**
- IV naloxone (opiate antagonist), 0.01 mg/kg, should be administered if opiate intoxication is suspected (coma, respiratory depression, small reactive pupils).
- Flumazenil (benzodiazepine antagonist), 0.2 mg IV, may reverse benzodiazepine intoxication, but its duration of action is short, and additional doses may be needed. Flumazenil should be used with caution in certain patient populations (e.g., epileptics) because it reduces the seizure threshold.
- In delirious patients, sedatives should be avoided if possible. If necessary, low doses of quetiapine (12.5–25 mg) or lorazepam (1 mg) can be used. **Remember to always consider comorbidities before administering these medications.**

Other Nonpharmacologic Therapies

If herniation is identified or suspected, treatment consists of measures to lower intracranial pressure while surgically treatable etiologies are identified or excluded. All of the listed measures are only **temporizing methods**. Consultation with neurosurgery should be performed concurrently.

- Elevate the head of the bed to at least 30 degrees.
- Endotracheal intubation is usually performed to enable hyperventilation to a partial pressure of carbon dioxide (PCO_2) of 25–30 mm Hg. This reduces intracranial pressure within minutes by cerebral vasoconstriction. Bag mask ventilation can be performed if manipulation of the neck is precluded by possible or established spinal instability. Reduction of PCO_2 below 25 mm Hg is not recommended because it may reduce cerebral blood flow.
- Administration of IV mannitol (1–2 g/kg over 10–20 minutes) osmotically reduces free water in the brain via elimination by the kidneys and does not require a central line for administration. Remember that, given its potent diuretic effect, mannitol can precipitate renal failure if volume is not adequately replaced. Hypertonic saline (5% or 23.4% saline) is an alternative option but also has side effects and requires central venous access.
- Dexamethasone (10 mg IV, followed by 4 mg IV q6h) reduces the edema surrounding a tumor or an abscess but is not indicated for diffuse cerebral edema or the mass effect associated with malignant cerebral infarcts.
- Coagulopathy should be corrected if intracranial hemorrhage is diagnosed and before surgical treatment or invasive procedures (e.g., LP) are performed. Each patient's circumstances should be carefully assessed before therapeutic anticoagulation is reversed.

Surgical Management

Surgical evacuation of epidural, subdural, or intraparenchymal (e.g., cerebellar) hemorrhage and shunting for acute hydrocephalus should be considered in the appropriate clinical circumstances. However, some structural lesions are not amenable to surgical treatment.

AUTOIMMUNE ENCEPHALITIS

Autoimmune encephalitis is increasingly recognized as an etiology of subacute confusion in certain patients. It is characterized by subacute onset of confusion, often with other neurologic signs/symptoms (e.g., seizures, movement disorders, psychosis).

Diagnostic Testing

- Patients in whom autoimmune encephalitis is suspected should undergo evaluation with LP, EEG, and MRI. A thorough investigation aimed at identifying other possible etiologies should also be pursued.
  - CSF often demonstrates findings consistent with inflammation (protein >50 mg/dL or lymphocytic pleocytosis >5 cells/μL) but can be normal.
  - MRI features consistent with encephalitis include T2/FLAIR hyperintensities restricted to one or both medial temporal lobes or multifocal in gray and/or white matter compatible with demyelination or inflammation with our without contrast enhancement.
  - Interictal EEG may demonstrate focal discharges or slowing in a patient with seizures.
- The Antibody Prevalence in Epilepsy and Encephalopathy (APE2) score (Table 27-2) is used to predict neural-specific antibody positivity. An APE2 score ≥4 is 99% sensitive and 93% specific in this regard.[4]
- The Mayo autoimmune encephalitis (not paraneoplastic) panel should be sent from both serum and CSF if an autoimmune encephalitis is suspected.

Principles of Treatment

- The initial treatment of choice, which is also used to determine response to immunotherapy, is IV methylprednisolone 1000 mg/d for 3 days.
- Other treatment considerations include IV immunoglobulin (IVIG), plasma exchange, azathioprine, mycophenolate mofetil, rituximab, and cyclophosphamide.

SEVERE BRAIN INJURY

- **Brain death** occurs from irreversible brain injury sufficient to permanently eliminate all cortical and brainstem functions. Because the vital centers in the brainstem sustain cardiovascular and respiratory functions, brain death is incompatible with survival despite mechanical ventilation and cardiovascular and nutritional supportive measures. Brain death is distinguished from persistent vegetative state (PVS) in which the absence of higher cortical function is accompanied by intact brainstem function. Patients in a PVS are unable to think, speak, understand, or meaningfully respond to visual, verbal, or auditory stimuli, yet with nutritional and supportive care, their cardiovascular and respiratory functions can sustain viability for many years.
- Brain death criteria vary by institution. Refer to your institution's policy for details. AAN prerequisite guidelines are summarized below[5]:
  - Declaration of brain death requires presence (clinical and radiographic) of CNS catastrophe.

TABLE 27-2	APE2 Score	
		Value
New-onset, rapidly progressive mental status changes that developed over 1–6 wk or new-onset seizure activity (within 1 y of evaluation)		+1
Neuropsychiatric changes; agitation, aggressiveness, emotional lability		+1
Autonomic dysfunction (sustained atrial tachycardia or bradycardia, orthostatic hypotension [≥20 mm Hg fall in systolic pressure or ≥10 mm Hg fall in diastolic pressure within 3 min of quiet standing], hyperhidrosis, persistently labile blood pressure, ventricular tachycardia, cardiac asystole or gastrointestinal dysmotility)		+1
Viral prodrome (rhinorrhea, sore throat, low-grade fever) to be scored in the absence of underlying systemic malignancy within 5 y of neurological symptom onset		+2
Faciobrachial dystonic seizures		+3
Facial dyskinesias, to be scored in the absence of faciobrachial dystonic seizures		+2
Seizure refractory to at least to two antiseizure medications		+2
CSF findings consistent with inflammation (elevated CSF protein >50 mg/dL and/or lymphocytic pleocytosis >5 cells/µL, if the total number of CSF RBCs is <1000 cells/µL)		+2
Brain MRI suggesting encephalitis (T2/FLAIR hyperintensity restricted to one or both medial temporal lobes or multifocal in gray matter, white matter, or both compatible with demyelination or inflammation)		+2
Systemic cancer diagnosed within 5 y of neurological symptom onset (excluding cutaneous squamous cell carcinoma, basal cell carcinoma, brain tumor, cancer with brain metastasis)		+2

APE2, Antibody Prevalence in Epilepsy and Encephalopathy; CSF, cerebrospinal fluid; RBCs, red blood cells.

- CNS depressant effect must be absent.
- Acid–base disturbances must be corrected.
- Patient must be normothermic.
- Systolic blood pressure must be >100 mm Hg.
- Prognostication after cardiac arrest utilizes a multimodal assessment including the clinical examination, EEG, somatosensory evoked potentials, and serum neuron-specific enolase (NSE).[6]
  - Key features of the clinical examination include pupillary response, corneal reflex, motor reaction to pain, and presence of early myoclonus.
  - EEG is used to identify certain patterns (such as burst suppression), but also to identify the presence of status epilepticus, which should be treated.
  - Serum NSE is not widely used given slow turnaround time and lack of availability.

ALCOHOL WITHDRAWAL

Alcohol withdrawal typically occurs when illness or hospitalization interrupts continued alcohol intake.

- Tremulousness, irritability, anorexia, and nausea characterize minor alcohol withdrawal. Symptoms usually appear within a few hours after reduction or cessation of alcohol consumption and resolve within 48 hours. Treatment includes supportive care with hydration and reassurance. **Thiamine**, 100–500 mg IM/IV, followed by 100 mg PO daily; multivitamins containing **folic acid**; and a balanced diet as tolerated should be administered. Serial evaluation for signs of major alcohol withdrawal is essential.
- Alcoholic hallucinosis occurs within 8–48 hours after cessation of alcohol and is distinguished from delirium tremens (DTs) by a clear sensorium.
- Alcohol withdrawal seizures, typically one or a few brief generalized convulsions, occur 12–48 hours after cessation of ethanol intake. **Antiepileptic drugs (AEDs) are not indicated for typical alcohol withdrawal seizures.** Other causes for seizures (see "Seizures" section) must be excluded. If hypoglycemia is present, thiamine should be administered before glucose.
- Severe withdrawal or DTs consists of tremulousness, hallucinations, agitation, confusion, disorientation, and autonomic hyperactivity (fever, tachycardia, diaphoresis), typically occurring 48–72 hours after cessation of drinking. DTs complicates 5%–10% of cases of alcohol withdrawal, with mortality up to 15%. Other causes of delirium must be considered in the differential diagnosis (see Table 27-1).[7]
- Mild withdrawal symptoms can be managed with chlordiazepoxide PO 25–50 mg q6–8h (maximum total daily dose 300 mg) with a subsequent dose taper or, preferably, with a symptom-triggered treatment protocol. This medication is hepatically cleared and should be avoided in patients with liver disease. In patients with severe hepatic failure, oxazepam (15–30 mg PO, q6–8h as needed), which is excreted by the kidney, is preferred. For patients with severe withdrawal symptoms, seizures, and/or DTs, diazepam or lorazepam IV are effective agents. Diazepam 10 mg IV every 5–20 minutes or lorazepam IV 2–4 mg every 15–20 minutes should be given until symptom control is achieved. Treatment can then be transitioned to a symptom-triggered or scheduled regimen.
- Maintenance of fluid and electrolyte balance is important. Alcoholic patients are susceptible to hypomagnesemia, hypokalemia, hypoglycemia, and fluid losses, which may be considerable due to fever, diaphoresis, and vomiting.

Alzheimer Disease

GENERAL PRINCIPLES

Alzheimer disease (AD) is the most common neurodegenerative disorder in older individuals (older than 60 years), typically characterized by memory problems and inability to independently perform activities of daily living.

Epidemiology

- Prevalence is <1% before age 65 years, 5%–10% at age 65 years, and approximately 45% by age 85 years. Approximately 5.7 million Americans have AD.
- Inherited forms of AD manifest typically before age 65 years and are associated with mutations in amyloid precursor protein (*APP*) gene on chromosome 21,

presenilin-1 (PSEN1) gene on chromosome 14, and presenilin-2 (PSEN2) gene on chromosome 1.

- The greatest risk factor for late-onset/sporadic AD is the presence of the apolipo-protein ε4 variant.
- Lifetime risk doubles if a sibling or parent is diagnosed with AD.
- It is common for AD patients to present at late stages of the disease after an unrelated medical illness unmasks signs and symptoms of the disease that had previously gone unrecognized by the family.
- Pseudodementia (cognitive impairment related to comorbid depression) should be considered in the appropriate clinical context.

Pathophysiology

Pathologic diagnosis requires presence of both neurofibrillary tangles due to tau and neuritic plaques composed of amyloid.

DIAGNOSIS

Clinical Presentation

- For a diagnosis of AD, the patient must exhibit cognitive impairment that is a change from baseline.
- Episodic memory for newly acquired information is impaired, whereas memory for more remote events is not affected.
- Declarative memory for facts and events is affected, whereas procedural memory and motor learning are spared in earlier stages of the disease.
- With progression of disease, language, visuospatial skills, abstract reasoning, and executive function deteriorate. Some patients will also develop apraxia, alexia, and delusions.

Differential Diagnosis

See Table 27-3.

Diagnostic Testing

Progression of disease can be assessed by the Mini-Mental State Examination, the Montreal Cognitive Assessment (MoCA), and the Clinical Dementia Rating Scale.

Laboratory Studies
- Definitive diagnosis of AD requires histopathologic confirmation (i.e., autopsy).
- Reversible causes of dementia such as B_{12} deficiency, neurosyphilis, HIV, and thyroid abnormalities should be ruled out.

Imaging
- Brain MRI can suggest potential alternative diagnoses.
- MRI may show diffuse atrophy with hippocampal atrophy that is seen with AD.
- [^{18}F]Fluorodeoxyglucose positron emission tomography (PET) or perfusion single-photon emission computed tomography (SPECT) may demonstrate hypometabolism and hypoperfusion, respectively, within the parietotemporal cortex.
- Amyloid PET tracers (florbetapir) can measure amyloid deposition in the brain and are approved for clinical use but are quite expensive. New PET tracers for tau are being actively developed.

TABLE 27-3	Differential Diagnosis of Alzheimer Dementia

Frontotemporal dementia
  Changes in personality, behavior, and executive functioning
Vascular dementia
  Stepwise course due to repeated strokes or strokelike events
Dementia with Lewy bodies
  Visual hallucinations, dream enactment behavior (i.e., REM behavior disorder), cognitive fluctuations, parkinsonism, sensitivity to neuroleptics
Normal pressure hydrocephalus
  Triad of dementia, urinary incontinence, and gait instability ("wacky, wet, and wobbly")
Vitamin B$_{12}$ deficiency
Neurosyphilis
Thyroid dysfunction
HIV
Creutzfeldt–Jakob disease
Autoimmune encephalopathies (including paraneoplastic syndromes)

REM, rapid eye movement.

Diagnostic Procedures
- Neuropsychological testing can establish a baseline cognitive status. This testing can sometimes differentiate dementia from depression (i.e., pseudodementia).
- Both structural MRI and PET imaging may assist in early diagnosis.
- CSF measures of reduced Aβ_{42} and increased tau can be obtained and may assist in the diagnosis.

TREATMENT

- Cholinesterase inhibitors including donepezil, rivastigmine, and galantamine can be considered for early AD.
- Memantine, a noncompetitive N-methyl-D-aspartate receptor antagonist, can be considered for moderate to severe dementia.
- A combination of the above medications is sometimes used in more advanced AD patients. Additional therapies (including antiamyloid agents) are being investigated.
- Aducanumab, an amyloid β-directed monoclonal antibody, was approved by the US Food and Drug Administration (FDA) in 2021 but its use remains controversial and will not be covered here.

Seizures

GENERAL PRINCIPLES

Definition
- Seizure: Stereotyped spells caused by abnormal electrical brain activity. A more complex definition is uncontrolled excessive electrical discharges in the brain that may produce a sudden change in brain function causing physical convulsion, minor physical signs, thought disturbances, or a combination of symptoms.

- Epilepsy is defined by recurrent seizures.
- Status epilepticus is defined by >5 minutes of continuous seizure activity or recurrent seizures without full recovery between episodes. Generalized convulsive status epilepticus (GCSE) is a medical emergency.
- NCSE is defined by electrographic seizures with clinically absent or subtle motor activity and impairment or loss of consciousness. NCSE should also be treated promptly to avoid irreversible cerebral injury.
- An epileptic aura is a simple partial seizure manifesting as sensory, autonomic, or psychic symptoms.
- A prodrome is a sensation or feeling that a seizure will soon occur. Distinguishing a prodrome from an aura can be clinically challenging.

Classification

- Focal seizures begin at a single locus in the brain. Provided are both the current seizure nomenclature (International League against Epilepsy, 2017) and the more classic nomenclature.
- **Focal onset seizure *without* impaired awareness (simple partial):** Awareness is not impaired. The symptoms can be motor (hand jerking), sensory (focal tingling, visual, auditory), autonomic (sensation of epigastric rising), or psychic (déjà vu).
- **Focal onset seizure *with* impaired awareness (complex partial):** Awareness is impaired. The symptoms vary based on whether they involve the temporal (automatisms such as lip smacking or picking at clothes, staring, behavior arrest), frontal (hypermotor behaviors, bicycling, pelvic thrusting, and automatisms), or occipital lobes (unformed images, visual hallucinations). Frontal seizures are often misdiagnosed as nonepileptic seizures (i.e., pseudoseizures) due to their often complex, sometimes bizarre semiology and the frequent absence of electrographic seizure activity on standard EEG.
- Generalized seizures originate from the bilateral hemispheres and, by definition, awareness is impaired.
  ○ May begin as a generalized seizure, or a focal seizure with secondary generalization.
  ○ Include motor and nonmotor (including absence).

Epidemiology

- Epilepsy is estimated to affect approximately 70 million people worldwide, and 3.4 million in the US, with the prevalence being twice as high in low-income countries.
- The median worldwide incidence of epilepsy is approximately 50 per 100,000 per year.[8]

Etiology

Etiologies for seizures include those listed in Table 27-4. For patients with a known seizure disorder presenting with an increase in seizure frequency, the most common causes are AED noncompliance, subtherapeutic anticonvulsant levels, or infection.

DIAGNOSIS

Clinical Presentation

History
- Ask about family history of epilepsy, developmental delay, trauma, and a thorough medical history including medical conditions, medications, allergies, recreational drugs, and possible precipitating events.

TABLE 27-4	Etiologies of Seizures

- CNS infections
- Fever
- Hypoxic brain injury
- Stroke (ischemic or hemorrhagic)
- Cerebral venous thrombosis
- Vascular malformations
- Tumors/carcinomatous meningitis
- Head injury
- Eclampsia
- Hypertensive encephalopathy/reversible posterior leukoencephalopathy
- Hyperthyroidism
- Congenital brain malformations
- Hereditary (Sturge–Weber, tuberous sclerosis, Dravet syndrome, and other channelopathies)
- Toxic metabolic (porphyria, uremia, liver failure)
- Drug withdrawal (alcohol, barbiturates, benzodiazepine, AEDs)
- Drug intoxication (TCAs, bupropion, clozapine, tramadol, cocaine, amphetamine)
- Electrolyte abnormalities/metabolic
  - Hyponatremia or hypernatremia
  - Hypocalcemia
  - Hypomagnesemia
  - Hypophosphatemia
  - Hypoglycemia/hyperglycemia

AEDs, antiepileptic drugs; CNS, central nervous system; TCAs, tricyclic antidepressants.

- Ask the patient about any prodrome/aura. An eyewitness account of the event is critical, and a video can be extremely helpful. Inquire about temporal lobe features (i.e., acute onset with a rapid crescendo), **incontinence**, **tongue biting**, and how the patient behaved after the event ended (e.g., confusion, somnolence) and for how long.

Physical Examination
- Vital signs and blood sugar should be obtained immediately on all patients. Empiric thiamine should be given when treating hypoglycemia. Ictal and/or postictal fever can occur.
- Look for nuchal rigidity, rash, asterixis, or signs of trauma.
- Convulsive seizures are usually easily identified.
- Features of the seizure can aid in identifying the ictal focus (e.g., complex automatisms in frontal lobe seizures, lip smacking and postictal nose wiping in temporal lobe seizures).
- Carefully observe for subtle signs of nonconvulsive seizures, such as automatisms, facial or extremity twitching, eye deviation, and fluctuating periods of awareness.
- Patients may present during the postictal period, before they return to baseline mental status. During this time, patients may act confused and obtunded and have amnesia for events. This period can typically last from minutes to hours, though can last days in the elderly and those with prior CNS injury.
- Postictal weakness (also called Todd paralysis) is a transient neurologic deficit that lasts for hours to days after a seizure.

Differential Diagnosis

Alternate diagnoses that may mimic seizures include:

- Syncope, especially convulsive syncope in which seizure-like motor activity is observed. The Calgary Seizure Syncope Score is a useful and reliable clinical tool in distinguishing these two entities.[9]
- Nonepileptic seizures ("pseudoseizures").
- Transient ischemic attack (TIA).
- Migraine with aura.
- Toxic-metabolic encephalopathy.
- Tremors, dyskinesias (episodic movement disorders).
- Nonepileptic myoclonus.
- Sleep disorders.
- Rigors.

Diagnostic Testing

Laboratory Studies

Initial laboratory studies should include blood glucose, electrolytes (sodium, calcium, magnesium, and phosphorus), CBC, urinalysis, urine drug screen, and AED levels if indicated.

Imaging

Neuroimaging is usually indicated to identify structural etiologies.

- Start with a noncontrast head CT in the acute setting.
- Brain MRI with and without contrast is almost always indicated in the evaluation of new-onset seizures and mandatory if focal features are present.

Diagnostic Procedures

- LP should be done if there is concern for CNS infection. Send for routine CSF studies as well as HSV viral testing.
- EEG is not required for initial diagnosis and management of GCSE. If mental status is not improving as expected after convulsive seizures stop, EEG may be necessary to exclude conversion to NCSE. Unless the patient is known to typically have an extraordinarily prolonged postictal period, NCSE should be considered in any patient who fails to return to baseline within an hour of a seizure. Approximately 50% of patients who present with GCSE will go on to develop NCSE within 24 hours of cessation of clinical seizure activity.
- Routine EEG is indicated for all new-onset seizure.
- Video EEG is the gold standard test for the evaluation of suspected nonepileptic seizures. A notable (30%–50% in some studies) number of patients with nonepileptic seizures ("pseudoseizures") will also have epileptic seizures.

TREATMENT

- **Initiation of AED therapy is usually not indicated after a single unprovoked seizure** because about two-thirds of patients who had a single seizure will not have seizure recurrence.[10] However, patients with a single unprovoked seizure and either an abnormal EEG or evidence of an ictal focus on head CT or brain MRI warrant initiation of AED therapy given a much higher likelihood of seizure recurrence.
- In general, AEDs should not be started in patients with provoked seizures.
- A diagnosis of epilepsy is made after two or more unprovoked seizures. AED treatment is generally started after the second seizure because the patient has a substantially increased risk (approximately 75%) for repeated seizures after two events.

- Treatment of status epilepticus must be prompt because efficacy of treatment decreases with increased seizure duration and GCSE carries an all-cause mortality of 30% (see Figure 27-1 for treatment of status epilepticus).[11] Within 5–30 minutes of GCSE onset, the body's homeostatic mechanisms begin to fail and patients' risk of permanent brain injury increases, as does risk of systemic complications including hyperthermia, pulmonary embolism, cardiovascular and respiratory insufficiency, and other life-threatening complications. Prolonged NCSE will also result in brain injury but on a timescale of days as opposed to minutes (see Figure 27-2).

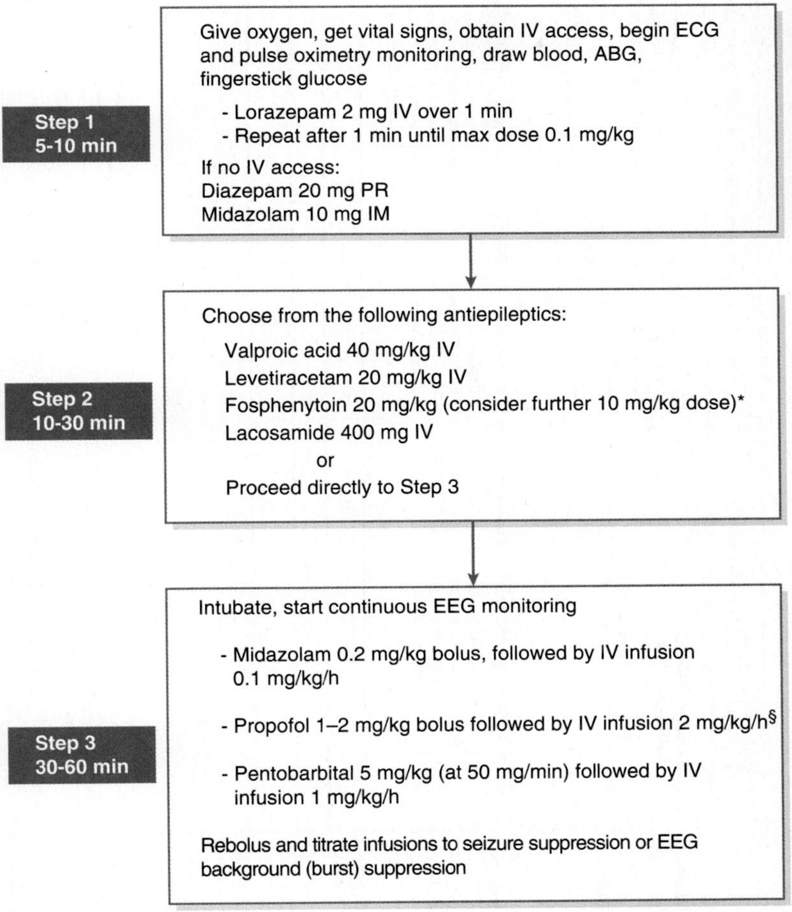

Step 1
5-10 min

Give oxygen, get vital signs, obtain IV access, begin ECG and pulse oximetry monitoring, draw blood, ABG, fingerstick glucose

- Lorazepam 2 mg IV over 1 min
- Repeat after 1 min until max dose 0.1 mg/kg

If no IV access:
Diazepam 20 mg PR
Midazolam 10 mg IM

Step 2
10-30 min

Choose from the following antiepileptics:

Valproic acid 40 mg/kg IV
Levetiracetam 20 mg/kg IV
Fosphenytoin 20 mg/kg (consider further 10 mg/kg dose)*
Lacosamide 400 mg IV
or
Proceed directly to Step 3

Step 3
30-60 min

Intubate, start continuous EEG monitoring

- Midazolam 0.2 mg/kg bolus, followed by IV infusion 0.1 mg/kg/h

- Propofol 1–2 mg/kg bolus followed by IV infusion 2 mg/kg/h§

- Pentobarbital 5 mg/kg (at 50 mg/min) followed by IV infusion 1 mg/kg/h

Rebolus and titrate infusions to seizure suppression or EEG background (burst) suppression

*Check phenytoin level 2 h after load. Level should be 20–25 μg/mL.
§Using propofol at high doses for >2 d may result in potentially lethal propofol toxicity.

Figure 27-1. Treatment of status epilepticus. ABG, arterial blood gas; EEG, electroencephalogram.[11]

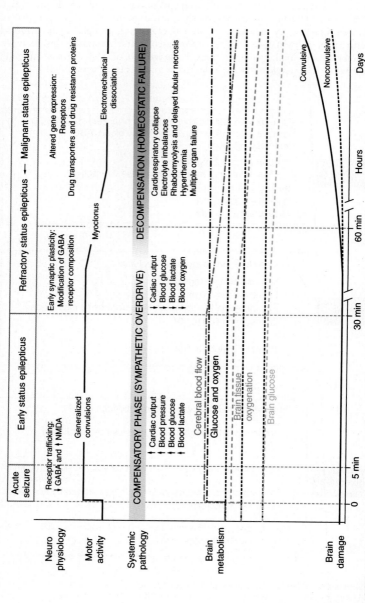

Figure 27-2. Brain and systemic pathology in prolonged convulsive and nonconvulsive status epilepticus. (Reprinted with permission from Hirsch LJ, Gaspard N. Status epilepticus. *Continuum.* 2013;19:767.)

Medications

- The selection of a specific AED for a patient must be individualized according to the drug effectiveness for seizure type(s), potential adverse effects of the drug, interactions with other possible medications, cost, and mechanism of drug action.[12]
- About half of all patients with a new diagnosis of epilepsy will be seizure free with the first AED prescribed.[13]
- Treatment should be started with a single drug that can be titrated until adequate control or until side effects are experienced.
- **In the outpatient setting, combination therapy (polytherapy) should be attempted only after at least two adequate sequential trials of single agents have failed.** Failure to control epilepsy with adequate trials of two drugs meets criteria for treatment-resistant epilepsy, and a referral for presurgical evaluation should be considered.[14]

Lifestyle Modifications

- Patients should not start other medications (e.g., over-the-counter medications or herbal remedies) without contacting their physician because drug interactions may occur.
- Patients should keep a seizure diary to identify possible seizure triggers. Screen patients for poor sleep hygiene. Women may have catamenial (perimenstrual) seizures.
- Women should ideally inform their physicians well in advance of any plans for pregnancy or at the very least immediately upon finding out they are pregnant given the teratogenicity associated with certain AEDs, the increased risk of teratogenicity with polytherapy versus monotherapy, and the potential need for medication adjustment during pregnancy.
- Patients should reduce alcohol intake because heavy consumption (three or more drinks per day) is associated with an increased risk of seizures.

REFERRAL

Neurologic consultation may be helpful for managing status epilepticus and for evaluation and management of new-onset seizures.

PATIENT EDUCATION

Patients with epilepsy, especially those left untreated, have a small risk of sudden death in epilepsy.[15] Patients with epilepsy should not swim unsupervised, bathe in a bathtub of standing water, use motorized tools, or be in position to fall from heights during a seizure (i.e., patients should avoid situations in which they could harm themselves or others if they were to have a seizure). Driver licensing requirements for patients with epilepsy vary from state to state. A complete listing of state laws can be found at https://www.epilepsy.com/driving-laws.

MONITORING/FOLLOW-UP

- Regular follow-up visits should be scheduled to check drug concentrations, blood counts, and hepatic and renal function. Side effects after initiating AED should be monitored.
- Again, correctable causes for seizures (e.g., hyponatremia, drug toxicity, alcohol withdrawal) do not require long-term anticonvulsant therapy.

CHAPTER 27

Multiple Sclerosis

GENERAL PRINCIPLES

Definition

- Multiple sclerosis (MS) is a chronic, progressive, immune-mediated disorder of the CNS, initially characterized by inflammatory demyelination followed later in its course by neurodegeneration.
- Although the disorder is presumed to be autoimmune in nature, the antigen(s) driving the immune response remains unknown.

Classification

- Types of MS
  - Relapsing-remitting MS (RRMS): Episodic neurologic dysfunction followed by a complete or partial recovery in between episodes. Most patients are initially diagnosed with RRMS.
  - Primary progressive MS (PPMS): Progressive neurologic dysfunction from onset without relapses or remissions. Less common.
  - Secondary progressive MS: Progressive neurologic dysfunction but follows an initial relapsing-remitting course.
- Classification is important in that progressive forms of the disease, in general, do not respond to many of the first-line disease-modifying therapies (DMTs) effective in RRMS (e.g., interferon-β) but do respond to other therapies (e.g., ocrelizumab in PPMS).

Epidemiology

- Approximately 500,000 patients carry a diagnosis of MS in the US.
- The worldwide prevalence is estimated at over 2.3 million and growing.

Etiology

The exact etiology of MS remains unknown. The pathophysiologic pattern of MS is characterized by inflammatory cell infiltration, demyelination, axonal damage, and gliosis culminating in neurodegeneration.

DIAGNOSIS

Clinical Presentation

At disease onset, symptoms are variable and can include visual dysfunction (i.e., optic neuritis), sensory abnormalities, motor dysfunction, ataxia, fatigue, and bowel/bladder dysfunction.

Differential Diagnosis

- The differential diagnosis of MS is too extensive to be covered here but is reviewed in great detail elsewhere.[16]
- Important differential diagnoses to consider include neuromyelitis optica (NMO), another immune-mediated demyelinating disorder of the CNS. NMO, in the majority of cases, is associated with antibodies against the aquaporin-4 antigen.
- Another autoantibody-mediated demyelinating disorder of the CNS that shares clinical features with MS and NMO is anti–myelin oligodendrocyte glycoprotein (anti-MOG) disease.

Diagnostic Testing

- A cornerstone of diagnostic testing and monitoring/follow-up is MRI of the brain and spinal cord (in many cases). It is worth noting that "MRI-negative" MS does not exist. Lesions on MRI are part of the diagnostic criteria (2017 McDonald criteria) for the disease. However, in patients unable to undergo MRI scans, additional laboratory studies (i.e., CSF analysis) can be used, in the appropriate clinical context, to support a diagnosis of MS.
- RRMS is a disease disseminated in space and time. Patients should have clinical or radiographic evidence of ≥2 attacks.
- CSF analysis is second to MRI in its value as a diagnostic marker of MS. Historically, CSF-specific oligoclonal bands have substituted for criteria of dissemination in time. More recently, CSF kappa free light chain has been demonstrated to have comparable performance with increased sensitivity and is therefore used as a screening test.[17]

TREATMENT

- Acute relapses are often treated with corticosteroids.
- There is no cure for MS. DMTs remain the cornerstone of treatment.
- In general, as DMTs increase in efficacy, the side effect profile increases. Lower efficacy medications (i.e., injectables) are preferred for less severe cases and higher efficacy medications are used for more severe cases.
- There has been a substantial growth in the number of DMTs available to treat MS in recent years.
- See Table 27-5 for more details.

REFERRAL

In general, all patients with suspected MS or MS should be referred to a neurologist for formal diagnostic testing and initiation of DMTs if indicated.

Cerebrovascular Disease

GENERAL PRINCIPLES

- Stroke is a medical emergency that requires rapid diagnosis and treatment. Remember that "TIME IS BRAIN."
- The hallmark of stroke is acute interruption of cerebral blood flow to a specific brain region, resulting in a **sudden-onset focal neurologic deficit.**
- Fluctuation of functional deficits after stroke onset or a brief deficit known as TIA suggests tissue at risk for infarction that may be rescued by reestablishing and/or maintaining perfusion.

Epidemiology

More than 795,000 strokes occur per year in the US (one stroke every 40 seconds in the US population), and it is the fourth leading cause of death in the US (one death every 4 minutes).

TABLE 27-5	Disease-Modifying Therapies Approved for Use in Relapsing-Remitting Multiple Sclerosis		
Drug	Mechanism of Action	Efficacy	Side Effects
Injectables			
Interferon-β preparations—IM or SC (Betaseron, Extavia, Avonex, Rebif, and Plegridy)	Modulates B- and T-cell function Reverses blood–brain barrier disruption Modulation of cytokine expression	30% reduction in relapses Reduction in disability Reduction in MRI lesions	Flu-like symptoms Injection site reactions Transaminitis (monitor HFP)
Glatiramer acetate (Copaxone, Glatopa)—SC	Stimulates regulatory T cells Potential neuroprotection and repair	30% reduction in relapses Reduction in disability Reduction in MRI lesions	Injection site reactions
Orals			
Fingolimod (Gilenya) Siponimod (Mayzent) Ozanimod (Zeposia)	Sphingosine-1-phosphate receptor modulators Inhibits egress of lymphocytes from lymph nodes toward CNS	Reduces annual number of relapses and MRI lesions Reduces the risk of disability progression	**First-dose bradycardia** (except ozanimod) Skin malignancies Herpes infection Cardiac arrhythmia Macular edema Lymphopenia
Teriflunomide (Aubagio)	Downregulation of T- and B-cell proliferation via de novo synthesis of pyrimidines (drug derived directly from leflunomide)	Reduces annual number of relapses and MRI lesions Reduces the risk of disability progression	Lymphopenia UTIs Elevated liver enzymes Teratogenicity (washout necessary)
Dimethyl fumarate (Tecfidera)	Shifts dendritic cell differentiation Suppresses inflammatory cytokine production	Reduces annual number of relapses and MRI lesions Reduces the risk of disability progression	Lymphopenia Abdominal pain Diarrhea Flushing

TABLE 27-5	Disease-Modifying Therapies Approved for Use in Relapsing-Remitting Multiple Sclerosis *(continued)*		
Drug	Mechanism of Action	Efficacy	Side Effects
Infusions			
Natalizumab (Tysabri)—IV	Humanized monoclonal antibody that blocks the interaction of α4β1 integrin on leukocytes with vascular cell adhesion molecules to prevent migration of leukocytes from the blood to the CNS	68% reduction in relapses Reduction in disability Reduction in MRI lesions by 92% relative to placebo	Infusion reactions including anaphylaxis Progressive multifocal leukoencephalopathy (need to monitor JCV antibodies/titers) Rebound if abruptly stopped
Alemtuzumab (Lemtrada)—IV	Humanized monoclonal antibody against CD52 Depletes circulating lymphocytes and monocytes	50% reduction in relapses relative to interferon-β Reduction in MRI lesions relative to interferon-β	Infusion reactions Infections (URI, UTI, oral herpes) Secondary autoimmune disorders
Ocrelizumab (Ocrevus)—IV Ofatumumab (Kesimpta)—SQ	Humanized monoclonal antibody against CD20 (B-cell depletion)	~50% reduction in relapses relative to interferon-β Reduction in MRI lesions relative to interferon-β First drug to slow disease progression in PPMS	Infusion reactions Avoid live vaccines Follow CD19 counts Baseline hepatitis serologies

CNS, central nervous system; HFP, hepatic function panel; PPMS, primary progressive multiple sclerosis; URI, upper respiratory tract infection; UTI, urinary tract infection.

Etiology

- **Ischemic stroke** can be subclassified into large artery atherothrombotic, small vessel, embolic, hypoperfusion, or hypercoagulable state (the latter being relatively rare).
  - **Atherothrombosis** results from reduced flow within an artery or embolism of thrombus into the distal segment of an artery.
    - Atherosclerosis is the most common etiology of thrombus formation in large vessels.
    - Less common etiologies include dissection, fibromuscular dysplasia, moyamoya, and vasculitis.
  - **Small-vessel disease** is due to lipohyalinosis, usually caused by hypertension.

○ **Cardioembolic** strokes account for about 20% of all ischemic strokes. High-risk cardiac sources include atrial fibrillation/flutter, rheumatic valve disease, cardiac thrombus, cardiomyopathy, prosthetic valves, bacterial endocarditis, nonbacterial endocarditis (antiphospholipid antibody syndrome, marantic endocarditis, Libman–Sachs endocarditis), sick sinus syndrome, and coronary artery bypass graft surgery.

○ **Hypoperfusion** occurs due to general circulatory problems and often results in bilateral symptoms. Infarction commonly occurs in border zones between large vessels resulting in watershed infarcts.

○ **Hypercoagulable states** may predispose to arterial thrombosis. These include sickle cell disease, polycythemia vera, essential thrombocythemia, thrombotic thrombocytopenic purpura, antiphospholipid antibody syndrome, hyperhomocysteinemia, and others. Factor V Leiden, protein C and S deficiency, and antithrombin III deficiency typically result in venous, not arterial, infarcts.

• **Hemorrhagic stroke** occurs in about 20% of all cases.

○ The location of an **intraparenchymal hemorrhage (IPH)** may suggest its etiology.

  ▪ Deep hemorrhage in the basal ganglia, thalamus, or pons is often due to chronic systemic hypertension.

  ▪ Amyloid angiopathy typically causes peripheral lobar hemorrhages and is a common etiology in the elderly.

  ▪ Head trauma, anticoagulants, drugs (cocaine or amphetamines), arteriovenous malformation (AVM), tumor, blood dyscrasia, hemorrhagic conversion of an ischemic stroke, and vasculitis are other possible hemorrhagic stroke etiologies.

○ **Aneurysmal subarachnoid hemorrhage** (for this section, SAH will refer to aneurysmal subarachnoid hemorrhage unless designated otherwise) is caused by the rupture of an arterial aneurysm resulting in bleeding into the subarachnoid space (which contains CSF). Hypertension, cigarette smoking, genetic factors, and septic emboli (resulting in mycotic aneurysms) can all contribute to aneurysm formation.

• **Cerebral venous sinus thrombosis** (CVST) is the occlusion of a venous sinus by a thrombus. It occurs in hypercoagulable states such as late pregnancy or postpartum, cancer, and thrombophilias, as well as with trauma and adjacent inflammation/infection. It may manifest with ischemic infarcts and/or hemorrhage.

Risk Factors

Major significant risk factors for ischemic stroke include hypertension, prior TIA/stroke, carotid stenosis, diabetes mellitus, dyslipidemia, heart failure, cigarette smoking, alcohol consumption, oral contraceptive use, obesity, genetics, and age.

DIAGNOSIS

Clinical Presentation

History

• Time of last known well is critical if thrombolytic therapy is to be administered. It is crucial to note that this is **not** when the patient was found with their deficit but when they were last observed to be at their neurologic baseline.

• Onset of symptoms is typically sudden. Ask about progression or fluctuation of symptoms.

• Inquire about cardiac arrhythmias and atherosclerotic risk factors.

- A history of neck trauma or recent chiropractic maneuvers warrants evaluation for arterial dissection.
- SAH commonly presents with sudden onset of a severe thunderclap headache (i.e., the "worst headache of my life"). Lethargy or coma, fever, vomiting, seizures, and low back pain may also be present.
- IPH presents with neurologic deficits accompanied by headache, vomiting, and possibly lethargy.
- CVST often presents with signs and symptoms of elevated intracranial pressure, such as a positional headache with diurnal variability (waking from sleep, worse in the morning), bilateral sixth nerve palsies, blurred vision (typically peripheral with sparing of central vision initially), and papilledema.

Physical Examination
- A careful neurologic examination can reliably establish the anatomic location of a stroke in most cases.
- In general, carotid artery distribution (anterior circulation) strokes produce combinations of functional deficits (hemiparesis, hemianopia, cortical sensory loss, often with aphasias or agnosias) contralateral to the affected hemisphere.
- Vertebrobasilar strokes (posterior circulation) produce unilateral or bilateral motor/sensory deficits, usually accompanied by cranial nerve and brainstem signs (vertigo, diplopia, ataxia).
- General physical examination should be focused on possible etiologic factors. Examine for abnormal pulses, arrhythmias, murmurs, carotid bruits, and embolic phenomena.

Differential Diagnosis
Mimics of stroke include postseizure paralysis (Todd paralysis), migraine with aura, and hypo- or hyperglycemia.

Diagnostic Testing
Laboratory Studies
- In the acute setting (e.g., acute evaluation for thrombolytic therapy), these should include blood glucose and may include CBC and coagulation studies (e.g., international normalized ratio [INR], partial thromboplastin time [PTT], antifactor Xa level, thrombin time).
- The following are indicated but not emergent: basic metabolic panel, troponin, lipid profile, and hemoglobin A1C. Tests such as erythrocyte sedimentation rate (ESR), C-reactive protein (CRP) and blood cultures (if endocarditis is suspected), rapid plasma reagin, antinuclear antibody, antiphospholipid antibodies, drug toxicology screen, and HIV are not part of a "standard screen" but may be indicated in certain clinical contexts.

Electrocardiography
ECG should be done to look for atrial fibrillation or ischemic changes.

Imaging
- **Noncontrast head CT** scan should be obtained acutely to rapidly differentiate hemorrhagic from ischemic strokes. It can identify acute hemorrhages in most cases. It is insensitive for acute ischemic strokes. It is often the rate-limiting step in making decisions on thrombolytic therapy. Head CT scan is diagnostic of SAH in 90% of SAH patients in the first 24 hours.

CHAPTER 27

- **Emergent vascular imaging** (typically **CT angiography** [CTA] with or without CT perfusion scanning) is now performed in all patients presenting with suspected large vessel occlusion (carotid, proximal middle cerebral artery, or basilar artery) in order to screen for lesions amenable to endovascular thrombectomy.
  - CTA is also obtained in patients with IPH to evaluate for the presence of an AVM or aneurysm warranting intervention.
- **MRI** scan is the most sensitive imaging study for stroke diagnosis. Diffusion-weighted images detect stroke the earliest. If a diagnosis of stroke is clear from clinical examination, MRI is not always necessary because it is unlikely to affect management in a great majority of cases.
- **Magnetic resonance angiography** (MRA) and **venogram** are useful noninvasive tests to evaluate large arteries and veins, respectively. MRA of the neck with contrast can serve as a screen for carotid stenosis.
- **Carotid Doppler** studies enable noninvasive estimation of carotid stenosis and should be done for **anterior** circulation strokes unless some form of angiography has already been performed for another indication.
- **Two-dimensional transthoracic echocardiography** is helpful to demonstrate intracardiac thrombi, valve vegetations, valvular stenosis or insufficiency, and right-to-left shunt (bubble study). In some patients, transesophageal echocardiography may be necessary to evaluate the left atrium for thrombi.

Diagnostic Procedures
- **Cerebral catheter angiography** is the definitive study for vascular malformations but may miss small aneurysms. Some surgeons prefer having this procedure performed before proceeding with carotid endarterectomy (CEA).
- If suspicion for SAH is high and head CT is negative, an **LP** should be performed.
  - Tubes 1 and 4 should be sent for cell count. If the number of red blood cells (RBCs) decreases dramatically from tube 1 to tube 4, a traumatic LP is more likely than SAH.
  - Bloody CSF should be centrifuged and examined for xanthochromia (yellow color). Xanthochromia results from RBC lysis and takes several hours to develop, indicating SAH rather than a traumatic LP.

TREATMENT

- Vital signs, including oximetry and continuous telemetry, should be monitored.
- Hypertension management after ischemic stroke:
  - Patients with acute stroke often present hypertensive. Blood pressure (BP) tends to fall on its own over several days following a stroke.
  - Aggressive lowering of BP has been associated with neurologic deterioration.[18]
  - Although management of hypertension in the setting of acute stroke remains controversial, BP should not be lowered acutely unless necessary for treatment of acute coronary syndrome, CHF, hypertensive crisis with end-organ involvement, or systolic BP >220 mm Hg or diastolic BP >120 mm Hg.[19] BP lowering should proceed cautiously, with 15% during the first 24 hours being a reasonable goal.
- Treatment of intracranial hemorrhage consists of supportive care, gradual reduction in BP, and elevation of head of bed by 15 degrees.
- Treatment of SAH depends on aneurysm anatomy and available resources (surgical clipping vs. intravascular coiling).
  - Supportive measures include bed rest, sedation, analgesia, and laxatives to prevent sudden increases in intracranial pressure.

○ Patients with SAH tend toward volume contraction, and although there is insufficient evidence to support a benefit for volume expansion, guidelines do emphasize the importance of maintaining euvolemia to avoid delayed cerebral ischemia (DCI).

○ Induced hypertension (unless contraindicated by cardiac comorbidities or in patients with baseline elevated BP) is still recommended in patients with vasospasm/DCI because it has been shown to improve cerebral blood flow in these patients.

○ Endovascular angioplasty is recommended in patients with symptomatic vasospasm of proximal cerebral arteries that fail to respond to induced hypertension. In many instances, endovascular therapies are combined with intra-arterial vasodilator therapies (e.g., calcium channel blockers).

○ Other nonpharmacologic (i.e., hemodilution) and pharmacologic (i.e., statins, endothelin receptor antagonists, magnesium) therapies have failed to demonstrate a definitive benefit in patients with SAH.

○ Future therapies for preventing and treating cerebral vasospasm hinge on gaining a better understanding of the mechanisms underlying cerebral vasospasm and DCI.

Medications

• Recombinant tissue plasminogen activator (t-PA) remains the only FDA-approved pharmacologic therapy for acute ischemic stroke.

○ Generally, administration of t-PA must commence within 4.5 hours of stroke onset but should be started as close to onset as possible (i.e., do not delay to see if the patient "gets better" if they present early in the window).[20] Some centers are now using perfusion imaging to administer t-PA up to 9 hours from stroke onset.

○ Hyperacute MRI may be used to estimate the time of onset for patients with strokes of unknown onset time in order to make decisions regarding thrombolysis.[21]

○ t-PA treatment increases the risk for symptomatic brain hemorrhage, compared to placebo, but without any significant impact on 3- and 12-month mortality rates.

○ Exclusion criteria differ by stroke center protocol (Table 27-6). The acute stroke team should be contacted emergently to evaluate **all** acute strokes because some patients ineligible for IV t-PA may be candidates for other interventions, such as thrombectomy.

○ Advanced radiology can assist with selection of patients with large vessel occlusions who would benefit from endovascular thrombectomy (Table 27-7).

○ Aspirin and anticoagulants should be held for the first 24 hours after t-PA.

• Aspirin reduces atherosclerotic stroke morbidity and mortality and is typically given at an initial dose of 325 mg within 24–48 hours of stroke onset. The dose may be reduced to 81 mg in the post–acute stroke period.

• Other antiplatelet-aggregating drugs (clopidogrel, aspirin/dipyridamole) are available and may be of benefit for certain patients. Both of these drugs have a significant advantage over aspirin in secondary stroke prevention. Dual antiplatelet therapy for secondary prevention may benefit select patients, though is also associated with increased risk of hemorrhage.

• Heparin, low-molecular-weight heparin (LMWH), and warfarin anticoagulation are **not** recommended routinely for acute ischemic stroke.

• Anticoagulation with a DOAC or warfarin is indicated to prevent recurrent embolic strokes due to atrial fibrillation. This is typically started after 4–14 days.

TABLE 27-6	Inclusion and Exclusion Criteria for t-PA for Acute Ischemic Stroke (Washington University Stroke Center Protocol)

t-PA Inclusion Criteria

1. Age ≥18 y
2. Clinical diagnosis of ischemic stroke causing disabling neurologic deficit
3. Onset of stroke symptoms well established to be <4.5 h before treatment would begin

t-PA Exclusion Criteria

1. Intracranial hemorrhage on noncontrast head CT
2. Serious head trauma within 3 mo
3. Active bleeding, or suspected underlying coagulopathy including thrombocytopenia (<100), INR >1.7, therapeutic anticoagulation (verify with coagulation testing)[a]
4. Sustained SBP >185 or DBP >110 at the time of treatment
5. Nondisabling or rapidly improving symptoms
6. Symptoms suggest subarachnoid hemorrhage despite negative CT scan
7. Infective endocarditis suspected as cause of stroke
8. For 3–4.5 h window, severe stroke (NIHSS >25)

Relative Exclusion Criteria

Balance potential benefit of t-PA in reducing long-term disability with risk of hemorrhagic complications. Consultation with a stroke team and other subspecialists is advised.

1. Major surgery or serious trauma within 30 d
2. Intracranial or spinal surgery within 3 mo
3. Serum glucose <50 mg/dL or >400 mg/dL (reassess after treatment for blood sugar)
4. Stroke within past 3 mo
5. History of intracranial hemorrhage
6. GI/GU hemorrhage within 21 d, or known structural GI malignancy at risk of bleeding
7. Primary or metastatic intracranial, intra-axial neoplasm
8. Seizure at onset (with deficits thought related to postictal paresis)
9. Recent arterial puncture at a noncompressible site
10. Large (>10 mm) unsecured intracranial aneurysm
11. Intracranial arteriovenous malformation
12. Extensive regions of clear hypoattenuation on CT (large subacute stroke)

DBP, diastolic blood pressure; GI, gastrointestinal; GU, genitourinary; INR, international normalized ratio; NIHSS, National Institutes of Health Stroke Scale; SBP, systolic blood pressure; t-PA, tissue plasminogen activator.

[a]Because time is critical, thrombolytic therapy should not be delayed while waiting for the results of the PT, PTT, or platelet count unless a bleeding abnormality or thrombocytopenia is suspected; the patient has been taking warfarin, heparin, dabigatran, rivaroxaban, or apixaban; or anticoagulation use is uncertain.

The current American Heart Association/American Stroke Association Guidelines can be found at: Powers WJ, Rabinstein AA, Ackerson T, et al. 2018 Guidelines for the Early Management of Patients With Acute Ischemic Stroke: A Guideline for Healthcare Professionals From the American Heart Association/American Stroke Association. *Stroke.* 2018;49(3):e46-e110.[22]

TABLE 27-7	Inclusion and Exclusion Criteria for Endovascular Thrombectomy (Washington University Stroke Center Protocol)

Endovascular Thrombectomy Inclusion Criteria

1. Age ≥18 y
2. Clinical diagnosis of ischemic stroke causing disabling neurologic deficit
   a. NIHSS ≥6 if <16 h from time last seen well
   b. NIHSS ≥10 if 16–24 h from time last seen well
3. Ability to initiate thrombectomy in appropriate time window (24 h based on current trials)
4. For posterior circulation strokes (e.g., basilar thrombus), time window is at the discretion of the stroke and neurointerventional attending physicians

Imaging Inclusion Criteria

1. Noncontrast head CT: absence of intracranial hemorrhage/mass/mass effect
2. Noncontrast head CT/MRI: absence of evidence of large, completed infarct
3. CT/MR angiography: large vessel occlusion, e.g., ICA, MCA (M1/M2), vertebral or basilar artery
4. CT perfusion within 6–16 h[a]: core infarct volume ≤70 mL, core–penumbra mismatch volume ≥15 mL, core–penumbra mismatch ratio ≥1.8
5. CT perfusion within 16–24 h[b]: core infarct volume ≤30ml (if age <80 y), core infarct volume ≤20 mL (if age ≥80 y)

Endovascular Thrombectomy Exclusion Criteria

1. Premorbid disability (mRS ≥2) or comorbidities that affect recovery potential
2. Intracranial hemorrhage, mass, or mass effect as cause of stroke symptoms
3. Current severe uncontrolled hypertension, SBP >185 or DBP >110, despite reasonable treatment
4. Active bleeding, or suspected underlying coagulopathy including thrombocytopenia (<30), INR >3, therapeutic anticoagulation (verify with coagulation testing)

DBP, diastolic blood pressure; INR, international normalized ratio; mRS, modified Rankin Scale; NIHSS, National Institutes of Health Stroke Scale; SBP, systolic blood pressure.
[a]Based on the results of the DEFUSE 3 trial.[23]
[b]Based on the result of the DAWN trial.[24]

- Nimodipine, a calcium channel blocker, improves outcome in SAH patients and may reduce the incidence of associated cerebral infarction with few side effects. However, the mechanism by which nimodipine offers neuroprotection remains unclear (i.e., no evidence that it prevents vasospasm).
- Anticoagulation with heparin/LMWH followed by warfarin is indicated for venous sinus thrombosis both with and without hemorrhagic infarcts. Trials of DOACs for this indication are ongoing. Boluses of heparin to correct the activated PTT (aPTT) should be avoided in the setting of hemorrhage. aPTTs should be closely monitored and maintained between 60 and 80 seconds.

Nonpharmacologic Therapies

- Published trials have demonstrated a clear benefit to endovascular thrombectomy in select patients with acute ischemic stroke. This may be combined with IV t-PA.
- CTA and CT perfusion scans may be used to select patients who will benefit from thrombectomy up to 24 hours after the time they were last known well.[24]

- These studies represent the first major breakthrough in acute ischemic stroke therapy since the introduction of IV t-PA in 1996.
- Physical, occupational, and speech therapy are extremely important in stroke rehabilitation and have a clear beneficial impact on poststroke outcomes.
- Stroke patients with obvious dysphagia, dysarthria, or a facial droop should be kept nothing by mouth until an experienced individual can assess their swallowing abilities.

Surgical Management

- CEA decreases the risk of stroke and death in patients with recent TIAs or nondisabling strokes and ipsilateral high-grade (70%–99%) carotid stenosis.[25]
  - The CREST (Carotid Revascularization Endarterectomy vs. Stenting) trial provides evidence to suggest that carotid stenting is of equal efficacy to CEA but carries a higher periprocedural stroke risk.[26]
  - Neurology and surgery recommendations should be sought before deciding between the two approaches.
- CEA for asymptomatic high-grade carotid stenosis (≥60%) reduces the 5-year risk of ipsilateral stroke in men, provided that the operator's surgical/angiography complication rate is <3%.[27,28]
- See the earlier section on Other Nonpharmacologic Therapies for information on endovascular therapies in acute ischemic stroke.
- Hemicraniectomy increases survival and can improve functional outcomes in select patients with large hemispheric infarcts and severe edema (e.g., "malignant" middle cerebral artery infarcts). Neurosurgical consultation should be obtained early in these cases.
- Cerebellar infarction or hematomas may result in brainstem compression or obstructive hydrocephalus and may also warrant urgent neurosurgical intervention.

Lifestyle/Risk Modification

Modifiable risk factors (Table 27-8) include the following:
- BP reduction even in normotensive stroke patients is beneficial.[29]
- Diabetes control is important with care taken to avoid hypoglycemia and hyperglycemia.
- Smoking cessation.
- Patients younger than 75 years with no concerns for safety of statin therapy should be placed on "high-intensity" statin therapy (e.g., atorvastatin 40–80 mg or rosuvastatin 20–40 mg), whereas patients older than 75 years or patients for whom there is

TABLE 27-8	Secondary Stroke Prevention ("BLASTED")

- **B**lood pressure
- **L**DL
- **A**SA (**a**ntiplatelet), **A**1C
- **S**troke management and rehabilitation team (varies from facility to facility)
  - PT, OT, ST, stroke educator, smoking cessation counseling
- **T**elemetry: cardiac rhythm monitoring
- **E**chocardiography
- **D**oppler for carotid stenosis, **d**iabetes (A1C, diabetes educator, etc.)

ASA, acetylsalicylic acid; LDL, low-density lipoprotein; OT, occupational therapy; PT, physical therapy; ST, speech therapy.

concern for safety of statin therapy should be placed on "moderate-intensity" statin therapy (e.g., atorvastatin 10–20 mg, rosuvastatin 5–10 mg, simvastatin 20–40 mg, pravastatin 40–80 mg).[30]
- Identify and treat obstructive sleep apnea.
- Oral contraceptives or hormonal therapies may need to be discontinued in women with stroke.

COMPLICATIONS

- Cerebral edema following ischemic stroke peaks at 48–96 hours after stroke, and patients need to be watched closely during this time.
- Hemorrhagic conversion of an ischemic stroke is more likely in patients who are receiving anticoagulation or in patients with large strokes, particularly those with embolic ischemic infarcts.

Headache

GENERAL PRINCIPLES

Classification

- **Primary headache syndromes** include migraines with or without aura, the hemicranias and indomethacin-responsive headaches, tension headaches, chronic daily headaches, and cluster headaches.
- **Secondary headaches** have specific etiologies, and symptomatic features vary depending on the underlying pathology (e.g., SAH, tumor, hypertension, posterior reversible encephalopathy syndrome, reversible cerebral vasoconstriction syndrome (RCVS), analgesic overuse, iatrogenic).
- **Migraine without aura:** At least five attacks that last 4–72 hours. Symptoms should include at least two of the following: unilateral location, pulsating or throbbing, moderate to severe in intensity, aggravated by activity, and at least one of these associated features: nausea/vomiting, photophobia, and/or phonophobia.
- **Migraine with aura:** Same as above, except at least two attacks with an associated aura that lasts from 4 minutes to 1 hour (longer than 60 minutes is a red flag). The aura should have a gradual onset, should be fully reversible, and can occur before, with, or after headache onset.
- **Cluster headache:** Unilateral orbital or temporal pain with lacrimation, conjunctival injection, nasal congestion, rhinorrhea, facial swelling, miosis, ptosis, and eyelid edema.
- **Rebound headache** (medication overuse headache) occurs in the setting of chronic use of analgesics or narcotics.
- **Trigeminal neuralgia** presents as episodic sharp stabbing pain that is unilateral. Rule out MS or an alternative etiology with MRI.
- **Temporal arteritis** presents as a dull unilateral headache with a thick tortuous artery over temporal region. The disease is almost exclusively limited to individuals older than 60 years with jaw claudication, low-grade fever, and an elevated ESR and CRP.

Etiology

Secondary headache etiologies include:
- Subdural hematoma (SDH), intracerebral hemorrhage, SAH, AVM, brain abscess, meningitis, encephalitis, vasculitis, obstructive hydrocephalus, and cerebral ischemia or infarction.

CHAPTER 27

- Idiopathic intracranial hypertension (commonly known as pseudotumor cerebri) presents with headache, papilledema, diplopia, and elevated CSF pressure (at least >20 cm H_2O in relaxed lateral decubitus position). CVST should be ruled out in all patients presenting with suspected idiopathic intracranial hypertension.
- Extracranial causes include giant cell arteritis, sinusitis, glaucoma, optic neuritis, dental disease (including temporomandibular joint syndrome), and disorders of the cervical spine (i.e., "cervicogenic" headache).
- Systemic causes include fever, viremia, hypoxia, carbon monoxide poisoning, hypercapnia, systemic hypertension, allergy, anemia, caffeine withdrawal, and vasoactive or toxic chemicals (e.g., nitrites).
- Depression is a common cause of long-standing, treatment-resistant headaches. Specific inquiry about vegetative signs of depression and exclusion of other causes help support this diagnosis.

DIAGNOSIS

Clinical Presentation
History
- The sudden onset of severe headache ("**the worst headache of my life**," also known as a "thunderclap headache") or a severe persistent headache that reaches maximal intensity within a few seconds/minutes warrants immediate investigation for possible SAH.
- Other headache syndromes that can present with a thunderclap headache include RCVS, posterior cerebral artery infarcts, CVST, arterial dissections, CNS vasculitis, pituitary apoplexy, intracerebral hemorrhage, and some of the indomethacin-responsive headache syndromes.
- History should focus on:
  ○ Age at onset
  ○ Frequency, intensity, and duration of attacks
  ○ Triggers, associations (menstrual cycle), associated symptoms (e.g., photophobia, phonophobia, nausea, vomiting), and alleviating factors
  ○ Location and quality of pain (e.g., sharp, dull)
  ○ Number of headaches per month, including number of disabling headaches
  ○ Family history of migraines
  ○ Sleep and diet hygiene (caffeine intake)
  ○ Use of pain medications, including over-the-counter medications.

Physical Examination
- On general examination, check BP and pulse, listen for possible bruits, palpate head and neck muscles, and check temporal arteries.
- If neck stiffness and meningismus (resistance to passive neck flexion) are present on examination, then consider meningitis.
- If papilledema is observed on examination, then consider an intracranial mass, meningitis, CVST, or idiopathic intracranial hypertension.

Diagnostic Testing
Imaging
Neuroimaging is generally not indicated for known primary headache syndromes but may be required to exclude secondary etiologies (listed earlier) in cases that have not been previously diagnosed or in patients presenting with new headaches, especially those who present with atypical features or abnormal examination findings.

Diagnostic Procedures

LP is indicated in a patient with severe headache with suspicion of SAH even if the head CT scan is negative. However, head CT is over 99% sensitive for detecting SAH if obtained within 6 hours of headache onset.

TREATMENT

- **Acute treatment of migraine,** the most common primary headache syndrome, is directed at aborting the headache. This is easier at onset and often very difficult when the attack is well established. Accordingly, the threshold for treating at the first sign of a headache should be low. Patients have often used nonprescription analgesics (acetylsalicylic acid [ASA], acetaminophen, NSAIDs) and oral prescription medications (butalbital with aspirin or acetaminophen), which are the first-line treatments and are most effective early in the course of an attack. Emergent treatments include serotonin agonists and other parenteral medications.
- Scheduled IV NSAIDs (e.g., ketorolac) in combination with antiemetics (typically prochlorperazine) and IV fluids are an effective first-line regimen in many cases.
- Antidopaminergic therapies including haloperidol and droperidol are also effective first-line therapies. A baseline ECG should be obtained to evaluate for a prolonged QTc.
- **Triptans** (serotonin receptor $5HT_{1B}$ and $5HT_{1D}$ agonists) are effective abortive medications available in multiple formulations and may be effective even in a protracted attack. Triptans should not be used in patients with coronary artery disease, cerebrovascular disease, uncontrolled hypertension, hemiplegic migraine, or vertebrobasilar migraine.
- **Dihydroergotamine** is a potent venoconstrictor with minimal peripheral arterial constriction. Cardiac precautions and a baseline ECG are indicated in all patients. This medication is contraindicated when there is a history of angina, myocardial infarction, or peripheral vascular disease. Alternative therapies should also be considered in elderly patients.
- **Ergotamine** is a vasoconstrictive agent effective for aborting migraine headaches, particularly if administered during the prodromal phase. Ergotamine should be taken at symptom onset in the maximum dose tolerated by the patient; nausea often limits the dose. Rectal preparations are better absorbed than oral agents. This medication is also contraindicated in patients with a history of angina, myocardial infarction, or peripheral vascular disease.
- Additional abortive therapies with less evidence supporting their use include IV valproic acid, IV/PO methylprednisolone, IM ziprasidone, and IV magnesium.
- Chronic daily headaches should not be treated with narcotic analgesics so as to prevent addiction, rebound headaches, and tachyphylaxis.
- Treatment of secondary headaches is directed at the primary etiology, such as surgical treatment of cerebral aneurysm causing SAH, evacuation of SDH, calcium channel blockers in RCVS, or shunting in obstructive hydrocephalus.
- **Prophylactic medications** should be considered if a patient has at least three disabling migraines per month.
  - It is important to review a patient's use of all medications and comorbidities because they may influence choice of medication and offer additional factors contributing to the headache syndrome.
  - Possible prophylactic medications include propranolol, topiramate, tricyclic antidepressants (TCAs) (amitriptyline, nortriptyline), and now, less commonly,

valproic acid. Second-line agents include verapamil, selective serotonin reuptake inhibitors (SSRIs), and serotonin-norepinephrine reuptake inhibitors. Weaker evidence exists for other AEDs and for calcium channel blockers.
  ○ Alternative (nonprescription) therapies for migraine prophylaxis include butterbur, riboflavin, magnesium, and acupuncture.
  ○ Botulinum toxin (onabotulinum toxin A) and anticalcitonin gene-related peptide therapies are approved for migraine prophylaxis in adult patients with chronic migraine (defined as ≥15 headache days per month for >3 months).

Lifestyle Modifications
• Patients should keep a headache diary to identify possible triggers.
• Patients should reduce alcohol, caffeine, and other triggers that may increase risk of migraines.

REFERRAL

Neurosurgical consultation is indicated for managing SAH, SDH, vascular malformations, tumors, and other space-occupying lesions resulting in mass effect. Neurologic consultation is indicated if a patient is not well controlled on a first-line prophylactic agent with appropriate use of an abortive therapy.

Head Trauma

GENERAL PRINCIPLES

Definition
• **Traumatic brain injury (TBI)** can occur with head injury due to contact and/or acceleration/deceleration forces.
• **Concussion:** Trauma-induced alteration in mental status with normal radiographic studies that may or may not involve loss of consciousness.
• **Contusion:** Trauma-induced lesion consisting of punctate hemorrhages and surrounding edema.

Classification
• Closed head injuries may produce diffuse axonal injury.
• Contusion or hemorrhage can occur at the site of initial impact, "coup injury," or opposite to the side of impact, "countercoup injury."
• Penetrating injuries (including depressed skull fracture) or foreign objects cause brain injury directly.
• Secondary increases in intracranial pressure may compromise cerebral perfusion.

Epidemiology
• Head injury is the most common cause of neurologic illness in young people.
• The overall incidence of TBI in the US population is estimated at approximately 750 per 100,000 (i.e., approximately 2.5 million per year with approximately 11% requiring hospitalization).[31]
• Two-thirds of TBIs are considered "mild," whereas 20% are severe and 10% are fatal. Note that although designated as "mild," mild TBI can still translate into significant disability (permanent in 15%).
• Rates of TBI are highest in the very young, adolescents, and the elderly.

DIAGNOSIS

Clinical Presentation

- Patients will often present with confusion and amnesia, including loss of memory for the traumatic event as well as inability to recall events both immediately before and after trauma.
- Patients may complain of nonspecific signs including headache, vertigo, nausea, vomiting, and personality changes.
- Intracerebral hematomas may be present initially or develop after a contusion.
- Epidural hematoma is usually associated with skull fractures across a meningeal artery and may cause precipitous deterioration after a **lucid interval.**
- SDH is most common in aged, debilitated alcoholics and/or in anticoagulated patients. Antecedent trauma may be minimal or absent.

Physical Examination
- Careful examination for penetrating wounds and other injuries.
- Hemotympanum, mastoid ecchymosis (Battle sign), periorbital ecchymosis ("raccoon eyes"), and CSF otorrhea/rhinorrhea are indicative of a basilar skull fracture.
- Neurologic examination should focus on the level of consciousness, focal deficits, and signs of herniation. The GCS should be used for an assessment. Serial examinations must be performed and documented to identify neurologic deterioration.
- Degree of impairment due to trauma can be classified using injury severity scores, with GCS being the most common.
- Treatment and diagnostic assessment of patients with severe head injury at admission are done according to the Advanced Trauma Life Support protocol.
- The Standardized Assessment of Concussion is a standardized tool for the sideline evaluation of athletes who suffer a head injury.

Diagnostic Testing

- Head CT should be considered for patients with GCS <15 2 hours after trauma, suspected skull fracture, repeated episodes of vomiting after trauma, age greater than 65 years, dangerous mechanism (e.g., pedestrian struck by motor vehicle, occupant ejected from motor vehicle, fall from ≥3 feet or ≥5 stairs), drug or alcohol intoxication, or persistent anterograde amnesia.
- Noncontrast head CT scan in the emergency room can rapidly identify intracranial hemorrhage and contusion.
  - A lenticular-shaped extra-axial hematoma is characteristic of epidural hematoma.
  - Bone window views may help to locate fractures, if present.
- Cervical radiographs with or without CT of the neck must be performed to exclude fracture or dislocation.
- MRI can assist in evaluation of TBI patients with persistent sequelae because it is more sensitive for demonstrating small areas of contusion or petechial hemorrhage, axonal injury, and small extra-axial hematomas.

TREATMENT

- Hospital admission is recommended for patients at risk for immediate complications from head injury. These include patients with GCS <15, abnormal CT scan, intracranial bleeding, cerebral edema, seizures, or abnormal bleeding parameters.
- When admitted, continuously monitor vital signs and oximetry. ECG should be performed. Arterial pressure monitoring in conjunction with intracranial monitoring may be indicated.

- Immobilize the neck in a hard cervical collar to avoid spinal cord injury from manipulating an unstable or fractured cervical spine.
- **Avoid hypotonic fluids** to limit cerebral edema.
- Steroids are not indicated for head injury.
- Avoid hypoventilation and systemic hypotension because they may reduce cerebral perfusion.
- Anticipate and conservatively treat increased intracranial pressure:
  - Head midline and elevated 30 degrees.
  - In the mechanically ventilated patient, modest hyperventilation (i.e., PCO_2 approximately 35 mm Hg) reduces intracranial pressure by cerebral vasoconstriction; excessive hyperventilation may reduce cerebral perfusion. Remember that these are merely temporizing measures and neurosurgical consultation is always warranted if there is concern for increased intracranial pressure due to head injury.
- Neurologic deterioration after head injury of any severity requires an immediate repeat head CT scan to differentiate an expanding hematoma that necessitates surgery from diffuse cerebral edema that requires monitoring and reduction of intracranial pressure.
- The use of AEDs in the acute management of TBI can reduce the incidence of early seizures but does not prevent development of epilepsy at a later time. Furthermore, certain AEDs can have adverse effects on cognition, and so these agents should only be used when clinically indicated, with careful consideration of the specific agent chosen. There is no evidence to support AED use for seizure prophylaxis.
- Because a second injury, referred to as the "second impact syndrome," may lead to severe complications including death, guidelines have been proposed for when individuals can return to play.[31]

Surgical Management
- Neurosurgical consultation is indicated for patients with contusion, intracranial hematoma, cervical fracture, skull fractures, penetrating injuries, or focal neurologic deficits.
- In cases of closed head injury complicated by increased intracranial pressure, intracranial pressure monitoring assists medical management.
- Evacuation of chronic SDH is determined by the symptoms and degree of mass effect.

Acute Spinal Cord Dysfunction

GENERAL PRINCIPLES

- Spinal cord dysfunction is demonstrated by a level below which motor, sensory, and autonomic functions are interrupted.
- **Traumatic spinal cord injury** (TSCI) may be obvious from history or examination but should also be considered in unconscious, confused, or inebriated patients with trauma or found down.
- **Spinal cord concussion** refers to posttraumatic spinal cord symptoms and signs that resolve rapidly (hours to days).

Etiology
See Table 27-9.

TABLE 27-9	Causes of Acute Spinal Cord Dysfunction

Structural
- Tumor (primary or metastatic)
- Herniated disk
- Epidural abscess or hematoma
- Osteomyelitis
- Trauma ± fracture of bony elements
- Atlantoaxial instability (e.g., rheumatoid arthritis)
- Fibrocartilaginous

Ischemia/infarction (particularly after aortic surgery)
- Aortic dissection or surgery
- Embolic (cardiogenic, gaseous embolus)
- Prolonged hypotension with underlying vascular disease
- Intravascular lymphoma

Toxic
- Nitrous oxide (typically in the setting of vitamin B_{12} deficiency)
- Heroin

Vascular malformations (e.g., AVM)

Inflammatory/infectious (transverse myelitis)
- Multiple sclerosis
- Neuromyelitis optica (classically longitudinally extensive, >three spinal segments)
- Anti–myelin oligodendrocyte protein disease
- Acute disseminated encephalomyelitis
- Parainfectious processes (e.g., after *Mycoplasma pneumoniae*)
- Sarcoidosis
- Paraneoplastic (amphiphysin and CRMP-5)
- Systemic lupus erythematosus
- Sjögren syndrome
- Behçet disease
- Viruses (e.g., enterovirus, HSV, HIV, VZV, CMV, WNV)
- Fungal (extremely rare)
- Lyme disease
- TB
- Syphilis

AVM, arteriovenous malformation; CMV, cytomegalovirus; CRMP-5, collapsin response mediator protein 5; HSV, herpes simplex virus; VZV, varicella-zoster virus; WNV, West Nile virus.

DIAGNOSIS

Clinical Presentation

- **Spinal cord compression** often presents with back pain at the level of compression, progressive walking difficulties, sensory impairment, urinary retention with overflow incontinence, and diminished rectal tone. Rapid deterioration may occur.
- Spinal shock with hypotonia and areflexia may be present soon after a traumatic event.
- **Transverse myelitis or myelopathy** can present with symptoms and signs similar to cord compression.

- Acute presentations suggest traumatic or vascular insults, whereas a subacute course suggests an enlarging mass lesion or infectious process. Autoimmune/inflammatory disorders can present in both ways.
- **Radicular signs** (lancinating pain, paresthesias, and numbness in the dermatomal distribution of a nerve root, with weakness and decreased tone and reflexes in muscles supplied by the root) suggest concurrent inflammation or compression of the corresponding nerve root. Tenderness to spinal percussion over the lesion may be present.
- **Spinal cord syndromes**
  - **Complete cord syndrome:** Bilateral flaccid paralysis (quadriplegia or paraplegia) and loss of all sensation (anesthesia) below a dermatomal level, initially with areflexia and sphincter dysfunction (urinary retention/loss of rectal tone). With time, patients develop spasticity and hyperreflexia caudal to the lesion with possible lower motor neuron signs (areflexia and flaccid paralysis) at the level of the lesion and extensor plantar responses (Babinski signs).
  - **Brown–Séquard syndrome:** Unilateral cord lesion resulting in contralateral pain and temperature loss, with ipsilateral weakness and proprioceptive loss.
  - **Anterior cord syndrome** often results from anterior spinal artery lesions and produces bilateral pain and temperature loss and weakness below the site of the lesion with preserved proprioception and vibratory sensation.
  - **Cauda equina syndrome** from compression of the lower lumbar and sacral roots produces sensory loss in a saddle distribution, asymmetric flaccid leg weakness, decreased reflexes, and urinary/bowel incontinence due to an areflexic bladder and loss of rectal tone.
  - **Conus medullaris syndrome** has similar features to cauda equina syndrome with one important difference being the presence of mixed upper and lower motor neuron signs due to involvement of the caudal spinal cord.
  - **Central cord syndrome** is often characterized by motor impairment in upper extremities more than lower extremities, bladder dysfunction, and variable degree of sensory loss at the site of the lesion. Trauma is a common cause.

Diagnostic Testing

Imaging
- The presence and extent of spinal cord injuries should be confirmed with neuroimaging.
- Plain radiographs of the spine may reveal metastatic disease, osteomyelitis, discitis, fractures, or dislocation.
- Emergent MRI scan of the entire cord can confirm the exact level and extent of the lesion(s). CT myelography may be necessary in individuals unable to undergo MRI.
- CT of the spine is not sufficient to "rule out" spinal cord compression.
- CT of the spine with and without contrast can also be used to evaluate for epidural abscess, osteomyelitis, and/or discitis in patients unable to undergo MRI.

Diagnostic Procedures
Inflammatory and infectious etiologies often require an LP with CSF analysis for pleocytosis, malignant cells, abnormal protein/glucose, oligoclonal bands, and IgG index; if indicated, tests for specific pathogens and cytology/flow cytometry can be considered. If possible, imaging should be performed prior to performing an LP to rule out abscess, tumor, or other structural contraindication to LP. Remember to always check an opening pressure when possible and save CSF for additional studies that may be deemed indicated once additional clinical data have been gathered.

TREATMENT

- Vital signs should be continuously monitored, and adequate oxygenation and perfusion should be ensured.
- Respiratory insufficiency from high cervical cord injuries requires immediate airway control and ventilatory assistance, without manipulation of the neck.
- Immobilization, especially of the neck, is essential to prevent further injury while the patient's condition is stabilized and radiographic and neurosurgical assessment of the injuries is performed.
- Autonomic dysfunction is common and can lead to fluctuating vital signs and BP. Bladder distension can cause sympathetic overactivity (headache, tachycardia, diaphoresis, and hypertension) as a result of autonomic dysreflexia.
  - Management of autonomic dysreflexia should incorporate the help of a spinal cord rehabilitation specialist. These patients require strict attention to bowel and bladder functions (e.g., manual disimpaction, promotility agents, straight catheterization) as a means to prevent an autonomic crisis.
  - Do not treat fluctuations in vital signs blindly because changes can occur precipitously with potential for iatrogenic injury. Always look first for a cause and treat fluctuations in heart rate or BP with caution.

Medications

- Treatable infections require appropriate antimicrobial therapies (e.g., acyclovir for varicella-zoster myelitis).
- **Dexamethasone**, 10–20 mg IV bolus followed by 2–4 mg IV q6–8h, is often administered for compressive lesions, tumors, or spinal cord infarction, although benefit has not been proven for all etiologies.
- For TSCI, **methylprednisolone**, 30 mg/kg IV bolus, followed by an infusion of 5.4 mg/kg/h for 24 hours when initiated within 3 hours of injury, and infusion for 48 hours when initiated within 3–8 hours of injury, may improve neurologic recovery.
- Pharmacologic deep venous thrombosis prophylaxis is extremely important. LMWH is superior to unfractionated heparin for prevention of venous thromboembolism and pulmonary embolism.

Surgical Management

Neurosurgical consultation should be obtained because in many cases, spinal cord compression can be decompressed and stabilized. Penetrating injury, foreign bodies, comminuted fractures, misalignment, and hematoma may require surgical treatment.

SPECIAL CONSIDERATIONS

Emergent radiation therapy combined with high-dose steroids is usually indicated for cord compression due to malignancy and generally requires a histologic diagnosis.

MONITORING/FOLLOW-UP

Long-term supportive care is important for patients with spinal cord dysfunction. Pulmonary and urinary infections, skin breakdown, joint contractures, spasticity, and irregular bowel and bladder elimination are common long-term problems.

Parkinson Disease

GENERAL PRINCIPLES

- Parkinson disease (PD) is a chronic, progressive neurodegenerative disease characterized by at least two of three cardinal features: resting tremor, bradykinesia, and rigidity. Often, postural instability is seen later in the disease.
- The neurologic examination remains the gold standard diagnostic test for PD.
- Cognitive dysfunction and dementia are common in PD (one-third of patients in most studies; six times higher than age-matched controls). Considerable overlap can occur between AD and PD.
  - One-third of PD patients are depressed.
  - Olfactory dysfunction, autonomic dysfunction, and sleep disorders are also common in PD and have a significant impact on quality of life.

Epidemiology
Approximately 1 million people in the US have been diagnosed with PD. Usually, the age at diagnosis is older than 50 years. Approximately 1% of the population older than 50 years has the disorder.

DIAGNOSIS

Clinical Presentation
- The parkinsonian tremor is a resting pill rolling tremor (3–7 Hz) that is often asymmetric.[32]
- Bradykinesia is characterized by generalized slowness of movement, especially in finger movement dexterity and gait (often shuffling).
- Cogwheel rigidity is often observed with a ratchety pattern of resistance and relaxation as examiner moves limbs ("cog wheeling" is due to the rigidity with a superimposed tremor).
- Postural instability can be assessed by the "pull" test, where the examiner pulls the patient by the shoulders while standing behind the patient, assessing the patient's ability to recover.
- Other signs that are often associated but not required for diagnosis include masked-like facies, decreased eye blink, increased salivation, hypokinetic dysarthria, micrographia, and sleep disorders, particularly rapid eye movement (REM) sleep behavior disorder.
- Dementia seen with PD is typically subcortical with psychomotor retardation, memory difficulty, and altered personality.

Differential Diagnosis
See Table 27-10.

Diagnostic Testing
MRI of the brain (or head CT with contrast in patients unable to undergo MRI) should be performed to exclude specific structural abnormalities.

TREATMENT

Medications
- **PD patients should not be given neuroleptics or any dopamine-blocking medications under any circumstances** (e.g., prochlorperazine, metoclopramide)

TABLE 27-10	Differential Diagnosis of Parkinson Disease

- Essential tremor
  - Action tremor
- Dementia with Lewy bodies
  - Visual hallucinations, fluctuating cognition, sensitivity to neuroleptics
- Corticobasal degeneration
- Multiple system atrophy
- Progressive supranuclear palsy
- Alzheimer disease
- Frontotemporal dementia
  - Changes in personality
- Huntington disease
- Wilson disease and other neurodegenerative disorders with metal accumulation
- Toxic/iatrogenic
  - Carbon monoxide, manganese, neuroleptics, other dopamine receptor antagonists

because this can have devastating consequences ranging from worsening PD symptoms to death.[33] If a neuroleptic is absolutely necessary, quetiapine and clozapine are the safest, but the risk/benefit profile needs to be considered. Pimavanserin has also been approved specifically for PD psychosis.
- Treatment of PD can be divided into neuroprotective and symptomatic therapy.
- Initiation of symptomatic treatment for a PD patient is determined by the degree to which the patient is functionally impaired.

First Line
- Carbidopa–levodopa (Sinemet, CD–LD) is the most effective symptomatic therapy for PD and is often considered when both the patient and the physician decide that quality of life of the patient is being affected by PD.
- Dopamine agonists (i.e., pramipexole, ropinirole) can be used as monotherapy or in combination with other PD medications. They are ineffective in patients who show no response to levodopa. They are often used in patients who develop significant dyskinesias or motor fluctuations on CD–LD, but these drugs are less efficacious and have more adverse effects.
- Many patients can be managed with CD–LD alone without the need for agonist therapy.

Second Line
- Amantadine and catechol-*O*-methyl transferase inhibitors can help supplement the effects of dopamine replacement therapy and are beneficial with regard to the dyskinesias and fluctuations, respectively, commonly experienced by patients.
- Anticholinergic drugs are used only in younger patients in whom tremor is the predominant symptom.

Third Line
Deep brain stimulation and Duodopa (intestinal infusion of carbidopa/levodopa gel) have benefit in PD patients who progress to develop motor fluctuations and dyskinesias unresponsive to oral medications. It is important to note that advanced therapies are not a cure for PD and patients will continue to progress.

CHAPTER 27

COMPLICATIONS

- Patients can develop neuroleptic malignant syndrome (NMS) after sudden withdrawal of levodopa or dopamine agonists and following exposure to neuroleptics or other antidopaminergic drugs.
- Serotonin syndrome can occur when monoamine oxidase inhibitors (MAOIs) are combined with TCAs or SSRIs.

NEUROMUSCULAR DISEASE

Guillain–Barré Syndrome

GENERAL PRINCIPLES

Definition

Guillain–Barré syndrome (GBS) is an acute polyradiculoneuropathy syndrome and a common cause of acute flaccid paralysis. There are many GBS subtypes with marked geographic variability in their prevalence. The clinical syndrome is classically characterized by back pain, ascending weakness, distal paresthesias, and areflexia. Classically, GBS follows a viral infection, vaccination, or surgery, but in many instances, no prodrome is identified.

Classification

- The acute immune/inflammatory demyelinating polyneuropathy (AIDP) variant is the most common GBS variant in North America. It is an acute immune-mediated polyneuropathy/radiculopathy with presumed autoantibodies (as yet unidentified) directed against myelin antigens.
- Axonal variants of GBS include acute motor axonal neuropathy (AMAN), acute motor and sensory axonal neuropathy, acute motor conduction block neuropathy (AMCBN), Miller Fisher syndrome (MFS), and pharyngeal–cervical–brachial (PCB) weakness. Many of these syndromes are associated with antiganglioside antibodies directed against gangliosides located in the axolemma near the nodes of Ranvier. These axonal variants are much more common in Japan, China, and third-world countries than they are in the US. Antibody associations include:
  - IgG anti-GM1 antibodies in AMAN and AMCBN
  - IgG anti-GQ1b and less commonly IgG anti-GT1a in MFS, a syndrome consisting of ophthalmoparesis, ataxia, and areflexia
  - IgG anti-GT1a and less commonly IgG anti-GQ1b in PCB weakness syndrome.

Pathophysiology

- GBS results from an attack of peripheral myelin or axons mediated by autoantibodies originally generated in response to an infection that typically precedes the onset of neuropathy symptoms by days to weeks. These antibodies cross-react with the myelin or nodal axolemma antigens via molecular mimicry.
- This concept is well established in the axonal variants where there is definitive evidence of molecular mimicry between *Campylobacter jejuni* lipooligosaccharides and the ganglioside antigens listed above.
- This concept is less well established in other AIDP variants, given the absence of a known autoantibody/myelin antigen. Prodromal infections commonly associated with AIDP include cytomegalovirus and Epstein–Barr virus.

DIAGNOSIS

Clinical Presentation

- AIDP typically presents with progressive, symmetric ascending paralysis.
- Mild asymmetries are common, but major asymmetries are a red flag suggestive of an alternative diagnosis.
- Reflexes are almost always hypoactive or absent. Exceptions exist, especially with the axonal variants (in particular with Fisher–Bickerstaff syndrome, which has elements of MFS along with hypersomnolence in the setting of concurrent brainstem encephalitis).
- Sensory symptoms, such as paresthesias in the hands and feet, are often present, but objective sensory loss is uncommon.
- Facial and/or oropharyngeal weakness occurs in about 70% of AIDP patients.
- Respiratory failure, necessitating intubation, occurs in 25%–30% of patients.[34]
- Pain in the back, hips, and thighs is common. Pain is one of the most common presenting symptoms of GBS in the pediatric population.
- Autonomic instability is common (approximately 60%) and potentially life threatening. Common manifestations include tachycardia/bradycardia, hypotension alternating with hypertension, and ileus.

Differential Diagnosis

See Table 27-11.

Diagnostic Testing

Imaging

MRI of the spine is indicated in atypical cases or in those with concern for one of the differentials listed earlier that could result in a myeloradiculopathy. Nerve root contrast enhancement and/or thickening can be seen with GBS.

Diagnostic Procedures

- **LP should be performed to narrow the differential and evaluate for albumino-cytologic dissociation.**
- CSF protein is usually elevated about 1 week after symptom onset. It may be normal if checked earlier (e.g., 85% of patients with normal CSF within first 2 days).
- CSF leukocytosis is uncommon, and if present (especially >25 cells/μL), an alternative diagnosis should be considered.
- Nerve conduction studies (NCS) and electromyography (EMG) are a very important part of the evaluation but should not delay initiation of treatment, particularly in severe cases. NCS should include evaluation of the proximal nerve segments via "late" responses (F waves and H reflexes). EMG–NCS performed early in the disease course may have very few abnormalities and can even be normal but serves an important role in the diagnostic evaluation, even when normal. A repeat study after a few weeks can be extremely useful for classification and prognostication, particularly when there is a baseline study available for comparison.

TREATMENT

- Follow **respiratory function closely**, including oximetry and frequent bedside measurements of vital capacity (VC) and negative inspiratory force (NIF).
- We use the "20/30" rule in identifying patients who will likely require ventilatory support: <20 mL/kg of forced VC (FVC) (approximately 1.5 L for an

CHAPTER 27

TABLE 27-11 Differential Diagnosis of Acute Immune Demyelinating Polyneuropathy

- Acute/initial presentation of chronic inflammatory demyelinating polyneuropathy
- Paraproteinemic/paraneoplastic ppolyradiculopathy/polyneuropathy
- Diabetic/nondiabetic lumbosacral radiculoplexopathies
- Sarcoidosis
- Mononeuritis multiplex (confluent)
- West Nile and polioviruses (usually has fever, CSF pleocytosis, and often asymmetric paralysis)
- HIV
- Lyme disease (if in endemic area)
- Postdiphtheric paralysis
- Tick paralysis and other neurotoxins
- Myasthenia gravis (MFS variant)
- Critical illness myopathy
- Prolonged neuromuscular junction blockade
- Periodic paralysis
- Thiamine deficiency (MFS variant in particular)
- Botulism
- Arsenic
- Lead
- Chemotherapy
- Acute intermittent porphyria
- Carcinomatous or lymphomatous meningitis with root involvement
- Functional weakness/conversion disorder

See http://neuromuscular.wustl.edu/time/nmacute.htm for further information. CSF, cerebral spinal fluid; MFS, Miller Fisher syndrome variant of Guillain–Barré Syndrome (associated with ataxia, areflexia, and ophthalmoparesis).

average-size adult) and an NIF >-30 cm H_2O. These parameters provide a more sensitive measure for impending respiratory failure than do the presence of hypoxia, dyspnea, and acidosis. The threshold for elective intubation should be low.
- If NIF/FVC testing is not available at the bedside, a quick and indirect measure is to ask the patient to count to as high a number as possible on one breath. Each number equals 100 mL of VC (e.g., a count to 10 = 1 L).
- Paroxysmal hypertension should not be treated with antihypertensive medications unless absolutely necessary (e.g., signs of end-organ injury or comorbid coronary artery disease). If necessary, extremely low doses of titratable short-acting agents are preferred.
- Hypotension is usually caused by decreased venous return and peripheral vasodilation. Mechanically ventilated patients are particularly prone to hypotension. Treatment consists of intravascular volume expansion; occasionally, vasopressors may be required (see Chapter 8, Critical Care).
- Continuous telemetry monitoring is necessary to monitor for cardiac arrhythmias.

• Prevention of exposure keratitis of the eye, venous thrombosis, and vigilance for hyponatremia, including syndrome of inappropriate diuretic hormone, should be priorities.

Medications

• **Plasma exchange (PLEX) and IVIG** are comparably effective in improving outcomes and shortening duration of disease when administered early to patients who cannot walk or have respiratory failure.[35] The decision between the two depends on the individual patient's comorbidities and medical history.
• **Corticosteroids are not indicated and may actually delay recovery.**
• Neuropathic pain medications may be needed.

Nonpharmacologic Therapies

Physical therapy to prevent contractures and improve strength and function should be started early.

COMPLICATIONS

Complications from prolonged hospitalization and ventilation may occur. These include aspiration pneumonia, sepsis, pressure ulcers, and pulmonary embolism.

PROGNOSIS

• The disease typically progresses over 2–4 weeks, with all patients, by definition, reaching their nadir by 4 weeks, followed by a plateau of several weeks.
• Recovery takes place over months.
  ○ Overall, about 80% of patients recover completely or have only minor deficits.
• About 5% of the patients die due to respiratory or autonomic complications despite optimal medical therapy.

Myasthenia Gravis

GENERAL PRINCIPLES

Definition

Myasthenia gravis (MG) is an autoimmune disorder that involves antibody-mediated postsynaptic dysfunction of the neuromuscular junction of skeletal muscle resulting in fatigable weakness.

Classification

• Generalized disease is most common and affects a variable combination of ocular, bulbar, respiratory, and appendicular muscles.
• Ocular MG is confined to eyelid and oculomotor function. It accounts for 10%–40% of all MG cases.

Epidemiology

Bimodal distribution with peak incidence in women in the second and third decades and in men in the sixth and seventh decades.

Pathophysiology

MG is an acquired autoimmune disorder resulting from the production of autoantibodies against the postsynaptic acetylcholine receptor (AChR) or, less commonly, against receptor-associated proteins, including muscle-specific receptor tyrosine kinase (MuSK) or low-density lipoprotein receptor-related protein 4. However, despite the identification of these additional antigens, "seronegative" forms still account for up to 10% of MG patients.

Associated Conditions

- MG is often associated with thymus hyperplasia; 10% may have a malignant thymoma. Hyperplasia is more common in those younger than 40 years. Thymoma is more common in MG patients older than 30 years.
- Autoimmune thyroiditis (hyper- more common than hypo-) is present in approximately 15% of patients with MG. MG patients also have an increased risk of other autoimmune diseases including lupus, rheumatoid arthritis, polymyositis, and pernicious anemia.

DIAGNOSIS

Clinical Presentation

History

- The cardinal feature of MG is fluctuating weakness that is worse after exercise or prolonged activity and improves with rest.
- More than 50% of patients present with ptosis that may be asymmetric.
- Other common complaints include blurred vision or diplopia, trouble smiling, and difficulties with chewing, swallowing, and speaking (e.g., winded at end of sentences, "staccato" [interrupted] speech, nasal speech, or weak voice).
- Weakness of neck flexors and extensors and proximal arm weakness are common. MG is one of the few neuromuscular disorders to cause prominent neck extensor weakness, creating a "head drop."
- **Myasthenic crisis** consists of respiratory failure or the need for airway protection and occurs in approximately 15%–20% of MG patients.[36] Patients with bulbar and respiratory muscle weakness are particularly prone to respiratory failure, which may develop rapidly and unexpectedly.
- Respiratory infection, surgery (e.g., thymectomy), medications (e.g., **aminoglycosides, quinine, quinolones, β-blockers, lithium, magnesium sulfate**), pregnancy, and thyroid dysfunction can precipitate crisis or exacerbate symptoms. However, it is important to note that none of these medications should be withheld if required to treat a concurrent illness. Anticholinergic medications are a notable exception to this rule for obvious reasons, and in the absence of a life-threatening indication, their use should be avoided.

Physical Examination

- Presenting signs include ptosis, diplopia, dysarthria, dysphagia, extremity weakness, and respiratory difficulty.
- Fatigability on examination is a useful diagnostic feature.
- Ptosis may worsen after prolonged upward gaze (usually by 60 seconds). Patients may also begin to develop diplopia after sustained gaze in one direction.
- Carefully evaluate the airway, handling of secretions, ventilation, and the work of breathing.
- NIF and FVC are useful at the bedside to assess for respiratory muscle weakness. The breath count test described earlier in the GBS section is also useful in this

population. The same general rules for ventilatory support (i.e., inability to protect airway or ventilate adequately) apply.

Differential Diagnosis

- Lambert–Eaton myasthenic syndrome (LEMS) is an autoimmune disease affecting the presynaptic voltage-gated calcium channels of the neuromuscular junction. It is frequently associated with malignancy (small-cell lung cancer). LEMS also presents with fluctuating weakness, but improves with exercise. Weakness in LEMS is classically more prominent in the legs relative to the arms, and unlike MG, oculobulbar deficits are uncommon. A quick bedside examination finding that may be present is to evaluate for facilitation of reflexes that are absent or diminished at rest but present or increased after 10 seconds of isometric exercise.
- Amyotrophic lateral sclerosis (ALS) may present with bulbar weakness and a "head drop." However, ALS can be differentiated from MG by presence of upper motor neuron signs in the former. Electrodiagnostic studies are also very useful in distinguishing the two.
- The differential also includes botulism (covered in more detail below), congenital forms of myasthenia, mitochondrial disorders (e.g., chronic progressive external ophthalmoplegia), and acquired and hereditary myopathies or other motor neuronopathies (other than ALS).

Diagnostic Testing

A good rule of thumb is to have two lines of diagnostic evidence (usually serologic and electrodiagnostic) in the appropriate clinical context to make a diagnosis of autoimmune MG.

Laboratory Studies
- Serum **AChR binding antibodies** are detected in 85%–90% of adult generalized MG patients and in 50%–70% of ocular MG patients.
- **MuSK antibodies** are detected in about 30%–70% of AChR antibody–negative MG patients.
- Thyroid function should be checked to evaluate for autoimmune thyroiditis.

Imaging
Chest CT is indicated to screen for a **thymoma**.

Diagnostic Procedures
Electrodiagnostic studies are an important step in diagnosing MG.
- Myasthenic weakness is often improved by cold. Although the history obtained from the patient may suggest this phenomenon, the "ice pack test" is an easy and safe, objective "bedside" measure of this phenomenon and is often helpful in the evaluation of ocular MG. Repetitive nerve stimulation typically shows a decrement in the amplitude of the compound muscle action potential in MG. If the patient is taking pyridostigmine, it should be held (if possible) because it could mask a decrement.
- In LEMS, the response is incremental.
- Single-fiber EMG has a sensitivity of >95% for both generalized and ocular MG when performed on facial muscles.
- Edrophonium testing is no longer routinely used.

TREATMENT

- Treatment of MG is individualized and depends on the severity of the disease, age, comorbidities, and response to therapy.

CHAPTER 27

- **Myasthenic crisis** requires prompt recognition and aggressive support.
  - Consider ICU level care and elective intubation for FVC <20 mL/kg or NIF >−30 cm H_2O (similar parameters to the "20/30" rule used for GBS).
  - Given the potential for fairly rapid improvement with acute immunomodulatory therapies (see below), noninvasive ventilation (e.g., bilevel positive airway pressure) can also be considered, in patients with adequate airway protection, as a means to avoid invasive ventilation.
  - Treat superimposed infections and metabolic derangements.
  - **Plasmapheresis** and IVIG are both used to treat MG crises/exacerbations and have equal efficacy with a similar rate of adverse effects.[37] However, expert guidelines support the use of plasmapheresis over IVIG in myasthenic crisis, given its greater short-term efficacy and quicker onset of action, unless there are comorbidities or elements of the individual's medical history that make IVIG the better option.[38]
  - Because the effects of PLEX or IVIG are relatively rapid in onset but short-lived, corticosteroids are typically started soon after initiating PLEX, usually at a dose of 10–20 mg/d and slowly titrated (e.g., by 5 mg every 3 days) to a dose of 50 mg/d.
  - Anticholinesterases should be temporarily withdrawn from patients who are receiving ventilation support to avoid cholinergic stimulation of pulmonary secretions.
  - Neuromuscular blocking agents should be avoided.

Medications

First Line

- Anticholinesterase drugs can produce symptomatic improvement in most forms of MG (anti-MuSK MG is frequently an exception).
- **Pyridostigmine** should be started at 30–60 mg PO tid–qid and titrated for symptom relief.

Second Line

- Immunosuppressive drugs are typically used when additional benefit is needed beyond cholinesterase inhibitors.
- High doses of **prednisone** (usually 50 mg daily) can be used to achieve rapid improvement. **However, up to 50% of patients experience a transient worsening of weakness on initiation of prednisone therapy.** Hence, it is important to start low and increase slow (see above), especially if the patient has not been or is not being treated with PLEX or IVIG.
- Azathioprine, mycophenolate mofetil, cyclosporine A, tacrolimus, and cyclophosphamide are steroid-sparing immunomodulatory agents that have all been used to treat MG with varying degrees of evidence to support their efficacy.
- There is strong evidence that rituximab (anti-CD20 chimeric monoclonal antibody) has great efficacy in treating anti-MuSK MG.[39]
- Eculizumab (Soliris), a humanized monoclonal antibody that binds with high affinity to human terminal complement protein C5, is approved for use in treatment-refractory anti-AChR MG.

Surgical Management

- Thymectomy is indicated in all patients with thymoma, regardless of age, and in patients with generalized MG who are aged 65 years or younger.[40]
- Thymectomy in ocular MG patients and generalized MG patients older than 65 years is considered on a case-by-case basis.

Other Neuromuscular Disorders

GENERAL PRINCIPLES

- **Myopathies:** Rapidly progressive proximal muscle weakness can be caused by many drugs including but not limited to ethanol, steroids, colchicine, cyclosporine, and cholesterol-lowering drugs (particularly in combination). Other common causes include HIV or HIV therapies, particularly zidovudine, and hypothyroidism.
  - **Critical illness myopathy** is increasingly recognized in patients with critical illness. **Myosin loss myopathy** accounts for a percentage of patients with critical illness myopathy and is commonly associated with clinical features of respiratory failure (e.g., difficulties weaning from the ventilator), severe weakness, and classic risk factors including exposure to high-dose corticosteroids and/or neuromuscular blocking agents. The diagnosis of myosin loss myopathy requires pathologic confirmation (i.e., a muscle biopsy must be performed).
  - **Polymyositis (PM) and dermatomyositis (DM)** fall into a class of diseases now referred to as the idiopathic immune and inflammatory myopathies. Most forms respond well to immunomodulatory therapy with a notable exception being the inclusion body myopathies. DM and PM can also be a component of a syndrome affecting multiple different organ systems. Perhaps the best examples are antisynthetase syndromes (e.g., Jo-1 myositis), which involve skin, joint, lung, and muscle. Patients suspected of having DM or PM should have myositis-specific and myositis-associated autoantibodies checked and should be screened for interstitial lung disease, which has a high degree of morbidity if left untreated (see Chapter 25, Arthritis and Rheumatologic Diseases).
- **Rhabdomyolysis** may produce rapid muscle weakness, leading to hyperkalemia, myoglobinuria (by definition true rhabdomyolysis causes myoglobinuria), and renal failure (for management, see Chapter 12, Fluid and Electrolyte Management, and Chapter 13, Renal Diseases). The potential etiologies include **M**etabolic (deficits of lipid or carbohydrate metabolism), **E**xcessive exercise/exertion (including seizures/dystonia), **D**rugs (abuse and prescribed), **I**schemic, **C**ompression/crush (trauma), **I**nfection/**I**nflammatory, **N**oxious (toxins), and **E**lectrolyte abnormalities (diabetic ketoacidosis, hyperosmolar hyperglycemic nonketotic syndrome, hypokalemia) (**"MEDICINE"**).
- **Botulism** is a disorder of the **neuromuscular junction** caused by ingestion of an exotoxin produced by *Clostridium botulinum*, acquired through a wound, or via an iatrogenic route.
  - The exotoxin interferes with release of acetylcholine from presynaptic terminals at the neuromuscular junction.
  - Classically, it is associated with ingestion of raw honey in infants, but inhalation/ingestion of soil-based spores and wound botulism from "skin popping" (i.e., injection of drugs of abuse underneath the skin) are likely more common means of absorption.
  - Symptoms begin within 12–36 hours of ingestion in food-borne botulism and within 10 days in wound botulism.
  - Symptoms include autonomic dysfunction (xerostomia, blurred vision, urinary retention, and constipation), followed by cranial nerve palsies, **descending weakness**, and **possibly respiratory distress.**

CHAPTER 27

- ○ **Serum assays for botulinum toxin** may aid diagnosis in adults.
- ○ Management includes removing nonabsorbed toxin with **cathartics, supportive care**, and neutralizing absorbed toxin with **equine trivalent (A, B, E) antitoxin** (more immunogenic because it contains both the Fab and Fc portions) or **heptavalent (A, B, C, D, E, F, G) antitoxin** (less immunogenic as Fc portion is cleaved off and has F(ab)$_2$ portions).
- ○ Recovery is slow and occurs spontaneously, but with appropriate ventilatory and supportive care, most make a full recovery.

Disorders With Rigidity

GENERAL PRINCIPLES

- **NMS** is associated with the use of neuroleptic drugs, certain antiemetic drugs (e.g., metoclopramide, promethazine), and sudden withdrawal of dopamine agonists (L-dopa in PD) and can even occur as an "off" phenomenon in PD patients experiencing severe "on–off" fluctuations.
  - ○ Features include hyperthermia, altered mental status, muscular rigidity, and dysautonomia.
  - ○ Laboratory abnormalities include a leukocytosis and a markedly elevated creatine kinase with myoglobinuria.
  - ○ Treatment includes discontinuing precipitating drug(s), restarting medications that were stopped (in the case of a PD patient), cooling and paralytics (if necessary), monitoring and supporting vital functions (arrhythmias, shock, hyperkalemia, acidosis, renal failure, and management of rhabdomyolysis), and administering **dantrolene and/or bromocriptine.** Treatment is essentially identical to that used for malignant hyperthermia (see the following text).
- **Serotonin syndrome** results from excessive serotonergic activity, especially following recent dosage changes of SSRIs, MAOIs, and TCAs.
  - ○ It presents as a **triad of mental status change, autonomic overactivity**, and **neuromuscular abnormalities.** Distinguishing features of serotonin syndrome from NMS include the degree of mental status change, seizures, and the marked **hyperreflexia.** However, in certain circumstances, the two can be difficult to distinguish from one another.
  - ○ Hyperthermia, tremor, nausea, vomiting, and clonus are common signs.
  - ○ Treatment includes removal of offending drugs, aggressive supportive care, cyproheptadine, and benzodiazepines.[41]
- **Malignant hyperthermia** is the acute development of high fever, obtundation, and muscular rigidity following triggering factors (e.g., halothane anesthesia, succinylcholine).
  - ○ The most common etiology is an autosomal dominant mutation in the ryanodine receptor (*RYR1*), making a screen of the family history a critical part of the preoperative evaluation. Abnormalities in this calcium channel predispose patients to an elevation in intracytoplasmic calcium triggered by certain anesthetics. Other ion channels have also been identified, and children with dystrophinopathies and other forms of muscular dystrophy are also at an increased risk.
  - ○ **Serum creatine kinase is markedly elevated.** Renal failure from myoglobinuria and cardiac arrhythmias from electrolyte imbalance can be life threatening.
  - ○ Successful management requires prompt recognition of early indicators of the syndrome (increased end-tidal carbon dioxide, tachycardia, acidosis, and/or muscle rigidity; note, hyperthermia comes later if at all); discontinuation of the offending

anesthetic agent; aggressive supportive care that focuses on oxygenation/ventilation, circulation, correction of acid–base, and electrolyte derangements; and administration of **dantrolene sodium**, 1–10 mg/kg/d, for at least 48–96 hours to reduce muscular rigidity.

- **Tetanus** typically presents with generalized muscle spasm (especially trismus) caused by the exotoxin (tetanospasmin) from *Clostridium tetani*, a gram-positive bacillus commonly found in intestinal flora and soil.
  - The organism usually enters the body through wounds. Onset typically occurs within 7–21 days of an injury.[42]
  - Patients who are **unvaccinated or have reduced immunity** are at risk, underscoring the importance of prevention by tetanus toxoid boosters following wounds. Tetanus may occur in **drug abusers who inject SC.**
  - Management consists of supportive care, particularly airway control (due to laryngospasm) and treatment of muscle spasms (benzodiazepines, barbiturates, analgesics, and sometimes neuromuscular blockade). Cardiac arrhythmias and fluctuations in BP can occur. Recovery takes months. Shorter incubation periods (≤7 days) portend more severe courses and a worse prognosis.
  - Specific measures include wound debridement, **penicillin G or metronidazole**, and **human tetanus immunoglobulin** (3000–6000 units IM).
  - **Active immunization** is needed after recovery (total of three doses of tetanus and diphtheria toxoid spaced at least 2 weeks apart).

REFERENCES

1. Douglas VC, Josephson SA. Delirium. *Continuum (Minneap Minn)*. 2010;16(2):120-134.
2. Douglas V, Hessler CS, Dhaliwal G, et al. The AWOL tool: derivation and validation of a delirium prediction rule. *J Hosp Med*. 2013;8(9):492-499
3. Hatta K, Kishi Y, Wada K. Preventative effects of ramelteon on delirium: a randomized placebo-controlled trial. *JAMA Psychiatry*. 2014;74(4):397-403.
4. Dubey D, Kothapalli N, McKeon A, et al. Predictors of neural-specific autoantibodies and immunotherapy response in patients with cognitive dysfunction. *J Neuroimmunol*. 2018;323:62-72.
5. Wijdicks EF, Varelas PN, Gronseth GS, Greer DM; American Academy of Neurology. Evidence-based guideline update. Determining brain death in adults: report of the Quality Standards Subcommittee of the American Academy of Neurology. *Neurology*. 2010;74(23):1911-1918.
6. Rossetti AO, Rabinstein AA, Oddo M. Neurological prognostication of outcome in patients in coma after cardiac arrest. *Lancet Neurol*. 2016;15(6):597-609.
7. Sarff M, Gold JA. Alcohol withdrawal syndromes in the intensive care unit. *Crit Care Med*. 2010;38(9):S494-S501.
8. Ngugi AK, Kariuki SM, Bottomley C, et al. Incidence of epilepsy: a systematic review and meta-analysis. *Neurology*. 2011;77(10):1005-1012.
9. Sheldon R, Rose S, Ritchie D, et al. Historical criteria that distinguish syncope from seizures. *J Am Coll Cardiol*. 2002;40(1):142.
10. Hauser WA, Rich SS, Lee JR, et al. Risk of recurrent seizures after two unprovoked seizures. *N Engl J Med*. 1998;338(7):429-434.
11. Arif H, Hirsch LJ. Treatment of status epilepticus. *Semin Neurol*. 2008;28(3):342-354.
12. Glauser T, Ben-Menachem E, Bourgeois B, et al. ILAE treatment guidelines: evidence-based analysis of antiepileptic drug efficacy and effectiveness as initial monotherapy for epileptic seizures and syndromes. *Epilepsia*. 2006;47(7):1094-1120.
13. Kwan P, Brodie MJ. Effectiveness of first antiepileptic drug. *Epilepsia*. 2001;42(10):1255-1260.
14. Kwan P, Arzimanoglou A, Berg AT, et al. Definition of drug resistant epilepsy: consensus proposal by the ad hoc Task Force of the ILAE Commission on Therapeutic Strategies. *Epilepsia*. 2010;51(6):1069-1077.
15. Ryvlin P, Cucherat M, Rheims S. Risk of sudden unexpected death in epilepsy in patients given adjunctive antiepileptic treatment for refractory seizures: a meta-analysis of placebo-controlled randomised trials. *Lancet Neurol*. 2011;10(11):961-968.
16. Solomon AJ. Diagnosis, differential diagnosis, and misdiagnosis of multiple sclerosis. *Continuum (Minneap Minn)*. 2019;25(3):611-635.
17. Leurs C, Twaalfhoven H, Lissenberg-Witte B, et al. Kappa free light chains is a valid tool in the diagnostics of MS: a large multicenter study. *Mult Scler*. 2020;26(8):912-923.

CHAPTER 27

18. Oliveira-Filho J, Silva SC, Trabuco CC, et al. Detrimental effect of blood pressure reduction in the first 24 hours of acute stroke onset. *Neurology.* 2003;61(8):1047-1051.

19. Adams HP Jr, del Zoppo G, Alberts MJ, et al. Guidelines for the early management of adults with ischemic stroke: a guideline from the American Heart Association/American Stroke Association Stroke Council, Clinical Cardiology Council, Cardiovascular Radiology and Intervention Council, and the Atherosclerotic Peripheral Vascular Disease and Quality of Care Outcomes in Research Interdisciplinary Working Groups. The American Academy of Neurology affirms the value of this guideline as an educational tool for neurologists. *Stroke.* 2007;38(5):1655-1711.

20. Hacke W, Kaste M, Bluhmki E, et al. Thrombolysis with alteplase 3 to 4.5 hours after acute ischemic stroke. *N Engl J Med.* 2008;359(13):1317-1329.

21. Thomalla G, Simonsen CZ, Boutitie F, et al. WAKE-UP Investigators. MRI-guided thrombolysis for stroke with unknown time of onset. *N Engl J Med.* 2018;379(7):611-622.

22. Powers WJ, Rabinstein AA, Ackerson T, et al; American Heart Association Stroke Council. 2018 guidelines for the early management of patients with acute ischemic stroke: a guideline for healthcare professionals from the American Heart Association/American Stroke Association. *Stroke.* 2018;49(3):e46-e110.

23. Albers GW, Marks MP, Kemp S, et al. Thrombectomy for stroke at 6 to 16 hours with selection by perfusion imaging. *N Engl J Med.* 2018;378(8):708-718.

24. Nogueira RG, Jadhav AP, Haussen DC, et al. Thrombectomy 6 to 24 hours after stroke with a mismatch between deficit and Infarct. *N Engl J Med.* 2018;378(1):11-21.

25. North American Symptomatic Carotid Endarterectomy Trial Collaborators, Barnett HJM, Taylor DW, et al. Beneficial effect of carotid endarterectomy in symptomatic patients with high-grade carotid stenosis. *N Engl J Med.* 1991;325(7):445-453.

26. Brott TG, Hobson RWII, Howard G, et al. Stenting versus endarterectomy for treatment of carotid-artery stenosis. *N Engl J Med.* 2010;363(1):11-23.

27. Endarterectomy for asymptomatic carotid artery stenosis. Executive Committee for the Asymptomatic Carotid Atherosclerosis Study. *J Am Med Assoc.* 1995;273(18):1421-1428.

28. Rothwell PM, Goldstein LB. Carotid endarterectomy for asymptomatic carotid stenosis: asymptomatic carotid surgery trial. *Stroke.* 2004;35(10):2425-2427.

29. PROGRESS Collaborative Group. Randomised trial of a perindopril-based blood-pressure-lowering regimen among 6,105 individuals with previous stroke or transient ischaemic attack. *Lancet.* 2001;358(9287):1033-1041.

30. Smith SC Jr, Grundy SM. 2013 ACC/AHA guideline recommends fixed-dose strategies instead of targeted goals to lower blood cholesterol. *J Am Coll Cardiol.* 2014;64(6):601-612.

31. McCrory P, Meeuwisse WH, Aubry M, et al. Consensus statement on concussion in sport: the 4th International Conference on Concussion in Sport, Zurich, November 2012. *J Athl Train.* 2013;48(4):554-575.

32. Tolosa E, Wenning G, Poewe W. The diagnosis of Parkinson's disease. *Lancet Neurol.* 2006;5(1):75-86.

33. Mena MA, de Yébenes JG. Drug-induced parkinsonism. *Expert Opin Drug Saf.* 2006;5(6):759-771.

34. van Doorn PA, Ruts L, Jacobs BC. Clinical features, pathogenesis, and treatment of Guillain-Barré syndrome. *Lancet Neurol.* 2008;7(10):939-950.

35. Hughes RA, Swan AV, Raphaël JC, et al. Immunotherapy for Guillain-Barré syndrome: a systematic review. *Brain.* 2007;130(pt 9):2245-2257.

36. Alshekhlee A, Miles JD, Katirji B, et al. Incidence and mortality rates of myasthenia gravis and myasthenic crisis in US hospitals. *Neurology.* 2009;72(18):1548-1554.

37. Barth D, Nabavi Nouri M, Ng E, et al. Comparison of IVIg and PLEX in patients with myasthenia gravis. *Neurology.* 2011;76(23):2017-2023.

38. Sanders DB, Wolfe GI, Narayanaswami P; MGFA Task Force on MG Treatment Guidance. Developing treatment guidelines for myasthenia gravis. *Ann N Y Acad Sci.* 2018 1412(1):95-101.

39. Hehir MK, Hobson-Webb LD, Benatar M, et al. Rituximab as treatment for anti-MuSK myasthenia gravis: multicenter blinded prospective review. *Neurology.* 2017;89(10):1069-1077.

40. Wolfe GI, Kaminski HJ, Aban IB, et al. Randomized trial of thymectomy in myasthenia gravis. *N Engl J Med.* 2016;375(6):511-522.

41. Boyer EW, Shannon M. The serotonin syndrome. *N Engl J Med.* 2005;352(11):1112-1120.

42. Brook I. Current concepts in the management of *Clostridium tetani* infection. *Expert Rev Anti Infect Ther.* 2008;6(3):327-336.

28 Toxicology

Jason Devgun, Kevin Baumgartner, and
Michael E. Mullins

THE POISONED PATIENT

GENERAL PRINCIPLES

- Patients who present to the hospital with an overdose or toxic exposure can be challenging for the clinician. This section will review the general approach to the poisoned or potentially poisoned patient. Specific toxins will be discussed in the sections that follow.
- When managing the poisoned patient, prioritize **basic supportive care measures**, including airway protection and support of respiration and circulation.

Definition

- A **toxidrome**, or toxic syndrome, is a **constellation of clinical examination findings** that assists in the diagnosis and treatment of the patient who presents following an exposure to an unknown agent.
- The toxidromes are generally defined by **vital signs, pupillary diameter, skin and mucous membrane findings,** and **mental status.** In certain cases, **bowel and bladder function** may also be relevant. See Table 28-1.

DIAGNOSIS

Diagnostic Testing

Diagnostic testing is typically guided by historical features of the exposure and physical exam findings. Very few diagnostic tests are helpful without history or physical exam findings to suggest an exposure.

Laboratories
- **Finger stick blood glucose (FSBG):** This test should be considered one of the vital signs in the patient with altered mental status.
- **Chemistry**: A basic metabolic profile should be ordered on any patient with a toxic exposure. The most important components of the basic metabolic panel (BMP) are the bicarbonate, anion gap, and creatinine.
  - **Bicarbonate:** The presence of acidosis is an important indicator of the presence and severity of poisoning by many important xenobiotics (e.g., toxic alcohols, salicylates, iron, and metformin).
  - **Anion gap:** An elevated anion gap acidosis in a poisoned patient should prompt testing for ketones, lactate, salicylates, and in certain select circumstances toxic alcohols.
  - **Creatinine:** Many important xenobiotics are renally excreted; impaired renal function may require treatments such as hemodialysis for toxin removal.
- **Blood gas:** In most cases of intoxication, pH rather than oxygenation is relevant. Therefore, it is reasonable to send **venous blood gases (VBGs)** rather than arterial

TABLE 28-1	Toxidromes						
		Vital Signs				Physical Exam Characteristics	
Toxidrome	Mechanism/ Pharmacology	HR	BP	Temp	RR	Mental Status	Pupils
Sympathomimetic	α and β adrenergic stimulation through increased secretion, impaired reuptake, or direct effect of an agent	↑	↑	↔ to ↑	↔	Excited ± delirium	Dilated
Cholinergic	Proximate effects on stimulation of ACh-mediated postsynaptic muscarinic receptors. Delayed effects on stimulation of presynaptic ACh-mediated nicotinic receptors	↓	↔	↔ to ↓	↓	Depressed or obtunded	Small/ pinpoint
Anticholinergic	Inhibition of postsynaptic muscarinic receptors	↑	↔ to ↑	↑	↔	Agitation with delirium, hallucinations, picking at surroundings	Dilated

Skin/Mucous Membranes	Motor Activity	Reflexes	GI Motility	Common Agents	Pearls
Diaphoretic/ flushed	Increased voluntary movement (psychomotor agitation)	↔	↔ to ↓ (with local GI exposure such as body "stuffers")	Cocaine, amphetamines, synthetic cathinones ("bath salts"), vasopressors, bupropion	Effective and timely management of excited delirium is potentially lifesaving. The combination of metabolic acidosis, physical restraint impairing effective ventilation, and chemical sedation impairing respiratory drive is dangerous
Excess oral/ respiratory secretions	Overall, decreased. Fasciculations/ seizures possible	↓	↑ (diarrhea, urinary incontinence)	Nerve agents, organophosphate/ carbamate pesticides, carbamate pharmaceuticals (e.g., neostigmine)	Early treatment of the "killer Bs," bradycardia, bronchorrhea, and associated respiratory impairment with atropine is imperative for nerve agent/pesticide poisoning
Dry (lack of axillary moisture)	Overall, decreased. Often fighting/ picking at surroundings	↔	↓ (decreased bowel sounds, urinary retention)	First-generation antihistamines, tricyclic antidepressants, jimson weed, atropine, scopolamine, hyoscyamine	Some cases may present with delirium absent other physical findings, "central anticholinergic syndrome"

CHAPTER 28

(continued)

TABLE 28-1	Toxidromes (continued)						
		Vital Signs				Physical Exam Characteristics	
Toxidrome	Mechanism/ Pharmacology	HR	BP	Temp	RR	Mental Status	Pupils
Opioid	Stimulation of μ-opioid receptors	↔ to ↓ (depending on degree of respiratory depression)	↔	↔ to ↓	↓↓	Depressed or obtunded	Small/ pinpoint
Sympatholytic	Stimulation of imidazoline receptors or in some cases alpha-2 agonism	↓	↓	↔ to ↓	↓	Depressed or obtunded	Small/ pinpoint

blood gases (ABGs) in most cases. However, if adequate oxygenation is a concern (e.g., cyanide, carbon monoxide poisoning, methemoglobinemia), then an ABG should be sent.

Co-oximetry (i.e., testing for dyshemoglobins such as methemoglobin or carboxy-hemoglobin) can be performed on arterial or venous samples.

- **Serum acetaminophen (*N*-acetyl-*para*-aminophenol [APAP]):** APAP is widely available and potentially life-threatening in overdose. Screening for acetaminophen should be performed in any patient presenting with an intentional overdose.
- **Serum salicylate:** The authors recommend universal screening for salicylates in patients with intentional overdoses (although other physical exam/chemistry findings may be also present).
- **Serum ethanol:** Routine or universal testing or ethanol is not helpful. Ethanol intoxication remains primarily a clinical diagnosis. Ethanol testing is necessary as part of the workup for toxic alcohol poisoning.
- **Urine drug screen (UDS):** This test is **rarely helpful** in the acute medical management of the poisoned or potentially poisoned patient. Clinical treatment should be guided by signs/symptoms of poisoning (toxidrome). The UDS is a test of exposure, not a test of intoxication. Appropriate UDS with confirmatory reflex testing may be useful for forensic purposes (e.g., drug-facilitated sexual assault, elder abuse). The UDS tends to vary between hospitals but often tests for the following substances:
  - **Amphetamines:** The assay for amphetamines commonly cross-reacts with over-the-counter cold medications. Many designer amphetamines will not be detected.

Skin/Mucous Membranes	Motor Activity	Reflexes	GI Motility	Common Agents	Pearls
↔	Decreased	↔	↓ (constipation with chronic use)	Opiates (morphine, codeine, diacetylmorphine [heroin]); opioids (fentanyl, oxycodone, hydrocodone, hydromorphone)	
↔	Decreased	↔	↔ to ↓	Imidazolines (e.g., oxymetazoline, dexmedetomidine, clonidine)	

CHAPTER 28

- **Opiates:** Detects only substances naturally derived from or metabolized to components of the opium poppy (morphine, codeine). Testing for specific synthetic opioids is typically performed as a separate test and may not be readily available.
- **Methadone:** Susceptible to false positives, particularly with psychotropic medications such as quetiapine and certain antidepressants.
- **Cocaine:** Almost all drug screening assays for cocaine are directed at the cocaine metabolite benzoylecgonine (BEG), as cocaine is rapidly metabolized by cholinesterases *in vivo*. This metabolite itself is also short-lived and a positive cocaine screen typically indicates exposure within the last 3–4 days.[1] The BEG immunoassay is not typically susceptible to false-positive results.
- **Cannabinoids:** Detection of tetrahydrocannabinol (THC) metabolites is a reliable indicator of cannabis use. Heavy cannabis users may continue to test positive for THC metabolites for several weeks after cessation. In general, synthetic cannabinoids will not cause a positive test result.
- **Benzodiazepines:** The detection of benzodiazepines most commonly relies on the detection of oxazepam (nordiazepam); therefore, commonly used benzodiazepines that are not metabolized to oxazepam (such as lorazepam, clonazepam, alprazolam) are not consistently detected. Some commercial screening assays do specifically test for benzodiazepines such as clonazepam or alprazolam, but this is not universal.
- **Phencyclidine (PCP):** Screening assays may cross-react with dextromethorphan, ketamine, and diphenhydramine to produce a false-positive result.

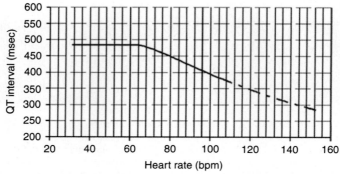

Figure 28-1. Qt interval nomogram (Adapted from Chan A, Isbister GK, Kirkpatrick CMJ, Dufful SB. Drug-induced QT prolongation and torsades de pointes: evaluation of a QT nomogram. *QJM.* 2007;100(10):609-615, by permission of Oxford University Press.)

Electrocardiography
- The ECG is a critical part of the toxicologic evaluation, as certain overdoses produce characteristic ECG changes that guide diagnosis and treatment.
- In general, cardiac toxins tend to prolong the PR interval (reflecting nodal blockade), the QRS (reflecting sodium channel blockade), or the QT interval (potassium channel blockade).
  - The specific prolongation of segment from the end of the ventricular depolarization to the end of repolarization ("JT" interval) is characteristic of toxic exposures that directly antagonize the IKr potassium channel. Toxins that antagonize the fast cardiac sodium channels will prolong the QRS interval; this will by definition impact the QT interval as well, as the QT interval includes the QRS interval.
  - Automatic correction of the QT interval for heart rate (e.g., by Bazett's method) may overestimate the risk of ventricular dysrhythmia in poisoning. An alternate means of correction such as the QT nomogram (Figures 28-1) may more accurately represent the risk of dysrhythmia from QT prolongation in poisoning.[2]

Imaging
- In general, diagnostic imaging has a limited role in toxicology.
- An abdominal radiograph may reveal radiodense material in the gastrointestinal (GI) tract of patients who have ingested certain radiopaque toxins, namely chloral hydrate, metals, certain antipsychotics, and enteric-coated or sustained-release pharmaceuticals.
- Occasionally, subtle abnormalities on the abdominal film will detect the presence of "rosettes" or elongated packets in the GI tract of body packers (patients who swallow hundreds of packets of drugs in an attempt to smuggle them). The abdominal film is of limited utility in body stuffers (patients who ingest small quantities of poorly packaged drugs to evade detection by law enforcement).

TREATMENT

- **Prevention of absorption:** GI decontamination should not be performed routinely or indiscriminately. It is most helpful in patients who present early, have ingested large quantities of xenobiotics, and/or have ingested dangerous xenobiotics without other effective treatments.

○ **Induction of emesis** (via ipecac or salt administration) is **never indicated.**

○ **Gastric lavage** is inefficacious in most cases and is uncomfortable for the patient and technically challenging to perform. It may have a limited role in the small subset of patients who present rapidly following ingestion of dangerous xenobiotics, liquid xenobiotics, or xenobiotics not adsorbed by activated charcoal. Lavage via a standard-bore orogastric or nasogastric tube is ineffective for solids/pill fragments. An Ewald tube is required, which may not be readily available.

○ **Activated charcoal (AC)** nonspecifically adsorbs most chemicals and xenobiotics, preventing their absorption into the circulation.

  ▪ The clinical utility of this method of decontamination is diminished if the ingestion occurred more than 1–2 hours before presentation in most ingestions. As such, most toxicologists do not routinely recommend the administration of AC.

  ▪ Patients at risk for decreased mental status or seizures should **not** be given AC owing to concerns for aspiration; patients whose airways are protected by intubation may be given AC per tube.

  ▪ AC should be dosed to produce a ratio of at least 10:1 AC to ingested drug by weight (g/g), with the caveat that 100 g of AC is typically the highest one-time dose an awake patient can tolerate.

○ **Whole-bowel irrigation (WBI)** involves the administration of massive quantities of polyethylene glycol with electrolytes (PEG-ELS) to clear the GI tract of ingested material by bulk action.

  ▪ WBI may be considered in patients who have ingested sustained-release medications, patients who have ingested metals that do not bind to AC (e.g., iron, lithium, lead), or in body packers.

  ▪ The optimal dose of PEG is 1–2 L/h until the rectal effluent is clear. It is usually necessary to place a nasogastric tube to administer this volume of fluid.

○ **Cathartics** have no role in the management of overdose. They are often present in the premixed AC solutions. If this is the case, only one dose should be administered.

○ All GI decontamination interventions are **contraindicated** in the presence of airway compromise, persistent vomiting, and the presence of an ileus, bowel obstruction, or GI perforation.

• **Enhanced elimination:** In certain circumstances, techniques to promote the rapid elimination of toxins may be helpful.

  ○ **Forced diuresis** with intravenous crystalloid is typically not useful. It may have a role in the treatment of lithium poisoning.

  ○ **Urinary alkalinization** with intravenous sodium bicarbonate enhances the elimination of weak acids and is useful in the setting of salicylate overdose and certain other poisonings.

  ○ **Multidose activated charcoal (MDAC)**, as opposed to single-dose AC discussed above, may enhance the elimination of certain xenobiotics that undergo enterohepatic recirculation (most importantly quinine, theophylline, carbamazepine, phenobarbital, and dapsone).

  ○ **Hemodialysis** and other extracorporeal elimination methods may be indicated in serious poisonings by specific dialyzable xenobiotics. Hemodialysis may also be used to correct acid-based disorders due to poisoning, even when it does not directly remove a significant amount of xenobiotic.

• **Antidotes:** Antidotal therapy is indicated only in specific circumstances and should not be administered indiscriminately.

CHAPTER 28

SPECIAL CONSIDERATIONS: SEIZURES IN POISONING

- Many poisonings and withdrawal syndromes produce seizures. Toxic seizures are usually generalized and tonic-clonic; nonconvulsive status epilepticus and focal seizure are rare in toxicology.
- Generally speaking, it is not necessary to preemptively or prophylactically treat patients at risk for toxic seizures. Exceptions include chloroquine and hydroxychloroquine and the cholinesterase inhibitor pesticides and nerve agents.
- Toxic seizures should be treated with agents that **directly enhance GABAergic tone.**
  - **Benzodiazepines** are the first-line agent of choice. They do not directly open the GABA-A chloride channel, but rather enhance opening in response to endogenous GABA binding.
  - **Barbiturates** may be used in patients refractory to benzodiazepines. Unlike benzodiazepines, barbiturates open the GABA-A chloride channel even in the absence of endogenous GABA, and thus may be particularly helpful in patients with impaired GABA synthesis (e.g., hydrazine poisonings, severe alcohol use disorder [AUD]).
  - **Propofol** also directly opens the GABA-A chloride channel. It is an excellent choice in intubated patients who are experiencing or at risk for toxic seizures.
  - Parenteral **pyridoxine** may be helpful in select cases, especially in hydrazine poisoning (isoniazid, *Gyromitra esculenta*, hydrazine fuels) and in malnourished patients.
- Anticonvulsants that are not directly GABAergic should not be used to treat toxic seizures.
  - Levetiracetam and other anticonvulsants used in epilepsy (e.g., valproate, carbamazepine, lacosamide, zonisamide) are likely ineffective in poisoned or withdrawing patients.
  - **Phenytoin may actually be harmful** in certain poisonings (e.g., theophylline) and should be avoided.[3]

ANALGESICS

Acetaminophen

GENERAL PRINCIPLES

Epidemiology

- APAP is available worldwide as an over-the-counter analgesic and antipyretic. It is a common component of cold and flu remedies and is often sold in combination preparation together with nonsteroidal anti-inflammatory drugs (NSAIDs), opioids, or sedatives.
- APAP is available in multiple formulations, including tablets, extended-release tablets, capsules, liquids, suppositories. An intravenous formulation is also available.
- In the US, APAP is the **most common pharmacologic agent** involved in **toxicologic fatalities** and the **most common cause of acute liver failure.**

Pathophysiology

- APAP is a centrally active cyclooxygenase (COX) inhibitor with analgesic and antipyretic effects.
- In therapeutic doses, APAP is primarily metabolized via phase II conjugation enzymes in the liver, which generates nontoxic conjugate products. Small amounts of APAP are metabolized by phase I enzymes (primarily cytochrome P450 2E1),

producing a toxic oxidizing metabolite, *N*-acetyl-*p*-benzoquinone imine (NAPQI). NAPQI is then detoxified by glutathione.

- In cases of APAP toxicity, the phase II conjugation enzymes are saturated, and a higher proportion of APAP is metabolized via oxidation to NAPQI. Conjugation of NAPQI by glutathione occurs until cellular glutathione is depleted, after which the toxic NAPQI and other free radicals accumulate and cause damage to the hepatocytes.
- Toxicity may occur after a large APAP overdose or after the repeated use of supratherapeutic amounts of APAP.
- Conditions that reduce glutathione stores (such as fasting, malnutrition, and chronic heavy alcohol use) or induce CYP 2E1 (chronic heavy alcohol use, phenytoin and other anticonvulsants, isoniazid) predispose patients to APAP toxicity.

DIAGNOSIS

Clinical Presentation

- **0–24 hours**—Asymptomatic (stage 1)
  - Early symptoms are nonspecific and primarily related to irritation of the GI tract by ingested tablets (nausea, vomiting, and anorexia).
  - This initial phase has few symptoms and patients generally appear clinically well. If a patient exhibits significant vital sign abnormalities or symptoms in the first 24 hours following ingestion, consider other co-ingestants.
  - In rare cases, patients who ingest supermassive quantities of APAP may present early with encephalopathy and metabolic acidosis, as APAP is a direct mitochondrial toxin at extremely high concentrations.
- **24–48 hours**—Hepatotoxic (stage 2)
  - Right upper quadrant abdominal pain is the most common symptom.
  - Transaminase elevations and elevated prothrombin time (PT)/international normalized ratio (INR) develop in this phase.
- **2–4 days**—Fulminant hepatic failure (stage 3)
  - Significant hepatic dysfunction, potentially including fulminant hepatic failure, develops. Jaundice, severe coagulopathy, thrombocytopenia, hypoglycemia, hepatic encephalopathy, and renal injury may be present.
- **4–14 days**—Recovery (stage 4): If stage 3 is survived, the hepatic dysfunction usually resolves over the following days/weeks. If renal injury occurred, it would typically resolve slowly during this phase.

History

- Obtain a **reliable time of ingestion** to accurately predict the risk of hepatotoxicity after acute overdose.
- Characterize the time course of poisoning—was there a single acute overdose, or was there repeated supratherapeutic use, chronic overdose, or a staggered overdose (occurring over the course of several hours)?
- Obtain as much information as possible about the amount of APAP that has been ingested, the formulation ingested (for example, combination preparations, extended-release form), and the period over which the overdose occurred.
- Obtain information about co-ingestants (alcohol, other medications, other drugs) and comorbid conditions (especially heavy alcohol use and hepatic disease).

Physical Examination

- As in all poisoned patients, assess airway, breathing, circulation, and mental status. These will generally be normal in isolated APAP poisoning, except in patients who present to medical care late (already in stage 3) or in the rare patients who ingest supermassive quantities of APAP.

• Right upper quadrant tenderness, jaundice, or evidence of hepatic encephalopathy (mental status changes, asterixis) may be present in those presenting late to medical care (in stage 2 or 3 of poisoning).

Diagnostic Criteria

• In general, an APAP dose of 150 mg/kg or higher is potentially toxic and may require therapeutic intervention. Unfortunately, the total dose ingested is frequently inaccurate or unknown.

• Use the **modified acetaminophen (Rumack-Matthew) nomogram** (Figures 28-2) to predict the risk for hepatotoxicity in acute APAP poisoning.[4] This nomogram is **not applicable** in cases of chronic poisoning, poisoning due to repeated supratherapeutic use, poisoning due to ingestions that are staggered over several hours, or poisoning by the extended-release APAP formulation.

  ○ Obtain a serum APAP concentration at **4 hours or later after ingestion.** APAP concentrations obtained before 4 hours postingestion have **no prognostic value.**

  ○ If the patient plots below the treatment line with an accurate time of ingestion, no further testing or treatment is necessary.

• It is challenging to predict hepatotoxicity in patients with staggered, subacute, or chronic APAP ingestions, or ingestions that cannot be accurately timed. These patients should generally be treated with NAC.

• During treatment of APAP overdose, it is important to assess the risk of liver failure that may require evaluation for hepatic transplantation. The King's College Hospital (KCH) criteria provide prognostic markers that help to predict the probability of developing severe liver damage (Table 28-2).[5]

  The decision to transfer a patient to a transplant center for evaluation is complex and should take into account local practice patterns, logistics, and risk tolerance in addition to the KCH criteria. Generally speaking, patients who meet *none* of the KCH criteria may be safely managed at a nontransplant center.

Diagnostic Testing

• **Serum APAP** at **four or more hours** after ingestion (see earlier discussion).

• **Hepatic function panel (HFP)** to assess for transaminase elevations that indicate the presence of hepatocellular injury.

• Testing for evidence of hepatic failure **(PT/INR, bilirubin, pH, lactate, phosphate, and renal function panel)** is not generally required at presentation in patients with acute overdose who present to medical care rapidly but may be necessary later in hospitalization or in patients who present late in the course of poisoning.

  NAC therapy can cause minor interference in the PT/INR assay; this does not indicate an *in vivo* coagulopathy and will not elevate the INR above 2.0.

TREATMENT

• GI decontamination is generally not required or useful in APAP poisoning. Some authors advocate for AC administration in patients who present within 1–2 hours of overdose and have no contraindications to AC.

• **N-Acetylcysteine (NAC):** NAC is the specific antidote to prevent APAP-related hepatotoxicity. NAC replenishes depleted glutathione stores, directly detoxifies NAPQI, and counteracts oxidative stress caused by NAPQI. It is most effective

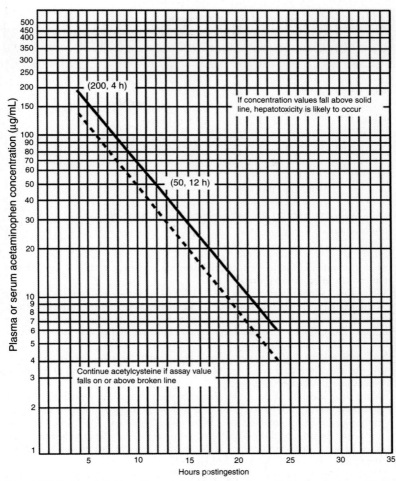

Figure 28-2. Acetaminophen (Rumack-Matthew) nomogram (Reproduced with permission from Rumack BH, Matthew H. Acetaminophen poisoning and toxicity. *Pediatrics.* 1975;55(6): 871-876. Copyright © 1975 by the American Academy of Pediatrics.)

TABLE 28-2	King's College Criteria	
pH < 7.3[a]		or
Lactate > 3.5 mmol/L at 4 h[a]		or
Lactate > 3.0 mmol/L at 12 h[a]		or
INR > 6.5, creatinine > 3.4 mg/dL, and severe hepatic encephalopathy (grade III or IV)		
Other prognostic factors		
Phosphate > 3.72 mg/dL on days 2–4		

[a]After fluid resuscitation.

TABLE 28-3	Dosing of N-Acetylcysteine		
	Oral	IV (Authors' One-Bag Protocol)	IV (FDA Package Insert)
Loading dose	140 mg/kg	150 mg/kg over 1 h	150 mg/kg over 1 h
Subsequent doses	70 mg/kg q4h ×17 doses (72 h)	12.5 mg/kg/h for 20 h or longer	12.5 mg/kg/h for 4 h
			6.25 mg/kg/h for 16 h
Comments	Sulfur taste, recommend lid with straw, antiemetics PRN. Use only if IV NAC not readily available	Less errors and stoppage with this method + programmable IV pump	Original FDA approval dosing used in many hospitals
When to stop IV NAC: 21 h + AST < 50% of peak, INR < 2.0, clinical improvement			

when administered within 8 hours after ingestion, although it will still have a hepatoprotective effect even beyond this time.[6]

- When dosed appropriately (Table 28-3), IV NAC is very safe. There is a small risk of rate-related anaphylactoid reactions (flushing, headache, nausea, pruritus), which typically resolve with antiemetics, antihistamines, and in some cases slowing the infusion rate of IV NAC. A one-bag method (Table 28-3) may help reduce administration delays and dosing errors.[7]
- **NAC indications:** NAC treatment should be started in the following circumstances:
  ○ Any patient after acute poisoning with a toxic APAP level according to the modified Rumack-Matthew nomogram.
  ○ If the determination of the initial acetaminophen level and potential initiation of treatment with NAC is anticipated to be delayed longer than 8 hours postingestion (e.g., due to late presentation or lab or pharmacy delays). In this circumstance, NAC may be stopped if the APAP level is ultimately determined to be nontoxic.
  ○ Patients who present more than 24 hours after acute ingestion and still have a detectable serum APAP level or elevated AST.
  ○ Patients with chronic supratherapeutic APAP exposure (i.e., >4 g/d or >2 g/d in patients with significant hepatic disease or heavy alcohol use) who present with elevated transaminases or unmetabolized APAP.
  ○ Patients with signs of fulminant hepatic failure, regardless of etiology. NAC has been shown to improve transplant-free survival of patients in fulminant hepatic failure.
  ○ Patients poisoned by other xenobiotics that cause oxidative hepatocellular damage, such as *Amanita phalloides* mushrooms, carbon tetrachloride, and eugenol.

Salicylates

GENERAL PRINCIPLES

- Salicylate toxicity may result from acute or chronic ingestion of acetylsalicylic acid (ASA). Toxicity is usually mild after acute ingestions of <150 mg/kg, moderate after ingestions of 150–300 mg/kg, and generally severe with overdoses of 300–500 mg/kg.

- Toxicity from chronic ingestion is typically due to intake of >100 mg/kg/d over a period of several days and usually occurs in elderly patients with chronic underlying illness. Diagnosis is often delayed in this group of patients, and mortality is approximately 25%. Significant toxicity due to chronic ingestion may occur with blood concentrations lower than those associated with acute ingestions.
- Topical preparations containing methyl salicylate or oil of wintergreen can cause toxicity with excessive topical use or if ingested.

Pathophysiology

- At toxic doses, salicylates disrupt aerobic respiration in the mitochondria. They uncouple oxidative phosphorylation from ATP production by disrupting the proton gradient in the intermembrane space.
- The resultant impairment of aerobic respiration produces an elevated anion gap metabolic acidosis, impairs effective glucose utilization, and leads to widespread cellular metabolic failure.

  The brain is particularly reliant on glucose as an energy source. Disruption of aerobic metabolism by salicylate poisoning leads to rapid depletion of central nervous system glucose through less effective anaerobic respiration.
- In the early stages of poisoning, salicylates directly stimulate the medullary respiratory centers, producing the characteristic early tachypnea and primary respiratory alkalosis. As poisoning progresses, metabolic acidosis worsens and the tachypnea becomes compensatory.

DIAGNOSIS

Clinical Presentation

- Patients with salicylate poisoning typically present with GI upset, tinnitus or hearing changes, tachypnea, tachycardia, and hyperpnea.
- Severe intoxication may produce lethargy, encephalopathy, coma, seizures, or hypoxemic respiratory failure (due to noncardiogenic pulmonary edema).
- **Chronic** salicylate poisoning, especially in elderly patients, may mimic sepsis, with tachycardia, tachypnea, alterations in mental status, and occasionally hyperthermia.

Diagnostic Testing

Laboratories

- Obtain a BMP.
  - Acidosis with an elevated anion gap is an important indicator of salicylate poisoning.
  - Some chloride analyzers may report **spurious hyperchloremia** in the presence of high salicylate concentrations, which falsely depresses the anion gap.
  - Maintenance of **eukalemia** is critical for treatment (see below).
- Obtain a blood gas (either venous or arterial). The acid–base pattern will depend on the phase of poisoning.
  - Early, patients exhibit a primary respiratory alkalosis (due to direct stimulation of the medullary respiratory centers, as above).
  - Later, a mixed picture develops, with a combined primary respiratory alkalosis and primary metabolic acidosis (the "classic" acid–base finding in salicylate poisoning).

- Patients in extremis or patients with a co-ingestion of a respiratory depressant may develop a mixed metabolic and respiratory acidosis.
- Obtain a serum salicylate concentration.
  - Salicylate concentrations >30 mg/dL are supratherapeutic and potentially toxic.
  - Salicylate concentrations >70 mg/dL at any time represent moderate to severe intoxication.
  - Salicylate concentrations >100 mg/dL are serious and often fatal.
  - Enteric-coated aspirin may have delayed absorption and delayed peak concentration.
  - **Chronic** salicylate poisoning can cause severe toxicity with lower serum salicylate concentrations.
  - **Be aware of units.** Most hospitals report salicylate concentrations in mg/dL. However, some hospitals still report concentrations in mg/L, which has caused multiple interpretation errors.
- **Frequent repetition** of laboratory tests is critical—the toxicokinetics of salicylates are unpredictable and erratic, and patients' lab results and clinical condition can change rapidly.
  Frequency of lab monitoring depends on the clinical condition—critically ill patients may require q2 hour monitoring of salicylate concentration, electrolytes, and blood gas, while mildly or moderately poisoned patients may have labs checked every 6–8 hours.

Imaging
Salicylate is known to produce large concretions or bezoars in overdose. Theoretically, imaging by computed tomography or endoscopy might reveal the presence of a bezoar, but imaging is almost never required for diagnosis or management.

TREATMENT

Medications

- Administer **AC** to patients presenting shortly after acute overdose with no contra-indications to AC. **Repeated doses of AC,** even many hours postingestion, may be useful in severe poisoning, especially in cases when salicylate concentrations fail to decline as expected (due to possible bezoar formation or pylorospasm leading to a prolonged absorption phase).[8]
- In an acute overdose, most patients will be volume depleted due to GI volume losses and insensible losses from tachypnea and will benefit from intravenous crystalloid resuscitation. Caution should be used in patients with renal failure or congestive heart failure (CHF).
- Enhanced elimination via **urinary alkalinization** with **sodium bicarbonate** is indicated for symptomatic patients with salicylate blood concentrations >30 mg/dL.
  - Initiate therapy with a bolus dose of ~1 mEq/kg sodium bicarbonate (typically about two standard 50 mEq ampules).
  - Continue therapy with an infusion of sodium bicarbonate (150 mEq sodium bicarbonate in 1 L of 5% dextrose in water) at twice the maintenance rate.
  - Monitor the success of urinary alkalinization by following the patient's clinical condition (target consistent improvement), salicylate concentrations (target consistent decline), and urine pH (target 7–8). Administer additional boluses of sodium bicarbonate and/or increase the infusion rate as needed to achieve these goals.
  - Avoid excessive alkalemia. **Pause or scale back bicarbonate therapy if serum pH exceeds 7.55.**

- Aggressively **replete potassium** to a target of >4 mEq/L. Even relative hypokalemia will impair appropriate urinary alkalinization, and bicarbonate therapy will induce hypokalemia via transcellular shift.
  - **Use caution with urinary alkalinization** in patients with significant renal impairment, heart failure with reduced ejection fraction, or volume overload.
  - **Sodium acetate** may be substituted for sodium bicarbonate during a drug shortage. Sodium acetate cannot be administered as a rapid IV bolus but may be infused in place of sodium bicarbonate.
- Administer **intravenous dextrose** to patients with altered mental status, **even if the peripheral blood glucose is normal.** Salicylate poisoning causes profound depletion of glucose in the central nervous system.
- Administer parenteral **benzodiazepines** (or other directly GABAergic antiepileptics such as barbiturates or propofol) to patients with seizures. These patients should also receive intravenous dextrose as noted above.

Nonpharmacologic Therapies

- **Avoid intubation and mechanical ventilation** if possible. Even the brief period of sedation and apnea required for rapid-sequence intubation will significantly worsen acidosis and promote the movement of salicylate into target organs.
  - The compensatory hyperpnea and tachypnea seen in severe salicylate poisoning often cannot be replicated by mechanical positive-pressure ventilation. Intubation and mechanical ventilation are associated with profound acidosis and death in salicylate-poisoned patients.
  - If intubation is **completely unavoidable** (e.g., refractory hypoxemia, gross aspiration, profound respiratory fatigue), push sodium bicarbonate before and during intubation, maximize tidal volume and respiratory rate on the ventilator, and arrange for emergent hemodialysis (see below).
- **Hemodialysis** effectively clears salicylates and corrects acid–base deficits. It is indicated in salicylate poisoning in the following situations:
  - Salicylate > 100 mg/dL, or >90 mg/dL in the presence of renal impairment
  - Any degree of altered mental status
  - New hypoxemia requiring supplemental oxygen
  - Failure of standard therapy with elevated salicylate concentrations (>90 mg/dL, or >80 mg/dL with renal impairment) or pH < 7.20

Nonsteroidal Anti-Inflammatory Drugs

GENERAL PRINCIPLES

NSAIDs are widely prescribed as analgesics and for the management of inflammatory diseases. There are many different agents available; the discussion here relates to ibuprofen and naproxen.

Pathophysiology

- NSAIDs exert their therapeutic effects by inhibiting COX and thereby preventing the formation of prostaglandins.
- This mechanism accounts for both their therapeutic effects and toxicities, which include ulceration of the GI mucosa and renal dysfunction.
- In most cases, *acute overdose* is benign. In rare cases of massive overdose, mental status changes, anion gap metabolic acidosis (from accumulation of acidic metabolites), and seizures may occur.

CHAPTER 28

DIAGNOSIS

Clinical Presentation
- Patients with acute NSAID overdose typically have no symptoms or signs or isolated GI distress.
- In **rare** cases of massive overdose, patients may present with encephalopathy, coma, seizures, and cardiovascular collapse.

Diagnostic Testing
- Obtain a **BMP** to evaluate renal function and acid–base status.
  - Large overdoses may cause an elevated anion gap metabolic acidosis.
  - Kidney injury is unusual in acute overdoses; if present, it typically resolves rapidly and spontaneously.
- Obtain an **APAP concentration**, as many patients confuse over-the-counter analgesics.

TREATMENT

Significant toxicity is extremely rare in NSAID overdose. Most patients require no treatment or symptomatic treatment only. In rare cases of massive overdose, substantial resuscitative care may be required.

Medications
- Patients with GI upset or dyspepsia may benefit from antiemetics and antacids.
- Intravenous fluid resuscitation for those with hypovolemia or hemodynamic instability.
- Treat seizures with benzodiazepines (or other directly GABAergic antiepileptics such as barbiturates or propofol).
- In rare cases, vasopressors and/or inotropes may be needed.
- As in most cases of elevated anion gap acidosis, indiscriminate use of sodium bicarbonate is not helpful.

Nonpharmacologic Therapies
- In rare cases, patients with massive overdoses resulting in coma may require intubation and mechanical ventilation.
- Hemodialysis may improve acid–base status but does **not** remove NSAIDs.

Opioids

GENERAL PRINCIPLES

Pathophysiology
- Opioids are naturally occurring or synthetic xenobiotics that act at the opioid receptors in the brain, spinal cord, and periphery.
- Most of the clinically relevant effects of opioids are related to mu-opioid agonism.

DIAGNOSIS

Clinical Presentation
- Patients with opioid poisoning present with a depressed level of consciousness (ranging from drowsiness to coma), respiratory depression, and miosis.

Miosis may be absent in patients who have seized, patients who are profoundly hypoxemic or acidotic, or patients poisoned by certain opioids (e.g., meperidine).
- Blood pressure and heart rate may be mildly decreased in opioid poisoning, but profound hemodynamic instability suggests an alternative etiology.

Diagnostic Testing

Laboratories
- Obtain a **point-of-care blood glucose** to rule out hypoglycemia, which may mimic opioid poisoning.
- Other laboratory tests (such as blood gases, electrolytes, UDS) are not generally helpful in acute medical management.

Electrocardiography
Obtain an ECG in cases of known or suspected methadone poisoning, as methadone may substantially prolong the QT interval.

TREATMENT

- The goal of treatment is to **maintain adequate respiration**, not to produce complete wakefulness.
- In many cases of mild opioid poisoning, close monitoring is sufficient, and no active treatment is required.
  - Continuous monitoring of end-tidal carbon dioxide ($ETCO_2$) is more sensitive for hypopnea, bradypnea, and apnea than pulse oximetry.

Medications

- **Naloxone**, a mu-opioid antagonist, is the antidote for opioid poisoning.
  - The **lowest effective dose** that restores normal respiration should be used. Excess naloxone will provoke opioid withdrawal in opioid-dependent patients.
  - The typical starting dose is **0.04 mg IV.** This dose may be repeated or increased as necessary to achieve sustained normal respiration. A patient who has not improved with 10 mg naloxone should prompt an alternative diagnosis.
  - Poisoning by long-acting may require a naloxone infusion typically started at two-thirds the effective reversal dose per hour titrated to adequate respiratory rate.[9]
  - If IV access is not available, naloxone may be administered by the intranasal, intramuscular, endotracheal, or intraosseous routes. Higher doses are required when using these alternate routes.

Nonpharmacologic Therapies

- Support of respiration by bag-valve mask may be required prior to naloxone administration.
- Endotracheal intubation is rarely indicated in isolated opioid poisoning (as respiratory depression should be reversed by naloxone) but may be necessary in cases of polysubstance intoxication or co-occurring major trauma or medical illness.

SPECIAL CONSIDERATIONS: OPIOID USE DISORDER

- Opioid use disorder (OUD) is a problematic pattern of opioid use leading to clinically significant impairment or distress. Patients appropriately taking prescribed opioids may develop tolerance or dependence, but this does not indicate the presence of OUD.

CHAPTER 28

TABLE 28-4	Medications for Opioid Use Disorder		
	Buprenorphine (Sublingual or IM)	Methadone	IM Naltrexone (Vivitrol)
Pharmacology on μ-opioid receptors	Partial agonist, very high receptor affinity	Full agonist, high receptor affinity	Antagonist
Estimated elimination half-life	24–42 h	13–47 h	5–10 d
Typical dosing	4–32 mg total daily dose, divided twice or three times daily	30–150 mg daily	380 mg monthly
Considerations	Can be prescribed in an acute care hospital without DEA waiver, outpatient Rx requires "X-waiver"	Outpatient administration only at a methadone clinic. Requires daily transport to clinic	Requires period of opioid abstinence and 7 d oral naltrexone prior to administration. Does not treat cravings or withdrawal symptoms

- There are two primary options for medication for opioid use disorder (mOUD): methadone and buprenorphine (Table 28-4). mOUD produces sustained remission, prevents relapse and overdose, improves quality of life, and prevents premature death.
- Symptomatic treatment of opioid withdrawal may be helpful in patients who decline mOUD or during the initiation of mOUD.
  - Clonidine (starting dose 0.1 mg PO q8 hours as needed) may help treat anxiety, psychomotor agitation, and malaise.
  - Symptomatic treatment of GI symptoms (e.g., antiemetics for nausea and vomiting, loperamide for diarrhea) may be helpful.
  - Hydroxyzine may be helpful for pruritus, anxiety, and insomnia.
- Patients taking mOUD may sometimes require opioids for the treatment of acutely painful medical conditions. Consultation with Pain Management and Addiction Medicine may be helpful in these circumstances.
- Patients with known or suspected OUD should be referred for outpatient evaluation and treatment and prescribed naloxone for use in case of accidental overdose.

ANTICONVULSANTS

Phenytoin and Fosphenytoin

GENERAL PRINCIPLES

Pathophysiology

- Phenytoin exerts therapeutic activity by binding to neuronal sodium channels and inhibiting reactivation.
- Phenytoin exhibits saturable kinetics, and at plasma levels >20 μg/mL, toxic effects become rapidly apparent.
- Fosphenytoin is a prodrug that is converted to phenytoin after IV or IM injection.

Risk Factors

- Patients with mutations of the cytochrome P450 system that impair phenytoin metabolism are at risk for toxicity even with therapeutic use.
- Coadministration of xenobiotics that inhibit CYP 2C9, 2C19, or 3A4 impairs the metabolism of phenytoin and may lead to phenytoin toxicity.
- Phenytoin is highly albumin bound; patients with hypoalbuminemia (e.g., those with malnutrition or cirrhosis) may have higher levels of free (active) drug and experience toxicity despite seemingly normal total phenytoin concentrations.

DIAGNOSIS

Clinical Presentation

- Patients with phenytoin poisoning will present with confusion, changes in mental status, and changes in gait and speech.
- At plasma phenytoin concentrations of >15 μg/mL, patients will exhibit nystagmus. Ataxia develops at concentrations of 30 μg/mL. Confusion, encephalopathy, and frank movement disorders occur at concentrations above 50 μg/mL.
- Severe poisoning may actually produce seizures.
- Rapid IV administration of phenytoin may produce bradycardia and hypotension due in part to propylene glycol and ethanol; these are **not** seen in chronic poisoning or acute oral overdose.[10]
- IV phenytoin may lead to severe tissue injury (typically with extravasation), "purple glove syndrome," which may require surgical debridement.[11]

Differential Diagnosis

- Phenytoin poisoning may mimic other poisonings with mental status depression.
- The nontoxicologic differential diagnosis for phenytoin poisoning should include Wernicke encephalopathy, meningoencephalitis, posterior circulation ischemic stroke, and intracranial hemorrhage and mass lesion.

Diagnostic Testing

Laboratories

- Obtain a **phenytoin concentration** on any patient with a potential phenytoin exposure, even if acute overdose is not suspected.
  - Most hospital laboratories report a total phenytoin concentration rather than free phenytoin. Correction for hypoalbuminemia is necessary.
  - The phenytoin concentration should be **trended over time**, as delayed absorption and delayed excretion are common in poisoning.
- Obtain a **complete blood count**, as phenytoin may cause agranulocytosis.
- Obtain an **HFP**, as phenytoin may cause drug-induced liver injury (DILI).

Electrocardiography

Electrocardiography and continuous cardiac monitoring are indicated only in cases of iatrogenic poisoning by intravenous phenytoin (see above).

TREATMENT

- Most patients will do well with cessation of phenytoin therapy and supportive care.
- **MDAC** is suggested by some experts to enhance phenytoin elimination.
- Treat seizures with benzodiazepines or other directly GABAergic agents.

CHAPTER 28

- Hypotension and bradycardia in the setting of IV phenytoin administration are typically self-limiting, but may occasionally require treatment with fluids, atropine, and/or vasopressors.
- Agranulocytosis should be treated with granulocyte colony-stimulating factor.
- DILI typically resolves with drug discontinuation.
- **Hemodialysis** effectively clears phenytoin and may be reasonable in cases of prolonged coma or prolonged and incapacitating ataxia.

Valproic Acid

GENERAL PRINCIPLES

Pathophysiology

- Valproic acid (VPA) is widely prescribed for the management of seizures and mood disorders. It exerts its effects in therapeutic dose and overdose by inhibiting the function of voltage-gated sodium and calcium channels as well as enhancing the function of GABA.
- VPA is metabolized by the hepatocytes through a complicated biochemical process that involves β-oxidation in the mitochondria.
  - VPA may produce profound DILI in overdose or therapeutic use. DILI due to VPA is characterized by microvesicular steatosis.
  - VPA metabolism may lead to significant ammonia accumulation (ammonia concentrations >80 μg/dL or >35 μmol/L), leading to profound encephalopathy, a condition called valproate-induced hyperammonemic encephalopathy (VHE). Many patients taking VPA may have mild ammonia elevations without systemic symptoms.

DIAGNOSIS

Clinical Presentation

- Patients with valproate poisoning may present with tremor, ataxia, sedation, altered sensorium, or coma.
- Patients with DILI due to VPA may complain of abdominal pain or present with jaundice or hepatic encephalopathy.
- Patients with VHE will typically be profoundly encephalopathic or comatose.

Differential Diagnosis

- Valproate poisoning is similar to poisoning by other anticonvulsants. Patients with carbamazepine poisoning typically exhibit antimuscarinic signs and/or cardiotoxicity, which are not seen in valproate poisoning.
- The nontoxicologic differential diagnosis for valproate poisoning should include Wernicke encephalopathy, meningoencephalitis, posterior circulation ischemic stroke, and intracranial hemorrhage and mass lesion.
- Other causes of hyperammonemia such as hepatic encephalopathy and inborn errors of metabolism should be considered.

Diagnostic Testing

Laboratories
- Obtain a **valproate concentration.** Therapeutic concentrations range from 50 to 10 mg/L. The valproate concentration should be **trended over time**, as delayed absorption and delayed excretion may occur in poisoning.

- Obtain a **complete metabolic panel** to assess for evidence of metabolic acidosis or hepatic injury.
- Obtain a **complete blood count**, as valproate poisoning has been associated with pancytopenia.
- Obtain an **ammonia concentration.**
  - Markedly elevated ammonia levels in a patient with encephalopathy or coma may suggest VHE.
  - Do not be alarmed by mild ammonia elevations in asymptomatic or minimally symptomatic patients.

TREATMENT

- Most patients will do well with cessation of valproate therapy and supportive care.
- Treat seizures with benzodiazepines or other directly GABAergic agents.
- Patients with VHE may benefit from **levocarnitine** therapy.
  - In patients who are critically ill (most hospitalized patients with VHE), levocarnitine should be administered IV: 100 mg/kg (up to 6 g) as a loading dose, followed by 15 mg/kg every 4 hours.
  - Levocarnitine therapy may be discontinued when the ammonia level has normalized and the patient is clinically improving.
- Therapy with **lactulose**, which is routinely used for the treatment of hepatic encephalopathy in cirrhosis, is **not thought to be effective** in VHE.
- **Hemodialysis** effectively clears valproate.
  - Hemodialysis is **recommended** in severe VPA poisoning when [VPA] is >1300 mg/L or when shock or cerebral edema is present.
  - Hemodialysis is **suggested** in severe VPA poisoning when [VPA] is >900 mg/L, coma or respiratory depression requiring mechanical ventilation is present, acute hyperammonemia is present, or the pH is <7.10.[12]

Carbamazepine and Oxcarbazepine

GENERAL PRINCIPLES

- Carbamazepine is an anticonvulsant that is structurally related to the tricyclic antidepressants (TCAs). It is also prescribed for trigeminal neuralgia and mood disorders.
- Oxcarbazepine is a prodrug that is converted to the active agent monohydroxy carbamazepine *in vivo*. The mechanism of action and toxicity of oxcarbazepine are generally similar to those of carbamazepine.

Pathophysiology

- Carbamazepine and oxcarbazepine exert their anticonvulsant effects via neuronal sodium channel blockade.
- Carbamazepine is structurally related to the TCAs.
- Carbamazepine is associated with the syndrome of inappropriate antidiuretic hormone release (SIADH).

Risk Factors

Coadministration of xenobiotics that inhibit the cytochrome P450 system (especially CYP 1A2, 2C8, 2C9, and 3A4) impairs the metabolism of carbamazepine and may lead to toxicity.

DIAGNOSIS

Clinical Presentation

- Patients with carbamazepine or oxcarbazepine poisoning present with tremor, nystagmus, ataxia, sedation, altered sensorium, or coma.
- Carbamazepine or oxcarbazepine poisoning may produce seizures in overdose.
- Carbamazepine produces **antimuscarinic** effects, including tachycardia, mydriasis, urinary retention, and delirium.
- The antimuscarinic effects of carbamazepine slow GI transit. Carbamazepine undergoes enterohepatic recirculation. This combined with active metabolites may create a "cyclical coma."
  In severe cases, **bradycardia and hypotension** may occur, due to direct myocardial toxicity.

Differential Diagnosis

- Carbamazepine poisoning is similar to poisoning by other anticonvulsants, including phenytoin, valproate, and lamotrigine.
  The antimuscarinic and cardiotoxic effects of carbamazepine are generally not seen in poisoning by other antidepressants.
- Other antimuscarinic xenobiotics (e.g., TCAs, first-generation antihistamines, and botanical toxins) generally do not produce cerebellar signs, which may help distinguish carbamazepine poisoning from other causes of the antimuscarinic toxidrome.
- The nontoxicologic differential diagnosis for carbamazepine poisoning should include Wernicke encephalopathy, meningoencephalitis, posterior circulation ischemic stroke, and intracranial hemorrhage and mass lesion.

Diagnostic Testing

Laboratories
- Obtain a **carbamazepine concentration.**
  ○ The therapeutic range is 4–12 mg/L.
  ○ Concentrations above 40 mg/L are associated with cardiotoxicity.[13]
  ○ The carbamazepine concentration should be **trended over time**, as delayed absorption and delayed excretion are common in poisoning.
- Obtain a **BMP** to evaluate for evidence of SIADH.

Electrocardiography
Obtain an ECG in all cases of known or suspected carbamazepine poisoning. In severe poisoning, carbamazepine prolongs the QRS complex and may cause atrioventricular conduction delays.

TREATMENT

- Treat seizures with benzodiazepines or other directly GABAergic agents.
- Patients with QRS prolongation should be treated with **sodium bicarbonate** as recommended in the discussion of TCAs below.
- **MDAC** enhances carbamazepine elimination and should be considered in patients without contraindication to AC.[14]
- **Hemodialysis** effectively clears carbamazepine.
  ○ **Recommended:** multiple seizures refractory to treatment or life-threatening dysrhythmias occur.
  ○ **Suggested:** prolonged coma or respiratory depression requiring mechanical ventilation is expected or failure of other therapies.

Other Anticonvulsants

See Table 28-5.

TABLE 28-5	Other Anticonvulsants			
	Mechanism of Action	Potential Effects in Overdose	Potential Treatments	Comments
Gabapentin	Ca^{2+} channel inhibition ($\alpha2$-δ subunit)	Sedation, ataxia, myoclonus	Supportive	Wide therapeutic index
Lamotrigine	Na^+ channel inhibition	Sedation, seizures, QRS prolongation	Supportive, benzodiazepines (seizures), sodium bicarbonate (QRS prolongation)	Long delay to reach steady state (esp. w/ VPA)
Lacosamide	(Slow) Na^+ channel inhibition	Sedation, ataxia	Supportive, benzodiazepines (seizures), sodium bicarbonate (QRS prolongation)	Excreted unchanged, attractive d/t lack of CYP interactions
Levetiracetam	Modulation of neurotransmitter release binding to SV2A	Sedation, bradycardia	Supportive	Limited data in overdose, significant toxicity reported at high levels 300–400 µg/mL
Topiramate	Na^+ and Ca^{2+} channel inhibition, AMPA/kainate inhibition	Sedation, ataxia, myoclonus, seizures	Supportive care, hemodialysis in severe poisoning	Impairs renal carbonic anhydrase → hyperchloremic metabolic acidosis
Zonisamide	Na^+ and T-type Ca^{2+} channel inhibition	Sedation, possible: hypotension, QRS prolongation, seizures	Supportive, benzodiazepines (seizures), sodium bicarbonate (QRS prolongation)	Severe toxicity in large overdoses reported (>4 g)

CHAPTER 28

PSYCHOTROPICS

Selective Serotonin Reuptake Inhibitors

GENERAL PRINCIPLES

- The selective serotonin reuptake inhibitors (SSRIs) are widely prescribed for major depressive disorder, anxiety disorders, posttraumatic stress disorder, and other psychiatric conditions.
- The SSRIs have generally supplanted older antidepressants as first-line agents in depression due to their safety profile in therapeutic use and overdose.
- Most SSRIs have similar pharmacologic and toxicologic profiles, with two important exceptions:
  - **Citalopram** is more dangerous in overdose than other SSRIs. Citalopram poisoning tends to produce more cardiotoxicity (QRS and QT prolongation) and seizures than poisoning by other SSRIs.
  - **Fluoxetine** has active metabolites and a very long half-life. Initiation of other serotonergic medications (especially MAO inhibitors—see below) too soon after fluoxetine discontinuation carries a risk of serotonin syndrome (see below).

Pathophysiology

The SSRIs inhibit serotonin reuptake via the SERT transporter on the presynaptic neuron terminal, thus increasing the amount and persistence of serotonin in the synaptic cleft and enhancing serotonergic signaling.

Unlike other antidepressants, the SSRIs have limited effects on any other receptor, channel, or pump.

DIAGNOSIS

Clinical Presentation

- Patients with poisoning due to SSRIs are generally well-appearing and minimally symptomatic. Patients may complain of GI upset and "shakiness."
- Patients with moderate toxicity may develop mild tachycardia, somnolence, and vomiting.
- Rare patients with severe toxicity may develop dysrhythmias and seizures.
- The development of serotonin syndrome following an acute overdose of a single serotonergic agent is uncommon but possible. Patients with SSRI poisoning should be assessed for evidence of serotonin excess (see below).

Diagnostic Testing

Electrocardiography
- The ECG will typically be unremarkable or demonstrate sinus tachycardia.
- SSRIs may prolong the QT interval in therapeutic use or overdose.
- Citalopram may prolong the QRS interval in significant overdose.

TREATMENT

- The vast majority of patients with SSRI poisoning **do not require medical interventions.**

- Patients with evidence of significant QT prolongation may benefit from observation on telemetry, supplementation of potassium and magnesium to normal levels, and avoidance of other QT prolonging agents.
  In the uncommon event that torsades de pointes does develop, treat as usual with magnesium and chemical or electrical overdrive pacing.
- Patients with QRS prolongation due to citalopram poisoning should be treated with **sodium bicarbonate** (see the discussion of TCAs below).
- Treat seizures with benzodiazepines or other directly GABAergic agents.
- Patients with evidence of serotonin excess should be treated as discussed below.

Serotonin Syndrome

GENERAL PRINCIPLES

- Serotonin syndrome is a clinical condition of neuromuscular abnormalities, mental status changes, and hyperthermia in patients exposed to serotonergic xenobiotics.
- Serotonin syndrome is a **spectrum of disease** that ranges from mild to life-threatening.[15]
  - Some authors prefer the term "serotonin toxicity" or "serotonin excess" for all but the sickest patients.
  - Mild serotonin excess may not require any treatment or medical evaluation.
- Serotonin syndrome classically develops when two or more serotonergic xenobiotics are coadministered, but it may also occur following an acute overdose of one or more serotonergic xenobiotics, dose titration of serotonergic xenobiotics, and initiation of therapy with a single serotonergic xenobiotic.

Pathophysiology

- Serotonin syndrome is thought to occur due to excessive stimulation of $5HT_1$ and $5HT_2$ receptors.
- Many classes of xenobiotics have been implicated in the development of the serotonin syndrome.
  - **Psychotropics**: SSRIs, TCAs, serotonin–norepinephrine reuptake inhibitors (SNRIs), MAO inhibitors, other atypical serotonergic antidepressants, bupropion, lithium, amphetamines, certain atypical antipsychotics
  - **Opioids:** meperidine, tramadol, dextromethorphan, and possibly fentanyl
  - **Other pharmaceuticals:** linezolid, triptans, valproate, lamotrigine, bromocriptine, methylene blue
  - **Recreational drugs:** methamphetamine and other amphetamines, cocaine, serotonergic hallucinogens (MDMA, psilocybin, tryptamine derivatives)

DIAGNOSIS

Clinical Presentation

History
- Consider serotonin syndrome in any patient who has been exposed to one or more serotonergic xenobiotics who presents with mental status changes, anxiety, tremulousness, GI upset, or abnormal extremity tone or movements.
- The onset of serotonin syndrome is typically very rapid (on the order of hours) following the culprit exposure. Delayed-onset serotonin syndrome generally does not occur.

Physical Examination
- Patients may present with mental status changes, neuromuscular abnormalities, and/or other serotonergic signs.
- Mental status changes may range from anxiety to coma.
- The neuromuscular abnormalities of serotonin syndrome typically consist of **hyperreflexia, tremor, and clonus.**
  - These findings are **predominantly in the lower extremities.** Prominent upper extremity findings should prompt consideration of an alternative diagnosis.
  - The "rigidity" of serotonin syndrome is due to profound hypertonia; the examiner will generally be able to passively range the patient's extremities with significant effort. Complete unmovable "lead-pipe" rigidity is not consistent with serotonin syndrome.
- Other serotonergic signs, such as **mydriasis, diaphoresis, flushing, shivering, and vomiting or diarrhea**, may also be present.[15]
- The presence of **hyperthermia** is a late and ominous sign and indicates severe serotonin syndrome. The absence of hyperthermia should never be used to rule out serotonin syndrome.

Differential Diagnosis
- The toxicologic differential diagnosis of serotonin syndrome includes neuroleptic malignant syndrome (NMS), malignant hyperthermia, alcohol or sedative-hypnotic withdrawal, sympathomimetic intoxication, and the antimuscarinic toxidrome.
  - The most important distinguishing factor is the **exposure history.**
  - NMS typically presents with lead-pipe rigidity of all four extremities and bradykinesia with subacute onset, over the course of days.
- The nontoxicologic differential diagnosis of serotonin syndrome includes sepsis of any source (especially in older patients), meningitis and encephalitis, thyrotoxicosis, and carcinoid syndrome.

Diagnostic Testing
Laboratories
- Laboratory testing is not routinely indicated in mild cases.
- In moderate or severe cases, laboratory testing may be helpful:
  - **BMP** and/or **blood gas** to evaluate for acidosis
  - **Creatinine kinase** to evaluate for rhabdomyolysis.
- Laboratory testing may be helpful in questionable cases to evaluate for alternative causes of symptoms, for example, CSF (cerebrospinal fluid) studies to rule out meningitis.

TREATMENT

- The first principle of treatment is to **discontinue the offending agent(s)** and avoid all serotonergic xenobiotics.
- **Benzodiazepines** and other directly GABAergic sedatives should be used liberally to treat psychomotor agitation and neuromuscular hyperexcitation.
  - Heat generation in serotonin syndrome is entirely peripheral; aggressive control of neuromuscular abnormalities and agitation prevents progress to life-threatening hyperthermia.
  - The goal of treatment is for the patient to be resting comfortably with normal neuromuscular tone and improving vital signs.

- In severe cases, intubation and deep sedation may be necessary to achieve this goal. **Paralysis** with nondepolarizing neuromuscular blocking agents may be used as a last resort if muscular rigidity is refractory to deep sedation.
- Patients with any **hyperthermia** should be rapidly and aggressively cooled in addition to appropriate sedation as above.
  - The most effective external cooling method is evaporative cooling—spray the patient with water and circulate air over them with large fans.
  - If evaporative cooling is unavailable, consider immersion in an ice water bath.
  - Antipyretic medications are **not effective.**
- Patients with **mild to moderate symptoms** may benefit from **cyproheptadine.** Cyproheptadine has no role in the treatment of patients with severe serotonin syndrome or patients who are critically ill.

Tricyclic Antidepressants

GENERAL PRINCIPLES

- TCAs have fallen out of favor as first-line treatment for major depressive disorder due to their significant toxicity in overdose.
- TCAs are still prescribed for depression as second-line agents and are also utilized for migraine prophylaxis, neuropathic pain, sleep, and pruritus.
- A number of other medications are structurally homologous to the TCAs and have similar effects in overdose: diphenhydramine and other first-generation antihistamines, cyclobenzaprine (does not cause cardiac toxicity or seizure in overdose), carbamazepine (cerebellar dysfunction also present in overdose).

Pathophysiology

TCAs antagonize a wide variety of receptors, ion channels, and pumps in overdose. Their actions on these molecular targets predict their clinical effects.
- **Serotonin and norepinephrine reuptake pumps:** may contribute to the development of serotonin syndrome
- **Cardiac sodium channel:** QRS prolongation, ventricular dysrhythmias, cardiogenic shock
- **IKr potassium channel:** QT interval prolongation
- **Muscarinic acetylcholine receptor:** antimuscarinic toxidrome
- **H1 histamine receptor:** somnolence
- **Alpha-1 adrenoceptor:** peripheral vasodilation, hypotension, tachycardia
- **GABA-A receptor:** seizures

DIAGNOSIS

Clinical Presentation

- Onset of toxicity is **rapid**—patients typically become ill within 1–4 hours of ingestion, and onset of toxicity after 6 hours is very rare. **Recovery** is also typically rapid (usually within 24 hours unless hypoxic end-organ injury has occurred).
- **Tachycardia** is invariably present unless there are co-ingestants that depress the heart rate, or the patient is moribund.
- Physical examination will demonstrate evidence of the antimuscarinic toxidrome: delirium, mydriasis (may be absent early in the clinical course), dry mucous membranes, anhidrosis, absent bowel sounds, and urinary retention.

CHAPTER 28

- **Seizures** are common in severe poisoning.
- **Hypotension, dysrhythmias,** shock, and cardiac arrest may occur.

Diagnostic Testing

Laboratories
- Serum TCA concentrations have no role in the management of acute TCA poisoning because they are not predictive of severity of illness.
- Obtain serial **blood gases and electrolytes** in patients treated with sodium bicarbonate (see below).

Electrocardiography
Electrocardiography is an essential tool in the risk-stratification of patients with TCA poisoning.
- A QRS interval of <100 ms suggests that the patient is not at risk of seizures or ventricular dysrhythmias.
- A QRS interval ≥100 ms—or, in patients with preexisting QRS prolongation due to conduction system disease, a significant increase in the QRS duration—indicates risk of seizures and/or dysrhythmias.[16]
- An RSR' pattern in aVR also predicts significant toxicity.[17]

TREATMENT

- The mainstay of treatment is **sodium bicarbonate.**
  - Sodium bicarbonate is indicated in patients with QRS > 100, seizures, dysrhythmias, or shock.
  - Sodium bicarbonate provides a **sodium load** to overwhelm cardiac sodium channel blockade, and also provides **alkalinization**, which may reduce TCA binding to cardiac sodium channels.
  - Sodium bicarbonate should be administered as a bolus or series of boluses of 1–2 mEq/kg, titrated rapidly to effect, followed by an infusion at twice the maintenance rate.
    - The goal is to **narrow the QRS to <100 ms** (or to the patient's baseline) and reverse shock.
    - **Avoid severe alkalemia** (pH > 7.55); if alkalemia becomes problematic and further treatment is required, **hypertonic saline** may be used.
- Treat **seizures** with **benzodiazepines** or other directly GABAergic agents.
- Patients with **shock or dysrhythmias** that do not immediately improve with sodium bicarbonate may benefit from additional interventions:
  - **Norepinephrine** and vasopressin may be used for hypotension that is unresponsive to sodium bicarbonate.
  - **Lidocaine** may be used for refractory shock or dysrhythmias at usual cardiac doses; this is thought to displace the TCA from the cardiac sodium channel.
  - **Intravenous lipid emulsion** (bolus of 1.5 cc/kg, max 100 cc, followed by infusion of 0.25 cc/kg/min ×20 minutes) may also be considered in patients with refractory shock or dysrhythmias.
- **Intubation and mechanical ventilation** is frequently necessary in critically ill TCA-poisoned patients with profound encephalopathy or repeated seizures.
- **VA ECMO** may be considered as a last resort for patients with refractory cardiovascular collapse.

Monoamine Oxidase Inhibitors

GENERAL PRINCIPLES

- Monoamine oxidase inhibitors (MAOIs) were the first class of effective antidepressants. They have fallen out of widespread use due to their numerous drug and food interactions and extreme toxicity in overdose.
- MAOIs may still be prescribed for treatment-resistant depression; one MAOI, selegiline, is used in the treatment of Parkinson disease.

Pathophysiology

- Monoamine oxidase is an enzyme responsible for the inactivation of biogenic amines such as epinephrine, norepinephrine, tyramine, dopamine, and serotonin. Inhibition of this enzyme results in an increase of synaptic concentrations of biogenic amines.
- As MAOIs affect an enzymatic pathway, there may be a **significant delay** in the development of toxicity after overdose.
- The duration of action of the MAOIs (especially the older irreversible inhibitors) **significantly exceeds their half-life.** A long washout period is necessary before other antidepressants can be safely administered.

DIAGNOSIS

Clinical Presentation

- **Acute overdose** of an MAOI initially produces a **sympathomimetic toxidrome**, with tachycardia, hypertension, diaphoresis, mydriasis, and agitation.
  - Onset of toxicity may be delayed for **24 hours or more after overdose.**[18]
  - **Hyperthermia, seizures,** and intracranial hemorrhage may occur in severe cases.
  - The excitatory phase may be followed by **coma and refractory cardiovascular collapse** if complete monoamine depletion occurs.
- Coadministration of **any serotonergic, dopaminergic, or adrenergic xenobiotic** with an MAOI (including **after discontinuation of the MAOI**) may precipitate a sympathomimetic crisis or serotonin syndrome.
- Consumption of foods rich in **tyramine** (aged cheeses, red wine, cured meats) while taking a MAOI may precipitate a **hypertensive crisis.**

Diagnostic Testing

Laboratories
- Obtain a **BMP** to evaluate for acidosis, hyperkalemia, and renal failure.
- Obtain a **creatinine kinase** to evaluate for rhabdomyolysis.
- Obtain **serial troponins** to evaluate for myocardial infarction.
- Obtain **coagulation studies** to evaluate for disseminated intravascular coagulation in severe cases.

Electrocardiography
Electrocardiography may demonstrate sinus tachycardia, evidence of myocardial ischemia, or ventricular dysrhythmias.

Imaging
Computed tomography of the brain should be obtained on any patient with MAOI poisoning who has an altered mental status or complains of a headache to evaluate for intracranial hemorrhage.

TREATMENT

- Strongly consider aggressive GI decontamination.
- Treat hypertension with **short-acting, titratable parenteral agents** (e.g., nicardipine, clevidipine, or nitroglycerin) given the risk of rapid fluctuations in blood pressure.
- **Avoid beta blockers (BBs)** due to the theoretical risk of unopposed alpha-adrenergic stimulation.
- Treat agitation and seizures with **benzodiazepines** or other directly GABAergic sedatives.

Lithium

GENERAL PRINCIPLES

Lithium is a mood stabilizer that is used in the management of bipolar disorder and other psychiatric disorders.

Pathophysiology
- The mechanism of action of lithium is poorly understood. Lithium is believed to enhance serotonergic signaling and has been implicated in cases of serotonin syndrome.
- Lithium has a narrow therapeutic index; many cases of lithium poisoning are accidental. Lithium is **exclusively renally cleared;** any impairment in renal function will lead to lithium accumulation and potentially to toxicity.
- Lithium poisoning primarily affects the central nervous system.
- Lithium may also cause nephrogenic diabetes insipidus, hypothyroidism, and in rare cases cardiotoxicity.
- Lithium follows multicompartment kinetics. Chronic and acute-on-chronic lithium poisoning are generally more dangerous than acute lithium poisoning because of the accumulation of lithium in the tissue compartment.[19]

DIAGNOSIS

Clinical Presentation
- Patients with an **acute overdose** (either acute or acute-on-chronic) of lithium will invariably present with GI upset, as lithium salts are very irritating to the mucosa of the GI tract.
  - This feature will be **absent** in **chronic lithium poisoning**, which occurs without a single acute overdose.
  - Profound GI volume losses may lead to hypovolemic shock.
- It is common for **chronic poisoning** to be provoked by a drop in the GFR due to a GI illness, decreased oral intake, or nephrotoxic medications.

- Lithium poisoning of any etiology may cause **neurotoxicity;** there is a wide spectrum of disease.
  - Mental status changes may range from subtle cognitive impairment to coma. When delirium occurs, it is typically **hypoactive.**
  - **Signs of cerebellar dysfunction**, including nystagmus, dysmetria, and ataxia, may be seen.
  - Peripheral neuromuscular abnormalities, including **hyperreflexia, clonus, rigidity, and tongue fasciculations**, also occur.
- In **acute overdose**, there is usually **delayed development of neurotoxicity.** In **chronic poisoning**, neurotoxicity may be the presenting complaints.
- It is common for the resolution of the clinical signs and symptoms of lithium poisoning to **lag behind the serum lithium concentration,** sometimes by days.

Diagnostic Testing
Laboratories
- Obtain a **serum lithium concentration.**
  - The therapeutic range is approximately 0.6–1.2 mmol/L.
  - Have a low threshold to check a lithium concentration in **any** patient taking lithium, given the narrow therapeutic index.
  - In poisoned patients, the lithium concentration should be **trended over time** to demonstrate clearance; additionally, in acute overdose, absorption may be delayed.
  - The lithium concentration must be checked on blood that has **not come into contact with a lithium-containing sample tube.**
- Obtain a **BMP** to evaluate renal function and assess for hyponatremia (which will impair lithium excretion) or hypernatremia (which should raise concern for diabetes insipidus).
  Significantly elevated lithium concentrations may produce a **low anion gap,** as lithium is an unmeasured cation.

Electrocardiography
The ECG may show nonspecific T-wave flattening or inversion or QT_c prolongation; however, cardiac dysfunction is unusual in this overdose.

TREATMENT

- **AC does not bind to lithium.** If GI decontamination is desired, WBI is the technique of choice. WBI may be appropriate in patients who present after ingestion a large amount of extended-release lithium preparations.
- The mainstay of treatment is **hyperhydration** to promote lithium excretion.
  - Patients with clinical or laboratory evidence of hypovolemia should be appropriately resuscitated with intravenous crystalloid.
  - All patients with lithium poisoning should be hydrated with **normal saline at 1.5-2× maintenance rate.**
    - Hypotonic fluids may promote lithium retention and should be avoided.
    - Generally, hyperhydration may be stopped when the lithium concentration is in the therapeutic range and the patient is clinically improved.
- Hemodialysis may be reasonable in cases of severe neurologic toxicity such as coma or seizures (especially in chronic poisoning), very high lithium concentrations (generally >5 mmol/L or >4 mmol/L in the presence of renal impairment), or the

failure of standard measures to rapidly (<1 mmol/L within 36 h) reduce the lithium concentration.[20]

- ○ Local practice patterns vary considerably, and early consultation with a medical toxicologist (or poison control center) and a nephrologist is reasonable.
- ○ If hemodialysis is performed, patients should be monitored for **rebound in serum lithium concentration** due to redistribution of lithium from tissue stores.

Antipsychotics

GENERAL PRINCIPLES

Pathophysiology

- Antipsychotic agents exert their therapeutic effect largely by antagonizing dopamine receptors in the central nervous system. Newer antipsychotic agents also modulate serotonergic tone.
  - ○ Dopamine antagonism unbalanced by muscarinic antagonism leads to extrapyramidal neuromuscular effects, such as acute dystonia, torticollis, oculogyric crisis, drug-induced Parkinsonism, and tardive dyskinesia.
  - ○ Generally speaking, the atypical or second-generation antipsychotics have significant antimuscarinic effects that mitigate (but do not eliminate) the risk of extrapyramidal symptoms.
  - ○ Dopamine antagonism in the tuberoinfundibular system may lead to gynecomastia and galactorrhea; risperidone is particularly problematic in this regard.
- The antipsychotics also have several well-known "off-target" effects on other receptors and ion channels that are relevant in therapeutic use and overdose.
  - ○ Muscarinic antagonism may produce sedation and an antimuscarinic toxidrome in overdose. Quetiapine is particularly antimuscarinic.
  - ○ Alpha-1 adrenoceptor antagonism may produce orthostasis and reflex tachycardia.
  - ○ Blockade of the cardiac sodium and potassium channels may produce prolongation of the QRS and QT intervals and predispose to dysrhythmias.
- Although each antipsychotic has its own unique pharmacologic profile, in general, first-generation agents (neuroleptics, e.g., haloperidol, droperidol, chlorpromazine) cause more cardiac toxicity and extrapyramidal symptoms than second-generation agents (atypicals, e.g., quetiapine, olanzapine, risperidone).
- Clozapine has unique adverse effects, including profound sialorrhea and agranulocytosis. Its use is closely monitored and restricted.

DIAGNOSIS

Clinical Presentation

- The predominant feature of an **acute antipsychotic overdose** is profound sedation.
- Other features of acute toxicity depend on the pharmacologic profile of the agent involved (Table 28-6): for example, quetiapine overdose will produce an antimuscarinic toxidrome.
- **Extrapyramidal symptoms** usually develop after therapeutic use, typically (although not invariably) following initiation or dose escalation.
  - ○ **Acute dystonia** may cause spasm of any muscle group, including the neck (torticollis) or extraocular muscles (oculogyric crisis). It may be life-threatening when it involves the laryngeal musculature.

TABLE 28-6	Effects of Selected Antipsychotics				
		I_{Na} Sodium Channel Anatagonism (QRS Prolongation)	I_{kr} Antagonism (QT Prolongation)	α_1 Anatgonism (Hypotension)	Muscarinic Antagonism (Anticholinergic Toxidrome)
Typical Antipsychotics	Haloperidol	↔	↑	N/A	N/A
	Fluphenazine	↔	↔	N/A	N/A
	Loxapine	↑	↔	↑↑	↑
	Chlorpromazine	↑	↑	↑↑	↑
	Pimozide	↔	↑	↔	N/A
Atypical Antipsychotics	Risperidone	N/A	N/A	↑	N/A
	Olanzapine	N/A	N/A	↑	↑↑
	Quetiapine	↔	↔	↑↑	↑↑
	Aripiprazole	N/A	N/A	↑	N/A
	Lurasidone	N/A	N/A	↔	N/A
	Ziprasidone	N/A	↑↑	↑	N/A
	Clozapine	N/A	↔	↑↑	↑↑

N/A, no significant effect in therapeutic dosing; ↔, may have effect in supratherapeutic dosing/overdose; ↑, antagonism; ↑↑, substantial antagonism.

○ **Akathisia** is a clinical syndrome of restlessness, anxiety, psychomotor agitation, and a compulsion to move.
○ **Drug-induced Parkinsonism** presents with bradykinesia and rigidity.
○ **Tardive dyskinesia**, a pattern of stereotyped movements of the lips, face, and tongue, usually develops later (sometimes after years of therapy) and may be irreversible.

Diagnostic Testing
Laboratories
Routine laboratory testing is not generally helpful.
Target laboratory testing based on the patient's clinical presentation and the agent ingested.

Electrocardiography
• All antipsychotics **prolong the QT interval**; the degree of prolongation varies among the available agents.
• Some antipsychotics, including first-generation agents and quetiapine, may **prolong the QRS interval** in overdose. The most problematic agents have been withdrawn from the market.

TREATMENT

• Treatment of acute overdose is generally supportive and symptom-targeted.
○ Intubation and mechanical ventilation are not typically required.
○ Treat seizures with **benzodiazepines** or other directly GABAergic agents.
○ Hypotension is unusual; if it occurs, treat with fluid resuscitation and vasopressors.
• In patients with **QT prolongation**, supplement magnesium, potassium, and calcium, and avoid other QT prolonging agents. If **torsades de pointes** develops, magnesium or overdrive pacing may be required.
• In patients with **QRS prolongation**, administer sodium bicarbonate as discussed above under tricyclic antidepressant poisoning.
• Treat **extrapyramidal symptoms** with **antimuscarinic agents**, typically diphenhydramine or benztropine.
○ Patients who require continued therapy with antipsychotics may require initiation of scheduled antimuscarinic agents to prevent extrapyramidal symptoms.
○ Tardive dyskinesia may be resistant to treatment.

SPECIAL CONSIDERATIONS: NEUROLEPTIC MALIGNANT SYNDROME

• NMS is a severe, life-threatening adverse effect of antipsychotics that is thought to be mediated by dopamine antagonism. NMS is **rare.**
• NMS may occur with exposure to any antipsychotic agent, not just with first-generation antipsychotics.
• The onset of NMS is **subacute** (over a period of days). It typically (but not exclusively) occurs in the days to weeks following the initiation of an antipsychotic.
• NMS classically presents with a triad of mental status changes, neuromuscular abnormalities, and hyperthermia.
○ Mental status changes may range from mild delirium to coma and catatonia
○ Neuromuscular symptoms typically consist of "lead-pipe" rigidity involving all four extremities and bradykinesia.

- Hyperthermia is a late finding and may be accompanied by profound autonomic instability.
- The most important principle of management is to **stop the offending agent** and avoid all antidopaminergic xenobiotics.
- **Aggressive resuscitative care** in the intensive care unit is required.
  - Administer **benzodiazepines** or other directly GABAergic sedatives with the goal of eliminating agitation (if present) and improving neuromuscular rigidity. In extreme cases, **paralysis** with nondepolarizing neuromuscular blockers may be required to control rigidity.
  - If hyperthermia is present, **aggressive external cooling** must be pursued.
  - Monitor for and treat **rhabdomyolysis** and electrolyte derangements.
- The role of putative antidotes such as bromocriptine (a dopamine receptor agonist) or dantrolene is **controversial** and their efficacy is unproven.

CARDIOVASCULAR AGENTS

Beta Blockers and Calcium Channel Antagonists

GENERAL PRINCIPLES

Beta-adrenergic antagonists (beta blockers, BBs) and calcium channel antagonists (CCAs) are widely prescribed for hypertension, atrial fibrillation and other dysrhythmias, and noncardiac indications such as essential tremor, migraine prophylaxis, Raynaud's, and situational anxiety.

Pathophysiology

- BBs antagonize beta-adrenergic receptors in the myocardium and pacemaker system, producing decreased chronotropy and inotropy.
  - **Sotalol** has BB activity and is also an IKr antagonist (class III antidysrhythmic). In overdose, it produces QT prolongation and bradycardia, which creates a high risk for torsades de pointes.
  - **Propranolol** has cardiac sodium channel antagonist properties in overdose and is also lipophilic enough to cross the blood–brain barrier and produce mental status changes and seizures in overdose.
- CCAs inhibit the entry of calcium into cells.
  - The **non-dihydropyridine** CCAs (diltiazem, verapamil) act primarily on cardiac myocytes and cells of the pacemaker system, producing decreased chronotropy and inotropy.
  - The **dihydropyridine** CCAs (amlodipine, nifedipine) act primarily on peripheral vascular smooth muscle, producing vasodilation.
  - In **significant overdose**, all CCAs lose channel selectivity and can affect all types of calcium channels.

DIAGNOSIS

Clinical Presentation

- The cardinal features of BB and CCA poisoning are **hypotension and bradycardia.** In certain cases of CCA poisoning in which vasodilation predominates, patients may initially present with a normal heart rate or tachycardia.

CHAPTER 28

• Mental status will typically be normal (even with profound shock) until late in the course of poisoning. This is not always true in the case of poisoning by **propranolol**, which is centrally active and may cause mental status changes or seizures.

Differential Diagnosis

Consider other conditions that may cause hypotension and bradycardia: digoxin/cardioactive steroid poisoning, sympatholytic poisoning, myxedema coma, hypothermia, high-grade heart block with cardiogenic shock, and shock with profound acidosis or hyperkalemia.

Diagnostic Testing

Laboratories
• **Blood glucose** may help distinguish BB from CCA poisoning: CCA poisoning tends to present with hyperglycemia, while BB poisoning typically presents with euglycemia or hypoglycemia.
• Obtain a **BMP** to assess for renal function and potassium, which have implications for the monitoring of some treatments for BB and CCA poisoning.

Electrocardiography
• All BBs and CCAs may produce sinus bradycardia and AV blocks.
• **Sotalol** will prolong the QT interval.
• **Propranolol** may prolong the QRS interval in overdose.

TREATMENT

• Mild poisoning may respond to **intravenous fluids** and **calcium.** If calcium is used as a primary treatment in moderate or severe cases, high doses may be required.
• BB poisoning, especially in mild cases, may respond to **glucagon.**
  ○ Large amounts of glucagon (typically 5–10 mg IV in an average adult patient) are required.
  ○ The duration of action of glucagon is very short. Patients responding to glucagon boluses should be started on a glucagon infusion (dosed at the effective bolus dose per hour, and titrated to effect).
  ○ Many hospitals do not stock enough glucagon for this indication.
  ○ Significant GI upset should be anticipated.
• Patients with significant toxicity should be treated with **vasopressors and/or high-dose insulin.**
  ○ **Vasopressors** may be more effective in patients with a predominantly vasodilatory phenotype (preserved ejection fraction, near-normal heart rate, profound systemic vasodilation).
    ▪ **Norepinephrine** and **vasopressin** are reasonable first-line agents; **epinephrine, phenylephrine,** and **dopamine** may also be added.
    ▪ Multiple agents at very high doses may be necessary.
  ○ **High-dose insulin** (also known as hyperinsulinemic-euglycemic therapy, HIET) may be more effective in patients with poor inotropy and chronotropy.[21]
    ▪ The initiation dose of HIET is a bolus of 1 unit/kg regular human insulin IV, followed by an infusion of 1–10 unit/kg/h. Onset of action may be delayed up to 20–30 minutes after initiation or rate changes.

- Aggressive dextrose supplementation and very frequent blood glucose checks are **mandatory** to avoid iatrogenic harm. Potassium should also be monitored closely. Patients with CCB poisoning may have profound insulin resistance and require little or no supplemental dextrose (frequent glucose checks still necessary).
  - In many cases, the **combination of vasopressors and HIET** is reasonable and effective.
- **Methylene blue** infusion (1–2 mg/kg/h) may reverse peripheral vasoplegia. Many hospitals do not stock enough methylene blue for this indication.
- **Intravenous lipid emulsion** (1.5 cc/kg bolus, max 100 cc, followed by infusion of 0.25 cc/kg/min for 20 minutes) may be considered for patients refractory to the above therapies.
- **VA ECMO** is effective and lifesaving in severe poisoning, although not without risks. Have a **low threshold** to transfer patients with significant poisoning to an ECMO-capable center.
- **Hemodialysis** may be used to enhance the elimination of select BBs only: nadolol, acebutolol, sotalol, and atenolol. It otherwise has **no role.**
- **Atropine** and **electrical pacing** are unlikely to be effective in significant poisoning.

Clonidine and Other Sympatholytics

GENERAL PRINCIPLES

- Clonidine belongs to the imidazoline class; these medications are also referred to as sympatholytics.
- Other commonly encountered members of this class include guanfacine, dexmedetomidine, tizanidine, and the topical nasal and ocular imidazolines (tetrahydrozoline, oxymetazoline, naphazoline, and brimonidine).

Pathophysiology

- Sympatholytics are centrally acting alpha-2 adrenergic agonists; they have a negative feedback effect on catecholamine release and thus decrease heart rate, blood pressure, and CNS excitation.
- Sympatholytics also interact with the less-understood imidazoline (I) receptor system; this system also has CNS depressant and antihypertensive actions.
- When used as intended, the topical nasal and ocular imidazolines act primarily as alpha-1 adrenergic agonists, and thus induce local vasoconstriction.
  In large overdose or when consumed by mouth, these agents act primarily as alpha-2 adrenergic agonists.
- Early in the course of sympatholytic poisoning, off-target effects on alpha-1 adrenoceptors may lead to peripheral vasoconstriction and transient hypertension.

DIAGNOSIS

Clinical Presentation

- Patients with sympatholytic poisoning present with **bradycardia**, normal or depressed **blood pressure**, **miosis**, and significantly **depressed mental status.**
  - Mental status changes in sympatholytic poisoning are usually characterized by **preserved response to physical stimulus** and a **waxing and waning course.**

CHAPTER 28

○ In severe poisoning, mental status depression may be profound enough to impair respiration, producing **apnea** or **ineffective respirations.**
• Onset of toxicity and recovery are typically **quite rapid.**

Differential Diagnosis

• In patients with bradycardia and hypotension, consider BB/CCA poisoning, digoxin/cardioactive steroid poisoning, myxedema coma, hypothermia, high-grade heart block with cardiogenic shock, and shock with profound acidosis or hyperkalemia.
• In patients with profound mental status depression, ineffective respirations, and miosis, consider **opioid** poisoning.

Diagnostic Testing
Laboratories
Routine laboratory testing is not usually helpful.

Electrocardiography
ECG will usually show sinus bradycardia.

TREATMENT

• In general, sympatholytic poisoning does not require treatment.
  ○ While striking, the bradycardia does not typically lead to profound hypotension or end-organ malperfusion.
  ○ The duration of sympatholytic poisoning is typically very short.
• **Atropine** will likely be effective in increasing the heart rate but is rarely truly indicated.
• In very severe cases, when effective respiration is impaired, **intubation and mechanical ventilation** may be necessary.
• Significant hypotension is unusual but will respond to low-dose norepinephrine.
• For patients with profound mental status changes, apnea, or hypotension, for whom critical care interventions such as intubation or vasopressors are being discussed, consider a trial of **high-dose naloxone.**[22]
  ○ A single dose of naloxone 10 mg IV may reverse sympatholytic poisoning.
    Repeated bolus doses or an infusion may be necessary due to the relatively short duration of action of intravenous naloxone.
  ○ Avoid high-dose naloxone in opioid-tolerant patients, in whom it may precipitate opioid withdrawal.

SPECIAL CONSIDERATIONS: SYMPATHOLYTIC WITHDRAWAL

• Patients who are chronically exposed to sympatholytics are at risk for **withdrawal** if sympatholytics are stopped abruptly.
  ○ The withdrawal syndrome consists of tachycardia, severe hypertension, and anxiety and agitation.
  ○ The profound "rebound hypertension" seen when patients miss a clonidine dose may represent early sympatholytic withdrawal.
  ○ Treat withdrawal by reinstituting sympatholytics and tapering them off gradually.
• Patients on **dexmedetomidine** infusions for sedation in the intensive care unit may develop sympatholytic dependence in as little as 72–96 hours.
  Clonidine tapers may be helpful in preventing withdrawal when dexmedetomidine is discontinued.

Other Antihypertensives

See Table 28-7.

TABLE 28-7	Other Antihypertensives			
	Mechanism of Action	Potential Effects in Overdose	Potential Treatments	Comments
Prazosin	α_1 adrenergic blockade	Sedation, postural hypotension	Supportive, IV fluids, vasopressin/phenylephrine/norepinephrine	May cause priapism
Hydralazine	Interferes with IP$_3$-mediated Ca^{2+} release from sarcoplasmic reticulum → arteriolar relaxation	Hypotension, tachycardia	Supportive, IV fluids, vasopressors	Myocardial ischemia reported in overdose
Minoxidil	ATP-K$^+$ channel opening, NO-mediated vasodilation	Hypotension, tachycardia	Supportive, IV fluids, vasopressors	Myocardial ischemia reported in overdose, direct myocardial toxicity in animal models
Nitroprusside	NO-mediated vasodilation	Hypotension, tachycardia, thiocyanate/cyanide toxicity	Discontinue offending agent. Consider sodium thiosulfate or hydroxocobalamin	Thiocyanate toxicity may occur due to impaired renal clearance
Thiazide diuretics	Primarily by inhibition of NaCl cotransporter in distal convoluted tubule	Altered mental status, hypotension, electrolyte abnormalities, hyperuricemia, hyperglycemia	Supportive (correction of electrolytes, volume status)	

CHAPTER 28

(continued)

TABLE 28-7	Other Antihypertensives (*continued*)			
	Mechanism of Action	Potential Effects in Overdose	Potential Treatments	Comments
Loop diuretics	Primarily by inhibition of Na-K-2Cl cotransporter in ascending loop of Henle	Altered mental status, hypotension, electrolyte abnormalities (hypokalemia, hypomagnesemia), ototoxicity		
K+ sparing diuretics	Aldosterone antagonists (spironolactone)/inhibition of epithelial sodium channel in collecting tubule (amiloride, triamterene)	Altered mental status, hypotension, electrolyte abnormalities (hyperkalemia)		
ACE inhibitors	Inhibition of angiotensin converting enzyme	Sedation, hypotension	Supportive, IV fluids, vasopressors	Reports of success using angiotensin II in ACE-I overdose. Reports of success in using methylene blue with cardiogenic shock
ARBs	Inhibition of angiotensin type 1 receptor			

Digoxin

GENERAL PRINCIPLES

- Digoxin is a cardioactive steroid that was previously used in the treatment of CHF and arrhythmias (typically refractory atrial fibrillation).
- Other cardioactive steroids with digoxin-like effects are found in many plants and animals, including foxglove, red squill, oleander, and the *Bufo* toad.

Pathophysiology

- Digoxin inhibits the sodium/potassium ATPase pump, producing a rise in the intracellular sodium concentration that indirectly leads to an increase in the intracellular calcium concentration.

- The overall effect of digoxin is thus to enhance vagal tone (therefore suppressing conduction of atrial impulses to the ventricles), increase cardiac excitability (which predisposes to arrhythmias), and enhance inotropy.
- Unfortunately, digoxin has a **very narrow therapeutic index**, and accidental poisoning is relatively common, especially in patients with fluctuating renal function.

DIAGNOSIS

Clinical Presentation

- Digoxin poisoning classically presents with **bradycardia, mental status changes, and GI upset.**
- Poisoning may occur after an acute overdose, but the more common scenario is chronic poisoning due to changes in renal function or pharmacokinetic interactions.

Diagnostic Testing

Laboratories

- Obtain a **serum digoxin concentration.** Have a low threshold to send this test in any patient taking or prescribed digoxin.
- Obtain a **BMP** to assess the potassium.
  - **Hyperkalemia** is a marker of severity in digoxin poisoning. In acute poisoning, a potassium over 5.0 mEq/L is an indication for antidote administration.[23]
  - **Hypokalemia** exaggerates the effects of digoxin and may lead to toxicity even at a therapeutic serum digoxin concentration.
  - Worsening **renal function** indicate a risk for digoxin toxicity, as digoxin is renally eliminated.

Electrocardiography

- Digoxin poisoning may cause essentially **any dysrhythmia** (with the exception of a conducted supraventricular tachycardia).
- Certain dysrhythmia patterns are particularly suggestive of digoxin poisoning:
  - Atrial fibrillation with a **slow** ventricular response
  - The combination of AV blocks and significant ectopy
  - Bidirectional ventricular tachycardia
- The "Salvador Dali mustache" sign (concave sloped ST segments) is an indicator of digoxin **effect, not poisoning.**

TREATMENT

- The treatment of choice for digoxin poisoning is **anti-digoxin Fab** (Digifab or Digibind), a monoclonal antibody fragment that binds digoxin.
  - Anti-digoxin Fab is indicated in the following circumstances:
    - Digoxin-related life-threatening dysrhythmia
    - Acute digoxin poisoning with K > 5.0 mEq/L[23]
    - Chronic digoxin poisoning with dysrhythmia or mental status changes
    - Digoxin concentration ≥15 ng/mL at any time or ≥10 ng/mL at 6 hours postingestion
    - Acute ingestion of ≥10 mg digoxin in an adult
  - The dosing of anti-digoxin Fab is controversial.
    - The classic approach (in accordance with the package insert) is to calculate the dose using the amount of digoxin ingested or the digoxin concentration, and to use very high doses for acute empiric treatment of critically ill patients.

CHAPTER 28

- Some experts advocate for the use of only 1–2 vials of anti-digoxin Fab in chronic toxicity.[24]
  ○ Do **not** recheck the serum digoxin concentration after the administration of anti-digoxin Fab; the test cannot distinguish between bound and unbound drug and is not clinically useful.
- Treatment of hyperkalemia in digoxin poisoning is controversial.
  ○ If hyperkalemia is being driven primarily by digoxin poisoning, it should resolve with administration of anti-digoxin Fab.
  ○ If hyperkalemia is due to renal failure or another etiology, usual hyperkalemia care may be necessary.
  ○ Some authors recommend avoiding administration of calcium salts to patients with digoxin poisoning; this is probably reasonable, but no high-quality data demonstrating harm exist.
- **Atropine** is a reasonable treatment for symptomatic bradycardia in digoxin poisoning, as digoxin directly enhances vagal tone.
  Atropine may be used to temporize patients while awaiting anti-digoxin Fab therapy, or it may be used as monotherapy in patients with isolated atropine-responsive bradycardia and no other indications for Fab.

SEDATIVE-HYPNOTICS

Benzodiazepines

GENERAL PRINCIPLES

- Benzodiazepines are widely used as sedatives, anxiolytics, hypnotics, and antiepileptics.
- Unfortunately, benzodiazepines are also widely misused and diverted.

Pathophysiology

- Benzodiazepines are positive allosteric modulators of the GABA-A chloride-channel linked receptor. Upon binding, they render the channel more likely to open in response to endogenous GABA binding.
  Benzodiazepines do **not** directly open the GABA-A chloride channel and are ineffective in the absence of GABA.
- Benzodiazepines generally have anxiolytic, sedative, hypnotic, and anticonvulsant properties.

DIAGNOSIS

Clinical Presentation

Acute overdose of **oral benzodiazepines without co-ingestants** produces sedation with normal vital signs and preserved respiration.
- Iatrogenic **parenteral** benzodiazepine overdose may produce respiratory depression.
- **Mixed overdoses** of benzodiazepines and other sedatives (especially opioids and ethanol) may produce respiratory depression.

TREATMENT

- Isolated benzodiazepine overdoses **rarely require treatment** beyond time and careful monitoring. **Mixed overdoses** involving benzodiazepines may produce respiratory depression requiring intubation and mechanical ventilation.

- **Flumazenil**, a benzodiazepine receptor antagonist, effectively reverses the effects of benzodiazepines, but is **rarely indicated** due to the relative safety of benzodiazepines in overdose.
  - **Avoid** flumazenil in patients with known or suspected benzodiazepine dependence, as it may precipitate withdrawal and seizures.
  - **Avoid** flumazenil in patients who have co-ingested agents that cause seizures.
  - **Consider** flumazenil for reversal of iatrogenic oversedation with benzodiazepines in benzodiazepine-naïve patients, or for treatment of patients with mixed ingestions including benzodiazepines with respiratory failure.
  - Flumazenil should be given at a low dose (typically 0.1 mg IV by slow push which may be repeated if necessary for titration to effect).

Barbiturates

GENERAL PRINCIPLES

- Barbiturates were once widely used as sedatives, anxiolytics, and hypnotics, but have generally been supplanted by the safer benzodiazepines.
- Barbiturates are still used in headache medications (Fioricet and Fiorinal), as anticonvulsants, in the treatment of alcohol withdrawal, and in certain limited circumstances for anesthesia and deep sedation.

Pathophysiology

- Barbiturates bind to the GABA-A receptor and directly induce opening of the chloride channel; this action is GABA-independent.
- Some barbiturates act as direct AMPA or NMDA glutamate antagonists.
- Barbiturates have anxiolytic, sedative, hypnotic, and anticonvulsant properties.

DIAGNOSIS

Clinical Presentation

- Barbiturate poisoning presents with coma, respiratory depression, and miosis.
- Hypotension and shock may occur in severe poisoning.
- Large cutaneous bullae called "barb blisters" may be present, especially when the patient has been down on a hard surface for a long period of time.

TREATMENT

- The mainstay of treatment is respiratory support, including intubation and mechanical ventilation in severe poisoning.
- If hypotension is present, treat with intravenous crystalloids and/or vasopressors.
- **MDAC** enhances the elimination of phenobarbital.[25]
  - Administer MDAC **only** to patients with a protected airway (either spontaneously protected or secured by intubation).
- **Urinary alkalinization** with sodium bicarbonate was historically recommended for phenobarbital poisoning, but its efficacy is unclear.
- **Hemodialysis** effectively clears barbiturates and may be considered if prolonged coma, fluid-refractory shock, or respiratory depression necessitating intubation is present. Hemodialysis may also be considered in patients who do not improve with MDAC.

CHAPTER 28

Other Sedatives

See Table 28-8.

TABLE 28-8	Other Sedatives		
Drug(s)	Description	Receptor Effects	Clinical Effects
Propofol	Sedative used for procedural sedation, anesthesia	GABA$_A$ agonist, NMDA antagonist	Deep sedation, short duration of action. Infusions >4–5 mg/kg/h >48 h may be associated with propofol-related infusion syndrome (rhabdomyolysis, cardiac dysrhythmias)
Etomidate	Short-acting sedative, primarily used as RSI induction agent	GABA$_A$ agonist	Deep sedation, short duration of action. Prolonged infusions may cause adrenal suppression
Meprobamate/ carisoprodol	Carbamate anxiolytic. Carisoprodol is metabolized to meprobamate	GABA$_A$ agonist	Profound sedation/coma possible in overdose. May cause myocardial depression
Chloral hydrate	Trichloroethanol metabolite has similar effects to ethanol at lower doses. Pediatric sedative (historical)	GABA$_A$ agonist	Deep sedation, variable elimination half-life. Myocardial sensitization to catecholamines; cardiac dysrhythmias possible
Zolpidem, eszopiclone, zaleplon	Non-benzodiazepine also binding at the benzodiazepine site. Decreases sleep latency. Used as sleep aid	GABA$_A$ agonist	Mild sedation. Respiratory depression rare in isolation
Ramelteon/ melatonin	Synthetic/natural melatonin analog. Used as sleep aid	Melatonin receptor (MT$_1$/MT$_2$) agonist	

SYMPATHOMIMETICS

Amphetamines

GENERAL PRINCIPLES

- Amphetamines and amphetamine derivatives are used medically in the treatment of attention-deficit hyperactivity disorderand to a lesser degree for narcolepsy and weight loss.
- Both pharmaceutical and nonpharmaceutical amphetamines and amphetamine derivatives are used for recreational purposes.

Pathophysiology

- Amphetamines induce the release of monoamine neurotransmitters (norepinephrine, serotonin, and dopamine) and inhibit their reuptake, creating an excitatory or sympathomimetic state.
- Amphetamines with oxygen or halogen substitutions, such as methylenedioxymethamphetamine (MDMA, "ecstasy"), tend to have more serotonergic effects.
- Methamphetamine is uniquely toxic and addictive. Its additional methyl group facilitates more rapid movement across the blood–brain barrier.
- Methamphetamine (and to a lesser degree other amphetamines) also cause a direct vasculopathy.

DIAGNOSIS

Clinical Presentation

- Amphetamine poisoning presents with the **sympathomimetic toxidrome** of tachycardia, hypertension, diaphoresis, hyperthermia, and mental status changes (ranging from anxiety to agitated delirium). This can cause **end-organ damage** including seizures, neurologic deficits from stroke or intracranial hemorrhage, or chest pain.
- Methamphetamine (and other amphetamines) may cause psychiatric derangements, including mania and psychosis. Methamphetamine-induced psychosis may **persist for weeks** after cessation of exposure.

Diagnostic Testing

Laboratories
- Urine drug testing is not useful in acute clinical management.
- Have a low threshold to obtain a **BMP, troponin,** and/or **creatinine kinase** to evaluate for end-organ damage, including renal injury, myocardial ischemia, and rhabdomyolysis.

Electrocardiography
Electrocardiography may demonstrate sinus tachycardia or ventricular dysrhythmias.

Imaging
- Imaging to evaluate for end-organ damage should be guided by the patient's complaints and physical examination.
  - Obtain **computed tomography of the brain** in patients with significant mental status changes or headache to evaluate for intracranial hemorrhage.
  - Obtain **computed tomography angiogram** of the chest in patients with chest pain that is clinically concerning for aortic dissection.

CHAPTER 28

TREATMENT

- The mainstay of treatment is **benzodiazepines** or other directly GABAergic sedatives, titrated to control of agitation and improvement of vital signs.
  Patients presenting with predominantly psychiatric symptoms (psychosis or mania) may benefit from **antipsychotics.**[26]
- Intravenous fluid resuscitation is reasonable and is mandatory in cases of rhabdomyolysis.
- Control of **blood pressure** and heart rate should be achieved by appropriate titration of benzodiazepines or other sedatives. When tight blood pressure control is required (e.g., aortic dissection, intracranial hemorrhage, acute MI), use agents that are rapidly titratable, such as nicardipine, clevidipine, or nitroglycerin.
- Patients with **hyperthermia** require aggressive external cooling in addition to aggressive sedation. **Paralysis** with nondepolarizing neuromuscular blockers may be required in severe cases.

Cocaine

GENERAL PRINCIPLES

- Cocaine was historically used as a topical vasoconstrictor and local anesthetic.
- Cocaine is used recreationally by a variety of routes—it may be insufflated, smoked, injected, or taken orally.

Pathophysiology

- Cocaine inhibits the reuptake of serotonin, norepinephrine, and dopamine, producing an excitatory or sympathomimetic state.
- Cocaine is also a local anesthetic with sodium channel antagonist properties and may produce cardiac conduction abnormalities.
- Cocaine is vasculotoxic, enhances platelet aggregation, and accelerates the development of atherosclerotic disease.[27]

DIAGNOSIS

Clinical Presentation

- Cocaine poisoning presents with a **sympathomimetic toxidrome** (see above, amphetamines). Cocaine may also cause choreoathetoid movements and psychomotor agitation.
- Patients may present with symptoms related to **end-organ damage** from the sympathomimetic toxidrome, including seizures, neurologic deficits from stroke or intracranial hemorrhage, or chest pain.
- The onset of action of cocaine by the usual routes of use is very rapid, and the duration of cocaine intoxication is typically short; symptoms due to cocaine intoxication should resolve within about 8 hours after use.

Diagnostic Testing
Laboratories
Have a low threshold to obtain a **BMP, troponin,** and/or **creatinine kinase** to evaluate for end-organ damage, including renal injury, myocardial ischemia, and rhabdomyolysis.

Electrocardiography
- Electrocardiography may demonstrate sinus tachycardia or ventricular dysrhythmias and may show ischemic changes in the ST segments or T waves.
- Cocaine may prolong the QRS complex or induce or unmask a Brugada-like pattern.[28]

TREATMENT

- The mainstay of treatment is **benzodiazepines** or other directly GABAergic sedatives, titrated to control of agitation and improvement of vital signs.
- Intravenous fluid resuscitation is necessary in cases of rhabdomyolysis.
- Patients with evidence of sodium channel blockade (QRS prolongation on ECG) should be treated with **sodium bicarbonate** (bolus of 1–2 mEq/kg followed by infusion, with the goal of normalizing the QRS duration).
- Management of **chest pain** and myocardial infarction may be complex.
  - Cocaine intoxication may cause **coronary vasospasm** leading to chest pain and myocardial infarction; this should be treated with benzodiazepines.[27]
  - Patients who use cocaine are **also** at risk of **type I myocardial infarction** due to accelerated atherogenesis and platelet adhesion.
    If this occurs, usual treatment with antiplatelet agents, anticoagulants, and potentially cardiac catheterization should be pursued.
  - Close discussion with a cardiologist is warranted if objective evidence of myocardial ischemia is present.
- Control of **blood pressure** and heart rate should be achieved by appropriate titration of benzodiazepines or other sedatives. When tight blood pressure control is required (e.g., aortic dissection, intracranial hemorrhage, acute MI), use agents that are rapidly titratable, such as nicardipine, clevidipine, or nitroglycerin. Consider avoiding beta-adrenergic antagonists due to a theoretical concern that "unopposed alpha" stimulation could cause severe peripheral vasospasm.
- Patients with **hyperthermia** require aggressive external cooling in addition to aggressive sedation. **Paralysis** with nondepolarizing neuromuscular blockers may be required in severe cases.

Bupropion

GENERAL PRINCIPLES

- Bupropion is an antidepressant that is also used for smoking cessation and weight loss.
- Bupropion is available in the US in three formulations: immediate-release, sustained-release (dosed twice daily), and extended-release (dosed once daily). The extended-release formulation is the most common.
- Bupropion is misused recreationally, especially by people with limited access to other recreational substances, such as prisoners.

Pathophysiology

- Bupropion is a cathinone, which is an amphetamine derivative with a ketone group on the alpha-carbon. Bupropion is the only cathinone in pharmaceutical use—all other cathinones are illicit recreational drugs (sometimes referred to as "bath salts").

CHAPTER 28

- Bupropion has amphetamine-like properties: it inhibits the reuptake of dopamine and norepinephrine and enhances their release.
  Bupropion is not directly serotonergic but may enhance serotonin signaling by indirect mechanisms and has been implicated in the development of serotonin syndrome.
- In overdose, bupropion is profoundly cardiotoxic—it is thought to antagonize myocardial gap junctions and may cause takotsubo-like myocardial stunning.

DIAGNOSIS

Clinical Presentation
- Bupropion poisoning produces a **sympathomimetic toxidrome** (see above, amphetamines).
- Bupropion poisoning causes **seizures.**
  - Seizures may be **delayed in onset** (up to **24 hours postingestion** in the extended-release formulation) and may occur in patients with **minimal or no other symptoms of poisoning.**
  - Seizures may occur even after **minimal overdose,** including accidental double doses in some cases.[29]
  - Status epilepticus may occur in severe poisoning.
- Severe bupropion poisoning may cause **shock** and **cardiovascular collapse.**

Diagnostic Testing
Laboratories
Have a low threshold to obtain a **BMP, troponin,** and/or **creatinine kinase** to evaluate for end-organ damage, including renal injury, myocardial ischemia, and rhabdomyolysis.

Electrocardiography
- ECG may demonstrate sinus tachycardia or ventricular dysrhythmias.
- Bupropion may **prolong the QRS duration** due to gap junction antagonism.[30]

TREATMENT

- The mainstay of treatment is **benzodiazepines** or other directly GABAergic sedatives, titrated to control of agitation, improvement of vital signs, and control of seizures if present.
- It is critically important to **observe patients in a medical setting** for seizures and cardiovascular complications for an adequate time period postingestion. For extended-release bupropion, most experts recommend a **full 24-hour observation period** before medical clearance.
- Patients with severe poisoning causing cardiovascular instability may require treatment with vasopressors, inotropes, and mechanical ventilation.
- Sodium bicarbonate is generally **not** effective in reversing QRS prolongation due to bupropion.[30]
- Administration of **intravenous lipid emulsion** (bolus of 1.5 cc/kg, max 100 cc, followed by infusion of 0.25 cc/kg/min for 20 minutes) may be reasonable in patients with status epilepticus, significant cardiovascular instability, or cardiac arrest.
- **VA ECMO** is lifesaving in severe poisoning. Have a low threshold to transfer patients with severe bupropion poisoning to an ECMO-capable center.

Methylxanthines

GENERAL PRINCIPLES

- The methylxanthines include caffeine, theophylline, and theobromine.
- Caffeine is widely consumed in the form of coffee or tea and is used medically in the treatment of headaches.
  Caffeine is commercially available in highly concentrated powdered form for use as a preworkout supplement or food additive.
- Theophylline was once commonly used to treat asthma and chronic obstructive pulmonary diseasebut has generally fallen out of favor with the emergence of safe and effective inhaled agents.

Pathophysiology

- The methylxanthines are **adenosine receptor antagonists** and **phosphodiesterase inhibitors.**
  - In combination, these effects lead to the enhanced release of catecholamines and enhancement of the receptor effects of catecholamines, especially at the beta-adrenoceptors.
  - Adenosine antagonism in the central nervous system promotes wakefulness and decreases fatigue.
- In poisoning, these effects lead to tachycardia (via beta-1 stimulation), hypotension (via beta-2 stimulation), hypokalemia (via beta-1 stimulation), and seizures (via central nervous system adenosine antagonism).

DIAGNOSIS

Clinical Presentation

- Methylxanthine poisoning produces **tachycardia, hypotension, GI upset, anxiety and agitation, and seizures.**
- Most severe caffeine poisoning involves the highly concentrated powdered form.
- Patients taking theophylline are at risk of accidental poisoning with abrupt smoking cessation (due to induction of CYP1A2 by smoking).

Diagnostic Testing

Laboratories
- Obtain a **BMP** to evaluate for **hypokalemia** and **hyperglycemia.**
  - Hypokalemia due to excessive beta-1 adrenergic signaling is **characteristic of methylxanthine poisoning.**
- In the case of theophylline poisoning, obtain a **theophylline concentration.**
  - Therapeutic concentrations are typically 5–15 µg/mL.
  - In the rare case of acute overdose, concentrations should be trended over time.
- Most hospital laboratories do not have access to rapid testing of caffeine concentrations.

Electrocardiography
- The ECG may show sinus tachycardia or atrial or ventricular dysrhythmias.
- Supraventricular tachycardia and atrial or ventricular ectopy are particularly common.

TREATMENT

- Treat **seizures** with benzodiazepines or other directly GABAergic agents such as barbiturates or propofol.

CHAPTER 28

- Significant **dysrhythmias** should be treated with **esmolol.** Adenosine will likely be ineffective.
- **Hypotension** refractory to fluid resuscitation should be treated with **esmolol** (if there is significant tachycardia impairing cardiac output) and **norepinephrine or phenylephrine** (for alpha-1 agonism mediating beta-2 peripheral vasodilation)**.**
- **MDAC** enhances theophylline elimination and should be considered in theophylline-poisoned patients without contraindication to AC.
- **Hemodialysis** effectively clears methylxanthines and may be indicated in certain circumstances.
  - In **theophylline poisoning,** indications for hemodialysis include high concentrations (>100 mg/L in acute poisoning or >60 mg/L in chronic poisoning), patient at extremes of age or with significant medical comorbidities, and the presence of life-threatening dysrhythmias, shock, and/or seizures.
  - In **caffeine poisoning,** indications for hemodialysis are not well-developed, but hemodialysis would be reasonable in cases of shock, dysrhythmias, or seizure refractory to medical management.

ALCOHOLS

Ethanol

GENERAL PRINCIPLES

Pathophysiology

- Ethanol enhances inhibitory signaling through the GABA-A receptor and suppresses excitatory signaling through the NMDA glutamate receptor.
- Over time, patients with chronic heavy ethanol use will develop profound **tolerance** to the effects of ethanol.
  This occurs via qualitative changes in GABA-A receptors which render them less sensitive to activation, and via quantitative upregulation of NMDA receptors.
- Ethanol is eliminated primarily by the alcohol dehydrogenase pathway; elimination follows **zero-order kinetics.**
- Acute and chronic heavy ethanol use have many deleterious health effects that are outside the scope of this chapter (e.g., alcoholic hepatitis, pancreatitis, cardiomyopathy, peptic ulcer disease, cancers).

DIAGNOSIS

Clinical Presentation

- Alcohol intoxication produces **mental status changes, slurred speech,** and **motor impairment**, with prominent **cerebellar dysfunction.**
- In cases of severe intoxication, airway protective reflexes and respiration may be impaired (although this is much more common in mixed ingestions with other sedatives such as benzodiazepines or opioids).
- **Tolerance** for ethanol varies considerably; a patient with a history of chronic heavy ethanol consumption may show **no clinically obvious signs of intoxication.**

Diagnostics

Laboratories
- Obtain a **blood glucose.** Hypoglycemia may mimic ethanol intoxication, and patients with chronic heavy ethanol use are at risk of hypoglycemia.

- It may be reasonable to check a blood ethanol concentration in a patient with mental status changes of unclear etiology.

TREATMENT

- Treatment for ethanol intoxication is **exclusively supportive**, with clinical monitoring for recovery to baseline and airway support in the rare patient with airway compromise.
- **Clinical reassessment for clinical sobriety** is a key component of treatment.
- It is **unusual** for patients to require intubation and mechanical ventilation for ethanol intoxication alone.
- Patients with any evidence of **Wernicke encephalopathy** (confusion or mental status changes not improving with time, ataxia or gait changes not improving with time, oculomotor abnormalities) should be treated with **high-dose intravenous thiamine** (500 mg IV tid ×3-5 days).

SPECIAL CONSIDERATIONS

Alcohol Withdrawal

- Alcohol withdrawal is a potentially life-threatening syndrome of central nervous system hyperexcitation that may occur when an alcohol-tolerant patient abruptly discontinues alcohol intake.
  - Not all patients with chronic heavy ethanol use will experience alcohol withdrawal.
  - The most important risk factor for alcohol withdrawal in the hospitalized patient is **previous episodes of alcohol withdrawal.**
- Alcohol-tolerant patients develop significant qualitative and quantitative changes in their GABAergic and glutamatergic signaling pathways that allow for significant alcohol tolerance, as described above.
  When the alcohol is removed, the patient's underlying unbalanced excitatory-inhibitory state is unmasked.
- Ethanol withdrawal may occur **anytime from hours to 4 or 5 days after the patient's last drink.**
- There are four primary manifestations of alcohol withdrawal:
  - **Acute uncomplicated alcohol withdrawal** presents with tremulousness, anxiety, nausea, flushing, tachycardia, and hypertension.
  - **Alcoholic hallucinosis** presents with visual and auditory disturbances that are more accurately termed illusions since patients typically retain reality testing.
  - **Alcohol withdrawal seizures** may occur seemingly at random, even in the **absence of any other signs of withdrawal.**
  - **Delirium tremens,** which is **life-threatening**, presents with significant dysautonomia (including hyperthermia), seizures, agitation, and psychosis.
- The treatment of alcohol withdrawal should consist of **protocol-based, symptom-triggered** administration of GABAergic sedatives typically benzodiazepines or phenobarbital. Agent selection varies with local patterns of practice.
  - Scheduled, fixed-dose treatment regimens are comparatively ineffective and may lead to undertreatment or overtreatment.
  - Sedatives may be given by mouth for mild symptoms; moderate and severe symptoms require intravenous treatment.
- **Dexmedetomidine** is generally not helpful; it does not target the GABAergic or glutamatergic systems, it may mask autonomic signs of alcohol withdrawal without preventing seizures, and it has generally not proven to improve patient-centered outcomes or length of stay in clinical trials.[31]

CHAPTER 28

Alcohol Use Disorder

- AUD is a problematic pattern of alcohol use leading to clinically significant impairment or distress. Patients with AUD may have overwhelming cravings for alcohol, use alcohol in dangerous situations or despite the knowledge that it is harming them, suffer social and legal consequences from alcohol use, and experience tolerance and withdrawal.
- Pharmacotherapy for AUD may be helpful in reducing drinking days, reducing the amount of alcohol consumed, and controlling cravings for alcohol.
  ○ Psychotherapy and social support are also key components of AUD treatment for many patients.
  ○ The goal of AUD treatment is **not always complete abstinence.**
- **Naltrexone** 50 mg daily may help reduce heavy drinking and cravings by interfering in the endorphin reward pathways that incentivize alcohol consumption.
  ○ Long-acting injectable naltrexone (Vivitrol) may enhance compliance compared to oral naltrexone; this should be administered only after the patient has tolerated oral naltrexone for at least 1 week.
  ○ Naltrexone is contraindicated in patients with a need for opioid therapy (including patients with comorbid OUD who benefit from treatment with buprenorphine or methadone) and in patients with hepatic impairment.
- **Gabapentin** may help reduce heavy drinking, although the existing evidence is somewhat equivocal.
  Various dosing regimens have been studied; 1200 mg daily in divided doses is reasonable.[32]
- Other agents including **acamprosate, topiramate,** and **baclofen** may be helpful.
- **Disulfiram** is ineffective and potentially dangerous and **should not be used.**

Toxic Alcohols

GENERAL PRINCIPLES

- The classic toxic alcohols are methanol, ethylene glycol, and isopropanol. Other agents include diethylene glycol, propylene glycol, and glycol ethers.
- Toxic alcohols may be found in automotive and household products, including brake and wiper fluid, antifreeze, coolant fluids, and hand sanitizer.
- Methanol is produced during the process of liquor distillation and may contaminate alcoholic beverages, especially when these are illicitly produced by people not familiar with the distillation process.

Pathophysiology

- Metabolism of toxic alcohols by alcohol dehydrogenase and aldehyde dehydrogenase generates **toxic organic acids** which are responsible for acidosis and end-organ damage.
  ○ Methanol is metabolized to **formic acid**, which is toxic to the retina.
  ○ Ethylene glycol is metabolized to **glycolic acid** (which is primarily responsible for the metabolic acidosis seen in this poisoning) and **oxalic acid** (which is nephrotoxic).
  ○ Isopropanol is metabolized to **acetone** (a ketone) and cannot be further metabolized by aldehyde dehydrogenase.

DIAGNOSIS

Clinical Presentation

The clinical presentation of toxic alcohol poisoning **varies depending on the time from ingestion to presentation.**

* Patients presenting relatively rapidly after ingestion will present with **inebriation** and may be mistakenly diagnosed with ethanol intoxication.
* Patients presenting late may have **tachypnea, tachycardia, mental status changes, or frank shock** due to acidosis. Patients presenting late after methanol poisoning may complain of **vision changes.**
* Suspect toxic alcohol poisoning in an **inebriated** patient who does not clinically improve over time as would be typical in ethanol intoxication.

Differential Diagnosis

Alcoholic ketoacidosis, sepsis, occult hemorrhage, and cardiogenic shock, poisonings by other xenobiotics that produce shock, mental status changes, and acidosis (metformin, iron, cyanide, salicylates, dinitrophenol, and nucleoside reverse transcriptase inhibitors).

Diagnostics

Laboratories

* **Rapid** laboratory testing for toxic alcohols and their metabolites is **not usually readily available in most institutions.** Send-out laboratories for methanol and ethylene glycol should be obtained.
* Because rapid reliable laboratory tests are not available, the initial diagnosis of toxic alcohol poisoning must frequently be made by **inference from other laboratory tests.**
  ○ A significantly elevated **osmolar gap**, which is the difference between the calculated osmolarity and the measured serum osmolarity, may indicate the presence of "unmeasured osmoles," which include toxic alcohols.
    ▪ A normal or low osmolar gap does **not** rule out toxic alcohol poisoning. There is significant interindividual variation in the normal or baseline osmolar gap.
    ▪ The osmolar gap **declines over time** as toxic alcohols are metabolized to organic acids; patients presenting late may have a normal osmolar gap.
  ○ A significantly elevated **anion gap** with metabolic acidosis may indicate the presence of "unmeasured anions," which include the organic acid products of toxic alcohol metabolism.
    ▪ The anion gap **increases over time** as organic acids are generated and accumulate; patients presenting early may have a normal anion gap.
    ▪ An **anion gap acidosis** that **worsens significantly over time** despite appropriate resuscitative care may suggest toxic alcohol poisoning.
    ▪ An **anion gap acidosis** that **improves with resuscitative care alone** (i.e., without antidote or hemodialysis) essentially **rules out** significant toxic alcohol poisoning.
* Obtain a **BMP** (to assess for renal function, anion gap, and acid–base status), **ethanol concentration** (to aid in calculation of the osmolar gap and in treatment decisions), and **serum osmolarity** (to aid in calculation of the osmolar gap).
* Certain **point of care lactate** analyzers misinterpret glycolic acid as lactic acid, whereas laboratory-based lactate testing typically does not suffer from this error.

A **significantly elevated point of care lactate** with a **normal laboratory-run lactate** may suggest the presence of glycolic acid, which suggests ethylene glycol poisoning.
- Urinalysis may show **calcium oxalate crystals** in ethylene glycol poisoning.
- Isopropanol poisoning classically produces **ketosis without acidosis.**

TREATMENT

- **Empiric treatment before laboratory confirmation** is **frequently required**, given the difficulties involved in obtain direct laboratory confirmation of toxic alcohol poisoning described above.
- The mainstay of treatment is **fomepizole.**
  - Fomepizole is an alcohol dehydrogenase inhibitor, which functionally blocks the metabolism of toxic alcohols into organic acids. It will not reverse acidosis or end-organ damage.
  - The initial dose of fomepizole is 15 mg/kg IV, followed by maintenance dosing of 10 mg/kg IV every 12 hours.
    - If more than 48 hours of therapy is required, the maintenance dose should be increased to 15 mg/kg IV every 12 hours, as fomepizole induces its own metabolism.
    - Fomepizole must be dose-adjusted if the patient undergoes hemodialysis.
  - Fomepizole therapy should be **continued** until the toxic alcohol concentration (methanol or ethylene glycol) is <20 mg/dL.
- **Ethanol** therapy was previously widely used to treat toxic alcohol poisoning, as ethanol is an effective competitive antagonist of alcohol dehydrogenase.
  Ethanol therapy is difficult to dose and titrate and has significant associated adverse effects; it is **not indicated** unless fomepizole is completely unavailable.
- **Hemodialysis** effectively clears toxic alcohols, clears the organic acid metabolites, and corrects acidosis.
  - Hemodialysis is indicated in any patient with toxic alcohol poisoning who has significant acidosis (pH ≤ 7.15), coma, seizures, shock, significant renal impairment, or evidence of end-organ damage (acute kidney injury in ethylene glycol poisoning or vision deficits in methanol poisoning).
  - Hemodialysis is frequently required in methanol poisoning because of the extremely prolonged half-life of methanol in patients being treated with fomepizole.
  - Hemodialysis may be more cost-effective than prolonged hospitalization and fomepizole therapy in patients with extremely high ethylene glycol concentrations.
- **Sodium bicarbonate** should be a temporizing therapy for severe acidosis only and does not directly treat or reverse toxicity.
- **Intravenous high-dose vitamin supplementation** may promote the metabolism of toxic alcohols via alternative metabolic pathways that produce nontoxic end products.
  - **Methanol** poisoning: administer folate or leucovorin 1 mg/kg (max 50 mg) IV q4-6 hours.
  - **Ethylene glycol** poisoning: administer thiamine 100 mg IV q4-6 hours and pyridoxine 50 mg IV q6-12 hours.
- Severely poisoned patients may require aggressive **resuscitative care**, including fluid resuscitation, vasopressors and inotropes for shock, and intubation and mechanical ventilation.
- **Isopropanol poisoning** rarely requires any treatment beyond close observation and supportive care.

ENVIRONMENTAL TOXINS

Carbon Monoxide

GENERAL PRINCIPLES

- Carbon monoxide (CO) is a colorless, odorless, and tasteless gas that is produced during incomplete combustion of carbon-containing fuels.
- Common sources of exposure include smoke inhalation in house fires, malfunctioning heaters and electric generators, automobile exhaust, smoking, forklifts, and chemicals such as methylene chloride.

Pathophysiology

- CO binds with hemoglobin to form carboxyhemoglobin, which causes a functional anemia and shifts the oxyhemoglobin dissociation curve to the left.
- CO inhibits cellular respiration by binding to mitochondrial cytochrome oxidase and disrupting the electron transport chain.
- CO poisoning also increases nitric oxide levels, producing vasodilation.

DIAGNOSIS

Clinical Presentation

- The diagnosis of CO poisoning is challenging because of its many vague signs and symptoms that can wax and wane depending on the patient's source of exposure.
- Patients with mild poisoning may present with **flu-like symptoms**, which include headache, myalgias, fatigue, lethargy, nausea, vomiting, and dizziness. If these patients remove themselves from the exposure, such as when they leave their house to seek medical attention, the symptoms **may improve before they are evaluated by a physician.**
- Patients with more severe poisoning present with symptoms of **end-organ damage**, which are predominantly **cardiac or neurologic.**
  These may include chest pain, myocardial infarctions, cardiac dysrhythmias, syncope, stroke-like symptoms, seizures, coma, and other psychoneurological symptoms.
- Patients may present late after significant exposure with delayed neurologic sequelae (DNS), which can occur anywhere between 2 and 40 days after the exposure.
- Have a low threshold to consider CO poisoning during the **winter months** (when patients may be exposed to malfunctioning heating systems) and in **groups of patients** living or working in the same environment who present with similar symptoms.

Diagnostic Testing

Laboratories

- **Carboxyhemoglobin (CO-Hgb) levels** are readily available. They can be obtained on either arterial or VBG specimens.
  - CO-Hgb levels **greater than 5%** generally indicate an exogenous CO exposure.
  - Levels do not always correlate well with a patient's symptoms or prognosis.
- **Standard pulse oximeters** may be **falsely reassuring** because they cannot detect a difference between oxyhemoglobin and CO-Hgb.
  Specialized handheld pulse co-oximeters can be used to noninvasively measure CO-Hgb; they are accurate in **ruling out** significant CO poisoning, but elevated values should generally be confirmed with blood gas testing.

- **Metabolic acidosis** and **elevated lactate concentrations** may suggest CO poisoning in the right clinical context but are not specific for this toxin.

Electrocardiography
- Obtain an ECG in any patient with known or suspected CO poisoning who has chest pain, tachycardia, palpitations, syncope, shock, coma, seizures, or neurologic deficits.
- ECG may demonstrate evidence of myocardial ischemia.

TREATMENT

- The mainstay of treatment is the administration of **oxygen**, which enhances the elimination of CO. Administration of 100% oxygen by nonrebreather face mask decreased the half-life of CO to about 60–90 minutes.
- The use of **hyperbaric oxygen** (HBO) therapy in CO poisoning is **controversial.**[33] The theoretical indication for HBO is to prevent DNS, not to facilitate more rapid CO elimination. Consider for end-organ dysfunction such as syncope, coma, CO-Hgb >25%, or in pregnancy.
- Additional care includes airway and ventilatory support, vasopressors for hypotension, and treatment of any concurrent injury or poisoning, such as if the patient has a burn, trauma, or cyanide toxicity from a house fire.

Cyanide

GENERAL PRINCIPLES

- The most common source of cyanide poisoning in the US and other western countries is combustion of plastics and other synthetic materials in **house fires.**
- Patients may also be exposed to cyanide in laboratory or industrial settings, during therapy with sodium nitroprusside, or by ingestion of compounds that liberate cyanide during metabolism (such as acetonitrile, the pits of stone fruits, and inappropriately processed cassava).

Pathophysiology
- Cyanide is a chemical asphyxiant. It induces **cellular hypoxia** by inhibiting complex IV (also known as cytochrome c oxidase or cytochrome oxidase aa_3) in the electron transport chain and thus **preventing the formation of adenosine triphosphate** which results in anaerobic metabolism and **metabolic acidosis.**
- Cyanide is also an **excitotoxin** in the central nervous system.

DIAGNOSIS

Clinical Presentation
- Poisoning by cyanide is typically **rapid in onset and not subtle:** patients are either critically ill or not poisoned.
  Patients who have **ingested cyanogenic substances** may have a more delayed onset of toxicity and initial complain of more mild symptoms.
- Cyanide poisoning causes **cardiovascular instability** (initial tachycardia and hypertension followed by cardiovascular collapse) and **neurotoxicity** (mental status depression, seizures, and coma).

- "Classic" textbook signs of cyanide poisoning such as the bitter almond odor and cherry red skin discoloration are **unreliable** and should not be used to make or exclude the diagnosis of cyanide poisoning.

Diagnostic Testing

Laboratories

- Blood cyanide concentrations are **not available** in a timely fashion and have no role in clinical decision making.
- A **profoundly elevated lactate** (8–10 mmol/L or higher) in the correct clinical context is suggestive of cyanide toxicity.
- **"Arterialization"** of venous blood (i.e., equilibration of the venous and arterial pO2) may suggest cyanide toxicity, as cyanide poisoning effectively halts extraction of oxygen from arterial blood by the tissue.

TREATMENT

- The treatment of choice for cyanide poisoning is **hydroxocobalamin.**
  - Hydroxocobalamin directly binds to cyanide, forming cyanocobalamin (vitamin B12).
  - Hydroxocobalamin is safe—the adverse effects are usually minor and transient hypertension and tachycardia and discoloration of the skin and body fluids (which may briefly interfere with pulse oximetry and colorimetric laboratory tests).
  - The dose of hydroxocobalamin is **5 g IV** over 15 minutes.
    - This dose may be repeated once if necessary based on clinical response.
    - Usually, repeated dosing is not necessary, except in patients who have ingested cyanogenic substances.
- If hydroxocobalamin is not available, the older **cyanide antidote kit** may be used.
  - First, **sodium nitrite** is used to induce **methemoglobinemia**; cyanide binds more avidly to methemoglobin than to complex IV, so methemoglobin formation encourages the dissociation of cyanide from the mitochondria.
  - Second, **sodium thiosulfate** is administered to accelerate the endogenous detoxification of cyanide, which relies on the presence of sulfur donors.
  - The antidote kit is **not preferred as first-line therapy** because the induction of methemoglobinemia can be dangerous in critically ill patients, nitrites cause hypotension, and the dosing of nitrites is challenging.
- The rest of care is supportive, including adequate volume resuscitation, airway support, and vasopressor and inotropic support as needed.

CHAPTER 28

REFERENCES

1. Ambre J, Ruo TI, Nelson J, Belknap S. Urinary excretion of cocaine, benzoylecgonine, and ecgonine methyl ester in humans. *Journal of Anal Toxicol.* 1988;12:301-306.
2. Chan A, Isbister GK, Kirkpatrick CM, Dufful SB. Drug-induced QT prolongation and torsades de pointes: evaluation of a QT nomogram. *QJM.* 2007;100:609-615.
3. Blake KV, Massey KL, Hendeles L, Nickerson D, Neims A. Relative efficacy of phenytoin and phenobarbital for the prevention of theophylline-induced seizures in mice. *Ann Emerg Med.* 1988;17:1024-1028.
4. Rumack BH, Peterson RC, Koch GG, Amara IA. Acetaminophen overdose. 662 cases with evaluation of oral acetylcysteine treatment. *Arch Intern Med.* 1981;141:380-385.
5. O'Grady JG, Alexander GJ, Hayllar KM, Williams R. Early indicators of prognosis in fulminant hepatic failure. *Gastroenterology.* 1989;97:439-445.
6. Smilkstein MJ, Knapp GL, Kulig KW, Rumack BH. Efficacy of oral N-acetylcysteine in the treatment of acetaminophen overdose. Analysis of the national multicenter study (1976 to 1985). *N Engl J Med.* 1988;319:1557-1562.

7. Johnson MT, McCammon CA, Mullins ME, Halcomb SE. Evaluation of a simplified N-acetylcysteine dosing regimen for the treatment of acetaminophen toxicity. *Ann Pharmacother.* 2011;45:713-720.

8. Vertrees JE, McWilliams BC, Kelly HW. Repeated oral administration of activated charcoal for treating aspirin overdose in young children. *Pediatrics.* 1990;85:594-598.

9. Goldfrank L, Weisman RS, Errick JK, Lo MW. A dosing nomogram for continuous infusion intravenous naloxone. *Ann Emerg Med.* 1986;15:566-570.

10. Mixter CG IIIrd, Moran JM, Austen WG. Cardiac and peripheral vascular effects of diphenylhydantoin sodium. *Am J Cardiol.* 1966;17:332-338.

11. O'Brien TJ, Cascino GD, So EL, Hanna DR. Incidence and clinical consequence of the purple glove syndrome in patients receiving intravenous phenytoin. *Neurology.* 1998;51:1034-1039.

12. Ghannoum M, Laliberté M, Nolin TD, et al. Extracorporeal treatment for valproic acid poisoning: systematic review and recommendations from the EXTRIP workgroup. *Clin Toxicol (Phila).* 2015;53:454-465.

13. Hojer J, Malmlund HO, Berg A. Clinical features in 28 consecutive cases of laboratory confirmed massive poisoning with carbamazepine alone. *J Toxicol Clin Toxicol.* 1993;31:449-458.

14. Neuvonen PJ, Elonen E. Effect of activated charcoal on absorption and elimination of phenobarbitone, carbamazepine and phenylbutazone in man. *Eur J Clin Pharmacol.* 1980;17:51-57.

15. Boyer EW, Shannon M. The serotonin syndrome. *N Engl J Med.* 2005;352:1112-1120.

16. Boehnert MT, Lovejoy FH, Jr. Value of the QRS duration versus the serum drug level in predicting seizures and ventricular arrhythmias after an acute overdose of tricyclic antidepressants. *N Engl J Med.* 1985;313:474-479.

17. Liebelt EL, Francis PD, Woolf AD. ECG lead aVR versus QRS interval in predicting seizures and arrhythmias in acute tricyclic antidepressant toxicity. *Ann Emerg Med.* 1995;26:195-201.

18. Linden CH, Rumack BH, Strehlke C. Monoamine oxidase inhibitor overdose. *Ann Emerg Med.* 1984;13:1137-1144.

19. Camus M, Henneré G, Baron G, et al. Comparison of lithium concentrations in red blood cells and plasma in samples collected for TDM, acute toxicity, or acute-on-chronic toxicity. *Eur J Clin Pharmacol.* 2003;59:583-587.

20. Decker BS, Goldfarb DS, Dargan PI, et al. Extracorporeal treatment for lithium poisoning: systematic review and recommendations from the EXTRIP workgroup. *Clin J Am Soc Nephrol.* 2015;10:875-887.

21. Engebretsen KM, Kaczmarek KM, Morgan J, Holger JS. High-dose insulin therapy in beta-blocker and calcium channel-blocker poisoning. *Clin Toxicol (Phila).* 2011;49:277-283.

22. Seger DL, Loden JK. Naloxone reversal of clonidine toxicity: dose, dose, dose. *Clin Toxicol (Phila).* 2018;56:873-879.

23. Bismuth C, Gaultier M, Conso F, Efthymiou ML. Hyperkalemia in acute digitalis poisoning: prognostic significance and therapeutic implications. *Clin Toxicol.* 1973;6:153-162.

24. Chan BS, Isbister GK, O'Leary M, Chiew A, Buckley NA. Efficacy and effectiveness of anti-digoxin antibodies in chronic digoxin poisonings from the DORA study (ATOM-1). *Clin Toxicol (Phila).* 2016;54:488-494.

25. Boldy DA, Vale JA, Prescott LF. Treatment of phenobarbitone poisoning with repeated oral administration of activated charcoal. *Q J Med.* 1986;61:997-1002.

26. Fluyau D, Mitra P, Lorthe K. Antipsychotics for amphetamine psychosis. A systematic review. *Front Psychiatry.* 2019;10:740.

27. McCord J, Jneid H, Hollander JE, et al. Management of cocaine-associated chest pain and myocardial infarction: a scientific statement from the American heart association acute cardiac care Committee of the Council on Clinical Cardiology. *Circulation.* 2008;117:1897-1907.

28. Robertson KE, Martin TN, Rae AP. Brugada-pattern ECG and cardiac arrest in cocaine toxicity: reading between the white lines. *Heart.* 2010;96:643-644.

29. Johnston JA, Lineberry CG, Ascher JA, et al. A 102-center prospective study of seizure in association with bupropion. *J Clin Psychiatry.* 1991;52:450-456.

30. Caillier B, Pilote S, Castonguay A, et al. QRS widening and QT prolongation under bupropion: a unique cardiac electrophysiological profile. *Fundam Clin Pharmacol.* 2012;26:599-608.

31. Yavarovich ER, Bintvihok M, McCarty JC, Breeze JL, LaCamera P. Association between dexmedetomidine use for the treatment of alcohol withdrawal syndrome and intensive care unit length of stay. *J Intensive Care.* 2019;7:49.

32. Myrick H, Malcolm R, Randall PK, et al. A double-blind trial of gabapentin versus lorazepam in the treatment of alcohol withdrawal. *Alcohol Clin Exp Res.* 2009;33:1582-1588.

33. Buckley NA, Juurlink DN, Isbister G, Bennett MH, Lavonas EJ. Hyperbaric oxygen for carbon monoxide poisoning. *Cochrane Database Syst Rev.* 2011;2011:Cd002041.

Appendix A

Immunizations and Postexposure Therapies

Carlos Mejia-Chew and Stephen Y. Liang

Introduction

- **Active immunization** promotes the development of a durable primary immune response (B-cell proliferation, antibody response, T-cell sensitization) directed toward a specific pathogen such that subsequent exposure to that pathogen results in a secondary immune response that protects against infection (Table A-1).
- **Passive immunization** involves the administration of immune globulin resulting in transient protection against infection. It is usually employed in a host with limited capacity to mount a primary immune response, when exposure to a pathogen occurs in a previously unvaccinated host, or to protect against toxin-mediated disease.
- **Postexposure prophylaxis** is therapy given following exposure to a pathogen to prevent the development of disease. This can include active immunization, passive immunization, and/or antimicrobial therapy (Tables A-2 and A-3).
- **Adverse events potentially related to vaccination** should be reported through the Vaccine Adverse Event Reporting System at http://vaers.hhs.gov/ or 1-800-822-7967.
- **More information,** including adult vaccination schedules, recommendations regarding travel, and up-to-date guidelines, can be found at the Centers for Disease Control and Prevention (CDC) website, http://www.cdc.gov/. Additional guidance for specific clinical questions can be obtained by contacting the CDC via https://www.cdc.gov/cdc-info/ask-cdc.html or by phone at 1-800-232-4636 (1-800-CDC-INFO).

Rabies Postexposure Prophylaxis

- For all suspected rabies exposures, consultation with local or state health officials is recommended. Contact information can be found at http://www.cdc.gov/rabies/resources/contacts.html.
- Postexposure prophylaxis is generally indicated only for bite wounds from mammals.[1]
  - Bites from bats, skunks, raccoons, foxes, and most other carnivores warrant immediate prophylaxis unless the animal is confirmed to be rabies negative by laboratory testing. Animals should not be held for observation but euthanized as soon as possible.
  - Bites from dogs, cats, and ferrets that are rabid or suspected to be rabid also warrant immediate prophylaxis. If the animal is healthy and can be observed for 10 days, do not begin prophylaxis but observe. If signs or symptoms of rabies develop in the animal, prophylaxis should begin immediately. For bites where the status of the animal is unknown, consult with public health officials.

- Bites from all other sources (e.g., rodents, hares, livestock) should be considered on an individual basis and prophylaxis initiated in consultation with public health officials.
- Postexposure prophylaxis consists of wound care, vaccination, and in certain situations, administration of human rabies immune globulin (HRIG) (Table A-4).[2]
  - All wounds should be cleaned thoroughly with soap and water and irrigated with a virucidal solution such as povidone-iodine.
  - Human diploid cell vaccine or purified chick embryo cell vaccine, 1 mL IM, should be administered in the deltoid region, the only acceptable site for vaccination in adults.
  - If HRIG is indicated, give 20 IU/kg IM once. Do not administer in the same syringe as the vaccine. When possible, infiltrate as much of the product around and into the wound(s). The remaining volume can be administered intramuscularly at any site anatomically distant from the site of vaccination. Subsequent vaccine doses at later dates can be given at the same site as previous HRIG.

TABLE A-1	Selected Adult Immunization Recommendations in the United States		
Vaccine, Dose	**Indications and Dosing**	**Contraindications**	**Precautions**
Haemophilus influenzae type b (Hib) Hib conjugate vaccine: 0.5 mL IM	**Unvaccinated adults with anatomic or functional asplenia (including sickle cell disease) or undergoing elective splenectomy (preferably 14 d before surgery):** Administer 1 dose **Hematopoietic stem cell transplant recipients 6–12 mo after successful transplant:** Administer three doses (4 wk apart)	Severe allergic reaction to any vaccine component or after a previous dose	Moderate or severe acute illness with or without fever
Hepatitis A Single-antigen hepatitis A vaccine (HepA; Havrix, Vaqta): 1 mL IM Combined hepatitis A/hepatitis B vaccine (HepA-Hep B; Twinrix): 1 mL IM	**Any adult seeking protection from hepatitis A virus (HAV)** **Specific indications:** travel to countries with high or intermediate HAV endemicity (including infants ≥6 mo); chronic liver disease; HIV infection; men who have sex with men (MSM); injection or noninjection drug use; persons experiencing homelessness; laboratory workers exposed to HAV; persons who anticipate close personal contact with an adoptee from a country with high or intermediate HAV endemicity during the first 60 d after arrival in the United States; pregnancy (if at risk for infection or a severe outcome from infection during pregnancy); healthy persons ages ≥12 mo recently exposed to HAV (adults >40 y may also receive HAV immunoglobulin). **Standard dosing:** Havrix: Administer two doses at 0 and 6–12 mo Vaqta: Administer two doses at 0 and 6–18 mo Twinrix: Administer three doses at 0, 1, and 6 mo	Severe allergic reaction to any vaccine component or after a previous dose	Moderate or severe acute illness with or without fever

(continued)

TABLE A-1	Selected Adult Immunization Recommendations in the United States	(continued)	
Vaccine, Dose	**Indications and Dosing**	**Contraindications**	**Precautions**
Hepatitis B Single-antigen hepatitis B vaccine a) HepB; Recombivax HB, standard (10 µg/mL) and high-dose (40 µg/mL) formulations: 1 mL IM b) HepB; Engerix-B (20 µg/mL): 1 mL IM Recombinant hepatitis B vaccine with an immunoadjuvant (Heplisav-B): 20 µg/0.5 mL Combined hepatitis A/hepatitis B vaccine (HepA-Hep B; Twinrix): 1 mL IM	**Any adult seeking protection from hepatitis B virus (HBV)** **Specific indications:** chronic liver disease; HIV infection; percutaneous or mucosal risk of exposure to blood (e.g., household contacts of persons with chronic HBV infection; persons age <60 y with diabetes mellitus and those ≥60 y at discretion of treating clinician; adults with ESRD including those receiving dialysis; injection drug users; healthcare and public safety workers at risk for exposure to blood or body fluids); sexual exposure risk (e.g., sex partners of persons with chronic HBV infection; sexually active persons not in long-term, mutually monogamous relationship; persons seeking evaluation or treatment for a sexually transmitted disease; MSM); persons receiving care in settings where risk of HBV infection is high (e.g., facilities providing STD treatment, HIV testing and treatment, or drug abuse treatment and prevention services; healthcare settings targeting services to injection drug users or MSM; correctional facilities; ESRD and hemodialysis programs; institutions for persons with developmental disabilities); travelers to countries with high or intermediate HBV endemicity; pregnancy (if at risk for infection or a severe outcome from infection during pregnancy) **Standard dosing:** Standard-dose Recombivax HB, Engerix-B, or Twinrix: Administer three doses at 0, 1, and 6 mo Heplisav-B: Administer two doses at 0 and 1 mo (not recommended in pregnancy) **HD patients or other immunocompromised:** High-dose Recombivax HB: Administer three doses at 0, 1, and 6 mo Engerix-B: Administer four two-dose (2 mL) injections at 0, 1, 2, and 6 mo	Severe allergic reaction to any vaccine component or after a previous dose	Moderate or severe acute illness with or without fever

Human papillomavirus (HPV) 9-valent vaccine (9vHPV; Gardasil 9): 0.5 mL IM	**All adults through age 26 y:** If age <15 y at initial vaccination, administer two doses at 0 and 6–12 mo If age ≥15 y at initial vaccination or immune compromised (any age), administer three doses at 0, 1–2, and 6 mo **Age 27 through 45 y (based on shared clinical decision making):** Administer two- or three-dose series as above	Severe allergic reaction to any vaccine component or after a previous dose	Moderate or severe acute illness with or without fever; **pregnancy**
Influenza Inactivated or recombinant influenza vaccine (IIV or RIV): 0.5 mL IM (5 mL if multidose vial used) Live attenuated influenza vaccine (LAIV): 0.2 mL intranasal	**Annual vaccination is recommended for all persons aged ≥6 mo without contraindications.** **Age 6 mo through 35 mo:** IIV (LAIV option for age ≥ 2 y) **Pregnancy:** IIV or RIV **Age ≥65 y:** IIV or RIV **All others:** IIV, RIV, or LAIV (if age 2 through 49 y) **Egg allergy:** RIV4 preferred if age ≥ 18 yr. *Cell culture-based IIV4 if age ≥4 y* **Healthcare personnel** who receive LAIV should avoid providing care for severely immune-suppressed persons (i.e., requiring protective environment) until 7 d postvaccination	Severe allergic reaction to any vaccine component or after a previous dose Persons with a history of egg allergy of any severity may receive any licensed, recommended, and age-appropriate influenza vaccine LAIV: **pregnancy, immune suppression** (includes close contacts), children aged 2–4 y with asthma, children/adolescents on salicylate therapy (aspirin), persons who have taken influenza antiviral medications within previous 48 h	Moderate to severe illness with or without fever; history of Guillain-Barré syndrome (GBS) within 6 wk of previous influenza vaccination LAIV: asthma; chronic medical conditions that may predispose to higher risk of influenza-related complications (e.g., lung disease, cardiovascular disease, diabetes, renal or hepatic disease)

(continued)

TABLE A-1	Selected Adult Immunization Recommendations in the United States *(continued)*		
Vaccine, Dose	**Indications and Dosing**	**Contraindications**	**Precautions**
Measles, mumps, rubella Live measles, mumps, and rubella (MMR) vaccine: 0.5 mL SC	**Anyone without evidence of immunity:** Administer one dose **Evidence of immunity:** • Born before 1957 (except for healthcare personnel) • Documented vaccination • Laboratory confirmation of immunity or disease **HIV infection with CD4$^+$ >200 cells/μL for at least 6 mo without evidence of immunity:** Administer two doses ≥28 d apart **Students in postsecondary educational institutions, international travelers, and household contacts of immune compromised persons:** Administer two doses ≥28 d apart **Women of childbearing age:** Rubella immunity should be determined. If no immunity and nonpregnant, administer 1 dose of MMR; **pregnant women with no rubella immunity:** administer 1 dose on completion or termination of pregnancy and before discharge from the healthcare facility **Healthcare personnel born in 1957 or later:** If no documentation of vaccination or laboratory confirmation of immunity or disease, administer two doses if measles or mumps nonimmune ≥28 d apart; one dose if rubella nonimmune) **Adults who previously received ≤2 doses of MMR identified to be at increased risk for mumps during an outbreak:** Administer one dose	Severe allergic reaction to any vaccine component or after a previous dose; current febrile respiratory or other febrile infection; known **severe immunodeficiency** (e.g., hematologic and solid tumors, receipt of chemotherapy, congenital immunodeficiency, long-term immunosuppressive therapy, HIV infection with CD4$^+$ <200 cells/μL); **pregnancy**	Moderate or severe acute illness with or without fever; recent (≤11 mo) receipt of antibody-containing blood product; history of thrombocytopenia or thrombocytopenic purpura; need for tuberculin skin testing within 4 wk of vaccination (measles component may temporarily suppress reactivity)

		Severe allergic reaction to any vaccine component or after a previous dose	Moderate or severe acute illness with or without fever

Meningococcal (*Neisseria meningitidis*)

Quadrivalent meningococcal conjugate vaccine–diphtheria toxoid carrier (MenACWY; Menactra, Menveo): 0.5 mL IM

Adults with anatomical or functional asplenia, HIV infection, persistent complement component deficiency, or complement inhibitor (e.g., eculizumab, ravulizumab) use: Administer two doses of MenACWY ≥8 wk apart; revaccinate with 1 dose of MenACWY every 5 y if risk persists

Adults traveling to living in countries where meningococcal disease is hyperendemic or epidemic, microbiologists routinely exposed to *N. meningitidis*, military recruits, first-year college students living in residence halls if no vaccination at age ≥16 y: Administer one dose of MenACWY; revaccinate with one dose of MenACWY every 5 y if risk persists

Meningococcal serogroup B vaccine (MenB-4C, Bexsero; MenB-FHbp, Trumenba): 0.5 mL IM

Adults with anatomical or function asplenia, persistent complement component deficiency, complement inhibitor use, microbiologists routinely exposed to *N. meningitidis*, or at risk for meningococcal disease outbreak attributed to serogroup B:

MenB-4C: Administer two doses ≥1 mo apart

MenB-FHbp: Administer three doses at 0, 1–2, and 6 mo

(continued)

TABLE A-1	Selected Adult Immunization Recommendations in the United States *(continued)*		
Vaccine, Dose	**Indications and Dosing**	**Contraindications**	**Precautions**
Pneumococcal (*Streptococcus pneumoniae*) 13-Valent pneumococcal conjugate vaccine (PCV13): 0.5 mL IM 23-Valent pneumococcal polysaccharide vaccine (PPSV23): 0.5 mL IM or SC	**Immunocompetent adults ≥65 y:** • Administer one dose of PPSV23 (if PPSV23 administered before age 65 y, administer 1 dose PPSV23 ≥5 y after previous dose) • Administration of PCV13 is based on shared clinical decision making. The highest benefit is in nursing home residents or settings with low or no pediatric PCV13 uptake. Administer one dose of PCV13 (if not previously received), followed by one dose of PPSV23 ≥1 y later **Adults 19–64 y with chronic heart disease (excluding hypertension), chronic lung disease, chronic liver disease, alcoholism, diabetes mellitus, or tobacco dependence:** Administer one dose of PPSV23. **Adults ≥19 y with immunocompromising condition, HIV infection, anatomic or functional asplenia, chronic kidney disease, or nephrotic syndrome:** Administer one dose of PCV13, followed by one dose PPSV23 at ≥8 wk and second dose at ≥5 y after first PPSV23. If last PPSV23 received before age 65 y, at age 65 y, administer another dose of PPSV23 ≥5 y after last dose **Adults 19–64 y with cerebrospinal fluid leak or cochlear implant:** Administer one dose of PCV13, followed by one dose of PPSV23 at ≥8 wk. If PPSV23 received before age 65 y, at age 65 y, administer another dose of PPSV23 ≥5 y after last dose	Severe allergic reaction after a previous dose or to a vaccine component PCV13: severe allergic reaction to any vaccine containing diphtheria toxoid	Moderate or severe acute illness with or without fever

Tetanus, diphtheria, pertussis Tetanus and diphtheria toxoids vaccine (Td): 0.5 mL IM Tetanus, diphtheria, and acellular pertussis vaccine (Tdap; Adacel, Boostrix): 0.5 mL IM Other formulations (e.g., diphtheria and tetanus toxoids and acellular pertussis [DTaP]) not recommended for adult use	**Everyone:** Td or Tdap: Administer every 10 y **Pregnant women**: Administer one Tdap every pregnancy (preferably at 27–36 wk gestation) **Adults not previously vaccinated:** Administer three-dose series consisting of Tdap followed by Td or Tdap 4 wk later and Td or Tdap 6–12 mo later **Postexposure prophylaxis:** See Table A-2	Severe allergic reaction to any vaccine component or after a previous dose Tdap: encephalopathy (e.g., coma, prolonged seizures) not attributable to other cause within 7 d of administration of previous dose	Moderate or severe acute illness with or without fever; GBS within 6 wk after previous dose of tetanus toxoid–containing vaccine; history of Arthus-type (type III) hypersensitivity reactions after previous dose of diphtheria toxoid–containing vaccine Tdap: progressive or unstable neurologic disorder, uncontrolled seizures, or progressive encephalopathy until treatment regimen established and condition stabilized

(continued)

TABLE A-1	Selected Adult Immunization Recommendations in the United States	*(continued)*	
Vaccine, Dose	**Indications and Dosing**	**Contraindications**	**Precautions**
Varicella (chickenpox) Live varicella vaccine (VAR, Varivax): 0.5 mL SC	**Anyone without evidence of immunity:** Administer two doses (4–8 wk apart); if one dose given previously, only give second dose **Evidence of immunity:** • Documented vaccination (two doses >4 wk apart) • US born before 1980 **except** if pregnant or healthcare personnel • Varicella or zoster infection documented by healthcare provider • Laboratory confirmation of immunity or disease	Severe allergic reaction to any vaccine component or after a previous dose; known **severe immunodeficiency** (e.g., hematologic and solid tumors, receipt of chemotherapy, congenital immunodeficiency, long-term immunosuppressive therapy, HIV infection with CD4+ <200 cells/μL); **pregnancy**	Moderate or severe acute illness with or without fever; simultaneous or recent (≤2 wk) receipt of antibody-containing blood product; receipt of specific antivirals (i.e., acyclovir, famciclovir, valacyclovir) 24 h before vaccination; avoid antiviral use for 14 d after vaccination
Herpes zoster (shingles) Recombinant zoster vaccine (RZV; Shingrix): 0.5 mL IM Zoster vaccine live (ZVL; Zostavax): 0.65 mg SC	**Adults ≥50 y:** Administer two doses of RZV 2–6 mo apart regardless of prior episode of herpes zoster or receipt of ZVL (give RZV at least 2 mo after ZVL) **Adults ≥60 y:** Administer either two doses of RZV as above (preferred) or single dose of ZVL	Severe allergic reaction to a vaccine component ZVL: known **severe immunodeficiency** (e.g., hematologic and solid tumors, receipt of chemotherapy, congenital immunodeficiency, long-term immunosuppressive therapy, HIV infection with CD4+ <200 cells/μL); **pregnancy**	Moderate or severe acute illness with or without fever ZVL: receipt of specific antivirals (i.e., acyclovir, famciclovir, valacyclovir) 24 h before vaccination; avoid antiviral use for 14 d after vaccination

COVID-19	Everyone:	
mRNA vaccine (Moderna; Spikevax) 0.5 mL IM (Pfizer-BioNTech; Comirnaty) 0.3 mL IM	Pfizer-BioNTech: Administer 2 doses three weeks apart in ages 12 and older Moderna: Administer 2 doses 4 wk apart in ages 18 and older J&J/Janssen: Administer 1 dose in ages 18 and older **People with moderate to severe immune compromise**[a]: consider an additional dose of mRNA vaccine at least 28 d after the initial two-dose primary series **Boosters:** Guidelines are in development, for most up-to-date recommendations please see cdc.gov/coronavirus/2019-ncov/vaccines/	Severe or immediate allergic reaction after a previous dose or to a component of an mRNA COVID-19 vaccine
Viral vector (Johnson & Johnson's Janssen) 0.5 mL IM		Moderate or severe acute illness; post marketing data demonstrated increased risks of myocarditis and pericarditis with a higher risk in males under 40 y of age, mostly with mRNA vaccines; a rare complication of thrombosis with thrombocytopenia syndrome (TTS) has been seen in women younger than 50 with J&J/Janssen[3]

Adapted from Centers for Disease Control and Prevention. *Advisory Committee on Immunization Practices recommended adult immunization schedule for ages 19 years or older—United States, 2020.* https://www.cdc.gov/vaccines/schedules/hcp/imz/adult.html

ESRD, end-stage renal disease

[a]Not limited to: moderate or severe primary immunodeficiency (e.g., DiGeorge syndrome, Wiskott-Aldrich syndrome); advanced/untreated HIV infection; active treatment for malignancies, solid-organ transplant; chimeric antigen receptor (CAR)-T-cell or hematopoietic stem cell transplant; immunosuppressive therapy (e.g., alkylating agents, antimetabolites, transplant-related immunosuppressive drugs, cancer chemotherapeutic agents, tumor-necrosis factor [TNF] blockers, and other biologic agents, and high-dose corticosteroids equivalent to prednisone ≥20 mg/day for ≥2 wk).

TABLE A-2	Selected Adult Postexposure Prophylaxis Recommendations
Disease	**Indications and Therapy**
Anthrax	Indicated for all contacts. Either ciprofloxacin 500 mg PO q12h (preferred for **pregnant women**), or doxycycline 100 mg PO q12h for 60 d and anthrax vaccine absorbed (AVA) SC series (obtained from the CDC): First dose administered as soon as possible, second and third doses administered at 2 and 4 wk after the first dose. (Alternative antibiotic regimens available; see CDC website.)
Botulinum toxin	Close observation of exposed person; treat with heptavalent botulinum antitoxin (equine immunoglobulin) at first sign of illness (obtained via consultation with state health department).
Diphtheria	Indicated for close (e.g., household) contacts: Benzathine penicillin G 1.2 million units IM once or erythromycin (base) 500 mg PO q12h for 7–10 d and tetanus and diphtheria (Td) booster vaccine (see Table A-1). Diphtheria antitoxin (DAT) 10,000 units IM/IV (after appropriate sensitivity testing) used for prophylaxis only in exceptional circumstances, obtained in consultation with the CDC (770-488-7100).
Hepatitis A	Indicated for unvaccinated household and sexual contacts of infected individual; persons who have shared illicit drugs with the infected individual; coworkers of infected food handlers; all staff and children at day care centers caring for diapered children where ≥1 case has occurred or when cases occur in ≥2 households of center attendees; only classroom contacts in centers not caring for diapered children. **For healthy persons <40 y**: Administer single-antigen hepatitis A vaccine (see Table A-1). **For persons ≥40 y, immune compromised, or with chronic liver disease:** Administer single-antigen hepatitis A vaccine (see Table A-1) and immune globulin (IG), 0.1 mL/kg IM, once **within 14 d of exposure.**
Hepatitis B	**Nonoccupational:** If exposure source is known surface antigen positive, unvaccinated or incompletely vaccinated persons should receive vaccine (see Table A-1) and hepatitis B immune globulin (HBIG) 0.06 mL/kg IM once. Vaccinated persons without serologic confirmation of immunity should receive one vaccine dose. If exposure source antigen status is unknown, unvaccinated persons should receive the vaccine series, and incompletely vaccinated persons should receive the remaining doses. Vaccinated persons require no further treatment. **Occupational:** See Table A-3.

TABLE A-2	Selected Adult Postexposure Prophylaxis Recommendations (*continued*)
Disease	**Indications and Therapy**
HIV	**Nonoccupational:** Indicated within 72 h of exposure to HIV-infected blood, urogenital secretions, or other body fluids (e.g., condomless sexual intercourse, needle sharing). Administer tenofovir-emtricitabine 300/200 mg (1 tablet) PO daily with raltegravir 400 mg PO q12h or dolutegravir 50 mg once daily for 28 d. Test for HIV at presentation and ensure follow-up for repeat HIV testing at 6 wk. See https://www.cdc.gov/hiv/pdf/programresources/cdc-hiv-npep-guidelines.pdf. If alternative regimens desired, recommend consultation with an HIV specialist. **Occupational:** See Table A-3.
Measles	**Nonoccupational:** If nonimmune (see Table A-1), give measles, mumps, rubella (MMR) vaccine within 72 h of initial exposure. For **pregnant women** (if nonimmune) or severely **immunocompromised** (regardless of prior immunity), give immunoglobulin 400 mg/kg IV (IVIG) once, within 6 d of exposure. Monitor for signs/symptoms for at least one incubation period. **Occupational:** See Table A-3.
Meningococcus (*Neisseria meningitidis*)	Indicated for close contacts of patients with invasive meningococcal disease, including household contacts, child care center contacts, and persons directly exposed to the patient's oral secretions. Administer ciprofloxacin 500 mg PO once, rifampin 600 mg PO q12h for 2 d, or ceftriaxone 250 mg IM once (preferred in **pregnancy**).
Pertussis (*Bordetella pertussis*, whooping cough)	Indicated for close contacts of symptomatic patients (face-to-face exposure ≤3 ft), persons with direct contact with infected respiratory or oral secretions, persons with high risk of severe illness (e.g., **immunocompromised**, third trimester of **pregnancy**, asthma), or those who will have contact with high-risk persons (including infants age <12 mo). Administer a macrolide antibiotic (azithromycin 500 mg PO day 1, 250 mg PO daily days 2–5; erythromycin 500 mg PO q6h for 14 d; clarithromycin 500 mg PO q12h for 7 d) within 21 d of onset of cough in exposure source.
Plague	Indicated for close contacts of pneumonic plague patients (face-to-face exposure ≤3 ft) that have received ≤48 h of effective antibiotic therapy or persons with direct contact with infected body fluids or tissues (for **pregnant women**, weigh prophylactic benefits with antibiotic risks). Administer doxycycline 100 mg PO q12h or ciprofloxacin 500 mg PO q12h for 7 d.

(continued)

TABLE A-2	Selected Adult Postexposure Prophylaxis Recommendations *(continued)*
Disease	**Indications and Therapy**
Rabies	See Rabies Postexposure Prophylaxis section of this Appendix.
Tetanus	**For clean, minor wounds:** If vaccination history unknown or <3 doses tetanus toxoid-containing vaccine, give Tdap and complete catch-up vaccination (see Table A-1). If ≥3 doses and >10 y since last dose, give Tdap (if not yet received) or Td. **For all other wounds:** If vaccination history unknown or <3 doses tetanus toxoid-containing vaccine, give tetanus immune globulin 250 units IM once, as well as Tdap (at separate site) and complete catch-up vaccination. If ≥3 doses and >5 y since last dose, give Tdap (if not yet received) or Td.
Tularemia	Routine prophylaxis not recommended. If exposure in bio-terrorism or mass casualty setting, give doxycycline 100 mg PO q12h or ciprofloxacin 500 mg PO q12h (preferred in **pregnant women**) for 14 d.
Smallpox	Indicated in setting of intentional release of smallpox (variola virus) for exposed persons and persons with contact with infectious materials from smallpox patients, weighing risks and benefits for those with relative contraindications. Administer smallpox (vaccinia) vaccine (ACAM2000; available from the CDC Drug Service at 404-639-3670) ideally within 3 d of exposure; vaccination 4–7 d after exposure may offer some protection.
Varicella	Indicated for exposed persons without evidence of immunity. Vaccinate (see Table A-1) within 3 d of exposure (possibly effective up to 5 d of postexposure). If contraindication to vaccination and at high risk of severe infection (e.g., **pregnant women, immunocompromised, malignancy**), give varicella-zoster immune globulin (VariZIG) 12.5 international units (IU)/kg IM once (minimum, 125 IU; maximum, 625 IU) within 10 d of exposure, which can be obtained from FFF Enterprises (800-843-7477, http://www.fffenterprises.com).

CDC, Centers for Disease Control and Prevention; Tdap, tetanus, diphtheria, pertussis.

TABLE A-3	Selected Postexposure Guidelines for Healthcare Personnel[a]
Pathogen	Treatment
HIV	Indicated for exposure to HIV-infected blood, tissue, or body fluids (e.g., semen, vaginal secretions, amniotic fluid)[b] via percutaneous injury, contact with mucous membranes, or contact with nonintact skin. Administer as soon as possible within 72 h after exposure (can consider up to 1 wk in very–high risk cases). Preferred regimen is tenofovir-emtricitabine 300/200 mg (1 tablet) PO daily and raltegravir 400 mg PO bid for 28 d or until exposure source tests negative for HIV (unless acute seroconversion is suspected).[c] Test exposed workers at baseline, 6 wk, 12 wk, and 6 mo for HIV (baseline, 6 wk, and 4 mo if using fourth-generation test). Assistance with choosing a regimen may be obtained by calling the National Clinicians' Post-Exposure Prophylaxis Hotline (PEPline) at 1-888-448-4911 (9 a.m.–2 a.m. ET) or consulting an HIV expert.
Hepatitis B	For percutaneous injury with blood or blood-contaminated fluids from known surface antigen–positive source: Unvaccinated healthcare worker: Administer hepatitis B immunoglobulin (HBIG), 0.06 mL/kg IM, within 96 h of exposure AND start hepatitis B vaccine series (see Table A-1). Vaccinated healthcare worker: Known responder (documented anti-HBs ≥10 mIU/mL): no treatment Nonresponder after one complete series: HBIG × 1 and repeat series Nonresponder after two complete series: HBIG × 2 doses 1 mo apart Antibody response unknown: check anti-HBs titer; if ≥10 IU/mL: no therapy; if <10 IU/mL: HBIG × 1 and vaccine booster.
Hepatitis C	Immunoglobulin and postexposure prophylaxis not effective. Ensure occupational health follow-up for baseline and subsequent follow-up testing.
Measles	If no documented evidence of immunity, give MMR vaccine within 72 h of initial exposure. For **pregnant women** (if nonimmune) or severely **immunocompromised** (regardless of prior immunity), give immunoglobulin 400 mg/kg IV (IVIG) once within 6 d of exposure. Monitor for signs/symptoms for at least one incubation period. Healthcare personnel without evidence of immunity should be off duty from day 5 after first exposure to day 21 after last exposure, regardless of whether prophylaxis was given.

[a]All blood and body fluid exposures should be reported to the occupational health department. Source patients should be tested for HIV (with consent), hepatitis B surface antigen (HbsAg), and hepatitis C antibody (anti-HCV).
[b]Body fluids not considered infectious include feces, urine, vomitus, saliva, and tears, unless these are visibly contaminated with blood.
[c]Multiple alternative antiretroviral regimens are available if exposed worker has contraindications to or is otherwise unable to use the preferred regimen, or if the exposure source is known to have resistant virus. See *Infect Control Hosp Epidemiol. 2013;34:875.* Consultation with an HIV specialist is recommended in such cases.

TABLE A-4	Rabies Postexposure Prophylaxis Recommendations	
	Therapy	
Vaccination Status	**Vaccine**	**HRIG**
Not previously vaccinated	Yes, on days 0, 3, 7, and 14	Yes, once on day 0
Previously vaccinated	Yes, on days 0 and 3	No

HRIG, human rabies immune globulin.

REFERENCES

1. Manning SE, Rupprecht CE, Fishbein D, et al. Human rabies prevention–United States, 2008: recommendations of the Advisory Committee on Immunization Practices. *MMWR Recomm Rep.* 2008;57(RR-3):1-28.
2. Rupprecht CE, Briggs D, Brown CM, et al. Use of a reduced (4-dose) vaccine schedule for postexposure prophylaxis to prevent human rabies: recommendations of the Advisory Committee on Immunization Practices. *MMWR Recomm Rep.* 2010;59(RR-2):1-9.
3. National Center for Immunization and Respiratory Diseases (NCIRD). *Selective Adverse Events Reported after COVID-19 Vaccination.* 2021. Accessed date September 28, 2021. cdc.gov/coronavirus/2019-ncov/vaccines/safety/adverse-events.html

Appendix B

Infection Control and Isolation Recommendations

Caline Mattar and Stephen Y. Liang

- **Standard Precautions** should be practiced on all patients at all times to minimize the risk of healthcare-associated infection.
  - **Perform hand hygiene** with an alcohol-based hand sanitizer before patient contact, before clean or aseptic procedures, after body fluid exposure, after touching a patient (including after gloves are removed), and after touching patient surroundings (Figure B-1, Table B-1). Soap and water should be used to clean visibly contaminated hands and after contact with patients with confirmed or suspected *Clostridioides difficile* infection if the alcohol-based preparation used is not active against *C. difficile* spores.
  - **Wear gloves** when direct contact with body secretions or blood is anticipated.
  - **Wear a gown** when clothing may be in contact with body fluids.
  - **Wear a surgical mask** when prolonged procedures, including lumbar puncture, are performed.
  - **Wear a surgical mask and protective eyewear** when splashes of body fluid are possible.
  - **Use proper respiratory hygiene and cough etiquette** (applies to all healthcare personnel, patients, and visitors). Mouth and nose must be covered when coughing, and tissues must be disposed of properly. Hand hygiene must be performed after contact with respiratory secretions.
  - **Safely dispose** of sharp instruments, needles, wound dressings, and disposable gowns.
- **Transmission-Based Precautions** supplement Standard Precautions for patients with documented or suspected infection or colonization depending on the major mode of microorganism transmission in healthcare settings.
  - **Contact Precautions** are used when microorganisms can be transmitted via direct contact between patients and healthcare personnel or by contact between patients and contaminated objects and/or environments. In addition to Standard Precautions, the following must be done:
    - Assign the patient to a **private room** if possible. Cohorting of patients with the same organisms is allowed if necessary.
    - **Wear gown and gloves** to enter the room; remove them before leaving the room.
    - Use a **dedicated stethoscope and thermometer.**
    - Minimize environmental contamination during patient transport (e.g., patient can be placed in a gown).
  - **Droplet Precautions** are used when microorganisms can be transmitted by respiratory droplets (>5 μm). Droplets remain suspended in the air for limited periods, and exposure of ≤3 ft (1 m) is usually required for human-to-human transmission. In addition to Standard Precautions, the following must be done:

Your 5 moments for
HAND HYGIENE

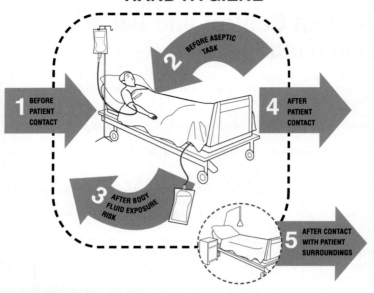

1	**BEFORE PATIENT CONTACT**	**WHEN?**	Clean your hands before touching a patient when approaching him or her
		WHY?	To protect the patient against harmful germs carried on your hands
2	**BEFORE AN ASEPTIC TASK**	**WHEN?**	Clean your hands immediately before any aseptic task
		WHY?	To protect the patient against harmful germs, including the patient's own germs, entering his or her body
3	**AFTER BODY FLUID EXPOSURE RISK**	**WHEN?**	Clean your hands immediately after an exposure risk to body fluids (and after glove removal)
		WHY?	To protect yourself and the health care environment from harmful patient germs
4	**AFTER PATIENT CONTACT**	**WHEN?**	Clean your hands after touching a patient and his or her immediate surroundings when leaving
		WHY?	To protect yourself and the health care environment from harmful patient germs
5	**AFTER CONTACT WITH PATIENT SURROUNDINGS**	**WHEN?**	Clean your hands after touching any object or furniture in the patient's immediate surroundings, when leaving—even without touching the patient
		WHY?	To protect yourself and the health care environment from harmful patient germs

World Health Organization

Figure B-1. World Health Organization's My Five Moments for Hand Hygiene. From World Health Organization's 5 Moments for Hand Hygiene in acute care settings. (Reproduced, with permission of the publisher, from *"Five Moments for Hand Hygiene,"* World Health Organization; 2009. Accessed February 2021. https://www.who.int/gpsc/tools/5momentsHandHygiene_A3.pdf?ua=1)

- Assign the patient to a **private room.** The door must be kept closed as much as possible. Rooms with special air handling systems are **not** required.
- Wear a **surgical mask** within 6 ft of the patient.
- Limit patient transport and activity outside their room. If transporting the patient outside the room is necessary, the patient must wear a surgical mask.
  - **Airborne Precautions** must be used when microorganisms can be transmitted by respiratory droplet nuclei (<5 μm). These droplet nuclei remain suspended in the air for extended periods. In addition to Standard Precautions, the following must be done:
    - Assign the patient to a **negative-pressure airborne infection isolation room.** Doors must remain closed.
    - Wear a **tight-fitting respirator** that covers the nose and mouth with a filtering capacity of 95% (e.g., N95 respirator) or powered air-purifying respirator (PAPR) to enter the room. Susceptible individuals should not enter the room of patients with confirmed or suspected measles or chicken pox. An N95 respirator should be fitted to the wearer.
    - Limit patient transport and activity outside their room. If transporting the patient outside the room is necessary, the patient must wear a surgical mask. Higher level respiratory protection (e.g., N95 respirator) is **not** required for the patient.

TABLE B-1	Healthcare Isolation Recommendations for Specific Infections	
Infection/Condition	**Type**	**Duration, Comments**
Adenovirus, pneumonia	Droplet, Contact	Duration of illness
		In immunocompromised hosts, extend duration of precautions owing to prolonged viral shedding.
Anthrax	Standard	Duration of illness
		Contact precautions indicated if wound with uncontained copious drainage. Alcohol hand rubs ineffective against spores; use soap and water or 2% chlorhexidine gluconate solution for hand hygiene. If aerosolizable spore-containing substance (e.g., powder) is present, wear respirator, protective clothing until decontamination is complete.
Botulism	Standard	Duration of illness
Burkholderia cepacia, pneumonia, or colonization	Contact	Unknown
		Recommendations will vary by institution. Avoid exposure to persons with cystic fibrosis. Private room preferred.

(continued)

TABLE B-1	Healthcare Isolation Recommendations for Specific Infections *(continued)*	
Infection/Condition	**Type**	**Duration, Comments**
Clostridioides difficile	Contact	Duration of hospitalization and future hospitalizations
		Recommendations for initiation and discontinuation of precautions will vary by institution.
Conjunctivitis, acute viral	Contact	Duration of illness
Diphtheria		
Cutaneous	Contact	Until off antimicrobial treatment and two cultures taken 24 h apart are negative
Pharyngeal	Droplet	Same as for cutaneous diphtheria
Hepatitis, viral	Standard	Duration of illness
		For hepatitis A and E, contact precautions are indicated for diapered or incontinent individuals.
Herpes simplex virus		
Encephalitis	Standard	Duration of illness
Mucocutaneous, recurrent (skin, oral, genital)	Standard	Duration of illness
Mucocutaneous, severe (disseminated or primary)	Contact	Until lesions dry and crusted
Herpes zoster		See Varicella
Human metapneumovirus	Contact	Duration of illness
Influenza	Droplet	Immunocompetent: 7 d after illness onset or until 24 h after resolution of symptoms, whichever is longer
		Immunocompromised: Duration of illness
		Respiratory protection equivalent to an N95 respirator is recommended during aerosol-generating procedures.
Lice		
Head (pediculosis)	Contact	Until 24 h after start of therapy
Body	Standard	Duration of illness
		Can be transmitted via infested clothing. Wear gown and gloves when handling clothing.
Pubic	Standard	Duration of illness

TABLE B-1	Healthcare Isolation Recommendations for Specific Infections *(continued)*	
Infection/Condition	**Type**	**Duration, Comments**
Measles (rubeola)	Airborne	Immunocompetent: 4 d after onset of rash Immunocompromised: Duration of illness[a]
Meningitis, *Haemophilus influenzae* type B or *Neisseria meningitidis*	Droplet	Until 24 h after start of therapy For other etiologies of meningitis, standard precautions can be used.
Meningococcal disease (*N. meningitidis*)	Droplet	Until 24 h after start of therapy If colonization without active disease, standard precautions can be used.
Middle eastern respiratory syndrome coronavirus (MERS-CoV)	Airborne, Contact	Determine on a case-by-case basis in consultation with local, state, and federal public health authorities.
Monkeypox	Airborne, Contact	Airborne: Until monkeypox confirmed and smallpox excluded Contact: Until lesions crusted
Multidrug-resistant organisms, infection or colonization (e.g., MRSA, VRE, ESBL)	Contact	Duration of hospitalization and future hospitalizations Recommendations for initiation and discontinuation of precautions will vary by institution and organism.
Mumps (infectious parotitis)	Droplet	Until 5 d after onset of symptoms[a]
Mycoplasma, pneumonia	Droplet	Duration of illness
Parvovirus B19 (erythema infectiosum)	Droplet	Immunocompromised patient: Duration of hospitalization Transient aplastic crisis or red cell crisis: 7 d
Pertussis (*Bordetella pertussis*, whooping cough)	Droplet	Until 5 d after start of therapy
Plague (*Yersinia pestis*)		
Bubonic	Standard	Duration of illness
Pneumonic	Droplet	Until 48 h after start of therapy
Poliomyelitis	Contact	Duration of illness

(continued)

TABLE B-1	Healthcare Isolation Recommendations for Specific Infections *(continued)*	
Infection/Condition	**Type**	**Duration, Comments**
Respiratory syncytial virus	Contact	Duration of illness
		In immunocompromised hosts, extend duration of precautions due to prolonged viral shedding.
Rhinovirus	Droplet	Duration of illness
		Add contact precautions if copious moist secretions.
Rubella (German measles)	Droplet	Until 7 d after onset of rash[a]
		Pregnant women who are not immune should not care for these patients.
Scabies	Contact	Until 24 h after start of therapy
		For Norwegian scabies: 8 d or 24 h after the second treatment with scabicide
Severe acute respiratory syndrome coronavirus (SARS-CoV)	Airborne, Droplet, Contact	Duration of illness plus 10 d after resolution of fever if respiratory symptoms are absent or improving
		Eye protection (goggles, face shield) also recommended.
Severe acute respiratory syndrome coronavirus 2 (SARS-CoV-2), COVID-19	Airborne (if performing an aerosol-generating procedure), Droplet, Contact	Duration of illness; at least 10 d and up to 20 d from symptom onset AND at least 24 h have passed since last fever (without use of fever-reducing medications) AND symptoms have improved. Recommendations may continue to evolve with the COVID-19 pandemic. Immunocompromised patients may shed virus longer. Expert consultation should be obtained.
Smallpox (variola)	Airborne, Contact	Duration of illness; until all scabs have crusted and separated (3–4 wk)[a]
		For vaccine complications, see Vaccinia.
Streptococcus group A	Droplet	Until 24 h after start of therapy
		For endometritis or limited skin, wound, or burn infection, standard precautions can be used.

TABLE B-1	Healthcare Isolation Recommendations for Specific Infections (continued)	
Infection/Condition	**Type**	**Duration, Comments**
Tuberculosis (*Mycobacterium tuberculosis*)	Recommendations regarding initiation and discontinuation of precautions will vary by institution.	
Extrapulmonary, draining lesion	Airborne, Contact	Until patient is improving clinically and drainage has ceased or there are three consecutive negative cultures of drainage Rule out active pulmonary disease.
Extrapulmonary, without draining lesion	Standard	Duration of illness Rule out active pulmonary disease.
Pulmonary or laryngeal disease, confirmed	Airborne	Until patient is on effective therapy, is improving clinically, and has three consecutive sputum smears negative for acid-fast bacilli collected on separate days
Pulmonary or laryngeal disease, suspected	Airborne	Until likelihood of infectious tuberculosis is deemed negligible and either there is another diagnosis that explains the clinical syndrome or the results of three sputum smears for AFB are negative Each of the sputum specimens should be collected 8–24 h apart, and at least one should be an early-morning specimen.
Tularemia	Standard	Duration of illness
Vaccinia	Standard	Duration of illness[a] Contact precautions recommended for eczema vaccinatum, fetal vaccinia, generalized vaccinia, progressive vaccinia, and blepharitis or conjunctivitis with significant drainage. If unvaccinated, only healthcare workers without contraindications to vaccine should provide care.

(continued)

TABLE B-1	Healthcare Isolation Recommendations for Specific Infections (continued)	
Infection/Condition	**Type**	**Duration, Comments**
Varicella		
Varicella disease (chickenpox)	Airborne, Contact	Until lesions dry and crusted[a]
		In immunocompromised host, prolong duration of precautions for duration of illness.
Herpes zoster, localized (shingles)	Standard	Duration of illness[a]
		In immunocompromised host, use airborne and contact precautions until disseminated disease ruled out.
Herpes zoster, disseminated	Airborne, Contact	Duration of illness[a]
Viral hemorrhagic fevers		
Ebola virus disease	Droplet, Contact	Discontinue only in consultation with local, state, and federal public health officials.
		In addition to droplet and contact precautions, a powered air-purifying respirator (PAPR) or N95 respirator, examination gloves with extended cuffs, and fluid-resistant or impermeable gowns, aprons, and boot covers are recommended. Detailed information and updated recommendations can be found at http://www.cdc.gov/vhf/ebola/healthcare-us/hospitals/infection-control.html.
Lassa, Marburg, and Crimean–Congo fever viruses	Droplet, Contact	Duration of illness
		Single-patient room preferred. Emphasize use of sharps safety devices and safe work practices, hand hygiene, barrier protection against blood and body fluids, including goggles or face shields, and appropriate waste handling. Use N95 or higher respirators when performing aerosol-generating procedures.

AFB, acid-fast bacilli; ESBL, extended-spectrum β-lactamase; MRSA, methicillin-resistant *Staphylococcus aureus*; VRE, vancomycin-resistant enterococcus.
[a]Susceptible healthcare workers should not enter room if immune caregivers are available.
Adapted from Siegel JD, Rhinehart E, Jackson M, et al. 2007 Guideline for isolation precautions: Preventing transmission of infectious agents in healthcare settings. *Am J Infect Control*. 2007;35:S65-S164. Copyright © 2007 Elsevier. With permission.

Appendix C

Advanced Cardiac Life Support Algorithms

Siri Ancha

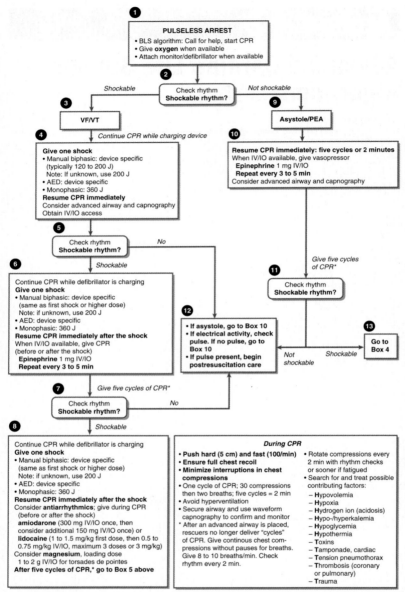

Figure C-1. Advanced cardiac life support pulseless arrest algorithm. AED, automated external defibrillator; BLS, basic life support; CPR, cardiopulmonary resuscitation; IO, intraosseous; PEA, pulseless electrical activity; U, unit; VF, ventricular fibrillation; VT, ventricular tachycardia. (Adapted from American Heart Association in Collaboration with the International Liaison Committee on Resuscitation. Guidelines 2010 for cardiopulmonary resuscitation and emergency cardiovascular care. *Circulation.* 2010;122:S729-S767 and 2015 American Heart Association guidelines update for cardiopulmonary resuscitation and emergency cardiovascular care. *Circulation.* 2015;132:S315-S518.)

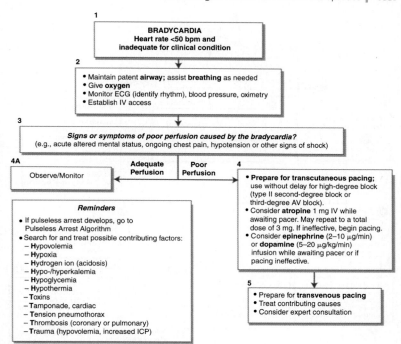

Figure C-2. Bradycardia algorithm. AV, atrioventricular; bpm, beats per minute; ICP, intracranial pressure. (Adapted from American Heart Association in Collaboration with the International Liaison Committee on Resuscitation. Guidelines 2010 for cardiopulmonary resuscitation and emergency cardiovascular care. *Circulation.* 2010;122:S729-S767 and 2015 American Heart Association guidelines update for cardiopulmonary resuscitation and emergency cardiovascular care. *Circulation.* 2015;132:S315-S518.)

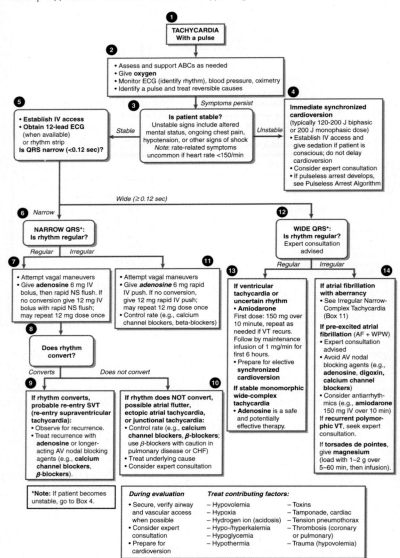

Figure C-3. Advanced cardiac life support tachycardia algorithm. AF, atrial fibrillation; AV, atrioventricular; CHF, congestive heart failure; NS, normal saline; SVT, supraventricular tachycardia; VT, ventricular tachycardia; WPW, Wolff–Parkinson–White syndrome. (Adapted from American Heart Association in Collaboration with the International Liaison Committee on Resuscitation. Guidelines 2010 for cardiopulmonary resuscitation and emergency cardiovascular care. *Circulation.* 2010;122:S729-S767 and 2015 American Heart Association guidelines update for cardiopulmonary resuscitation and emergency cardiovascular care. *Circulation.* 2015;132: S315-S518.)

Index

Note: Page numbers followed by "f " indicate figures and "t" indicate tables.